W9-BLY-993

Respiratory Care

Contributing Authors

Edgar L. Anderson, Jr., Ph.D., R.R.T., C.R.N.A.
Gail A. Banasiak, R.R.T., R.-C.P.T.
Jacqueline Ryan Barrascout, M.A., R.P.T.
Robert H. Bartlett, M.D.
A. Jay Block, M.D.
Roger C. Bone, M.D.
Michael H. Bonnet, Ph.D.
George G. Burton, M.D.
Sandra L. Caldwell, M.B.A., R.N., R.R.T.
Clarence A. Collier, M.D.
Linda J. Corcoran, R.R.T., R.-C.P.T.
James J. Couperus, M.D.
Daniel B. Cress, B.S., R.R.T., C.R.T.T.
Thomas J. DeKornfeld, M.D.
David A. Desautels, M.P.A., R.R.T.
James R. Dexter, M.D.
Harvey A. Elder, M.D.
Robert J. Fallat, M.D.
Michael J. Farrell, R.R.T.
Linda Feenstra, M.S., R.-C.P.T.
Mary Ann Fletcher, M.D.
Philip M. Gold, M.D.
Laura S. Gray, R.N., R.R.T.
H. Frederic Helmholz, Jr., M.D.
Donald W. Herrmann, M.D.
John E. Hodgkin, M.D.
David Hoover, R.R.T., R.-C.P.T.
Robert R. Kirby, Col. USAF, MC
Kevin B. Lake, M.D.
Suzanne C. Lareau, M.S., R.N.
Steven E. Levy, M.D.
Glen A. Lillington, M.D.
Mitchell Litt, D. Eng. Sc.
Ray Masferrer, R.R.T.
David L. McLean, M.P.H., R.R.T.
Michael McPeck, R.R.T.
Edward J. O'Connor, M.D.
John J. Osborn, M.D.
Gene G. Ryerson, M.D.
Howard G. Sanders, Jr., B.S., R.R.T.
Craig L. Scanlan, Ed.D., R.R.T.
Robert A. Smith, R.R.T.
Charles B. Spearman, B.S., R.R.T.
Myron Stein, M.D.
Hugh E. Stephenson, Jr., M.D.
Kent N. Sullivan, M.D.
David L. Swift, Ph.D.
Gennaro M. Tisi, M.D.
James M. Webb, B.S., R.R.T.
Rodney A. Wertz, M.D.
Dale J. Wilms, M.D.
Alan R. Yee, M.D.
Irwin Ziment, M.D.
Eileen G. Zorn, M.S., R.N.

Respiratory Care

A Guide to Clinical Practice

Second Edition

Edited by George G. Burton, M.D.

DIRECTOR, KETTERING INSTITUTE OF RESPIRATORY DISEASES,
KETTERING MEDICAL CENTER, KETTERING, OHIO

FORMERLY, PROFESSOR OF MEDICINE, SCHOOL OF MEDICINE,
LOMA LINDA UNIVERSITY, LOMA LINDA, CALIFORNIA;
CHIEF, PULMONARY SECTION, AND MEDICAL DIRECTOR,
RESPIRATORY CARE SERVICES, WHITE MEMORIAL MEDICAL CENTER,
LOS ANGELES, CALIFORNIA

John E. Hodgkin, M.D.

CLINICAL PROFESSOR OF MEDICINE, UNIVERSITY OF CALIFORNIA, DAVIS;
MEDICAL DIRECTOR, CENTER FOR HEALTH PROMOTION AND REHABILITATION;
MEDICAL DIRECTOR, RESPIRATORY CARE AND PULMONARY REHABILITATION,
ST. HELENA HOSPITAL AND HEALTH CENTER, DEER PARK, CALIFORNIA

WITH 54 CONTRIBUTORS

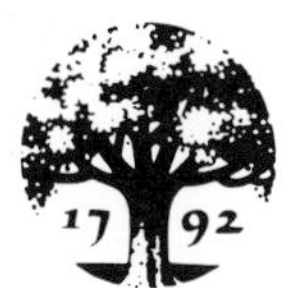

J. B. Lippincott Company

Philadelphia • London • Mexico City
New York • Saint Louis • São Paulo • Sydney

Acquisitions Editor:
Lisa A. Biello
Sponsoring Editor:
Sanford J. Robinson
Manuscript Editor:
Leslie E. Hoeltzel
Indexer:
Barbara Littlewood
Art Director:
Maria S. Karkucinski
Designer:
Pat Pennington
Production Supervisor:
Tina K. Rebane
Production Coordinator:
Susan A. Caldwell
Compositor:
Hampton Graphics
Printer/Binder:
The Murray Printing Company

The authors and publisher have exerted every effort to ensure that drug selection and dosage set forth in this text are in accord with current recommendations and practice at the time of publication. However, in view of ongoing research, changes in government regulations, and the constant flow of information relating to drug therapy and drug reactions, the reader is urged to check the package insert for each drug for any change in indications and dosage and for added warnings and precautions. This is particularly important when the recommended agent is a new or infrequently employed drug.

Second Edition

5 6 4

Library of Congress Cataloging in Publication Data

Main entry under title:
Respiratory care.

Bibliography: p.
Includes index.
1. Respiratory therapy. I. Burton, George G.
II. Hodgkin, John E. (John Elliott), 1939–
[DNLM: 1. Respiratory tract diseases—Therapy. WF 145 R434]
RC735.I5R47 1984 616.2′0046 83-11250
ISBN 0-397-50548-5

This book is dedicated to our children,
who constantly bring joy and gladness to the hours of our lives.

Joan, David, Kevin, Janelle, Jon
Steven, Kathryn, Carolyn, and Jonathan

Contributors

Edgar L. Anderson, Jr., Ph.D., R.R.T., C.R.N.A.
Associate Professor of Health Sciences and Director, Respiratory Therapy Education, School of Allied Health Professions, State University of New York at Stony Brook, Stony Brook, New York (Chapter 6)

Gail A. Banasiak, R.R.T., R.-C.P.T.
Supervisor, Pulmonary Function Laboratory, Veterans Administration Hospital, Loma Linda, California (Appendix C)

Jacqueline Ryan Barrascout, M.A., R.P.T.
Physical Therapy Consultant, Los Angeles, California (Chapter 26)

Robert H. Bartlett, M.D.
Professor of General and Thoracic Surgery, University of Michigan; Head, Section of General Surgery and Director, Surgical Intensive Care Unit, University of Michigan Medical Center, Ann Arbor, Michigan (Chapter 37)

A. Jay Block, M.D.
Chief, Division of Pulmonary Medicine, College of Medicine, University of Florida, Gainesville, Florida (Chapter 18)

Roger C. Bone, M.D.
Professor of Medicine and Chief, Pulmonary Division, University of Arkansas for Medical Sciences, Little Rock, Arkansas (Chapter 35)

Michael H. Bonnet, Ph.D.
Assistant Professor of Medicine, School of Medicine, Loma Linda University; Director, Sleep Laboratory, Veterans Administration Hospital, Loma Linda, California (Appendix C)

George G. Burton, M.D.
Formerly, Professor of Medicine, School of Medicine, Loma Linda University, Loma Linda, California; Chief, Pulmonary Section and Medical Director, Respiratory Care Services, White Memorial Medical Center, Los Angeles, California; Currently, Director, Kettering Institute of Respiratory Diseases, Kettering Medical Center, Kettering, Ohio (Chapters 4, 9, 13, 25, 31, Appendix F)

Sandra L. Caldwell, M.B.A., R.N., R.R.T.
Respiratory Care Consultant, Seattle, Washington (Chapter 21, Appendix H)

Clarence A. Collier, M.D.
Formerly Professor of Medicine and Physiology and Biophysics, School of Medicine, University of Southern California; Associate Director, Pulmonary Physiology Laboratory, Los Angeles County/University of Southern California Medical Center, Los Angeles, California (Chapter 12)

Linda J. Corcoran, R.R.T., R.-C.P.T.
Supervisor, Sleep Laboratory, Veterans Administration Hospital, Loma Linda, California (Appendix C)

James J. Couperus, M.D.
Associate Professor of Medicine, School of Medicine, Loma Linda University, Loma Linda, California (Chapter 19)

Daniel B. Cress, B.S., R.R.T., C.R.T.T.
Chief Therapist, Pulmonary Rehabilitation Department, Loma Linda Community Hospital, Loma Linda, California (Appendix D)

Thomas J. DeKornfeld, M.D.
Professor of Anesthesiology and Postgraduate Medicine and Health Professions Education, School of Medicine, University of Michigan, Ann Arbor, Michigan; Chairman, Joint Review Committee for Respiratory Therapy Education (Chapters 2, 3, 5, 8)

David A. Desautels, M.P.A., R.R.T.
Director, Respiratory Therapy Department, Shands Teaching Hospital and Clinics, College of Medicine, University of Florida, Gainesville, Florida (Chapter 24)

James R. Dexter, M.D.
Medical Director, Sleep Laboratory and Medical Director, Pulmonary Function Laboratory, Veterans Administration Hospital, Loma Linda, California (Appendices B, C)

Harvey A. Elder, M.D.
Professor of Medicine, School of Medicine, Loma Linda University; Chief, Infectious Disease Section, Veterans Administration Hospital, Loma Linda, California (Chapter 19)

Robert J. Fallat, M.D.
Medical Director, Pulmonary Medicine and Associate Research Member, Institute of Biomedical Engineering Sciences, Presbyterian Hospital of the Pacific Medical Center; Associate Clinical Professor of Medicine, School of Medicine, University of California, San Francisco, San Francisco, California (Chapter 39)

Michael J. Farrell, R.R.T.
Director, Respiratory Therapy Section, Veterans Administration Hospital, Loma Linda, California (Chapter 32)

Linda Feenstra, M.S., R.-C.P.T.
Cardiopulmonary Technician, Pulmonary Function Laboratory, Loma Linda Physicians Medical Group, Inc., Loma Linda, California (Appendices B, C)

Mary Ann Fletcher, M.D.
Associate Professor of Child Health and Development, and Obstetrics and Gynecology, School of Medicine, George Washington University; Associate Director, Newborn Service, George Washington University Medical Center, Washington, D.C. (Chapters 28, 29, 30)

Philip M. Gold, M.D.
Medical Director, Department of Respiratory Care, Loma Linda University Medical Center, Loma Linda, California (Chapter 32)

Laura S. Gray, R.N., R.R.T.
Director, Pulmonary Rehabilitation Program, St. Helena Hospital and Health Center, Deer Park, California (Chapter 25)

H. Frederic Helmholz, Jr., M.D.
Emeritus Associate Professor of Physiology, Mayo Graduate School of Medicine, Rochester, Minnesota (Chapter 17, Appendix F)

Donald W. Herrmann, M.D.
Assistant Professor of Medicine, School of Medicine, Loma Linda University; Director, Pulmonary Laboratories, Loma Linda University Medical Center, Loma Linda, California (Appendix A)

John E. Hodgkin, M.D.
Clinical Professor of Medicine, University of California, Davis; Medical Director, Center for Health Promotion and Rehabilitation; Medical Director, Respiratory Care and Pulmonary Rehabilitation, St. Helena Hospital and Health Center, Deer Park, California (Chapters 10, 11, 12, 25, 27; Appendices B, D, E, G)

David Hoover, R.R.T., R.-C.P.T.
Program Analyst, Department of Clinical Systems, Loma Linda University Medical Center, Loma Linda, California (Appendix A)

Robert R. Kirby, Col. USAF, MC
Clinical Professor of Anesthesiology, University of Texas Health Sciences Center; Chairman, Department of Anesthesiology, Wilford Hall USAF Medical Center, Lackland Air Force Base, San Antonio, Texas (Chapter 24)

Kevin B. Lake, M.D.
Associate Clinical Professor of Medicine, School of Medicine, University of Southern California, Los Angeles, California; Medical Director, Department of Respiratory Therapy, Methodist Hospital of Southern California, Arcadia, California (Chapter 36)

Suzanne C. Lareau, M.S., R.N.
Clinical Nurse Specialist, Pulmonary Section, Veterans Administration Hospital, Loma Linda, California (Chapter 32)

Steven E. Levy, M.D.
Associate Clinical Professor of Medicine, School of Medicine, University of California, Los Angeles, Los Angeles, California; Co-Director, Department of Pulmonary Medicine, Brotman Medical Center, Culver City, California (Chapter 33)

Glen A. Lillington, M.D.
Professor of Medicine and Chief, Division of Pulmonary Medicine, School of Medicine, University of California, Davis, Sacramento, California (Chapter 14)

Mitchell Litt, D.Eng.Sc.
Professor of Bioengineering and Chemical Engineering, University of Pennsylvania, Philadelphia, Pennsylvania (Chapter 16)

Ray Masferrer, R.R.T.
Associate Executive Director, American Association for Respiratory Therapy, Dallas, Texas (Chapter 1)

David L. McLean, M.P.H., R.R.T.
Clinical Coordinator, Pulmonary Rehabilitation, Loma Linda University Medical Center, Loma Linda, California (Chapter 27)

Michael McPeck, R.R.T.
Assistant Clinical Professor, Cardiorespiratory Sciences Program, Health Sciences Center, State University of New York at Stony Brook; Director, Department of Respiratory Therapy, University Hospital, Stony Brook, New York (Chapter 6)

Edward J. O'Connor, M.D.
Assistant Clinical Professor of Neurology, School of Medicine, University of California, Los Angeles; Chief, Division of Neurology, White Memorial Medical Center, Los Angeles, California (Chapter 34)

John J. Osborn, M.D.
Director, Bothin Heart Laboratory; Director, Institute of Biomedical Engineering Sciences, Presbyterian Hospital of the Pacific Medical Center, San Francisco, California (Chapter 39)

Gene G. Ryerson, M.D.
Assistant Professor of Medicine, College of Medicine, University of Florida; Director, Medical Intensive Care Facilities, Veterans Administration Hospital, Gainesville, Florida (Chapter 18)

Howard G. Sanders, Jr., B.S., R.R.T.
Chairman, Department of Respiratory Therapy, School of Allied Health Professions, Loma Linda University, Loma Linda, California (Chapter 7)

Craig L. Scanlan, Ed.D., R.R.T.
Associate Director, Graduate Program in Allied Health Education, School of Health Related Professions, University of Medicine and Dentistry of New Jersey, Newark, New Jersey (Chapter 2)

Robert A. Smith, R.R.T.
Director, Critical Care Medicine Animal Research Laboratory, Memorial Medical Center, Jacksonville, Florida (Chapter 24)

Charles B. Spearman, B.S., R.R.T.
Instructor, Department of Respiratory Therapy, School of Allied Health Professions, Loma Linda University, Loma Linda, California (Chapter 7)

Myron Stein, M.D.
Clinical Professor of Medicine, School of Medicine, University of California, Los Angeles, Los Angeles, California; Co-Director, Department of Pulmonary Medicine, Brotman Medical Center, Culver City, California (Chapter 33)

Hugh E. Stephenson, Jr., M.D.
Professor of Surgery and Chief, Division of General Surgery, School of Medicine, University of Missouri, Columbia, Missouri (Chapter 38)

Kent N. Sullivan, M.D.
Clinical Associate Professor of Medicine, School of Medicine, University of Washington, Seattle, Washington (Chapter 21, Appendix H)

David L. Swift, Ph.D.
Professor of Environmental Health Sciences, School of Hygiene and Public Health, The Johns Hopkins University, Baltimore, Maryland (Chapter 16)

Gennaro M. Tisi, M.D.
Associate Professor of Medicine, School of Medicine, University of California; Director, Education and Clinical Services, Division of Pulmonary and Critical Care Medicine, University Hospital, San Diego, California (Chapter 22)

James M. Webb, B.S., R.R.T.
Director, Respiratory Care Services, Florida Hospital, Orlando, Florida (Chapter 15)

Rodney A. Wertz, M.D.
Research Fellow, Section of Pulmonary and Intensive Care Medicine, Department of Medicine, Loma Linda University Medical Center, Loma Linda, California (Appendix D)

Dale J. Wilms, M.D.
Assistant Professor of Medicine, School of Medicine, Loma Linda University; Medical Director, Medical Intensive Care Unit, Veterans Administration Hospital, Loma Linda, California (Chapter 32)

Alan R. Yee, M.D.
Assistant Professor of Medicine, School of Medicine, Loma Linda University; Assistant Medical Director, Pulmonary Rehabilitation, Loma Linda University Medical Center, Loma Linda, California (Chapter 27)

Irwin Ziment, M.D.
Professor of Medicine, School of Medicine, University of California, Los Angeles, Los Angeles, California; Chief of Medicine and Director, Department of Respiratory Therapy, Olive View Medical Center, Van Nuys, California (Chapters 20, 23)

Eileen G. Zorn, M.S., R.N.
Director, Critical Care Nursing, Loma Linda University Medical Center, Loma Linda, California (Chapter 27)

Preface

In the 7 years that have passed since the first edition of Respiratory Care, the education of respiratory care workers has continued apace. Despite some predictions to the contrary, there has not been a decrease in JRCRTE-approved schools of respiratory therapy or the total number of students enrolled therein. Three national studies have refined the scope of practice of respiratory therapists, resulting in a clearer concept of what knowledge and skills base are required of school graduates *upon entry into the field*. Unfortunately, that data base has not contracted sufficiently to allow any shortening of *Respiratory Care!* Indeed, the opposite has occurred, and some observers see, on the not-too-distant horizon, the demise of the 12-month-long curriculum for technician educational programs.

Our readers will recall the original pattern of organization of the first edition of *Respiratory Care:* [1] respiratory care service and education in the modern hospital; [2] a rational, scientific basis for respiratory therapy; and [3] respiratory care in critical illnesses. The same general outline is followed in the second edition.

The current cost-consciousness of health care providers at all levels has caused us to expand portions of Section One. The reader concerned and *willing to do something constructive about* the recent bad press that the respiratory care profession has endured would *do well to review this section again, because much of it has been rewritten*. What we hope emerges from the new Section One is a conviction that cost-containment is as much a part of departmental efficiency and productivity as it is of the kind and number of modalities employed.

We had expected that Section Two of this edition would likewise have needed expansion by a plethora of studies that were expected to follow the conferences in Sugarloaf (1974) and Atlanta (1979). Except for data on the effects of long-term oxygen therapy and IPPB in patients with chronic obstructive pulmonary disease, other data generated by studies spawned by the Sugarloaf Conference have not yet been published or, unhappily, were never begun. The reader will recall that the Sugarloaf Conference dealt with the effects of outpatient and domiciliary modalities, whereas the studies proposed in Atlanta were to have concerned themselves with in-hospital use of respiratory care services. To our knowledge, *none* of the studies proposed in Atlanta have yet been published, and most were never started. Thus, there is less new information to present in Section Two, "A Rational, Scientific Basis for Respiratory Therapy," than we would have liked. Nonetheless, the reader will doubtless discern new concepts and technological improvements in most of the chapters. A chapter on pulmonary rehabilitation has been added, acknowledging the proven benefits of comprehensive care programs for patients with chronic obstructive lung disease.

Section Three has been enhanced, we believe, by

a free-standing chapter on acute respiratory failure, which presents a classification of acute respiratory failure and discusses general principles of treatment.

Our appreciation is extended to our secretaries, Roberta Hoyos and Carol Lewis, whose forbearance with the quirks of contributors and editors can never be fully appreciated. Our personal thanks are also extended to our authors, not only for their contributions, but also for their patience and the license with which they allowed us to process their chapters into the larger framework of a comprehensive textbook.

We wish to thank our friend and mentor, Dr. H. Frederic Helmholz, for his constructive criticism of the first edition and his contribution to the second edition.

GEORGE G. BURTON, M.D.
JOHN E. HODGKIN, M.D.
Los Angeles and St. Helena, California
January, 1984

Preface to First Edition

Medicine and nursing are the oldest of the health professions. Before the relatively recent advances in knowledge and technology, the skill of physicians and nurses alone was sufficient to care for the needs of people with respiratory illnesses, considering the limited nature of the means at hand. Now, however, "total patient care" is complex enough to require the cooperative efforts of many groups of health professionals.

In the 25 years since its emergence as a new allied health profession, the field of respiratory care has developed its own systems of education, credentialing, politics, and economics. Some of this early growth was haphazard, as in any emerging profession. As the years progressed, the effect of stabilizing and maturing influences was felt and a profession worthy of the name emerged. Had the "bread and butter" aspects of respiratory therapy remained simply the pushing of oxygen tanks and giving of IPPB treatments, the field would probably have withered by now. Actually, these tasks were but a beginning, and much, much more was to come.

What has followed can be epitomized by the work of therapists and nurses who now find themselves involved in total respiratory support of the patient; acceptance of the modalities used by the field can be appreciated by the large numbers of hospitalized patients who receive some service from respiratory care departments. While early growth patterns are now stabilizing, problems in effective respiratory care delivery still remain. Two of the most serious problems are treated in the first two sections of this book.

The first problem involves the uncoordinated, non-parallel, and often competitive work activities of members of the so-called respiratory care team. Rather than complementing each others' efforts in a true colleague relationship, in some sectors physicians, therapists, nurses, and technicians seem bent only on fragmentation, rather than unification and clarification of purpose and activity. The patient, and the economy, clearly suffer in this role-playing confrontation, as do the team members themselves. Teamwork failure has slowed the application of sound respiratory care principles in a manner not universally appreciated, though certain voices now are being heard in protest.

Our goal in the organization of Section One was to set in perspective the common needs, purposes, qualifications, and concerns that can unify the team, and to place in focus the needs of patients rather than the real or imagined needs of individuals or facilities.

Section Two reflects our concern with the generally poor understanding of the principles of respiratory therapy. Most readers of this volume will recall trying to learn physiologic principles at a time when they had yet to see their first patient! Consequently, the principles of the gas laws or of the significance of shifts in the oxyhemoglobin dissociation curve are often misapplied.

There is growing concern that many respiratory care modalities have little or no basis in scientific fact. Some of this concern is justified. Therapists and nurses should realize that the current medical literature is replete with reports of untoward effects of many of the modalities they employ. Cardiac arrhythmia, infection, hypoxia, pneumothorax, and reduced cardiac output complicating the use of some of these modalities all have been reported in the medical literature in the recent past. These reports, in general, have not been balanced by testimonials of efficacy. It is our hope that workers in the field of respiratory care will initiate studies leading to the accumulation of objective data that will place respiratory therapy modalities on a sound scientific footing.

A concern of this volume is that many respiratory care workers do not understand in sufficient detail the scientific basis for many modes of treatment and so are unable to respond correctly when such criticisms arise. How many therapists, for instance, can discuss cellular oxygen and carbon dioxide metabolism, or know where various-sized aerosol particles are deposited? What does airway humidification actually accomplish? Such information is in the literature but, unfortunately, not always in the readily accessible "mental files" of respiratory care workers. Section Two, then, is meant to serve as a review and update of the academic training of respiratory care workers, so that they may appreciate the principles and applications in the light of their experience and apply them better.

Section Three is concerned with respiratory care of critically ill patients. It has grown out of a syllabus prepared by us for use in a course for senior respiratory therapy students and new employees in our institutions. This section focuses on common illnesses wherein intensive respiratory services are mandatory and enlarges on the principles and methods outlined in Section Two. Several chapters on pediatric pulmonary disease are included.

Readers may not recognize the initials R.R.T. (Registered Respiratory Therapist) following the names of many contributors. In June, 1977, this designation officially replaced the old A.R.R.T. (American Registered Respiratory Therapist) credential. We have used the new title wherever it is appropriate. It was not used in the chapter co-authored by Jimmy Young, who died before the new designation came into use. In addition, the change has not been made in chapter content in the early portions of Section 1, dealing with the American Registry of Respiratory Therapists, which were written and submitted prior to the effective date of this change.

Our appreciation is extended to our secretaries, Lois Rockwell, Sandra Howl, Cheryl Herr, Jeanie Walker, and Barabara West, who bore the brunt of multiple typings and retypings of the manuscript, and to Lewis Reines, Editor-in-Chief, Medical Books, of the J. B. Lippincott Company for his patient understanding and helpful advice. Also our thanks are extended to the many contributors who so kindly allowed us to process their words and thought into what we hope is a cohesive, cogent, and helpful volume.

GEORGE G. BURTON, M.D.
GLEN N. GEE, R.R.T.
JOHN E. HODGKIN, M.D.

Contents

APPENDICES—John E. Hodgkin, M.D., Editor

Respiratory Care

Section One

RESPIRATORY CARE SERVICE AND EDUCATION IN THE MODERN HOSPITAL

1

History of the Inhalation Therapy–Respiratory Care Profession

Ray Masferrer

And he put his mouth upon his mouth . . . and the flesh of the child became warm.

II Kings 4:34

In that manner 28 centuries ago, in the Biblical story of the prophet Elisha who restored to life the son of a Shunammite woman, the principle was recognized that respirable air was necessary for human life. Nevertheless, the unraveling of the mysteries of respiration was to take many centuries and to engage the minds of some of the world's greatest scientists. Pythagoras (580–489 B.C.), a mathematician and philosopher, developed a philosophy based on the mystical power of numbers. He believed that matter and life comprised four basic elements: earth, fire, water, and air. Corresponding to these four elements were the qualities of dryness, heat, cold, and moistness. Air was considered to be hot and moist. The Greek physician Hippocrates (460–370 B.C.) introduced and developed the doctrine of *essential humors*. He attributed all diseases to humoral disorders within the body fluids and taught that an essential, yet undefined, material derived from the inspired air entered the heart and was then distributed throughout the body systems.

Aristotle (384–322 B.C.), in probably the first recorded scientific experiment in respiratory physiology, observed that animals kept in airtight chambers soon died. The correct interpretation escaped him, for he ascribed the death to their inability to cool themselves. He further incorrectly assumed that the heart was the organ that provided the source of heat for the blood. Galen (A.D. 131–201) envisioned a system of physiology that combined the humoral doctrines of Hippocrates and the Pythagorean theory of the four elements with his own conception of spirit, or *pneuma*, penetrating all the parts. Galen postulated that arterial blood (charged with "natural spirits" in the liver) flowed back and forth in its various channels, which were not interconnected except for some imaginary pores in the cardiac ventricular septum. He further assumed that the arteries took in and cast out air in diastole and systole, just as the lungs did in the course of respiration. As the lungs were ventilated, he envisioned that the heart and blood were cooled and that the pulsations of the arteries cooled the body.

The author and editors wish to acknowledge the contribution of Jimmy A. Young (deceased), past president of the American Association of Respiratory Therapy, to the content and form of this chapter. Mr. Young, in collaboration with Winfield S. Singletary, Jr., authored this chapter in the first edition of RESPIRATORY CARE. The authors also wish to acknowledge the contributions of H. Frederic Helmholz, M.D., and Phillip Porte, President, Phillip Porte & Associates, Arlington, Virginia.

Leonardo da Vinci (1452–1519) concentrated on the anatomical structure of the body and concluded, importantly and correctly, that fire consumed a component within air and that animals could not live in an atmosphere that could not support flame. Andreas Vesalius in 1542 passed a reed into the trachea of an animal whose thorax had been opened and blew into it intermittently. He observed that this procedure caused the lung to expand and the heart to recover its normal pulsation. He also observed that if the lungs were allowed to remain collapsed, the pulsation of the heart and arteries became wavelike and wormlike (our understanding of what is now known as ventricular fibrillation). Michael Servetus (1509–1553) finally discovered that blood in the pulmonary circulation, after mixing with air in the lungs, returned to the heart.

Not until 75 years later did thinking in regard to the physiology of the circulation become clarified. By meticulous dissections, William Harvey (1578–1657) proved that the heart acted as a muscular pump, propelling the blood, and that the blood's motion was continual and cyclic. In 1628 he published his important treatise *An Anatomical Disquisition on the Motion of the Heart and Blood in Animals.*

In 1666 Robert Boyle suspected that there were in the air

> numberless exhalations of the terraqueous globe .... The difficulty we find in keeping flame and fire alive ... without air renders it suspicious that there may be dispersed through the rest of the atmosphere some odd substance, either of solar, astral, or other foreign nature; on account whereof the air is so necessary to flame.

In his note in the *Philosophical Transactions* (12 September 1670), Boyle surmised that the lack of oxygen or a similar substance was also a destructive factor, and recorded the production of aeroembolism by subjecting animals to low pressure.

One hundred years later, in 1774, Joseph Priestley reported the discovery of oxygen produced by heating the red oxide of mercury. His remarks after this magnificent discovery bear repetition.

> My reader will not wonder that, having ascertained the superior goodness of dephlogisticated air by mice living in it, and the other tests above mentioned, I should have the curiosity to taste it myself .... I have gratified that curiosity by breathing it, drawing it through a glass syphon, and by this means, I reduced a large jar full of it to the standard of common air, but I fancied that my breath felt peculiarly light and easy for some time afterward. Who can tell but that in time this pure air may become a fashionable luxury. Hitherto, only two mice and myself have had the privilege of breathing it.

Joseph Black (1728–1799) discovered that carbon dioxide was the by-product of respiration and that it was given off by the lungs. Between 1775 and 1794, the brilliant French scientist Antoine Laurent Lavoisier showed that oxygen was absorbed from the lungs and consumed in the body, carbon dioxide and water were given off during the exhalation phase of ventilation, and an inert substance in the air (nitrogen) was unchanged. Although each of these scientists made notable contributions to physiology and medicine, Lavoisier is generally thought to have formulated the fundamental principles of respiratory gas exchange as we know them.

In 1800 Thomas Beddoes, using the knowledge gained from the discoveries of Priestley, Lavoisier, and Black, established the Pneumatic Institute in Bristol, England, where he began the therapeutic use of oxygen to treat heart disease, asthma, and opium poisoning. In most textbooks Beddoes is thought of as "The Father of Inhalation Therapy." However, not until 1920 was a firm physiological basis for the inhalation of oxygen established, largely owing to the studies of John Scott Haldane and Joseph Barcroft on the effects of oxygen deficiency in humans.

In 1920 Barcroft performed a crucial experiment when he lived for 5 days in a chamber filled with 15% oxygen, thus simulating the decreased ambient oxygen tension of high altitudes. He became sick with nausea, headache, visual disturbances, rapid pulse, and lassitude. In another experiment, Haldane exposed himself to an even lower inspired oxygen concentration and became disoriented. He probably would have died had not his assistants removed him from the exposure chamber.

CLINICAL USE OF OXYGEN THERAPY

With the development of methods of administering oxygen (face mask, rubber catheter, oxygen chamber), clinical studies gradually clarified the role and value of oxygen in the treatment of hypoxia. The most rapid advancements, however, came only in the 20th century. In 1907 Sir Arbuthnot Lane advised that oxygen be administered by means of a nasal catheter. In 1918 Haldane perfected an oxygen mask that was used successfully to treat patients with combat gas-induced pulmonary edema. In 1920 Sir Leonard Hill developed an oxygen tent for treating a patient with a chronic leg ulcer. The tent was designed to be fitted over the patient in bed but had no provision for eliminating heat and moisture. The general concept, however, stimulated numerous attempts to design a more practical method of delivering oxygen while removing carbon dioxide and eliminating heat buildup.

In 1926 A. L. Barach devised an oxygen tent in which carbon dioxide was removed by soda lime, water vapor was removed by calcium chloride, and heat was removed by flowing the oxygen-enriched air over chunks of ice contained in a refrigeration cabinet. This was a major development. Oxygen chambers, where the patient could reside without any appliance over his face, were then devised by Barcroft in England and W. C. Stadie at the Rockefeller Institute; gas circulation in these chambers was accomplished by motor-driven blowers. At the Presbyterian Hospital in New York, Barach developed entire rooms in which oxygen-enriched air was circulated from pipes that contained circulating ice water or brine on one side of the room and a steam radiator on the other.

At about this time, J. S. Haldane developed a method for diluting gases with room air, using the "Carbetha" apparatus to administer carbon dioxide. Barach used this method to develop his "meter mask." He also developed a positive pressure mask which, by initiating a disc mechanism in front of an expiratory valve, produced pressures up to 4 cm of water on exhalation. This mask was found to be advantageous for administering helium-oxygen mixtures.

In 1938 Drs. Boothby, Lovelace, and Bulbulian devised the BLB mask at the Mayo Clinic, which allowed for high concentrations (80–100%) of oxygen to be inhaled with minimal rebreathing. The mask was also used to administer oxygen to pilots flying at high altitudes. Soon appliances and new procedures were developed to augment breathing in patients who were hypoventilating, to administer gas mixtures under pressure, and to ventilate patients during cardiopulmonary resuscitation.

Intermittent positive pressure ventilation (IPPV) was first described by Guedel in 1934 after he clinically observed the apnea that followed hyperventilation during deep ether anesthesia. Further development of mechanical devices for artificial ventilation with IPPV followed the use, during World War II, of continuous positive pressure breathing as a means of increasing altitude tolerance in flight crews. During these years "safe" combinations of inspired oxygen concentrations and mask pressures for flight crews at altitudes up to 45,000 feet were developed, as were pressure-tight face masks and valving mechanisms still in use today (Figs. 1-1, 1-2).[2] In 1947 Motley and his coworkers[4] suggested IPPV for certain clinical conditions other than apnea, such as the treatment of acute pulmonary edema and postoperative atelectasis.

From 1934 to 1947 the techniques of oxygen therapy and inhalation therapy were carried to the bedsides of many patients with various diseases.[3] As the demand for more skilled manpower to administer these modalities increased, an appropriate concern developed for an organized approach to the education and clinical training of adequate numbers of personnel to provide respiratory care for patients.

ORGANIZATION AND INCORPORATION OF THE INHALATION THERAPY ASSOCIATION

During the mid-1940s a group of interested and enterprising physicians and "oxygen technicians" in Chicago organized a series of meetings to discuss oxygen therapy, its rationale, and possible means of improving the care of patients requiring the administration of medical gases. Drs. Albert Andrews, Edwin Levine, and Max Sadove were among the prime movers in recognizing the need for an organization to provide education to those persons involved in administering medical gases to patients. They held their first meeting in 1946 at the University of Chicago and decided to form the Inhalational Therapy Association (ITA). On 15 April 1947 a nonprofit charter was obtained by the ITA from the State of Illinois. The incorporators were George A. Kneeland, Richard E. Goss, Vincent T. McCue, Brother Roland Maher, and Brother Sulverius Case. The stated purposes of the Association were

1. to promote higher standards in methods and professional advancement of members of the association;
2. to create mutual understanding and cooperation between the technician, the physician, and all others who were employed in the interest of individual or public health through the Tri-State Hospital Assembly;
3. to advance the knowledge of inhalation therapy through institutes, lectures, and other means given under the sponsorship of doctors of the Society of Anesthesia; and
4. to grant certificates of qualification to individuals who had successfully completed the prescribed requirements.

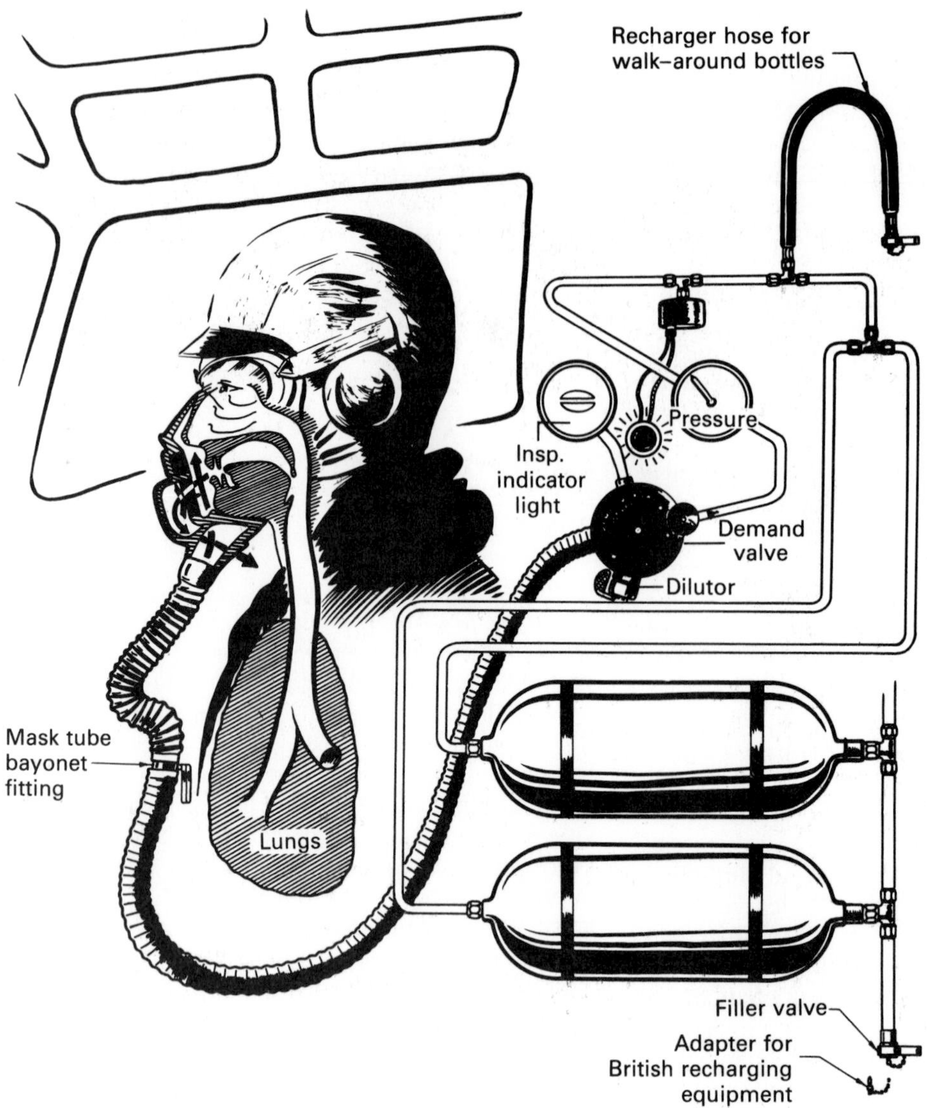

Fig. 1-1. Composite diagram of demand oxygen system assembly as used by fighters and bomber pilots during World War II. (From a course given to aviators between 1943 and 1945 by H. Frederic Helmholz, Jr., M.D.)

The Association at that time consisted of 59 members, nine of whom were honorary members.

Within the ensuing months numerous plans were laid and promotional attempts made to advance the newly formed Association. In 1948 the name of the Association was changed to the Inhalation Therapy Association. During its initial years the Association had been supported entirely by membership dues, and in 1950 the Board of Directors passed a resolution to develop a journal that was to be supported by advertisements. The *Bulletin* was to be mailed quarterly and sent free of charge to 1500 hospitals throughout the United States. In the first issue Brother Roland Maher, then president of the ITA, discussed the Association's rapid growth and the interest in its activities by people outside the Chicago area. Several lecture courses and meetings had already been held by the Board of Directors, and there was a demand for more. On 19 December 1950, 31 certificates were issued to those members of the Association who had participated in the series of 16 lectures and workshops.

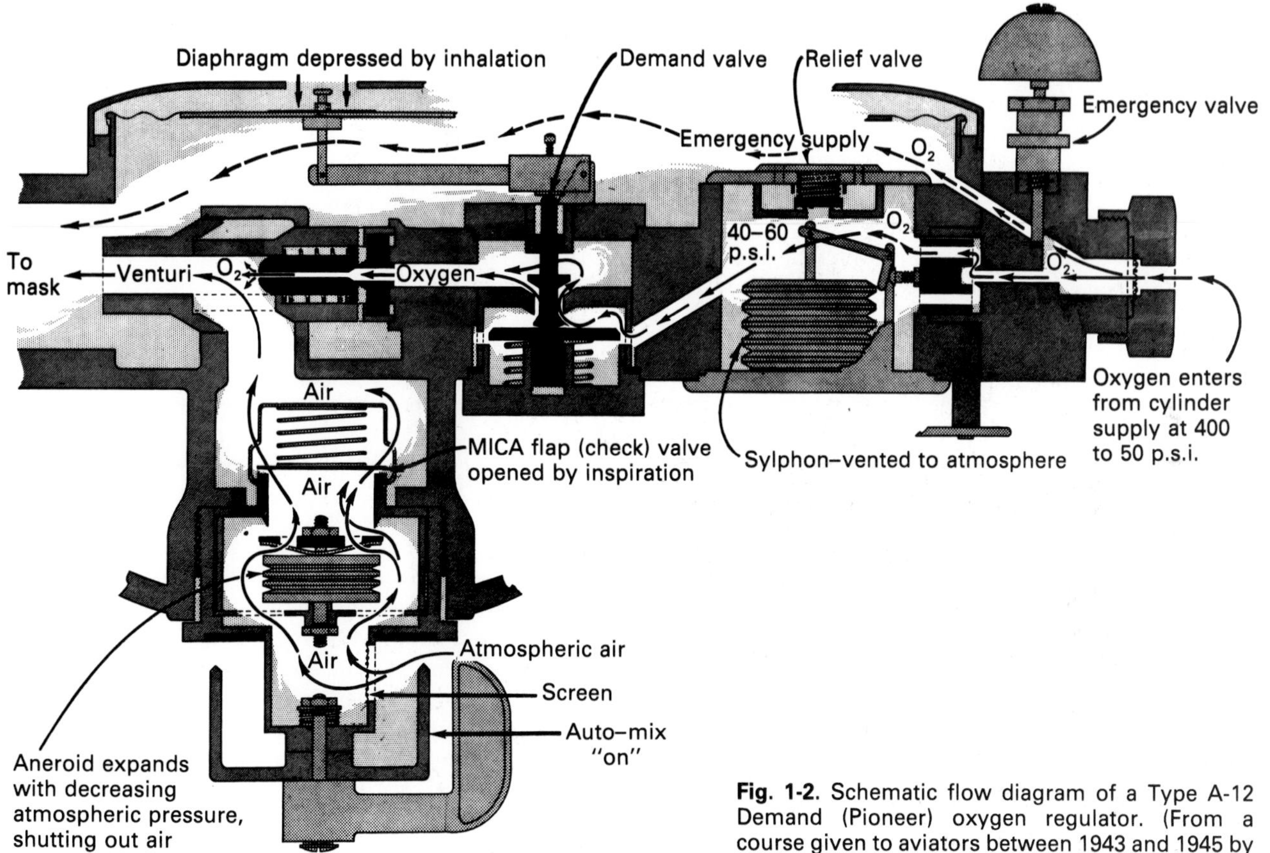

Fig. 1-2. Schematic flow diagram of a Type A-12 Demand (Pioneer) oxygen regulator. (From a course given to aviators between 1943 and 1945 by H. Frederic Helmholz, Jr., M.D.)

This was a historic event in the growth of the Association and the profession. From then on, great emphasis was placed on formal education and credentialing of those persons practicing inhalation therapy (respiratory care). In 1951 the ITA voted to sponsor a 5-day program in conjunction with the American College of Chest Physicians. The announcement that the American College of Chest Physicians was officially sponsoring the ITA was made in the 1953 summer edition of the ITA *Bulletin*.

With the increasing interest evidenced by convention attendance from 14 states and Canada, the Association expanded to one of nationwide scope. A proposal was made that the name be changed to the American Association of Inhalation Therapists (AAIT) at the November 1953 annual convention. The ITA Board of Directors, at their 3 May 1954 meeting held at the Palmer House in Chicago, discussed reorganization and prepared new plans. The name of the new association—American Association of Inhalation Therapists—was adopted.

THE AMERICAN ASSOCIATION OF RESPIRATORY (INHALATION) THERAPISTS

The new organization began by electing new officers and a Board of Directors. Sister Borromea was elected the first president. Mr. J. Addison Young was appointed to serve as acting executive director until a permanent director had been hired. At the 3 May 1954 meeting it was proposed to change the name of the Inhalation Therapy Association *Bulletin* to the *AAIT Monthly Newsletter*. It was first published in July 1955 and continued to appear until December 1968, at which time it became the *AAIT Bulletin*.

In 1954 a central office in Chicago was proposed and local and state chapters began organizing. Letters were sent to all hospitals within the United States to outline membership qualifications and to recruit new members for the Association. Plans were also formalized to outline the requirements for the education of future respiratory therapists.

During the next few years better equipment and more advanced therapy techniques were introduced. Those practicing in the profession began to adopt the title "inhalation therapist" and joined the AAIT local chapters being formed. By 1960 there were 21 local chapters, which increased to 31 in 1966 and 48 in 1972; at present there are 48 chapters now called chartered affiliates.

Current sponsoring organizations of the AAIT (now the American Association for Respiratory Therapy) are the American College of Chest Physicians, the American Society of Anesthesiologists, and the American Thoracic Society.

THE BOARD OF MEDICAL ADVISORS (BOMA)

One of the most important reasons for the rapid and orderly growth of the respiratory therapy profession has been its relationship to physicians' groups. Unlike many other health disciplines, a peer relationship has developed at almost every level, especially concerning the administrative aspects of the organization locally and nationally.

Initially, the BOMA comprised six physicians, three of whom were appointed by the American College of Chest Physicians and three by the American Society of Anesthesiologists. In 1966, with the revision of the bylaws, the BOMA comprised 16 member physicians: four from the American College of Chest Physicians; four from the American Society of Anesthesiologists; two from the American Academy of Pediatrics; two from the American Thoracic Society; and two from the American College of Allergists. In 1972, with another bylaws revision, the BOMA membership was increased to 18 physicians after two members were added from the American Thoracic Society. Still later, members were added from the American Academy of Pediatrics, the American College of Allergists, the Society for Critical Care Medicine, and the Society of Thoracic Surgeons. By 1982, 21 physicians composed the BOMA.

In 1975 a bylaws revision approved by the AART membership stated that appointees to the BOMA must be physicians who have identifiable roles in clinical, educational, or investigative respiratory therapy. This revision was intended to emphasize the importance of effective and responsible medical leadership within the profession of respiratory therapy in order to enhance its dynamic growth in future years.

CHANGES IN ASSOCIATION CONSTITUTION AND BYLAWS

The professional organization for respiratory therapy has undergone various changes in its constitution and bylaws. Several of the more significant changes occurred in 1972 with a name change of the Association to the American Association for Respiratory Therapy (AART) and full sponsorship by the American Thoracic Society.

The American Respiratory Therapy Foundation (ARTF) was incorporated on 18 November 1970 in California. The purposes of the ARTF were

- to further clinical, epidemiologic, basic scientific, social, and other studies in all aspects of respiratory diseases;
- to promote and support allied health professional education in the field of respiratory diseases at all levels, including approved schools of respiratory therapy, universities, colleges, hospitals, training programs for the registered therapist, the certified technician, the pulmonary function technician, and the nurse;
- to promote and support model demonstration care projects to the extent required by research and teaching;
- to promote and support community education in the field of respiratory diseases with particular emphasis on prevention;
- to provide leadership for all allied health professionals in interpreting the scope and importance of all respiratory diseases;
- to serve as a consultant to government agencies, community service organizations, and voluntary health organizations concerned with control of respiratory diseases;
- to promote international educational programs and exchange of ideas on the study and control of respiratory diseases.

The Board of Trustees of the Foundation comprises seven members appointed by the AART, the BOMA, the House of Delegates of the AART, and the general membership of the AART. Each member of the Board of Trustees is elected for a 3-year nonrecurring term. The Foundation has only elected officers. The AART has worked closely with the Foundation and has supported its endeavors in an effort to provide the necessary "seed monies" to make the

Foundation financially viable. The membership of the Association has donated to, and has benefited from, the activities of the Foundation.

MEMBERSHIP

The membership of the AART has grown tremendously since 1947. Three name changes, one in 1954 to the American Association of Inhalation Therapists, another in 1967 to the American Association for Inhalation Therapy, and the last in 1972 to the present American Association for Respiratory Therapy, indicate that the membership has become national in scope, with members in each state, and that the Association has broadened its areas of activities in promoting high professional standards, achievements, goals, and opportunities for respiratory therapy personnel.

As of 1983 the Association had a membership of more than 25,000. There are 48 chartered affiliates in the United States. A 1982 manpower survey conducted by the AART indicated that more than 100,000 persons were involved in the profession.

The number of educational programs has paralleled the membership growth of the AART. There are more than 400 approved schools for the education and clinical training of technicians and therapists.

CURRENT ORGANIZATIONAL STRUCTURE

The AART functions under the leadership of the Board of Directors, which is elected by, and is responsible to, the membership. The Board of Directors supervises all the business and activities of the Association. The executive committee of the Board of Directors are the AART officers who are elected by the general membership. Under the chairmanship of the AART president, the executive committee is responsible for the day-to-day operations of the executive director and the Association office staff. The Board of Directors is responsible for reviewing and directing the decisions of the executive committee and for final decision-making in areas that do not require a vote of the membership according to the AART bylaws. Personnel of the standing and special committees are the working groups from which dynamic changes have come about within the profession.

ANNUAL MEETING AND OTHER EDUCATIONAL MEETINGS

The Association holds a national convention each fall to conduct Association business and to educate its members. Attendance at this annual meeting has grown from 400 in 1963 to more than 6400 in 1981. The scientific and educational exhibitions at the annual meetings present the latest advancements in the profession. The educational programs are prepared by the nine membership sections of the Association representing special member interests. The sections are clinical practice; critical care; education; cardiopulmonary; perinatal–pediatric; clinical research; management; and rehabilitation-continuing care.

In addition to the annual meeting the Association presents an annual Summer Forum and other symposia addressing topics of interest to the entire membership. Each chartered affiliate also conducts annual meetings for educational and business purposes.

THE BOARD OF SCHOOLS AND THE JOINT REVIEW COMMITTEE FOR RESPIRATORY THERAPY EDUCATION

As the need for formal educational programs became more evident, it was necessary to organize and develop a formal approach to accreditation of all educational programs. As a result the Board of Schools for Inhalation Therapy was organized in 1956 as an advisory committee to the Council on Medical Education of the American Medical Association. It was sponsored by the American College of Chest Physicians, American Society of Anesthesiologists, and the American Association of Inhalation Therapy. The stated purpose of the Board of Schools was to maintain high standards within the educational programs of inhalation therapy and to encourage future development of the profession.

Chapter 2 discusses in considerable detail the education and credentialing of respiratory care professionals. However, a few historical notes on the manner in which these processes became formalized should be mentioned at this point. While organizational processes were developing in the political sphere of inhalation therapy in the 1950s, a group of physicians in New York, spearheaded by Alvin Barach,[1] published an article entitled "Minimum Standards for Inhalation Therapy." In 1950 the Committee on Public Health Relations of the New York Academy of Medicine prepared a report entitled "Standards of Effective Administration of Inhalation Therapy" that also underscored the need for trained people at the technical level.

Pursuing the recognized general educational deficiencies of the technicians, another group of New York physicians, led by Edwin Emma and Vincent Collins, began work on plans for an educational program in inhalation therapy. Their endeavors took the form of recommendations to the AMA.

In 1957 a resolution to develop *schools* of inhalation therapy was introduced into the AMA's House of Delegates by the Medical Society of the State of New York and, after approval, was referred to the Council on Medical Education. An exploratory conference was held in October 1957, and afterward a report entitled "Essentials for an Approved School of Inhalation Therapy Technicians" was proposed. The following 3 years were a trial period to test the adequacy of the school system and the curriculum. The experience was good, and the Council on Medical Education recommended adoption of the proposed "Essentials." Approval was given by the AMA House of Delegates in December 1962. To implement the "Essentials," the Council on Medical Education called sponsoring organizations together in January 1963. The organization of the Board of Schools for Inhalation Therapy was refined and approved to function as an inspecting, surveying, and reporting agency.

The "Essentials" for approved educational programs have been revised four times, first by the Technician Certification Board (now the NBRT) and later by the Joint Review Committee for Respiratory Therapy Education (JRCRTE). "Essentials" to provide for training of persons to perform as technicians with approximately 1 year of formal training were approved in 1972. As of this writing, "Essentials" are being rewritten yet again to reflect more accurately the demands of the profession and the workplace. They will not be in effect until about 1988.

The Board of Schools for Inhalation Therapy, a body duly organized to survey educational programs and to make recommendations to the AMA Council on Medical Education, was reorganized and incorporated in 1970 as the Joint Review Committee for Inhalation Therapy Education (JRCITE). In 1972, with the approval of the three sponsoring bodies and the Council on Medical Education, the American Thoracic Society became a sponsor as well. The group was renamed the Joint Review Committee for Respiratory Therapy Education (JRCRTE) in 1974. Since 1977, the JRCRTE has been functioning in association with the Committee on Allied Health Education of the AMA.

FORMATION AND INCORPORATION OF THE AMERICAN REGISTRY OF INHALATION THERAPISTS

In 1960 another landmark in the growth of the inhalation therapy profession was achieved when the Articles of Incorporation for the formation of the American Registry of Inhalation Therapists were filed in the office of the Secretary of the State of Illinois. The stated purposes for the organization were

1. to advance the art and science by promotion of the understanding and utilization of Inhalation Therapy in the prevention and treatment of human ailments;
2. to assist in developing and maintaining educational and ethical standards in Inhalation Therapy for the public good; for the advancement of medical care; and for the professional guidance of registrants of the registry;
3. to encourage the establishment of high standards by which the competency of Inhalation Therapy under the prescription, direction, and supervision of licensed physicians [could] be determined;
4. to prepare, conduct, and control investigations and examinations to test the qualifications of voluntary candidates; and
5. to do and perform any and all things necessary or desirable to accomplish the foregoing specified purposes.

Twelve examinees received their registration in 1961; there are now more than 16,700 registered respiratory therapists. During the years of its existence the Registry Board has steadily encouraged the profession to improve its fund of basic and clinical knowledge by requiring increasingly higher qualifications for admission to the examination system.

The primary function of the now-renamed National Board for Respiratory Care, Inc., is to examine those eligible persons who voluntarily seek to be tested on their knowledge and competency in the area of respiratory care. The examination procedure is currently twofold: A written examination is taken as a prerequisite to a second more comprehensive test, the written "Clinical Simulation" examination.

THE NEED FOR CREDENTIALED ENTRY-LEVEL PERSONNEL AND THE FORMATION OF THE TECHNICIAN CERTIFICATION BOARD

The rapid growth of technology and the increasing need for credentialed personnel in the field challenged the profession in the late 1960s to develop a much-needed group of qualified, entry-level personnel. This objective was accomplished by preparing a suggested set of curricular guidelines that could be used to initiate uniform educational programs to prepare respiratory therapy technicians.

During 1968 and 1969 the AAIT planned and organized what is now the certification system for respiratory therapy technicians. At the 1969 Annual Meeting of the AAIT in Kansas City, the proposed Technician Certification Program was approved and the first pilot certification examination administered. Subsequent to that meeting the AAIT Board of Directors had approved a definition of respiratory therapy that had considerable bearing on the proposal. The statement assigned to respiratory therapy a broadly defined role that closely parallels the activities of other allied health professionals, such as nurses and physical therapists.

DEFINITION OF RESPIRATORY THERAPY

> Respiratory Therapy is an allied health specialty employed with medical direction in the treatment, management, control, diagnostic evaluation, and care of patients with deficiencies and abnormalities of the cardiopulmonary system.
>
> Respiratory Therapy shall mean the therapeutic use of the following: medical gases and administration apparatus, environmental control systems, humidification, aerosols, medications, ventilatory support, bronchopulmonary drainage, pulmonary rehabilitation, cardiopulmonary resuscitation, and airway management.
>
> Specific testing techniques are employed in respiratory therapy to assist in diagnosis, monitoring treatment, and research. This shall be understood to include measurement of ventilatory volumes, pressures, flows, blood-gas analysis, and other related physiologic monitoring.

Specific job definitions based on this statement were also approved in 1969 by the AAIT Board of Directors, relative to a therapist's education, experience, and the credentialing examinations he had successfully completed.

THE NATIONAL BOARD FOR RESPIRATORY CARE, INC.

From 1969 to 1974 the examination system for certifying technicians was a function of the AART. In 1972 the concept of a single national credentialing organization for both technicians and therapists was proposed by AART president James A. Liverett, Jr., to the Board of Trustees of the American Registry of Inhalation Therapists (ARIT). Following that meeting, the two organizations formed a joint committee to study the feasibility of merging the credentialing functions of the AART's Technician Certification Board and ARIT.

During the deliberations of this committee it became evident that simply transferring the functions of the Technician Board to the American Registry of Inhalation Therapists would not serve the future of the profession. The committee, and subsequently the Boards of the two organizations, agreed to form a new organization around the modified structure of the American Registry of Inhalation Therapists. The final plans for setting up the National Board for Respiratory Care, Inc. (NBRT), were approved by the two organizations in early 1974. The NBRC has bylaws and a Board of Trustees that comprises representatives of its sponsoring organizations, the AART, the American College of Chest Physicians, the American Society of Anesthesiologists, and the American Thoracic Society.

In December 1974 the AART ratified the transfer of the technician certification examination system to the NBRC, thus making possible the credentialing of all respiratory therapy personnel under one organization.[5] There are now some 33,800 certified respiratory therapy technicians.

PUBLICATIONS

The official publications of the AART have undergone several changes since the first *Bulletin* of the Inhalation Therapy Association appeared in April 1950. The initial intent was to present material "in the interest of students of inhalation therapy." The publication was printed quarterly. Until 1954, very little was published about the Association and its activities.

In 1955 the *Bulletin* was replaced by the *Newsletter*, which was written in its entirety by the Association president and published monthly. The *Newsletter* was a mimeographed sheet addressed simply "Dear Member" and signed "Very sincerely" by the president. Its content was devoted entirely to Association news, thus leaving a void in the publication of articles regarding the scientific aspects of respiratory care.

As an economic measure the monthly *Newsletter* became a bimonthly by mid-1956. The following year only four issues were published. Quarterly publication of the *Newsletter* continued until 1967, when it again became a bimonthly publication.

To fill the gap created by discontinuation of articles on the practice of respiratory therapy in the *Bulletin-Newsletter*, the AART developed a journal. *Inhalation Therapy*, the official journal of the Association, was first published in February 1956. It was a 30-page, 6- by 9-inch magazine. James F. Whitacre served as the first editor, a position he held for the next 10 years. The new journal included news and information pertinent to the profession, including materials, research, operative techniques, and practical administration of therapy.

A major change in editorial policy occurred in January 1967 in accordance with a revision of the AAIT bylaws and the appointment of an editorial board. Operating policy for the *Newsletter* stated that it would be published six times a year in alternate months with the journal. Further, it would be the means of communication from the Board of Directors, the House of Delegates, and national committees to the membership. The *Newsletter's* intent was to keep the membership informed of all activities of their Association.

The journal was well conceived at its outset and has had staff stability as a hallmark; only three individuals have served as editor, with three publishers, in 26 years of publication. Its name was changed to *Respiratory Care* in 1971, and it began as a monthly publication in January 1974.

The journal today is widely recognized as the best scientific publication of the respiratory care profession. The editorial board and the journal's assistant editors and associates are people who speak with authority and recognition in the field of pulmonary medicine. Articles have followed the growth, improving status, and development of professionalism of the field. From a meager beginning *Respiratory Care* has evolved into a highly sophisticated publication reporting original investigations, new therapeutic concepts and equipment evaluations, modifications and review of equipment and procedures, and discussions of the management and philosophy of respiratory care.

In July 1977 the Association decided to publish a new magazine to keep the members informed of all activities affecting the profession. *AARTimes* has been well received and accepted by its readers and is considered essential for those who wish to be informed of all happenings within the profession.

Finally, the AART in early 1982 began publishing the AART Report with the purpose of reporting fast-breaking important news items.

EFFECTS OF LEGISLATION ON THE RESPIRATORY THERAPY PROFESSION

Federal legislation in October 1972 recommended adoption of a system of proficiency examinations to upgrade health personnel in connection with the Medicare and Medicaid programs. Known as Public Law 92-603, this act required the Secretary of Health, Education, and Welfare to develop a national credentialing system to determine qualifications of health personnel in relation to payment for services provided through Medicare and Medicaid. The task of establishing some sort of credentialing system was given to the Division of Medical Care Standards, Health Services and Mental Administration, a component of the Department of Health, Education, and Welfare. However, the responsibility of actually developing a credentialing mechanism was given to the Bureau of Health Manpower Education of the National Institutes of Health.

This legislation had definite implications for the field of respiratory therapy as well as for other allied health professions. In 1972 the Division of Allied Health Manpower awarded the AART a research contract designated to delineate the roles and functions of respiratory therapy workers, to develop proficiency examinations that would measure individual competency, and to establish a uniform mechanism for administering the examinations. Despite the fact that this work was performed, aside from the above-mentioned credentialing examination administered by the NBRT, the actual *role* of proficiency examinations in credentialing has yet to be determined, 11 years after the enabling legislation!

The federal government has increased its direct involvement in the practice of respiratory therapy directly proportional to the growth of the Medicare and Medicaid programs. Enacted in 1965, these two programs alone accounted for more than $70 billion in the 1982 federal budget. The federal government's involvement has been direct, with a pervasive attitude that if the taxpayer is paying the bill, the taxpayer ought to have some influence over the care delivered. This has sometimes resulted in formulation of ill-advised policies. Fortunately, through the efforts of the AART and its physician advisor groups, several important pieces of legislation have favorably modified the federal government's involvement in the practice of respiratory care. In 1980, as part of Public Law 96-330, the Veterans Administration was forced to conduct a survey to determine whether respiratory therapists should be shifted out of the traditional federal pay scales and into the special pay authorizations given to physicians and nurses employed within the Veterans Administration. Another section of that law, in fact, gave the Administrator of the Veterans Administration the authority to increase the salaries of respiratory therapists within a particular community if the therapists could verify that their salaries were below community norms for therapists in the private sector.

That same year another important piece of legislation, Public Law 96-499, was enacted by the Congress of the United States. The legislation established, for the first time, the words "respiratory therapy" as an integral part of the Medicare statutes. The actual statute created respiratory therapy as a reimbursable service when provided by a comprehensive outpatient rehabilitation facility. This important step was coupled with another section of that same law that required the Department of Health and Human Services to conduct a study to determine the conditions under which respiratory therapy should be reimbursed in the home. That study is clearly the first step toward full reimbursement for respiratory therapy services in the home setting.

The National Institutes of Health has been involved in important research in pulmonary medicine. A 6-year study of IPPB is to be completed shortly, and a recent study examining the benefits of continuous oxygen versus nocturnal oxygen brought dramatic results indicating the real value of continuous oxygen.

FUTURE OF RESPIRATORY THERAPY AND RESPIRATORY CARE

The respiratory therapy profession continues to attract many dedicated young people, while some people are beginning to question the challenge offered by the discipline. Is there to be a decline in future needs for respiratory care practitioners? Not likely, since analysis of death rates indicates that more than 10% are attributed to respiratory diseases; deaths caused by traumatic injuries also continue to rise; and respiratory problems as the result of smoking and, recently, drug abuse are a persistent major problem in the health status of our society.

Problems in health care delivery identified in the 1970s still remain as such in the 1980s. We still have a general maldistribution of health manpower; that is, adequate numbers of able workers possess many skills but are not directing them to where the need is greatest. A fundamental manpower issue in the respiratory therapy profession is the disparity between need and expectation on the one hand and available resources on the other. For example, the better-educated and increasingly urban population is demanding access to more and better health services, including respiratory care. Such services are neither ubiquitous nor uniformly available. Can the profession do anything to encourage better distribution of its own members?

The extraordinary growth of medical and technical knowledge in the last 30 years has made it nearly impossible for a complete range of services to be supplied except in highly sophisticated settings. Specialization has resulted, and the physician has become increasingly dependent on allied health professionals to assist him in the best and most efficient performance of his work.

The role and function of the respiratory care professional in highly specialized areas still remains to be clearly defined. The effectiveness of the health care delivery system could be enhanced by adequately educating allied health and medical professionals and by providing for health care teams. The word "adequately" is the key here: It would be as harmful to overtrain and overpopulate any of these professions as it would be to undertrain and underpopulate.

Efforts by the AART have helped define much of the role and scope of respiratory therapy and have produced some consensus as to what is adequate and effective education for the respiratory care practitioner. However, a few questions still must be answered.

1. The current system allows two different levels of training (certification and registry) at entry. There is considerable overlap in tasks performed by both groups. Is the two-level system practical any longer?
2. Who should monitor the performance of the system as a whole?
3. Who should plan?
4. What is the appropriate role of the public, and how can it be structured?
5. What should be the role of specific professional organizations and health care institutions?
6. How can given institutions or professions be induced to play the roles and undertake the

A CHRONOLOGICAL HISTORY OF THE RESPIRATORY THERAPY PROFESSION

1800 Beddoes uses oxygen therapeutically.
1918 Haldane studied effects of oxygen deficiency in humans and treats pulmonary edema.
1926 Oxygen tents first used by Barach.
1938 BLB mask used to supply oxygen for pilots at high altitude.
1947 IPPV used by Motley and coworkers for pulmonary atelectasis and acute pulmonary edema.
Inhalational Therapy Association organized.
1948 Official name changed to Inhalation Therapy Association.
1950 First *Bulletin* published.
First certificates of education in respiratory therapy issued.
1953 American College of Chest Physicians becomes official sponsor of the Inhalation Therapy Association.
1954 Official name changed to American Association of Inhalation Therapists.
1956 Board of Schools for Inhalation Therapy organized.
1960 American Registry of Inhalation Therapists incorporated.
1962 "Essentials" for approved schools developed.
1966 Board of Medical Advisors constituted.
1967 Official name changed to American Association for Inhalation Therapy.
1969 First Technician Certification Program approved and a pilot examination administered.
1970 American Respiratory Therapy Foundation incorporated.
Joint Review Committee for Inhalation Therapy Education established.
1972 Official name changed to American Association for Respiratory Therapy.
"Essentials" adopted by the American Medical Association.
American Thoracic Society becomes official sponsor of the American Association for Respiratory Therapy.
1974 National Board for Respiratory Therapy, Inc., established.
1981 Vigorous attempts at obtaining state legal credentialing (*e.g.,* licensure bills) begun nationwide.
1982 "Nontraditional" educational methods are accepted by the Joint Review Committee for Respiratory Therapy Education.

functions that would make sense in an effective plan?

7. How should continuing education in respiratory therapy be structured, and should it be mandatory for the professions?
8. Should there be mandatory recredentialing in respiratory therapy?
9. Is there an adequate supply of respiratory therapy manpower?

Many believe that the health care system in the United States will be characterized by provision of comprehensive services to all people. Greatly increased attention will be given to health maintenance and disease prevention. This is the result of [1] health maintenance being grossly neglected by the present system of health care; [2] new scientific developments in preventive medicine that will contribute to this trend; and [3] the fact that health professionals, as well as the general public, feel responsible for the health system and have recognized that prevention of illness is a less expensive undertaking than treatment of acute or chronic disease.

The respiratory therapy profession must strive for the best and for less expensive treatment for the patient. At the same time, it must be prepared to accept results of well-planned studies and be willing to abandon previously held opinions, and thereby alter established practice routines.

Additionally, the profession should develop guidelines for proper use of therapy and should serve as an educational and regulatory agency. Finally, the profession must see that research is encouraged and done within its own and the medical community to ensure that the principles and practices of the profession develop and retain a more solid scientific basis.

REFERENCES

1. Barach AL et al: Minimum standards for inhalation therapy. JAMA 144:25, 1950
2. Boothby WM: Effects of high altitudes on the composition of alveolar air: Introductory remarks. Proc Staff Meet Mayo Clin 20:209, 1945
3. Hinshaw HC et al: Clinical applications of oxygen therapy. Arch Phys Ther XXIII:598, 1942
4. Motley HL et al: Observations on the use of positive pressure. J Aviat Med 18:417, 1947
5. Tomashefski JF: The National Board for Respiratory Therapy: Past, present and future. Bull Am Coll Chest Physicians 14:9, 1975

BIBLIOGRAPHY

Miller WF: The future of respiratory therapy. Hosp Adm Can Sept: 31, 1973

Pierce AK: Respiratory therapy: State of the art. Respir Care 26:746, 1981

2

Education of Respiratory Care Personnel

Thomas J. DeKornfeld • Craig L. Scanlan

The word "education" is defined in Webster as "the act or process of imparting or acquiring general knowledge or skill, developing the powers of reasoning and judgment and generally of preparing oneself or others intellectually for maturity."

Our purpose in this chapter is to discuss the history and present status of education in respiratory care and to place it into context with health education generally. A brief historical overview is followed by a more detailed description of the current status of education in respiratory care, with a special look at nontraditional educational activities and their relation to the accreditation process. Separate sections are devoted to the developmental problems of schools of respiratory therapy, to credentialing, to continuing education, and, briefly, to the economics of respiratory care education. In a final section we make an "educated" guess as to the directions in which education in this important health field is likely to move. A glossary to assist with the educational jargon and a bibliography are appended.

Initially, we wish to make a few brief philosophical comments on education generally. A rather general misconception equates education with knowledge. Confounding the process with the product is easy, and it is very tempting to assume that if the process is sound, the product is bound to be competent. In an ideal world this may be true, but in a system governed by human frailties, administered by imperfect human beings and directed toward young people of widely varying abilities, interests, aims, and integrity, the system is bound to be marred by inconsistencies, weaknesses, and shortcomings. This is true for any educational system, and the problems are significantly increased if the students need, by the nature of their chosen field, not only knowledge but competence, not only information and problem-solving ability but psychomotor skills and empathy.

The goal of the educational process in respiratory care, as indeed in all health professions, is to take an amorphous pool of human raw material and, in a brief time, transform it into learned, competent, concerned, dedicated health professionals. The highest praise that can be bestowed on the present system is that it succeeds in accomplishing this goal in a remarkable number of instances.

HISTORICAL OVERVIEW

HEALTH EDUCATION

Health education is probably almost as old as mankind inself. Still mixed heavily with magic, health education began to assume more formal shape in the days of Hammurabi (20th century B.C.), when a considerable amount of health information was available and undoubtedly passed on from generation to generation. In classic Greece, the school of Hippocrates in Delos, associated with the temple of Apollo, assumed a major role in the gathering of ancient information, in the development of new knowledge, and in the education of young men who wished to devote their lives to the practice of the healing arts. The Hippocratic school, bolstered and perpetuated by the writings and teachings of Galen (2nd century A.D.), survived well into the middle ages of the Christian era, when formal schools of medicine were first established in Europe. The School of Salerno was followed over the next 2 centuries by the development of numerous medical schools, associated with the great universities of Italy, France, and Germany: Padua, Montpelier, Paris, and, later, Leyden, the sources from which medical education flowed to all parts of the western world. This knowledge was much augmented by early contacts with Arabic medicine, which at that time was more advanced than its counterpart in the West.

Besides medicine, the only other healing art that has a longstanding history is nursing. Practiced primarily by religious orders, nursing fell into some disrepute during the 18th and 19th centuries when, following the Crimean War, it was reestablished on a high level by Florence Nightingale in Great Britain.

Both medical and nursing education, once formally established, developed very slowly and were hampered by tradition and by the massive conservatism of organized medicine. In fact, medical education was a morass until its weaknesses were demonstrated by Abraham Flexner in the first years of the 20th century. Following the appearance and acceptance of the Flexner Report, medical education assumed the shape that we see today. The apprentice system was abandoned except as part of a structured curriculum, science education became an integral part of medical education, and medical educators became academicians, both in the basic and clinical sciences. This era was also characterized by an explosive increase in research and an exponential increase in medical information.

Nursing education lagged behind medical education for reasons we need not examine. Suffice it to say that nursing education remained a largely hospital-based apprenticeship training function until the 1950–1960s, when the proliferation of 4-year baccalaureate programs and the gradual, slow development of graduate programs changed this major branch of health education into a modern educational system. It is both interesting and pertinent that the general acceptance of formal undergraduate education for nurses was followed rapidly by the development of a lower level, formal, educational system based in community colleges and culminating in an Associate in Arts degree. Thus, at the present writing, nursing training still takes place at three levels, although hospital-based, 3-year programs are diminishing rapidly and the 2-year, associate-degree programs are under attack.

The educational systems in the other health professions followed similar patterns, practically without exception. Recognition of a need for specialized knowledge and skills was followed by a self-selection of small numbers of interested people who may or may not have had hospital experience in another field. If the validity of the "new" profession could be demonstrated, training programs emerged. A purely apprenticeship level training was followed rapidly by the establishment of more formal systems, first based in hospitals and later based in educational institutions. The accreditation of the programs and the credentialing of the graduates followed as a matter of course. The next step in almost all the allied health professions was a fragmentation of the educational system and the establishment of two or more levels of training and formal recognition. The results of these developments are too recent to be fully tested, although this has not prevented a continued drive for more and more formal education and the voicing of noisy and usually highly subjective criticism of the existing system.

RESPIRATORY CARE EDUCATION

The developmental patterns outlined above apply, with very minor modifications, to the history of respiratory care education.

The need for specially trained nonmedical personnel to manage patients with respiratory problems was recognized in the years immediately after World War II. The formation of the Inhalation Therapy Association in 1947 was followed very shortly by the first formal educational program. In 1950, a course was presented in Chicago of 16 weeks' duration, and a total of 31 participants received a Certificate of Completion.

That same year two publications, originating in New York City, dealt with the standards required for the safe and effective administration of inhalation therapy. These two publications, by Barach and his associates and by the Committee on Public Health

Relations of the New York Academy of Medicine, established the basis for most of the early educational activities in this field.[4,33]

In rapidly developing health fields, the supply of trained personnel often lagged behind the number of positions available in the major metropolitan and academic health centers. The only form of training was apprenticeship or on-the-job training (OJT). In effect the technologists who entered the field, usually from the ranks of orderlies and aides or, rarely, from the ranks of nursing, were instructed by physicians interested in respiratory problems. This, of course, meant that the instruction was highly individualized and reflected the likes or dislikes, knowledge or ignorance, idiosyncracies or prejudices of the individual mentors.

After several years of this method, two anesthesiologists in New York, Drs. Edwin Emma and Vincent Collins, initiated a process that led to the formation of an advisory committee to the Council on Medical Education (CME) of the American Medical Association (AMA) in 1956. This advisory committee represented the three organizations most concerned with respiratory care education: the American Society of Inhalation Therapy, the American College of Chest Physicians, and the American Society of Anesthesiologists.

The process, once began, moved through the administrative maze with surprising dispatch. The New York delegation to the House of Delegates of the AMA introduced a resolution at the annual meeting in 1957 to develop schools of inhalation therapy. This resolution was referred for action to the CME which, that same year, issued a document entitled "Essentials for an Approved School of Inhalation Therapy Technicians." After a trial period of 3 years the CME formally endorsed these "Essentials" and submitted them to the House of Delegates of the AMA for formal approval. This was granted by the House in December 1962, and thus the early development of respiratory care education had reached its initial plateau.

To assure implementation of, and compliance with, the "Essentials," a group of "experts" was needed who would be willing to assume the responsibility for this task. Thus in January 1963, on invitation by the CME and under its auspices, the first Board of Schools for Inhalation Therapy was established. Its membership comprised four physicians (two representing the ASA and two representing the ACCP) and three therapists (representing the AAIT). The Board was formally charged with the responsibility of reviewing applications, performing on-site evaluations, and making recommendations to the CME on the formal accreditation of programs in respiratory care. The members of the Board of Schools were appointed by the presidents of the organizations they represented, and, initially, there was no time limit on the length of service of the members.

The initial "Essentials" were weak, but the enthusiasm and devotion of a large group of physicians and therapists ensured that sound programs could develop in the absence of really meaningful guidelines. The Board struggled valiantly to perform their very difficult task. Prominent among its early members were Vincent Collins (ASA), Edwin R. Levine (ACCP), H. Frederick Helmholz, Jr. (ACCP), Vincent Kracum, James Whitacre, and Easton Smith (AAIT).

The Board worked in close cooperation with the AMA and was strongly and ably supported by Don Lehmkuhl, Ph.D., the AMA staff person assigned to the Board. During the first few years of the Board's existence the number of schools increased slowly. The first program to receive accreditation was at Cook County Hospital in Chicago in June 1964.

The "Essentials" were revised in 1966, and the revision was approved by the House of Delegates of the AMA in June 1967. These "Essentials" were an improvement over the first set and required a training period of 18 months. The Board officially still opposed academic orientation in respiratory care education and was unwilling to recommend accreditation for programs sponsored by postsecondary educational institutions. This policy, reflecting the personal bias of the Chairman, was not shared by most members. It was therefore decided to disband the Board of Schools, to establish immediately the Joint Review Committee for Inhalation Therapy Education under the chairmanship of H. F. Helmholz, Jr., and to give parity to the therapist members. Accordingly, and with AMA approval, the Joint Review Committee was incorporated under the laws of the State of Minnesota on 15 January, 1970. The first members of the Joint Review Committee were H. F. Helmholz, Jr., and E. R. Levine (ACCP), P. E. Dumke and L. H. Ruttle (ASA), and G. L. Davis, V. F. Kracum, E. R. Smith, and J. F. Whitacre (AAIT).

The new Joint Review Committee immediately undertook the revision of the "Essentials," which were finally approved by the AMA in June 1972. The new "Essentials" made significant contributions to respiratory care education: They recommended academic sponsorship for the therapist level programs, and for the first time recognized a second level of education in respiratory care. This was the result of the establishment of the Technician Certification Board by the AAIT and the formal recognition by the professional organization that the field of respiratory care required health professionals functioning, and therefore requiring training, at two levels.

Also in 1972 the Joint Review Committee expanded by admitting the American Thoracic Society (ATS) as a sponsor. To maintain parity, the number of therapist members was increased to six. In 1974, in conformance with proper usage, the name of the committee was changed to Joint Review Committee for Respiratory Therapy Education. At the same time a public representative was added to the membership of the committee.

Because the field of respiratory care was changing rapidly, it was necessary to revise the "Essentials" again in 1977. These new "Essentials" mandated that therapist level programs be sponsored by the educational institutions and that technician programs, which for the first time had separate "Essentials," had to be at least "affiliated" with educational institutions. The 1977 "Essentials" also made significant advances in recognizing the need for "advanced standing," for proper experience and training for the key personnel of the programs, for an expanded curriculum, and for relevant laboratory experience before clinical contact for the students.

The last few years have seen a number of changes in the formal structure of respiratory care education and its evaluation. The AMA has transferred final authority from the House of Delegates to the CME. The CME in turn has established a Committee on Allied Health Education and Accreditation (CAHEA) as the accrediting agency, which has been recognized by the United States Department of Education and by the Council on Postsecondary Accreditation. The Joint Review Committee has also seen a number of changes. Dr. Helmholz resigned as Chairman in 1976. He had been instrumental in leading the Joint Review Committee into the era of modern health education—that is, from largely apprenticeship training in hospitals to the legitimate educational activities performed by educational institutions. Respiratory care education owes more to Dr. Helmholz than to any other person. The change in chairmanship brought a number of other changes, the most important of which were the establishment of an Executive Office, the selection of an Executive Director, the limitation of terms of office for the officers, the establishment of an executive committee and a number of other committees, and the establishment of a new process for handling applications.

The foregoing is a brief overview of the development of respiratory care education. It has been an almost explosive development, certainly not free of strife and agitation. It was guided and shaped by two organizations, the Joint Review Committee and the National Board for Respiratory Care. The current status of respiratory care education described in the following section is the result of the activities, usually harmonious and always vigorous, of these two organizations.

CURRENT STATUS OF RESPIRATORY THERAPY EDUCATION

Respiratory therapy education currently represents the third largest allied health occupational category accredited under CAHEA (radiography and medical laboratory sciences being first and second in size, respectively). Some 430 accredited programs in 48 states enroll in excess of 15,000 students, graduating close to 14,000 new respiratory therapy practitioners each year.[8] About half of these graduates complete their education in respiratory technician programs. Since the adoption of "Essentials" for accredited educational programs for respiratory therapy technicians (1972), technician education has undergone remarkable growth and change. In the short period between 1974 and 1984, the number of accredited technician programs has increased more than thirtyfold (Table 2-1). Whereas most of the early technician programs were hospital sponsored, the majority of those currently active now operate under the auspices of postsecondary educational institutions (junior col-

Table 2-1. CAHEA Accredited Respiratory Therapy Programs

YEAR	TECHNICIAN	THERAPIST
1983	203	227
1982	192	178
1980	194	192
1978	155	165
1976	55	147
1974	5	126
1972	0	125
1970	0	56
1968	0	44
1966	0	21
1964	0	

leges, community colleges, or vocational–technical schools). This trend in sponsorship changeover from hospital to college is due to the general change in health education and was catalyzed by the 1977 revision of the JRCRTE "Essentials." It now ensures that all students enrolled in technician programs are exposed to an academic milieu and receive at least some college credit for their educational experience. Concomitant with this growing emphasis on the academic component of technician training has been a noticeable trend toward increasing the length of the educational programs beyond the 12-month minimum now required in the "Essentials." Approximately 15% of the extant technician programs exceed 12 months; a small number of programs have curricula of 18 months or more. Few, however, provide an Associate's Degree or its equivalent. Most graduates receive a certificate of completion and are eligible to take the Certification Examination offered by the National Board for Respiratory Care (NBRC), provided all other criteria for eligibility are met. Successful completion of the Certification Examination results in credentialing as a Certified Respiratory Therapy Technician (CRTT).

The other respiratory therapy graduates complete their preparation for entry into the field through one of the approximately 200 accredited respiratory *therapist* educational programs. Whereas technician programs must be *affiliated* with a credit-granting institution of higher education, therapist programs must be *sponsored* by a properly accredited postsecondary vocational–technical school, college, or university. In such a setting, students who receive therapist-level education are granted full credit for both the academic and clinical components of their course work, receiving, upon completion of their education, both a certificate and a degree. The vast majority of therapist programs offer an Associate's Degree, although a small but growing number of programs provide opportunities for students to receive a baccalaureate degree. Graduate therapists are eligible for a two-level examination system offered by the NBRC. Upon successful completion of the second level of the NBRC examination system, individuals are credentialed as Registered Respiratory Therapists (RRT).

TYPICAL PROGRAM STRUCTURE

Although there is a diversity of organizational arrangements among the educational programs and no structural framework is truly "typical," we have attempted to portray the most common organizational pattern in Figure 2-1. The figure depicts the organizational chart of a 2-year therapist program sponsored by a community college. With minor variations it could be applied to both community-college-sponsored technician programs and to 2- or 4-year programs located in a university setting. As a generic model, it provides the basis for describing the institutional relationships that characterize a well-conceived respiratory therapy educational program and the functions of the key personnel.

Institutional Administration

Typically, college-based respiratory therapy programs function under a major academic division of the institution, usually administered by a dean. The dean is responsible for the overall organization, planning, controlling, and budgeting of the material and personnel resources necessary to operate the various programs and courses offered by that division. Although respiratory therapy program personnel may be directly responsible to this administrative officer, it is more common to find a middle-level administrator overseeing such operations, especially where multiple allied health programs are offered. If the allied health programs are organized as a school (typical of academic health science centers), this person may, in fact, hold a dean-level position. If there is no School of Allied Health, the "Director of Allied Health" reports to the dean of the academic division and is delegated major responsibilities for administering the health-related programs. These responsibilities include fiscal planning, budget administration, faculty recruitment, selection and evaluation, curriculum assessment, student selection, admissions, and the implementation of the contractual clinical affiliations. The Director of Allied Health may also be responsible for the supervision of the nonacademic support staff such as secretaries, clerical aides, and laboratory personnel.

Program Faculty

Typically, two key, full-time faculty are directly responsible for the operation of the program: the Program Director and the Director of Clinical Education (Clinical Coordinator).

Operating under the administrative supervision of the Director of Allied Health, the Program Director is responsible for the overall organization, administration, periodic review, continued development, and effectiveness of the educational program. In addition,

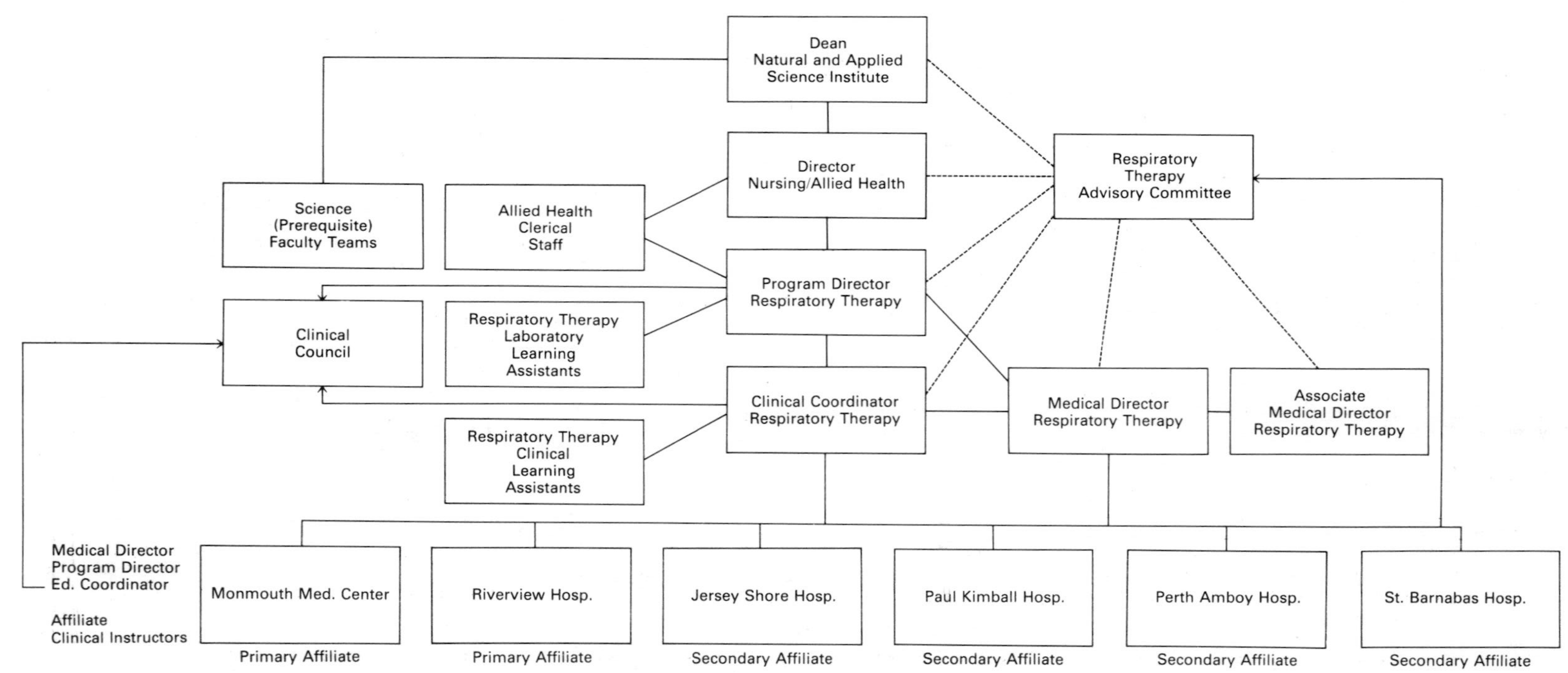

Fig. 2-1. Organizational chart of a typical respiratory therapy educational program.

the Program Director typically assumes major responsibility for coordinating (and providing) the didactic and preclinical or laboratory components of the curriculum and for ensuring that an appropriate evaluation system is used and that comprehensive records of student performance and proficiency are maintained. Competent coordination of these many and diverse functions requires that the Program Director collaborate fully with other program faculty, with the Medical Director of the Program, and with other supportive and contributing personnel. Fulfilling such a role requires strong administrative support from the institutional sponsor of the program.

The Director of Clinical Education (Clinical Coordinator) is typically responsible to the Program Director for the overall coordination, supervision, and evaluation of the clinical component of the program, to include [a] the establishment and implementation of policies and guidelines for clinical instruction and evaluation; [b] the supervision, coordination, and evaluation of the clinical affiliate staff providing instruction for the program; and [c] the development and maintenance of the students' clinical performance and proficiency records. In addition, the Director of Clinical Education serves as the primary liaison between the program and the clinical affiliate service departments and may be responsible for the ongoing evaluation of the contribution and effectiveness of the clinical affiliates in regard to meeting the program needs and the accreditation standards. In collaboration with the Medical Director, the Director of Clinical Education additionally may assume responsibility for scheduling and coordinating the physician input at each of the program's clinical affiliates.

Medical Director

Although usually not a full-time faculty member of the sponsoring institution, the Medical Director assumes a crucial role in the overall success of the program. Typically, the Medical Director holds a staff position or attending appointment at one or more of the program's clinical affiliates and commonly serves simultaneously as Medical Director of an affiliate's Respiratory Care Service Department. In assuming ultimate responsibility for the medical quality of the program, the Medical Director must take an active role not only in the didactic and clinical instruction of students, but also in the ongoing planning, implementation, and evaluation of the entire program of instruction. Particularly critical is the Medical Director's responsibility in ensuring that all students receive pertinent instruction from physicians in each phase of their clinical experience and at all clinical sites. The Medical Director must gain the active collaboration of interested physicians in the bedside or classroom instruction of the students to assure the quality of the program and to contribute significantly to the skills and knowledge of its graduates. Where possible, or necessary, an Associate Medical Director can provide support and assistance to the Medical Director of the program. Such a role is particularly appropriate when multiple, primary clinical affiliates are used and when a second physician (at an affiliate other than that at which the Medical Director holds staff appointment) has an especially strong interest in contributing to the program.

Clinical Affiliates

Clinical sites, their personnel, and material resources are the lifeblood of the respiratory therapy educational programs. Ultimately, the quality of a program, the knowledge, skills, and sensitivities of its graduates are contingent upon the soundness of the clinical component of the educational process. No other aspect of program structure and function is as important or consequential as the development and nurturing of strong collaborative efforts to provide and maintain quality clinical education.

Clinical educational sites should be selected, developed, and evaluated according to the degree to which they meet the standards of accreditation (the "Essentials"), the appropriate standards of national agencies (JCAH, AOA), and the extent to which they fulfill program needs. An example of such programmatic criteria for clinical site selection, developed and adapted from similar guidelines promulgated by the American Physical Therapy Association, follows.[27]

CRITERIA FOR EVALUATION AND SELECTION OF CLINICAL AFFILIATES

1. The clinical agency's philosophy and objective for patient care and education must be similar to, and compatible with, those of the educational institution.
2. The clinical agency must demonstrate support of, and interest in, the educational programs.
3. Communication within the clinical agency itself should be effective and positive.
4. The affiliate service department should provide an active, stimulating environment ap-

propriate for the learning needs of the student.

5. The affiliate service department should have an active and viable process of internal evaluation of its own affairs and should be receptive to procedures of review approved by appropriate external agencies.
6. Consumers should be satisfied that their needs for the designated service are being met.
7. Selected support services should be available to affiliating students.
8. Adequate space for study, conferences, and patient treatment should be available to affiliating students.
9. Programs for affiliating students should be planned to meet the specific objectives of the curriculum and the student.
10. The clinical agencies must have a sufficient variety of learning experiences available to affiliating students.
11. The staff of the clinical agency must maintain ethical standards of practice.
12. The roles of the various affiliate departmental personnel must be clearly defined and distinguished from one another.
13. There should be an active staff development program for the clinical agency.
14. The staff of the affiliate service department should be interested and active in professional associations.
15. The staff of the affiliate service department must possess the expertise to provide quality patient care and, where required, be of adequate size to provide appropriate supervision/instruction.
16. One staff member of the affiliate service department should be designated to coordinate the activities of the students at the clinical agency.
17. Selection of clinical instructor/supervisors must be based on specific criteria.
18. Clinical instructor/supervisors must be able to apply the basic principles of education to clinical learning.
19. The special expertise of the various clinical agency staff members should be shared with the affiliating students.
20. The clinical agency must be committed to the principles of equal opportunity and affirmative action as required by federal legislation.

To ensure that the rights, obligations, and responsibilities of the collaborating parties and of the students are clearly defined and protected, cooperative arrangements between the sponsor and the health care agencies that provide the clinical component of education *must* be formalized. Such formalized arrangements, in the form of written contracts, are the prerequisites to establishing good interinstitutional relationships. To the extent that the formalized arrangements provide for a meaningful *quid pro quo* relationship, the strength and continuity of the collaborative efforts are enhanced. Guidelines for the development of formal interinstitutional arrangements for clinical education are provided by Moore, Parker, and Nourse.[19]

Clinical agencies participating in the education of respiratory therapy personnel may generally be classified according to the scope and the intensity of experience they provide. *Primary affiliates* characteristically provide a comprehensive experience in a variety of clinical respiratory care procedures and services, conforming in quality and type to national standards. *Secondary affiliates* provide limited, specialized learning experiences in selected areas of respiratory care or in related service departments. As the scope of practice broadens and as increasing technological sophistication creates the demand for new and more specialized skills, the need for providing students with such specialized experience, and the need for carefully selected and rationally used secondary affiliates, is likely to grow. Secondary affiliation should never be misconstrued as an excuse for a second-rate clinical experience. In fact, the use of a good secondary affiliate implies that the experience provided there is better in scope or in intensity than what would otherwise be available.

Since most clinical instruction and supervision, in most educational programs, is provided by service departmental staff, their input to and collaboration with, the full-time program faculty and medical director is crucial to the success of the program. In college-sponsored programs, it is incumbent upon the administration to recognize formally the contribution of these personnel by granting them adjunct faculty status or some other title and, where possible, the rights and privileges normally granted to such members of the academic community. Equally important is the involvement of such personnel in the development, implementation, and evaluation of program policies and procedures, particularly those related to clinical instruction and to the evaluation of clinical progress and proficiency. In our experience, nothing is less appropriate or potentially more divisive than giving service departmental staff the responsibility for the instruction and supervision of students without granting them some authority in making the judgments and decisions necessary to determine student progress. To the extent that such decision-making authority is shared, the likelihood of cooperation is increased. Establishment of a *clinical council* (Fig. 2-1), organized by the Director of Clinical Education and with representation from each participating clinical affiliate, is one method of sharing both responsibility and authority for implementing clinical policies and procedures. Whether formally established by affiliate contractual agreement or informally organized by consensus of those with a vested interest in the clinical component of the educational program, the clinical council can provide invaluable assistance to key program personnel in coordinating clinical activities, monitoring student progress, and assessing the overall quality of clinical instruction and supervision.

Advisory Committee

Whereas the clinical council oversees the day-to-day operations of the clinical components of the educational program and may be instrumental in developing and enacting policy decisions, the advisory committee serves to assist the program staff and its institutional sponsor in maintaining program responsiveness to professional, community, and agency needs. Typically, the advisory committee includes [a] representatives from each of the affiliated institutions; [b] health professionals not associated with the program; [c] one or more public representatives; and [d] an enrolled student or program graduate. College administrative personnel (if the program is college sponsored) and program faculty should not be members of the committee. As representatives of the sponsoring institution, such personnel are *seeking* the counsel and advice of the committee members, not giving it.

Advisory committees, in our experience, are successful only to the extent that their role in the program is clearly defined. All too often, operating without goals or direction, advisory committees drift aimlessly between two extremes: those that dogmatically seek to control program policies and operations and those that tacitly "meet and eat." Neither role is, of course, appropriate. That advisory committees can play a vital role in the development and maintenance of quality education for respiratory care personnel is clear; how well they perform that role is contingent upon both the care with which the members are selected and the degree to which their function is deliberately planned.[7]

FUNCTIONAL ASPECTS OF PROGRAM OPERATIONS

No organizational chart or description of personnel and material resources can portray adequately the functional complexities encountered in operating a respiratory therapy educational program. Such programs are not static; they are dynamic systems of interacting components operating within complex organizational and social environments to which they must be constantly attuned and responsive. How well extant components are integrated, and how well the various resources and transactions necessary to the program are orchestrated, will largely determine both the soundness of the educational endeavor and the benefits accrued to its participants.

A helpful perspective, by which the complex operational aspects of a dynamic educational program can be better understood, is that of *systems theory*. An elaboration of this approach, employed as a mechanism to administer and control efficiently the interacting components of the educational process, is described by DeLapp.[11] Simply, an educational program is perceived as an open system of definable inputs (students, tangible program resources), processes, or transactions (mainly the teaching–learning activities) and outputs (graduate practitioners with specific knowledge, skills, and sensitivities). As depicted in Figure 2-2 the system is "open" to the extent that its function is subject to the influence of, and interaction with, its environment. The environment provides the program with its inputs (students, resources), affects the nature and characteristics of the teaching–learning activities, and ultimately serves as the consumer of the program's output (graduate practitioners). An abstract but important input from the environment is the community's *expected* output from the system. Thus program planners must match the expected output from the community with those of the evolving program and provide the frequent modulation of both processes as experience accumulates. This modulation may well be achieved by an active and interested "Advisory Committee." Key environmental influences affecting a respiratory therapy program include its parent organization; its applicable accrediting and credentialing agencies; federal, state, and local gov-

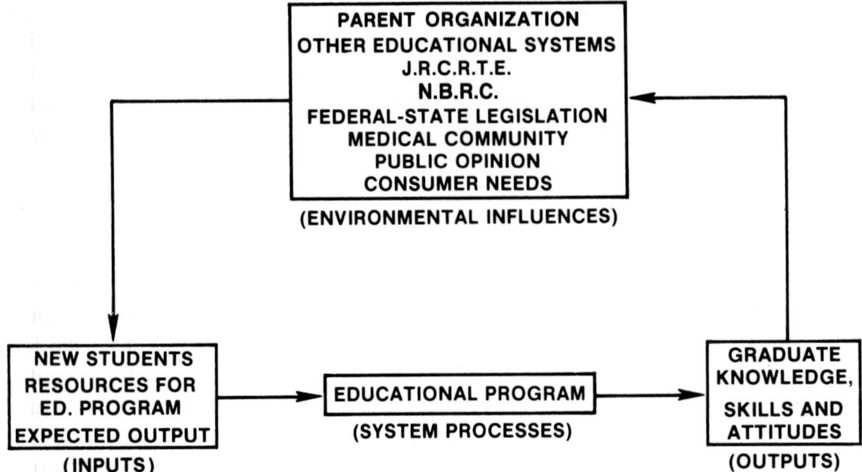

Fig. 2-2. An "open system" respiratory therapy educational program. (This material is reproduced, with permission, from DeLapp GT: The systems approach for administration of respiratory therapy education programs. Respir Care 24:514, 1979.)

ernments; the medical and allied health professional and education communities; health care provider agencies; health care consumers; and the public at large.

Although it is beyond the scope of this chapter to detail the components and complex interactions that characterize the "dynamics of function" of a respiratory therapy program, certain key elements demand scrutiny. Foremost among these are two input processes (student selection and curriculum development), two transactional processes (curriculum integration and student evaluation), and one general systems process (program evaluation).

Student Selection and Admission

The nature of the teaching–learning activities of an educational program and, to a large extent, the quality of its output depend on the entering characteristics of its students. With many more applicants than can be accommodated by limited class capacities, respiratory therapy programs have not only the right but also the duty to implement selection processes that assure, with a high degree of accuracy, that those admitted to the program will succeed in achieving its goals and objectives. Unfortunately, the relatively high attrition rates encountered in respiratory therapy programs indicate that such processes, even where used, do not provide such assurance.

Good admission processes—that is, those that exhibit high predictive validity—must focus on prospective student characteristics that can reasonably be shown to relate to the necessary aptitude, skill, and sensitivity required of the successful practitioner. These should include selection criteria from the cognitive domain, the affective domain, and the psychomotor domain. Sole reliance on grade point average (GPA) or academic aptitude tests is no longer acceptable because, while these have some predictive value for student performance, they have practically no predictive value for practitioner performance.[14] Those characteristics developed as a result of the instructional process are logically excluded as admission criteria. Other attributes should be subject to "internal validation" to determine how effectively they do predict success in the program. Where no standardized mechanism exists to assess the characteristics or traits identified as prerequisite to successful achievement, it must be developed locally according to acceptable psychometric procedures. Finally, the selection process, its policies, and procedures must be clearly delineated to all concerned with its implementation. Particular care must be exercised to ensure that the process accommodates all federal statutes and regulations related to discrimination and due process. The result of such efforts—that is, a valid and legally defensible selection mechanism—should enable the program to achieve its goals and improve the quality of its output (the professional competence of its graduates).

Curriculum Development

A program's curriculum is the body of experiences and activities selected and arranged for instruction and learning. Curriculum development is the ongoing process of selecting, organizing, and evaluating the effectiveness of the instructional experiences and activities of the system.

The efficacy with which this process is able to identify and incorporate relevant learning experiences within the program will largely determine the degree to which the knowledge, skill, and sensitivity of the program's graduates will meet those expected or required of the entry-level practitioner. Learning experiences are relevant to the extent that they facilitate the students' development of the competencies necessary to discharge their professional roles. *Competency-based* curriculum development identifies the professional roles students will assume upon completing their program and determines exactly what constitutes effective performance within these roles.[31]

Unfortunately, the process of curriculum development in respiratory therapy education has been based, until recently, on often parochial notions of the competencies expected of graduate practitioners. With only the topical outlines provided in the "Essentials" as a guide, it is little wonder that program graduates have varied widely in both range and level of their proficiency. Recent developments in the profession, however, are beginning to exert a significant influence on respiratory therapy program curricula. Under contract with the Health Resources Administration (HRA), the AART completed, in 1977, a project to delineate the roles and functions of respiratory care personnel.[2] Although the major findings and recommendations of the study continue to provoke heated debate, its major conclusion—that a single, generalist position for credentialing practitioners at entry level would be most appropriate for the field—has been adopted by the National Board for Respiratory Care as the basis for developing its new credentialing examination process. More recently, the University of Texas Health Science Center at Dallas, also under HRA contract, has completed a curriculum guide for respiratory therapy that incorporates the major and minor responsibilities identified in the 1977 AART role delineation study as the basis for selecting and organizing the learning experiences of the instructional component of the educational process.[12] As of this writing, it is too early to judge the full impact of these developments on the educational system. Similar trends in other allied health disciplines suggest that the long-term ramifications are likely to be far-reaching.

Curriculum Integration

Even sound curriculum content cannot guarantee effective or efficient student learning. Learning experiences must be organized purposefully to establish meaningful interrelationships between the essential concepts and activities of the program's curriculum. The process of purposefully organizing and articulating the various elements of the curriculum into a unified framework is called *integration*.

Of particular importance in respiratory therapy programs is the integration of the didactic and clinical components of the curriculum. When properly implemented, such integration facilitates the transfer of conceptual knowledge and comprehension to the professional realities of application, problem-solving, and synthesis. Lacking a unifying framework, learning occurs in discrete and unrelated episodes of little immediate value to the student or future value to the practitioner.

One of us (CLS) has elaborated a systematic planning and evaluation model designed to promote the articulation of the curricular and course elements into such a unified or integrated framework. According to the model, the full integration of didactic and clinical learning experiences depends on the successful implementation of three concurrent strategies: administrative integration of program components; curriculum integration; and course integration. Although the details of the model are beyond the scope of this chapter, certain key elements are relevant and worthy of emphasis. Those interested in pursuing the concept in depth should consult the primary source, *Clinical Education for the Allied Health Professions*.[27]

Administrative strategies that facilitate the integration of didactic and clinical education are based on the institutional/programmatic philosophy and goals; the selection and use of clinical resources; and the distribution and development of personnel resources. Many of the discrete administrative strategies have already been discussed. Additional administrative mechanisms to promote the integration of the didactic and clinical components of the curriculum follow.

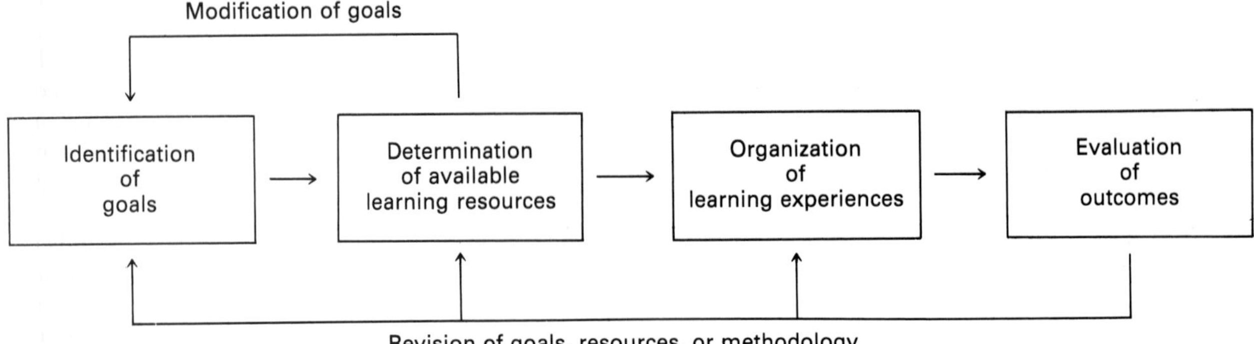

Fig. 2-3. Curriculum development model.

Two major categories of curriculum integrative strategies are evident: those related to the derivation and specification of program, course, and unit goals and objectives; and those related to the selection and organization of the learning experiences that constitute the curriculum. Derivation and specification of goals and objectives should be based on a systematic planning model such as that of Tyler[35] (Fig. 2-3). Objectives, once derived, can promote integration if they contribute to satisfying a learner need; the relation between enabling objectives and the general goals of the learning episode is made clear; overspecificity is avoided; and the integration of learning experiences is itself revealed as an objective.[23]

In terms of the selection and organization of learning experiences, the model uses a three-dimensional curriculum perspective that provides not only integration, but also sequence and continuity. Within such a framework, *integration* organizes learning experiences to provide for horizontal relationships between curricular elements; *continuity* establishes a vertical relation between different levels of the same skills or proficiencies; and *sequence* organizes learning experiences at progressively higher and more diverse levels of competency.

STRATEGIES FOSTERING INTEGRATION

Administrative Strategies

Institutional and Programmatic Philosophy and Goals

- should be determined by sponsoring institutions
- should be based on identified competencies
- should be compatible with needs and characteristics of the learners

Designation of Clinical and Didactic Components

- clinical resources should be selected according to identified criteria
- primary and secondary affiliate selection should be based on identified need
- clinical sites should be in proximity to the sponsoring institution
- liaison and advisory committees should assist in coordinating interinstitutional arrangements

Distribution and Development of Personnel Resources

- the role of the director of clinical education (clinical coordinator) should be delineated
- faculty assignment (clinical and didactic) should be rotated
- clinical staff development programs should be implemented
- clinical staff should be recognized and acknowledged for their input

Curriculum Strategies

Identification of Goals and Objectives

- a systematic curriculum planning and evaluation model should be used
- objectives should be derived from identified practitioner competence
- objectives should be specified in a manner that fosters integration

Selection and Organization of Learning Experiences

- a three-dimensional curriculum perspective (integration, sequence, and continuity) should be used
- organizing elements (general goals) should be consistent with overall objectives of long-range utility to learners

- the skills or practice laboratory should be integrated within a clinical mastery sequence
- a concurrent curriculum design with full-time clinical asignments toward the end of the program should be used
- clinical experience should be organized in three phases: initial exposure and observation, learning and reinforcement, and minimally supervised experience

Course Strategies

- content should be organized in appropriate units
- individualized, flexible clinical scheduling should be provided
- team teaching should be encouraged
- problem-solving and seminars should be emphasized and correlated with later phases of clinical experience
- instructors should model integrative behavior

Articulating the didactic and clinical experience within this three-dimensional curriculum perspective is facilitated by the incorporation of a practice or skills laboratory as an integral component of the students' learning experiences; the logical patterning of didactic, laboratory, and clinical instruction; and the use of organizing centers.

The development and use of a respiratory therapy learning laboratory has been previously described by one of us (CLS)[30]; subsequently the JRCRTE has emphasized its importance in the curriculum and made it a requirement in the 1977 "Essentials." The JRCRTE also provides programs with a generic laboratory equipment list as part of its *Current Standards*.[16]

The patterning of didactic, laboratory, and clinical instruction is an equally critical curriculum integrative strategy. Unfortunately, there is a dearth of research in this area. Until evidence appears to the contrary, however, the arrangement most logically promoting integration appears to be weekly clinical assignments throughout the curriculum (correlated with the didactic and laboratory experience), culminating in full-time clinical assignment scheduled in the late phases of the program. Within such a framework, the student ideally progresses through three stages of clinical experience: initial exposure and observation; learning and reinforcement; and minimally supervised experiential learning.

Once the administrative components of the program have been coordinated and the various elements of the curriculum purposefully articulated, the program faculty is in a position to implement selected integrative strategies within the courses for which it is responsible. Such strategies, summarized in the list above, include unit or modular organization of content; flexible clinical scheduling; team teaching; case studies or patient management problems; and seminars. Details on the implementation of these strategies are provided elsewhere.[27]

The success of such course strategies depends on the ability of the program's faculty to establish a learning environment that fosters the integrative behavior of the students. Clearly, faculty who expect students to integrate the diverse experiences in even the best organized respiratory therapy program's curriculum must themselves be models of integrative behavior.[17]

Student Evaluation

The evaluation of student achievement is one of the most important processes of the teaching/learning component of the educational system. An ongoing evaluation process, objectively based on prespecified proficiencies in the cognitive, psychomotor, and affective domains, is the prerequisite to the implementation of a competency-based curriculum. In addition, a well-conceived evaluation system can greatly facilitate the integration of the didactic and clinical components of the program and ultimately provides the basis for assessing the efficacy of the instructional process itself.

Evaluation includes both measurement and judgmental processes. Sound judgments require reliable and valid measures. A *system* of evaluation incorporates reliable and valid measures of student achievement within the sequence of the curriculum, providing both formative and summative assessment of knowledge, skills, and behavior in such a way as to facilitate student mastery of the applicable goals and objectives. Figure 2-4 depicts a mastery sequence that integrates an evaluation component within the progression from classroom instruction to laboratory demonstration and practice through the development of clinical skills proficiency. *Two* evaluative frames are used: preclinical and clinical. Outcomes at each stage of evaluation determine the student's progression in the sequence. Satisfactory performance is the necessary prerequisite for sequential advancement; unsatisfactory performance mandates the remediation of deficiencies before progressing to higher levels of skills mastery.

The measurement tools used in a sound evaluation system are designed according to the type of per-

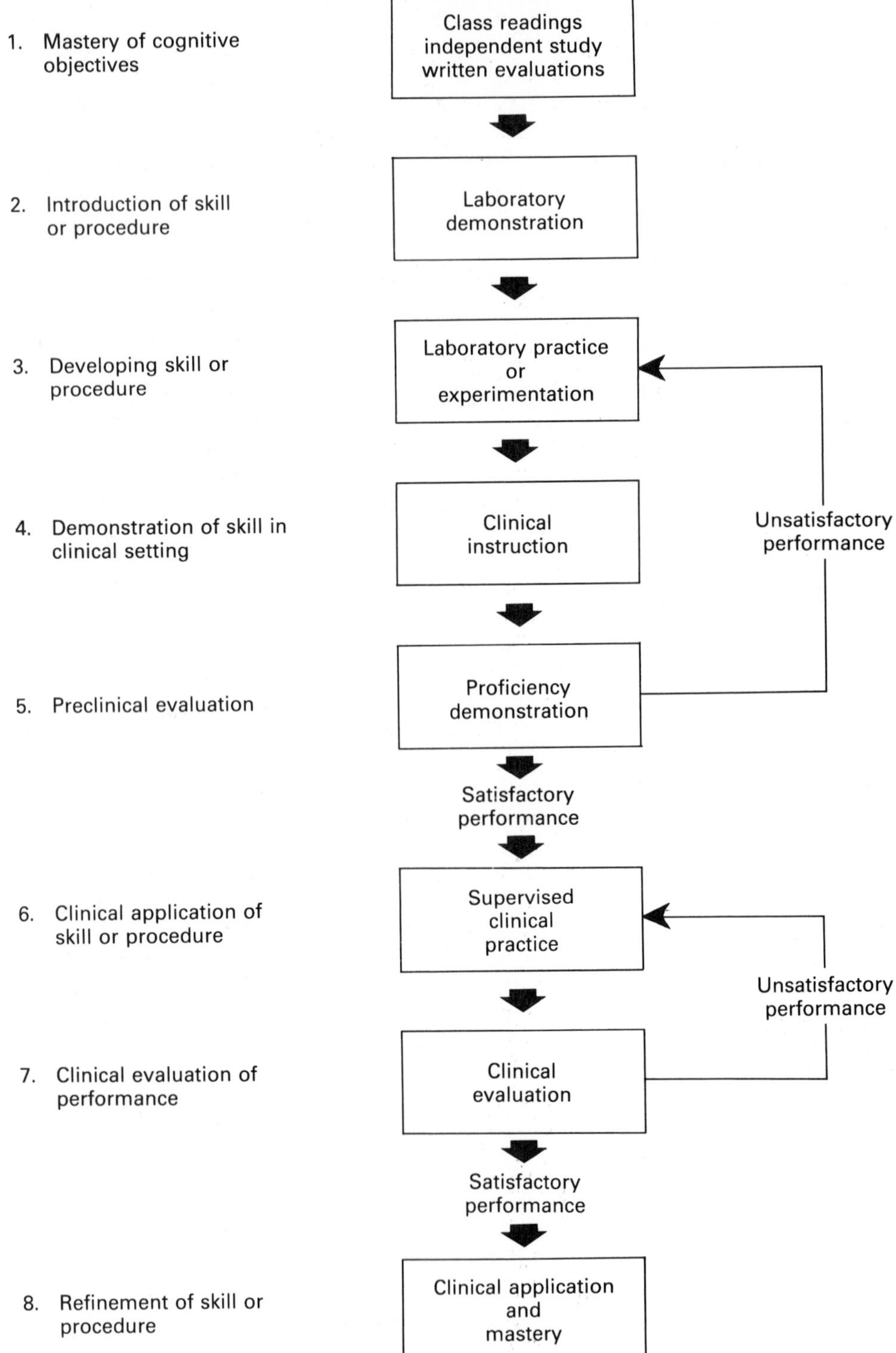
RESPIRATORY THERAPY PROGRAM
CLINICAL MASTERY SEQUENCE
1. Mastery of cognitive objectives
Class readings independent study written evaluations
2. Introduction of skill or procedure
Laboratory demonstration
3. Developing skill or procedure
Laboratory practice or experimentation
4. Demonstration of skill in clinical setting
Clinical instruction
Unsatisfactory performance
5. Preclinical evaluation
Proficiency demonstration
Satisfactory performance
6. Clinical application of skill or procedure
Supervised clinical practice
Unsatisfactory performance
7. Clinical evaluation of performance
Clinical evaluation
Satisfactory performance
8. Refinement of skill or procedure
Clinical application and mastery

Fig. 2-4. Mastery learning and evaluation sequence.

formance being assessed. If the proficiency involves the observable performance of a technical skill or procedure that can be described in terms of a sequence of discrete steps or elements, the checklist is generally the most appropriate means of assessment (Fig. 2-5). If the specified performance involves the student's exhibition of behavioral traits rather than technical skills, a rating scale should be used (Fig. 2-6). Other types of assessment tools commonly used to evaluate clinical skills, proficiency, and behavior include anecdotal records, product evaluations, and simulations or patient management problems. The consistency (or reliability) with which such instruments discriminate between various levels of performance depends less on the design of the instrument itself than on the training of those responsible for their use. The validity of judgments derived from using such assessment tools depends mainly on the degree to which the performance measured is congruent with the objectives of learning or instruction. Details on the selection, design characteristics, strengths, limitations, and appropriate use of clinical assessment tools are provided by Morgan and Irby.[20]

In summary, a well-designed evaluation system, incorporated within the curriculum of a respiratory therapy program, should provide the following.

1. A method for *documentation* of students' clinical activities (e.g., procedures performed and observations).
2. A mechanism for *evaluating* and *judging* student progress toward mastery of both specified procedural competencies and desired behavioral or attitudinal outcomes.
3. A means of providing *formative* feedback to assist students in understanding performance strengths and deficiencies.
4. A mechanism for *remediation* of identified weaknesses that assists students in resolving procedural or behavioral deficiencies.

Program Evaluation

Program evaluation is the ongoing process of assessing the degree to which an educational system's intents are indeed realized. The strength of the system's perspective lies in its ability to assist program personnel in the collection and interpretation of information relevant to evaluating the efficacy of the various components of the program. Typically, an open system provides informational feedback useful in assessing the degree to which its intended inputs, processes, and outcomes are congruent with those that are observed. Such feedback includes, but is not limited to, prospective student applications and requests for information, the characteristics and attributes of prospective students, the reasons for accepted candidates not enrolling, the results of summative didactic and clinical evaluation, student attrition, student evaluations of instruction, student evaluations of instructors, peer and supervisor evaluations, complaints, resource use and needs reports, accreditation recommendations, performance of graduates on credentialing examinations, graduate follow-up evaluations of the program, and postgraduation employer performance evaluations.

Incorporating such information into a meaningful evaluative framework is not easy. Often the sheer volume or complexity of informational feedback precludes its rational use in assessing the efficacy of the program as a whole. The most common pitfall is to screen the information deluge selectively and to apply only that which is immediately understandable or, worse, positively supportive of one's expectations. As an example, high pass rates on the national credentialing examination are often cited as a measure of program quality. Placed in the context of 60% student attrition and employer dissatisfaction with the graduates' clinical performance, the interpretation of such a statistic and inferences as to the quality of the program would be substantially different.

Program evaluation, of course, involves more than collecting information. Feedback on the various components of the educational system is useful only when it assists program personnel in making informed decisions and implementing change. The ability to identify logically and respond rationally to needed changes in the structural or operational aspects of a program is one of the most important skills that a respiratory therapy educator can possess. The success with which such skill is exercised will largely determine the quality of the educational experience a program offers to its students and, consequently, the service it can provide in meeting the needs of the health care community.

Nontraditional Education

No other aspect of the education of respiratory therapy personnel is less well understood or more controversial than the diverse program structures, educational methods, and delivery systems grouped under the rubric of "nontraditional" education.

Nontraditional education may best be understood

STUDENT:	DATE:

BROOKDALE COMMUNITY COLLEGE
RESPIRATORY THERAPY PROGRAM
PROFICIENCY EVALUATION

PROCEDURE (TASK): AEROSOL/HUMIDITY THERAPY – DIRECT APPLICATION

☐ THERAPEUTIC PROCEDURE:	☐ NONTHERAPEUTIC PROCEDURE
☐ CLINICAL ☐ NEW PATIENT ☐ REPEAT PROCEDURE ☐ COLLEGE LABORATORY ☐ PEER APPLICATION ☐ MANIKIN/ANALOGUE	☐ COLLEGE LABORATORY ☐ CLINICAL EQUIPMENT UTILIZED:

	STEPS IN PROCEDURE OR TASK	SATISFACTORY	UNSATISFACTORY	NOT OBSERVED	NOT APPLICABLE
	EQUIPMENT AND PATIENT PREPARATION				
1.	*Selects, gathers, and assembles appropriate equipment. Ensures asepsis.*				
2.	*Verifies, interprets, and evaluates physician's order*				
3.	*Identifies patient, self, and department*				
4.	*Explains procedure and confirms patient understanding*				
	IMPLEMENTATION AND ASSESSMENT				
5.	*Adds appropriate solution aseptically and in correct amount*				
6.	*Connects humidifier/aerosol generator to appropriate gas source*				
7.	*Initiates gas flow/aerosol generation*				
8.	*Tests equipment for proper function*				
9.	*Applies modality to patient, ensuring maximum comfort/safety*				
10.	*Ensures gas flow and oxygen concentration appropriate to order/objectives*				
11.	*Adjusts humidity (aerosol output), temperature appropriate to order/objectives*				
12.	*Gives additional instructions, where necessary, to maximize therapeutic benefit*				
13.	*Assesses patient response (objective and subjective)*				
14.	*Modifies technique to deal with adverse response*				
	FOLLOW-UP				
15.	*Maintains proper equipment function*				
16.	*Records pertinent data in chart and department records*				
17.	*Notifies appropriate personnel*				

Fig. 2-5. Respiratory therapy program proficiency evaluation.

PERSONAL ATTRIBUTES

INITIATIVE	
	A. Exhibits enthusiasm and initiative in performing assigned tasks: continually seeks out new learning experiences beyond those scheduled or planned.
	B. Readily accepts assigned activities and constructively exploits their learning potential; generally seeks out new or additional learning experiences.
	C. Keeps pace with regular work assignments and occasionally seeks out new activities.
	D. Requires occasional prodding to keep up with delegated tasks, rarely uses time constructively.
	E. Must be continuously prodded to meet responsibilities; completes assigned activities only because they are required; does not seek out new learning experiences.
	F. At present there is insufficient information available to provide a valid rating; or, this scale is not applicable (circle appropriate statement).
Comments (cite specific incidences from which the above conclusions were drawn):	

Fig. 2-6. Attribute rating scale (example).

as an educational philosophy rather than a specific method or technique of teaching and learning. The philosophy of nontraditional education places a major emphasis on the *outcomes* of learning, with minor attention to the structural inputs and processes traditionally associated with educational systems. What is most disconcerting to educational purists is the fact that such philosophy tends to refute many of the basic tenets on which traditional education systems are founded—that is, that learning requires physical presence, that the accumulation of credits certifies achievement or proficiency, and that education is typically the learner's major (if not only) activity.[10]

Three basic perspectives are helpful in refining the concept of nontraditional education: the student perspective; the institutional (or program) perspective; and the accrediting agency perspective.

Nontraditional students are generally defined by default—that is, they are *not* 18- to 24-years-old and they do *not* pursue education as a full-time activity. In addition such students typically possess experiences often directly applicable to their educational needs. A nontraditional program offers education designed for nontraditional students, provides learning experiences in unusual locations or designs, and delivers its experiences in novel ways. The degree to which an institution is nontraditional is determined by the extent to which its operational components (admission, counseling, curriculum, educational methods in scheduling, completion requirements) vary from the norms of traditional educational structure and function or (from an accrediting agency perspective) from the standards of accreditation.

Nontraditional education in respiratory therapy is not new. One of the oldest and most established therapist programs in the country has been operating a nontraditional component for more than a decade and has graduated more students, to date, than any other school. What is new, however, is the recent growth and proliferation of nontraditional practices in respiratory therapy education. Based on its 1980 survey of educational programs, the JRCRTE estimates that as many as 3000 persons, or about 25% of the total student population, are involved in some form of nontraditional study in respiratory therapy.

Although the reasons for such growth are manifold, demand for upward career mobility has played the most significant role. Based on the American Association for Respiratory Therapy's 1977 *Uniform Manpower Survey*,[1] some 30% to 35% of the total work force of respiratory therapy personnel (about 17,000 people) lacked formal training and were consequently ineligible for the credentialing examination system of the NBRC. Little wonder, then, that perceptive programs foresaw the need to develop mechanisms designed to meet the special requirements of this large population of prospective learners. Many educational institutions have implemented processes that accommodate the learning requirements of this group without requiring them to forgo employment or to relocate. The experiential competencies developed by this group of learners are becoming increasingly recognized, measured, and codified, and thus provide access to the credentialing system.

Not surprisingly, a diversity of nontraditional program formats have evolved. Understanding how such programs function to meet the needs of their students can be facilitated by addressing three key operational questions.

1. Does the program presume that the student has previously developed some or all of the competencies included in the curriculum?
2. Are the teaching–learning activities provided by the program delivered on or off campus?
3. Does the program integrate experiential learning into its curriculum sequence?

Answers to these key operational questions create a design matrix that categorizes nontraditional program formats according to eight generic types (Table 2-2). For example, the type IV nontraditional program format may be described as one that presumes previous development of competencies (advanced standing), employs an outreach delivery system (perhaps correspondence or home-study), and does not integrate clinical experiential learning into its curriculum sequence. Some program formats may in fact represent more than one typologic category, and variants of the descriptive matrix may now exist or may be developed. Currently there is no evidence to determine which of the various formats may be most appropriate for which type of students. There is also no substantive, empirical evidence that indicates which of the formats may be most effective or efficient in facilitating student achievement.

Nontraditional education in respiratory therapy is not without its problems. Foremost is the fact that the development of mechanisms to assure the quality of such educational formats has lagged behind the rapid growth in nontraditional program activity and student enrollment. A second significant problem, related to the first, is the real potential for charlatanism and student exploitation by unethical persons, programs, or institutions having motives other than providing quality education. A final problem is the credibility of the degree or certificate provided by such nontraditional programs.

Cognizant of the need to address such problems, the JRCRTE has taken a leadership role in developing guidelines and administrative mechanisms whereby programs that offer nontraditional formats must demonstrate accountability to their students, the respiratory therapy educational community, and the profession as a whole. Such efforts represent one aspect of the competency assurance mechanisms discussed below.

Development of a New Program

The unprecedented growth of a new allied health specialty has led to unprecedented growth in the number of programs designed to produce an educated manpower pool for the new specialty. Fortunately the

Table 2-2. Design Matrix for Nontraditional Program Formats

	DOES THE PROGRAM PRESUME PRIOR EXPERIENTIAL DEVELOPMENT OF COMPETENCIES?			
	Yes		*No*	
	On Campus	*Off Campus*	*On Campus*	*Off Campus*
Integrated experiential learning	Type I	Type III	Type V	Type VII
Experiential learning not integrated	Type II	Type IV	Type VI	Type VIII

JOINT REVIEW COMMITTEE FOR RESPIRATORY THERAPY EDUCATION GUIDELINES TO ESSENTIAL VIII, C

The JRCRTE defines advanced standing mechanisms as those nontraditional approaches to education that recognize or combine applicable work experience and previous knowledge with a structured learning and evaluative process. The approach is nontraditional in that it varies from the didactic, laboratory and clinical method normally used—hence from the "Essentials" applicable to program operation.

Although the JRCRTE encourages the development and implementation of such advanced standing mechanisms, it firmly believes that the processes employed must ensure that persons completing the nontraditional program component have the same competencies as those completing the regular curriculum. To assist educators in achieving this goal, the committee recommends that programs offering an advanced standing component adhere to the following guidelines.

Sponsorship: The JRCRTE will recognize only those advanced standing mechanisms that operate within the context of functional and accredited educational programs.

Statement of Purpose and Objectives: Programs offereing advanced standing mechanisms should provide a definition of purpose and a description of how the mechanism varies from its traditional approach, with reference to the "Essentials"; and a statement of how the program variations meet the needs of students, the profession, and the community or region served.

Disclosure: The sponsoring institution should clearly delineate (in writing) all differences in eligibility, cost, instructional methods, academic regulations, and criteria for completion to prospective students *before* their actual enrollment.

Curriculum: The units of instruction *available* to those seeking the alternate route of completion should be equivalent to, and correspond fully in content to, those offered in the regular curriculum.

Staffing: Such staff responsible for the nontraditional component should meet the same qualifications applied to the regular faculty. In addition, the program should demonstrate that the number of staff is sufficient to ensure appropriate attention to individual learning needs and adequate access to personal direction and guidance. When the educational methods used differ substantially from those normally used or where representatives external to the institution provide instructional support or guidance, the program must ensure that such people are trained in the unique aspect of program function and the basic principles of nontraditional education.

Instructional Strategies: The instructional strategies implemented in the nontraditional program components should be structured to accommodate the individual learning needs of students who select such alternative routes.

Educators who implement alternative learning strategies should provide individual enrollees pursuing nontraditional routes with substantive feedback on performance strengths and weaknesses. Where deficiencies in knowledge or skills are identified by the program staff, program personnel should provide learners with ready access to the full scope of learning resources available in the regular program—that is, to both the didactic and *clinical resources* of the program.

During the course of the learner's progress through the curriculum, program personnel should further ensure that students have direct *in-person* access to those responsible for facilitating their acquisition or demonstration of knowledge and skills. Such people should have a direct relationship to, and defined role within, the sponsoring institution.

In addition, program personnel should maintain comprehensive and cumulative records (where applicable) of assessed needs, knowledge acquisition, and skills proficiency appropriate to the program methodology.

Validation of Mechanism: Program personnel should provide evidence of equivalence of the methods used and demonstrate comparable outcome relative to the accredited traditional program.

Compliance with Regulations: Because many nontraditional educational formats are not bound to a specific geographical locale, the JRCRTE insists that program personnel demonstrate compliance with any and all local, state, and federal statutes, laws, and regulations applicable to their full scope of operation.

years during which this need was recognized coincided with the rapid growth and development of the community college system and with an unprecedented availability of federal and state funds devoted to higher education. The establishment of health programs became a status symbol, a source of revenue, and a major attraction for new students, while at the same time filling a perceived societal need. The haste with which new health programs were started, the dearth of properly trained key personnel, and the lack of any national or regional control mechanism led to many ill advised, poorly conceived, and generally unsatisfactory programs. The Joint Review Committee was the only structure that had both the responsibility and the power to eliminate the programs that did not meet the minimum standards set by the "Essentials." Unfortunately, the Joint Review Committee had absolutely no legal power to prevent the establishment of programs and, until the adoption of the 1977 "Essentials," did not not even have solid, sufficiently high criteria that could reasonably assure that the "minimal standards" were acceptable standards.

This situation has changed markedly during the past few years, and the recession of 1979–1980 has stemmed the free flow of new funds for education. It also seems unlikely that there will be a major change in the foreseeable future. Higher education, even in health, has lost its magic, and a number of existing programs may be forced to close their doors over the next 5 years. It seems likely also that few new programs will start and that considerably more thought will be devoted to the elements necessary for the careful planning and successful launching of a new program.

The authors do not envisage this section to serve as a blueprint for starting a new program in respiratory care. Nevertheless, we do outline the steps that must be taken to have a reasonable likelihood of starting a successful program.

The first step, without doubt, must be a careful needs assessment in the geographic region that the educational institution serves, and from which it receives its primary economic support. This assessment is difficult to perform because it has all the difficulties that have bedeviled manpower surveys in all health fields. The critical question that must be answered is the number of existing unfilled positions in the respiratory care departments of hospitals in the educational institution's catchment area. The next question must be the number of additional positions for which a management commitment has been made and for which the hospital has made allowances in its long-range budget planning. Additionally important information is the existence of other respiratory care training programs that obtain a significant percentage of their student body from the area under study and to where the graduates of the existing programs are likely to return. Finally, a study of the demography of the existing manpower, its distribution, level of training, age, work history, and turnover rate must be performed. An analysis of the data thus obtained will suggest whether a program is needed, whether a significant percentage of eventual graduates are likely to have job opportunities in the area, commensurate with their training, and, assuming normal attrition in the area, how many graduating classes of what size are likely to be accommodated in the area.

If the answer to these questions is unfavorable, following an honest and unbiased evaluation, the process should stop, and the efforts of the institution should be directed toward a more rewarding project.

If the answer is favorable, the planning of the program may begin. This process is also stepwise, with several points at which a "yes–no" decision must be made before too much time and effort have been expended in a desirable but impossible effort.

The first step in the planning process has to be taken by the executive officers of the educational institution, since at this point an initial commitment to identify and to secure funds must be made. Taking this as a given, a program planner should be engaged, preferably one who is a respiratory therapist with the necessary qualifications to be eligible under the "Essentials" to fulfill the role of Program Director. It is not absolutely necessary, although it is highly desirable, that the first director of the program should have participated in the planning process and thus be thoroughly familiar with the educational institution and with the community that it serves.

Once the planner has been hired, he must do a "feasibility study" to evaluate the health care facilities that will serve as the clinical affiliates for the program. This implies extensive discussions with respiratory care department heads, medical directors, and hospital administrators. The planner must be sure that the medical and respiratory care community are willing to support the program and make substantial contributions in time and effort. The completion of this survey is one of the decision points where the planner must make a formal recommendation to the Chief Executive Officer of the educational institution to continue or to abandon the planning.

If the decision is to "go," then the "advisory committee" must be assembled. This committee is essential to the successful planning process, and its existence, during the establishment of the program, is an "Essential" requirement. The members of the planning advisory committee may be the same ones as the members of the committee once the program has been established. We believe that there is considerable merit in having continuity between the planning and operating phases of the program, although periodic changes are needed to avoid decreasing interest and usefulness of the members. During the planning phase, the committee should have representation from all the health care facilities in the area, preferably by persons in a decision-making position in these institutions. The medical community must be represented by several influential members, one of whom is a prospective medical director of the program. Obviously the educational institution must be represented by one or more senior administrators and by one or more faculty members familiar with curriculum planning and the mobilization of institutional resources. The members of the advisory committee must become familiar with the precise purpose of their existence as a group, and they must agree to contribute time and effort to the program. The committee should become familiar with the results of the need assessment and feasibility studies. With this information, the committee can determine the adequacy of the institutional and community resources and decide on the nature of the program and the size of the first and subsequent classes. Once the committee agrees on this initial point, it must make a formal recommendation to the educational institution.

This is another "go–no go" point, since a favorable recommendation will initiate the final phase of the planning process—the phase of economic planning. In this phase, the planner, in cooperation with the fiscal officers of the educational institution, must prepare a tentative budget that considers not only salaries and fringe benefits for key personnel, secretarial support, and clinical instructors, but also space, equipment, library and other requirements of the program. When this budget is prepared, the final "go–no go" point will have been reached, and the institution must make the final decision whether to establish the program at that time.

Assuming that the final decision was to go ahead, the detailed planning of the program can begin. This phase primarily comprises designing the curriculum and evaluation tools. In addition, the laboratory equipment, audio–visual material, books and journals should be ordered and the classroom, laboratory, and office space identified and prepared. The faculty must be identified for all phases of the curriculum and be made thoroughly familiar with the objectives of the program. This is extremely important, particularly in the basic science courses, but also in the clinical phase of the program. This is the point where the identification and employment of the Director of Clinical Education becomes essential. He is the person who must design the clinical courses, identify, train, and coordinate the clinical instructors, assist in the preparation of the agreements between the educational institution and the clinical affiliates, and, in cooperation with the medical director and the program director, arrange adequate and appropriate medical input.

Having accomplished this, some items still must be considered and decided: Among these, the entrance requirement into the program, the method of selecting students, and the offering of advanced standing are the most important. Most educational institutions have firm policies or traditions in all three of these areas. We feel very strongly, however, having considerable experience with a large number of programs and with the accreditation process, that rigid and high entrance requirements are among the surest guarantees for a successful program, that student selection should be based on past performance and demonstrated ability, and that a sound and well-designed advanced standing mechanism for both cognate and clinical courses contributes greatly to the usefulness and success of the program.

We wish to make three more general comments.

1. Throughout the planning process, the appropriate "Essentials" and "Guidelines" should be studied with attention to minute details. It is the hallmark of a good program that it exceeds the "Essentials" in all significant areas.
2. It is not necessary for each new program planner or director to invent the educational process in all its details from scratch. Most established and accredited programs are pleased to share their written materials and can save the planners of the new program an infinite amount of time.
3. The planning process should include an initial contact with the Joint Review Committee. In this way, the Joint Review Committee can assist by recommending a list of consultants, by making accreditation materials available to facilitate the preparation of the application, and by answering all questions that pertain to accreditation.

COMPETENCY ASSURANCE OF RESPIRATORY THERAPY PERSONNEL

Competency assurance derives from a combination of regulatory mechanisms and procedures designed to hold the health professions accountable for the activities and practices of their members. Demands for such accountability are based on the fundamental tenet that the public has the right to competently delivered health care and to practitioners proficient in the services they render.[28]

As in most other health professions, competency assurance in respiratory care is a joint venture. The educational and credentialing systems *and* the individual practitioners, constituting the work force, must share the responsibility for demonstrating accountability to the public interest, safety, and welfare. Mechanisms that currently regulate the quality of practice in respiratory therapy include accreditation, certification, and legal recognition. Complementing these mechanisms, and designed to assure the continued competency of practitioners, is continuing education. A description of the nature of each of these competency assurance mechanisms and their strengths and limitations follows.

Accreditation

Accreditation is the process by which a private, nongovernmental agency or association grants public recognition to an institution or specialized program of study that meets certain established qualifications and educational standards.[21] The primary purpose of the accreditation process in allied health is to provide a professional judgment as to the quality of the educational process and to encourage its continued improvement, thereby protecting the public against the professional or occupational incompetence of its graduates.

Institutional accreditation applies to a total institution and means that the organization as a whole is satisfactorily achieving its goals and objectives. *Programmatic* accreditation applies to specialized programs of study and means that the instructional resources and the learning experiences provided comply with the standards or criteria of accreditation.[8] Respiratory therapy educational accreditation is, appropriately, conducted at the program level, with institutional accreditation of program sponsors subsumed within the standards of accreditation.

Respiratory therapy programs are accredited by the Committee on Allied Health Education and accreditation (CAHEA) in collaboration with the Joint Review Committee for Respiratory Therapy Education. CAHEA is a quasi-independent, broadly representative agency responsible for the accreditation of some 26 allied health occupations. CAHEA assumed the accreditation responsibilities, formerly held by the Council on Medical Education (CME) of the AMA, in January 1977, and has subsequently gained recognition as an "umbrella" accrediting agency for allied health educational programs by the U.S. Department of Education (Office of Education) and the Council on Postsecondary Accreditation (COPA). CAHEA currently collaborates with about 46 organizations which, in turn, sponsor the discipline-specific accreditation review committees. Collaborating organizations also develop and adopt standards of accreditation or "Essentials" for their respective review committees. The American Medical Association maintains its role as a collaborating organization in the accrediting of allied health educational programs through its CME. The CME is responsible for formal recognition of emerging allied health occupations; formal recognition of other collaborating organizations that sponsor review committees; and adoption of "Essentials," new or revised.

Accreditation Process

The JRCRTE is the agency responsible for the logistics of the accreditation process and for the formulation of accreditation recommendations for all educational programs in respiratory therapy. It is sponsored by the American Association for Respiratory Therapy (AART), the American College of Chest Physicians (ACCP), the American Society of Anesthesiologists (ASA), and the American Thoracic Society (ATS). The AART appoints six representatives to the JRCRTE, and each physician sponsor organization appoints two representatives. One nonhealth professional voting member represents the general public. The program review, evaluation, and accreditation processes are administered by an Executive Office staff consisting of an Executive Director, Executive Secretary, and support personnel.

The accreditation process for respiratory therapy technician programs and respiratory therapists programs is identical, except for differences in the "Essentials." The process whereby a new program gains accreditation status is depicted in Figure 2-7. The reaccreditation process differs only in that established programs undergoing periodic reevaluation do not receive a letter of review or support.

As summarized in Figure 2-7, programs seeking accreditation voluntarily submit a self-study docu-

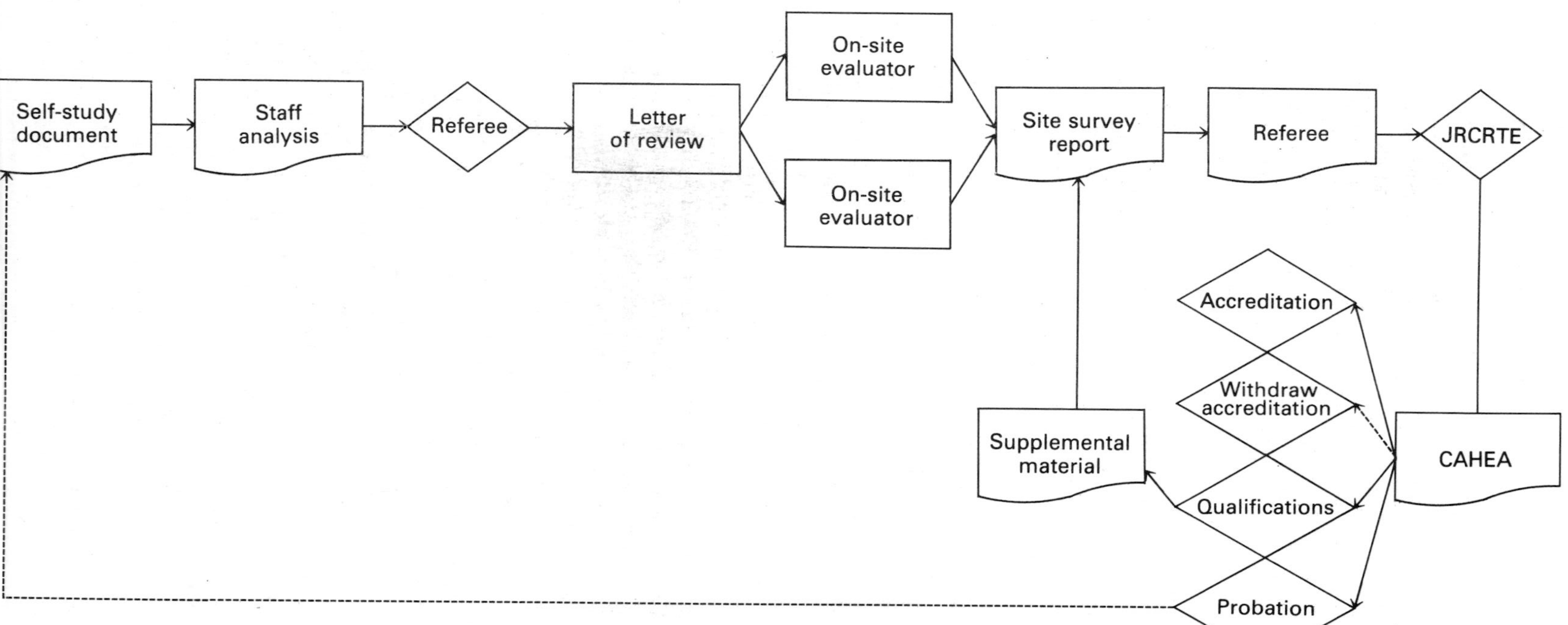

Fig. 2-7. Joint Review Committee for Respiratory Therapy Education programmatic evaluation flowsheet.

ment to the JRCRTE. The self-study document represents a detailed analysis of a program's instructional resources and educational processes as they relate to the applicable "Essentials." Normally, program faculty, administrative personnel, and students provide input to the analysis and assist in the identification of programmatic strengths and weaknesses.

Self-study documents, once submitted, are reviewed for completeness and clarity by the Executive Office staff. If staff analysis of the document indicates that all pertinent information has been included, the self-study is forwarded to a committee member serving as a referee. The referee is the program's ombudsman, communicating with the program's officials to clarify or correct potential violations of the "Essentials" and working with the JRCRTE Executive Office and the Committee as a whole to facilitate the program's progress through the accreditation process.

Once the referee is satisfied that the documentation provided by the program indicates substantial compliance with the "Essentials," a "Letter of Review" is issued to the program by the Executive Office. The Letter of Review indicates that analysis of the written program documentation provides preliminary evidence of compliance with the "Essentials." Upon issuance of a Letter of Review, the JRCRTE also communicates with the National Board for Respiratory Care, recommending that future program graduates be considered eligible for their respective credentialing examinations.

Following issuance of a "Letter of Review," an on-site evaluation of the program is scheduled and a site-visit team selected. The site-visit team comprises two members: a physician qualified to be Medical Director of the program being evaluated; and a therapist with the experience and education necessary to fulfill the role of Program Director. The on-site evaluators confer with responsible members of the sponsoring institution's administration, the program faculty, staff, and students. Both the instructional resources of the program and the clinical resources of its affiliates are inspected and all necessary documentation and records reviewed. Finally, the team provides an overview of the perceived strengths and weaknesses of the program (in relation to the "Essentials") and, where applicable, makes recommendations for improvement. A written report, summarizing the team's observations and conclusions, is subsequently forwarded to the JRCRTE Executive Office. The sponsoring institution receives a copy of the report and may respond to it with appropriate supplemental documentation.

After the sponsoring institution has been given the opportunity to respond to the site-visit report, the referee presents the program to the full Committee for an accreditation recommendation. For new programs, one of three accreditation recommendations can be made: full accreditation; accreditation with qualifications, or withholding of accreditation. Accredited programs seeking reaccreditation may be recommended for full accreditation; accreditation with qualifications, or probation. Programs coming before the Committee with extant qualifications to accreditation that have not been remediated (or accredited programs with a significant number of serious deficiencies noted on reevaluation) may be recommended for probation. Programs holding probationary status and failing to remedy "Essential" violations in the allotted time are recommended for withdrawal of accreditation.

Recommendations for program accreditation status are forwarded from the JRCRTE to CAHEA. CAHEA has the final authority for accreditation action. Programs awarded *full accreditation* by CAHEA are those that have demonstrated substantial compliance with all the applicable "Essentials." Programs granted accreditation with *qualifications* have deficiencies or violations of the standards of accreditation that JRCRTE and CAHEA believe to be readily correctable. These programs must provide progress reports that document the means by which the deficiencies noted are being addressed and are usually given 1 year to fully remediate such shortcomings. *Probationary accreditation* status indicates the existence of significant violations of the "Essentials" that threaten the program's ability to provide acceptable educational experiences for its students. Programs holding probationary status must normally submit a new self-analysis, addressing the identified deficiencies, and may be required to undergo a new on-site evaluation to demonstrate compliance with the "Essentials." Programs from which *accreditation* has been *withheld* are new programs that do not fulfill several major requirements of the "Essentials" when such deficiencies are significant and not easily correctable. Programs that have their accreditation withheld may appeal directly to CAHEA or may, if they desire, reapply for accreditation later. *Accreditation* may be *withdrawn* voluntarily (at the request of the institutional sponsor) or be mandated by failure of the program to provide evidence of compliance with the "Essentials" within the specified probationary period. Programs that have their accreditation involuntarily withdrawn may likewise appeal to CAHEA.

STRENGTHS AND LIMITATIONS OF THE ACCREDITATION PROCESS

The strengths and limitations of the current process for accreditation of respiratory therapy educational programs are best assessed in terms of its two major elements: the standards of accreditation themselves (the "Essentials"); and the evaluative/judgmental process by which compliance with the "Essentials" is determined and accreditation actions are taken.

A generic outline of the 1977 "Essentials" appears in Table 2-3. The current accreditation standards represent the third revision for therapist programs (originally adopted in 1962) and the first revision for technician education programs. The "Essentials" represent *minimum* requirements for CAHEA accreditation and have been developed after extensive collaborative efforts between respiratory therapy educators, respiratory therapy practitioners, and physicians. Accompanying each "Essential" are guidelines. Guidelines clarify or amplify the letter of the standards and provide justification of, and direction for, meeting the criteria. Both the "Essentials" and their guidelines generally correspond to CAHEA's

Table 2-3. Essentials of an Accredited Educational Program for the Respiratory Therapist and Respiratory Therapy Technician—A Generic Outline*

PREAMBLE

Objective
Description of the Occupation(s)

REQUIREMENTS FOR ACCREDITATION

I. *Sponsorship (Site of Educational Programs)*

- **A.** Public or private postsecondary vocational or technical schools, community or junior colleges or universities (*all* therapist programs)
- **B.** Accredited hospitals with college affiliations (some technician programs)

II. *Clinical Facilities*

- **A.** Primary affiliate criteria
- **B.** Secondary affiliate criteria
- **C.** General clinical affiliate criteria
  - **1.** Geographic proximity
  - **2.** Key personnel access
  - **3.** Cooperation to assure student learning
  - **4.** Written agreements/contracts
  - **5.** Equipment and supplies

III. *Program Facilities*

- **A.** Classroom, laboratory, and support services
- **B.** Laboratory facilities and equipment
- **C.** Library resources
- **D.** Self-instructional/audio–visual materials

IV. *Finances*

- **A.** Adequacy of financial support
- **B.** Reasonable fees for students
- **C.** Disallowance of student stipends
- **D.** Disallowance of student substitution for paid clinical personnel

V. *Faculty*

- **A.** Key personnel
- **B.** Program director qualifications and responsibilities
- **C.** Director of clinical education qualifications and responsibilities
- **D.** Medical director qualifications and responsibilities
- **E.** Other instructional staff qualifications and responsibilities
- **F.** Change of key personnel (administrative notification)
- **G.** Advisory committee purpose, constituency, and documentation of activity

VI. *Students*

- **A.** Selection processes and minimum criteria
- **B.** Student health
- **C.** Enrollment and student–faculty ratios
- **D.** Counseling

VII. *Records*

VIII. *Curriculum*

- **A.** Length of educational program
- **B.** Units of instruction
  - **1.** Basic units of instruction (prerequisite science and clinical topics units)
  - **2.** Respiratory therapy units of instruction
- **C.** Advanced standing

ADMINISTRATION OF ACCREDITATION

*Joint Review Committee for Respiratory Education, 1977.

Recommended Standard Format for such documents.[8]

The strengths of the "Essentials" lie in their rational demand for adherence to sound principles of organizational structure and educational process. The need for quality institutional sponsorship, adequate clinical and program resources, qualified key personnel, a comprehensive curriculum, and effective strategies of student progress monitoring and evaluation are clearly delineated and logically defensible. Although such criteria are traditionally acceptable as accreditation standards, there is growing concern that continued focus solely on the inputs and processes of an educational program is no longer appropriate as a measure of quality. Such concern is founded on the lack of evidence showing a clear relation between the program's compliance with accreditation standards and the quality of their output—that is, graduate practitioners. That the hypothesis remains untested is, as any good scientist knows, insufficient grounds for its rejection. Recent research by the Department of Allied Health Education and Accreditation of the AMA tends consistently to support the face validity of the "Essentials" between and among members of the allied health educational community, employers of allied health program graduates, and those responsible for implementing the accreditation system. The JRCRTE itself is currently in the process of determining the degree to which compliance with the "Essentials" can be expected to result in quality program outcomes. Ultimately such research will provide answers to the most fundamental questions about the accreditation process and will, we hope, assist the educational community in developing more thorough and efficient systems of preparing students for their subsequent professional roles.

The evaluative and judgmental processes by which program compliance with the "Essentials" is determined have strengths and limitations. The strength of the existing system is based on multiple checks and balances that generally ensure both consistency and fairness in accreditation decision-making. Recognizing that the information gathered during on-site evaluation is crucial to its decision-making process, the JRCRTE has expended considerable time and effort to train its cadre of on-site evaluators. New policies for their selection, training, evaluation, and reappointment, based on specific performance criteria, have recently been implemented and will be continuously monitored for effectiveness. Notwithstanding such continued efforts at self-analysis and improvement, the accreditation process is and will always be, a human process. That the system has generally succeeded in upgrading and promoting quality educational practices in respiratory therapy has not been seriously questioned—a tribute to the concerted efforts of those who believe that the sound basic education of practitioners provides the necessary foundation for a strong, viable profession.

CERTIFICATION

Certification is the process by which a nongovernmental agency or association grants recognition to a person who has met predetermined qualifications, including graduation from an accredited program; completion of a given amount of work experience; and acceptable performance on a qualifying examination or series of such examinations.[26] A similar term, *registration*, is often used synonymously with certification, although it more properly describes the process by which qualified persons are listed on an official roster maintained by a governmental or nongovernmental agency. The functions of certification and registration are commonly performed by a credentialing body or agency. The awards based on examination or recognition of qualified persons by such agencies are thus designated as *credentials*.

Historical Background

The credentialing process for respiratory care practitioners began in 1960 when the American Registry of Inhalation Therapists (ARIT) incorporated as a not-for-profit agency in the state of Illinois. Then sponsored by the American College of Chest Physicians (ACCP), the American Society of Anesthesiology (ASA), and the American Association of Inhalation Therapy (AAIT), the fledgling organization ambitiously set out to achieve the following major objectives.[13]

1. To assist in developing and maintaining educational and ethical standards in inhalation therapy for the public good, for the advancement of medical care, and for the professional guidance of registrants of the Registry.
2. To prepare, conduct, and control investigation and examinations to test the qualifications of voluntary candidates.
3. To encourage the establishment of high standards by which the competency of inhalation therapists to administer inhalation therapy under the prescription, direction, and supervision of licensed physicians may be determined.

The ARIT administered its first written examination in April 1961 to 33 candidates, 29 of whom passed what was, by today's standards, a rather unsophisticated test of basic knowledge. Eligibility for the early examinations offered by the ARIT could be satisfied by either work experience (3 years) or completion of formal schooling. Support for the formal educational preparation of candidates was finalized in 1970 when the Registry changed its eligibility policies to exclude work experience alone as a basis for admission to the examination system.

Before 1969, the credential "ARIT" (American *Registered* Inhalation Therapist) was the only national award that recognized proficiency in the field. At that time only 700 persons were so credentialed, and concern over an apparent manpower shortage of qualified people began to grow. Although an ad hoc committee of the Registry recognized the need for a second level of credentialing, the ARIT was reluctant to initiate a new system of examination and recognition that did not require formal education. The burden of responsibility for the development and administration of what became the Certification examination system was assumed by the AAIT in 1969 with the formation of the Technician Certification Board (TCB).

The first TCB examination was administered in November 1969 to 88 candidates. Eligibility for the certification examination then required candidates to document 2 years' experience in the field or graduation from an accredited educational program. Eligibility by work experience alone was subsequently ended in 1975, with those applying under the "Grandfather Clause" required to complete successfully the certification process by 1977.

Concern over the existence of dual credentialing processes administered by separate agencies (ARIT and TCB) and the clear potential for conflict of interest in the AAIT's involvement in certification of its own members provoked efforts toward combining the functions of registration and certification under a single agency. With approval of their respective Boards, the ARIT and TCB merged in 1974, creating the National Board for Respiratory Therapy (NBRT). With the opening of its new Executive Office in Kansas City in mid-1974, the NBRT accepted the American Thoracic Society (ATS) as its fourth sponsor, expanded its Board to 24 members (4 each from the three sponsoring physician organizations and 12 representatives from the renamed American Association for Respiratory Therapy) and changed the credential designations of ARIT and CITT to ARRT and CRTT, reflecting the change in nomenclature of the field from "inhalation therapy" to "respiratory therapy." Subsequent litigation between the American Registry of Radiologic Technologists (also claiming the use of the initials ARRT) and the NBRT resulted in the 1976 change of the official designation for registered therapists to "RRT."

Current Status

When the NBRT became the credentialing board in 1974, there were about 8,500 CRTTs and 2,400 RRTs. As of June 1980, there were about 27,000 certified technicians and almost 11,000 registered therapists nationwide.[13] Concurrent with this rapid growth in credentialed manpower have been several significant changes in the credentialing process. In 1977, a mechanism was established whereby Certified Technicians with appropriate experience and college credit could become eligible for the Registry examination process. In 1979, the oral examination component of the Registry was replaced by a sophisticated clinical simulation examination that allowed for simultaneous and reliable testing of large numbers of candidates in multiple centers. The clinical simulation examination currently comprises ten branching-logic, patient–management situations designed to assess the candidates' ability to gather and interpret clinical data and to analyze and solve patient problems according to acceptable standards of judgment and decision-making. The care and deliberation with which such tests have been developed and the strict adherence of the NBRT to sound psychometric procedures of validation and reliability assessment have been recognized. The NBRT was among the first of many national health certifying agencies to be granted unconditional Category A membership status in the National Commission for Health Certifying Agencies (NCHCA), a voluntary not-for-profit organization formed to develop and encourage high standards of professional conduct among health certifying organizations. To meet future requirements for membership in the NCHCA, the NBRT will appoint a consumer representative to its Board of Trustees and plans to develop a recertification program to assure continued competency of its certified and registered members.[13]

In 1979, the NBRT Board approved perhaps the most ambitious and far-reaching change ever in its credentialing process: the development and implementation of an entry level examination for respiratory care practitioners. The goal of the entry-level examination (administered initially in 1983) is to test for and certify those competencies necessary to *begin* practice in the field. (The current CRTT and RRT examinations may not be taken at entry into practice.)

Although the full justification for such examination is beyond the scope of this chapter, the NBRT has provided five basic reasons for the development and implemention of its entry-level examination process.[21]

1. A common core of knowledge and skills is needed by all practitioners when they enter clinical respiratory therapy.
2. There is an increasing trend by third-party payers to reimburse for health care services only if they are rendered by credentialed practitioners.
3. Because of posteducational clinical experience requirements, large numbers of respiratory care practitioners remain uncredentialed for substantial periods of time.
4. The federal government has increasingly supported and encouraged credentialing agencies to provide mechanisms to certify health care providers at entry-level.
5. Existence of an entry-level examination should encourage the establishment of uniform standards for state legal recognition, avoid problems in reciprocity, and discourage dual-level recognition.

The implementation model of the entry-level examination system is depicted in Figure 2-8. According to the model, graduates of all CAHEA accredited respiratory therapist *and* respiratory therapy technician programs will be eligible for the entry-level examination immediately after completing their program requirements.[21] The entry-level examination, offered for the first time in March 1983, was designed to assess the proficiency of candidates within the domain of the major and minor responsibilities of the 1977 AART Role Delineation, as subsequently analyzed by the Educational Testing Service for the NBRT.[2,22]

Upon successful completion of the entry-level examination, all persons, regardless of the nature or length of their academic preparation (*i.e.*, technician or therapist; 1-year, 2-year, or 4-year programs) will be awarded the CRTT credential. Under the new system, only those who have successfully completed the entry-level examination will be eligible for advanced credentialing at the Registry level (RRT). Therapist program graduates (those with certificates of completion from 2-year or 4-year CAHEA-accredited programs) with 1 year of clinical experience under medical direction (and credentialed as CRTTs) will be eligible for a revised Registry examination comprising *both* a standard written multiple-choice component and the clinical simulation management problems. Once graduates of CAHEA-accredited technician programs have attained certification status (CRTT), they will have to accumulate 62 college credits (with the appropriate mix of basic sciences) *and* 4 years of clinical experience to qualify for the Registry examination. Certified Technicians with a baccalaureate degree and appropriate credit in the basic sciences will require only 2 years' postcertification clinical experience as a prerequisite for Registry eligibility.

Those persons "in the middle" of the current Registry process at the time of implementation of the entry-level examination (*i.e.*, those having passed the written RRT examination only) will be awarded the CRTT credential and be given 5 years to pass the clinical simulation component of the new combined

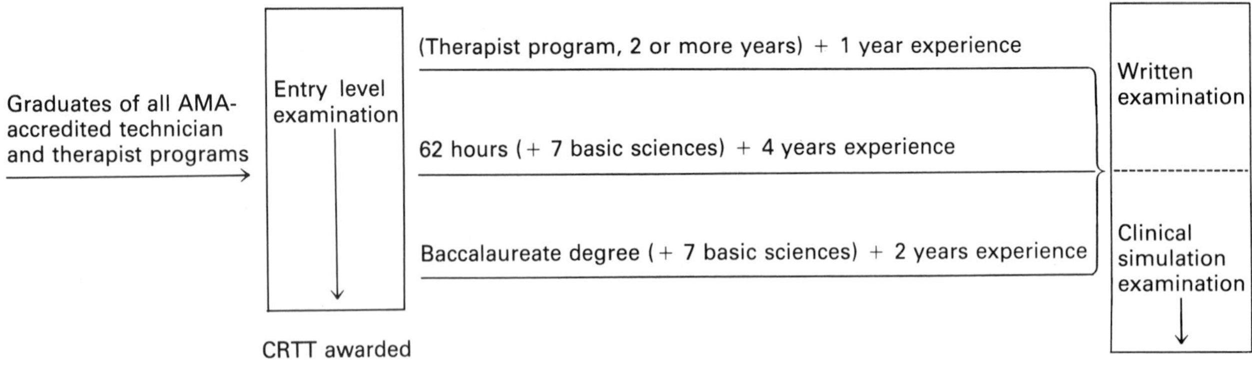

Fig. 2-8. Implementation model of the entry level examination system. (Modified, with permission, from NBRT Ad Hoc Committee for the Study of Entry Level Examinations: The entry level examination proposal. NBRT Newsletter 5(6)(suppl):3, 1979.)

Registry Examination, thereby qualifying as Registered Respiratory Therapists. Failure to do so in the alloted time period will require those unsuccessful in completing the Registry process to sit for the entire new Registry Examination.

Clearly, it is impossible to predict the full impact of this new system on the field. For the 5,000 or more practitioners currently "in limbo" between the written Registry and the Clinical Simulation Examination, the awarding of the CRTT credential will certainly be beneficial. The availability of professional certification immediately upon completion of the educational requirements would additionally seem to benefit the profession itself and help satisfy the many requirements and regulations and the growing expectations of both governmental agencies and institutional health care providers. At this time, however, several important questions remain unanswered. Will there be significant differences between the performance of therapist program and technician program graduates on the entry-level examinations? If so, to what extent (and in what direction) will such differences affect the current educational system? How will employers distinguish between persons with the same credential (CRTT) but distinctly different levels of educational preparation? Will the need for an advanced-level generalist examination (RRT) continue, or will it be supplanted by specialty examinations? Will the entry-level system make state licensure so appealing and easy to implement that it will replace voluntary credentialing entirely?

Such questions will no doubt be addressed during and after the full implementation of the new credentialing system. The ability of the profession to address such issues will largely determine their successful resolution. If the historical perspective is accurate, the voluntary NBRT* credentialing process for respiratory care practitioners will weather the changes, grow justifiably stronger, and continue to represent exemplary practices in the certification process of health care practitioners.

Limitations

Notwithstanding the strengths of the present and projected certification processes of respiratory care personnel, the extant credentialing system has several distinct weaknesses. Foremost among these is the voluntary nature of the system. No legal sanctions exist in voluntary certification processes to prevent noncredentialed persons from practicing in the field. In the absence of such sanctions, many people may seek and maintain gainful employment as health care practitioners without having undergone either formal training or credentialing. Such is the case in respiratory therapy; as recently as 1977, the AART reported that an estimated 71% of the basic practitioner groups and 49% of the advanced practitioner groups had no respiratory therapy credentials whatsoever.[1] Because of a dramatic increase in the number of credentialed personnel and an apparent slackening of the manpower shortage in respiratory care, such figures are likely to decrease significantly. As long as the system of credentialing is voluntary, however, the door will remain open for the uncredentialed, untrained, and potentially unqualified respiratory care practitioner to enter the field.

Another weakness of a voluntary credentialing system is that, although descriptions of respiratory care practice do indeed exist, the voluntary process is unable to assure that those it qualifies can indeed assume such practice roles. Further, there are no legal means to prevent other health professions from encroaching upon the role of the voluntary credentialed respiratory care practitioner. Where such other professions are licensed by an agency of the government, their practice acts can restrict the functions of those responsible for the delivery of respiratory care services. Encroachment of this sort, although currently isolated in occurrence, may play an increasingly important role in the future of voluntary credentialing in respiratory care.

The last major criticism of the existing credentialing process is the commonly voiced public concern over peer control and restricted entry into the field. Such concerns are legitimate only if the system either capriciously controls supply in the manpower marketplace or arbitrarily excludes qualified persons from practice. Neither assumption can be supported in reality. Qualified manpower shortages do indeed exist, but efforts to remedy the situation (nontraditional education, the entry level examination process, and others) are clearly evident. Arbitrary exclusion of qualified persons is equally fallacious. The NBRC is one of only a handful of health certifying agencies to have demonstrated the ability of its examinations to discriminate between the practitioners' levels of clinical proficiency (concurrent validity). Unfortunately, as long as some health professions do, in fact, restrict entry and control manpower for their own benefit,

*In January 1983, the National Society for Cardiopulmonary Technology became the fifth sponsor of the NBRT, and the name of this organization was changed to the National Board for Respiratory Care (NBRC).

such concerns will continue to be generalized to the respiratory care community. In the meantime, practitioners who are justifiably proud of their credentialing system (and its demonstrable impact on the quality of personnel who provide respiratory care services) should make every effort to educate the uninformed.

LEGAL RECOGNITION: LICENSURE

Licensure is the process whereby an agency of the government grants permission to an individual to engage in a given occupation after verification that the applicant has demonstrated the *minimum* degree of competency necessary to protect the public health, safety, and welfare.[22] Under constitutional law, licensure represents one of many "police powers" delegated to the states, and it is therefore through state legislative processes that licensure laws are enacted.[18]

Medical practice acts were generally the first licensure laws adopted by the states to regulate health professionals. Subsequent legislative efforts to assure the minimal competency of other health occupational groups have tended to use the medical practice acts as models.[18] Typically a licensing law defines the profession and delimits its scope of practice, it also describes the requirements and qualifications for obtaining a license and the grounds for revocation of the right to practice. Generally, the administrative mechanism by which the act has been implemented is detailed (including the formulation and responsibilities of a licensure board), and legal penalties for practicing without a license are specified.

Licensure laws may be either permissive or mandatory.[18] Permissive or voluntary licensure laws permit unlicensed persons to work in the occupation as long as they do not use the title recognized by the state. Mandatory or compulsory licensure requires that all persons engaged in the profession be licensed. Health professional licensure laws are characteristically mandatory, although exceptions do exist. Permissive licensure laws typically become mandatory with time.[32]

Historical Perspective

The past 10 years have seen the respiratory therapy community, under its professional association leadership, vacillate between adamant opposition to state licensure laws and the current strong, political thrust to support legal statutes recognizing the profession.[3,34]

Early opposition to licensure of respiratory care personnel was in concert with the 1971 HEW recommendations for the states to observe a moratorium on the licensure of additional categories of health personnel.[26] HEW's major concerns at that time were related to the proliferation of health professional occupational categories and to the questionable efficacy of the extant mechanisms of assuring the competency of health care practitioners. The respiratory therapy national leadership was also concerned about regulation since this was perceived to lead to the potential loss of peer control, dilution of standards of proficiency, and restrictions to practice. The effect of such forces (both the federal wariness and the professional reticence) was predictable, and through the mid-1970s licensure activity in respiratory therapy was minimal: Where activity did occur it was generally *not* supported by the profession, and only one state (Arkansas) enacted licensure laws for respiratory care personnel.

Several changes that occurred during the second half of the decade combined to shift the perspective from opposition to support for respiratory therapy licensure. First, a general increase in the political awareness of the profession as a whole sensitized its leaders to the need for "legitimization" of the occupation in the eyes of the government, both state and federal. Second, sporadic but disconcerting evidence of encroachment of other health professions on the "domain" of the respiratory care practitioner created, in the minds of many, the need to define legally an occupational scope of practice, and thereby to protect the interests of the profession as a whole. Hand-in-hand with this "territorial imperative" was a continued effort toward professionalization of the work force and the concurrent desire to protect the public from the untrained, uncredentialed, or otherwise unqualified practitioner.

Licensure activity for respiratory care personnel has been particularly spirited since the withdrawal of the HEW moratorium in 1975. As of this writing, at least 10 states are actively engaged in pursuing respiratory therapy licensure acts. The AART has recently published guidelines to assist states in writing legislation that would facilitate reciprocity and ensure unrestricted definitions of the scope of practice.[3] Notwithstanding the end of the moratorium, most states have, and are continuing to adhere to, subsequent HEW guidelines cautioning them to entertain licensure proposals *only* under the following conditions:[29]

1. If unregulated practice clearly endangers the health, safety, and welfare of the public in an easily recognizable way;

2. if licensure will ensure professional competence;
3. if licensure is the only way to protect the public effectively;
4. if licensure is the most appropriate form of regulation;
5. if the newly licensed category will not have a negative impact on the scope of practice of categories previously licensed by the state;

In light of such a perspective and in view of the current political trend of loosening governmental authority and increasing reliance on private-sector regulation, the future of state licensure in respiratory therapy is unclear.*

Strengths and Limitations

Notwithstanding doubt on the future of licensure in respiratory therapy, those responsible for addressing the issue must understand its strengths and limitations.[32] Licensure is one of several mechanisms that can prevent unqualified personnel from practicing within the field. As we have seen, voluntary credentialing mechanisms such as certification and registration cannot preclude such persons from entering into or practicing respiratory care. In addition, licensure does indeed give public recognition to an occupation and can protect an occupation from encroachment by related disciplines. Last, licensure is one of the mechanisms that can *require* practitioners to demonstrate continued competency (see section below).

Licensure is, however, fraught with limitations. Depending on how a licensure act is written, occupations may actually find themselves more restricted and with less control over their practice than before its enactment. Licensure generally attempts to assure minimal competency only, and, without other controls or mechanisms to assure quality health care, mediocrity can result. Licensure acts, once in place, are difficult to change or to amend, and thus in fields subject to rapid technological changes (like respiratory therapy) immutable laws could restrict innovative and progressive expansion of practitioner roles and functions. Finally, licensure laws can result in parochial standards of practice that are deleterious to the profession as a whole and that can preclude meaningful national progress toward generic standards of quality care.

*The only recent licensure act for respiratory care personnel was enacted in California in 1982. Several other states have licensure or registration actions pending before their legislative bodies.

OTHER FORMS OF LEGAL RECOGNITION

Although licensure is by far the most common form of legal recognition, the state has several other approaches through which a health professional may gain legal recognition. These include the already mentioned noncompulsory licensure or "registration," institutional licensure, practice act modification, and certification by one of the State Regulatory Agencies.

Noncompulsory licensure is much less confining than regular licensure and is essentially a protection for the title of the health profession. In any state that has such recognition, only persons who meet the educational and other requirements of the statute may call themselves respiratory therapists or respiratory technicians. This form of regulation, called "registration" in Michigan, does not prevent any person from performing the functions usually associated with respiratory care as long as they do not call themselves respiratory therapists or technicians. This form of regulation has merit because it is less expensive to administer and it provides both formal recognition of the professional and some protection to consumers.

Institutional licensure is another form of governmental regulation in which the state delegates the recognition process to the health care facility that employs the health professional. Under this regulation it becomes the responsibility of the hospital to assure competence of its health care workers, and it is the institutional license that is in jeopardy if the hospital employs personnel who do not meet the prescribed standards.

Nonphysician health care practitioners may also be legally recognized by a statutory inclusion into the medical or nursing practice art. Under this scheme, the legislature amends the appropriate practice act and permits the medical or nursing board to establish and implement standards for the recognition (certification) of the new health care profession. Physicians' assistants have been recognized by this mechanism in a number of states.

Finally, the legislature may delegate this power to one of the state agencies, such as the Department of Licensing and Regulation or the Department of Public Health. Under this system, the state agency will set the standards and implement them.

CONTINUING EDUCATION

The competency assurance mechanisms thus far discussed (accreditation, certification, and licensure) share two major characteristics: They represent *institutionalized* approaches to the issue of professional accountability, and they are directed at demonstrating such accountability only on the practitioners' *entry* into practice.

Continuing education is an accountability mechanism based on *individual* responsibility, which, in theory, should assure the continued competency of practitioners *after* entry into the field and throughout a lifetime of practice. Continuing education may thus be broadly defined as any purposeful, systematic, and sustained effort conducted by professionals, after completion of their entry-level education, to update, maintain, or expand the proficiency, knowledge, skill, and sensitivity necessary to discharge their occupational roles effectively.[29]

Continuing education may be broadly divided into two major categories; that which is self-directed (individually planned and pursued) and that which is other-directed (formal activities planned and organized by an educational agent other than the learner). Evidence gleaned from other health disciplines indicates that all professionals regularly engage in some form of continuing education, with self-directed activity generally predominating.[29] Other-directed continuing education (sponsored by professional associations, educational institutions, and health care agencies) generally attract only a portion of the active work force unless, of course, participation is mandated by licensure requirements. What is not generally appreciated is that professionals engage in organized, other-directed, continuing education activities for a variety of reasons. Such "motives for participation" may include professional advancement, learning for its own sake, acquisition of new credentials, compliance with formal requirements or expectations, escape from the routine of work and home, and social interaction.[29]

Although continuing professional education represents the fastest growing segment of postsecondary education in the United States, it has generally failed to develop in a coordinated manner and has recently come under criticism for its questionable effectiveness in assuring the continued competency of its target population. Of particular concern in health professions continuing education is the general lack of empirical evidence demonstrating the effect of educational intervention on the quality of health care.[29] Respiratory therapy is archetypical of both the problems and the promise of continuing health professions education.

No one involved in respiratory care over the last decade can argue with the need for mechanisms to assist practitioners in updating and maintaining their clinical knowledge and skills. Changes in both theory and practice have been so dramatic that practitioners educated in 1970 would today be functionally obsolete without continued and recurrent efforts to keep informed. There is, however, less agreement on exactly how the diverse learning needs of the respiratory care work force can best be met.

Organized, formal, other-directed continuing education opportunities for respiratory therapy personnel are generally provided through three organizational systems: professional associations, educational institutions and health care agencies. By far the most active and visible component of the formal continuing educational delivery system has been the professional association (AART). Through its national office and in conjunction with its chartered affiliates, the AART has regularly provided formal continuing education activities for clinicians, educators, and management personnel in the field. The National Convention annually attracts more than 5,000 participants and offers a diversified fare of lectures, workshops, and related activities. A smaller but more highly focused activity is the annual "Education Forum," also sponsored by the AART. At the chartered affiliate level, activity is directed at serving regional, state, or local needs; monthly educational meetings and annual statewide or regional conferences are typical of such activity. Related formal learning opportunities are provided by other health professional associations, and cosponsorship arrangements are not uncommon.

Recognizing that such diverse activities were of variable educational quality and that no mechanism existed to either assure quality or document participant learning activity, the AART ambitiously set out to establish a mechanism that could [a] guide the development of continuing education programs appropriate for respiratory care personnel; [b] approve and grant credit equivalents for participation in such programs; and [c] maintain cumulative records of continuing education activity for subscribers to the system. Introduced to the membership in 1975, the system, called PROCEED (Professional Recognition Of Continuing Education Experience and Development), combined a sophisticated program review and approval process with a computerized records system capable of transcripting both formalized, other-directed, and self-directed educational activities.[6] Credit equivalents in the system were based on a standardized national measure of participation (the CEU); credit granting authority was limited to programs that demonstrated sound educational design (through the review process), and only those participants who demonstrated achievement of the programs' prespecified outcome (by post-test) were awarded CEUs.

Strangely, the system never got off the ground. Initial membership enrollments fell far short of expectations, and less than 10% of the membership subscribed. The applications for program review and approval represented only a small portion of the known continuing educational opportunities being offered nationwide. Changes were suggested during 1978 to make enrollment in the system more appealing, to award a Certificate of Recognition such as the "Physicians Recognition Award" in medicine, and to ease the burdensome program approval process by recognizing institutional sponsors rather than only discrete programs. These suggestions, however, were never implemented, and the future of the PROCEED system is in doubt.

That such a system failed to achieve its goals indicates specific respiratory therapy problems and also the general problems of other small health professional groups who try to address the continuing educational needs of their practitioners. Unlike nursing and medicine, whose continuing education systems are more highly developed, respiratory therapy practitioners tend to be distributed geographically in small groups and usually lack a concentration of members in their institutional work settings. The logistics of providing cost-effective educational opportunities for such groups, and of meeting learning needs, are staggering. Compounding the logistic problems encountered by providers are the many situational, institutional, and informational obstacles to participation that hamper the busy respiratory care professional. Perhaps most important is the current lack of positive incentives for participation in organized continuing education. Extrinsic incentives alone (credits, certificates) are insufficient, and, unless the practitioners are able to assume responsibility for translating new knowledge and skills into practice, there is little likelihood for a growing commitment to participate in formal continuing education.

Logistic problems should and can be alleviated. Educational institutions that provide entry-level educational programs currently represent an untapped geographical network for the delivery of quality continuing education opportunities for practitioners. Such programs must not assume that their responsibility ends with the graduation of their students. These programs already have the personnel and material resources necessary to provide quality organized continuing education to meet the needs of working practitioners in their community or region. What is needed is a reorientation of priorities that acknowledges the importance of the role of such educational institutions in continuing education and that provides program personnel to fulfill such responsibilities. Institutional administrators cognizant of the potential fiscal benefits of such reordered priorities (successful continuing education can offset the cost of entry-level programs) will be generally supportive, if not enthusiastic. The sharing of costs with cooperating clinical affiliate agencies can increase both the efficiency and effectiveness of such efforts.

Hospitals themselves need to assume more leadership in providing continuing educational opportunities for respiratory care personnel. The work setting is the ideal location for the translation of new theory into practice. Unfortunately and too often, "staff development" and "in-service education" are directed at meeting institutional or departmental needs rather than the real or perceived needs of the professional staff. Meeting the learning needs of the individual staff members can serve as a potent incentive for improved work performance and can often provide the catalyst for increased educational activity congruent with institutional or departmental needs.

Lastly, more and better efforts to facilitate the self-directed learning activities of respiratory care practitioners are direly needed. Journals, the old standby of self-directed learning, need to develop innovative ways of providing not only information, but also instruction. Such efforts have been phenomonally successful in other health professions and need now be applied to respiratory care. Publications such as *Current Reviews in Respiratory Therapy*, geared specifically to the individual, self-directed learner, are noteworthy, but wider dissemination, at lower cost, could be achieved through the not-for-profit journals of the professional association.

Fulfilling the needs of learners during a lifetime of practice must become a higher priority of the educational and professional community in respiratory care. To the extent that such efforts are successful, benefits will accrue to practitioners themselves, to the profession as a whole, and ultimately to health care agencies and to the public they serve.

In 1982, PROCEED was replaced by Continuing Education in Respiratory Therapy (CERT). This system, also sponsored by the AART, shows considerable promise and may significantly improve the continuing education climate in respiratory care.

THE ECONOMICS OF EDUCATION

Education, stripped from its philosophic and sociologic trappings, is a business and must therefore be conducted in a businesslike way.

In the past, three types of educational programs were considered from a fiscal point of view: the hospital-based programs, the programs based in a proprietary school, and the programs based in a community college or university. The hospital-based program, now largely a matter of history, funded its educational activities from its general revenue sources, most of which were generated from the patients who used the services of the hospital. In most areas, third-party payers recognized that educational activities, at least those controlled by the hospital, were reimbursable legitimate expenses. Further, hospital-based programs had relatively few direct costs related to these programs, and by far the largest item was the time spent with the students by salaried hospital employees. The hospital-based program usually charged no tuition, or only a very nominal tuition, and paid no stipend to the students. In most programs, the students generated income for the hospital by performing tasks somewhat beyond the capacity of the regular department. Thus, the hospital-based programs, although educationally weak in many instances, were certainly the most cost-effective and allowed students to get an education with a relatively modest outlay of money.

The proprietary schools, relatively few in number, operate on an entirely different principle. These programs are operated for profit, and the owner of the school expects to make a living by showing a profit at the end of the fiscal year. The tuition paid by the students is usually the only revenue these schools have, although a few may have modest endowments or gain revenue from noneducational business activities. Since tuition must generate enough income to cover the expenses and to provide income for the owner, the cost for the students is obviously formidable. A tuition rate of $2,500 to $3,500 per year is not unusual, and some programs charge tuition well above these rates. It is, we believe, legitimate to ask, "What does the student buy with this substantial investment?" The answer is simple. In most proprietary schools, the student buys a good education, albeit at a considerable price. In other schools the students buy a diploma or a certificate of completion. It is obviously the accrediting agency's responsibility to see that the fortunately few programs that fit into the second category be eliminated. The National Association of Trade and Technical Schools (NATTS) does a careful and very thorough job of investigating the financial status of the proprietary schools it accredits. Because of NATTS and programmatic accrediting agencies such as the Joint Review Committee, the dishonest schools usually have a very brief existence. Unfortunately, this will not protect the first or second class of students from paying a huge premium for a shoddy education.

Proprietary schools have a real economic problem because their only defense against rising costs is to continuously raise tuition. Further, proprietary schools frequently have to pay higher salaries and buy more services than do their nonproprietary competition. Not surprisingly, particularly in times of economic retrenchment, a number of these schools are closing their doors entirely or eliminating the expensive health programs and concentrating on those programs where the cost per student is the most favorable.

The third type of system is the not-for-profit private or public college or university. These schools differ from the proprietary schools in that they pay no taxes, and the profits, if any, must accrue to the institution, not for the benefit of any individual. The private and public schools differ from each other in that the latter receive a substantial portion of their operating funds from taxes collected in the community that they serve. This community may be a school district, a county, a state, a town, or a city. The tax support allows the schools to have lower tuition rates, but also mandates certain admission policies, certain procedural limitations, and occasionally curricular restrictions. Since the community supports the educational institution with tax revenues, there is usually a two- or three-tiered tuition rate depending on the legal residence of the students.

Private schools, more dependent on tuition, tend to have much higher tuition rates, smaller enrollments, higher entrance requirements, and a perceived haughty attitude that may or may not be warranted by the superiority of its faculty and facilities. Private schools also depend heavily on endowments and donations from alumni, grants, contracts, and other sources. Private schools tend to be more flexible and more likely to be innovative, whereas public schools are more rigid and more likely to be traditional in their approach to education.

In respiratory care, most programs are sponsored by public colleges and universities, and the majority of these are 2-year community colleges, awarding an Associate in Arts or Science degree.

Table 2-4 reviews the fiscal year 1980–1981 budget for a 2-year community-college-sponsored program that had been in existence for several years. The program has four clinical affiliates and 20 students in each of the 2 years.

Table 2-4. Typical Budget for Medium-Sized 2-Year Respiratory Therapy Education Program*

Salaries, instruct full time	$50,250
Salaries, instruct part time	$30,000
Salaries, overload	$4,500
Salaries, substitute	$2,000
Salaries, other	$15,523†
Fringe benefits	$8,177
FICA and retirement	$20,835
Contractual services	$33,000‡
Supplies and materials, instructional	$10,907
Supplies and materials, general	$200
Duplicating and printing	$4,000
Rental equipment	$1,000
Conference expense	$450
Local travel	$500
Professional dues	$400§
Activity expense	$200‖
Account total	$181,942
Source of revenue	
Tuition	17.7%
State aid	27.0%
Local property taxes	55.3%
Total	100.0%

*There is no capital equipment budget item, since this program has been in operation for several years at the time this budget was prepared.
†Clinical instructor.
‡Clinical faculty contracts.
§Accreditation.
‖Field trips.

We wish to draw particular attention to the cost of clinical education. This is discussed also in another chapter but is of sufficient importance to be repeated. Traditionally the cost of clinical education is borne by the clinical affiliate where the clinical experience is provided and the educational institution provides no money, or only a token payment to defray the indirect cost of this educational experience. This arrangement is, of course, very advantageous for the educational institution that collects tuition for all phases of the program but has expenses only for the didactic, laboratory, and administrative phases. The cost of the clinical phase is really provided by the patients, directly or through third-party payers. This we believe to be wrong for several reasons: First, it contributes to the high cost of health care; second, the patients who contribute to the cost of education may derive no benefits from it; and last, the educational institution, by making no contribution toward it, has less control over the quality and intensity of the clinical instruction.

We deeply believe that the cost of the clinical instruction must be, to a large extent, part of the budgeted cost of the entire program, and that the educational institution must reimburse the health care facility for at least the major portion of the cost. It is the school's responsibility to plan for this and to build this cost into the budget over a period of 3 to 5 years. Thus, the change will be gradual and will give the school the opportunity to adjust its financial commitment over time.

We are aware that this problem is a complex one. In the present economic climate, a substantial increase in the cost of the program may prove an intolerable burden to the educational institution and may force the discontinuation of this type of activity. It is also true that some studies have suggested that the cost of the clinical education is offset by the contributions the students make to patient care. Although we do not question the validity of these studies, it seems likely that if the students generate substantial income to the hospital, student exploitation may result.[15,24]

A solution to this vexing problem is urgently needed. It may best be accomplished if the financial officers of the educational institution and of the health care facility were to examine the issues together, were to obtain accurate cost and benefit estimates, and were to reach a mutually satisfactory economic agreement. Any arrangement is satisfactory, provided that the patients are not burdened improperly and the students are not exploited.

FUTURE PERSPECTIVES

With more than three decades of combined experience in respiratory care and respiratory therapy education, we feel justified in speculating on the shape of things to come. Such prognostication is based on a firm belief that future events are the result of deliberate planning and not of fortuitous happenstance. We believe that careful consideration of alternative futures is a necessary and desirable means of controlling our collective destiny.

RESPIRATORY THERAPY PRACTICE

The future of respiratory therapy education is inextricably linked with the future of respiratory therapy practice. If, as historians claim, past events portend future circumstances, tomorrow's practice of respiratory care will be very different from what we see today. Dramatic increases in knowledge and in its technological application are a given. Concomitant with such changes, significant alterations in the nature of the health care delivery system are most likely. An aging population will require both institutional and ambulatory health care services of a different nature than those currently available. Chronic diseases will eventually largely supplant acute disorders, and increasing emphasis will be placed on ambulatory and domiciliary care and on patient education. Changing reimbursement mechanisms are likely to encourage this and will further deemphasize the role of the acute care facility in all but the most life-threatening maladies. High technology will continue to flourish, however, as the care of the acute illness becomes ever more sophisticated and concentrated in regionalized tertiary care facilities. In such facilities, specialized respiratory care practice will be commonplace. Although governmental intervention in cost-benefit and quality of care issues may decline, health care agencies and practitioners alike will be expected to demonstrate the efficacy and economy of their methods. The quality of care issue will intensify as the barriers to access decrease and the distributional problems are alleviated.

In such context, the respiratory therapy practitioners of the future (if indeed that is what we will call ourselves) will find their role expanded outside the acute care institutions and will become increasingly responsible for extending the physician's role into the community and into the homes of the health care consumers. Proficiency in patient education will become a necessary component of the respiratory care practitioner's repertoire of skills, as will sophisticated rehabilitative, health promotional, and health maintenance activities.

The acute care setting will continue, however, to remain the major focal point for most respiratory care practitioners. Within such a setting technology will have its greatest impact on both the nature and type of care provided and on the providers themselves. Foremost among the technological changes will be the growth of noninvasive monitoring and diagnostic systems and the relentless increase of computer application in assessment *and* treatment. The "knob-turner" of the past will become the computer systems analyst of the future, as physiological functions are monitored and controlled by sophisticated patient–machine interfaces. Such changes will demand that practitioners acquire technological expertise well beyond the scope of what is currently required. Ironically, however, in such settings, psychosocial skills will be at a premium.

The issues of quality and efficacy will be increasingly addressed by practitioners skilled in basic and applied research methods working in conjunction with other members of the health care team. Such research will increasingly focus on less esoteric health care problems, and it is not inconceivable that the respiratory care researcher of the future may attempt to unravel the mysteries of the common cold and its attendant ailments! Research will extend beyond the pathophysiology and therapy of disease into investigation of the efficacy of various behavior modification techniques dealing with the continued problems of our own improprieties.

RESPIRATORY THERAPY EDUCATION

Concomitant with changes in the scope and pattern of respiratory care practice will be changes in the nature of the educational systems that prepare people for entry into such practice. These changes will be evolutionary rather than revolutionary and will hopefully be in tune with the needs of the health care system.

Setting and Levels

In the near future sponsorship of respiratory care education will shift completely from the hospital setting to the academic environment. In this setting, two distinct levels of education will emerge: technical and professional respiratory care that requires the associate and baccalaureate degree, respectively.[5] Baccalaureate program curricula will become less diverse as accrediting standards are developed for 4-year educational programs and as a core of advanced clinical skills becomes clearly defined. Baccalaureate curricula will accommodate articulation with the lower division technical programs, thereby facilitating the upward career mobility of those who desire to pursue advanced academic preparation. As manpower needs stabilize, the total number of educational programs will decrease and stabilize according to regional planning demands. Professional educational programs at the baccalaureate level will represent an increased proportion of the total program complement, with at least one program in each state. Training in specialized areas of clinical respiratory care will be provided mainly by structured postgraduate learning experiences offered in academic health science centers that have the necessary clinical resources. Graduate education will be reserved for training in clinical research and teacher training.

Teaching/Learning Process

The teaching/learning process, not unlike clinical practice, will feel the impact of technology. As the cost of microprocessor hardware decreases and sophisticated instructional software becomes readily available, the laborious process of inculcating basic knowledge will be increasingly accomplished by computer-assisted instruction.[25] With cognitive testing, student progress monitoring, and instructional management efficiently handled by computer, educators will be better able to address the needs of clinical skill development and performance evaluation. Both cognitive and performance evaluations will become increasingly sophisticated, with computer and laboratory simulations providing reliable and valid measures of problem-solving ability and procedural expertise. The dream of true competency-based education will become a reality when standardized measures of proficiency become the criteria for unit, course, and program completion. With instructors freed from the more mundane and necessarily time-consuming elements of rote transfer of knowledge, record-keeping, and cognitive testing, attention to individual student needs will be facilitated, and the creative side of the educational enterprise will be significantly enhanced.

Accreditation and Credentialing

With valid and continuously updated delineations of the roles and functions of both entry-level practitioners and specialists in respiratory care, the accreditation and credentialing systems will become fully integrated and mutually complementary.

The accreditation process for respiratory therapy educational programs will shift in emphasis from the assessment of input and process standards to the evaluation of the content validity of the curriculum—that is, the degree to which the curriculum content and organization coincides with the competencies requisite to entering practice and to multiple criterion measures of student learning outcomes. The few input and process standards that remain will be those demonstrably related to achieving successful program outcomes and ensuring institutional probity and fair educational practices. The length of accreditation will be increased to 10 years, and the programmatic on-site evaluation process will become integrated with institutional or school-wide accreditation. Annual and interim report mechanisms will increasingly place the burden of responsibility on institutional sponsors and program personnel to provide empirical evidence of the quality and ongoing improvement of their program processes and outcomes. Accreditation mechanisms will be developed to ensure that specialized postgraduate experiences do indeed accomplish their goals.

Implementation of the entry-level examination process will cause minor upheavals in the educational community but will quickly gain acceptance and catalyze the transition to a tiered technical and professional system. The advanced generalist credential (RRT) will probably survive, but increasing emphasis will be placed on specialty credentialing examinations designed to assess competencies in discrete and focused domains of clinical practice. Licensure, in some form, will become a reality when and if the scope of respiratory care practice regularly extends outside the confines of the acute care setting. Such systems will initially mandate continuing education participation for renewal but will eventually require periodic proof of continued competence. Eventually, licensure or its equivalent will supplant voluntary credentialing at entry level; such credentialing will, however, continue to recognize individuals at advanced and specialized areas of clinical practice.

GLOSSARY OF TERMS*

ACCREDITATION, INSTITUTIONAL. Accreditation granted to an entire educational institution by a national accrediting body recognized by the U.S. Department of Education (ED) or the Council on Postsecondary Accreditation (COPA) after a comprehensive evaluation of governance, organization, financing, academics, faculty, instructional resources, student services, physician facilities, development, and admissions, among others, as related to the institution's educational mission.

ACCREDITATION, PROGRAM. Applies to a particular program of specialized study and signifies that the institution sponsoring the program, along with any necessary affiliates, provides the instructional resources and planned learning experiences specified in the educational Essentials.

ACCREDITATION, SPECIALIZED. A status of affiliation accorded a unit or program by a professional accrediting agency. The unit accredited may be a school, department, program, or curriculum. It may be part of a total educational institution, an independent, specialized institution, or an educational unit within a primarily noneducational institution (e.g., a hospital).

*Excerpted, with permission from the Committee on Allied Health Education and Accreditation: *Allied Health Education Directory*, 9th ed. Chicago, American Medical Association, 1981.

ACCREDITATION STATUS. Formal recognition given an institution or specialized program for meeting established standards of educational quality, as determined by regional or national institutional and specialized nongovernmental accrediting agencies.

ACCREDITATION, VOLUNTARY (ALSO PRIVATE). A peer process whereby a private, nongovernmental agency or association grants public recognition to an institution or specialized program of study that meets or exceeds certain established qualifications and educational standards, as determined through periodic evaluations. Because the process is voluntary, review committees and CAHEA do not begin the process of program review until the Chief Executive Officer or designee for the institution sponsoring the program requests accreditation evaluation.

ADMISSION POLICY. The rationale that determines the applicants who qualify for admission to an institution. Consideration is given to the role assigned to the institution by its governing body; the programs, resources, and facilities of the institution; and the qualifications and goals of the applicant.

ADVANCED STANDING. Credit given on the basis of transferable credit, equivalency examination, or developmental experiences, where appropriate. Appropriate assessments and documentation are made part of the student record. The certificate or diploma granted by the program should be the same for all students, regardless of whether advanced standing has been granted.

AFFILIATION AGREEMENT. A formal exchange of written understanding between an institution sponsoring the program and a second independent facility that agrees to provide appropriate clinical learning experiences for students, or between a hospital sponsor and an educational affiliate.

AFFILIATION CONTRACT. A formal document consisting of written agreements, signed by both parties, that reflect the contractual relationship. CAHEA recommends that all affiliation contracts be reviewed annually.

ALLIED HEALTH. A large cluster of health-care-related professions and personnel whose presence in the national workforce fulfills necessary functions and roles that are supportive of, supplement, or otherwise facilitate the work of the fully licensed physician, and who prefer to be identified as allied health personnel. The cluster embodies various interrelationships: related (sometimes overlapping) occupations; mutual members of a team function; and distant or even remote occupations. All meet established needs within the system of medical care in which the physician has final medical responsibility. Definitions of "allied health" vary due to its changing nature and to the differing perspectives of those who attempt its definition and because certain medically related but traditionally parallel or independent occupations prefer identities independent of allied health: nursing, podiatry, pharmacy, and clinical psychology, among others. Other occupations may regard themselves as "allied health," depending on their varying circumstances—for example, nutritionists, speech pathologists, audiologists, public health specialists, licensed practical nurses, and medical research assistants.

APPEALS PROCEDURE. Review of an adverse accreditation decision, on the grounds that it was arbitrary, capricious, not in accord with CAHEA's accreditation standards and procedures, or not supported by substantial evidence. CAHEA maintains a written procedure for processing appeals that may be requested by institutions whose programs have been the subject of an adverse accreditation decision by CAHEA.

CAREER LADDER. A sequence of lateral or vertical steps that link jobs related in the same job family permitting an employee to build from education and experiences in order to move to an advanced position or to a related occupation.

CERTIFICATE OF COMPLETION. Written documentation that provides a declaration that a person has completed a course of prescribed study and is qualified to be so cited; usually awarded by the institution that sponsors the course of study.

CERTIFICATION. The process by which a nongovernmental agency or association grants recognition to a person who has met certain predetermined, usually quantitative, qualification specified by that agency or association and who voluntarily seeks such recognition.

CLINICAL EDUCATION (ALSO DIRECTED CLINICAL EXPERIENCE/FIELD WORK/PRACTICUM). The portion of a structured educational program provided in a health care facility and usually specifically related to previous or ongoing didactic education. In some instances, the terms "directed clinical experience/field work/practicum" may be more appropriate than "clinical education." Although a sharp distinction cannot be made between clinical experience and clinical education, the word "education" implies major focuses on gaining knowledge, skill, and aptitude through instruction, whereas the word "experience" implies that the major focus is on gaining knowledge, skill, and aptitude through direct participation in events.

In any event, the term refers to the planned learning experiences assigned as an integral part of, or complement to, didactic courses, designed to provide initial and basic experiences in direct observation and then in participation in selective practical activities under the supervision of qualified, competent personnel.

Clinical education or experience involves scheduling students to participate during specific blocks of time in planned activities that provide them with opportunities to apply academically acquired knowledge in an actual work situation applicable to their field of preparation. Emphasis is on gaining skill and performing the basic procedures used in the occupation in various situations likely to be encountered on the job.

COMMITTEE ON ALLIED HEALTH EDUCATION AND ACCREDITATION (CAHEA). An allied health program accreditation agency in the voluntary sector, listed by the Secretary, U.S. Department of Education and recognized by the

Council on Postsecondary Accreditation (COPA). CAHEA is known as an "umbrella" accreditation agency inasmuch as it works cooperatively with externally located review committees to accredit educational programs in 26 or more fields of postsecondary allied health education.

COMPETENCY-BASED EDUCATION. A course, program, or curriculum based on what the student is supposed to learn to do or on demonstrable outcomes.

COMPETENCY OBJECTIVES. The specific level or nature of competence to be achieved by the learner/performer. Such objectives ordinarily are prepared in written form and provided both to faculty and to students and are available to site visitors during a site visit to the program.

COMPLIANCE, SUBSTANTIAL. That degree to which a program meets the standards (or *Essentials*) established as minimum qualifications for accreditation. To comply, a program may have weaknesses but must largely conform with the fundamental characteristics of the *Essentials.*

CONSORTIUM. Two or more institutions that have agreed formally to sponsor the development and continuation of an educational program.

CONTINUING EDUCATION. A structured educational activity pursued by the individual practitioner or other health system specialist for the purpose of upgrading, extending, or expanding a person's skill and knowledge base. Generally, its purpose is to keep the individual practitioner current with the technology and techniques of the field of practice or to prepare the practitioner to assume responsibilities as an educator or a manager.

CONTINUING EDUCATION UNIT (CEU). Educational unit consisting of 10 contact hours of participation in organized continuing education experience under responsible sponsors, capable direction, and qualified instruction.

COUNCIL ON MEDICAL EDUCATION (CME). Standing council of the AMA delegated the traditional prerogative of the House of Delegates to adopt the allied health Essentials for the AMA. The CME approves petitions of new and emerging allied health occupations to be recognized by the AMA and approves petitions for recognition of organizations to collaborate with the AMA in accreditation of allied health programs.

COUNCIL ON POSTSECONDARY ACCREDITATION (COPA). A national, nonprofit organization, the major purpose of which is to support, coordinate, and improve all nongovernmental accrediting activities conducted at the postsecondary educational levels in the United States. In this role, COPA assumes a unique "balance wheel" function in relation to the various groups involved in, or affected by, accreditation.

COURSE (DISCRETE). An orderly series of instructional activities dealing with a subject, in which learning experiences are structured to the established educational objectives. A structure in which each subject matter area or segment is taught as an entity without special effort and articulation or correlation with other subject matter areas or segments.

CREDENTIALING BODY. An agency, usually in the private sector, engaged in the examination and recognition of qualifying persons for the award designated as credentials. A credentialing body may be engaged either in certification or registration of individuals and may or may not conduct examinations of the competence of these persons. When the credentialing body is engaged in licensure, it will then be an agency of state government.

CREDENTIAL(S). [1] A certificate stating that the student has graduated from a certain curriculum or has passed certain subjects; [2] a statement signed by a proper authority certifying that a person is authorized to perform certain functions or has been designated as an official representative; [3] a detailed record of an applicant for a position, usually including transcripts of academic records and testimonials relative to previous experience, performance, and character; or [4] the confidential file of an applicant sent to prospective employers.

CRITERION-REFERENCED. Designed to ascertain a person's status with respect to a well-defined behavioral domain, which consists of a set of skills that an examinee displays in a testing situation. Examinees are compared to a single standard rather than to the performance of other examinees. *Also see* Norm-Referenced.

CURRICULUM. A set of courses offered by an educational institution or one of its branches. Curriculum is associated with the planned interaction of students with the instructional resources in achieving the instructional education objectives.

DEPARTMENT OF ALLIED HEALTH EDUCATION AND ACCREDITATION (DAHEA). A staff department within the AMA that conducts the day-to-day business of program accreditation, including staff support of CAHEA and of the development and maintenance of educational standards, liaison with review committees and collaborating organizations, and support to the Council on Medical Education.

ELIGIBILITY, FEDERAL. Certification by an agency of the federal government that an educational institution or program qualifies for participation in certain federal funding programs. Accreditation by an agency recognized by the Secretary of the United States Department of Education (ED) is a factor in the eligibility certification process.

EQUIVALENCY TESTING, ACADEMIC. The comprehensive evaluation of a person's knowledge, skills, and personal attributes acquired through alternate experiences as they compare to those developed through the formal program of the educational institution.

ESSENTIALS. The minimum standards by which educational programs are reviewed, surveyed, or evaluated for purposes of accreditation. Essentials tend to be general statements so that they may be widely applicable to varieties of programs and yet avoid provisions that may be seen as arbitrary. Essentials also incorporate terms requiring mandatory conditions or actions such as must, will, shall, require, and so forth. Revisions to Essentials are usually effected within a 5-year period.

EXPERIMENTAL/INNOVATIVE PROGRAM. Courses of study containing approaches or methodologies that vary substantially from the traditional didactic or laboratory method and hence from the Essentials applicable to such programs. The experimental/innovative components include the potential for alternate, improved, or otherwise desirable nontraditional means of achieving knowledge and skills than those applied within the usual or traditional didactic environment. CAHEA provides appropriate procedural review for such departures under its document entitled Procedure, Criteria, and Suggestions Regarding Experimental and Innovative Programs.

EXTERNAL DEGREE. An academic award earned through one or more of the following means: prior learning, extrainstitutional learning, credit by examination, specially devised sponsored experiential learning programs, self-directed study, and satisfactory completion of campus or noncampus courses.

EXTRAINSTITUTIONAL LEARNING. Learning attained outside the sponsorship of legally authorized and accredited postsecondary institutions. The term applies to learning acquired from work and life experiences; from independent reading and study; from the mass media; and from participation in formal courses sponsored by associations, business, government, industry, military, unions, and other social institutions, such as hospitals.

FACULTY, INSTRUCTIONAL. Refers to instructors in allied health programs, but not to librarians, administrators, counselors, or others who may have faculty rank.

Full-time: Faculty employed by the institution, the majority of whose assignments are class or course instruction but which may also include institutional nonclass-related faculty responsibilities such as academic advisement, curricular development and review, faculty selection and evaluation, and other. Those performing these functions may also be considered full-time faculty if a portion of their assignment is research service or academic administration.

Part-time or adjunct: Faculty whose major responsibility is not related to the institution in question and who are customarily assigned one or two classes with class-related responsibilities only.

FAIR PRACTICES IN EDUCATION. A CAHEA statement for implementation by institutions and programs to assure fair and objective treatment of students and, in general, to protect the welfare of the student.

HEALTH PRACTITIONER. A person who applies the skills of one or more specific occupations within the entire range of health systems services.

HOSPITAL BASED PROGRAM. An educational program sponsored by a hospital.

JOINT REVIEW COMMITTEE (JRC). Applicable to all review committees sponsored by two or more collaborating organizations other than the AMA, whether or not so named. *Also see* Review Committee.

LICENSURE. The process by which an agency of government grants permission to persons meeting predetermined qualifications to engage in a given occupation or to use a particular title; or grants permission to an institution to perform specified functions otherwise prohibited.

MEDICAL DIRECTOR. An appropriately qualified physician, as defined by the Essentials, who provides medical direction to the allied health educational program, particularly with respect to the medical content of the curriculum and the medically related activities of students in the clinical phase of their educational program.

MODULE. A unit of learning that deals with a specific topic or concept that may be used in one or more courses.

NONDISCRIMINATORY PRACTICES. Practices for the institution and the program, specified within CAHEA's Fair Practices in Education, that prohibit discrimination with respect to race, color, creed, sex, age, handicap, or national origin.

NONTRADITIONAL EDUCATION. Educational practices generally recognized as varying from the traditional didactic and clinical procedures. *Also see* Experimental/Innovative Program.

NORM REFERENCED. Examinations and other evaluation tools keyed to an established norm, such as a "90% pass rate." *Also see* Criterion Referenced.

OUTCOME EVALUATION, ACCREDITATION. Accreditation evaluation that focuses on the graduates of a program or institution rather than on (or only on) the process through which students pass during the course of their education.

PERFORMANCE OBJECTIVES. The interim competencies achievable by students within the course of their training and the terminal competencies to be achieved by students by the end of the program. Assessment frequently includes verification of written performance objectives and their application within the curriculum and the clinical phase of training.

POSTSECONDARY EDUCATION. The array of educational opportunities available to post-high-school adults, including educational programs of postsecondary educational institutions and extrainstitutional learning experiences.

PRACTICUM. An extended period of full-time experience (weeks or months) in professional practice during which students test and reconstruct the theory they have learned and during which clinical education proficiency is developed. The practicum, usually a type of internship, provides opportunities for the students to assume major responsibility for the full range of duties in a real health care situation under the guidance of qualified personnel from the educational institution and from the affiliating health care facility or agency. It presupposes the learning experience included in all other professional studies and is a more complete and concrete learning activity than laboratory and clinical education or directed field work. *Also see* Clinical Education.

PROCESS EVALUATION. The practice of evaluating educational programs by examining the process through which the learner passes; to be contrasted with product, or outcome, evaluation.

PROGRAM. An educational structure designed to provide students with the knowledge and skills needed to work in a specific job or to improve their competence in that job. Program includes the curriculum as well as the administrative support required to implement the sequence of educational and skill development experiences identified in the program plan.

PROGRAM DIRECTOR. The person in charge (perhaps designated as program or department chairman) of developing and maintaining an educational program within an institution, hospital, or other sponsoring agency, in accordance with the qualifications and responsibilities delineated in the Essentials.

PROGRAM EVALUATION, ON-SITE. A specifically evaluative approach to site visitation, followed by peer review by a review committee (which may involve a special critique by designated readers) and the review activities undertaken by CAHEA and its staff. In contrast to site visit or survey, program evaluation implies judgment-making and interim conclusions on site by visiting team members. *Also see* Site Visit, Site Survey, Site Evaluation.

PROPRIETARY. A school or system of schools constituted for profit.

RECERTIFICATION. Periodic renewal or revalidation of certification, based on reexamination, continuing education, or other methods developed by the certifying agency.

REGISTERED PRACTITIONER. Status of a professional whose name appears on a list of practitioners or others who are registered.

REGISTRATION. The process by which qualified persons are listed on an official roster maintained by a governmental or nongovernmental agency. Historically, this term has been used synonymously with the current definition of certification.

REGISTRY. A published list of those who are registered or an agency that publishes a list of those registered.

RELIABILITY. The consistency with which an instrument or tool measures each time it is used. In controlled studies, reliability is usually expressed as a numerical index of the extent to which consistency has been demonstrated.

REVIEW COMMITTEE. A generic descriptor of the various committees that cooperate with CAHEA in the review and evaluation of programs for initial or continuing accreditation. When programs apply for accreditation, the review committee makes arrangements for an on-site visit, selects the team, evaluates the team's report after the site visit, and forwards a recommended accreditation status to CAHEA.

Review committees vary in size and in the number of times they meet, but they all perform the same generic functions. The CAHEA document "Policies and Procedures for Review Committees" provides information on the establishment, structure, and staffing of review committees, as well as on policies and procedures relating to the interaction of CAHEA and the review committees in the accreditation process. The Statement of Basic Principles also contains a section entitled "Function and Mechanism for Establishment of Review Committees."

SCHOOL OF ALLIED HEALTH. For CAHEA accreditation purposes, an administrative unit with responsibility for three or more accredited or accreditable allied health educational programs. Such schools may exist within various institutions, including, but not limited to, universities, colleges, community colleges, academic medical centers, and hospitals.

SELF-ANALYSIS. The final portion of self-study/self-assessment/self-evaluation in which the program or institution examines its strengths and weaknesses and formulates recommendations to assist in planned improvements.

SELF-STUDY/SELF-ASSESSMENT/SELF-EVALUATION. Equivalent and interchangeable terms denoting detailed institutional or programmatic self-review of internal policies and functions and external relationships. The purpose of this self-review is the ongoing improvement of the institution or program; it also serves as the basis for external (peer) evaluation. Results of the self-review are presented in a self-study report, which is used by accrediting agencies, review committees, and site visitors. Programmatic self-study/self-assessment/self-evaluation may go beyond the needs of the accreditation process, but only the findings necessary to demonstrate substantial compliance with the Essentials need be documented in the self-study report. *Also see* Self-Analysis, Self-Study Report.

SELF-STUDY REPORT. A documented written account of the self-study/self-assessment/self-evaluation outcomes necessary to indicate substantial compliance with the Essentials. Such reports usually reflect an organized study-assessment/evaluation effort involving program officials, faculty, administrators, directors of support services, clinical supervisors, students, graduates, and an advisory committee. It is the prerogative of the program or institution to determine the nature and scope of the self-study, but the report itself should be limited. See CAHEA document "Standard Format for Self-Evaluation Reporting."

SIMULATION. An object, process, system, or a combination of these equivalent to an actual situation.

SITE VISIT. A visit to the site of a specialized educational program undergoing accreditation review by a team of two or more qualified persons appointed by a review committee to collect information as to how closely a program meets requirements for quality as mandated by Essentials.

SITE SURVEY. A site visit during which the accreditation team observes the program components in order to verify information obtained from the self-study and other sources. Team members do not make evaluative judgments as to how closely the program complies with the Essentials.

SITE EVALUATION. A site visit during which the accreditation team forms evaluative judgments as to how closely the program complies with the Essentials.

SITE VISIT REPORT. A confidential formal written report prepared by a site visit team signed by the team members, which may or may not include recommendations regarding accreditation. The report or summary is forwarded to the proper review committee for evaluation. A copy is then sent to the institution and program for correction of any inaccuracies in its factual content.

SITE VISIT TEAM. Two or more persons composing a visiting team that surveys or evaluates an educational program on site at a sponsoring institution, and perhaps in related clinical facilities. Site visit teams usually comprise at least two people, whose span of competence in educational experience and practitioner experience assures thorough assessment of the program.

SPONSOR, PROGRAM OR INSTITUTIONAL. An institution having primary responsibility for designing and conducting an allied health educational program.

STANDARDS. The criteria by which programs or institutions are reviewed for accreditation purposes. *Essentials* are minimum standards for allied health educational programs.

SUPERVISOR, CLINICAL. The person or persons, qualified through education and practitioner and clinical experience, who supervise the students in the clinical phase of their program, in special laboratory settings, during field projects, and the like. Other terms may be used to designate the person who performs in this capacity.

UNITED STATES DEPARTMENT OF EDUCATION (ED) (FORMERLY U.S. OFFICE OF EDUCATION). The federal agency authorized by federal statute to publish, through its secretary, a list of nationally recognized accrediting agencies and associations that are reliable authorities on educational quality.

VALIDITY. The extent to which an instrument or tool measures or performs in the manner in which it was intended. Validity is usually expressed as a numerical coefficient. *Also see* Reliability.

REFERENCES

1. American Association for Respiratory Therapy: Respiratory Therapy Uniform Manpower Survey. Dallas, American Association for Respiratory Therapy, 1977
2. American Association for Respiratory Therapy/Health Resources Administration: Delineation of Roles and Functions of the Entry-Level Generalist Respiratory Therapy Practitioner (Subproject I, HRA #231-75-0213, Final Report). Dallas, American Association for Respiratory Therapy, 1978
3. American Association for Respiratory Therapy, Ad Hoc Committee on Licensure Planning: Guidelines for writing a licensure bill for the practice of respiratory therapy. AARTimes 4(12):36, 1980
4. Barach AL et al: Minimum standards for inhalation therapy. JAMA 144:25, 1950
5. Barnes T: Baccalaureate programs in respiratory therapy: Introduction. An argument for the future of baccalaureate programs. AARTimes 4(5):17, 1980
6. Chuntz H: Proceed: A year's experience reported. Respir Care 21(10):960, 1976
7. Cochran LH et al: Advisory Committees in Action. Boston, Allyn and Bacon, 1980
8. Committee on Allied Health Education and Accreditation: Allied Health Education Directory, 11th ed. Chicago, American Medical Association, 1983
9. Credentialing Health Manpower. Washington, Department of Health, Education and Welfare, publication #(05) 77-55057, 1977
10. Cross KP et al: Planning Non-traditional Programs. San Francisco, Jossey–Bass, 1974
11. DeLapp GT: The systems approach for administration of respiratory therapy education programs. Respir Care 24 (6):514, 1979
12. Department of Allied Health Education, School of Allied Health Science, University of Texas Health Science Center: Curriculum Guide for Respiratory Therapy Education (HRS # 232-79-0098). Dallas, University of Texas Health Science Center, 1981
13. Eyler PB: NBRT's first twenty years. NBRT Newsletter 6(11):1, 1980
14. Ford CW et al (eds): Teaching in the Health Professions. St Louis, CV Mosby, 1976
15. Halonen RJ et al: Measuring the cost of clinical education in departments utilizing allied health professional. J Allied Health 5(4):5, 1976
16. Joint Review Committee for Respiratory Therapy Education: Description of Current Standards for Selected Essentials of the Accredited Educational Program for the Respiratory Therapist and Respiratory Therapy Technician. Dallas, Joint Review Committee for Respiratory Therapy Education, 1980
17. Krathwohl DR: The psychological bases for integration. In Henry NB (ed): The Integration of Educational Experiences—Fifty-Seventh Yearbook of the National Society for the Study of Education, part 3. Chicago, University of Chicago Press, 1958
18. Mishoe SC: Current and future credentialing in respiratory therapy. Respir Care 25(3):345, 1980
19. Moore ML et al: Form and Function of Written Agreements in the Clinical Education of Health Professions. Thorofare, NJ, CB Slack, 1972
20. Morgan MK et al: Evaluating Clinical Competence in the Health Professions. St Louis, CV Mosby, 1978
21. NBRT Ad Hoc Committee for the Study of Entry Level Examinations: The entry level examination proposal. NBRT Newsletter (Suppl)5(6):3, 1979
22. Nettles S: A National Study of the Practice of the Entry Level Respiratory Therapy Practitioner. Princeton, Educational Testing Service, 1981
23. Pace CR: Educational objectives. In Henry NB (ed): The Integration of Educational Experiences—Fifty-Seventh Yearbook of the National Society for the Study of Education, part 3. Chicago, University of Chicago Press, 1958
24. Porter RE, Kincaid CB: Financial aspects of clinical education to facilities. Phys Ther 57(8):16, 1977
25. Rau JL: Computer-assisted instruction: A solid-state Socrates. Respir Care 22(6):581, 1977

26. Report on Licensure and Related Health Personnel Credentialing. Washington Department of Health, Education and Welfare, publication #(HSM) 72-11, 1971
27. Scanlan CL: Integrating didactic and clinical education—high patient contact. In Ford CW (ed): Clinical Education for the Allied Health Professions. St Louis, CV Mosby, 1978
28. Scanlan CL: Professional accountability and competency assurance. Respir Care 24(1):12, 1979
29. Scanlan CL: Encouraging professionals to continue their education. In Darkenwald GG, Larson GA (eds): Reaching the Hard to Reach Adult (New Direction for Continuing Education Series, No. 8). San Francisco, Jossey–Bass, 1980
30. Scanlan CL, Clark DW: A respiratory therapy learning laboratory. Respir Care 19(5):347, 1974
31. Segall AJ, Vanderschmidt H, Burglass R et al: Systematic Course Design for the Health Fields. New York, John Wiley & Sons, 1975
32. Shapiro BA: Traditions and possibilities of licensure in respiratory therapy. Respir Care 25(3):345, 1980
33. Standards of Effective Administration of Inhalation Therapy. New York Academy of Sciences, 1950
34. State Licensure of Inhalation Therapy Practice. Position Paper of the ARIT Board of Directors, 13, Nov 1970. Respir Care 10:249, 1971
35. Tyler RW: Basic Principles of Curriculum and Instruction. Chicago, University of Chicago Press, 1950

3

Ethical Considerations and Interpersonal Relationships in Respiratory Care

Thomas J. DeKornfeld

Ethics may be defined as a branch of philosophy that deals with the fundamental values in life, both in the abstract and in the way in which these values affect, or should affect, human behavior in the concrete. Good and bad, right and wrong are the central concepts of the ethicist, and through the ages ethicists have struggled to define and to apply these concepts. Every society, from the most primitive to the most sophisticated, every religion, from the most austere to the most permissive, and indeed every learned profession has evolved some set of rules, some moral precepts, or some "ethical" standards to regulate individual and interpersonal behavior.

Medical ethics has only recently come to be viewed as a subset of general ethics that governs the nontechnical interphase between the health professional and the patient both individually and as a society. The ethics literature of the 19th and early 20th centuries accepted that physicians were governed only by a "professional ethic" that allowed them to do what others, following ordinary ethics, could not.

The revelations of the Nuremberg trials, the exponential growth of scientific knowledge, and the increasingly sophisticated technical and pharmacologic armamentarium led to the realization that general ethical principles had to apply to all, regardless of profession. This realization has been followed by an outpouring of literature that is both confused and confusing. It seeks to be objective and yet fails in this effort. Facts are treated as assumptions and assumptions as fact. Ethical concepts and legal concepts are commonly confounded, and patient management problems are often treated naively and with an obvious lack of familiarity with bedside problems. A few writers have tried to find workable solutions to very difficult personal and societal problems, but there has been little agreement among them, and the thoughtful reader is left with the uneasy feeling that perhaps no answer can satisfactorily resolve these awesome problems of life and death, truth and falsehood, right and wrong.

An exhaustive examination of the ethical and interpersonal issues in health care delivery and in respiratory care is not possible here. Instead, I shall give a brief overview of the major trends in contemporary ethics, indicating those areas in health care where ethical issues have become highly significant. Further, I shall discuss some specific ethical problems in the interpersonal and interprofessional relationships of the health care team. Finally, I shall present a series of specific, concrete, clinical situations in which decision-making ceases to be purely scientific and where nonscientific, ethical, and behavioral considerations must enter.

MAJOR TRENDS IN ETHICAL THOUGHT

The history of Western ethical thought starts in the 4th century B.C. in Greece with the efforts of Socrates, Plato, and Aristotle. Their attempts to distinguish right from wrong objectively and to find a rational explanation for human motivations and human behavior have influenced ethical thought to this day.

Roman Catholicism held almost universal sway during the first 16 centuries of the Christian era and impressed its own ethical views on Europe. The Church equated right and wrong, good or bad with whatever was pleasing or displeasing to a remote Deity and recorded in writings directly or indirectly attributed to Him. Catholic philosophers from Ambrose to Aquinas tried to harmonize natural law with divine will and put a rational base under the "Golden Rule." Interestingly, Catholic ethicists and philosophers have been pre-eminent in contemporary medical ethics with the same respect for logic and reason that characterized the great early thinkers of the Church.

The questioning spirit of the 18th century crystalized the two major directions of modern ethical thought, which had been present in a more diffuse fashion in the writing of Pagan and Christian ethicists. These two major strands of ethical thought may be termed utilitarianism and formalism or deontologism.

Utilitarianism, most clearly defined in the writings of Jeremy Bentham[2] and John Stuart Mill,[19] holds that an act is good if its results are good and bad if its results are bad. Thus an act in itself neutral or even harmful to an individual is good if its long-term results benefit a larger group or humanity itself. Even though it carries overtones of the allegedly Jesuitical "the end justifies the means," a modified utilitarianism is one of the basic principles of medical ethics.

Formalism or deontologism largely disregards the result of an act and looks at the act itself as being either good or bad. According to formalistic thinking, wrongful acts, such as telling lies, are never permissible even though the results may be most beneficial. The foremost proponent of this ethical theory was the German philosopher Immanuel Kant.[17]

Three contemporary ethical theories of the West will be discussed very briefly since they deal primarily with general social issues and have less relevance to specific health care problems than do the classical ethical theories.

John Rawls[21] in 1971 proposed the concept of "justice as fairness" by which totally objective observers are obliged to resolve all moral issues on behalf of the least advantaged in society, provided that this solution does not conflict with each person's equal right to liberty. Roderick Firth[24] in 1970 presented the concept of the "ideal observer." This mythical person, endowed with almost divine attributes, will make the "right" decision almost as a matter of course. William Frankena[11] in 1973 established the theory of "obligation." According to this theory, we have the obligation to do good, to prevent harm, to remove evil, and to refrain from doing either harm or evil. Frankena contends that if his principles are applied properly, both individual and public conflicts can be resolved satisfactorily.

Vigorous and protracted debates over the relative merits of these ethical theories have little practical effect on the real issues confronting the health care provider at the bedside. Obviously, neither Bentham nor Kant, nor even Aristotle or Aquinas, have provided complete and generally applicable answers for us, and the so-called ethical issues in daily health care practice must be approached on a largely individual basis. Some decisions have a utilitarian justification, others are decided on a deontologic basis, and others use neither, or perhaps a combination of the two.

In numerous situations adherence to theoretical concepts of ethics will lead to legal entanglements and to awkward interpersonal confrontations. It is, I believe, one of the major emotional problems in modern health care delivery that so many of the situations we encounter in our daily activities do not lend themselves to simple theoretical solutions. No rule can be applied universally, and the more closely a health professional attempts to be strictly "ethical" according to one of the major ethical philosophies, the more likely he will wind up in a morass of dilemmas. In fact, most of the so-called ethical issues in health care delivery can be resolved by remembering some basic principles and applying them with suitable modifications to the specific issue or to the individual situation. The ancient precept "primum non nocere" (first of all do no harm), expanded by the Golden Rule, "do unto others . . .," will resolve most problems.

It may be appropriate at this point to quote two brief passages from the oldest of all medical ethics texts, the "Hippocratic Oath."

> In purity and holiness I will guard my life and act.
>
> If I fulfill this oath and do not violate it, may it be granted to me to enjoy life and art, being honored with fame among all men for all times to come; if I transgress it and swear falsely, may the opposite of all this be my lot.

One other point fundamental to all interpersonal relationships must be emphasized: Good manners, courtesy, and respect for others' feelings and rights are the keystones that keep the edifice of society from collapsing.

ETHICAL DYNAMICS OF INTERPROFESSIONAL RELATIONSHIPS—THE TEAM CONCEPT

Traditional interprofessional relationships in health care delivery were predicated on a rigid caste system, with the physician on top followed, in descending order, by nurses, technologists, aides, and orderlies. A parallel structure existed in the administrative ranks, where the administrator was on top and the unskilled or semiskilled workers in the bowels of the hospital were on the bottom. Similar stratification was present in the various services, and each service or department had a rigid hierarchy determined on the basis of rank, although occasionally skewed to some extent by seniority.

These relationships were paternalistic and authoritarian. Personal relationships were held to a minimum and were actively discouraged, except among persons on the same level in the professional, administrative, or corporate structure.

This system clearly was not designed for personal contentment, and it is a tribute to human resilience that it was not only quite efficient, but also that its different components functioned competently and appeared reasonably satisfied with their role. In these relationships there was little reciprocal respect; what held the system together was discipline and an unquestioning acceptance of traditional authority.

During the past 20 years the emotional and behavioral relationships have undergone a gradual but accelerating change. Many factors have contributed to this change, including a decline in the perceived stature of the medical profession, a dramatic improvement in the educational sophistication of the nonphysician health care providers, and a realization that nonphysicians could make major contributions to the health care system; an increasing awareness of the importance of the nonscientific aspects of patient care; a sharp improvement in the ego assessment of the nursing and technical professions; and an almost universal democratization of society as a whole. One significant result of these different movements has been the slow evolution of the team concept in health care delivery.

The fundamental tenet underlying the team concept is that its members have specific contributions to make that are of comparable value and that all must function harmoniously for the end result to be optimal. There has been a definite blurring of lines of responsibility. A number of functions traditionally considered nursing functions have been assumed by technical specialists, and there has even been some exchange among the technical specialist groups.

Not all these transitions were smooth, and some conservative health professionals viewed all invasions of sacred turfs with profound misgivings, and predicted the most dire results.

Of course, these prophets of doom were wrong, and, even though not all changes proved to be totally satisfactory, the end result has been an improved personal fulfillment of the health care providers and an improved quality of health care. Changes are far from complete, however, and the next decade will bring further modifications in the system and in the relationship among the components of the system.

A brief inspection of the system as it exists at present reveals that, indeed, the tightly structured caste system in health care delivery has largely disappeared; each group within the system has now assumed a quasicollegial relationship vis-a-vis the other groups. These changes have also had a profound effect on the emotional relationships within and between the health professions. The caste system required a great deal of respect from the lower orders in return for authoritarian paternalism, quite similar to the structure of the Victorian family. There the father (physician) made all decisions and bestowed praise or punishment as he saw fit. The mother (nurse) backed the father's authority and contributed a certain humanizing influence. The children (technologists, aides, orderlies) were to be seen but not heard. They were to "behave" at all times, "do as they were told," and be grateful for every small kindness shown to them by the Jovian parent.

This type of organizational structure pervaded society at many levels. The family was the model, but industry, agriculture, government, and, indeed, society as a whole functioned largely along similar lines.

Changes came slowly but inexorably. Industrial relationships were the first to change under the leadership of the great founders of the labor movements. Two world wars made their contribution, and since about 1950 there has been an accelerating trend toward the "democratization" of all forms of social organizations from the family to the armed forces. Health care could not remain immune, and the changes described above finally reached this almost unique survivor of the paternalistic, quasifeudal model of interpersonal relationships. In line with other democratizing trends, there appeared in the health care system a lowering of the position of the "upper classes" and a raising of the "lower orders." The physician ceased to be the unquestioned "ruler of all he surveyed." His word was no longer law, except in a very limited area, and his instructions, although still formally labeled "orders," have been made both legally and ethically subject to questioning by those members of the health care team charged with executing those "orders."

These changes, spurred by both external and internal forces, have led to the gradual evolution of the health care team. The concept is certainly not new. Small teams have functioned in some areas for many years. Psychiatric hospitals have led in this area, and even 30 years ago teams of physicians, nurses, social workers, occupational therapists, and, rarely, some non healthprofessionals met to plan the management of individual patients. Similar teams became active in the mangement of emergency situations, cardiopulmonary resuscitation, and in the care of critically ill patients. These teams were still under the nominal leadership of the physician, although individual team members were frequently placed into decision-making roles depending on the requirements of specific problems.

Unfortunately the team concept, while receiving much verbal support, failed to achieve general acceptance for two major reasons: First was the already mentioned turf protection and the unwillingness of most people to recognize their own limitations or the abilities of others. The second, and perhaps equally important cause for the failure of the team concept must be attributed to our educational institutions. For a group to function well as a team, the individual members must have a thorough understanding of each other's roles, duties, and abilities. This is impossible unless the team members receive much of their training jointly and are exposed to both basic educational experiences and clinical learning situations as a group. To date, attempts to provide such joint learning opportunities and experiences have been few and largely unsuccessful. Even though some attempts to cluster medical students and nursing students in joint learning experiences have shown considerable promise, few, if any, of these endeavors have survived for economic, administrative, or emotional reasons.

Even continuing educational activities when planned for multidisciplinary audiences have proved to be failures. Planning sessions have been characterized by polarization between the health provider groups, primarily based on educational background. Baccalaureate-trained health care providers have been reluctant to share educational experiences with associate-level trainees, and even groups holding the same type of degree have been reluctant to join in planning and presenting courses. The reason for this was unclear for some time, but ultimately has been revealed to be jealousy, snobbery, and general "meow."

It seems unlikely that these emotional barriers can be eliminated administratively, and I believe that no substantial, rational advance in education or formal team development will take place until there is a strong societal mandate enforced by economic sanctions for failure to comply. This is likely to take years. What posture, then, should the individual health care provider assume now vis-a-vis colleagues in the other health professions? More precisely, what should the attitude of the respiratory therapists be in their relationship to physicians, nurses, physical therapists, and others who may have direct input into the management of patients served by respiratory therapy?

Foremost, the roles that each plays in the care of the patient must be understood. This knowledge must be both theoretical and practical. The respiratory therapist who aims to be more than a mechanic must have a good working knowledge of the medical problems of pulmonary patients and must have a thorough understanding of the diagnostic and therapeutic considerations that the physician brings to bear on the problem. The respiratory therapist must understand the contribution nurses have to make both in the narrow sense, as providers of bedside care, and in the broader sense, as consumer educators and coordinators of the health care team. The same principles apply to working with physical therapists, occupational therapists, and others.

The keys to this complex relationship are respect, good manners and equanimity, humor, humility, and, most important, a singleminded, inflexible devotion to the well-being of the patient.

These goals and behavior patterns are not easily accomplished. Human frailties and deep-seated personal and professional prejudices will remain recurring stumbling blocks in achieving this ideal. Nevertheless, both as human beings and as dedicated health professionals, we must heed the simplest and yet most difficult command: "Do unto others . . . ." and to follow the poets' plea to "make a stepping stone of every stumbling block."

MAJOR CONTEMPORARY PROBLEMS IN HEALTH ETHICS

In this section, I shall present what I perceive to be the major ethical issues that confront the health professional in the United States in the 1980s. My personal judgments will become manifest but should be viewed with the same skepticism with which all recommendations in ethical dilemmas must be approached. The readers are free to select their own solutions to these dilemmas, based, hopefully, on careful thought and common sense.

Most of the ethical issues to be discussed have been the subject of extensive litigation. It would be both unwise and dangerous for the health care provider to ignore legal precedents, even though we are dealing with areas of personal conscience or religious beliefs. This does not mean that legislatures or courts incorporate all the wisdom necessary to navigate these dark waters, but once a legislature or a court has spoken we must adhere to their rulings or be willing to take the consequences of civil disobedience or contempt of court.

PROBLEMS OF LIFE AND DEATH

Subsumed under the somewhat pretentious title of "problems of life and death" are such ethical problems as abortion, the management of the defective newborn, the problems of death and dying, and the problem of euthanasia.

Few, if any, of the ethical issues are as replete with emotional content, personal and religious prejudices, and attempts to resolve the insoluble as the issue of abortion. Recent Supreme court decisions (Roe v. Wade[23] and Doe v. Bolton[9]) have settled some of the legal aspects of the dispute without having resolved any of the ethical or moral issues involved.

The two sides of the argument can be stated briefly. The extreme antiabortionists believe that human life begins at the moment of conception, that is, at the time the fertile human ovum is entered by viable human sperm and the chromosomal pattern characteristic of human cells is established. It necessarily ensues then that interference with this "human" with intent to destroy must be considered murder and is thus forbidden by divine and human law. The only exception most of the proponents of this view are willing to allow falls under the heading of self-defense; the fetus may be "destroyed" if its continued existence seriously jeopardizes the mother's survival. Tubal pregnancy or removal of the cancerous pregnant uterus would be examples of such exceptions. Conservative antiabortionists may still consider this "homicide" but are willing to concede that it is "justifiable homicide," or that it is but a "side-effect" of a primarily ethical "life-saving" action. This latter idea is known as the "Doctrine of Double Effect."

At the other end of the spectrum, the most liberal proabortionists claim that the fetus *in utero* is not a person but an integral part of the mother's body, and as such the mother has the right to dispose of it until the moment of delivery. The arguments raised by this group include both ethical and legal ones and include references to the constitution and to the moral right of a person to the pursuit of happiness and to complete control over her own body.

Both of these extremes are difficult to defend rationally; indeed, such extreme views are held by only a relative minority of the opposing groups. The somewhat more enlightened antiabortionists concede that the mother's survival is not the only justification for abortion, but that pregnancy ensuing from forcible rape or incest may also be terminated. A further concession, although usually the last one made by the most liberal of the anti-abortionists, is the recognition that medically proven serious physical or emotional disturbances occasioned by pregnancy may, under certain circumstances, be acceptable as a reason for terminating the pregnancy.

Proabortionists commonly base their views on the principle that there is a point in the intrauterine development of the fetus when it changes from a "nonperson" to a "person," and thus may be aborted before this point at the mother's discretion. Abortion after this critical turning point must be governed by compelling medical reasons only. Cultural, historic, and even scientific arguments are marshalled to determine when this change takes place and when a crude assembly of cells suddenly becomes a human being entitled to all the rights and protections that society has traditionally granted to human beings. The early Catholic church, curiously, taught that "animation" or "ensoulment"—that is, the acquiring of "human" attributes—occurred 40 days after conception for males and 80 days after conception for females. English criminal law, until 1967, used a recognizable intrauterine movement, the so-called quickening, as evidence of "animation" that transformed the fetus to a "person." Other groups have emphasized "viability"—that is, the ability to survive outside the uterus—as the distinction between humanity and nonhumanity.

All of these distinctions are arbitrary. The time of "viability" changes dramatically with changes in life-support technology and with the availability of competent neonatal care facilities and personnel. Arguments have been proposed for and against all of the above "viabilist" positions, but, thus, far, I believe that none of these arguments have been entirely convincing.

Societal arguments on abortion are even more difficult to defend. Some opponents of abortion argue that once this type of "murder" is sanctioned, we are all embarked on a "slippery slope" that leads inevitably to a total disintegration of social mores and to a chaos of unimaginable brutality. Some proponents of abortion cite overpopulation, the mental health of the unhappy mother and the unwanted child, and numerous other irrelevant considerations in their attempts to justify abortions entirely at the discretion of the mother and her attending physician.

Although I have definite views on the matter, I am willing to accept the Supreme Court's decision in *Roe*, according to which first trimester abortions are at the discretion of the mother and her physician, whereas second trimester or later abortions are subject to regulation by state legislatures. Readers wishing to investigate this matter further are referred to the bibliography.

Respiratory therapy personnel have little, if any, role in decisions on abortion other than in reference to their own personal and family life. In the next ethical dilemma, the problem of the severely handicapped neonate, they do become involved professionally.

Despite the availability of intrauterine diagnostic techniques and legally available abortion services, many infants are born with severe congenital deformities that would prove fatal unless corrected surgically or that would make impossible a decent quality of life with or without therapy. The second group presents a relatively minor ethical problem. Any newborn, regardless of how grotesque or how severely damaged, who would survive with standard care cannot be willfully and intentionally put to death without incurring the appropriate prosecution for willful homicide. The problem becomes much more complex when sophisticated life-support machinery is required to maintain this infant alive or if surgical intervention becomes necessary to prevent the infant's inevitable death.

As with most ethical problems, this one cannot be discussed intelligently without a reasonable understanding of the legal issues involved. Two fairly recent cases illustrate this problem. In the "Johns Hopkins case,"[12] which was not submitted to a court for decision, an infant was born with intestinal atresia and with what appeared to be severe mongolism (Down's syndrome). The intestinal atresia was surgically correctible, and it was likely, with modern medicine, that this mentally deficient infant could be physically rehabilitated. The parents, after much discussion and agonizing, refused permission to operate, and the infant was allowed to die of starvation in about 2 weeks. During this time it was given minimal supportive care and was the center of considerable emotional turmoil among the nurses and other health professionals who were forced to stand by and watch it die. Much has been written about this case by writers representing a wide spectrum of philosophical and political orientations. Surprisingly, the condemnation of the parents and the Hopkins' physicians was practically unanimous.

The second case did involve a court decision in Maine[14] concerning a neonate who suffered from many grossly deforming congenital defects and who also had a tracheoesophageal fistula (TEF). This was the most immediately life-threatening deformity, although other defects were such that it was impossible to suppose a satisfying quality of life for the infant. The parents refused to consent to the TEF repair. The physicians at the Maine Medical Center petitioned the court to assume guardianship over the child and to authorize the surgery. The court ruled that surgery should be performed because ". . . the most basic right enjoyed by every human being is the right to life itself." The court also found that this right started with the moment of birth. Pursuant to this decision, the operation was performed.

Such decisions surrounding the crib or incubator on whether to save a profoundly damaged "life" or whether to let it die are among the most difficult ethical and moral issues. There are no clear guidelines at present, and responsible thinkers have doubted whether such guidelines are possible. The argument again ranges from the doctrinaire "we always must do everything to maintain life" to the nihilistic "we must save only those who are likely to be fulfilled and fulfilling human beings."

I believe that there is a minimal quality of life below which existence is, at best, humanoid. No newborn should be willfully and arbitrarily sentenced to live its life in pain, misery, and discomfort while placing an enormous emotional and economic burden on its family and on society as a whole. The parents have the right both legally and ethically to refuse extraordinary means to salvage what in their opinion would be an unacceptable quality of life. The obvious and, unfortunately, unanswerable question is that of the level below which the quality of life is not acceptable. There is no generalization that can be universally applied to this situation; this is the most excruciating dilemma with which parents can be confronted. All thinking and feeling parents must resolve this question for themselves and would be well advised to seek assistance in this decision from physicians involved in the care of the infant and from whoever is serving as a spiritual advisor to the family. If a conflict arises between the family and the physicians, the only resource is to refer the matter to a court. It seems likely that courts, just as in the Maine case cited above, will assume guardianship of the infant and will instruct the physicians to proceed with whatever is necessary to keep the infant alive.

This judicial action may have the virtue of appearing dispassionate, but it tends to disregard the burden it may place on the family or on society for many years to come. Seemingly, there should be a minimum standard below which no extraordinary means of support should be used. At the least the newborn must show some evidence that it is likely to have the cardinal human characteristics of cognition and emotion. Without these, whatever the newborn is, it is not a human being, and neither law nor morality would be served by maintaining it in a vegetative state.

A similar and yet distinct ethical and legal problem arises at the opposite end of human existence. The normal process of aging inevitably leads to physical, mental, and emotional deterioration, which is usually gradual but may, on occasion, be sudden and dramatic. When it occurs, its manifestations may be primarily physical, as in many terminal illnesses, or mental, as when brain damage occurs because of trauma, hypoxia, or various external or internal causes such as senility and chronic brain syndrome.

The problem is similar to that of the severely damaged newborn, but there are some significant differences. These differences flow from the fact that adults may be in a position to make decisions for themselves or may have left instructions about their desires for a certain course of action to be taken should such a catastrophe occur. Further, there are significant economic and emotional differences between letting a baby die or letting an old person die. Babies rarely have substantial estates; inheritance is rarely a consideration. Babies, at least ideally, have the possibility of a long and happy life before them. Old people can look forward only to death as a relief from the burden of life. Let us examine some of these differences.

In the conscious adult the situation is simple. Under constitutional guarantees a person has the unquestioned right to determine whether diagnostic and therapeutic manipulation shall be performed, and every adult has the right to refuse health care even though such refusal will inevitably lead to death. Both court decisions and the overwhelming weight of ethical writing clearly distinguishes between such a refusal to be treated for a terminal illness and suicide. Catholic theologians have taught and are teaching that while suicide is a deadly sin, refusal to engage in any extraordinary activity to prevent death cannot be considered suicide, and thus is not banned by the Church. The emphasis is on the word "extraordinary." Theologians and ethicists generally contend, although for different reasons, that the person has a duty to maintain the body in good health and to do everything reasonable and proper to avoid illness or to regain health. Where "reasonable and proper" ends and "extraordinary" begins has never been accurately defined, is subject to individual interpretation, and is likely to change with the development of new technology.

Fifty years ago the use of a respirator would have been most extraordinary; 25 years ago coronary bypass surgery was extraordinary; 10 years ago the balloon pump was extraordinary, as was the Swan–Ganz catheter. Obviously every patient must decide what is "extraordinary" for himself. Legally each has very great freedom to do so; ethically the constraints are only moderately more restrictive. From a practical point, however, an intelligent choice may be difficult. Owing to the increasingly complex instrumentation, to the very real potential for complications, and to the unfortunate fact that "extraordinary" means are usually offered only to critically ill patients, the burden of choice is a very heavy one.

Freedom of choice, however, is not absolute. The state has the right, through legislation and judicial decisions, to set some limits to constitutional guarantees. Just as it was held that yelling "fire" in a crowded theater could not be excused under the guarantee of "free speech," the state also has the right to quarantine and to treat patients with infectious diseases, to insist on the immunization of school children, to demand premarital blood tests, and to allow other "invasions of privacy" if these steps are in the evident interest of society as a whole.

If the adult patient is unconscious or otherwise incompetent to make a decision, the situation becomes more complicated, particularly if there are no real indications as to the wishes of the person involved.

Some states have enacted (or are now considering) "right to die" legislation.[28] According to these statutes a person of sound mind may formally request that no extraordinary means be used to prolong life should that person be unable to make the decision. In a proposed Michigan statute, part of this "living will" is the appointment of a relative or other person with the power of attorney to make this decision for the testator. The conditions under which this will is to go into effect and the circumstances under which the designated person may assume the decision-making power may be carefully specified. If this legislative proposal is enacted, it may be possible for the designated executor of the "living will" to make decisions for the incompetent (comatose) person. These decisions will be just as binding as if the patient had made them in the full power of consciousness. The Concern for Dying Council in New York has proposed a model "Living Will" (Fig. 3-1).

I strongly favor such legislation and trust that it will mitigate, to some extent, the number of dreadful scenarios enacted in so many hospitals too frequently. To die with dignity is just as much an inalienable right as living in dignity. Yet thoughtful and kind physicians, other health practitioners, and family members regularly and commonly deny this right to their patients or relatives. These are deep, dark waters that must be investigated with the utmost care, since the choices range from euthanasia to the indefinite maintenance of the living dead.

To kill another human being willfully is homicide. Euthanasia or "mercy killing" is homicide even though performed with the purest and most humane motives. Whether there are circumstances in which an outright positive act designed solely to produce death may ever be justified is difficult to answer.

The proponents of euthanasia feel strongly that the answer to this question is yes! There are situations, they believe, in which a conscious adult may reasonably request to be "put to sleep" or even where parents are entitled to make this decision for a badly damaged infant.

The opponents of euthanasia claim that the answer is a categorical and unalterable no! Opponents admit that some people may be better off dead and that an unqualified denial of euthanasia condemns some patients or infants to a degrading, quasihuman, or subhuman existence for an indefinite period. The arguments against euthanasia usually fall into one of two broad categories. It is claimed that both divine and human law demand that life not be taken except in war, in self-defense, or (perhaps) as the punishment for certain heinous crimes. It is also claimed by those who do not necessarily insist on the total sanctity of life that permitting euthanasia is wrong primarily because it is the thin edge of the wedge that leads inevitably to the elimination of increasing numbers and groups of undesirables. Ultimately it may even lead to political or racial mass murder. This group inevitably uses the events in Nazi Germany as an example and suggests that if euthanasia had not earlier been permitted for defective newborns, the horrors of the concentration camps might not have ensued.

I find it very difficult to accept such reasoning. Those who truly believe in the divine mandate, "Thou shalt not kill" should oppose killing absolutely in every form, including self-defense, judicial execution, and war. Once one is willing to accept one form of homicide, it appears illogical to deny categorically the potential appropriateness of another form of equally justifiable homicide. The second argument about the thin edge is even more more specious. Making the leap from carefully circumscribed voluntary euthanasia to political genocide is an absurd *non sequitur*. Mass murder has happened repeatedly in recorded history: in Nazi Germany, in Communist Russia, and, more recently, in at least one Southeast Asian country. It may happen again, but its recurrence is totally unrelated to the presence of legalized euthanasia.

Whatever the arguments may be, it is quite evident that American society is not prepared to accept euthanasia as an option. Let us therefore examine the next level of activity designed for the terminally ill and for those who are suffering gravely and irreversibly. Is there anything short of active euthanasia that is acceptable legally and ethically, that will benefit hopeless sufferers, and that has the support of the health care community?

Several suggestions have been made. Most common are those related to "making the patient comfortable" and to "not doing anything" that may pro-

To My Family, My Physician, My Lawyer and All Others Whom It May Concern

Death is as much a reality as birth, growth, maturity and old age—it is the one certainty of life. If the time comes when I can no longer take part in decisions for my own future, let this statement stand as an expression of my wishes and directions, while I am still of sound mind.

If at such a time the situation should arise in which there is no reasonable expectation of my recovery from extreme physical or mental disability, I direct that I be allowed to die and not be kept alive by medications, artificial means or "heroic measures". I do, however, ask that medication be mercifully administered to me to alleviate suffering even though this may shorten my remaining life.

This statement is made after careful consideration and is in accordance with my strong convictions and beliefs. I want the wishes and directions here expressed carried out to the extent permitted by law. Insofar as they are not legally enforceable, I hope that those to whom this Will is addressed will regard themselves as morally bound by these provisions.

Signed______________________________

Date ______________________________

Witness______________________________

Witness______________________________

Copies of this request have been given to ______________________________

____

____

____

Fig. 3-1. A living will. (Reprinted, with permission, from Concern for Dying, 250 West 57th Street, New York, NY 10019.)

long the patient's life. In the first category are such things as the very liberal use of narcotics. Morphine and the other narcotic analgesics are indicated in patients with pain. How much is given and how often is a medical decision. In a patient with severe pain, 15 mg of morphine would not be considered excessive. Given to elderly patients regularly, morphine is likely to keep the patient quite comfortable and, indeed, may ease and speed the transition from "this world to the next."

Is this euthanasia? Most ethicists will argue that it is not, whereas some maintain that in some respects it is just that. Most thoughtful health care providers will agree, however, that this method of managing the desperately, terminally, and painfully ill is not only ethically permissible but often mandated. Legally it is very unlikely to be questioned.

Withholding medication or other therapeutic modalities is a related but more difficult issue. Pneumonia was once referred to as "the old person's friend" because it was one of the most frequent and gentle causes of death in elderly patients in the preantibiotic era. The introduction of penicillin in the late 1940s and the tremendous proliferation of other antimicrobial agents in the past 30 years have made most pneumonias readily treatable. Now old patients who wish for death and who do get pneumonia can be "treated" and given weeks, months, or even years of existence that they do not really want. The question once again arises, "Is it permissible, ethically and legally, to withhold antibiotics from these patients, thus allowing them to die, without interfering artificially in a natural process"? I believe most physicians would treat these patients, since antibiotics have become a basic tool of the trade and can certainly not be considered extraordinary.

Taking this line of reasoning a step further, the question may arise whether major surgery—for example, a modified, radical mastectomy—should be performed on an 86-year-old senile patient confined in a nursing home. Valid consent cannot be obtained from the patient, and the family does not wish the procedure performed. May life-prolonging therapy be withheld from an incompetent patient? Fortunately in this situation there is case law to guide us. The Massachusetts Supreme Court has ruled in the case of *Belchertown State School v. Saikewicz*[26] that only a probate court could rule in such a situation (see Chap. 5).

The list of possible extensions of the interpretation of "extraordinary" could be enlarged indefinitely. One more example will serve. Let us assume that a 6-year-old child with Down's syndrome has acute appendicitis. The parents refuse consent for the operation. What should a responsible physician do? This child will almost certainly die unless operated on. Society will not lose by having one less mentally deficient person to support. The parents do have the right to refuse consent. There is considerable urgency since the mortality of appendectomy after rupture is significantly increased. Legally the physician is not compelled to operate in the absence of a valid consent.

In this situation, I believe the physician must apply to the appropriate court to remove the child from the custody of the parents and for permission to perform the appendectomy. Almost certainly the court will act quickly and the operation will be performed. The very real problem of then returning this child to parents who would have let it die must also be considered, and social workers or other appropriate agencies may have to get involved. As a last resort this child may have to be made a permanent ward of the court and either institutionalized or placed in a foster home. In a somewhat similar situation, a California court recently ruled differently and found that the parents had the right to withhold permission to perform a ventricular septal defect repair on an 11-year-old child with Down's syndrome. This ruling has been criticized very sharply even though the judgment was upheld by the California Supreme Court.[15]

A related issue concerns the problem of cardiopulmonary resuscitation. To resuscitate or not to resuscitate is a medical decision. Writing "no code" orders is legally permissible and ethically sound[14] and has been upheld by one of the most conservative jurisdictions.[13] Health care providers must remember that it is easier not to start resuscitation and not to connect a patient to a ventilator than to stop. Resuscitation should be started only if the victim can be reestablished as a functional human being, and should be discontinued when obvious evidence of significant central nervous system damage appears. It is very easy to be righteous in this area, but those of us who have resuscitated decerebrate patients and then were involved in their care are inclined to be pragmatic even to the point of therapeutic nihilism.

PROBLEMS OF BEHAVIOR MODIFICATION AND GENETIC ENGINEERING

Few areas of medical intervention are fraught with more promise and more potential danger than behavior control and its prospective application: genetic screening and genetic engineering. Behavior control is psychologic, pharmacologic, or surgical intervention to eliminate or reduce the likelihood of dangerous, inappropriate, or socially unacceptable activity on the part of emotionally disturbed patients.

Historically, such procedures, in their crudest form, were used as punishment. Castration for sex offenders, amputation of one or both hands for robbers, and whipping, chaining, near-drowning, or placement in snake pits for the violently insane were considered not only acceptable but desirable and salutary. In our allegedly more enlightened era, this form of behavior modification is no longer permissible and has been replaced by more sophisticated techniques, with emphasis on psychologic and pharmacologic manipulations.

Psychosurgery had its vogue some 25 years ago, and a number of psychotic patients had prefrontal lobotomy performed to make them more manageable and to enable them to be discharged from mental institutions. More recently psychosurgery has been advocated by Mark and his associates[18] in Boston and has been used in selected patients not amenable to any other form of therapy. The problem with even this more selective form of psychosurgery is the danger of significant personality change beyond the desired result, and the obvious difficulty of obtaining free and informed consent in this group of patients.

Currently this form of surgery is in abeyance, since the landmark case of *Kaimovitz v. Department of Mental Health*.[16] Kaimovitz, a Michigan Legal Services attorney, learned of a planned psychosurgical experiment on an 18-year-old psychopath committed to a Michigan Mental Institution. Both the patient and his parents had agreed to the procedure. After very careful consideration of all sides and listening to many hours of testimony, the court found that [1] patients involuntarily committed in state institutions are legally incapable of giving competent, voluntary, knowledgeable consent to experimental psychosurgery; [2] the first amendment freedoms of speech and expression presuppose a right to generate ideas that could be destroyed or impaired by psychosurgery, and [3] the constitutional right to privacy would be frustrated by an unwarranted medical intrusion into the brain. Although the Kaimovitz decision has binding power only in Michigan, the court's findings were worded broadly enough to halt similar intrusive brain surgery elsewhere in the United States.

There has been little fuss over psychotherapeutic or pharmacologic behavioral control. Admittedly these routes are less dramatic, are usually reversible, and are unlikely to cause much broader changes than those intended. There are few violent or potentially dangerous mental patients who are not subjected to some form of psychotherapy and to the administration of various psychoactive drugs during voluntary or involuntary commitments to a mental institution. Both psychotherapy and psychopharmacology are not without hazard, and their long range effectiveness has been greatly exaggerated, as evidenced by the frequent reports in the daily press relating the violent crimes committed by treated and released former mental patients. It is difficult to understand a system that protects the mentally ill but is unable to protect their innocent victims. Legalists and civil libertarians are rarely around when the victims of their protegees are brought to the emergency room raped, beaten, stabbed, shot, mutilated, or dead. Constitutional freedoms are important, and governmental or individual excesses must be controlled, but there must be a balance where individual rights and societal rights are placed into proper perspective.

This same balance should be achieved in genetic counseling and genetic engineering. It is well known that a considerable number of serious diseases are transmitted from parent to child: sickle cell anemia, hemophilia, thalassemia, Down's syndrome, Klinefelter's syndrome, cystic fibrosis, Morton's syndrome, retinoblastoma, some forms of muscular dystrophy, phenylketonuria, and others. These genetically linked illnesses present two major problem areas: the identification and counseling of the carriers; and the statutory enforcement of preventive sterilization, amniocentesis, and abortion.

Both areas are fraught with the greatest dangers to individual liberties, while at the same time the societal cost of total nonfeasance in this area is enormous. As usual, a compromise will have to be found. Few people will object to voluntary screening for the carrier state in adults who may be heterozygotes, and only those who object to all abortions will find fault with the decision to terminate a pregnancy when amniocentesis reveals a homozygote fetus. It is the duty of the family practitioner and the obstetrician to be fully aware of the family history of their patients and to counsel them on the principles of mendelian genetics and the statistical likelihood of affected offspring. The patients then can make a rational decision on marriage and procreation.

Those who advocate compulsory screening and forceful intervention—for example, the denial of a marriage license or mandatory abortion—are on extremely shaky ground. Their arguments are primarily economic, although disguised as a concern with human happiness and an endeavor to decrease human misery of both the parent and the child. The economic arguments are not convincing. The cost of maintaining badly damaged children is great, but it is extremely unlikely that the funds so spent would be available for more useful activities, and thus the argument that the damaged take away from others is, at best, specious. Mandatory mass screening may be constitutional but is very expensive and serves little, if any, useful purpose unless the condition it tries to identify is amenable to therapy. This is not the case in genetically linked congenital deformities. Here the only remedy, at the moment, is sterilization or abortion. Statutory enforcement of these "remedies" is unacceptable on both ethical and legal bases. The burden of proof for the desirability of such drastic invasion of privacy must lie with its advocates, and the proof must be compelling indeed before it can be even tentatively considered. I am not impressed with the "slippery slope" argument in general, but I do recognize that giving the state the authority to sterilize or abort against the wishes of the person involved and without the most careful safeguards may indeed set dangerous precedent.

Keeping the area of genetic counseling voluntary seems appropriate. Prospective brides and grooms should be concerned with the odds of having "normal" children and should take chances in this area only after careful and reasoned deliberation. Amniocentesis should be performed if there is a high index of probability for a genetically malformed fetus. Abortion should be discussed with the prospective parents and should be made available in a timely and medically proper fashion. Not to do so is to deprive the parents of their right to make decisions and may indeed leave them and the medical advisors open to the dangers of "wrongful life" litigation, such as the recent Curlander case in California.[7] In this case a child was born with Tay–Sachs disease even though a laboratory had claimed that the parents were not carriers of recessive Tay–Sachs genes. The court, after reviewing "wrongful life" cases in other jurisdictions, which generally did not recognize the child's right to litigate on its own behalf, has found that the child indeed has the right to sue for the negligence of others that led to its being born.

Lastly, a new area of controversy has emerged concerning the new methodologies of genetic engineering. It has become possible in recent years to make changes in the genetic patterns of certain bacteria and even certain higher-order animals that allow scientists to create hitherto unknown forms of life. A case in point is the so called "recombinant DNA" research project. New technology has made it possible to split the DNA helix carrying the genetic messages, splice in DNA fragments from other organisms, and reintroduce the "new" DNA into a host. In this way it may become possible to develop new strains of microorganisms that could, for example, make insulin, decrease the incidence of cancer, and make vast amounts of nutrient protein. It may, of course, be possible to create a Frankenstein's monster and let loose on an unsuspecting world new life forms of unimaginable tenacity and ferocity.

For this reason, thoughtful scientists and philosophers have argued vigorously against pursuing studies in this field. The arguments have been both objective and emotional. It was believed that the possible dangers of this work were so great and so unpredictable that they outweighed the possible benefits. Others argued that there were areas of possible knowledge that were best left unknown. Yet others condemned any research in this area as being contrary to the desires of the Creator.[25]

None of these arguments appears to be convincing. The benefits of creating new life forms may be substantial, and may indeed herald a new and better life for mankind. The dangers may be real but can be minimized and should not be allowed to influence the new technologies. The theological arguments are unanswerable and need no answer. If the Creator does not wish mankind to work in this area, it is safe to assume that the Creator will make his will known in no uncertain terms.

PROBLEMS OF ALLOCATION OF SCARCE HEALTH RESOURCES—TRIAGE

Two issues must be discussed. The first one deals with national or societal allocations and the second with individual allocations.

It is a generally accepted principle that all residents of the United States are entitled to health care, and it is an unfortunate, but inevitable, corollary of this principle that not all citizens can be furnished optimal health care at all times. There are manifold reasons for both the principle and the corollary. In its simplest terms, it has become a political necessity, and indeed an electioneering slogan, that all health care is a right and that every man, woman, and child is "entitled" to health care. Whether it is considered a constitutional guarantee or whether simply something on which all decent people agree is immaterial.

The fact remains that for the past half century, at least, there has been an increasing tendency to provide optimal health care to all who need it at all times and in all geographic locations.

Desires once again outran performance, and in fact there were major discrepancies both in the availability and in the quality of health care. These differences were geographic and economic. Rural areas and inner cities were underserved, as were the poor, regardless of geographic distribution. All efforts to the contrary, both the quantity and quality of health care services were superior in medium-sized towns, in the more affluent suburbs, and in those areas where health care delivery was associated with academic health centers. Even in this wealthiest of all countries, it has been impossible to assure optimal health care to all. There are insufficient facilities, insufficient personnel at all levels, and insufficient money to provide everything to everybody.

The most often cited reasons for this set of circumstances include the tightly organized, profit-oriented health professionals, governmental priorities that rank health below defense, and the general tendency of a society that would like to get something for nothing but which is not willing to make major sacrifices or efforts to obtain it. If we define optimal health care as providing to every person the benefit of the most advanced scientific and technological facilities, combined with the services of the most highly trained and highly skilled health professionals, it must be obvious to all that this simply cannot be done. It is not the improper priorities, or the greed of the health professional, or even the societal sloth that is to blame. It is simply that no society, no country, no population can afford to provide these things to everybody at all times.

A reasonable alternative appears to be to provide at least minimal acceptable health services to all people at all times and to work, slowly, gradually, but deliberately toward raising these minimal standards. It appears that these minimal standards have been largely achieved. Few areas of the country are deprived of some form of health service, and even the residents of the most deprived slums have access to the facilities of city hospitals. In fact, the urban poor are more fortunate in this respect than are the agricultural proletariat, which in some areas of the country have probably the least available and lowest quality health care facilities and health care providers. This has been well demonstrated by several studies, including the California State Health Plan 1980–1985.[5]

The solutions to this problem are almost entirely economic, and only to a limited extent personal and professional. Governmental priorities must be adjusted so that not only a larger share of the budget is devoted to health but that within the health budget a larger share is devoted to health care delivery where it is most urgently needed. The full weight of the federal and state governments must be applied on this issue, and a network of nurse practitioners and physicians' assistants must be established to provide entry into the health care system to every person in the country. Physicians, individually or in small clinics, will serve at the focal points of these networks to provide consultation to the nonphysician practitioner and to serve as the next step on the ladder leading to regional tertiary care facilities. To man these outposts, a modified form of health professional draft may have to be introduced, and young graduates of subsidized educational programs may have to be assigned for limited periods to these rural and urban facilities. It will not be optimal health care, but it will meet minimal health care standards.

Other concerns that confront health planners on the national level are the problems of allocating limited resources. Health care is an enormous arena composed of numerous related and yet quasi-independent segments. Having accepted the fact that resources are limited and that the first priority must be the provision of minimally acceptable health care to all, how should the remainder of the resources be allocated? Numerous options are available. Most of the funds could be devoted to research in the hope that the major contemporary scourges—cancer, heart disease, and chronic respiratory ailments—can be eliminated, or at least significantly reduced. The funds could also be used to continue to provide the most sophisticated scientific technology to the relatively few who would benefit the most from them. Such items as open heart surgery, organ transplant, chronic renal dialysis, computer tomography, and other similar "luxuries" come to mind immediately. Another solution would be to devote most of the remaining funds to preventive medicine and health maintenance. (Interestingly, in this context Medicare and Medicaid do not pay for preventive manipulations, vaccines, preoperative respiratory therapy, and so forth.) Health education is yet another option, as is the establishment of geriatric facilities, hospitals, drug treatment centers, chronic care facilities, and the like.

None of the above can possibly be singled out as uniquely deserving support, and the societal funds will have to be divided among all of them. The relative importance of the various areas and the sums allocated to them must be decided immediately. How these decisions are made and what the ultimate outcome of this decision-making process is concerns us all. They are not, strictly speaking, ethical or moral decisions, and yet they clearly have a major ethical component. To direct funds away from open heart surgery and toward rehabilitation centers for drug addicts, to take money from diabetes research and spend it on chronic care facilities for retarded children, to stop funding health education and establishing hospitals or hospices for the terminally ill are ethical concerns. Society in general and the health care provider community in particular cannot delay making such choices.

Some few brave and enlightened groups have already entered this battleground. Rather recently, the Governors of the Massachusetts General Hospital (MGH) decided against authorizing the establishment of a single organ transplant program in that august institution. For this decision they were taken to task by some very prominent medical groups and people who claimed that it was improper for nonmedical groups to make medical decisions. The Governors of MGH stood firm and have ignored the advice and abuse heaped on them. I am convinced that the Governors acted responsibly and prudently. The decision they made is precisely the kind of decision that must be made at the institutional level and, more significantly, on the regional and national levels. Medical groups have not demonstrated leadership in this area and appear still to be committed to the unlikely concept that American medicine can, and does, provide the best possible medical care to all who need it. In view of this, and unpleasant though the idea may be, major allocation decisions affecting large groups will be made by consumers through legislatures and through governmental agencies. Mistakes will be made and resources wasted. Nevertheless, societal decisions will be made by society and not by small, self-serving pressure groups.

The second major allocation of resources issue involves individuals and decisions made at the local level. Triage is a term well known in military medicine and used in civilian practice almost exclusively in major emergency situations where health care facilities are suddenly confronted with large numbers of injured or otherwise acutely ill patients. Under these circumstances triage implies a rank-ordering of casualties on the basis of injury severity, the amount of time and effort required to repair the injury, and the likelihood of reasonably rapid rehabilitation and return to duty or work. Contrary to the usual civilian practice, military or emergency triage gives precedence to the most lightly injured over those who have penetrating injuries or whose injuries are likely to result in permanent and severe disability. In that situation the ethics of triage are strictly utilitarian. The purpose is to devote limited resources to the benefit of the largest possible number of patients and to serve those first who need the least and who will be able to function as soldiers again. Those likely to require major surgery and lengthy rehabilitation and probable discharge have to wait and may even be "sacrificed" to allow their more fortunate comrades access to care.

In civilian practice triage usually takes a very different form. The issue is rarely one of emergency management of large groups but is usually one of selecting small groups from a large pool for treatment modalities or drugs that are available in limited quantity. When penicillin first became available in very limited amounts, physicians had to make choices in their allocation of the "miracle drug." Should they treat the mayor of the town who had gonorrhea or the principal of the high school who had pneumonia? Should the youngster with otitis media be given preference over the waitress with an infected hand?

The first renal dialysis unit established in Seattle was a similar sphere for decision-making.[1] The number of patients with terminal renal failure was much larger than the number that could be accommodated in the limited facilities of the dialysis unit. Choices had to be made, and these choices were matters of life and death. The question is obvious: "Who should make this choice, and on what basis?" The answer unfortunately is not obvious and involves some of the most complex ethical issues. It deserves a somewhat more detailed examination.

The basic ethical dilemma can be stated simply: "If not all can be saved, who shall be saved?" To answer this dilemma, a fundamental value judgment must be made. If we assume that all human beings have the same value and that there is no difference between a child with Down's syndrome and a Nobel Laureate in Medicine from the point of view of intrinsic "humanness," the selection process must be made by chance. Random selection by some form of lottery or selection on a "first come, first served" basis may well be the most appropriate. This method has advocates among the major ethicists of our time.

A highly respected contemporary ethicist has taken a diametrically opposite position. Admittedly in a somewhat different context, Edmund Cahn held that, if not all could be saved, none should be saved. Cahn finds a recourse to chance unacceptable because it abrogates responsibility and rationality.[4]

The less radical opponents of the random selection approach advocate a selection system based on "merit" or "value," in combination with the highest probability of success. Selection would first be made on the basis of life expectancy and likelihood of cure. A second consideration would be given to such factors as the number of family members who depend on the patient. Finally past societal services rendered or potential future societal contributions would be weighed in making choices between individuals.

The medical choices and the family choice are relatively clear. Given the limited nature of the resources, preference may well be given to those in whom the treatment is likely to be successful and who, by virtue of age, would benefit for the longest time. In the family criterion, the provider for a group of small children may well be awarded preference over the lonely bachelor or spinster. The societal value choices are much more complex. Past services rendered have generally been recognized as meritorious, and indeed both a logical and ethical case can be made for rewarding those who have already made contributions to society. More difficult to assess is a person's potential future value. Is a promising artist, athlete, or politician worth more than a skilled mechanic, promising physician, or brilliant engineer? Should there be a premium on "scarcity," or should "utility" be a primary determinant? If we accept the proposition that value judgments of this type are acceptable on ethical grounds, who is to make the selection, and how can the selection process be freed from subjective factors?

Because of their proximity to the problem, physicians have traditionally been in a position to make the selections, and indeed have done so in many instances. Yet nothing in the training or education of the physician qualifies him for making such choices in any area except the strictly medical one. Physicians as a group are no more qualified to make societal value judgments than are lawyers, merchants, or housewives, as groups. Who, then, should make the selection, and how should the selection be made? In the absence of any agreement between providers and consumers, a scheme that has considerable appeal has been suggested by Rescher.[22] Selection for life-saving therapy would be performed as a three-tiered process. The first level of selection would be done by health care personnel on medical grounds. The likelihood of success and the life expectancy of the candidate would be evaluated according to the best available estimate, and those who fall below a minimally acceptable level would be eliminated from further consideration. The next level of selection would be done from the reduced group by a lay panel using the criteria of familial and social value. From these two selection processes, a more or less homogeneous group would remain in whom the medical indications and the social indications are both favorable. The final selection from this group would then be made by chance, by lottery, and not on a first-come, first-serve basis. This scheme does not pretend to be "optimal," but it may well be "acceptable" and does attempt to let health providers make medical decisions, society make societal decisions, and chance make the final decision. In a related context, triage in the intensive care unit has been discussed by a number of critical care specialists. The reader is referred to the interesting papers by Tagge and colleagues[27] and Cullen and associates.[6]

In summary, the problem of allocating scarce medical resources is currently, in this country, a somewhat academic one. For all practical purposes no patient is denied access to life-saving technology. Renal dialysis, which initiated the allocation concern, is now available to all who need it. No other life-saving or life-prolonging technology is in such scarce supply as to mandate formal selection criteria. Nevertheless, the problem may surface again, and it behooves the health care community to be prepared to cope with it. In the interim the national allocation problems should be paramount, and the ethical and economic issues of health policy must be tackled at the highest and broadest levels of society.

PROBLEMS OF EXPERIMENTATION

Experimentation in medicine is as old as medicine itself. Any "first" in therapy—from the first incantation of a neolithic shaman to the first transplantation of a human heart—is an experiment, since there is no previous experience to serve as a predictor of result. The entire field of contemporary health care is based on experiments that were performed on patients by healers who tried a new method to treat illness. All of us are the beneficiaries of previous human experimentation, and indeed many of us would not be alive if we had not been treated with a drug or with a surgical procedure that was "experimental" at one time. It is therefore absurd to maintain that human experimentation is wrong; that it is always an invasion of the sanctity of the human body; and that it should not be permitted under any circumstances.

Other critics maintain that human experimentation is justified only if the experiment is designed to benefit the specific patient on whom the experiment is performed. These same critics deny the validity of any experiment on humans if the purpose is to increase physiologic or therapeutic knowledge, but not to benefit the patient directly. Yet others maintain that no experimentation should ever be done on minors, prisoners, or the mentally incompetent.

Until the end of World War II in 1945, very few questioned the ethics of "human experimentation" seriously and the pioneers of biologic knowledge were universally hailed as the benefactors of humanity. It may be interesting and useful to examine the reasons for this change in attitude and to review the current regulations and practices under which human experimentation may be conducted ethically. Some of the concerns and controversies will be discussed in the context of these regulations and practices.

The findings of the international tribunal that tried the major Nazi war criminals sent a wave of shivers around the world already numb with the horrors discovered in the German concentration camps. Not only were millions of racially or politically undesirables put to death, but there was irrefutable evidence that brutal and frequently fatal experiments had been conducted by medical practitioners on hundreds of prisoners. To prevent a repetition of such barbaric acts, the tribunal announced a code of ethics for human experimentation known as the Nuremberg Code (1946–1949).[20] The Code states that no person shall ever be used as an experimental subject unless he consents voluntarily; that there be no other way to gain the same information; that risks never outweigh the benefits; that the experiments be conducted only by experienced and careful scientists fully aware of their responsibilities to the subject; and that the subject be free to withdraw from the experiment at any time and for whatever reason.

Considerable amplification of this code was provided by the Declaration of Helsinki, a statement by the World Medical Association. This declaration, issued in 1964 and revised in 1975, lays down the basic principles of ethical medical research and distinguishes, for the first time, between clinical research and nontherapeutic biomedical research on human subjects.[8]

Following the discovery of some scandalous experimentation in an allegedly reputable hospital, the Surgeon General of the United States issued a set of guidelines[10] governing human experimentation in the United States. These guidelines, since expanded, now regulate all research done under federal grants or in federal institutions. Indeed, most health care facilities have voluntarily expanded the scope of these regulations and now insist that all investigations involving human subjects conform with the regulation regardless of funding source. The core of these regulations is the establishment of an institutional committee that is charged with reviewing and monitoring all projects that involve human subjects.

These committees are composed of senior members of the medical staff representing various disciplines and varied research backgrounds. Other nonmedical members also must participate. Careful minutes are kept and reviewed periodically by federal inspectors. The committees have considerable authority to request modifications in the proposed investigations and may even refuse permission to engage in certain types of "research."

I had the opportunity to serve as secretary of this committee at the University of Michigan for the past 14 years and have found it an interesting and rewarding experience. The committee meets weekly and reviews between 10 and 15 requests for new studies or renewals at each session. It was gratifying to see how the quality and format of the proposals had changed over this period. Occasionally we still see some inappropriate studies, but generally the investigators have become very much more aware of their responsibilities to the patients or to the healthy volunteers. The consent forms have shown a steady and dramatic improvement, and the number of the frivolous, useless, or dangerous experiments have decreased almost to the vanishing point.

The following is an excerpt of the instructions that accompany the application form to be used by the investigator.

> The Committee to Review Grants for Clinical Research and Investigation Involving Human Beings has been established partly to meet the requirements of granting agencies, but, in the main, to safeguard the welfare of the patient and also to protect as far as possible both the investigator and the University from legal action. While very few applications have been disapproved, many had to be revised or amplified, resulting in delay which was time consuming and unprofitable to the investigator. The following problems have been encountered most frequently and are among the major causes for delay in approval. They are therefore presented in an effort to expedite review:
>
> 1. If blood is drawn, the total amount at any one time and the total amount likely to be drawn over the entire period of study must be stated. The American Association of Blood Banks provide guidelines of permissible limits.
> 2. The use of minors and mentally incompetents in any study not entirely designed for the benefit of the patient raises major legal problems. Occasionally special steps may be necessary to pre-empt the

possibility of legal action at a later date. The applicant should state why the study cannot be done on any other population and should emphasize the benefits likely to accrue in relation to the risks involved.

3. The "Informed Consent" should be written in language a layman can understand. Risks should be spelled out clearly, and it should also be stated which part of the procedure, if any, is to the benefit of the patient and which is not.
4. The application to the Committee must, in all cases, be accompanied by the research protocol. While the Committee will not evaluate scientific merit per se, it should have enough information to be able to weigh the risks in relation to the scientific benefits.
5. If a participant may receive a placebo he must, almost invariably, be told about the possibility. If the availability of this information to the patient makes it impossible for the study to be carried out, approval may still be granted but only if failure to make this disclosure is either demonstrably harmless or in the best interest of the patient.
6. Some volunteers participate in multiple studies. This may modify the reliability of the data to be obtained and may be hazardous to the volunteer. The investigator is responsible for ascertaining that no additive hazards are likely to be encountered.
7. Any study involving the use of an experimental (nonapproved) drug or the use of a marketed drug for a purpose not yet authorized must have FDA approval. In each instance the drug brochure should accompany the form of application sent to the committee.
8. All studies involving radioisotopes in humans must have prior approval of the radioisotope committee.
9. The cost of a procedure which is not of direct benefit to the patient should not be born by the patient. Hence the research support must be identified. Sometimes these cost data are obvious, sometimes they are less obvious, e.g., if an operative procedure is significantly prolonged resulting in increased charges for the use of the operating room.
10. Many drugs are contraindicated in certain diseases, in certain age groups, or in women during the reproductive period. The application should therefore state what steps are being taken to exclude such individuals.
11. In annual applications for renewal of a grant, it would be helpful to the Committee to have a specific reference made to any changes from the original protocol.

Individual members of the Committee will be happy to discuss applications with the investigator prior to submission, if this appears to serve a useful purpose.

Generally, human experimentation takes two major forms: therapeutic or physiologic. Therapeutic experimentation, in turn, may have two major subsets: the testing of drugs or techniques on patients who may benefit from the new drug or technique, or the testing on healthy volunteers before introduction into the clinical area. The Food and Drug Administration requires that all new drugs have initial testing performed in healthy adults to ascertain the safety of the new agent. These are usually small-scale studies that involve a small number of volunteers in whom very elaborate laboratory and other studies are performed and to whom the new drug is administered in increasing doses, usually to the limits of tolerance. Traditionally many of these so called phase-I studies, were performed on prisoners in state penitentiaries. This was, in many ways, an ideal arrangement because there were usually a large number of volunteers, the experimental conditions could be rigidly controlled, and costs of the studies were relatively low.

In recent years serious questions have been raised about the ethics of experimentation on prisoners. It was claimed that prisoners were not in a position to give free consent, that there was a real possibility of coercion, and that prisoners volunteered for dangerous experiments to escape from the intolerable tedium of lengthy incarceration or in the hope of early parole. Long lists have been compiled of dangerous, painful, and generally dubious investigations that have been carried out in prisons, and these arguments were used to stop all studies that involved inmates in penitentiaries. Generalizations about the kind of research done in prisons and about the prisoners themselves have been quoted widely in "scientific" and popular publications.

These well-intentioned comments are wide of the mark. No experimentation should be carried out in prisons that could not, or should not, be performed on the outside. Conversely, legitimate, carefully controlled studies with a favorable cost-benefit ratio should be permitted in prisons provided that precisely the same precautions and controls are excercised as in a university student population or any other nonprisoner groups.

The second step in therapeutic testing is the use of the new drug or technique in a small and carefully selected groups of patients. Initially these studies are controlled with extensive laboratory tests. They serve to establish an approximate effective dosage range while checking for changes in laboratory variables.

The third phase is larger in scale, involves more patients, uses less laboratory control, and introduces a standard drug for the sake of comparative effectiveness. If the experimental drug still looks promising and has an acceptable incidence of side-effects, it enters the final phase of testing. In this phase, large, multicenter studies are conducted to reaffirm the effectiveness of the new agent and to look for the rare complication that may appear only after widespread use.

Fundamental to all these studies is valid, free, and informed consent. Assuming that such consent is obtained, few will argue that therapeutic trials are immoral or unethical.

Generally the same principles apply to therapeutic experiments conducted on minors or others who cannot give valid consent. If the new agent or technique clearly shows potential benefit for the patient in the study, the parent or guardian need not have ethical scruples in consenting for the child or ward. In the case of the older child, it is desirable, although not legally required, that assent to the study be obtained from the youngster.

Even though the therapeutic study is less controversial than other forms of human experimentation, some serious ethical questions can be raised. Let us assume that a new antimicrobial agent is to be tested that is allegedly effective against a certain type of serious infection. We already have agents effective against this particular microorganism. Is it justifiable to subject patients in life-threatening situations to a drug of unproven value when the patient could be treated effectively with a known agent? The answer I believe, is a highly qualified yes. This type of study is permissible only if the new drug shows *unusual* promise. It must be safer—that is, have fewer side-effects, be more effective, or be cheaper. Lacking these potential benefits, a strictly "me too" study is ethically highly suspect.

Another area of real doubt is in therapeutic studies where the nature of the agent requires the introduction of a placebo control. The ground rules should be the same. If consent can be obtained and if the participant's life is not threatened by being randomly assigned to the placebo group, the study may go forward. If the patient may be seriously jeopardized, even the best consent is insufficient, and such studies should not be performed. This may sound harsh, but in many years of reviewing research applications I have never encountered a situation where this type of study could not be redesigned and the risk to the participants reduced to acceptable levels. All that has been needed was to counsel the investigators and direct them to look at the experimental design from a somewhat different perspective.

The problem is entirely different if the proposed study is not therapeutic but where the purpose of the investigation is to obtain better understanding of physiologic or pathophysiologic principles. Occasionally these studies may benefit successive generations of patients, but in most other instances they serve only to increase the fund of human knowledge without any foreseeable benefits to anyone except the investigator.

Some ethicists believe that such studies are never permissible. The extreme position, like all extreme positions, is indefensible in my view. Experiments that increase our understanding of physiology and pathophysiology are not only permissible but even desirable, provided certain very rigid conditions are met in the experimental design. These conditions can be stated as follows:

1. The risk of the study to the participants must be minimal and may at no time include the possibility of permanent harm of any kind.
2. The design of the study must be such that results, positive or negative, have statistical validity. Badly designed, predictably inconclusive studies are never justified.
3. Physiologic studies should not be performed on patients and should be performed only on healthy volunteers. Pathophysiologic studies must be performed on patients but are legitimate only if there is minimal or no risk and if the patients understand very clearly that no benefit will accrue to them.
4. Such studies are probably never justified on minors or incompetents.
5. Inducement to participate should never be of a nature to make a rational decision difficult. Offering a large sum of money to a poor person to participate in a dangerous experiment automatically invalidates the freedom of the consent and must be condemned as unacceptable coercion. To give an extreme example, few of us could resist an offer of 1 million dollars to have a foot amputated so that a new orthopedic appliance could be tested. Yet such a study is clearly unethical. (The legal problems of "consent" are discussed in another chapter.)
6. Studies may produce psychological damage as well as physical damage, and emotional trauma is more difficult to predict and much more difficult to correct. If there is any doubt, the experiment should not be performed.

A special area of concern involves experimentation on the unborn fetus. This problem has generated considerable discussion in recent years, and some very interesting and potentially important proposals have been denied on the grounds of ethical unacceptability. These are very complex issues, and the interested reader is referred to the publications of the National Commission for the Protection of Human Subjects of Biomedical and Behavioral Research.

To summarize the ethical considerations of human experimentation, such studies are not only ethically permissible but even desirable if the guidelines established by the Surgeon General[10] are scrupulously enforced, if an honest assessment of risks and benefits is made, if individual freedom of choice is always respected, and if the ancient precept of "don't do unto others . . ." is always first and foremost in the mind of the investigator. Respiratory therapists, as a group, are just now expanding their research potential. They have a splendid opportunity to develop a model research program that combines the highest ethical principles with sound scientific methods.

THE PROBLEMS OF "WHAT THE HELL DO I DO NOW?"

Discussed herein are a number of ethically relevant but unrelated situations that the respiratory therapist must recognize and deal with.

The Impaired Health Professional

The problem of the impaired health professional is becoming a major issue, and all health care providers must learn to cope with it. All of us have colleagues or associates who are becoming incompetent because of senescence, alcoholism, drug abuse, emotional instability, or chronic illness. What is our ethical and, perhaps, legal obligation when we recognize that a physician, nurse, respiratory therapist, or other hospital worker no longer functions as well as he did in the past. His behavior becomes erratic, his moods show wide swings, he is forgetful, may become slovenly in his appearance, or may show other evidence of emotional or physical deterioration. The surgeon whose tremor is no longer controllable, the respiratory therapist who "forgets" what treatments have to be given, the nurse who makes repeated mistakes in scheduling patients or who makes errors in medication are all people who need help and who constitute a real or potential menace to the patient. Yet many of these people are our friends, our superiors, our colleagues. What is our duty, what do we have to do?

It is very easy to be categorically righteous and say that the impaired colleague must be reported to the proper hospital authority and must be removed from any patient care situation. Actually it is very difficult to do this. Very few of us relish the thought of "reporting" or "squealing" on a fellow health worker. There is the fear of reprisals, there is the possibility of error, there is the very real possibility that our motives will be misunderstood. At the very least, we are almost certain to lose the friendship of the person whose failings we bring to the attention of the administration. The obverse of the coin is equally awkward. If we do or say nothing and if because of this a patient is hurt, we have a heavy burden of responsibility to carry and may even be legally liable. To me, this latter is the greater of two evils, and I believe that we must not, and cannot, stand by in splendid inactivity and hope that all will come out well. We must take active steps to assure the safety of the patients and must do this in a way that will cause the least pain or stress to the health professional involved.

If it is an employee, the first step is a private session to make friendly inquiries, to offer assistance, and to make the individual aware that his problem has become known and that there is every intent to be supportive and helpful. Suggestions can be made for early retirement, for professional assistance, or for referral to appropriate local agencies. In many instances, this type of informal action will suffice, and the employee will voluntarily seek assistance or, if necessary, ask for leave of absence or reassignment to a less sensitive position. Some employees will not have been aware of their problem and will honestly be grateful for help and advice. If the employee denies any problem or becomes defensive or even abusive, the good supervisor will pursue the matter through the proper established channels, making certain that all allegations are fully documented and that the employee is given every possible assistance.

The problem is more complex if the impaired person is in a different health profession and particularly if that person is higher in the organizational structure of the institution, either by seniority or by the nature of his profession. I believe the obligation is still clear. If a respiratory therapist believes that a nurse or a physician is impaired and may be dangerous to patients, the respiratory therapist must not console himself that it is "not his business." In his situation the medical director of the respiratory therapy department is the appropriate recipient of a documented report. It is then the medical director's task to bring this matter to the attention of the hospital administration or of the appropriate person in the medical staff organization.

What if it is the medical director who becomes impaired? In this case much depends on the interpersonal relationship that exists between the technical director and the medical director. If this relationship is a good one, the technical director may be able to have a frank and friendly discussion with the medical director and indicate the concerns that have been raised by members of the department. If the relationship is such that a conversation of this type is not possible, then the technical director has no choice but to report to the hospital administrator. This is a tough step to take, and it is possible that the technical director who chooses this route may encounter serious criticism and even threats. It takes a good, strong person to have the courage of his convictions and to do the right things, even at the price of personal inconvenience and risk.

Society is beginning to recognize this dilemma, and some states, notably California, have given formal recognition to it in the form of "Impaired Physician" regulations.[29] These regulations offer immunity to the informant and make arrangements to help the impaired physician. No such activity exists yet for the nonphysician health care provider, but all of us will undoubtedly have this protection under the law soon.

The Dishonest Employee

Somewhat akin and yet sufficiently different is the problem of the dishonest employee and the ethical and legal burden this places on us all. There must be few of us indeed who, on occasion and in a usually very minor way, have not failed to distinguish between the property of the employer and the perquisites of the employee. The list of such minor peccadilloes is long and includes such items as using hospital stationery for personal correspondence, making personal telephone calls and even long distance calls from hospital telephones, snitching food in the cafeteria, swiping a few aspirin tablets at a nursing station, taking a bottle of hand lotion home, and so forth. More significant thefts include books from the library, surgical instruments for home workshops, scrub suits to be used as pajamas, and patients' robes and slippers. Finally there are the "serious" thefts that include money and other valuables, major equipment, and indeed almost anything that is not a structural component of the building.

Everyone will agree that stealing a patient's pocketbook or a hospital television set is wrong, and yet most people will see little if anything wrong with the "minor thefts." From a purely ethical point of view there is no difference between a sheet of stationery and a television set, even though the law does distinguish on the basis of monetary value and even the most strict employer is likely to ignore the pettiest of petty pilfering.

As employees, we do have a clear and binding duty to protect our employer's property, both from others and from ourselves. The excuses that "it does not matter" or "they'll never miss it" or "it's just a few cents' worth" are, at best, shabby. Whether we should take any action for the sake of a roll of tissue paper is another question. It is ethically wrong, but it may be practical if we look the other way and do not antagonize everybody for trivia. It would almost certainly accomplish nothing, make a lot of enemies, and place us into the invidious position of intolerable righteousness.

The situation is quite different if the thefts involve more costly items. Here, I believe, our duty is clear. We must report it with the awareness that apprehension of the thieving coworker will lead to loss of his employment, probably criminal prosecution, and possible incarceration.

The Wrong Order

In respiratory care it is quite common to find orders that are incomplete, incorrect, or even potentially harmful. Most departments have policies that address this issue, but in many departments this situation is left to the discretion of the individual practitioner. The temptation is great to ignore the wrong order and to do what is deemed appropriate. This I believe to be ethically unsound and legally tenuous. An order should not be willfully ignored or capriciously modified. The proper way to deal with this situation is to contact the physician who wrote the order and request a clarification or correction. If the physician is not available, the medical director of respiratory care should be contacted and asked to assume the responsibility for the evaluation of the situation and to endorse, cancel, or modify the existing order. If the medical director is also unavailable and no other physician is willing or able to assume responsibility, the respiratory therapist does have a dilemma. Should he follow the order, or should the order be modified or ignored? I believe that in this situation the therapist should use his best judgment and do what, by training and experience, appears to be the right course of action. It is absolutely essential, however, that the action taken be carefully documented in the record and that a written justification be given for the decision. If the therapist decides to follow an order that appears to be excessive, it is critical that the patient be observed continuously and that treatment be discontinued at the first sign of side reactions. Again full documentation of the action is necessary.

These problems test the system and quickly show up weaknesses. The unavailable medical director and the careless ordering physician are not uncommon. The lack of a written policy for handling improper orders is probably true for most hospitals. The good training and mature judgment of the therapist are tested and may be found wanting. The reaction of the physician whose order was changed may be indicative of his education or personality. An incorrect order may happen anywhere and at any time. Handling it properly, and with no bad feelings on any side, indicates mature professional relationships and is a good measure of the professional ethics of the health care providers.

Sexual Harassment

An ethical problem as old as mankind is the relationship of the sexes. In recent years this problem has become accentuated by the increasing entry of women into the job market and the appearance of women in occupations and careers that were previously considered exclusively male domains. Women entering these fields have to overcome prejudice, hostility, and humiliation. They are the target of abuse and discrimination, are considered easy prey for the predatory male, and are frequently the subject of covert or overt sexual harassment. This may take many forms from the smutty joke and "accidental" body contact to the frank sexual advances, including crass sexual blackmail.

The increasing permissiveness of the 1960s and 1970s has brought many of these previously camouflaged activities into the open, and the burgeoning feminism of the same period has drawn increasing attention to this problem.

From an ethical point of view the issues are relatively simple. No woman should ever be made to suffer discrimination or humiliation because she is a woman. Employees or coworkers must be treated with the same courtesy, consideration, and respect regardless of whether they are male or female.

Unfortunately, matters that may be ethically obvious and simple are very complex and perhaps even unresolvable in real life. Sexual impulses are among the strongest known urges, and to expect that all intersexual problems can be eliminated by regulations is absurd. Once again the issue is one of degree. Unquestionably sexual favors should never be demanded in exchange for retention in a job or promotion. All women should be able to have effective grievance procedures and receive the full protection of the administrative system in case of sexual harassment or abuse. The predominantly female occupations, such as nursing, physical therapy, occupational therapy, and clerical and secretarial work, must have the same formal recognition, job description, salary potential, and general consideration as the still primarily male occupations.

Once we proceed beyond these areas, however, we rapidly reach an area where ongoing contact between young or not so young males and females will inevitably lead to behavior that some will consider offensive, some flattering, some amusing, and some with righteous indignation.

There is no ready answer to this problem, and it is the function of the department managers to keep interpersonal behavior within decorous bounds. As in so many other situations, good manners and good taste will accomplish more than rigid rules or the loftiest ethical principles. Although sexual harassment has a peculiarly and distressingly male connotation, much trouble can be avoided if the females' behavior is also kept within the same decorous bounds. Unnecessarily provocative behavior or dress is an invitation to trouble, and the woman who flaunts her femininity or who tries to use it for advantages is just as guilty of sexual harassment as the male who is weak enough or stupid enough to fall for it.

Another area of ethical concern is the relationship between therapists and patients. Although sexual misbehavior between health professionals is regrettable, sexual misbehavior between health professionals and patients is intolerable. Occasionally the patient will be the aggressor, and these aggressions, verbal or manual, must be politely but firmly rejected. Occasionally the health professional will be the aggressor, and the patient may find herself in a very difficult and unpleasant situation. A general disinclination toward "causing trouble," a fear of forfeiting future care, or a weakened physical and mental state makes patients very vulnerable. Some health "professionals" have been known to take advantage of this, and both physicians and other health professionals have had their careers justifiably ended for the sake of what must have been a short and dubious pleasure.

A different, but still related, issue is the way health professionals address patients of the same or opposite sex. Customs change, and it has become quite common that coworkers, even of widely differing age and opposite sex, address each other by their first name. This is alleged to foster camaraderie and promote cheerfulness and cooperation. Perhaps so, and perhaps it is quite acceptable between members of the health team. I do not believe it is acceptable between health professionals and patients. To address an adult patient, particularly a middle-aged or elderly patient as Mary or Jane is not only rude but condescending and suggests a feeling of superiority. Even more objectionable are terms of endearment. "Honey, cutie, or dearie" have no place at the bedside. Patients appreciate being treated with courtesy, and a proper form of address is certainly part of elementary courtesy.

Regrettably a serious textbook directed at a major health care provider specialty has yet to address such matters. It was under the pressure of numerous complaints and many unfortunate personal observations that I have broached it. I approach the remainder of this chapter with undisguised relief.

PROBLEMS OF CONFIDENTIALITY

Chapter 5 discusses in some detail the problem of the privileged relationship that exists between the patients and *all* the personnel who participate in their care. A major component of this relationship is the confidentiality with which all data pertaining to the patient must be handled. This confidentiality is not only a legal obligation but also an ethical one. Health care providers are the repository of much information, not all of which is related to the particular health problem that brings the patient to the hospital or the health care provider to the patient's home. Generally, all information pertaining to the patient, the patient's family, or the patient's life must be treated with absolute discretion. Yet there are exceptions to this rule, and it is in the area of these exceptions that ethical problems arise.

Some are relatively simple. Quite regularly the patient's care requires consultation, and the consultant or other health care providers have a "need to know" all the information available on the patient. The patient's record must be reviewed not only by all members of the health care team but also by medical records personnel, quality assurance committees, and other hospital bodies that have a legitimate reason for reviewing charts, assembling statistical information, compiling data, and so forth. All these persons are bound by the same ethical restraints as the primary physician, and all information obtained by these people must be handled confidentially.

Somewhat more difficult is the issue of using information obtained from the patient or from the record for educational or scientific purposes. It is generally accepted that the health care providers may use patient information in the education of other health professionals or in the dissemination of important information to the scientific community by means of scholarly publications. The ethics of this particular activity requires that the patient's anonymity be strictly observed and that every effort be made to render identification of particular individuals impossible. Names must be withheld; even the use of initials is undesirable. Photographs or drawings may not be used if they can serve to identify individuals without the patient's specific, written permission. If the patient volunteers to participate in clinical investigations, he must be told that his record may be inspected by the sponsor of the research or by some federal or state regulatory agencies.

There are certain situations where a breach of confidentiality is mandated by statute, and ethical issues are not taken into consideration. Certain contagious conditions must be reported to the public health authorities, and injuries suffered through violence have to be reported to the police. In this latter situation there is sometimes a real ethical dilemma. To distinguish between accidental and intentional injuries is not always easy, and the health professional must decide whether or not to report. To report inevitably results in police involvement, awkwardness, and hard feelings. Not to report may lead to exposure of an innocent child or adult to further injury and to an unrecognized and unpunished crime. No rigid rules can be set. My recommendation is that when in doubt, report. Not to report is a cop-out that may be disguised by lofty rhetoric but is a cop-out nevertheless.

Even more difficult problems arise if health care providers have to decide between civic duty and their duty to patient. Let us suppose that a person whose picture appears on the wall of the local post office as a suspect in a felony seeks medical assistance and is recognized by the physician or by a respiratory therapist as a "wanted" person. Do you call the police? Ethicists argue this question at tedious length, and indeed it is not an easy question to answer. I have never been in such a situation, and it is thus easy for me to say that I would call the police if the "patient" were wanted for a crime of violence. Whether I would report an income tax evader or a confidence trickster is something I would have to decide at the time. I rather suspect that I would report it, but not without considerable reluctance and a great deal of soul-searching.

Problems arise also when minors are involved and when the question of whether to inform parents must be answered. Courts have spoken in some specific situations. Parents need not consent to contraceptive information or assistance being given to minors. Similarly, pregnancy need not be revealed. But what if a youngster is found to be a drug addict? Must we inform the parents? May we inform the parents? Should we inform the parents? Again ethicists differ. My feeling is that addicts desperately need help that a minor addict probably will not be able to obtain without parental assistance and support. I believe, therefore, that in this situation the health professional must inform the parents and that this action is not a violation of the ethical requirements of confidentiality.

These are all exceptional situations that require much thought and are the subject of much controversy. This is not the case with the routine patient in the ordinary performance of our health care delivery. There the confidentiality rule is absolute and inviolable, even though all of us have violated it. I do not believe that there is, or ever has been, a health care provider who has not violated this ethical mandate by relating a funny story involving patients, an interesting case, an unusual finding, a major therapeutic thriumph, or any other of the many trivia that make up the conversation whenever two or more health professionals get together. Just because an ethical mandate is regularly violated makes it no less an ethical mandate. It is something all health professionals should think about.

THE PROBLEMS OF THE "CODE OF ETHICS"

The Oath of Hippocrates, already quoted, in contemporary parlance would qualify as a code of ethics. It sufficed for centuries, and it was only when the revolution of manners and morals changed both interpersonal behavior and the authority "cascade" that a need appeared for new codes for the new professions and the new professionals. This trend has progressed to the extreme where every professional organization feels obliged to have a code of ethics. Even an otherwise reasonable and level-headed organization like the American Hospital Association (AHA) has found it necessary to publish a document entitled "A Bill of Rights for Patients."[3] In this "Bill of Rights" the AHA grandiloquently, patronizingly, and magnanimously grants "rights" to patients that every human being has long been granted by both statute and common law.

Less absurd are the professional codes of ethics of the AART, the AMA, the ANA, and others. They are all neat compilations of the obvious, which form a bridge between Amy Vanderbilt and the Ten Commandments. What they all fail to see is that unless the rules of behavior can be enforced, codes of ethics do not lead to ethical behavior. Since no professional organization has the power to enforce its "code" and since the worst "punishment" is expulsion from the organization, it is easy to see why the codes of ethics are nothing but straw men. In fact, codes that are continously broken are worse than useless, since many young graduates, filled with lofty ideals, seeing their elders acting unethically lose all respect for propriety and vie with each other in becoming just as unethical as their "role models." Having ethics and behaving ethically is terribly important, but codes of ethics do not assure ethical behavior, and the only code of ethics that has any real meaning is the one backed by the police power of the state and one that can enforce penalties ranging from the assessment of fines to the loss of license or personal freedom.

Obviously many persons are ethical because that is the only way their conscience allows them to be. Some are ethical because of religious convictions, whereas others may follow the path of virtue and righteousness for other reasons. The future of the profession is in their hands. If a code of ethics helps them, then perhaps there is indeed a need for such a code and my skepticism reflects only my age and cynicism.

SUMMARY

I have tried to do three things in this chapter: [1] outline a history of Western ethical thought; [2] discuss the ethics of interpersonal and interprofessional relationships; and [3] present a series of major contemporary ethical concerns as they relate to the health professional. Obviously a chapter cannot make people ethical; all that can be hoped is that people will start to think about ethical concerns.

I wish to express my deep appreciation to Ms. Cynthia B. Cohen, Ph.D., to Calvin E. Williams, M.D., and to Thomas J. DeKornfeld, Jr., M.A. (Litt.), for their many valuable suggestions regarding both content and format.

REFERENCES

1. Anonymous: Scarce medical resources. Columbia Law Rev 69:620, 1969
2. Bentham J: In LeFleur J (ed): An Introduction to the Principles of Morals and Legislation. New York, Hatner Press, 1948
3. Bill of Rights for Patients. Hospitals 4(4), 1973
4. Cahn E: The Moral Decision. Bloomington, Indiana University Press, 1955

5. California State Health Plan 1980–1985. Sacramento, Office of Statewide Health Planning and Development, 1979
6. Cullen DJ et al: Therapeutic intervention scoring system: A method of quantitative comparison of patient care. Crit Care Med 2:57, 1974
7. Curlander v. Bioscience Labs. 165 Cal. Rep. 477 CA, 1980
8. Declaration of Helsinki. Toyko, World Medical Assocation Revised Edition, 1975
9. Doe v. Bolton. 410 U.S. 179, 1973
10. Federal Register 46:8366, January 1981
11. Frankena WK: Ethics. Englewood Cliffs, New Jersey, Prentice–Hall, 1973
12. Gustafson JM: Mongolism, Parental Desires and the Right to Life. Perspect Biol Med 16:229, 1973
13. In re Dinnerstein, 380 N.E., 2nd 134, MA, 1978
14. In re Houle. 74–145, Supreme Court, Cumberland Co. MA (February 14, 1974)
15. In re Phillip B. 92 California Representative, 3rd 796 CA 1979—Certified Denied 100 S. Court 1597, 1980
16. Kaimowitz v. Department of Mental Health. N.E. 73–19434, A. W. Circuit Court, Wayne Co. MI, 1973
17. Kant I: Groundwork of the Metaphysics and Morals. New York, Harper & Row, 1964
18. Mark VH et al: Violence and the Brain. New York, Harper & Row, 1970
19. Mill JS: Utilitarianism and Other Writings. Cleveland, Meridian, 1962
20. The Nuremberg Code: Trials of War Criminals Before the Nuremberg Military Tribunals Under Control Council Law No. 10, Vol. II, Nuremberg, 1946–1949
21. Rawls J: A Theory of Justice. Cambridge, Harvard University Press, 1971
22. Resher N: The allocation of exotic medical life saving therapy. Ethics 79(3):173, 1969
23. Roe v. Wade. 410 U.S. 113, 1973
24. Sellons W et al: Readings in Ethical Theory. Englewood Cliffs, New Jersey, Prentice–Hall, 1970
25. Sinsheimer R: Troubled dawn of genetic engineering. New Scientist (Lond) 68, 1975
26. Superintendent of Belchertown State School v. Saikewicz. 370 N.E. 2nd 1234, MA 1978
27. Tagge GF et al: Relationships of therapy to prognosis in critically ill patients. Crit Care Med 2:61, 1974
28. Veatch RM: Death, Dying and the Biological Revolution. New Haven, Yale University Press, 1976
29. What You Need to Know About Impairment in Physicians. California Medical Association, Division of Scientific and Educational Activities, 731 Market Street, San Francisco, 94203, 1980

BIBLIOGRAPHY

Beauchamp TL, Walter L (eds): Contemporary Issues in Bioethics. Belmont, CA, Wadsworth Publishing 1978

Beauchamp TL: Principles of Biomedical Ethics. Cambridge, Oxford University Press, 1979

Brain Death: Interrelated Medical and Social Issues. Ann NY Acad Sci 315, 1978. Symposium issue on multiauthor conference.

David AJ, Aroskar MA: Ethical Dilemmas and Nursing Practice. New York, Appleton–Century–Crofts 1978

Glover J: Causing Death and Saving Lives. Harmondsworth, Middlesex, Penguin Books, 1977

Hastings Center Reports, 360 Broadway, Hastings-on-Hudson, NY 10706. Anyone seriously interested in bioethics should read these reports regularly.

Humber JM, Almeder R (eds): Biomedical Ethics and the Law. New York, Plenum Press, 1979

National Commission for the Protection of Human Subjects for Biomedical and Behavioral Research, DHEW Superintendent of Documents, Washington, DC, 1978, 1979

4

The Physician and the Respiratory Care Team

George G. Burton

Respiratory therapy has been defined as "an allied health specialty employed with *medical direction* in the treatment, management, control, diagnostic evaluation, and care of patients with deficiencies and abnormalities of the cardiopulmonary system."* This definition implies, but does not actually state, that respiratory care is much too complex to expect any one health worker to provide entirely comprehensive quality care services.

Such care requires the cooperative efforts of several groups of health professionals who must have knowledge of the patient as a whole and of the services necessary to meet those needs. Such professionals must appreciate each other's knowledge and skills, recognize their own competencies and limitations, and seek appropriate consultation, referral, or assistance as indicated. Placing the primary focus on the needs of *patients* rather than on the needs of individual professionals facilitates comprehensive respiratory care.[2]

The physician well trained in respiratory care, whether a pulmonary internist, anesthesiologist, or surgeon, is the natural leader of the health care team. The team includes nurses, respiratory therapists, physical therapists, and, in some instances, social workers, psychologists, and dietitians. Construction and maintenance of such a care team is a difficult, never-ending task that challenges the cooperative spirit and the scientific resources of all concerned.

This chapter is written for the physician involved in the care of patients with respiratory disease, and specifically for those physicians who direct or desire to direct allied nonphysician specialists in the care of the sick. Although most such physicians are well and reasonably uniformly trained, their training has rarely included instruction in the medical direction of respiratory care departments or in the day-to-day optimum use of a health care team.[4] While each physician who cares for the respiratory patient should use the available modalities and team members with some expertise, this requirement falls particularly heavily on the medical directors of respiratory care departments and services. Other physicians should learn by his example.

THE GENERAL PHYSICIAN AND THE RESPIRATORY CARE TEAM

SPECTRUM OF PHYSICIAN TRAINING AND COMPETENCE

Respiratory care requires a certain core skills–knowledge base that includes a current knowledge of applied pulmonary physiology, an understanding

*Definition prepared by the American Association for Respiratory Therapy (italics mine).

of the pathophysiology of many cardiopulmonary conditions, and a thorough comprehension of the indications for, and limitations and contraindications of, the various respiratory care modalities that the physician oversees. Fortunately, many national associations now address themselves to the problem of keeping physicians *au courant* by means of the program content of their annual meetings. In addition, pertinent postgraduate courses are held in many sections of the country so that it is usually not difficult for a physician to attend at least one or two such courses each year. In some states, associations of medical directors of respiratory therapy have been formed to further the continuing education of their members, but these efforts have been few and the efforts questionable. The National Association of Medical Directors of Respiratory Care (NAMDRC) has, in recent years, stepped in to fill this leadership vacuum.

The degree to which a nonspecialist physician can understand all the technological aspects of respiratory care delivery varies considerably. To a certain extent, his deficiencies in this area can be met by well-trained nurses, technicians, and therapists whose educational backgrounds are stronger than his in the areas of equipment operation, maintenance, and performance characteristics. He should not, however, delegate *entire* responsibility for operation of such equipment to the respiratory therapy technical staff. The physician who finds it impossible to maintain a working knowledge of current respiratory care techniques should make full use of a pulmonary physician's consultative service, rather than rely excessively on the knowledge and capabilities of respiratory therapy technical personnel and nurses. The hierarchical difficulties this may create should be self-evident.[3]

THE RESPONSIBILITY OF THE ATTENDING PHYSICIAN

Most attending physicians assume that once an order is written in the patient's chart it will automatically be carried out. They have learned to expect this in diet orders, medication orders, intravenous fluid orders, and so forth. Although they should expect that respiratory therapy and chest physical therapy orders will be carried out faithfully, such is not always the case, usually because of the patient's lack of cooperation in accepting the therapy ordered, and because of the occasional inability of therapy staff to deliver all the treatments in a given time. A brief list of common "reasons" for treatments not given appears in Table 4-1. These are often inexcusable lapses in quality care that require prompt identification by the attending physician. Complacency in thinking that precisely what he has ordered is actually being carried out may well be dangerous. Simple discussion with the patient on rounds each day will ascertain if treatments ordered are being missed, or are being given poorly or haphazardly. Such attention to detail will often result in rapid improvement in the patient's condition.[7] Far from the contrary, such feedback will usually be appreciated by the respiratory care team.

Table 4-1. Reasons for Therapy Being Missed

- **I.** *Unavailability of Patient*
  - **A.** Temporary: Patient still in room
    - **1.** Bath, meals, toilet
    - **2.** Clinical laboratory, ECG, or x-ray technicians in room, doctor with patient, nurses or physical therapists working with patient, family with patient
    - **3.** Patient asleep
  - **B.** Protracted: Patient out of room
    - **1.** Patient in x-ray department, pulmonary function laboratory, radiation therapy, surgery
    - **2.** Patient visiting family in lobby
- **II.** *Patient Refusal*
  - **A.** Nausea or vomiting
  - **B.** Fatigue
  - **C.** Pain
  - **D.** Previous adverse reaction
  - **E.** Patient confused
  - **F.** Patient combative
  - **G.** Patient unable to cooperate (*e.g.,* neuromuscular problems)
  - **H.** Occupied with visitors
  - **I.** No reason
- **III.** *Unavailability of Therapist*
  - **A.** Stat calls elsewhere
  - **B.** Priority treatments
  - **C.** Unrealistic treatment load
  - **D.** Insufficient equipment
- **IV.** *Miscellaneous*
  - **A.** Unclear treatment order
  - **B.** "Catch-up" treatment too close to next scheduled treatment

WRITING ORDERS

Many physicians (including those recently trained) have no real comprehension of how to write complete and effective respiratory care orders. For the various modalities used, the following advice may be helpful.

Oxygen Therapy

The liter flow or desired inspired oxygen concentration should be stated. If the patient is ambulatory or has varying metabolic needs for oxygen, the order should reflect different flow rates for sleep, daytime rest, and exercise. The equipment to be used (*e.g.*, cannula) should be stipulated.

Intermittent Positive Pressure Breathing Orders

There is considerable ambiguity in the writing of many intermittent positive pressure breathing (IPPB) orders (*see* Chap. 23). Too often orders simply read "IPPB q.i.d."! In precise orders, the time of day IPPB is to given, inspired oxygen concentration to be used, exact dosage of medications to be employed, and maximum inspiratory pressures not to be exceeded should be listed as a minimum. Yanda has made the excellent recommendation that all respiratory care orders be accompanied by a statement on the *expected results* of such therapy.[7] The standards issued by the Joint Commission on Accreditation of Hospitals (JCAH) generally reflect the same opinion (*see* Chap. 5). The procedure manual in the respiratory care department should reflect that incomplete or inappropriate orders will not be honored and that when this occurs the therapist or nurse giving the therapy must clarify the situation, perhaps substituting departmental "standing orders" (appropriately countersigned by the physician) before she proceeds.

When alternating medications are used, for instance, a mixture of isoproterenol and acetylcysteine alternated with isoproterenol and saline, such orders should be particularly explicit. Labeling one combination "A" and the other "B" is a simple expedient that can be codified in the institution's procedure manual.

The physician should be aware that most q.i.d. orders do not include treatment during the night. If he desires that therapy be spread out through the entire 24 hours, he should so indicate by writing orders for q. 3 h., q. 4 h., or q. 6 h. therapy. Advance p.r.n. orders for medication may be convenient at night but will require closer than usual scrutiny of the nursing and therapy charts to see exactly what has been given.

If IPPB is to be followed by *humidity* or *high-density aerosol therapy* or *chest physical therapy*, this should be stated in the complete respiratory care orders. Similarly, if the patient is identified as at particularly high risk, orders should be written to discontinue therapy if the heart rate exceeds a given frequency, if arrhythmias occur, or if chest pain (such as may indicate a pneumothorax) develops.

Orders for Patients on Volume Ventilators

It is surprising how cavalier many orders for total respiratory support are. I have seen more than a few orders stating "place patient on MA-1 respirator" with absolutely no other indication of what should be done. Here again the precise inspired oxygen concentration to be used is absolutely vital. In addition, the following variables must be prescribed: tidal volume, frequency, sigh rate (number and volume), peak pressure not to be exceeded during inspiration, use of negative inspiratory pressure (if indicated), positive end-expiratory pressure, IMV rate and volume, inspiratory:expiratory length ratio, and added dead space, if any. "Standard ventilator protocols" may be substituted if their obvious limitations (*i.e.*, relative inflexibility) are recognized (*see* below).

A frequent oversight is the omission of aerosolized bronchodilator therapy once the patient has been placed on a volume ventilator. For this purpose it is usually most convenient to disconnect the ventilator temporarily and to preoxygenate the patient with 100% oxygen via IPPB device or manual resuscitation bag. The intubated or tracheostomized patient usually requires less drug than does the patient who receives aerosolization through the mouth, where aerosol "rain out" occurs in the oropharynx.

Weaning

Specific orders for weaning from the respirator are more difficult to write, since there must be some flexibility for the sake of efficiency. Guidelines for such procedures are listed in Chapter 25.

As the physician gains sophistication and expertise, his order-writing will improve in quality, as will the care of his patients. His competence can be assimilated by the therapy and nursing staff, who will require less and less instruction in minutiae as their relationship grows.

Standing or Routine Orders

Except for ventilator protocols, standing or routine orders for respiratory care are mentioned here only to be, in general, condemned. Although standard operating procedures and procedure manuals are valuable for operating an intensive care unit or a respiratory care department, the use of "standard respiratory care orders" for individual patients is discouraged by most physicians active in respiratory care. Each patient has individual cardiopulmonary problems that may cause or complicate his course. I urge each physician to write specific orders in each instance. The above notwithstanding, departmental medical directors should work to ensure that the staff does not follow orders slavishly when their educated opinion reveals something inappropriate or inadequate in the physician's order.

It is a JCAH requirement that the effects of a patient's respiratory treatment be evaluated and recorded in the chart. The therapist (or nurse) should be taught how to do this effectively, and the attending physician's progress note should acknowledge his evaluation of such charting (see Chap. 6).

Automatic stop orders are an exception to the above statements. Therapy orders should not be left to run on and on when no longer necessary, and many hospitals have now adopted procedures whereby the physician is notified to review his prescription for therapy at periodic intervals (48–72 hours). Indeed, recent third-party reimbursement trends indicate that payment may be withheld if orders are not rewritten on a frequent, periodic basis.

Another situation that may justify implementing "standing" orders in specific disease-states is when little pulmonary expertise exists in a hospital or community. Under these conditions, a "cookbook" approach to therapy may be needed. The "cookbook" should be designed by the most knowledgeable members of the medical staff, preferably the person acting as medical director and the department technical director, and then submitted for criticism to a qualified specialist before implementation. This approach should be used with decreasing frequency as the pool of qualified respiratory care physicians enlarges.

STAT OR "CODE BLUE" CALLS

Physicians who have had training in cardiopulmonary resuscitation are particularly valuable when a stat or "code blue" call is flashed through the hospital. Chapter 38 describes in detail the various functions to be performed during cardiopulumonary resuscitation. In many cases, many categories of allied health personnel are better trained in actual procedures such as intubation and ventricular defibrillation than is the average physician. If this is so, and hospital policy allows it, allied health personnel should be permitted to perform these procedures in the absence of someone more qualified.

Whenever a physician is in the hospital, he should not assume, however, that the director of respiratory therapy or "someone else" will be the first to respond to the STAT call, and he himself should hasten to the area to see if he can assist. Indeed, there is often a hospital policy that requires any physician who is a member of the hospital staff or who has admitting privileges to respond to such emergencies when he is in the hospital. Therefore, *all* physicians should be knowledgeable in the current techniques of resuscitation. As is mentioned in Chapter 38, "Cardiopulmonary Resuscitation," a "stat team" should be formed in every hospital and specific responsibilities for the resuscitation procedure assigned.

COMMUNICATION

With the increasingly large number of health professionals involved in the delivery of respiratory care, all-important communication between these groups can be achieved to some extent by staff meetings, patient care conferences, and in-service education. The most important communication of all, however, is that which centers around the patient. "Walking rounds" should be considered by all involved. Here the patient's care is discussed daily with nurses, therapists, and physicians, and responsibilities are assigned. This is ideal, however, and is not possible in every setting. It certainly should be carried out in the intensive care unit, where vigorous respiratory care is being performed. It is not always necessary that the attending physician make all such rounds, although obviously the responsible physician should communicate with other team members at the patient's bedside at least once a day. My colleagues have found joint nursing and respiratory rounds at shift-change time to be particularly beneficial; although physicians do not participate in such rounds, their interests are not overlooked, and the exchange of ideas often results in a timely telephone call to the physician in charge.

It is the physician's responsibility to provide the patient with competent medical diagnosis and therapy. Until a physician becomes available, the nurse, whose training is generally broader than that of the therapist, should assess and manage the patient's overall care. In life-threatening situations, the person best qualified by education and training may assume the responsibilities of any member of the health care team, *including those of the physician*, in the physician's absence.

Efficient distribution of responsibilities can be accomplished if certain essential steps are taken. A basic step toward this goal is continuing joint education for all members of the team. JCAH standards mandate an ongoing program of theoretical as well as practical, formal as well as informal, instruction, including frequent physician–nurse–therapist team conferences where diagnostic and therapeutic problem cases are discussed by the health professionals involved. These sessions will help shape attitudes, reinforce motivations, allow better interpersonal relationships, and result in improved use of individual skills and in better patient care.

THE PHYSICIAN AND THE PULMONARY LABORATORY

Most hospitals that claim to be competent in caring for the respiratory patient now have either on the premises or in proximity to them a pulmonary physiology laboratory for complete and thorough evaluation of respiratory illnesses. Such laboratories are usually under the direction of physicians skilled in pulmonary testing procedures. Despite the availability of computers that are now sophisticated enough to enable provisional interpretation of much of the test data, a physician is needed to direct the overall medical and quality control aspects of the laboratory's function.[1]

As in the overall direction of respiratory therapy departments, the "committee approach" to quality control in the pulmonary laboratory is far from satisfactory. One person may, and often does, supervise both departments; if so, this is a full-time responsibility in general hospitals with more than 300 beds. The function of the physician–director of the pulmonary laboratory includes quality control and interpretation of the tests done, qualification of personnel, setting of appropriate charges, and policy and procedure determinations with hospital administration. Ideally, the director will be able to ascertain which patients require formal consultative evaluation to complement the physiological assessment. Pulmonary function testing alone does not provide specific diagnosis, but the data can be correlated with clinical and other laboratory findings to provide a comprehensive evaluation of the patient's problems: In complex cases, a pulmonary specialist is best suited to provide a total analysis and care plan.

Early in the development of a pulmonary laboratory, much of the medical director's time is devoted to quality-control aspects of the operation. Later, spot checks of various test procedures will usually suffice. The quality control technique that exists by comparing the physiological data with the patient's condition should not be underestimated. Venous blood, for instance, may be inadvertently sampled and appropriately analyzed but will not reflect the patient's need, or lack of need, for supplemental oxygen. For this reason it is advisable, if possible, for the physician in charge of the laboratory to be involved actively in the care of patients on the respiratory disease service of the hospital. Whether this is done as part of his routine work or as an additional consultative service depends on factors such as the complexity of the illness and the time required for the physician to help optimize the patient's management.

THE MEDICAL DIRECTOR OF RESPIRATORY CARE SERVICES

Convention, practicality, and, recently, JCAH standards have dictated that involved medical input is needed in all hospital departments concerned with specialized diagnostic and therapeutic procedures. Nursing services have established the general practice of functioning without direct physician control, although certain specialized nursing areas (such as coronary care and hemodialysis units) may be directed by a physician who has ultimate control over all personnel assigned to the unit.

When respiratory therapists and technicians (then called inhalation therapy technicians or "oxygen tank pushers") first began to appear in the hospital hierarchy, they were often under the direction of the nursing service. The distinctive qualities of today's respiratory therapists, however, in terms of education, mechanical aptitudes, and close working relationships with specialized physicians have resulted in an almost universal separation of respiratory care departments from nursing services.

Although the need for medical direction was long apparent and required by groups such as the American Association for Respiratory Therapy, it only became essential to the hospitals when the JCAH issued standards for respiratory care services in late 1973. Standard I directly and II and III indirectly require competent and involved medical direction, a requirement now being enforced.

Another reason for competent medical direction may be found in the nonuniform training of physicians who routinely order respiratory care services. Still another reason lies in the nonhomogeneous training of the respiratory therapy work force itself. Although the various accreditation bodies (see Chap. 2) are now bringing more uniformity into the training and skills background of the entering workers, there is still a broad spectrum of abilities among those involved. It is one of the duties of the medical director, in cooperation with the technical director, to define such skills and abilities and to deploy the workers in his department efficiently.

Hospital malpractice considerations also require medical scrutiny of respiratory therapy services by periodic audit, particularly because in most states respiratory therapists and technicians are unlicensed by state regulatory bodies (*see* Chap. 5). Coordination of these quality-assurance processes is the direct responsibility of the medical director of respiratory care services.

1983 JCAH STANDARDS PERTINENT TO MEDICAL DIRECTION FOR RESPIRATORY CARE SERVICES

Standard I, in its interpretation, states

> The relationship of the respiratory care department/service to other units and departments of the hospital shall be specified within the overall hospital organizational plan. The responsibility and accountability of the respiratory care department/service to the medical staff and hospital administration shall be defined.

Knowledgeable and interested physician members of the hospital staff should clearly identify the objectives of respiratory care. Input into the objective-setting process should also come from senior members of the respiratory therapy staff. Although a committee may formulate such objectives, a staff physician with appropriate training and knowledge in respiratory diseases must be responsible for assurance that the objectives of the respiratory care service are met.

Further, Standard I, in its interpretation, states,

> Medical direction of the respiratory care department/service shall be provided by a physician member of the active medical staff who has special interest and knowledge in the diagnosis, treatment, and assessment of respiratory problems. Whenever possible, this physician should be qualified by special training and/or experience in the management of acute and chronic respiratory problems. The physician director shall designate a qualified physician member of the active medical staff to act in his absence. The physician director or his qualified designee shall be available to provide any required respiratory care consultation, particularly on patients receiving continuous ventilatory or oxygenation support. The physician director shall have the authority and responsibility for assuring that established policies are carried out; that overall direction in the provision of respiratory care services in the inpatient, ambulatory care, and home care settings is provided; and that a review and evaluation of the quality, safety, and appropriateness of respiratory care services is performed.

Again, in another section of the interpretation of Standard I, we read that

> Respiratory care services shall be provided by a sufficient number of qualified personnel under *competent medial direction* [italics mine].

The implication is that the staff should be adequate in number and in competence to carry out all orders for respiratory therapy prescribed by the physician. Further, the lines of authority are clearly established in the interpretation, including the concept that the medical director should participate in the appointment of a technical director who will assume responsibility for the various functions of the department.

All these considerations and the uncertainty regarding the current legal status of the respiratory technologist necessitate the professional availability of, and direction by, a medical director who has ultimate responsibility for the activities of the technical staff of his department. This state of affairs is likely to persist regardless of the professional pathway over which respiratory care services may evolve; even the emergence of a "respiratory physician's assistant" will not change these fundamental relationships. Respiratory training, extensive as it may be, cannot be regarded as a shortcut into the practice of medicine by even the best trained and most experienced respiratory therapist. Although he may be degreed, licensed, registered, certified, or otherwise endowed with authority, he will not be a physician unless he has a doctorate in medicine.

Buried in the now-mandated concept of medical direction is the old role of the physician as *medical advisor*. The physician's role as advisor to the respiratory care team should not be forgotten; it was, and is, a viable means for improving patient care. Such advice may, and should, be requested by all members of the respiratory care team in such matters as individual patient problems, interpersonal problems, equipment purchase, or departmental policy.

QUALIFICATIONS OF THE MEDICAL DIRECTOR

As has been mentioned, the medical director should have a comprehensive background in respiratory pathophysiology and critical care medicine. Usually he will be a Board-certified or -eligible internist or anesthesiologist; often he will have subspecialty training in pulmonary disease. Egan has discussed the relative merits of one type of medical specialist over another.[5] Whatever his training background, the medical director should have ability and experience in teaching, cost accounting, inventory, budgeting, and administration. He will be a consultant on intensive care techniques and procedures. In some settings he may have a research background or a background in computer application.

Foremost, he must be an *interested* physician, willing to assume the responsibility given him by the medical staff. In addition to the knowledge, skills, and technical background that are basic requirements, perhaps the most outstanding personality characteristic of the medical director is that of enthusiasm and dedication to the overall operation of the program. He must have *time* to devote to the development, education, and maintenance of the team. The amount of time needed for these activities is extremely variable, as will be discussed later. Experience has shown that such direction cannot be delegated to a committee of the medical staff, although the medical director may delegate various selected responsibilities to qualified persons in his department.

FUNCTIONS OF THE MEDICAL DIRECTOR

General functions of the medical director as described in the JCAH standards are now becoming accepted as common practice. The general functions of the medical director are largely educative in nature.

1. He must provide a knowledgeable medical perspective of good practices in respiratory therapy and be responsible for the introduction and regulation of such practices for the benefit of patients. He may fulfill this function by providing in-service education, by one-to-one discussions with the respiratory care team, or, most important, by precept in the care of his own patients. To be able to introduce new practices that may benefit patients, he must be abreast of current developments in the field. He must be continually aware of the total hospitalized respiratory patient population at any given time to be able to bring these new procedures to bear orderly and uniformly. In addition, his role as an educator may become an extremely demanding one. Apart from organizing an ongoing (usually weekly) in-service educational program for respiratory therapists, he often will be required to provide periodic seminars or symposia for other members of the health care team. There is an ever-increasing need for medical directors to participate in respiratory therapy training programs in the community, and it may be desirable for the interested physician to assume a formal role as an educator in a local junior college program. Most medical directors who are strongly committed to their role will also participate in various professional educational meetings for therapists, physicians, and others, and additional committee work inside and outside the hospital may make further inroads into his time.
2. He must provide overall supervisory control of the respiratory care department as the JCAH standards state. He may delegate some of this responsibility to the technical director, but the ultimate responsibility for operating the department must be his. Accordingly, he must participate in many, if not most, of the executive decisions, particularly in the hiring and firing of key personnel. He also takes part in developing policies and procedures of the department. Another specific duty of the medical director is to develop procedure manuals and treatment protocols. Such manuals are required by accrediting agencies and serve a real, although often unused, function in day-to-day practice.
3. He must relate to the medical staff as a specialist in respiratory care. This is a professional task that must be approached with great delicacy: Many older physicians, for example, resent the intrusion of a brash young "know-it-all" who brings with him an armamentarium of machinery entirely foreign to their way of practice. In this critical area the medical director's public relations skills will be tested. If an individual physician orders unusual or unclear forms of therapy not in the procedure manual, the department employees should bring this to the attention of the medical director before giving treatment. Whenever possible, the medical director must not be arbitrary in his decision-making; yet at the same time he bears responsibility to the other staff and administration for aberrant or outmoded practices by his colleagues. The obvious basis of intelligent, even-handed performance in this area is a thorough knowledge of the procedures and techniques of respiratory care. Again, some degree of direct patient involve-

ment by the medical director is necessary if he is to fulfill this function adequately.

4. The medical director must relate to the hospital administration as the ultimate authority in the application and future practice of respiratory care in the medical facility in which he functions. He needs a sense of great prescience, in concert with his technical director, to be able to foresee the needs of an expanding department. Departments today are widening the scope of their activities, reaching into such areas as intensive care units, emergency care, pulmonary rehabilitation, hyperbaric oxygen therapy, home care services, and the development of contract services in nearby hospitals.
5. Because he is often the most knowledgeable local resource on pulmonary conditions, the medical director has a general responsibility to the *community* served by the hospital. He must educate various groups in preventive medicine (conditions such as those caused by smoking, industrial exposure to toxic inhalants, and air pollution) and must be willing to explain the hospital's function in the care of the respiratory patient to the community at large when called on to do so. In this function, he enhances the hospital image as well as that of his own department.

Although many of these duties in their fine detail can appropriately be delegated to the chief therapist, the medical director's role as an overseer is necessary. In summary, little about the day-to-day operation of a department under good medical direction should be surprising to the medical director. He should know the skills and limitations as well as the day-to-day work problems of his employees; he should be aware of all respiratory care activities in the hospital; he should be aware of the limitations and expertise of the medical staff; he should be alert to the role that his department plays in the overall operation of the hospital; and he should play a part in relating the hospital's role in respiratory care and concern to the community at large.

DIRECT PATIENT CARE BY THE MEDICAL DIRECTOR

The medical director may become directly involved in the care of patients through informal consultation or formal requested consultation. My preference is the former because many more patients can be cared for in this manner. All patients on continuous ventilator support need some review by the medical director unless they are under the care of physicians who have special skills in respiratory care. An audit of patients on ventilator support will quickly reveal the need, or lack of necessity, for the medical director's involvement in this arena.

Because of these responsibilities to the medical and patient community, departmental coverage in the absence of the medical director is mandated by the JCAH in Standard I, which states that "a qualified physician member of the active staff [must] act for him in his absence." Although no job can demand 168-hour-a-week availability, the medical director does have that responsibility 52 weeks a year. Malpractice considerations discussed in Chapter 5 further dictate that the medical director clarify the nature of his departmental coverage with the hospital administration, and that adequate provision be made for continuous medical coverage of the respiratory therapy service.

REMUNERATION

Generally, a yearly stipend should be paid to the medical director for the activities described above. Situations in which a percentage of gross departmental income is paid to the medical director are not generally satisfactory and lend themselves to accusations of "feathering one's own nest." Recent legislation will probably clarify the nature and extent of such remuneration.

DUTIES OF THE MEDICAL DIRECTOR IN FORMAL SCHOOLS OF RESPIRATORY THERAPY

The need for medical direction in respiratory therapy educational programs has been reviewed in detail in Chapter 2. The position of the medical director is most critical to the operation of an approved school of respiratory therapy. The most common reason for failure of schools to pass review by the Joint Review Committee on Respiratory Therapy Education (JRCRTE) is inadequate medical input by the program's medical director and other physicians at either the primary or affiliated institutions. The designated medical director of the program is the medical executive officer, who must take full responsibility for the scientific content and clinical operation of the program. He will need the help of an advisory committee in this regard, but he is responsible for the quality of instruction given by physicians, therapists, technicians, and other persons in all courses that have medical content. His detailed responsibilities are outlined in the "Essentials" of the JRCRTE.[6]

REFERENCES

1. ATS Respiratory Care Committee: Position paper—director of the pulmonary function laboratory. ATS News 4:6, 1978
2. Beck GJ et al: Physician and nurse responsibilities on the respiratory care team. Am Rev Respir Dis 108:392, 1973
3. Burton GG: The respiratory therapist as a behavioral change agent: Modification of physician activity as a social science. Educational Module, California College of Respiratory Therapy, 1810 State Street, San Diego, CA 92101
4. Chusid EL: Respiratory therapy education for the pulmonary physician trainee. Cardiopulmonary Med 20:26, 1981
5. Egan DF: Fundamentals of Respiratory Therapy, 2nd ed, pp 462–463. St Louis, CV Mosby, 1973
6. Essentials of an Approved Educational Program for the Respiratory Therapy Technician and the Respiratory Therapist. Chicago, Council on Allied Health Education, American Medical Association, 1977 (current revision in progress)
7. Yanda RL: Quality control of inhalation therapy. Chest 66:61, 1974

BIBLIOGRAPHY

Newsletters, National Association of Medical Directors of Respiratory Care (NAMDRC), P.O. Box 10832, Chicago, IL 60610. This association, founded in 1978, addresses itself to the peculiar needs of medical directors of respiratory care.

Shapiro AG, Kernaghan SG: JCAH standards—learn to use the tool. Hospitals 48:100, 1974. A lucid interpretation of valuable guidelines.

Yanda RL: The need for leadership in hospital respiratory services. Chest 68:81, 1975. The need for managerial skills in the control of respiratory services is illustrated by a series of interesting case reports. Methods of remuneration are also discussed.

Yanda RL: The Management of Respiratory Care Services. New York, Projects in Health, 1976

5

Legal Implications of Respiratory Care

Thomas J. DeKornfeld

The changing patterns in medical practice in the United States, the long overdue and increasing concern with the protection of the consumer (patient), and the increasing number of litigations in the health field make it not only desirable but necessary to include a chapter on medicolegal problems in a textbook on respiratory care. The rapid expansion of the scope and complexity of respiratory care is coupled with the ever-increasing level of educational requirements for the respiratory therapy technologist and for the respiratory care unit nurse. It is becoming apparent that the respiratory therapy technologist, and particularly the registered therapist, is expected to function in many hospitals as a highly specialized "physician's assistant" in the care of the respiratory patient. This changing relationship brings increased responsibilities to the technologist, particularly in view of the fact that the respiratory therapy technologist, at this time, in most states has no standing in law as a licensed health professional. The respiratory therapy technologist is probably the only unlicensed allied medical professional whose activities include not only the application of sophisticated equipment directly to the patient but also the compounding and dispensing of drugs and whose activities, if improperly applied, may significantly contribute to patient morbidity and even patient mortality. No other unlicensed allied health practitioner has this level of potential for causing injury to patients, and therefore no other allied health professional should be more informed about the medicolegal implications of their activities for themselves, for the physician under whose supervision they function, and for the hospital by which they are employed.

In recent years, the traditional role of the nurse has undergone significant changes. A general dissatisfaction with the underuse of the skills and knowledge of the nurse led to a drive for an expanded role that has now become a reality and constitutes a major improvement in the delivery of highly sophisticated health care. The "nurse practitioner" and the "clinical nurse specialist" are being given an opportunity to participate much more actively in the diagnostic and therapeutic aspects of patient care, and, indeed, a number of activities previously considered to be physicians' prerogatives have been transferred to these specially trained nurses. The first major area of such high level specialization was in the coronary care units. It was with some initial reluctance but subsequent admiration that the medical profession has recognized the ability of the nurse to function well beyond the archaic limitations imposed by tradition and by the general conservatism of physicians. The development of intensive medical and surgical care units and, particularly, the introduction of respiratory care units have led to increased use of the nurse in such expanded roles. Although the training and roles of the respiratory therapist and the respiratory care nurse obviously are different, and the legal position of the nurse is somewhat different from the respiratory therapy technologist by virtue of the nurse practice acts and licensing regulations, the general concepts of this chapter apply to both groups in most areas of activity.

Any discussion of the legal problems of respiratory care therefore must include a careful review of relationships between the health practitioners and the hospital, and also the legal relationships of the members of the health care team to each other. It is also of importance to review state and federal legislation on health care and the most important recent court decisions dealing with the health team.

In addition, a brief discussion of the anatomy of the liability (malpractice) suit should be pertinent. The best ways of avoiding medicolegal entanglements will be presented. Finally, the legal implications of employment will be discussed to clarify some common misconceptions about the responsibilities of employers and employees toward each other. In this context, a brief discussion of collective bargaining, its advantages and problems, seems appropriate.

In much of the following discussion, the legal role of the physician is emphasized because, under our present system of health care delivery, the physician is still the primary *contractor*, and most other health care practitioners function as *"assistants"* or *"legal servants"* of the physician or as *employees* of the hospital. There are, of course, exceptions to this, and some nurses and other health practitioners, including respiratory therapy technologists, function as independent contractors.

The purpose of clarifying the legal role and responsibilities of the physician in some detail is to place the functioning of most nurses and respiratory therapy technologists in the proper perspective and to assist these groups to better understand the legal constraints under which physicians function.

One of the great attractions of legal matters is the precision of terms and the clarity and logic of the legislative and judicial process. In this era of rapid change in the social and scientific structure of our life, language becomes one of the variables, and words change their meaning with distressing frequency and at a rapidly accelerating rate. The almost continuous harping on "communications" and the attribution of many of the world's ills to a lack of communication can be explained partly by the regrettable tendency to use terms incorrectly and by the lamentable lack of precision of language. The legal profession is one of the few learned fields where words have a specific meaning, and it is therefore appropriate that a glossary of terms be presented at the end of the chapter.

LEGAL RELATIONSHIPS

PHYSICIAN–PATIENT RELATIONSHIP

The physician–patient relationship is the basis of all medical practice. Any time an individual contacts a physician and the physician agrees to provide a service to that person, a legal relationship is established that cannot be dissolved by the physician unilaterally or without certain clearly defined conditions. This does not mean that in the first instance the physician must "accept" every patient. In fact, the physician is quite at liberty not to accept any patient, and no reason need be given for such a refusal to establish a physician–patient relationship. Even under emergency conditions, no legal requirement forces a physician to render a service if the physician chooses not to do so. There are some exceptions to this rule: A physician employed by a hospital to provide medical services in the emergency room or a "walk-in clinic" does not have this option and must render appropriate services to all patients who come to the emergency room or clinic. Similar principles apply to all employed physicians whose conditions of employment imply or indeed specify that they must render services to certain groups of hospitalized patients or to certain groups of outpatients or employees who have individual or collective contractual arrangements for such services. Physicians working in public institutions may not refuse any patient in violation of constitutional or statutory mandate.

Obvious ethical considerations make it grossly improper for a physician to refuse his services to a patient in need, but no legal constraints force him to do so. As soon, however, as the physician even indicates a willingness to see a patient or listen to a complaint, a legal relationship has been established. The physician is now legally responsible to act with due care and provide this patient with the proper information or services appropriate to the situation. To encourage physicians to render emergency care to accident victims, many states have enacted "Good Samaritan" laws that grant immunity to physicians and occasionally to nurses from prosecution for ordinary negligence, provided the health care practitioner has acted in good faith and the deviation from the standard of care was not capricious. Actually this matter is primarily academic since there has been no successful litigation arising from first aid rendered to accident victims. Further, the existence of Good Samaritan laws will not make those physicians stop at the site of an accident who would not have stopped in the absence of such legislation.

Generally the physician–patient relationship can exist under one of two legal theories. Under the *contract theory,* a direct or implied contract exists between the two parties. The physician agrees to provide a service for a fee. This theory is not a very good one because it applies poorly to emergency situations, when the patient is unconscious, or to situations when the service is rendered without the expectation of a direct fee. The second theory, more appealing both legally and emotionally, holds that accepting a patient creates a *professional relationship* in which the physician accepts the responsibility for rendering due care. This professional relationship, legally, falls under the *law of tort,* and, indeed, courts generally view the physician–patient relationship in this light. A contract exists primarily if the physician promises certain results or if, indeed, a written agreement exists between the health care provider and the health care consumer.

Personal contact is not necessary for establishing a professional relationship. A telephone consultation is sufficient, and, for instance, a radiologist viewing x-ray films or a pathologist examining a surgical specimen has a professional relationship with the patient and owes the patient due care as a professional obligation, although his duty to report the findings need not include a direct report to the patient.

This relationship will remain in effect until either the patient chooses to select a different physician or the physician withdraws from the case or the course of care is ended by discharge or death. The physician can withdraw only if he becomes physically or emotionally disabled, leaves the practice of medicine, or believes that he is no longer able to provide care for the patient and there is another physician who is able and willing to assume responsibility for the patient's care. If the physician unilaterally decides to discontinue medical care of the patient without adequate and appropriate provision for replacement and this results in injury to the patient, it constitutes *abandonment* and can serve as the basis for *action* on the part of the patient. The fact that a patient does not follow the physician's instructions may constitute adequate reason for a physician to withdraw from the care of the patient, but only provided that reasonable notice is given, there is an equally competent replacement available, and the patient understands and agrees.

Thus the first component of the physician–patient relationship is that the relationship has, in fact, been established. Secondly, the physician must use *reasonable skill and care* in providing his services. This is the fundamental consideration of health care and probably the most difficult one to define or quantify. No physician or other health care provider is expected to function perfectly or even consistently above the average. The general standard, however, to which all health care providers must conform has been nicely stated by the court in *Blair* v. *Eblen:*[1]

> A physician is under a duty to use that degree of skill which is expected of a reasonably competent practitioner in the same class to which he belongs, acting in the same or similar circumstances.

This definition does not exclude the honest difference of opinion quite common in health care. If there are two or more options by which a condition can be diagnosed or treated, any one of these options can be chosen provided that at least a respectable minority of the profession supports that choice. Even if, in retrospect, another option may have been better, the *standard* has not been violated if the choice was "reasonable."

The profession generally has no written standards and has been reluctant to establish such. For this reason, deviations from the standard have to be determined by the *jury.* Since the jury probably has inadequate knowledge to make such decisions, expert testimony is required to educate the jury by explaining the medical facts and by giving testimony on the standards of care. In the past, these standards of care had to conform to the standards of the community and to the level of care appropriate to the training and experience of the physician who provided the care. Recently the "*locality rule*" has been rejected by some courts, and several decisions have been rendered which indicate that, at least for medical specialists, standards of care reflect national rather than regional or local standards.

In Michigan, the case of *Naccarato* v. *Grob*[15] established that, among specialists, local customs were no longer an acceptable yardstick for standards of care. This case deals with the failure of a board-certified pediatrician to administer a phenylketonuria (PKU) test to a newborn child. Although three Detroit pediaticians testified that PKU tests were not performed regularly at that time in the Detroit area, two nationally recognized experts held that knowledge about PKU testing in 1960 was widely disseminated in the literature and that ". . . a practicing board certified pediatrician . . . should have included a test for phenylketonuria."

In reversing an appeal court decision in favor of the defendants, Mr. Justice Kavanagh of the Michigan Supreme Court opined that

> It is unnecessary to consider in this opinion whether a standard of parochial negligence can obviate the requirement of reasonable care by a local practitioner.

And further,

> The reliance of the public upon the skills of a specialist and the wealth and sources of his knowledge are not limited to the geographic area in which he practices . . . .

The standard of care for a specialist should be that of a reasonable specialist practicing medicine in the light of present-day scientific knowledge. Therefore, geographic conditions or circumstances control neither the standard of specialist's care nor the competence of an expert's testimony. Subsequently the Michigan legislature codified the rule by saying that experts had national standards but generalists had local standards.

Most recently some courts have swung back toward a more rigid interpretation of the locality rule and require either that the expert be thoroughly familiar with the community where the alleged negligence has taken place or that he practice in the same or a similar community. A 1975 Tennessee statute requires that the expert

> . . . be licensed to practice in the state or a continuous bordering state . . . and had practiced this profession or speciality in one of those states during the year preceding the date that the alleged injury or wrongful act occurred.[22]

This retrogressive step is regrettable because it will be difficult for plaintiffs to secure competent expert testimony on their behalf.

A third component of the physician–patient relationship is that the patient must give free and informed *consent* to any and all procedures and to all diagnostic and therapeutic manipulations. The necessary components of consent are that it must be free, that it must be informed, and that the patient must be legally able to grant the consent.

The freedom of consent principle applies primarily, although not exclusively, to experimental work and was first formulated in the *Nuremberg Declaration*, following World War II, as a consequence of the experimentation performed on prisoners in German concentration camps. More recently in the United States serious questions have been raised about the freedom of consent of prisoners in penal institutions to "volunteer" for medical experimentation. Under ordinary circumstances the freedom of consent has pertinence in children or in those adults mentally or physically unable to give consent. In these situations, the legally responsible parent or guardian can give consent, but, under current use, the child or adult for whom the consent was given may try to contest it after he becomes of age or is otherwise legally competent to grant consent.

In the case of life-threatening emergencies when consent cannot be obtained, physicians may proceed with life-saving measures. Courts have decided that this is entirely proper in those situations where it can be reasonably assumed that the patient would have given consent had he been able to do so.

The problem of *"informed" consent* is considerably more complicated. Obviously a patient is entitled to the opportunity to make an intelligent choice between treatment and no treatment or between two different types of treatment, but this is not accomplished easily in a substantial percentage of all cases. It is impossible to detail all the possible complications that might ensue from the administration of a drug or from a surgical or medical procedure, and the law does not require this. Nevertheless, all health care deliverers must make a reasonable effort to explain in lay language the major hazards of any drug or treatment to which a patient is going to be exposed. In addition, a patient must be given the opportunity to ask questions or seek advice from an outside source. No patient should ever be misled, and serious hazards, if known, should always be explained in as much detail as is needed to enable the patient to make a choice or at least to understand the hazards to which he will be subjected. Any procedure undertaken without consent technically constitutes *assault* for which the patient can claim legal recourse. This may include even such relatively harmless procedures as oxygen administration, humidity therapy, or intermittent positive pressure breathing.

I know of no case where a respiratory therapist or nurse was held liable for "assault" for any procedure performed under a physician's order. Nevertheless, before any "treatment" is given it is very important that the patient understands what the treatment is, its purpose, its risks, the availability of reasonable alternatives, and the benefits that should be derived from it. Any questions must be answered, and, if the patient refuses the treatment, under no circumstances should it be administered. It is the patient's absolute and unquestionable privilege to refuse a diagnostic or therapeutic procedure, and even if consent is obtained the patient has the right to withdraw such consent at any time and without having to state any reason for so doing. If a patient refuses consent, the possible hazards of this decision must also be explained. The recent decision in *Truman* v. *Thomas*[23] concludes that

> If a patient indicates that he or she is going to refuse a risk-free test or treatment, then the doctor has the additional duty of advising of all material risks of which a reasonable person would want to be informed before deciding not to undergo the procedure.

In most instances, patients grant *"implied consent"* by not questioning or objecting to any procedure performed in the routine management of their problem, but all health practitioners must be fully aware of the patients' rights in these matters and must be very sure that these rights are not violated.

This free and informed consent should have documentary evidence. The consent form should be signed by the patient, by the person obtaining the consent, and, if possible, by a witness not involved directly in that patient's care. The simple, all-inclusive consent form that patients used to sign at admission and that gave "permission" to a physician to do anything and everything is no longer considered sufficient. The consent form must specify the diagnostic or therapeutic manipulation to which the patient consents and should have a space for the likely complications, particularly if these complications are serious, disfiguring, disabling, or life-threatening.

A special problem in the general field of consent is the "right to die," an issue that has received increasing attention in recent years but that still remains somewhat unresolved. Many thoughtful physicians agree that patients should have the privilege of deciding when they no longer wish to have their life extended by extraordinary means. To die with dignity should be the prerogative of every human being, and one of the regrettable consequences of the improvement of our life support technology is that with respirators, pacemakers, and a whole panoply of drug and fluid therapy, we can postpone the inevitable by hours, days, weeks, or even months. Whether these enormously costly manipulations are justified when there is no hope for recovery is unfortunately not just a medical problem. Ethical and religious factors must also be considered, and it is not possible to promulgate specific rules that cover all these areas. Although the decision to "let somebody die" is no different in principle from the decision to prolong life, the average patient's desire to continue living and the family's usual desire to keep their relative alive tend to influence us in the direction of sacrificing the patient's dignity and the family's emotional and financial resources far beyond the reasonable limits set by charity and common sense. I should hope that the patient's "right to die" be considered most seriously and that, when so indicated, artificial support not be instituted or withdrawn, even though these two issues are quite different (*see* Chap. 3).

Without specific legislation on this matter, it is difficult to generalize about such an extremely sensitive area of health care. Nevertheless, certain basic principles have been generally accepted by the medical community and by consumers, including that life support, once started, should not be discontinued unless there is solid evidence of irreversible brain death and support for the proposed action by the next of kin. This was also the decision of the New Jersey court in the case of Karen Ann Quinlan.[10] In Massachusetts a court ruled quite differently in *Superintendent of Belchertown State School* v. *Saikewicz*.[21] The court opined that only a probate court could decide whether life-prolonging therapy could be withheld from an incompetent patient and that every such instance would have to be argued in court in an adversarial relationship. The Saikewicz decision was widely quoted and just as widely misunderstood. The court was careful to limit the decision to withholding life-prolonging therapy from the mentally incompetent.

In two other equally important decisions, the Massachusetts court ruled first in *Lane* v. *Candura*[11] that a competent patient had the right to refuse any life-saving and life-prolonging therapy regardless of what the physicians and the family had recommended or what an ordinary prudent person may or may not have done. In the second case involving *Shirley Dinnerstein*,[10] the court found that physicians had the right to write a "no code" or "do not resuscitate" order for a terminally ill, incompetent patient. The court in this case distinguished sharply between withholding from an incompetent patient life-prolonging therapy and writing a "no code" order on any patient. The matter was left to the discretion of the attending physician.

The situation is substantially more complex when considering the termination of life-support options. The New Jersey court, in the case of Quinlan, reached a clear conclusion for a patient who was irreversibly "brain dead." A number of other jurisdictions have reached similar conclusions, and it now appears reasonably safe to disconnect the respirator of patients who are demonstrably without any brain activity and where the chances for any recovery are negligible. The family in such a case has no legal standing, but prudent physicians will not "pull the plug" when there are obvious or highly probable strong objections from the family. The precise methodology whereby "brain death" is established may vary between institutions. A commonly followed pattern is the absence of any cortical activity on two successive electroencephalograms, 24 hours apart, provided that the patient is not severely hypothermic or suffering from an overdose of any CNS depressant drug. In many hospitals a panel of physicians, not directly involved in the care of the patient, is designated to provide consultation to the primary physician in making the appropriate determinations. If the patient is conscious and competent, he may demand that life support be discontinued. A recent Florida case involving Abe Perlmutter[10] has upheld this concept.

The only case where continued life support has been mandated by a court for a conscious, competent patient was in *Commissioner of Corrections* v. *Myers*,[4] where the Supreme Judicial Court of Massachusetts ruled that Myers, a prisoner in a penitentiary, could be forced to undergo continued renal dialysis against his wishes ". . . in the interest of upholding orderly prison administration." As indicated earlier, the problems of death and dying are not purely legal ones. Ethical and moral problems are discussed in Chapter 3.

A final legal aspect of the physician–patient relationship is the *confidentiality* of the information that the physician obtains. Everything a patient confides in his physician, everything that forms part of the patient's record must remain absolutely confidential and cannot be revealed without the patient's permission. This includes not only the physician's notes but also the nurses' notes, respiratory care notes, laboratory data, and all personal, technical, or other information that may be contained on the patient's chart. The observations made by the nurse or by the respiratory therapy technologist are just as much a part of the confidential legal document and must be handled with the same concern for confidentiality as the admission diagnosis, history, or physical finding.

From a practical viewpoint, all persons who may need information about the patient's care must have access to the record, including nurses, respiratory therapists, and others who participate in the patient's care. The rule of confidentiality is therefore extended to this group as well and must be respected strictly and without exception. It is an inexcusable breach of this rule to discuss a patient's problems in public, and even discussion among professionals should be limited to the nature of the problem without identification of the patient. Although it is common practice to discuss "an interesting case" with colleagues, unless this is done for the purposes of consultation or teaching and unless the patient's anonymity is preserved or his consent for disclosure is obtained, this is a breach of confidence that is actionable.

THE PATIENT–HOSPITAL RELATIONSHIP

Until recently, the relationship of the patient to the hospital was quite similar to that of a guest to a hotel. The hospital was obligated to provide a safe, salubrious environment, room and board, and the facilities and personnel necessary for a physician to practice his trade. The hospital was further obligated to provide safe and usable equipment and personnel who either participated with the physician in the care of the patient or who were responsible for the proper functioning of the building as a hotel and restaurant. The hospital did not have any responsibility for the quality of medical care being practiced in the facility although, traditionally, it participated with the medical staff in administrative decisions pertaining to practice privileges and to other similar items. Although the hospital employed and compensated the nurses and other health practitioners and was responsible for their actions, they were frequently held to be under the control of the physicians. It was the physician who was responsible for the employee's error under the *doctrine of the borrowed servant*.

Before *Darling* (see below), the hospital was liable only for harm to the patient caused by personnel, equipment, or circumstances under its control. This situation has now changed dramatically. The celebrated case of *Darling* v. *Charleston Community Hospital*[5] has established the principle, at least in Illinois, that the hospital, through its lay governing board, is responsible for the standards of medical care practiced in the hospital. This means that the hospital, as a corporate entity, may be held responsible if it permits the physicians on its staff to practice below acceptable standards and the hospital had the ability to prevent the harm. In other words, the hospital board of trustees must make sure that there is a suitable medical staff organization, that there are bylaws governing the activities of the medical staff, that the standards set by the Joint Commission for the Accreditation of Hospitals are met, and that the medical staff properly polices itself according to stated specific procedures. Although the Darling principle has been contested and the final word on the hospital's full responsibility toward the patients has not been determined, it is safe to assume, on the basis of several more recent decisions, that the hospital will continue to have a major role in making certain that the physicians and other practitioners it allows within its walls meet the appropriate standards of care.

The most important case since Darling on this matter has been *Gonzales v. Nork*,[8] which was decided by the California Supreme Court in 1978. This is a case in which the issue of the hospital's corporate responsibility was carefully investigated and in which Mr. Justice Goldberg, in a most convincing and literate opinion, states that

> the hospital by virtue of its custody of the patient, owes him a duty of care; this duty includes the obligation to protect him from acts of malpractice by his independently retained physician who is a member of the hospital staff, if the hospital knows, or has reason to know, or should have known that such acts were likely to occur.

Mr. Justice Goldberg awarded the plaintiff $2,000,000 in punitive damages and $1,710,447 in compensatory damages, the payment of which was to be divided between Mercy Hospital and Dr. Nork. Similar decisions against hospitals have been returned by courts in Arizona, Nevada, and Ohio.

THE PHYSICIAN–HOSPITAL RELATIONSHIP

In the United States, with few exceptions, all practicing physicians have some form of hospital affiliation that can take one of two basic forms: The physician may be employed by the hospital, or the physician may be granted practice privileges in the hospital without being in any way compensated by the hospital or in the hospital's employ. The former arrangement is still relatively rare, although the number of hospital-based and hospital-paid physicians is increasing steadily. In this system, physicians function legally as employees of the hospital, receive all or most of their compensation from the hospital, and perform specific tasks for the hospital that may be administrative, educational, patient care, or a combination of these. The full-time hospital-based physician must meet all the requirements for a regular staff position as stipulated by the bylaws of the hospital and of the medical staff organization.

In this situation, the source of professional incomes is either a salary from the hospital or a salary from an agency or organization that operates the hospital and employs the physician. An example of this latter situation is the federal or state government that employs physicians in the Armed Forces, Public Health Service, Veterans Administration, or other federal or state organizations. Certain nongovernmental organizations may also employ physicians who then perform all or most of their work in a hospital with which they have no financial relationship. Examples of this type of practice are the hospitals maintained by industrial or labor organizations and major prepaid hospital plans like the Kaiser-Permanente group in California and the proliferating health maintenance organizations (HMOs).

Another type of hospital-based practice is that of the full-time medical director of the respiratory care department, emergency room physicians, and medical director of intensive care units, among others.

The most common form of practice in the United States is still the private "fee-for-service" practice where the physician bills the patient for services rendered and where payment is made by the patient or by a third-party payer, (*i.e.*, an insurance company).

The legal situation differs depending on which of the above relationships exists between the physician and the hospital. If the physician is a full-time employee of the hospital, the relationship is simple and clear and the hospital is responsible for the action of the physician as long as he is performing his duties within the context of his employment. If the physician, however, is granted only "hospital privileges" (*i.e.*, he is admitted to the hospital staff and has the prerogative of admitting patients to the hospital and directing their care while in the hospital), the legal situation is much more complex.

Every hospital staff, comprising all the physicians with privileges in the hospital, traditionally establishes its own bylaws which are then approved by the hospital's governing body. These bylaws specify the categories of staff privileges and the conditions under which physicians are eligible for staff positions. In addition, the bylaws also establish the staff organization and deal with such matters as continuing education requirements, quality assurance, meetings, elections, and the steps for *due process* to be followed for admission to and dismissal from the staff.

The medical staff bylaws may also limit certain physicians, on the basis of training, to the performance of certain patient services. For instance, in a number of hospitals only trained obstetricians are permitted to perform forceps deliveries or cesarean sections, whereas family practitioners may perform uncomplicated manual deliveries. In others the care of patients who require ventilatory support may be limited only to those physicians trained and experienced in such activity (ventilator privileges). The bylaws may also specify the requirements for mandatory consultation. In one hospital, for example, no patient may be given continuous respirator care without the approval of a chest physician or an anesthesiologist.

Until the *Darling* decision, the hospital had no control over the physicians who enjoyed staff privileges in the hospital. As long as the physicians were willing to abide by the bylaws of the medical staff and maintained their license to practice medicine, the only controls over the quality of their practice were the elasticity of their conscience and the very mild peer-pressures exerted by their colleagues. The fear of a suit for negligence may also have contributed to the quality of care. It has certainly forced most practitioners to practice a more defensive type of medicine that may have benefited the patient's health but that most certainly has affected his pocketbook.

Changing attitudes toward the hospital's legal liability have made it imperative that the hospital's bylaws and medical staff regulations be carefully reviewed and conform with current practices. The steps for admission to the medical staff and particularly the disciplinary mechanisms whereby physicians can be corrected by their peers or can be dismissed from the staff must be specific and in accordance with due process. Highly desirable disciplinary measures have been frustrated when the physician or employee to be disciplined could show that due process had not been followed. In the 1970s concern for individual professional rights was allowed to outweigh the rights of society. Whether this is desirable or not is disputable.

The *Darling* and *Gonzales* decisions raise some particularly awkward problems not only for the formally constituted medical staff organizations of the hospital but also for all hospital employees, particularly nurses and respiratory therapists. The operative phrase in both the above cases was that ". . . the hospital knew or should have known . . ." that a physician was incompetent. The only way the hospital can know this is when somebody tells them. The implication is obvious: The hospital administration must establish quality assurance, credentials, and tissue committees and must make sure that these committees report regularly on any staff member who appears to violate the standards set for the institution; also, any employee who has information suggesting professional incompetence has the obligation to bring this matter to the attention of the hospital administration in a formal way—by an appropriate reporting mechanism. This may take various forms but is usually an "incident report" addressed to the hospital administration that outlines the alleged incident, identifies the persons involved, and, most important, identifies the person filing the report.

Thus the employees' duty is clear: They must report the negligent or incompetent physician even though this duty leaves them with a painful and potentially dangerous dilemma. Very few people enjoy "blowing the whistle" on a colleague, and the traditional relationship between physicians and nonphysicians makes it very difficult for the latter to "rat" on the former. Further, the suggestion of professional incompetence will have to be substantiated before the medical staff organization, and failure to do so may leave the complainant liable to disciplinary action, possible dismissal, and even legal action for damages. The decision to report or not to report observed deviations from the standard of care must therefore remain an individual decision. To report is an ethical and probably legal requirement, but one not without individual hazard; not to report is a "cop out" that may also have legal implications, since the withholding of such information may very well implicate the person as sharing in the responsibility for future damages. When does one "blow the whistle" on one's colleague, friend, or particularly on one's superior? It is an easy question to ask and an extremely difficult one to answer. Mr. Justice Goldberg has stated,

> As for the doctors on the Mercy Staff, two thoughts keep going through my mind. The one is from Dr. Jones (physician on the Mercy Staff), "No one told anyone anything." The other is from Edmund Burke (an 18th Century English politician), "The only thing necessary for the triumph of evil is for good men to do nothing."

THE PHYSICIAN–TECHNOLOGIST RELATIONSHIP

Under the bylaws of the American Association for Respiratory Therapy, the National Board of Respiratory Care, and, most recently, under the new standards published by the Joint Commission of Accreditation of Hospitals (January 1974), respiratory therapy technologists must work under competent medical supervision. Although there have been many unfortunate exceptions, this relationship between physician and technologist has generally been mutually beneficial, and the medical director concept has worked well whenever there was a concerned, competent physician to serve in this capacity.

The relationship between the technologist and the medical director or any other physician is composed of personal, professional, and legal elements. I shall discuss below only the legal elements of this relationship; the personal and professional relationships have been discussed in Chapter 3.

The legal relationship between a physician and a technologist depends largely on whether the technologist is employed by the physician. If an employer–employee relationship exists, then the legal liability that the physician has for the actions of the technologist is clear and well established in law. The doctrine of *respondeat superior* states that the "*master*" is responsible for all damages caused by the "*servant*." The terms master and servant, although not current in their social connotation, are still very much a feature of current legal practice. Nevertheless, to be liable for the actions of an employee, certain legal requirements must be met. It must be shown that the employee acted within the scope of his employment; that he was in fact negligent; and that this negligence was the proximate cause for the alleged injuries. Of these, the first one needs some additional comment.

A physician employer of a respiratory therapy technologist would not be responsible if the technologist drove a car under the influence of alcohol while on vacation and caused damage to person or property. This situation is clear, but in other instances a jury would have to decide the limits of liability. If, for example, a respiratory therapy technologist in the hospital administers IPPB therapy to a patient and at the end of treatment decides to adjust a surgical dressing or an orthopedic appliance, thereby causing some injury to the patient, this act is clearly outside the professional competence of the respiratory therapy technologist, does not form part of his usual and customary activities, and it would thus be a matter for a jury to decide whether the employer was responsible for this action of the employee.

Another delicate area in the physician-technologist relationship is the legal situation that arises when a technologist executes an order that is clearly improper and where the technologist, by virtue of his training, could or should have known that the order, if followed, was likely to lead to an injury to the patient. The classic example is the misplaced decimal point. Let us assume that the physician wishes to order 0.5 ml of Isuprel for an IPPB treatment, but, because of haste or carelessness, the order reads 5.0 ml. What is the responsibility of the technologist charged with delivering the treatment? Should he go ahead? Should he refuse to administer the potentially harmful dose, or should he arbitrarily change the dose to what he considers safe and appropriate? Few, if any, legal precedents give a clear answer in this dilemma in respiratory care.

In the relationship of the physician and the pharmacist, the situation is clear. If the pharmacist is instructed to fill a prescription that is clearly wrong, the pharmacist is obliged legally to check with the physician and not to dispense the medication. If he fails to do so and the patient suffers injury from the excessive dose, the pharmacist is held liable for damages.

In the case of the respiratory therapy technologist who is operating without a license and whose administration of drugs is questionable anyway, the situation is nebulous. If the technologist knowingly administers a dose that is clearly in excess of the usual and customary dose, he may be held responsible as the direct *tort feasor*, even though the primary responsibility is still the physician's who issued the incorrect order. I believe that, under the circumstances, the technologist has the duty to contact the responsible physician or, in his absence, the medical director of respiratory therapy and seek clarification or correction of the unusual order. The technologist should neither carry out nor willfully ignore or modify a physician's order without taking all necessary steps to have the situation clarified. I feel that carrying out an obviously dangerous and probably erroneous order places the technologist in legal jeopardy. Willfully ignoring or modifying an order without seeking competent advice may place the technologist in jeopardy as far as his employment is concerned. A technologist can certainly refuse to carry out any order but by so doing may leave himself open to severe and justifiable criticism if it should turn out that the order was indeed appropriate for that particular patient who suffered injury in consequence of the technologist's refusal to carry out the order. It may be prudent for the technical director and the medical director of each department of respiratory therapy to discuss this eventuality and to specify in the procedure manual of the department the method whereby such problems should be handled. Generally, it seems a wise policy to have technologists question all orders that they do not fully understand. With few exceptions, physicians will appreciate the opportunity to rectify an error or to explain the reason for orders that may appear unusual or excessive.

Human errors in writing orders will always occur despite all efforts to the contrary. Unfortunately, at present, too many physicians who write orders for respiratory therapy are inadequately trained in this field and therefore write orders that are incomplete, incorrect, or call for improper or unnecessary forms of therapy. The only way to improve this unfortunate situation is by improved physician education, by strengthening the role of the medical director of respiratory therapy, and by the increasingly stringent requirements of peer review, quality control, and the justification of all procedures in advance. Curiously enough, marked improvements in practice are being observed in many areas by the insistence of third-party payers on adequate justification and documentation of all procedures for which compensation is expected.

If the technologist is hired and paid by the hospital, the physician may still be liable under the doctrine of the *"borrowed servant."* This doctrine, which has been generally applied for many years, states that the physician who fully controls the activities of a hospital employee is responsible for the actions of this employee even though the physician did not hire the employee, may have no part in the employment process, and has no input into the job description or salary of the employee. The *"borrowed servant"* rule has its most general recognition in the *"captain of the ship"* concept. Courts have found that the surgeon in the operating room has the right to control the hospital employees in the performance of their duties and is thus liable for any injury caused by these hospital employees. The "captain of the ship" doctrine is a poor form of vicarious responsibility because there is reason to believe that the surgeon does not have the real power to control even though, perhaps, he may have the legal right to do so.

In the view of a prominent legal authority, the "captain of the ship" doctrine was introduced primarily to give the patients in charity hospitals an opportunity to obtain compensations for injuries.[19] Nonproprietary hospitals, until quite recently, were protected against suit by the so-called *charitable immunity concept,* which stated that charity hospitals could not be sued for damages because they had no funds other than those granted in trust and, therefore, even if found guilty had no resources from which to pay damages. Two important cases, *Moore v. Moyle*[14] and *Molitor v. Kaneland Community Unit District,*[13] effectively disposed of "charitable immunity," and in fact this argument was specifically dealt with in *Darling.* With the disappearance of the charitable immunity excuse, the "captain of the ship" doctrine will probably disappear also, except in those situations where the technologist clearly acts under the physician's control and supervision and where the *"borrowed servant"* doctrine may continue to operate.

Being held liable for injury caused by an employee or "borrowed servant" is not malpractice and should not be so considered. Although this may be small consolation to the insurance carrier, it avoids the professional or ethical stigma unavoidably attached to a physician found guilty of his own negligence.

Some additional implications of the general employer–employee relationship between physician employer and technologist employee will be discussed later in this chapter under "Legal Implications of Employment." Although rarely is the technologist directly employed by a physician, it occurs sufficiently enough to warrant discussion. Even though I shall discuss primarily the hospital as the employer, the same principles are valid in those cases where the employer is an individual physician, a group of physicians, or a service organization.

THE TECHNOLOGIST–HOSPITAL RELATIONSHIP

From the above, obviously there are two levels of relationship between a respiratory therapy technologist and the hospital in which he works and by which he is employed. One level relates to the professional activities of the technologist, and the other level relates simply and exclusively to the nonprofessional employer–employee interaction that is not different from the relationship of any employee to any employer.

Under current legal practice, the hospital, as a corporate entity, will be responsible for the technologist's negligence under *"respondeat superior,"* a responsibility that may or may not be shared by the nonemployer physician, as discussed above. It therefore behooves the hospital to insure, and insure adequately, against claims for damages because of the negligence of its employees. Whether technologists should carry their own liability insurance is a much debated issue. The argument in favor of employees carrying their own liability insurance is promoted primarily by insurance companies that collect the premiums and by employers who may, in some instances, decrease their financial liability by dividing the damages between two insurance carriers—their own and the employees. An additional argument in favor of employees having their own insurance is that at present the premiums are still relatively low, and employee peace of mind may be worth the expense.

The sole, but most effective, argument against the employee having his own insurance is simply that it is not necessary, since the employee is always protected under the "respondent superior" doctrine. In my opinion, the weight of these arguments is clearly against technologists carrying their own liability insurance unless they wish to do so as a favor to their employer, as a "sleep-aid," or as an "ego-stroke."

ANATOMY OF A MALPRACTICE SUIT

Physicians and other health professionals are considered in law the same as any other person. They are responsible for their actions, and, if their actions result in injury, the injured party may turn to the courts to obtain damages for the injury they have suffered. The basis of these suits is that the health professional was negligent in the performance of his duties.

The malpractice suit is a suit conducted under the general law of *negligence* against a professional. It is by far the most common but by no means the only reason a patient may start legal action against a health professional. Less common causes for legal action are *assault and battery, breach of contract, defamation, invasion of privacy*, and *fraud*. *Assault and battery* usually involves the problem of consent, whereas *breach of contract* almost invariably involves a guarantee by the health professional of a certain result that is not fulfilled. Fraud is a relatively rare cause for suit and must involve a deliberate misleading of the patient for monetary gain as, for example, unnecessary surgery or charges for services not performed. The elements of a suit for negligence will be discussed below, and the steps will be described that lead from the injury to the final disposition of the case.

If a patient believes that a health professional, in the performance of his duties, has caused an injury due to negligence, he may consult an attorney to start proceedings against the negligent party, the "tort feasor." There are, in most larger communities, attorneys who specialize in negligence cases, and these attorneys are usually referred to as the "plaintiff's bar." The usual practice among the plaintiff's bar is to accept such cases on a contingency fee basis, which means that the attorney's compensation will be derived from the damages awarded to the plaintiff at the termination of the action. The contingency fee is a percentage of the settlement or award usually determined by statute and may range from 25% to 50% depending on the size of the settlement or award. The contingency fee has been the subject of much criticism since the attorney is paid in proportion to the size of the settlement or award. The plaintiff's bar has been accused of claiming damages entirely out of proportion to the injury to increase their own share of the proceedings. Although some members of the plaintiff's bar may in fact be unethical, the contingency fee system does have distinct advantages for the potential defendant. The cost of preparing a suit for trial is very high, and the plaintiff's attorney will receive nothing for his time or expenses unless he can carry the case to a successful conclusion. In view of this, most attorneys will not accept a liability case unless they are reasonably certain that they will win it. Thus, while the contingency fee system tends to increase the size of the individual claims and may even increase the settlement and awards, it also tends to decrease the number of nuisance suits.

The contingency fee system has one other rather unfortunate effect: It makes it very difficult for a plaintiff with a minor, but very real, injury to recover damages. Since it costs $4000 to $5000 to prepare a case, most attorneys will not accept a case unless their share of the proceeds is in the range of several thousand dollars. Thus the plaintiff who has only a few hundred dollars worth of damages must depend on the generosity of the health professional or the hospital for recovery.

Once an attorney accepts the plaintiff as a client, the attorney is in complete charge of the proceedings. The first step is to attempt to obtain the pertinent hospital records; to do so, written authorization from the plaintiff is needed. If the hospital complies, a good attorney will submit the record to one or two physicians considered knowledgeable in the particular area for an opinion. If this opinion is favorable to the plaintiff, the attorney will proceed to file a "*complaint and (usually) demand for jury trial*" with the appropriate state trial court having jurisdiction in the area. If the experts' opinion was unfavorable to the plaintiff, responsible attorneys will so advise their client and will withdraw from the case. When the attorney is not able to obtain the record without a court order or if the time allowed to initiate action is about to expire, a complaint will be filed first and the records will then be procured by a mandate of the court.

The complaint must be detailed and should specifically state all the allegations made against the defendant. It must claim that injury has occurred, that the injury was due to negligence, and that the negligent act was the proximate cause for the injury. The complaint will also contain a number of subsidiary allegations attempting to include the hospital and any other physician or health professional who may have had anything to do with the case under litigation.

A very important consideration of the complaint is that action must be started within the time specified by the "*statute of limitations.*" Historically, in civil complaints, a specific time limit was established beyond which no action could be initiated. Thus if the patient did not start legal action within the time period allowed by the statute of that particular state from the time of injury, the physician or other tort feasor could no longer be held accountable. Recent court decisions have very significantly modified the "statute of limitations" concept as applied to medical malpractice, and, although the statute of limitation still refers to a specific period of years, the time when this period begins is no longer necessarily the time when the injury has originally occurred. In *Dyke v. Richard*,[6] the Supreme Court of Michigan has ruled that the statute of limitation begins

1. two years after time of last treatment;
2. when the patient discovers the alleged malpractice; or
3. when the patient should have discovered the alleged malpractice.

In another case ("*Cates v. Bald Estate*"[3]), the Michigan Court of Appeals further extended the time when the statute of limitation begins. In this case a needle was left in the patient during a hysterectomy performed in 1949. The patient knew that the needle had been left in her. She had numerous complaints and consulted a number of physicians during the years 1962 to 1969 only to be told to "forget about it" and "your trouble is nothing but nerves." Finally, in 1970, she went to a doctor who discovered the needle by himself and called in a surgeon, who removed the needle in April 1971.

In a court deposition, a psychiatrist stated that Mrs. Cates had been "programmed out" of taking any action "even though in the ordinary sense she knew" that something was wrong. On this basis the Appellate Court found that the statute of limitations had not expired, and reversed a lower court decision and remanded the case to the lower court for further proceedings.

The problem of statutes of limitation is different in the case of minors. If a minor suffers injury but his parents or guardian does not start any action for recovery of damages, the minor may do so in his own right within 1 year after he reaches legal age. Thus a physician may be sued 18 years after an alleged negligence that has occurred at the time of the claimant's birth.

This change in the interpretation of the statute of limitation places an extraordinary burden on the health care practitioner and on the insurance carrier. In fact, Justice Coleman, in a dissenting opinion in *Dyke v. Richard*, states:

> Public policy is poorly served by this decision which would leave open forever the possibility of suit for real or imagined injuries. Memory might dim, and witnesses be lost to the defense. Records would have to be maintained until the death of the doctor or later. . . . Our extension can be expected to serve Michigan poorly. It is anticipated that this "open season" on doctors and hospitals will further discourage the medical practitioner from coming to or remaining in this state, to the detriment of the public.

Not surprisingly an eminent attorney has felt free to state at a "Medicine and Law" symposium in 1974 that

> Probably the most nonsensical, unreasonable, and illogical legal decisions that have been rendered in recent years have related to the field of medical practice.[19]

Filing of a complaint consists of assigning it to a judge who has then an officer of the court deliver it to each of the defendants named in the complaint. The defendants must respond to the complaint in writing, within a specified period, and admit or deny the allegations made against them.

The next step may be that the plaintiff's attorney submits to the defendants a written "interrogatory"—that is, a series of specific questions on the matter at hand that the defendants must answer. In turn, the defendants have the right to submit interrogatories to the plaintiff. The purpose of this step is to acquaint both sides with the general direction that the plaintiff and defendant plan to pursue during the trial. In addition to the interrogatories, the plaintiff's attorney may take "depositions" from the defendants and from expert witnesses. These depositions are taken in the presence of a court reporter and are given under oath and in the presence of attorneys for both sides. Appropriate parts of the depositions may be introduced at the time of the trial in court subject to the court's ruling on their admissibility.

Expert witnesses may be granted the courtesy of giving their testimony in the form of a deposition—which may be in writing or on videotape—that is taken under oath in the presence of a court reporter.

At a deposition all questions must be answered, but, if challenged, the court will rule whether that particular part of the deposition may be presented to the jury.

There is considerable confusion on the role of expert witnesses in a negligence suit. Ordinarily, a witness in any trial is permitted to testify only to the facts of which he has direct and personal knowledge. He is not allowed to convey an opinion or refer to the experience or statements of other persons. The expert witness, however, is allowed to state opinions derived from his personal experience or knowledge of the field, and not necessarily his personal knowledge of the particular case at issue. In other words, the expert witness is permitted to interpret complex medical issues to a lay jury so that this jury may form an opinion as to the facts and render an informed judgment on guilt or innocence.

In fact, the most important role of the expert witness is to educate the jury on the basic medical (physiologic, psychologic/psychiatric, or pathologic) principles involved. A good trial attorney will use his "expert" in such a fashion that the lay jury will be able to make an intelligent decision based on the facts rather than on the reputation or credibility of the expert witness.

Expert testimony is not required in those cases in which the jury needs only common sense to arrive at a decision about the presence of negligence. If, for example, the surgeon operates on the wrong extremity or leaves a sponge in the abdominal cavity, the jury needs no expert to point out that this is not according to the expected standards of care. In the case of *Gary v. Wienstein*,[7] the court held that

> The absence of medical testimony disapproving the treatment or lack of it is not perforce fatal to the case. Many known and obvious facts in the realm of common knowledge speak for themselves, sometimes even louder than witnesses, expert or otherwise.

In such cases, the doctrine of "*res ipsa loquitur*" (the thing speaks for itself) is invoked, and the burden of proof is on the defendant to show that he has not acted negligently. All that the plaintiff must show is that the defendant or his servant was the direct cause of the injury and that without negligence the "accident" would not have happened. The "*res ipsa*" doctrine was established in 1863 in England in the celebrated case of *Byrne v. Boadle*.[2] This case is sufficiently important to be presented both for its content (declaration) and for its disposition.

> Declaration: For that the defendant, by his servants so negligently and unskillfully managed certain barrels of flour . . . that by and through the negligence of the defendant, by his said servants, one of the said barrels of flour fell upon and struck against the plaintiff, whereby the plaintiff was thrown down, wounded, lamed and permanently injured, to wit, thence hitherto, and incurred great expense for medical attendance, and was otherwise damnified.

On appeal from a verdict for defendant, the Court of the Exchequer ruled that

> There are certain cases of which it may be said, res ipsa loquitur, and this seems one of them.

Baron Pollock further stated that

> It is the duty of persons who keep barrels in a warehouse to take care that they do not roll out, and I think that such a case would, beyond all doubt afford prima facie evidence of negligence. A barrel could not roll out of a warehouse without some negligence and to say that a plaintiff who is injured by it, must call witnesses from the warehouse to prove negligence seems to be preposterous . . . The present case upon the evidence comes to this, a man is passing in front and there falls down upon him a barrel of flour. I think it apparent that the barrel was in the custody of the defendant . . . and who is responsible for the acts of his servants who had control of it; and in my opinion the fact of its falling is prima facie evidence of negligence and the plaintiff who was injured by it is not bound to show that it could not fall without negligence but if there are any facts inconsistent with negligence it is for the defendant to prove them.

This case, in addition to setting an extremely important legal precedent, also illustrates the "respondeat superior" doctrine very handsomely because clearly the owner of the warehouse is being held responsible for the injury and not the employees who were in charge of storing the barrels.

From a purely legalistic viewpoint, the "*res ipsa*" doctrine is actually contrary to the fundamental Anglo–Saxon concept of law where the plaintiff has to prove his case and the defendant is assumed to be innocent. Thus, courts are usually reluctant to shift the burden of proof of innocence to the defendant and will permit it only in limited situations. The simple fact that results of medical treament have been unsatisfactory to the plaintiff are insufficient cause for invoking "*res ipsa*." In some jurisdictions (e.g., Michigan and South Carolina), "res ipsa" cannot be invoked at all.

Many cases never proceed beyond the stage of depositions, and attorneys for the plaintiff may drop the case at this point, or attorneys for the defendants may decide to reach an "out of court" settlement.

If no settlement is reached, the suit is tried in court before a judge and jury. The mechanics of a jury trial vary slightly from one state to another, but the general outline is quite similar in all jurisdictions.

After the opening statements by counsel for the plaintiff and defendant, the plaintiff's witnesses are questioned by the plaintiff's attorney (direct examination) and by the defendant's attorney (cross-examination). The same procedure is followed in reverse for the defendant's witnesses. The concluding statements by the counsels follow, and then instructions to the jury by the judge. The judge is entirely impartial, and his instructions must be limited to the exposition of the law as it pertains to the specific case. The jury must then decide on the basis of the evidence whether negligence has been established and whether the negligence was the proximate cause of injury. The jury also sets the damages, which, at least theoretically, should bear some relation to the injury suffered by the plaintiff. Such items as cost of care, loss of earning capacity, education of minor children, pain and suffering, and support of parents are all considered. Unfortunately, the damages occasionally seem to bear little relation to the magnitude of injury or loss. Although most rational people agree that injured patients or the estate of the wrongfully dead should make suitable recovery, to use malpractice litigation to establish a major estate for future generations seems unreasonable and indefensible.

In civil suits, the judge has considerable authority to modify the amount of damages assessed by the jury. In fact, the judge may, if he so chooses, decrease the amount of damages or even assess only nominal damages if, in his opinion, the jury acted unreasonably and returned damages in excess of what could be considered reasonable and appropriate. If either side to the litigation is unhappy with the results, they may appeal to a higher tribunal. This appeal must be based on improper conduct of the trial or on improper interpretation of the law by the judge. It deals exclusively with matters of law and not with the interpretation of facts.

The foregoing is an overview of the anatomy of a malpractice suit and does not mention many of the legal or technical steps and options available to both plaintiff and defendant and which are beyond the scope of this chapter.

Recently an entirely new dimension was added to professional liability. In Orange County, California, a physician and a licensed vocational nurse were indicted on a charge of second-degree murder in connection with the death of a patient after cosmetic plastic surgery. The district attorney was quoted as saying, "We feel the practice of medicine he was engaged in involving a licensed vocational nurse administering anesthesia results in such danger to human life. . . . that he should be charged with the full consequences of the resulting death." Almost simultaneously a nurse in Maryland was charged with a criminal offense after discontinuing life support on a patient.

The implications of criminal action, as compared to civil action, for the health care professions are immense. It is no longer a matter of rising malpractice premiums and of tarnished reputations. We are now confronted with possible loss of a license to practice and spending years in a penitentiary. This clearly is a complex issue that needs to be discussed and debated in medical and legal circles; it is difficult to predict the outcome of these deliberations, but if criminal prosecution increases in cases of gross professional negligence, the impact on practice will be profound. I view this development with mixed emotions. Without question it will further restrict experimental and innovative procedures and will increase the cost of defensive health care delivery, but, on the whole, the benefits may ultimately outweigh the disadvantages. The possibility of going to prison will discourage careless, incompetent practitioners. It is difficult to defend on logical grounds why abuse of a drivers' license should be a criminal offense, whereas abuse of a professional license should be only a civil offense.

THE AVOIDANCE OF LEGAL ENTANGLEMENTS

A suit for malpractice is at best a nuisance and at worst a professional and financial disaster. Whether innocent or not, the defendant's reputation suffers by the mere fact of being sued, and even complete legal vindication is insufficient to wash away the stigma entirely. Although I feel strongly that patients not only have the right to sue if they are injured by professional negligence but also the obligation to do so, it is the responsibility of the health professional to avoid such suits whenever possible and proper.

Several ways are discussed below in which the likelihood of malpractice litigation can be decreased significantly.

IMPROVED CONSUMER–PROVIDER RELATIONSHIPS

By far the most important single factor is the establishment of good consumer–provider relationships and by a scrupulous attendance to the ethics and practice of the profession. Being a careful, conscientious, concerned practitioner may not grant immunity from litigation but will most certainly be the strongest bulwark against it. It would be presumptuous to try to discuss the details of "good health care" in the framework of this chapter, but it is certainly appropriate to point out that the major elements of good care are concern and competence. Concern incorporates such intangibles as caring for the patient as a human being; approaching all problems with humility and respect; wanting to do the "right thing"; and striving to live up to the best traditions of a noble profession.

Competence is defined as being duly qualified, answering all requirements, and having sufficient ability. Thus competence incorporates far more than the minimum legal standards under which a professional is permitted to practice. It includes an ongoing educational process, a "keeping up" with the field, a recognition of one's limitations, and the courage of one's convictions, provided these are based on erudition and not on stubbornness and pride. Continued competence is a quality that the consumer has the right to expect. Although it is impossible to know all new developments in a rapidly expanding field of knowledge, we must continue the educational process from the first day in school to the last day of practice. The moment this continuum stops, the professional begins to deteriorate. Even the medical giants of the previous generation would be charlatans if judged by contemporary standards. Continued education is and has been an ethical requirement for all health professionals; it has now become a legal or quasilegal one in most states.

Since the first edition of *Respiratory Care* in 1977, the area of mandatory continuing education has made rapid and impressive progress. Following the "malpractice crisis" of the 1970s, a number of states have enacted legislation requiring a certain amount and a certain type of continuing education from all physicians and from some other health care providers each year. This is a major step in the right direction, and making relicensure dependent on documented continuing education has at least forced the exposure of all affected health professionals to a certain amount of review and updating on a regular and recurring basis. Unfortunately, the required continuing education has been made much too easy to obtain, and, as usual, the enforcement agencies have not been provided with the personnel and budget to police compliance by all health professionals effectively. Further, there is a real question as to the effectiveness of continuing education. Numerous studies have shown that attendance at conferences, lectures, seminars, workshops, and the like may, at least temporarily, increase the knowledge of the participants, but there is little if any evidence that such attendance changes established practice patterns. It is a truism in adult education that the ones who benefit most are the ones who need it least and that the ones who need it most benefit little or not at all.

The most recent development in the health field is the issue of "continued competence." Several professional organizations have developed written tests that may be taken by specialists in these fields for the purpose of self-evaluation. It is only a matter of a few years before the credentialing agencies and the licensing bodies will require the satisfactory passing of such examinations in order to continue practice. This is the typical case in which it is impossible to argue against it, and yet its implementation will open a Pandora's box of yet unimagined and unimaginable problems. For instance,

1. What is meant by "competence" and how can it be determined by a single examination?
2. Are we going to accept "knowledge" and equate it with the ability to perform?
3. How are we going to measure such unmeasurable quantities as devotion, kindness, concern, availability, and so forth?
4. What are we going to do in communities with one or two physicians if these physicians fail the test? Are we going to deprive the population of that community of any medical care?
5. In the case of specialists and subspecialists, are we going to require general competence, or will we be satisfied with "competence" in the speciality? Will this lead to the introduction of a "limited licensure"?

This list can be protracted considerably, but, because it is easier to raise these questions than to answer them, I abandon this topic gratefully and gain considerable satisfaction from the thought that by the time my competence would be questioned by statute, I will be standing before a stricter Tribunal than any licensing board is likely to be.

IMPROVED COMMUNICATION

The second important factor is good communication between provider and consumer. "Communication" is a much abused word, and "lack of communication" has been blamed for everything from the decline and fall of the Roman Empire to the unseasonable weather that appears to afflict all regions most of the time. Certainly lack of adequate communication is indeed responsible for much misunderstanding in the field of health care delivery and consumer–provider relationships. Communication in this context means an exchange of ideas between the provider and consumer leading to a thorough understanding of the problem, of the proposed plan of diagnosis and treatment, and of the probabilities of cure or complications. With few exceptions, patients are reasonable and do not expect miracles provided they understand the issues involved in their disease and realize that the health professional is sincerely concerned and committed to do his best. No patient will tolerate being misled, few patients will tolerate being ignored, and most patients wish to be informed about their health care management. Unfortunately, this participatory management is foreign to the training of most health professions and is contrary to the "Divine Physician" image that many physicians like to create for themselves. In addition, it also takes considerable time that many health professionals do not have or do not wish to give.

Regardless of the reasons for it, poor communications between provider and consumer are responsible for a significant percentage of all actions under the law of negligence. It is well known that the most likely patient to sue is an angry patient, and patients usually feel anger not because of bad result but because of a real or perceived lack of understanding of the issues involved. These patients are "mad" at their doctor or other health care provider because of lack of courtesy, lack of adequate time spent with the patient, the appearance of always being in a hurry, the feeling that the doctor "doesn't care," that the patient is only "a case," and, worst, that the doctor considers the patient as a silly nuisance to be gotten rid of as quickly as possible. This is also the reason why the doctor with impeccable bedside or office manners gets away with terrible things, whereas the highly competent but rude and overbearing physician is a common target for litigation. Health care providers have obligations to their patients beyond competence and skill. They must be able to communicate with the patient at the patient's level of understanding and must make the time available to satisfy the reasonable patient. Ten minutes spent with a patient may save 10 days spent in a court room.

IMPROVED RECORDS

The third most important feature in the avoidance of legal troubles is the maintenance of good records. Most people, including health care practitioners, feel a general contempt for records and record-keeping. They settle for the minimum acceptable and begrudge every moment they spend or should spend in recording their observations, actions, conclusions, and results. Most physicians consider it beneath their dignity to keep detailed, meticulous records, and many of them consider it contrary to their freedom of action if the hospital or a peer group insists that records be kept fully, accurately, and informatively. Yet most negligence suits won by plaintiffs are won because of poor records, and most of the suits won by defendants are won because there was documented evidence of everything that happened in the case of the plaintiff patient.

Review of many hospital or office records reveals an appalling lack of pertinent information, and it is a rare record, indeed, that permits an outsider to reconstruct precisely the patient's problems, the events in the hospital, the justification for these events, and the results of diagnostic and therapeutic manipulations.

Worse even than the incomplete record is the record that a physician or other health worker considers as the suitable medium for witticisms or, worse, unfounded or unjustified comments on the actions of other health professionals. There is no excuse for any professional to use a legal document, such as a medical record, for the ventilation of personal criticism or petty jealousies. The medical record is not the suitable medium to try to correct errors in management. This purpose is best served by the "incident report," a confidential internal document that will bring problems to the attention of the hospital administration without directly imperiling the defense in subsequent litigation.

There is even less excuse for making incorrect entries on a medical record. This constitutes not only a complete breach of professional ethics but also is *fraud*, and thus subject to legal action. I have found, in reviewing many records, repeated evidence of treatments recorded but not given and of laboratory tests being entered without their ever having been performed. This despicable practice not only reflects the dishonesty of the so-called health professional but may also have catastrophic results for the patient. It is impossible to find strong enough words to condemn this despicable practice.

The requirement for keeping good records is not only a legal and professional one but has become a financial one as well. Third-party payers require that the record show evidence of the care provided in order that compensation be made. Certain procedures, for example, the "routine" preoperative chest x-ray, is no longer reimbursed unless there is documented medical rationale for it. The same is true for other procedures, and it is likely that this list will grow in view of the increasing concern about escalating hospital and medical costs.

INSURANCE

Since the purpose of malpractice action is to collect damages, all health professionals who provide health care as independent contractors should carry malpractice insurance so that patients may be adequately compensated for injury without financial ruin for the health professional. For many years the malpractice insurance business was stable, and many insurance companies issued policies to cover professional negligence. In recent years, partly in consequence of increasingly large judgments and settlements but mainly because of general economic problems in the insurance business, the insurance premiums have increased enormously. In fact, this problem has become a national crisis. A number of insurance companies have discontinued writing this type of policy, and even those that continue to do so have increased the premiums to exorbitant levels.

This malpractice crisis of the mid 1970s was largely due to the losses incurred by some insurance companies during the stock market decline, which made heavy inroads on the financial reserves of these companies. Because of these fiscal constraints the insurance companies started increasing the premiums in the area of professional liability insurance even though there was little, if any, documented justification for these increases based on losses suffered in that particular branch of the insurance business. In fact, investigations conducted by the insurance commissioners of several "crisis" states have found no evidence that the dramatically increased premiums or the withholding of insurance from young physicians could be justified on any valid actuarial basis. The reader interested in this dubious manipulation is referred to Law and Polan.[12]

This problem, unfortunately, is not amenable to any simple solution. Several remedies have been suggested and have been implemented in several areas, including legislative action in some states that more closely regulates the liability of insurance companies and establishes medical-society-sponsored mutual insurance companies. In addition, the most commonly mentioned approaches to this problem are compulsory arbitration and "no fault" health insurance. Under the first one, both parties agree to submit the case to an expert panel and abide by its decision. Where this approach has been tried, it has been moderately successful in decreasing both the number and the size of settlement. It is significantly more expeditious and less costly than formal court proceedings and does not permit the use of legal "tricks" that can delay cases almost indefinitely. The second approach, "no fault," has been tried successfully in automobile insurance but presents real difficulties in the health area. What "no fault" means is that the patients insure themselves against injury and thus receive compensation for bad results, regardless of whether it was the consequence of negligence. The advantage of this approach would be an enormous expansion of the actuarial base. The disadvantage is that in health care the results frequently fall short of the expectations of the patient and thus, particularly in chronic or incurable diseases, the "no fault" concept would lead to an exponential rise in claims, many of which would be unjustifiable on any basis.

A more sensible approach may be a limitation of the contingency fee, a rational limitation of the damages, and, most important, an effective policing of the medical and legal professions either from within or without. The insistence on continuing education and continuing competence in combination with the ruthless elimination of incompetent health care providers would go a long way toward keeping the malpractice problem within acceptable bounds. Unfortunately, at present, it seems unlikely that effective policing can be instituted for lack of adequate funds and against the opposition of those segments of organized medicine who thus far have steadfastly denied that there is room for improvement in the quality of medical care provided by physicians and other health care providers.

Once again, physicians are featured in this discussion because they are the primary target of malpractice litigation and because most nurses and other health professionals function as employees and thus do not need professional liability insurance of their own. If, on the other hand, the nurse or respiratory therapy technologist is in practice for himself and does not work under a physician's supervision or as a hospital employee, he becomes an independent contractor and is liable in exactly the same way as the physician. At present, it is still quite rare to have nurses or respiratory therapy technologists work in entirely independent roles. There are some, however, and their numbers are likely to grow. Thus all the above points are pertinent to all independent health care providers.

THE LEGAL IMPLICATIONS OF EMPLOYMENT

Employment is a contract that establishes a legal relationship between employer and employee. In an earlier section of this chapter, I discussed the problems of liability that an employer assumes for the negligence of the employee. In this section I shall discuss the duties and obligations that employer and employee owe to each other. The discussion seems particularly pertinent because respiratory therapists and other technological-level hospital employees have been frequently accused of disregarding their obligations toward their employer.

In the simplest terms, the offer of a job to an applicant and the acceptance of that job by the applicant establish a contractual relationship between the two parties that entails clear and binding conditions that both parties to the contract must respect and which, if broken by either party, open the door to legal remedies.

Under federal and state regulations, all offers for employment must be made in good faith, and the job must be available to all qualified applicants regardless of age, sex, race, religion, age, or national origin. There are some few exceptions to this rule where the nature of the job is such that it demands certain physical characteristics that can be met only by males or females. In addition, child labor laws clearly specify the conditions both in difficulty and in duration that minors, and particularly minor females, can assume.

Under the present regulations of the Fair Employment Practice Act, each job vacancy in any public institution must be advertised in suitable and appropriate media, giving a description of the job, the qualifications for employment, the approximate salary range, and any other pertinent data that would enable potential candidates to determine their interest in, or suitability for, the job.

Applicants must then complete a formal application for the job outlining their vital statistics, previous work record, and references for past performance. These references are to be sent directly to the employer and are usually handled in a completely confidential manner. Recently, however, serious questions have arisen whether a prospective employee is entitled to see the letters of recommendation and have an opportunity to refute any derogatory statement made therein.

For many positions, a personal interview is required, and for certain types of technical jobs an examination has been devised that all applicants must complete to show evidence of at least minimal competence in their area of training.

From this information, the employer or his representative makes a decision and selects the most suitable candidate for the job, preparing written justification both for selecting that particular candidate and also for turning down the other candidates whose basic qualifications conformed with the advertised job specifications.

Once the candidate is selected and the appropriate salary has been agreed on, the employee is processed through various initial stages of employment, including the completion of much paperwork that serves to establish the new employee as a full-fledged member of the organization. This paperwork includes such items as health forms, tuberculosis testing, tax withholding statements, insurance forms, and so on.

New employees, with some exceptions, are placed on probation for 3 to 6 months, during which orientation and in-service training take place and during which the employer is at liberty to discharge the probationary employee if it becomes evident that the job and the employee are not well suited. After the probationary period, the employee becomes a "regular" and is entitled to the elaborate and often cumbersome mechanism designed to protect the employee against any capricious and arbitrary actions on the part of his employer.

This discussion has avoided any consideration of the many clauses and conditions of collective bargaining agreements. This omission was not motivated by any disapproval of the collective bargaining process, and, in fact, I generally support the concepts of collective bargaining. The reason why union negotiations have been omitted from consideration is that these vary widely from union to union and from job family to job family. In addition, they are highly specific and cover all eventualities in such detail that they are clearly beyond the scope of any discussion in this section. Suffice it to say that the union contracts are most specific in the areas of grievance procedures and detail the various steps open to the employee in gaining redress for real or fancied inequities or injustices. The original intent of all these steps and the most rigid insistence on due process were desirable and even necessary during the time of sweatshop employers and capitalistic exploiters of the largely defenseless and frequently newly immigrated, unskilled, or semiskilled labor force. However, the situation has now developed to the point where the management prerogatives of employers and supervisors are seriously jeopardized, and employers have lost many of their managerial prerogatives. Protection of the employee has arrived at the point where incompetence, except in the grossest form, may no longer be a valid reason for dismissal and where even flagrant dishonesty has to be documented and redocumented far beyond the evident and obvious. In fact, the protection of the employee has proceeded to a point where the employer is frequently at a disadvantage in attempting to operate efficiently and economically.

As indicated above, collective bargaining units have accomplished much good and remedied many abuses. Unfortunately, an unforeseen consequence of this salutary development has been a decrease in the emotional ties that connect the employee to the employer and to the organization that they jointly represent. To put it somewhat differently, the total formalization of the employee–employer relationship has been largely responsible for decreasing, or even eliminating, much of the pride that employees used to take in their work and in the total performance of the organization. The "career" has become the "job," and although employees have become increasingly aware of the obligations the employers owe to them, there appears a parallel decrease in the responsibility that the employees feel toward the employer and the organization. The relationship tends to become an adversary one, and the employees, with obvious exceptions, tend to lose their sense of loyalty toward their organization.

For a respiratory technologist to accept a position offered in good faith and to agree to a level of compensation constitutes a contract that is just as binding on him as it is on his employer. Breaking this contract and walking away from a job, particularly in a supervisory position, is a breach of contract under the law and a reprehensible act by any civilized standard of behavior. It places a significant burden on the hospital and on the remaining members of the department. It also affects patient care, and thus infringes quite clearly on the principles of ethics that must guide all health professionals.

In fact, one of the most common complaints of hospital administrators and medical directors has been the extreme mobility of respiratory therapists. Even in a state respiratory therapy chapter the maintaining of an accurate mailing list has become a herculean task. It is a fundamental human endeavor to improve one's economic and occupational status, and every serious attempt to grow in one's chosen field is both laudable and in the best interests of the profession as a whole. Nevertheless, "job-hopping" places an extreme hardship on individual departments, particularly those whose salary structure is relatively inflexible because of the funding mechanism under which they operate.

In general terms the employer, by accepting an employee, commits himself to the conditions discussed below.

SALARY

Every employee is entitled to financial compensation commensurate with the type of employment that he is expected to assume and with the training and experience of the employee. Salary should be negotiable within certain ranges established by the employer's salary and wage officers.

The salary may be calculated on an hourly, monthly, or annual basis, and payments may be made weekly, biweekly, or monthly.

FRINGE BENEFITS

In almost all employment situations, except for part-time or temporary employees, the salary package includes a variety of fringe benefits, including social security benefits, retirement programs, health and accident insurance, life insurance, vacation and sick time, occasional financial support for continuing education, and others.

WORKING CONDITIONS

The employer is obliged to provide adequate working areas that meet the requirements of fire and occupational safety. Increasing concern over exposure to low-level toxic substances and the traditional lack of protection against dust and other pulmonary irritants have led to significant improvements in environmental controls. Much still needs to be done in this area, and the rapidly increasing number of identified carcinogens and teratogens makes the environmental protection process of employees an expensive and complex matter.

GRIEVANCE MECHANISM

Most employers establish written policies for handling complaints even if collective bargaining agreements do not extend to all employees. The due process of law discussed earlier clearly applies to all grievance procedures, and most employees are entitled to have their complaints heard and adjudicated by an orderly and well-established mechanism.

EQUAL OPPORTUNITIES IN EMPLOYMENT

Under existing federal and state legislation, all employers are legally bound not to discriminate in employment on the basis of race, sex, national origin, or religion. Generally, discrimination on the basis of age is also forbidden, although most states have specific statutes dealing with the employment of minors and the hours or type of work minors are permitted to perform.

The legal obligations of the employee are much more difficult to categorize with any degree of precision. Basically, employees commit themselves to perform their legitimately assigned duties satisfactorily so that they will keep their employer's interests at heart and perform "an honest day's work." Employees must also protect the employer's property as far as possible, maintain a clear distinction between "mine and thine," and give the employer adequate notice so that a replacement can be obtained without a major disruption of work schedules or patient services.

LAWS AFFECTING HEALTH CARE DELIVERY

LICENSING

The right to practice medicine has been interpreted to be a guarantee made to all citizens by the U.S. Constitution. Interpretation of the Constitution over the years, however, has also clearly established the principle that the states have the right to protect the public and to enact laws to promote the public welfare. This prerogative of the states has been upheld by the Supreme Court in a number of decisions, and it is today a generally accepted principle in law that the states through appropriate and legally constituted boards have the prerogative to regulate the practice of medicine and other modalities of health care. Thus, all states have enacted laws to establish legal bodies and boards to determine the minimum requirements that health professinals must meet before they are admitted to the particular practice of their choice.

The prototype of these bodies is the "State Board of Medical Examiners," which comprises physicians, surgeons, and consumers who are charged with establishing the criteria for practice in the state. These criteria usually include graduation from an approved school, a certain period of practical experience after graduation, and the satisfactory completion of a number of written or oral examinations, or both. Certain states also require United States citizenship or at least permanent residence in the state. In the past other requirements have included such variables as good moral character and not having been guilty of a felony involving moral turpitude.

Some boards of medical examiners have also considered such factors as age, type of practice, and racial or national origin. In fact, state boards have been accused in the past of using their powers to exclude from practice in the state any person whom the board considers to be controversial or undesirable. This, if true, is clearly an abuse of a board's constitutional powers, and it is gratifying to be able to say that in recent year the boards have become scrupulously honest in the interpretation of their rights and obligations.

The only real criticism still to be leveled against some boards is that although they are fair and equitable in admitting qualified physicians to practice in the state, they often do not exert their powers in supervising the quality of medical care rendered and in revoking the license of those practitioners who through age, physical, mental, or moral deterioration are no longer able to provide medical care at an acceptable level. The two major reasons for this lack of enforcement of the police powers of the state boards of medical examiners are lack of resources and the already mentioned general reluctance of physicians to sit in judgment over fellow physicians and possibly deprive them of their only means of livelihood. The economic factors are by far the more important ones, since most boards operate on an inadequate budget and can barely meet their responsibilities in examining candidates for licensure. They have neither the funds nor the trained manpower to investigate all complaints against physicians, and thus the boards generally limit their police powers to those few cases that cause a major scandal or where a physician is found guilty of a felony involving actions clearly in violation of the basic ethics of medicine.

An additional problem confronting state boards of medical examiners is the rapid development of the "physician extender" concept. Physicians' assistants, now licensed, in many states are placed under the general supervision of the board, and their license is issued under some revised form of the Medical Practice Act of the state. This introduces yet another factor to strain the already meager resources of the boards.

To regulate, supervise, and fully enforce the licensing regulations in medicine and in other health fields, the boards must be strengthened, properly financed and staffed, and be given every fiscal, legal, and political support that they need to perform their difficult mandate. Although peer reviews, societal forces, and the federal government all contribute to quality control in health care and toward the improvement of health services, the true power remains with the state licensing boards. Only these boards can effectively stop bad practitioners by revoking their license to practice. It seems most appropriate indeed that the boards exert this power fairly but vigorously, and that they be given the means to do so.

The medical practice acts were the first ones to be established, but the last few decades have seen significant proliferation of licensing bodies for health professions. Nurse practice acts, pharmacy practice acts, and dental practice acts are now established in all 50 states. A number of states have also established licensing regulations for some of the so-called technical specialties, and in some states radiological technicians, physical therapists, and others are required to obtain a license to perform their chosen profession.

These acts are similar in general form and intent to the medical practice acts and serve to establish the criteria that have to be met before a license is issued to an applicant in that particular phase of health care. Many of these acts are out of date and fail to recognize the enormous changes that have taken place both in the content and form of health care. Even some of the recent revisions of the practice acts or, worse yet, some of the new acts for new specialties are very deficient and do not really meet the needs of the particular specialty or of the consumer whom these health practitioners are supposed to serve. In addition, they all suffer from the same problems that bedevil the medical practice acts—that is, lack of adequate staff and a general reluctance to use the police powers granted to them by the state against a fellow practitioner.

Some years ago, there was great concern about the uncontrolled proliferation of licensing bodies for the rapidly increasing number of health care specialties, and, under the leadership of the United States Department of Health, Education, and Welfare (HEW), a moratorium on licensing was agreed to in 1971. This was a salutary development since it tended to eliminate, or at least decrease, the development of 50 different sets of regulations governing the practice of the many health professions.

It is not difficult to conceive the chaos that would result from having several hundred regulations that, while generally similar in content, vary sufficiently in detail to make training difficult and to limit sharply the mobility of health practitioners from one state to another. Because of this, the moratorium on licensing for new health practitioners was agreed upon under the stimulus of state boards and with the approval of HEW. In the meantime, considerable efforts are being made to develop a national licensing system that will ensure both uniformity in at least the basic requirements and also facilitate the mobility of health practitioners across the state lines.

In addition, it would be most desirable if all licensing agencies within a state or at the national level were to cooperate fully in facilitating career mobility, in enforcing proper standards of professional behavior and care, and in ruthlessly eliminating the fortunately few who cannot or will not live up to their calling and who, because of their professional or ethical shortcomings, taint the entire profession.

As far as the licensing of respiratory care personnel, there has been a reversal in the official position of the AART, which now not only supports licensure for its membership but also has thrown its considerable economic and political powers behind the chartered affiliates trying to obtain licensure in their respective states. As of spring 1983, this endeavor had been successful only in California. A licensure act in New Jersey had passed the legislature but was vetoed by the governor. In Michigan, a very major effort failed to achieve licensure but is likely to result in "registration," a significant albeit lower level of formal recognition.

The issue of licensure for respiratory therapy practitioners is complex and vexing, comprising many political, emotional, economic, and professional elements. The arguments in favor of licensure appear to be more compelling than the arguments against licensure. Unfortunately, both the economic climate and the lack of convincing evidence that licensure would materially contribute to consumer protection make it unlikely that many licensure laws for respiratory therapy will be enacted in the near future (see Chapter 2).

ACCREDITATION AND CERTIFICATION

The problems of accreditation and certification are tightly bound with the problem of licensing. The term accreditation is usually limited to evaluating the adequacy of a hospital or of the educational institution that prepares students to practice their chosen profession. At the moment, this area is also in considerable flux, and major changes in accreditation will likely take place during the next decade. Currently various bodies are charged with the inspection and accreditation of one or more phases of the health care system. These are voluntary bodies granted recognition by the states or by the federal government.

The allopathic hospitals are accredited by the Joint Commission on Accreditation of Hospitals (JCAH). This voluntary organization was incorporated in 1952 and is jointly sponsored by The American Hospital Association, The American Medical Association, The American College of Surgeons, and The American College of Physicians. Its fundamental purposes are to

1. Establish standards for the operation of hospitals and other health care facilities and services; and
2. Conduct survey and accreditation programs that will encourage members of the health professions, hospitals, and other health care facilities and services voluntarily to
   - a. promote high quality of care in all aspects in order to give patients the optimal benefits that medical science has to offer;
   - b. apply certain basic principles of physical plant safety and maintenance, and of organizational and administrative functions for efficient care of patients; and
   - c. maintain the essential services in the facilities through coordinated effort of the organized staffs and the governing bodies of the facilities.

Although the JCAH is a voluntary organization and has no formal regulatory powers, its standards and accreditation mechanism have assumed very major "clout" since the enactment of Public Law 89–97 (Medicare), which limits federal payments for health care services to those health care facilities that have been accredited by the JCAH. The JCAH has a full-time staff of inspectors who visit about 2000 hospitals each year. These hospital accreditation visits carefully examine whether the hospital meets the standards set by the Commission, and these standards are revised periodically to keep abreast of developments in the health field. In January 1974, the first standards dealing with respiratory therapy were issued by the JCAH and now form an integral part of the JCAH Accreditation Manual. These Standards are quite specific and, if properly implemented and enforced, will contribute enormously to the improvement of respiratory care provided by the hospitals. The original Standards state that

1. the objectives of the hospital's respiratory care service shall be clearly formulated;
2. an organizational plan designed for the effective implementation of the objectives of the services shall be established and appropriately documented;
3. respiratory care services in the hospital shall be provided by an appropriate number of qualified staff who receive competent medical direction;
4. written policies and procedures shall be developed for effectively implementing the objectives of the respiratory care services;
5. respiratory care services shall be provided in accordance with the written prescription of the responsible practitioner;
6. space, facilities, and equipment for the service shall be appropriate for the effective and timely care of the patient; and
7. reports of all respiratory care services provided to the patient shall be part of the patient's medical record.

For an interpretation of these sweeping regulations, the reader is referred to the excellent paper by Shapiro and Kernaghan.[20] The 1983 Standards and their interpretation appears on page 122.

The osteopathic hospitals are accredited by the Committee on Hospitals of the American Osteopathic Association (AOA). The final approval is granted by the Board of Trustees of the AOA, and this organization enforces its standards at least as rigidly as does the JCAH.

The 2- and 4-year colleges are under the jurisdiction of regional accrediting bodies that periodically inspect the educational institutions and place their stamp of approval on the educational institution as a whole.

The individual allied health educational programs are subject to *accreditation* by their own specialty accrediting bodies. Respiratory therapy education, for instance, utilizes the Joint Review Committee for Respiratory Therapy Education (JRCRTE), which is charged with inspecting and evaluating the individual programs. The Joint Review Committee comprises members who represent The American Association for Respiratory Therapy, The American Society of Anesthesiologists, The American College of Chest Physicians, The American Thoracic Society, and a member of the general public. Inspection by this body results in a recommendation that JRCRTE makes to the Committee on Allied Health Education and Accreditation (CAHEA) of the American Medical Association (AMA), which then makes the final decision concerning the approval of the respiratory therapy program. CAHEA, in this instance, acts under the approval of the United States Department of Education, which has thus far recognized the AMA as the final arbiter in determining the adequacy of the education process in most health profession educational programs at all levels, from the 1-year technician programs to 4-year programs that lead to a doctorate in medicine. Separate bodies, but with a somewhat similar basic structure, serve to accredit the educational process in other major areas of health care such as nursing, dentistry, pharmacy, and public health.

The educational accrediting process is reasonably well fixed for the so-called major health professions—medicine, dentistry, and nursing—but the process for the newly developing allied health professions is still very much in flux. A commission established some years ago published a report in 1972 entitled "Study of Accreditation of Selected Health Educational Programs." This report, usually referred to as the *SASHEP Report*,[17] has investigated this entire matter in considerable depth and has made some sweeping recommendations that may, if implemented, have far-reaching effects on the entire field of accrediting allied health educational programs. Interested readers are urged to study this report with great attention.

The third phase of the educational process in health education is the *credentialing process* in which a testing agency, through a series of examinations, recognizes the competence of the individual practitioner to perform his special tasks safely and effectively. Although superficially the licensing process and the credentialing process are similar, some fundamental differences must be clearly understood. The licensing process is a function of a sovereign state, whereby the state, through a legally constituted board, establishes minimal competency levels and on this basis grants permission to a health practitioner to perform certain functions specified in the licensing act and within the confines of the state. The licensing act also incorporates certain controls as to the quality of practice and usually has some mechanism whereby a license can be revoked if the practitioner fails to live up to the requirements under which the license was originally granted.

A credentialing body is an expert panel that conducts examinations on a purely voluntary basis and that has no legal standing in the eyes of the state or the federal government. All such a body can do is to administer one or more examinations and then verify that a candidate has successfully passed these examinations. Having achieved this status, the candidate can claim a certain expertise in a given area, but this expertise has no legal standing and does not affect the licensing process. It obviously has some economic implications and may well have some legal implications if the skill level of the practitioner is ever questioned in a court of law, but I must emphasize that certification as a specialist in a medical or allied health area is a voluntary activity that may have significant consequences on employment or earning potential but has no legal standing as far as the states' regulatory powers are concerned.

Recognition by a specialty board in medicine or by a credentialing board in one of the allied health specialties may be significant in the future in the context of national health insurance, professional standards review organizations (PSROs), or health maintenance organizations (HMOs). Currently, possession of such credentials is just a recognition of having passed certain examinations, and the likelihood but not guarantee, of increased competence over those who have fulfilled the educational requirements but who have not chosen to submit themselves to the credentialing examinations.

FEDERAL HEALTH LEGISLATION PAST, PRESENT, AND FUTURE

The rights of the states to license certain purveyors of services has been a well-established legal principle, and some of the problems of licensing in the health delivery field have been discussed above. This section will comment on recent federal laws and on some projected health legislation that will profoundly modify the practice of medicine and the entire system of health care delivery.

The first major health legislation in recent years was the *Harris–Kefauver Amendment* to the Food and Drug Act of 1962. Under this amendment, the methods whereby new drugs could be put on the market were defined, and the manufacturers of drugs were forced to prove both effectiveness and safety of the literally thousands of different pills, lotions, and other concoctions with which the public was "treated" by physicians and also by pharmacists in the so-called over-the-counter business. Although some of the regulations of the Drug Act of 1962 were cumbersome and the enforcement mechanism entrusted to the Food and Drug Administration was inadequate to do the job fully, I believe that the benefits of the Act were significant indeed. It controlled the frequently unscientific and shoddy methods whereby new drugs were put on the market and also tended to decrease the appearance of useless or harmful substances under the guise of medication.

More recently, amendments to the Social Security Act of 1935 have profoundly affected the practice of medicine and have not only established the principle that health care is a right, at least, for large parts of the population but also that the quality of care is a legitimate concern of the government that provides a very significant portion of the cost of this health care. Particular reference is made to *Public Law 92-603*, the so-called Professional Standards Review or PSRO law that stipulates very clearly the right of government to supervise and, where necessary, to regulate the standard of medical care, at least in those areas where the cost of this medical care is borne by the public through social security funds.

Other laws that affect the health and well-being of the population include *Public Law 91-596*, enacted in 1970, known as the Occupational Safety and Health Act (OSHA). This Act, not for the first time, but more effectively, attempts to regulate the working conditions of the millions of men and women whose health is seriously jeopardized by the disinclination of industry to expend the necessary funds for the creation of a salubrious working environment.

A companion piece to this law is *Public Law 92-573*, known as the *"Consumer Product Safety Act"* and which states, among its purposes, to protect the public against unreasonable risks of injury associated with consumer products, and to assist consumers in evaluating the comparative safety of consumer products.

These four acts have made giant strides in assuring the American public of a high standard of medical care, better drugs, safer products, and decent working conditions.

Additional laws such as the *Controlled Substances Act* of 1970, which regulated the distribution and use of potentially addicting or otherwise harmful drugs, have attempted to improve and update the regulations of the *Harrison Narcotics Act*. These old regulations were no longer suitable to deal with the dramatically changing drug-abuse scene of the post-World War II generation and which viewed the drug problem from a fiscal rather than a medical viewpoint.

These statutes are now "on the books" and are indeed the law of the land. Unfortunately, the laws must be enforced by imperfect human beings, and thus the lag is usually significant between the enactment of a useful piece of legislation and its satisfactory implementation for the common good. Frequently, Congress fails to provide adequate funds for enforcement of the legislation, and occasionally the best-intentioned laws fail because special-interest groups have enough power to block the enactment of laws that may decrease the profits of their industries or the earning power of certain persons.

A number of major health bills are being considered as of this writing; they deal with health manpower training and distribution, national health insurance, better environmental control, increased safety, and other subjects.

Nonstatutory regulation of the health industry has been undertaken by several federal agencies. The Federal Trade Commission has repeatedly involved professional organizations in extensive and costly litigation. The Department of Health and Human Services, through the Health Care Financing Administration, has issued several "transmittals" which become, unless contested speedily, regulations that profoundly affect the economics of health care, and thus the practice of health care.[16] The most recent (Spring 1983) regulations, known as TEFRA (Tax Equity and Fiscal Responsibility Act, 1983) and DRG (Diagnosis Related Groups), are likely to have tremendous impact on the health care system. They are discussed in some detail in Chapter 8.

The only prediction that can be made with a reasonable degree of certainty is that governmental regulatory activities will continue and are likely to increase. Consumers will continue to demand ready access to quality health care, and the health care industry will be expected to provide this. Judging from past experiences, this is unlikely to happen unless the education and control of the health professionals and the regulation of the health care industry become truly societal responsibilities.

SUMMARY

Respiratory therapy technologists, respiratory care nurses, and all other health care providers are governed by an ever-increasing pressure on the health professions to set their house in order, to assure quality care, and to eliminate the few bad practitioners. The laws and regulations reach deeply into the practice of health care at all levels, and even though the physician is still the most highly visible and most highly vulnerable member of the health team, the principles apply to all. No health care professional is immune either in his practice or in his relationship to the hospital in which he practices or to the other members of the health team with whom he practices.

I have attempted to clarify some of these relationships both from a legal and a personal viewpoint. In addition, I have discussed in some detail the main legal concern in health care delivery—the professional liability of the health care practitioner—with illustrations from court decisions and with considerable emphasis both on the anatomy of a malpractice suit and on the best ways of staying out of legal trouble. In this latter aspect, I have emphasized the importance of better provider–consumer relations, better standards of care, and better record-keeping.

I have also discussed the problems of health legislation, licensure, accreditation, and credentialing in their relationships to the individual, to hospitals, and to the public.

I have always profoundly respected and admired the law and those who write and interpret the law. A general condemnation of the legal profession is just as absurd as (the now fashionable) condemnation of the health profession. We both are beset with serious difficulties that have lowered our esteem with the general public. We must realize that both the law and the healing arts, both lawyer and health professional, have a single common purpose—to serve the public. The health professions must learn more about the law, and the legal profession must assist, rather than hamper, the health professions, all for the benefit of our common consumer, the American public.

GLOSSARY OF LEGAL TERMS

Most terms in this glossary are taken or paraphrased from Black's Law Dictionary. Readers are referred to this unique resource for citations and further information.

ABANDONMENT—When a physician intentionally and unilaterally terminates the existing relationship of physician and patient while the patient still requires treatment.

ACT OF GOD—A natural event, proceeding from physical causes alone, without the intervention of man. It is an accident that could not have been occasioned by human agency but proceeded from natural causes alone.

ACTION—In its usual legal sense means a suit brought in a court, a forward complaint within the jurisdiction of a court of law.

ACTIONABLE—That for which an action will lie, punishing legal ground for an action.

AJUDICATION—The formal giving or pronouncing of judgment or decree in a cause.

ADMINISTRATOR—A person appointed by a court to administer the assests and liabilities of a decedent (*i.e.*, the deceased).

ADMINISTRATOR AD LITEM—A special administrator appointed by the court to supply a necessary party to an action in which deceased or his estate is interested.

ADULT—One who has attained the legal age of majority, that is, acquires full capacity to make his own contracts or commit other legal acts.

ADVERSARY SYSTEM—The network of laws, rules, and procedures characterized by opposing parties who contend against each other for a result favorable to themselves.

AGENT—A person authorized by another to act for him.

AGREEMENT—A coming together of minds; a concord of understanding and intention between two or more parties with respect to the effect on their relative rights and duties, of certain past or future facts or performances.

APPEAL—The complaint to a superior court of an injustice done or legal error by an inferior court, whose judgment or decision the higher court is called upon to correct or reverse.

APPEARANCE—A coming into court as a party to a suit either in person or by attorney, whether as plaintiff or defendant.

ARBITRATION—The reference of a designate to an impartial (third) person chosen by the parties to the case who agree in advance to abide by the arbitrator's award issued after a hearing at which both parties have an opportunity to be heard.

ASSAULT AND BATTERY—The actual offer to use force to the injury of another person is assault; the use of it is a battery, which always includes an assault; hence, the two terms are commonly combined in the term "battery" regardless of its results, and it is excusable only when there is express or implied consent by the patient. The slightest touching of another, or of his clothes or anything else attached to his person, can be construed as battery.

ASSISTANT—A deputy, agent, or employee. Ordinarily refers to an employee whose duties are to help his superior to whom he must look for authority to act.

BORROWED SERVANT—An employee, "servant" who is under the complete and sole control and supervision of another individual not the employer. Under the doctrine, the person in charge of the employee is held accountable for the actions of the employee, even though no master–servant relationship exists.

BREACH OF CONTRACT—Failure, without legal excuse, to perform any promise that forms the whole or part of a contract.

BREACH OF DUTY—Generally, any violation or omission of a legal duty, whether willful and fraudulent or done through negligence or arising through mere oversight or forgetfulness.

BURDEN OF PROOF—In the law of evidence, the necessity or duty of affirmatively proving a fact in dispute on an issue raised between the parties in a case.

CAPTAIN OF THE SHIP—The captain-of-the-ship doctrine states that under certain conditions, the person in charge of a group of persons is responsible for their action even though no master–servant relationship exists (*see also* Borrowed Servant). It usually relates to the surgeon and operating room personnel.

CARE, ORDINARY—That degree of care that persons of ordinary care and prudence are accustomed to use and employ under the same or similar circumstances.

CAUSE—Something that precedes and brings about an effect or a result (*see also* Probable Cause and Proximate Cause).

CHARGE TO JURY—The final address of the judge to the jury in which he sums up the case and instructs the jury as to the rules of law that apply to its various issues and which they must observe.

CHARITABLE IMMUNITY—A doctrine that relieves a "charity" of liability in tort. This immunity was claimed by nonproprietary hospitals. Most states have abandoned or curtailed such immunity.

CHARITABLE INSTITUTION—One that dispenses charity, earns no profits or dividends, and derives its funds mainly from public and private charity.

CLASS ACTION OR REPRESENTATIVE ACTION—A legal method whereby, if a large group of persons is interested in a matter, one or more may sue as representatives of the class without needing to join every member of the class. In a class action there must be a community of interest (*q.v.*) in the questions in law, and the name representatives must truly represent the class.

COMMUNICATION, CONFIDENTIAL—A class of communication passing between persons who stand in a confidential relationship (*q.v.*) to each other which the law will not permit to be divulged or allow them to be inquired into a court of justice for the sake of public policy and the good order of society. Examples of such privileged relations are those of husband and wife, attorney and client, physician and patient (*see also* Privileged Communication).

COMMUNITY OF INTEREST—Basically a group of two or more persons or organizations that have a common concern in an issue affecting them all. For example, in respiratory care, the "community of interest" would be the therapists, the physician, and the patient.

CONCEALMENT—A withholding of something that one knows and that one, in duty, is bound to reveal.

CONFIDENTIAL RELATIONSHIP—A fiduciary relationship. It is a peculiar relation that exists between patient and physician, attorney and client, parent and child, and so forth. It covers every form of relation between parties wherein confidence is reposed by one in another and former relies and acts upon representation of the other.

CONSENT—A concurrence of wills. Consent is an act of reason accompanied with deliberation. It means voluntary agreement by a person in the possession and exercise of sufficient mentality to make an intelligent choice to do something proposed by another.

CONSENT, IMPLIED—That manifested by signs, actions, or facts or by inaction or silence which raises a presumption that the consent has been given.

CONSENT, INFORMED—A person's agreement to let something happen (such as surgery) based on full disclosure of facts needed to make a decision intelligently, that is, knowledge of risks involved, alternatives, and the risks of withholding consent.

CONTEMPT OF COURT—Any act calculated only to embarass, hinder, or obstruct a court in administration of justice or calculated to lessen its authority.

CONTINGENT FEE—Arrangement between attorney and client whereby attorney agrees to represent client, with compensation to be a percentage of the amount recovered. Such fees are often regulated by court rule or statute.

CONTRACT—A promissory agreement between two or more persons that creates a legal relation. An agreement upon sufficient consideration to do or not to do a particular thing.

CONTRACT, IMPLIED—An implied contract is one not created or evidenced by the explicit agreement of the parties but inferred by the law as a matter of reason and justice from their acts or conduct, the circumstances surrounding the transaction making it a reasonable or even necessary assumption that a contract existed between them by tacit understanding.

CONTRACTOR—One who in pursuit of independent business undertakes to perform a job or piece of work, retaining in himself substantial control of means, method, and manner of accomplishing the desired results.

CREDENTIAL—Commonly a letter license or certificate indicating the authority and capacity of the bearer.

DAMAGES—A pecuniary compensation that may be recovered in the court by any person who has suffered loss, detriment, or injury through the negligence or breach of contract or another.

DAMAGES, COMPENSATORY—Such as will compensate the injured party only for the injury sustained.

DAMAGES, PUNITIVE OR EXEMPLARY—Damages assessed to punish the defendant for his behavior or to make an example of him and to deter future transgressions.

DEATH—The cessation of life; permanent cessations of all vital functions or signs.

DEATH, BRAIN—In recent years a number of states have adopted "brain death" as equivalent to "death." The usual criteria are [1] no response to painful stimuli; [2] no spontaneous respiration; [3] no reflex activity; [4] two flat EEG tracings 24 hours apart; [5] the absence of drug ingestion, hypothermia, or other reversible condition.

DEFENDANT—The person defending or denying; the party against whom relief or recovery is sought in an action or suit.

DEFENSE—That which is offered and alleged by the party proceeded against in an action or suit as a reason in law or fact why plaintiff should not recover or establish what he seeks.

DEPOSITION—The testimony of a witness taken not in open court but intended to be used upon a trial. The testimony will be recorded word for word by an officer of the court and may further be recorded on television tape.

DILIGENCE, ORDINARY—That degree of care which men of common prudence generally exercise in their affairs in the country and the age in which they live.

DILIGENCE, REASONABLE—A fair, proper, and due degree of care and activity measured with reference to the particular circumstances; such diligence, care, or attention as might be expected from a man of ordinary prudence and activity.

DIRECTED VERDICT—In a case in which the party with the burden of proof has failed to present a prima facie case, the trial judge may order the entry of a verdict without allowing the jury to consider it because as a matter of law there can be only one such verdict.

DISCOVERY—Pretrial devices that can be used by one party to obtain facts and information about the case from the other party in order to assist the party's preparation for trial.

DISCOVERY RULE—Refers to the statute of limitations *(q.v.)* in medical malpractice cases and states that the cause of action will not be held to accrue until the patient knows or, in exercise of reasonable diligence, should have known of the alleged malpractice.

DUE PROCESS—The essential elements of "due process of law" are notice and opportunity to be heard and to defend in orderly proceeding, adopted to nature of case, and a guarantee of due process requires that every man have protection of day in court and benefit of general law. It is a constitutional guarantee to protect against unreasonable, arbitrary, or capricious proceedings.

DUTY—A human action exactly conformable to the laws that require us to obey them. An obligation to do a thing.

EMERGENCY DOCTRINE—When medical services are required in an emergency situation and the patient is unable to give consent physically or legally, the law implies the consent required to administer the required services.

EMPLOYEE—One who works for an employer; a person working for salary or wages. Servant is synonymous with employee.

EMPLOYER—One who employs the services of others; one for whom employees work and who pays their wages or salaries.

ERROR—A mistake in judgment or incorrect belief as to the existence or effect of matters of fact.

ETHICS—What is generally called the "ethics" of the profession is but consensus of expert opinion as to necessity of professional standards of conduct.

EVIDENCE—Any species of proof of probative matter legally presented at the trial of an issue by the act of the parties and through the medium of witness, records, documents, and so forth, for the purpose of inducing relief in the mind of the court or jury as to their contention.

EXPERT TESTIMONY—Testimony given in relation to some scientific, technical, or professional matter by experts, that is, persons qualified to speak authoritatively by reason of their special training, skill, or familiarity with the subject.

EXPERT WITNESS—One who by reason of education or specialized experience possesses superior knowledge of respecting a subject about which persons having no particular training are incapable of forming an accurate opinion.

FELONY—A crime of a more serious nature than those designated as misdemeanors. Usually an offense punishable by imprisonment for a period exceeding 1 year.

FINDING—The result of the deliberations of a jury or a court.

FRAUD—A general term, of multivarious means which human ingenuity can devise and which includes all surprise, trick, cunning, dissembling, and any unfair way by which another is cheated.

GRANDFATHER CLAUSE—Provision in a new law or regulation exempting those already in or part of the existing system being regulated. Part of all licensing regulation.

GUARDIAN—A person lawfully invested with the power, and charged with the duty, of taking care of the person, and managing the property and rights of another person, who for defect of age, understanding, or self-control is considered incapable of administering his own affairs.

HYPOTHETICAL QUESTION—A combination of assumed or proved facts and circumstances, stated in such a form as to institute a coherent and specific situation of facts upon which the opinion of an expert is asked by way of evidence on a trial.

INDEPENDENT CONTRACTOR—A person who contracts with another to do something for him but who is not controlled nor subject to control with respect to his conduct in the performance of the undertaking.

INSURANCE—The contract whereby for stipulated consideration, one party undertakes to compensate the other for loss on a specified subject by specified perils.

INTERROGATORIES—A set or series of written questions drawn up for the purpose of being propounded to a party or a witness whose written answer is received on his position. Written questions propounded by one party and served an adversary who must serve writ and answer to under oath.

INTERVENING CAUSE—An independent cause that intervenes between the original wrongful act or omission and the injury and produces a result that would not otherwise have occurred. Thus the original negligent actor is not liable for an injury that could not have been foreseen.

JUDGMENT—The official and authentic decision of a court of justice on the respective rights and claims of the parties to an action or suit therein litigated and submitted to its determination.

JURY—From the Latin "jurare"—to swear; a certain number of people selected according to law and sworn to inquire of certain matters of fact and declare the truth upon evidence laid before them.

LAW—That which is laid down, ordained, or established. That which must be obeyed and followed by citizens subject to sanctions or legal consequences.

LAYING FOUNDATION—In law of evidence the practice or requirement of introducing evidence of things necessary to evidence relevant, material, or competent.

LEGAL AGE—The age of which the person acquires full capacity to make his own contacts and deeds and transact business generally. Usually 18 years of age (*see also* Adult).

LEGAL DUTY—An obligation arising from a contract of the parties . . . the breach of which constitutes negligence.

LIABLE—Bound or obliged in law or equity; responsible, chargeable, agreeable, compellable to make satisfaction, compensation, or restitution.

LIABILITY—A broad legal term that includes almost every character, hazard, or responsibility, absolute, contingent, or likely.

LICENSE—Certificate or the document itself that gives permission. Permission by some competent authority to do some act that without such permission would be illegal, that is, permission to pursue calling of physician and surgeon.

LIMITATION, STATUTE OF—A statute describing limitations to the right of actions on certain described causes of action; that is declaring that no suit shall be maintained on such causes of action unless brought within a specified period after the right accrued.

LITIGATION—A lawsuit; legal action including all proceedings therein.

LOCALITY RULE—A limitation of the standards of care to a community or region.

MALICE—The intentional doing of a wrongful act without just cause or excuse.

MALPRACTICE—Any professional misconduct, unreasonable lack of skill or fidelity in professional duties. In a more specific sense, as applied to physicians and surgeons, it means bad, wrong, or injudicious treatment of a patient, professionally and in respect to the particular disease or injury, resulting in injury, unnecessary suffering, or death to the patient, and proceeding from ignorance, carelessness, want of proper professional skill, disregard of established rules or principles, neglect, or a malicious criminal intent.

MALTREATMENT—In reference to the treatment of his patient by a surgeon or physician, the term signifies improper or unskillful treatment; it may result either from ignorance, neglect, or willfulness, but the word does not necessarily imply that the conduct of the surgeon or physician in his treatment of the patient is either willfully or grossly careless.

MASTER—A principal who employs another to perform service in his affairs and who controls or has a right to control physical conduct of others in performance of the service.

MASTER AND SERVANT—The relation of master and servant exists where one person for pay or other valuable consideration enters into the service of another and devotes to him his personal labor for an agreed period. It usually contemplates employers right to prescribe, end, and direct means and methods of doing work.

MEDIATION—The act of a third person in intermediating between two contending parties with a view of persuading them to adjust or settle their dispute. A required step in labor disputes.

MEETING OF MINDS—The meeting of the minds required to make a contact is based on purpose and intention which has been made known or which from all circumstances should be known.

MENTAL ANGUISH—When connected with a physical injury, this term includes both the resultant mental sensation of pain and also the accompanying feelings of distress, fright, and anxiety. In other connections and as a ground for damages or an element of damages, it includes the mental suffering resulting from the excitation of the more poignant and painful emotions such as grief, severe disappointment, indignation, wounded pride, shame, public humiliation, and despair.

MINOR—An infant or person under the age of legal competence.

MISREPRESENTATION—Any manifestation by words or other conduct by one person to another that, under the circumstances, amounts to an assertion not in accordance with the fact.

MOTION—An application made to a court or judge for purpose of obtaining a rule or order directing some act to be done in favor of the applicant.

NEGLIGENCE—The omission to do something that a reasonable man guided by those ordinary considerations that ordinarily regulate human affairs would do or the doing of something that a reasonable and prudent man would not do.

NEGLIGENCE, CONTRIBUTARY—The act of omission amounting to want of ordinary care on part of the complaining party which concurring with defendant's negligence is proximate cause of injury.

NEGLIGENCE, CULPABLE—Failure to exercise that degree of care rendered appropriate by the particular circumstances and that a man of ordinary prudence in the same situation and with equal experience would not have omitted.

NEGLIGENCE, GROSS—The intentional failure to perform a manifest duty in reckless disregard of the consequences affecting the life or property of another.

NON COMPOS MENTIS—Not sound of mind, insane. This is a very general term embracing all varieties of mental derangements.

NUREMBERG CODE—The first codification of conditions under which experimentation involving human patients is permissible. It ensued from the Nuremberg trials investigating atrocities committed under the guise of experimentation during World War II by Nazi Germany. The principles established by the Nuremberg code were strengthened by the so-called Helsinki Declaration and were fixed in the United States by the Surgeon General's regulations of 1962 and following years.

OATH—Any form of assertion by which a person signified that he is bound in conscience to perform an act faithfully and truthfully.

OUT-OF-COURT SETTLEMENT—Agreements and transactions in regard to a pending suit that take place between the parties privately and without being referred to the judge or court for approval.

PAIN AND SUFFERING—Term used to describe not only physical discomfort and distress but also mental and emotional trauma recoverable as elements of damage in torts.

PARAMEDICAL—A bad term connoting nonphysician health practitioners. Considered to be synonymous with allied health or allied medical professions.

PARTY—A technical term in legal parlance meaning those by whom or against whom a legal suit is brought.

PATIENT–PHYSICIAN PRIVILEGE—The right of a patient to release, to divulge, or to have divulged by his physician the communication between him and the physician. This privilege belongs to the patient and hence may be waived by the patient.

PERSONAL INJURY—A hurt or damage done to the man's person such as a cut, bruise, or broken limb, as distinguished from an injury to his property or reputation. The term is also used in a much wider sense as including any injury that is an invasion of personal rights, and in this signification it may include such injuries as libel or slander, criminal conversation with a wife, seduction of a daughter, and mental suffering.

PHYSICIAN—A practitioner of medicine; a person duly authorized or licensed to treat diseases, one lawfully engaged in that practice of medicine without reference to any particular school.

PLAINTIFF—A person who brings an action. The party who complains or sues in a personal action and is so named on the record.

PLEA—Common law practice of pleading; any one in a series of pleading, more particularly the first pleading on the part of the defendant. In the strictest sense, the answer that the defendant in an action at law makes to the plaintiff's declaration and in which he sets up matter of fact as defense, thus distinguished from a demurrer, which interposes objections on ground of law.

POWER OF ATTORNEY—An instrument authorizing another to act as one's agent or attorney.

PRIMA FACIE—At first sight; on the face of it; a fact presumed to be true unless disproved by some evidence to the contrary.

PRIMA FACIE EVIDENCE—Evidence good and sufficient on its face. Such evidence, in the judgment of the law, as is sufficient to establish a given fact or a group of chains of facts constituting the party's claim or defense and which, if not rebutted or contradicted, will remain sufficient.

PRIVILEGED COMMUNICATION—Statements made by certain persons within a protected relationship that the law protects from force disclosure on the witness stand. The extent of the privilege is governed by state statutes.

PROBABLE CAUSE—Reasonable cause; having more evidence for than against.

PROFESSION—A vocation, calling, occupation, or employment involving labor, skill, education, special knowledge, and compensation of profit, but the labor and skill involved are predominantly mental and intellectual rather than physical and manual.

PROFESSIONAL CORPORATION OR P.C.—A legal entity organized by those rendering personal service to the public of a type that requires a license. Tax benefits are the primary reasons for professional incorporation. It does not alter professional liability.

PROXIMATE—Immediate, nearest, direct, next in order. In its legal sense, closest in causal connection.

PROXIMATE CAUSE—That which is a natural and continuous sequence unbroken by any efficient intervening cause, produces the injury, and without which the result would not have occurred.

RECORD—A written account of some act, transaction, or instrument drawn up under authority of law by a proper-officer and designed to remain as a memorial or permanent evidence of the matters to which it relates.

RECOVERY—The obtaining of a thing by the judgment of a court as the result of an action brought for that purpose. The amount finally collected or the amount of judgment.

RELEASE—Abandonment of a claim to party against whom it exists. Is a surrender of a cause for action and may be gratuitous or for consideration.

RES IPSA LOQUITUR—The thing speaks for itself. Rebuttable presumption that the defendant was negligent which arises upon proof that instrumentally causing injury was in defendant's exclusive control and the accident was one that ordinarily does not happen in absence of negligence.

RESPONDEAT SUPERIOR—Let the master answer. This maxim means that the master is liable in certain cases for the wrongful acts of his servants and the principal for those of his agent. Under this doctrine, master is responsible for want of care on servant's part toward those to whom master owes duty to use care provided failure of servant to use such care occurred in course of his employment.

RESPONSIBILITY—The obligation to answer for an act done and to repair or otherwise make institution for an injury it may have caused.

RISK, ASSUMPTION OF—Exists where no fault for injury rests with plaintiff but where plaintiff assumes consequences of injury occurring through fault of defendant, third person, or fault of no one. It is based on the legal maxim "volenti non fit injuria," which means that to which a person consents is not regarded in law as an injury.

RULE—An established standard, guide, or regulation. A principle or regulation set up by authority, prescribing or directing action or forebearance, as, for instance, the rules of the courts; of the law; of ethics.

RUNNING OF THE STATUTE OF LIMITATIONS—A metaphysical expression that means the time mentioned in the statute of limitations is considered as having passed.

SKILL—Practical and familiar knowledge of the principles and processes of an art, science, or trade combined with the ability to apply them in practice in the proper and approved manner and with readiness and dexterity.

SKILL, REASONABLE—Such skill as is ordinarily possessed and exercised by persons by common capacity engaged in the same business or employment.

SKILLED WITNESS (EXPERT WITNESS)—One possessing knowledge and experience as to a particular subject that are not required by ordinary persons. Such witness is allowed to give evidence of matters of opinion and abstract fact.

SPECIALIST—In this context, the health professional who has received training in addition to the basic requirements for licensure or practice and whose particular qualifications in a field of medicine have been recognized by a certifying board.

STANDARD—Stability, general recognition, and conformity to established practice; a type, model, or combination of elements accepted as correct or perfect.

STATE POLICE POWER—Every state has power to enact laws for the protection of its citizens' health, welfare, and safety, and such power is derived from the 10th Amendment to the U.S. Constitution. All licensing acts are issued under this power.

STATUTE—An act of the legislature declaring, demanding, or prohibiting something; a particular law enacted and established by the will of the legislative department of government. The written will of the legislature solemnly expressed according to the forms necessary to constitute the law of the state. This word is used to designate the written law in contradistinction to the unwritten law.

STIPULATION—The name given to any agreement made by an attorney engaged on the opposite sides of a case, for example, stipulation as to expertise of a witness.

SUBPOENA—The process to cause a witness to appear and give testimony commanding him to lay aside all pretenses and excuses and appear before a court or magistrate therein named at a time therein mentioned to testify for the party named under penalty therein mentioned.

SUBPOENA DUCES TECUM—A process by which the court, at the insistence of a suitor, commands a witness who has in his possession or control of some document or paper pertinent to the issues of a pending controversy to produce it at the trial.

SUIT—A generic term referring to any proceeding by one person against another in a court of justice.

SUMMON—Instrument used to commence a civil action. Upon the filing of the complaint the clerk of the court is required to issue a summons that will notify the person named that an action has been begun and that he is required to appear on a day named and answer the complaint in such action.

TESTIMONY—Evidence given by a competent witness under oath or affirmation as distinguished, derived from writing and other sources.

TESTIMONY, EXPERT—Identical with expert evidence. Testimony given in relation to some scientific, technical, or professional matters by experts or persons qualified to speak authoritatively by reason of their special training, skill, or familiarity with the subject.

THIRD PARTY COMPLAINT—A complaint filed by the defendant against a person not currently a party to the law suit. This complaint alleges that the third party is, or may be, liable for all or part of the damages that the plaintiff may win from the defendant.

TORT—A private or civil wrong or injury. A wrong independent of contract. A violation of a duty imposed by general law or otherwise upon all persons occupying the relation to each other that is involved in a given transaction. The three elements of every tort action are existence of legal duty from defendant to plaintiff, breach of duty, and damage as proximate result.

TORT FEASOR—A wrongdoer. One who commits or is guilty of a tort.

TRESPASS—Doing of unlawful act or of lawful act in unlawful manner to injury of another person or property. In practice, a form of action at the common law that will ask for redress in the shape of money damages for an unlawful injury done to the plaintiff in respect either to his person, property, or rights by the immediate force and violence of the defendant.

TRIAL—A judicial examination and determination of issues between parties to action.

TRIAL BY JURY—A trial where the issues of fact are to be determined by the verdict of a jury. The Seventh Amendment to the U.S. constitution provides that "In suits at common law, where the value in controversy shall exceed twenty dollars the right to trial by jury shall be preserved."

UNLICENSED PRACTITIONER—A health professional who performs his activities without having obtained a license from the state to do so. This is a criminal act and is not subject to malpractice litigation if no injury has ensued from the unlicensed but properly performed activity.

WARRANTY—A guarantee that a position of fact is true.

WARRANTY OF FITNESS—Warranty by seller or provider that goods sold are suitable for their anticipated use. Warranty may be stated, expressed, or implied. This concept is of particular significance for drugs or medical equipment that the manufacturer provides with at least the implied warranty that it will perform the actions for which it is being used.

WITNESS—Generally, one who being present, personally sees or perceives a thing; a beholder, spectator, or eyewitness. One who testifies to what he has seen, heard, or otherwise observed.

WITNESS, EXPERT—May be man of science educated in the art, or a person possessing peculiar knowledge acquired from practical experience. One who gives result of process or reasoning that can be mastered only by special scientists. Witnesses who have acquired ability to deduce correct inferences from hypothetically stated facts or from facts involving scientific or technical knowledge.

WRONGFUL ACT—Any act that in the ordinary cause will infringe upon the rights of another to his damage, unless done in the exercise of an equal or superior right.

WRONGFUL DEATH STATUTE—A statutory provision that operates on the common law rule that the death of a human being may not be complained of as an injury in a civil court. The cause of action for wrongful death is for the wrong to the beneficiaries.

The author wishes to express his sincere appreciation to Lawrence S. Charfoos, Esq., for his many helpful suggestions in the first edition and to Edward B. Goldman, Esq., for his equally valuable and most generously given assistance in this edition.

REFERENCES

1. Blair v. Eblen. S.W. 2nd 370, 373, Ky, 1970
2. Byrne v. Boadle. 175, 2 HAC 722–195, England Rep 229, 1863
3. Cates v. Bald Estate. Michigan Court of Appeals. Unpublished, Aug 13, 1975
4. Commissioner of Correction v. Myers. No. S. 1963, Mass, 1978
5. Darling v. Charleston Community Hospital. 200 N.E. 2nd 149, 211 N.E. 2nd 253, Ill, 1975
6. Dyke v. Richard. 390 Mich 739, 213 N.W. 2nd 185, 1973
7. Gary v. Wienstein. 227 NC 463, 42 S.E. 2nd 616, 1947
8. Gonzales v. Nork. 131 Cal. Reporter 717, Calif, 1976
9. In re Dinnerstein. 380 N.E. 2nd 134, Mass. App., 1978
10. In re Quinlan. 70 N.J. 10, 355 A 2nd 647, 1976
11. Lane v. Candura. 376, N.E. 2nd, 1232, Mass. App., 1978
12. Law S et al: Pain and Profit: The Politics of Malpractice. New York, Harper & Row, 1978
13. Molitor v. Kaneland. Community Unit District, 18, Ill 2nd 11
14. Moore v. Moyle. 405, Ill 555
15. Naccarato v. Grab. 180, N.W. 2nd, 788, Mich, 1970
16. Porte P: Government policy affecting respiratory therapy. Curr Rev Respir Ther 3:43, 1980
17. SASHEP Commission Report: Washington DC, National Commission on Accrediting, 1972
18. Satz v. Perlmutter. 362 So. 2nd, Fla, 1978
19. Schwartz VE: New Developments in Law. Ann Arbor, Institute for Continuing Legal Education, 1974
20. Shapiro GA et al: JCHA standards learn to use the tool. Hospitals 48:1, 1974
21. Superintendent of Belchertown State School v. Saikevicz. 370, N.E. 2nd 417, Mass, 1977
22. Tennessee Statute C.T.C.A. 23-3414 (B) Suppl 1975
23. Truman v. Thomas. 611 P. 2nd 902, Calif, 1980

BIBLIOGRAPHY

The Health Practitioner and the Law—Major Textbooks

Black HC: Black's Law Dictionary, 5th ed. St Paul, West Publishing, 1979

Charfoos LS: The Medical Malpractice Case: A Complete Handbook. Englewood Cliffs, NJ, Prentice–Hall, 1974

Haney DM: Medical Malpractice. Indianapolis, Allen Smith, 1973

Hayt E et al: Law of Hospital, Physician and Patient. Berwyn, IL, Physician's Record 1972

Holder AR: Medical Malpractice Law, 2nd ed. New York, John Wiley & Sons, 1978

King JH: The Law of Medical Malpractice. St Paul, West Publishing, 1977

Morris GH et al: New Development in Law/Medicine. Detroit, The Wayne University School of Law and Medicine, 1973

Morris RC et al: Doctor and Patient and the Law. St. Louis, CV Mosby, 1971

Sadler AM et al: The Physician's Assistant Today and Tomorrow. New Haven, Yale University School of Medicine, 1972

Shapiro DE (ed): Medical Malpractice, Personal Injury Library #3. Ann Arbor, Institute for Continuing Legal Education, 1966

Wasmuth CE: Law for the Physician. Philadelphia, Lea & Febiger, 1966

For the public laws indicated in the text, the reader is referred to the appropriate issues of the *Federal Register* and the *U.S. Code of Congressional and Administrative News*. These may be obtained from the Superintendent of Documents, Government Printing Office, Washington, DC 20402

The Health Practitioner and the Law—Current References

Alsobrook HB: Informed consent: A right to know. A J Public Health 63:37, 1973

Cayer P: Some perspectives concerning federal health legislation. Arch Surg 106:761, 1973

Holder AR: The importance of medical records. JAMA 228:118, 1974

Holder AR: Standard of care for specialists. JAMA a, 226:261–352, b, 226:395–396, 1973

Mitchell JH et al: Informed consent: A doctor's dilemma. J Maine Med Assoc 64:94, 1973

Mumme JL: Seven surefire ways to lose a malpractice case. RN Magazine, 49:60, 1977

Rubsamen DS: Medical Malpractice. Sci Am 235:18, 1976

Sackett WW: Death and dignity: A legislative necessity. J Fla Med Assoc 61:366, 1974

Saypal GM: Medical malpractice mediation. NY State J Med 74:1648, 1974

Accreditation, Licensure, and Certification

Accreditation Manual for Hospital, July 1973 and Jan 1981. Joint Commission, 645 N. Michigan Ave., Chicago, IL 69611

Dean WJ: State legislation for physician's assistants: A review and analysis. Health Serv Rep 88:3, 1973

Dolan AK: Challenging licensing laws: Who has the burden of proof. PRO Forum 3, No. 2, 1980

Essentials of an Approved Educational Program for the Respiratory Therapy Technician and the Respiratory Therapist. Chicago, Committee of Allied Health Education and Accreditation, AMA 535 North Dearborn Street, Chicago, IL 60610

Mosow S et al: Changing state laws regulating health manpower. Am J Public Health 63:37, 1973

Report of Licensure and Related Health Personnel Credentialing. DHEW Publication #72–11, 1973

Study of Accreditation of Selected Health Education Programs (SASHEP), One Dupont Circle, N.W., Washington, DC 20036
Part I Working Papers, Oct 1971
Part II Commission Report, May 1972

ACCREDITATION MANUAL FOR HOSPITALS, JOINT COMMISSION ON ACCREDITATION, 1983: RESPIRATORY CARE SERVICES

Principle

Respiratory care services that meet the needs of patients as determined by the medical staff shall be available at all times.

Standard I

The respiratory care department/service shall be well organized, properly directed, and appropriately integrated with other units and departments of the hospital. Staffing shall be commensurate with the respiratory care needs of patients and the scope of services offered.

INTERPRETATION

The relationship of the respiratory care department/service to other units and departments of the hospital shall be specified within the overall hospital organizational plan. The responsibility and accountability of the respiratory care department/service to the medical staff and hospital administration shall be defined.

Scope of Services The scope of the diagnostic and therapeutic respiratory care services provided to inpatients, ambulatory care patients, and home care patients shall be defined in writing. There shall be written guidelines for the transfer or referral of patients who require respiratory care services that are not provided by the hospital.

Pulmonary function studies and blood gas analysis capability shall be appropriate for the level of respiratory care services provided and shall be readily available to meet the needs of patients.

Hospitals providing any degree of respiratory care services, either from within the hospital or from an outside source, shall be evaluated for compliance with all applicable requirements of this section of the *Manual.* A hospital that provides continuous ventilatory support to patients shall comply with all requirements of this section of the *Manual.* A respiratory intensive care unit shall be evaluated for compliance with the requirements of this section and the Special Care Units section of this *Manual.*

Outside Sources When respiratory care services are provided to any extent from outside the hospital, the source(s) shall be approved by the medical staff through its designated mechanism, provide services whenever needed, meet all safety requirements, abide by all pertinent rules and regulations of the hospital and medical staff, document the quality control measures to be implemented, and meet all applicable requirements of this and related sections of the *Manual.*

Direction Medical direction of the respiratory care department/service shall be provided by a physician member of the active medical staff who has special interest and knowledge in the diagnosis, treatment, and assessment of respiratory problems. Whenever possible, this physician should be qualified by special training and/or experience in the management of acute and chronic respiratory problems. The physician director shall designate a qualified physician member of the active medical staff to act in his absence. The physician director or his qualified designee shall be available to provide any required respiratory care consultation, particularly on patients receiving continuous ventilatory or oxygenation support. The physician director shall have the authority and responsibility for assuring that established policies are carried out; that overall direction in the provision of respiratory care services in the inpatient, ambulatory care, and home care settings is provided; and that a review and evaluation of the quality, safety, and appropriateness of respiratory care services is performed.

Staffing Respiratory care services shall be provided by a sufficient number of qualified personnel under competent medical direction. When the scope of services warrants it, respiratory care services shall be supervised by a technical director who is registered or certified by the National Board for Respiratory Therapy, Inc., or has the documented equivalent education, training, and/or experience. The technical director's duties shall include responsibility for assuring the supervision of respiratory personnel in the performance of respiratory therapy and any designated related laboratory procedures; the care, maintenance, and disinfection or sterilization of all ventilatory equipment, accessories, and, as required, supplies; and the maintenance of appropriate records and reports. Additional responsibilities may be designated to the technical director by the physician providing medical direction for the respiratory care services.

Other qualified respiratory care personnel shall provide respiratory care services commensurate with their documented training, experience, and competence. Such personnel may include registered respiratory therapists or certified respiratory therapy technicians, or individuals with the documented equivalent in education, training, and/or experience; qualified cardiopulmonary technologists; and appropriately trained licensed nurses. This does not preclude the provision of respiratory care services by trainees or students supervised by qualified respiratory care personnel.

Personnel providing respiratory care services shall comply with all applicable federal, state, and local regulations.

The training of respiratory therapy students shall be carried out only in programs accredited by the appropriate professional educational organization. Individuals in student status shall be directly supervised by a qualified respiratory therapist or technician, particularly when engaged in patient care activities. When the hospital provides clinical facilities for the education and training provided by an outside program, the respective roles and responsibilities of the respiratory care department/service and the outside educational program shall be defined.

(Continued)

Other Manual References Refer also to related requirements in the following section of this *Manual:* Functional Safety and Sanitation, Infection Control, Medical Record Services, Medical Staff, Nursing Services, Pathology and Medical Laboratory Services, Pharmaceutical Services, and Special Care Units.

Standard II

Personnel shall be prepared for their responsibilities in the provision of respiratory care services through appropriate training and education programs.

INTERPRETATION

The education, training, and experience of personnel who provide respiratory care services shall be documented, and shall be related to each individual's level of participation in the provision of respiratory care services. A formal training program may be required as a prerequisite. Nonphysician respiratory care personnel shall perform patient procedures associated with a potential hazard, including arterial puncture for obtaining blood samples, only when authorized in writing by the physician director of the respiratory care department/service acting in accordance with medical staff policy. The director shall maintain documentation of the qualification of such personnel to perform these procedures. New personnel shall receive an orientation of sufficient duration and content to prepare them for their role in the provision of respiratory care services.

As appropriate, and prior to providing respiratory care services, individuals shall receive instruction and demonstrate competence in:

- fundamentals of cardiopulmonary physiology, and of fluids and electrolytes;
- recognition, interpretation, and recording of signs and symptoms of respiratory dysfunction and medication side effects, particularly those that require notification of a physician;
- initiation and maintenance of cardiopulmonary resuscitation and other related life-support procedures;
- prevention of contamination and of transfer of infection through appropriate aseptic techniques;
- mechanics of ventilation and ventilator function;
- principles of airway maintenance, including endotracheal and tracheostomy care;
- effective and safe use of equipment for administering oxygen and other therapeutic gases, and for providing humidification, nebulization, and medication;
- pulmonary function testing and blood gas analysis (when such procedures are performed within the respiratory department/service);
- methods that assist in the removal of secretions from the bronchial tree, such as hydration, breathing and coughing exercises, postural drainage, therapeutic percussion and vibration, and mechanical clearing of the airway through proper suctioning technique;
- procedures and observations to be followed during and after extubation; and
- recognition of, and attention to, the psychological and social needs of patients and their families.

All personnel providing respiratory care services shall participate in relevant in-service education programs. The director or his qualified designees shall contribute to the in-service education of respiratory care department/service personnel and other personnel who provide respiratory care services.

In-service education shall include instruction in the safety and infection control requirements described elsewhere in this *Manual.* Cardiopulmonary resuscitation training for personnel performing respiratory care services shall be conducted as often as necessary, but not less than annually, except for individuals who can otherwise document their competence. Education programs for respiratory care services personnel shall be based, at least in part, on the findings from the review and evaluation of respiratory care services provided. Outside educational opportunities shall be provided as feasible, at least for supervisory personnel. The extent of participation in continuing education shall be documented, and shall be realistically related to the size of the staff and the scope and complexity of the respiratory care services provided.

Standard III

Respiratory care services shall be guided by written policies and procedures

INTERPRETATION

There shall be written policies and procedures specifying the scope and conduct of patient care to be rendered in the provision of respiratory care services. Such policies and procedures must be approved by the medical staff through its designated mechanisms, and shall be reviewed at least annually, revised as necessary, dated to indicate the time of the last review, and enforced. The policies and procedures shall relate to at least the following:

- Specification as to who may perform specific procedures and provide instruction, under what circumstances, and under what degree of supervision. Such procedures include, but are not limited to, cardiopulmonary resuscitation; the obtaining of blood samples and their analysis; pulmonary function testing; therapeutic percussion and vibration; bronchopulmonary drainage; coughing and breathing exercises; mechanical ventilatory and oxygenation support for infants, children, and adults; and aerosol, humidification, and therapeutic gas administration.
- Assembly and sequential operation of equipment and accessories to implement therapeutic regimens.
- Steps to be taken in the event of adverse reactions, based on established criteria for the identification of undesirable side effects.
- Procurement, handling, storage, and dispensing of therapeutic gases.
- Pertinent safety practices, including the control of electrical, flammable, explosive, and mechanical hazards.
- Infection control measures to minimize the possibility of contamination and transfer of infection. These shall include changing equipment, accessories, and solutions according to an established schedule; and the methods of cleaning, disinfecting, and sterilizing reusable equipment.
- Administration of medications in accordance with the phy-

(Continued)

sician's order and the requirements of the Pharmaceutical Services section of this *Manual.*
- An established method of response to the absence of adequate, explicit instruction within the prescription for respiratory care services.

The respiratory care department/service shall have equipment and facilities to assure the safe, effective, and timely provision of respiratory care services to patients. **Standard IV**

INTERPRETATION

Sufficient space shall be provided for the respiratory care department/service to store, decontaminate, clean, disinfect or sterilize, maintain, and repair equipment; to store supplies; and to perform the administrative work related to the volume of services provided. There shall be sufficient space and equipment to perform any pulmonary function studies or blood gas analyses provided in the hospital. All requirements relating to the performance of pulmonary function studies or blood gas analyses must be met regardless of which hospital department is responsible for performing them.

All equipment shall be calibrated and operated according to the manufacturer's specification, and shall be periodically inspected and maintained according to an established schedule as part of the hospital's preventive maintenance program. A pin-index system, a diameter-index system, or another approved equivalent safety system shall be used with a therapeutic gas. Where piped-in gas supply system are installed, an evaluation shall be made prior to use to assure identification of the gas and its delivery within an established safe pressure range. Oxygen analysis of the therapeutic gases delivered by the ventilators and aerosol units using the piped-in gas supply should be made at regular intervals and recorded. After cleaning and reassembling equipment delivering therapeutic gases to the patient, and prior to patient use, an assessment of the gas flow shall be made to assure that it is within established safe limits. The temperature of inspired gas shall be measured at intervals that assure the temperature is not excessive, and shall be recorded. Ventilators used for continuous assistance or controlled breathing shall have operative alarm systems at all times.

Resuscitation, ventilatory, and oxygenation support equipment shall be available for patients of all sizes served by the hospital.

Respiratory care services shall be provided to patients in accordance with a written prescription of the responsible physician, and shall be documented in the patient's medical record. **Standard V**

INTERPRETATION

The prescription for respiratory care shall specify the type, frequency, and duration of treatment, and, as appropriate, the type and dose of medication, the type of diluent, and the oxygen concentration. A written record of the prescription and any related respiratory consultation shall be maintained in the respiratory care department's/service's files, shall be incorporated into the patient's medical record, and shall include the diagnosis. When feasible, the goals or objectives of the respiratory therapy should also be stated in the medical record. All respiratory care services provided to a patient shall be documented in the patient's medical record, including the type of therapy, date and time of administration, effects of therapy, and any adverse reactions. The responsible physician shall document in the patient's medical record a timely, pertinent clinical evaluation of the overall results of respiratory therapy.

Prior to discharge of the patient, instructions should be given in all aspects of pulmonary care relevant to the respiratory problem. This may include instruction to the patient or the patient's family on postural drainage, therapeutic percussion, and other measures. The need for long-term oxygen therapy should be adequately documented in the medical records of patients discharged on such therapy. When appropriate, such need should be based on arterial blood gas results at rest and/or exercise.

Standard VI

The quality and appropriateness of patient care provided by the respiratory care department/service shall be regularly reviewed, evaluated, and assured through the establishment of quality control mechanisms.

INTERPRETATION

The physician director of the respiratory care department/service shall be responsible for assuring that a review and evaluation of the appropriateness and effectiveness of such services is accomplished in a timely manner, including respiratory care provided to inpatients and, when applicable, to ambulatory care patients and home care patients. The review and evaluation shall be performed at least quarterly, and shall involve the use of the medical record and the use of preestablished criteria, including indications for use, effectiveness of treatment, and adverse effects requiring discontinuance of treatment. The review and evaluation shall include input from the medical staff and personnel of the respiratory care department/service. This review and evaluation should be performed within the overall hospital quality assurance program. Particular attention shall be given to evaluation of the necessity for those respiratory care services having the highest utilization rate. The quality and appropriateness of respiratory care services provided by outside sources shall be included in the review and evaluation on the same regular basis. Refer also to the Quality Assurance section of this *Manual.*

6

The Modern Respiratory Care Department

Edgar L. Anderson, Jr. • Michael McPeck

In the first edition of this book, this chapter began by stating that "A modern department of respiratory care is a highly developed, comprehensive service, delivering quality patient care; it must be acutely and continually aware of the dynamically changing environment within the institution and be prepared to deal with new needs as they arise. The challenge to departmental leadership, whether the department be large or small, is to be able to predict change or even to initiate it."

As we move through the 1980s, however, it is becoming clear that not only is the departmental leadership being challenged, but respiratory therapy practitioners themselves are being asked to become increasingly more responsible in shaping the direction of the continuing evolution of respiratory therapy. One example of that evolution is the current development of respiratory care subspecialties such as critical care respiratory therapy workers.

Modern, comprehensive respiratory care should not be limited to large departments; it should be available in any department, regardless of size, that is conscious of all the problems involved in delivering general respiratory care. Areas and functions that reflect the services of an extensive and sophisticated respiratory care department are listed on page 129. Although responsibility for many of these specialty service functions may fall to one person in a small department, in a large department each service must be considered a distinct, but not separate, entity.

Simple provision of the services listed in no way guarantees a "modern" department. In a dynamically changing environment, a constant search must be made for innovative approaches, development of new techniques, and new areas and efficiencies that will result in excellence of care. One of the most important resources of such a department is the people involved, not necessarily the pieces of equipment available. Critical factors include the administrative leadership in the institution, the involvement and innovation of the technical and medical directors (*see* Chap. 4), the remainder of the department management, and the knowledge, skills, and enthusiasm of the practitioners in the department itself. It is to these practitioners that this chapter is devoted, for without them the respiratory care department does not function.

It is hoped that, in the 1980s and beyond, *all* respiratory therapy practitioners will become involved in improving the ways in which respiratory care services are organized and managed. This is a task that should not be restricted solely to the departmental management. To accomplish this goal, experienced managers may have to change their tactics, learn new methods of management, and adapt to, or personally initiate, contemporary models of departmental organization. At the same time, the "rank and file" practitioners may be likened to the new respiratory therapy department head who will be expected to learn organization and management from the ground up but apply them in a contemporary sense. Either way, the implicit goal is for all respiratory therapy practitioners to evolve a new and improved organizational plan and mode of management that fits comfortably within their institutional structure and which, at the same time, allows extensive growth, development, and maturation of the respiratory therapy profession.

The organizational and managerial concepts described herein are derived from the traditional managerial (administrative) sciences but are discussed in terms that relate specifically to respiratory therapy.

DEPARTMENT MANAGEMENT AND ORGANIZATION

Organization and management are integrally related yet distinct concepts that relate to the manner in which departmental functions are carried out. Organization refers to the *structure* of the department, its anatomy. Management includes achieving the objectives of an organization through the organization itself and the *coordinated efforts* of the practitioners in the department.

Respiratory care department *organization* comprises a number of factors, including planned services and general philosophies of the hospital as well as specific services and philosophies of the respiratory care department, physical facilities, and equipment resources devoted to respiratory care and personnel allocation and deployment. Obviously, the most successful respiratory care department will be one in which these factors complement each other to the greatest possible extent.

All respiratory care practitioners must realize and understand their hospital's orientation and the range of services it wishes to deliver. This is as important to the incumbent department manager as it is to the person who aspires to become a respiratory therapy department head. The entire respiratory care staff must be aware of the population area the hospital serves and be sensitive to the types of services or number of beds the hospital wishes to devote to certain kinds of patients or surgical procedures.

SERVICE AND ACTIVITY CATEGORIES USUALLY PROVIDED BY LARGER, COMPREHENSIVE RESPIRATORY CARE DEPARTMENTS*

Respiratory intensive care unit (RICU)
General medical/surgical intensive care unit (MICU/SICU)
Coronary care unit (CCU)
Pediatric intensive care unit (PICU)
Neonatal intensive care unit (NICU)
Specialty ICUs (burn, neurosurgery, and others)
Emergency department and trauma service
Critical care transport
Home care and rehabilitation programs
Sleep apnea programs
Infant apnea home monitoring programs
Chest physiotherapy services
Cardiopulmonary resuscitation
Pulmonary function and blood gas laboratories
Materials management (equipment procurement and inventory)
Biomedical engineering (equipment repair, maintenance, and documentation)
Computer applications and physiologic monitoring group

*Day-to-day services in the rest of the hospital are not mentioned for lack of a satisfactory descriptive term.

CONCEPTS AND LEVELS OF MANAGEMENT

The management functions of a respiratory care department, as those of a hospital, can be divided into several areas, all of which require supervision, planning, and control. These areas include the following.

1. Finances
2. Auditing
3. Technical services
4. Education
5. Personnel
6. Records and reports

The general scope of these management functions is the same in all departments regardless of size; the only difference is in the number of *people* needed to carry out the functions.

Two basic modes of management and several "variations on the theme" exist for use by respiratory care department directors. First is the concept of *centralized management* for the purpose of control. It is a natural outgrowth of the "pyramidal" type of departmental organization (Fig. 6-1). The second concept is *decentralization* of control and the delegation of authority and responsibility. In actual practice, the

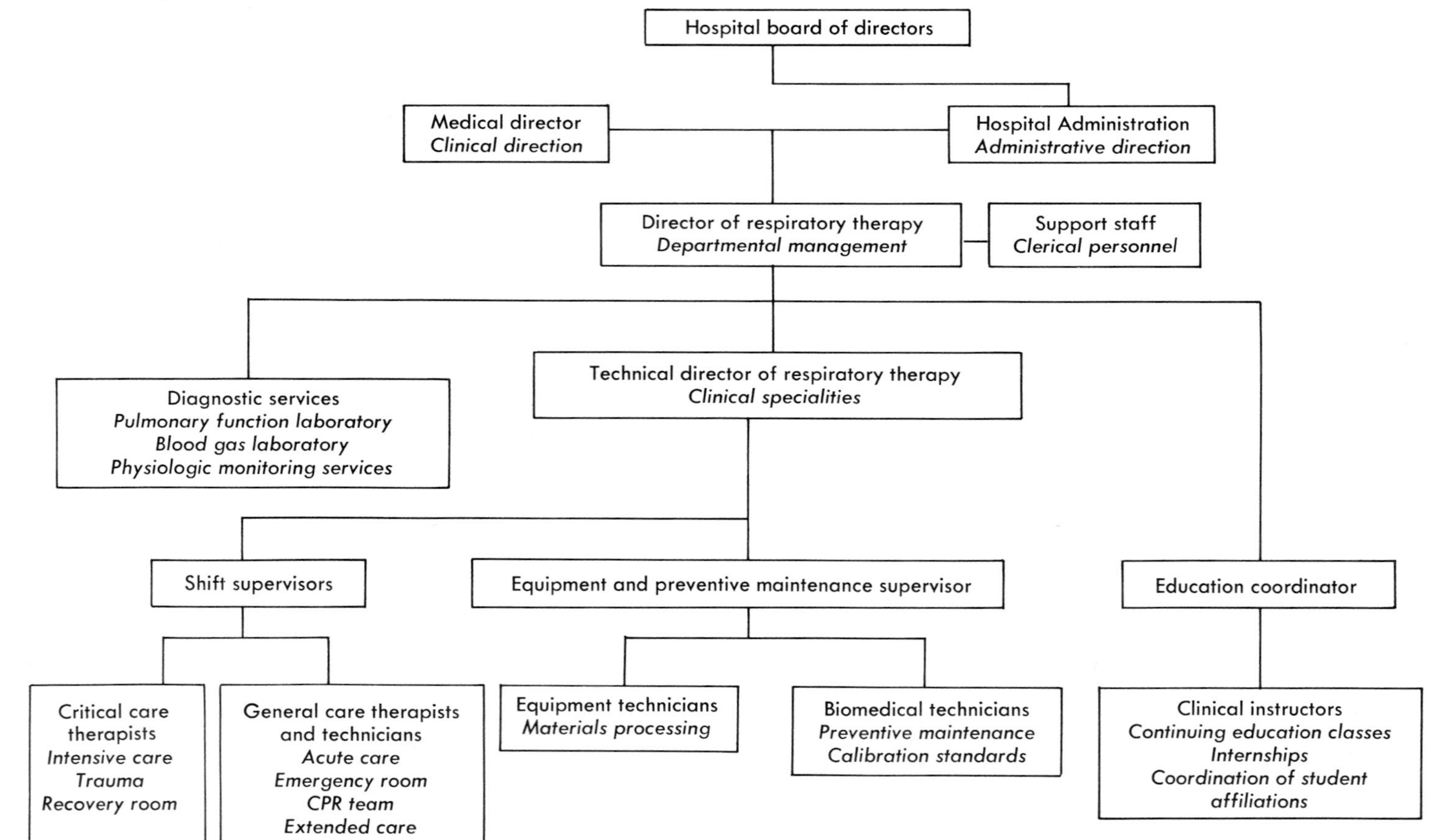

Fig. 6-1. The traditionally organized, centrally managed and controlled respiratory care department. (McDonald PM: The organization and service of a respiratory therapy department. In Spearman CB, Sheldon RL, Egan DF: Egan's Fundamentals of Respiratory Therapy, 4th ed. St. Louis, CV Mosby, 1968)

director may have as an ultimate goal the decentralization of control, but in certain segments of the department he may find it necessary to use a centralized concept until suitable personnel become available. Each method has its own inherent problems, advantages, and disadvantages; the effectiveness of either concept is influenced by the size of the department and the director's own personal style of management.[6]

Centralized Management

The concept of centralized management is historically the oldest. It is a concept of hierarchy, with the technical and medical directors personally setting all policies, goals, and objectives and making all the critical decisions (Fig. 6-2). Centralized management is used successfully in small departments of respiratory care (less than 20 full-time employees), as well as in many small businesses. In such cases, one of the reasons for using centralized management is to lessen the possibility that the organization will become administratively "top heavy."

Although efficiency and morale may be extremely good in such departments, two criteria are essential for success:

1. The department must be small enough to allow the director to supervise the performance of *all* staff members.
2. The director must have time to make decisions as well as to supervise the staff.

The deficiencies of this concept become apparent when either criterion is not met.

There is no arbitrary departmental size wherein centralized management is no longer possible. The "controllable critical mass" varies with the skills of the director and the success of the intradepartmental and interdepartmental communications networks he establishes. Not infrequently, management moves prematurely into the decentralized mode (see p. 132) when what really is needed is a strengthening of the basic communications network.

Difficulties clearly arise when the director either fails or refuses to recognize that the leadership of the department has grown beyond the point of a one-man operation. Disastrous results may be expected when those in authority do not understand the two essential criteria stated above and attempt single-handedly to administrate an overly large operation. The resulting situation usually results in failure. When the sheer size of the operation becomes so large that effective communication is no longer possible, then a more decentralized form of management clearly needs to be employed.

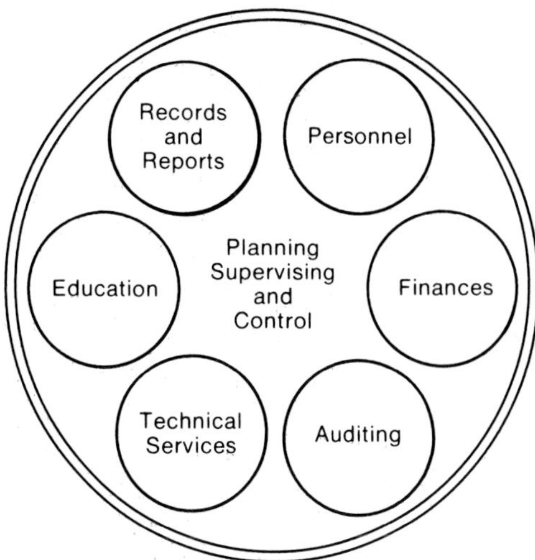

Fig. 6-2. Centralized management. In a department operated in this fashion (a rearrangement of Fig. 6-1 into a Venn diagram), one person plans, supervises, and controls, essentially carrying out all management functions himself. The external circle represents the total sphere of his influence.

Decentralized Management

In decentralized management, areas of specific responsibility are defined for other staff members, and authority is delegated to individuals in order to achieve results. As Dinsmore has pointed out,

> Department directors are finding that they can cope with increasing pressures on them personally and on their departments only by having more people with character and ability in the management group. They are seeing quite clearly the increasingly important role throughout the department of managers capable of individual thinking and initiative.[7]

In the department of respiratory care, the delegation of *responsibility* is easy, but the delegation of *authority* deters some directors from using this concept. There is always the possibility of authority being delegated to someone who proves unsuitable. In addition, some directors may believe, albeit incorrectly, that the delegation of authority to others results in either loss or unacceptable dilution of their own power. In practice, however, delegation of responsibility without authority is usually both unworkable and dangerous.

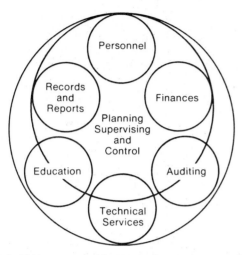

Fig. 6-3. The metamorphic state of management. As the department expands and the centralized administrative structure (*see* Fig. 6-2) becomes inadequate to handle increasing job pressures, additional staff will be given authority by the director to supervise those functions that have evolved to a point requiring semiautonomy.

Decentralization should not imply that the director is unaware of what is going on in the department, that he has given up whole areas of responsibility, or that he has lost or is losing his authority or control in any area. On the other hand, the concept *does* imply that those delegated authority are expected to make decisions on their own within the framework and according to the intent of the director's management policies. Each person is expected to seek counsel in those areas of concern about which he is unsure or when a decision affects the operation of some area other than his own. The "letting go of the reins" will at first be slow, as some functions are gradually moved outside the director's minute-to-minute supervision. This state of affairs might be described as the "*metamorphic state of management*" (Fig. 6-3).

The director must be able to choose supervisory personnel who he feels are capable of exercising authority wisely; thus, selected persons should demonstrate leadership qualities. They should perform beyond the level of achievement and quality of work that is consistent with the standards of the department. They should be logical, fair, decisive, communicative, equitable, and honest. These leadership personnel must share most of the ideas and goals of the director. If, in addition, their area of responsibility is large, they must develop lines of communication and authority within their own areas to accomplish the goals that have been established.

The director must spend a considerable amount of time with these people, developing philosophies and concepts and stimulating their imaginations, teaching them the techniques of management, encouraging and counseling them in difficult periods, and helping to set goals and objectives. It is *essential that the director be given feedback* in all situations in order to stay aware of current department functions and development.

Each person of authority should be anxious to work toward the overall success of the department, even though the ultimate responsibility for the department rests with the director. All these considerations emphasize the need for mutual confidence and respect between the members of the departmental management team and the director himself.

In addition to developing and advising managers, the director in the decentralized management format assumes the key role of creating programs and policies and of *directing, planning,* and *maintaining control.* The director also sets goals and objectives, obtains funds, and keeps a balance of strength throughout the department. In short, his job is to keep the operation running smoothly and in a coordinated fashion.[12] Eventually, more and more functions will move away from his direct supervision but not his entire responsibility. Simultaneously, these functions begin to overlap, underlining again the need for communication at all levels (Fig. 6-4).

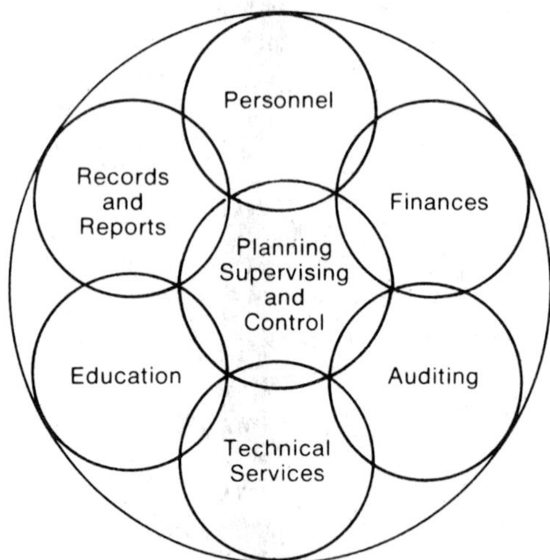

Fig. 6-4. Decentralized management. As the department continues to expand to its fullest potential and adds additional management staff, the director will continue to maintain his role of delegating authority to those functions, although the interrelationships become more complex.

The decentralized mode of management certainly offers a fertile training ground for young, talented managers and an opportunity to try middle-level managing before possibly moving on to begin departments of their own. Although there is nothing wrong with this of itself, the adroit director will view the satellite positions in his department as ends in themselves and will attempt to surround himself with a *stable* core of administrative and supervisory colleagues.

In studying Figures 6-2, 6-3, and 6-4, the reader is urged to realize that the degree to which any given sphere of influence may be removed from the director will depend on both his own personal talents and interests and the expertise of those who surround him.

Levels of Management

To achieve ideal departmental organization, three levels of management are usually necessary.

1. Top-level management, represented by the director and his senior associates, who *develop* policy.
2. Middle management, consisting of section heads who *interpret* policy.
3. Supervisory management, consisting of those who have the responsibility of seeing that tasks are carried out within the framework of the policies (*i.e.*, those who *translate* policy into action).

Although in a small department these three levels may be indistinct for reasons of economy and organization, the *functions* of all three levels must be assigned to someone in the department.

In the best organization, people see themselves working in a circle as if around a table. One of the positions is designated "director" because somebody has to make all the tactical decisions that enable an organization to keep working. In such a configuration, leadership easily passes from one to another, depending on the particular task being undertaken. Speaking of business organizations, Robert Townsend has observed,

> Organization Chart—rigor mortis—they have uses: for the annual salary reviews; for educating investors on how the organization works and who does what. But draw them in pencil. Never formalize, print, and circulate them. Good organizations are living bodies that grow new muscles to meet challenges. A chart demoralizes people. Nobody thinks of himself as below other people. And in a good company he isn't. Yet on paper there it is. If you have to circulate something, use a loose-leaf table of organization (like a magazine masthead) instead of a diagram with the people in little boxes. Use alphetical order by name and by function whenever possible.[16]

No matter what management format is eventually selected, communication is the key to its success. Effective communication is a two-way street; there must be communication from the top down and from the bottom up. Only in this fashion will plans and policies be relayed effectively throughout the organization.

PERSONNEL

Staffing

Joint Commission on Accreditation of Hospitals (JCAH) Standard I requires that a respiratory care department have ". . . staffing (that) shall be *commensurate with the respiratory care needs of patients and the scope of services offered*" (italics ours). In the JCAH Guidelines for this Standard, the words "sufficient numbers" are used. Since the first edition of this book, the use of manpower has become more science than art, beginning with the concept of employee task/training matching and culminating in the AARTs systematized hospital uniform reporting (SHUR) project. From this has emerged a clear understanding that what constitutes "sufficient" staff in one 300-bed hospital is woefully inadequate in another, based on patient mix, productive hours of work per day versus nonproductive hours of work per day, and other variables.

The following section attempts to describe a "first brush" analysis of the staffing needs of a hospital. Hopefully, it will allow the prospective director or employee a semiquantitative overview of the institution's commitment to follow the mandate of the JCAH. Some definitions follow.

Full-time Equivalents (FTEs): the total number of employees budgeted for by the administration for the department, including the administrative (technical) and medical director, servicing and cleaning personnel, secretaries, aides, inservice personnel, and shift supervisors. In some centers, these workers are known as *support and ancillary* staff. It will naturally include the core of the department that has hands-on working experience with patients (*i.e.*, technicians and therapists).

Nonproductive Work Time: the amount of time per day spent in activities related to, but not directly involved in, "hands-on" care. Such activities include the following.

1. Time spent preparing to do a task (e.g., obtaining equipment, medication, and needed supplies)
2. Report time
3. Break time
4. Department in-service time
5. In-hospital travel time
6. Allowance for language barriers, poor patient cooperation, and other considerations
7. Teaching time (if affiliated with a school of respiratory therapy)

These activities may easily consume 1 to 1.5 hours per day.

Lunch: usually figured in the total work day as a separate item. Allow at least 0.5 hours daily.

Benefit Hours: amortizes all vacation, compassionate and sick leave, and holidays over 2080 hours. This comes out to a surprising 0.75 hours/day if one works an 8.5-hour day. For example, suppose a hospital figures on an 8.5-hour day, including lunch. How much *productive work time* can one expect from therapists and technicians?

Total work time:		8.50 hours
Allowances:		
Nonproductive work time	(−1.50)	
Lunch	(−0.50)	
Benefit hours	(−0.75)	
		−2.75 hours
Time for productive work:		5.75 hours

One may get an idea of how well a hospital is staffed by inquiring as to the number of productive hours worked per year by the department and dividing by the productive hours of *one worker* (260 work days × 5.75 hours/day = 1495 hours/year). Thus, if the hospital and department did 73,000 hours of productive work per year, their staff should be $\left(\frac{73{,}000}{1495}\right)$, or approximately 48.

Productivity: most hospitals expect that a given number of procedures be done per hour of work. From this has derived the concept of various tasks as "units" (e.g., IPPB taking 30 minutes might be rated as 0.5 units—in a 1.0 unit hour). In these fiscally conscious times, productivity in excess of 100% is looked upon favorably by many administrators, and, accordingly, estimating work load by units of time has its advantages.

Selection

The organizational plan of the respiratory care service largely influences the selection of personnel and their utilization and deployment. Department heads must decide whether to employ technicians or therapists, or a combination of both. In some areas of the country, on-the-job-trained personnel, nurses, and nursing aides must also be included in the available candidate pool because of a scarcity of qualified respiratory therapy practitioners from traditional training programs.

Frequently one finds that the smaller community hospital with only a few, if any, ICU beds may select technician-level practitioners, whereas the large, multibed university-affiliated hospital with a half dozen or more specialized ICUs will preferentially select therapist-level respiratory therapy practitioners. In either case, the ultimate selection of personnel is mediated by a combination of factors, including training and qualifications desired, complexity of the job function, availability of qualified personnel, and particular regional influences.

Job Descriptions

A clear, concise job description is a valuable adjunct in defining a department's organization and an employee's function in it. The job description should be regarded as the one definitive explanation of what an employee's role is in the organization and what is expected of him from management. There should be a job description for every title in the department.

A large degree of employee dissatisfaction may arise either when the employee does not function according to management's expectations or when additional duties or tasks are given to an employee who does not believe that such additional work is warranted. While the complaint, "It isn't in my job description," is often heard, the fact is that most employees do not know what is or is not in their job description. Many employers fail to make job descriptions available to their employees.

A well thought-out and clearly written job description can serve many purposes and should not merely be regarded as an unpleasant cursory secretarial chore. The optimal job description should be

1. used by hospital and department management to define not only a particular job title's role, but also to define the scope of available respiratory therapy services based on task listing;
2. used by the department manager to describe job openings to job seekers;
3. used during the orientation and training of newly hired practitioners;
4. used to define various levels of education, skill, experience, and longevity within the department (see section on promotional ladders later in this chapter);
5. used to describe definitively a practitioner's expected performance level and tasks that he is allowed to perform;
6. tied into in-house "certification" programs (e.g., intubation, arterial puncture);
7. tied into routine performance evaluations (in fact, any type of employee rating or evaluation system should be directly related to the job description);
8. used in disciplinary measures; and
9. used by new employee or any employee at any stage of the "promotional ladder" to gauge progress, record achievements, and plan upcoming professional endeavors.

Employee Orientation

A comprehensive yet stimulating orientation for newly hired practitioners is essential. The orientation should include hospital and departmental policies, procedures, and rules, as well as a certification protocol for operating critical equipment and performing critical procedures. The length of the orientation period for new employees is at the prerogative of the department's management but should be long enough to allow the new employee to learn the physical layout of the facility, to intermingle and become comfortable with fellow staff members, and to seek answers to questions that have formed during the orientation period.

The orientation period is the ideal time in which to acquaint a new employee with his job description and to interpret it with respect to *actual* working conditions. By some accounts, the orientation period may also provide the manager with a crucial examination of a new employee's ability to learn and function during the probationary period. Sometimes a new employee's weaknesses and strengths become evident during the orientation period.

The observation of apparent educational weaknesses can suggest the subject matter for remedial assistance to the new employee as well as for continuing education for the entire department. The discovery of particular strengths or talents, especially with respect to certain complex devices, procedures, or concepts, can suggest a participatory function for the new employee in the department's in-service education schedule or other teaching programs. That any employee can be weak in one area yet strong in another should be no surprise. It is best for all concerned to deal with this natural phenomenon at the earliest time in the employee's tenure.

Finally, during each new employee's orientation period the department management should take the time to "get to know" that practitioner. The establishment of *human relations* between an employee and his manager is an invaluable aid in promoting good employee–employer relationships. Such relationships often ward off certain labor-specific employee-related problems. In addition, the departmental leadership should, during the "give-and-take" that occurs during orientation, use the opportunity to learn as much as possible from the newly hired employee. Fresh graduates, for example, may provide details with respect to current course content in the respiratory therapy programs; "veterans" of other hospitals can provide information on special programs, equipment, and procedures and can often be the source of new or updated information.

The schema listed on p. 136 could serve as a readily adaptable model of an "orientation checklist" that can be used by the employee and management alike in the development of the employee's personnel file.

Promotional Ladder

Workers in professional jobs have come to expect upward mobility as a sort of implied benefit. It is not uncommon for job candidates to inquire as distinctly about promotional opportunities as they do about salaries. Fully staffed, contemporary respiratory therapy departments generally cannot provide a great deal of upward mobility. This is unfortunately reflected in the high degree of lateral mobility that seems to exist—practitioners moving from one hospital to the next in search of higher salaries and improved benefits. In fact, there are few upper level positions avail-

ORIENTATION CHECKLIST

I. Policies and Rules
   1. Shift and hours
   2. Sick leave notification
   3. Staffing schedule
   4. Attendance records
   5. Payroll
   6. Leave request system
   7. "On call" system
   8. Receipt of job description
   9. Telephone and paging
   10. Department policy/procedure manual review
   11. Computer system ID and password/security
   12. Other: ______(specify)______

II. Equipment Operation Certification
   1. (brand) Adult ventilator
   2. (brand) Infant ventilator
   3. (brand) Transport ventilator
   4. (brand) Transport incubator
   5. (brand) Heated humidifier
   6. (brand) Oxygen analyzer
   7. (brand) Oxygen/aerosol tent
   8. (brand) Blood gas analyzer
   9. (brand) Transcutaneous oxygen monitor
   10. (brand) Oximeter
   11. (brand) Programmable calculator
   12. (brand) Computer system/terminal
   13. (brand) Other

III. Procedure Competency Certification
   1. Basic arterial puncture/sampling
   2. Arterial catheter installation
   3. Arterial catheter sampling
   4. Swan–Ganz catheter sampling
   5. "Arterialized" capillary sampling
   6. Transcutaneous electrode application
   7. Blood gas analyzer quality control
   8. Blood gas analyzer routine maintenance
   9. Blood gas analyzer electrode maintenance
   10. Allen ulnar artery patency test
   11. Oral endotracheal intubation
   12. Peak flow measurement
   13. Inspiratory force measurement
   14. Bedside pulmonary function testing
   15. Administration of IPPB
   16. Administration of medication by nebulizer
   17. Administration of chest physiotherapy
   18. Tracheal suctioning
   19. Tracheotomy tube change
   20. Swan–Ganz assistance
   21. Fiberoptic bronchoscopy assistance
   22. Basic cardiac life support
   23. Other: ______(specify)______

able in most respiratory therapy departments, although there are numerous candidates waiting to be promoted to shift supervisor, assistant technical director, education coordinator, and so on. The success of a respiratory care service largely depends on the number of available *practitioners*, not managers; thus the likelihood for many promotions to managerial positions in any given department is small.

In some departments, however, the implementation of an *in-grade* promotional ladder may be the method by which a promotional system can be established. The promotional ladder should be developed as an improved internal method for classifying and remunerating respiratory therapy practitioners according to the extent of their education, postgraduate experience, status with respect to credentialing, and longevity with the institution. Although only a few practitioners might be elevated to a management-level position, many more could enjoy title and salary increases within their grade.

The establishment of a promotional ladder where none previously existed might be justified by some or all of the following factors, depending on local circumstances.

1. Prevailing regional practice. Neighboring hospitals may have similar promotional systems for the same or similar classes of employees.
2. Recruiting aid. Promotional programs are useful aids in attracting qualified persons to apply for open positions.
3. Incentive to remain. A well-defined, predictable promotional program entices incumbents to remain on the job rather than to seek advancement elsewhere.
4. Increased morale. A predictable program of title and salary advances promotes employee morale and satisfaction.

One particular promotional ladder that was recently adopted in a respiratory care service in a state-budgeted university hospital is shown in Table 6-1. Many facets of this schema can be readily changed to fit the specific needs of individual services. One will note the impact of "task-to-training" matching in this schema.

Specialization Versus Rotation

Inasmuch as many large hospitals, and even some of the smaller ones, have developed a variety of intensive care units or a number of *specialty programs*,

Table 6-1. Qualifications for Employment as a Respiratory Therapy Practitioner at University Hospital, Stony Brook, New York*

	"THERAPIST"		"CLINICIAN"	
CRITERIA	*I*	*II*	*III*	*IV*
MINIMUM "TRAINEE" CRITERIA				
AA or higher college degree in respiratory therapy, cardiorespiratory sciences, or the equivalent	Yes	Yes	Yes	Yes
Graduate (defined as a "holder of a 'certificate of completion'") of an AMA-approved respiratory therapy *therapist level* educational program	Yes	Yes	Yes	Yes
Eligibility to sit for the written portion of the Registry examination given by the National Board for Respiratory Therapy (NBRT)	Yes	Yes	Yes	Yes
Experience: no less than that associated with the clinical rotations required by the candidates' AMA-approved RT educational program	Yes	Yes	Yes	Yes
ADVANCED PLACEMENT CRITERIA				
Additional postgraduate experience: at least 1 year but not more than 2 years of postgraduate clinical experience in a hospital setting	No	Yes	Yes	Yes
Successful completion (pass) of the written portion of the NBRT Registry examination	No	No	Yes ↑	Yes
Further postgraduate experience: at least 2 years but not more than 4 years in a hospital setting that must include ICU exposure	No	No	or Yes	Yes
Successful completion of the clinical simulation portion of the NBRT Registry examination and receipt of the "RRT" credential and registry number	No	No	No	Yes/No
Specialty experience and/or 4+ years of clinical experience in a hospital and/or ICU setting of which 6 months must be at University Hospital/SB	No	No	No	Yes

*Example of a "promotional ladder" implemented at a medium-sized university-affiliated teaching hospital. The yes/no format identifies for the personnel department and equal employment opportunity committee those qualifications that a candidate must possess to be considered for a particular shift. Thus, the promotional ladder is useful in placement of newly hired personnel and for promotion of incumbent personnel.

The distinction between "therapist" and "clinician" is for in-house titling purposes used to quickly identify personnel according to grade and experience. Rather than place the titles grade I, grade II, grade III, or grade IV on identification badges, personnel are designated in an abbreviated fashion as either respiratory therapists or respiratory therapy clinicians. Other designations such as technician, junior therapist, senior therapist, lead therapist, and so on are used in other institutions for the same purpose. The promotional ladder concept is readily adaptable to individual modification.

there has evolved a parallel development of specialized respiratory care practitioners. To name a few, respiratory care practitioners have specialized in the neonatal and pediatric areas, as well as in trauma, emergency medicine, and adult critical care areas. Specialization for its own sake should be avoided, but specialization, when it appears to offer substantial improvement in the quality or quantity of appropriate respiratory care services rendered, should be given consideration. On the positive side a specialist arguably provides better care than a generalist. Specialists may be a "happier" group of employees because they are doing only what they want to do (presuming they are specializing by their own choice), and thus are not required to do the tasks that do not satisfy them. On the negative side, it could be argued that specialists are difficult to find and difficult to replace. They may become aloof and place distance between themselves and the department's generalists. That, in turn, makes it difficult to find an adequate substitute for the specialist during absence. Additionally, specialists may become more prone to "burnout" and stress-related problems than generalists.

Rotation of practitioners through different clinical and nonclinical sections of a department has long been a very common practice in large and small hospitals alike. The root reasons are often cited as fairness and democracy. Rotation in place of specialization can be justified on the basis of its allowing other practitioners to develop special skills and, if properly administered, as a stress-relieving mechanism. Rotation is not without its drawbacks. Most frequently nurses, who tend to develop team relationships with, and confidence in, a certain practitioner, complain about having to deal with different therapists rather than a specific practitioner with whom they often work.

The Critical Care Respiratory Therapy Practitioner

An evolution toward "critical care respiratory therapy" as a distinct specialty may be occurring. There is as yet, however, no official definition of the *critical care respiratory therapy practitioner*. Perhaps the role delineation described below could be taken as a model on which individual respiratory care services could formulate job descriptions.

This role delineation seeks to answer the rhetorical question, "What *might* a critical care respiratory therapy practitioner do?" It does not suggest any privilege to monopolize skills that may also be required in any other specialty area of respiratory therapy. Although we do not expect all entries described herein to be appropriate for every respiratory care service, this listing should serve as a compendium of potential job functions for therapists who practice in critical care areas. Four categories are recognized as distinct from one another in theory but integrated in actual clinical practice. Many of these skills can be included in job descriptions or performance programs for practitioners whose principal responsibilities lie in intensive care units. They are psychomotor (mechanical) skills; decisional (cognitive) skills; educational (learning and teaching) skills; and management (administrative) skills.

Psychomotor (Mechanical) Skills. The critical care respiratory therapy practitioner should possess a wide range of psychomotor, or mechanical, skills so that decisional, educational, and administrative skills requiring eye–hand coordination, manual dexterity, and sensory perception can be applied efficaciously in diagnosing and treating the critically ill patient. These psychomotor skills include, but are not limited to, the following.

1. Ability to perform physical assessment of the patient through the use of a stethoscope, blood pressure apparatus, respirometer, pressure manometer, and other instruments in addition to the use of the practitioner's tactile, auditory, and olfactory senses. Visual recognition of common signs of illness and distress is paramount.
2. Ability to perform arterial puncture successfully, expeditiously, and atraumatically for the purpose of determining the arterial blood gas/acid–base status.
3. Ability to insert successfully and expeditiously an indwelling radial arterial catheter.
4. Ability to use safely indwelling arterial, venous, and intracardiac or intrapulmonary catheters to obtain blood samples for analysis or vascular pressure measurements.
5. Ability to correctly maintain, operate, calibrate, and troubleshoot blood gas analyzers, oximeters, capnographs, and related instrumentation.
6. Ability to assist the physician with insertion of balloon flotation pulmonary-artery catheters through the preparation, calibration, and operation of hemodynamic monitoring instrumentation.
7. Ability to maintain, calibrate, and operate

hemodynamic pressure monitoring, electrocardiographic monitoring, cardiac output monitoring, and other directly related instrumentation, including appropriate record-keeping.

8. Ability to perform endotracheal intubation successfully, expeditiously, and atraumatically under emergency and selective circumstances.
9. Ability to perform efficacious and atraumatic nasotracheal or tracheal suction and tracheal lavage to maintain bronchopulmonary hygiene.
10. Ability to perform basic life support maneuvers efficaciously, such as maintenance of a patent anatomical airway, external cardiac compression, and artificial ventilation by way of mouth-to-mouth, bag-and-mask, and related ventilatory techniques.
11. Ability to maintain, monitor, measure, and adjust mechanical lung ventilators appropriately to assure proper function and to ascertain therapeutic effectiveness.
12. Ability to measure, using appropriate available instrumentation, the following variables of ventilatory, gas exchange, and hemodynamic function: respiratory rate; tidal and minute ventilation; dead space ventilation; alveolar-to-arterial PO_2 gradient; intrapulmonary shunt fraction; respiratory mechanics, including total resistance and static and dynamic compliance; hemodynamic variables that may include pulse rate, blood pressure, pulmonary artery pressure, pulmonary wedge pressure, cardiac output, vascular resistance, and ventricular stroke work; and oxygenation variables that may include arterial and mixed venous oxygen contents and total systemic oxygen transport.
13. Ability to perform routine respiratory therapy procedures that include, but are not limited to, administration of oxygen by various modalities; administration of aerosolized pharmaceuticals by IPPB and medication nebulizers; administration of aerosol and heated humidification therapies and performance of various modalities of chest physiotherapy.
14. Ability to maintain, monitor, and operate chest tube drainage and suction devices.

Decisional (Cognitive) Skills. The critical care respiratory therapy practitioner should have a wide range of decisional, or cognitive, skills applicable to a large variety of clinical situations and disease states. These skills should enable the critical care respiratory therapy practitioner to take immediate therapeutic or diagnostic action, if necessary, or should, at the least, allow the critical care respiratory therapy practitioner to communicate effectively his observations or findings and recommendations to the responsible physician. Cognition is defined in one dictionary as "the act or process of knowing, including both awareness and judgment." Accordingly, decisional skills in actuality are antecedent to the psychomotor (mechanical) skills referred to above.

Education (Learning and Teaching) Skills. The critical care respiratory therapy practitioner should possess educational skills commensurate with the expected job performance. Educational skills are a "two-way street": Practitioners should be capable of learning and comprehending new knowledge as well as teaching already known facts, concepts, and procedures to others. The very process of teaching, when done effectively, often provides the additional benefit to the instructor of learning, relearning, or reinforcing his own knowledge of the subject matter that he is teaching.

Because a list of specific teaching skills is beyond the scope of this chapter, it should be reiterated that a critical care respiratory therapy practitioner's education skills should be commensurate with the expected job performance. If, for example, the practitioner's job role requires manipulation of Swan-Ganz catheters, he should be capable of enhancing his own knowledge-base regarding that procedure, and he should likewise be capable of passing on that information, through some educational process, to his peers and junior coworkers. Educational skills generally should probably be decided on by the managerial and medical directors of a practitioner's department.

Management (Administrative) Skills. The intensive nature of respiratory therapy practice in a hospital's critical care areas requires mature personnel who fully understand their hospital and departmental organization and their own role therein. A department's administrative and medical management group should make every effort to involve the critical care practitioners, if not all practitioners the department employs, in the majority of administrative plans, projects, and decisions. Likewise, the critical care practitioners, as well as the entire departmental staff (if such a distinction exists), should be obliged to participate fully in such activities. Participatory management is a concept often discussed in literature directed toward managers. But managers, in turn, must alert their staff to their concurrence with this approach and must teach their staff what is expected of them, if participatory management is to be worthwhile. Thus, critical care respiratory therapy practitioners should try to develop an awareness relative to the following generalized areas.

1. Development, implementation, and maintenance of departmental record keeping systems
2. Development, implementation, and maintenance of departmental quality assurance programs and audits
3. Development, implementation, and maintenance of departmental equipment maintenance, repair, and operational verification records
4. Equipment evaluation and selection processes, including applications and budgetary considerations
5. Budget planning, including the forecasting of equipment, supply, and personnel requirements using accepted techniques
6. Policy and procedure manual development, revision, implementation, and application
7. Maintenance of detailed statistical records on departmental operations, procedures performed, man-hours rendered, and billing rendered, among others
8. Continuing reevaluation of patient care priorities (when faced with constraints of staffing or equipment availability)
9. General and specific medicolegal considerations
10. Considerations about ethical issues
11. Liaison relations with other hospital departments and services (especially nursing)
12. Planning and program development with respect to departmental continuing education and in-service

Alternative Staffing Patterns

Alternative staff scheduling patterns and systems have recently been introduced in respiratory therapy departments to relieve stress, provide more balanced coverage, and promote improved employer–employee relations, in addition to or instead of other benefits. The 3-day and 4-day work weeks are an outgrowth of the desire of managers to allow nontraditional personnel scheduling in response to employee preferences. Another innovation known as "flex time" (flexible work schedules) has also been introduced in other industries but not yet to any significant degree in respiratory therapy or the health care industry.

The major attractions of alternative staffing patterns to respiratory care service managers have been that they reportedly reduce excess absenteeism, increase employee morale, and reduce employee turnover rate. To employees, the various methods of alternative staffing are said to result in increased free time, diminished commuting costs, and increased job satisfaction. In a field in which qualified manpower is scarce and practitioners are apt to change jobs readily, job satisfaction, and innovative contemporary methods that achieve it, should be a prime concern of all respiratory therapy practitioners.

RECORD KEEPING

The evolution and expansion of respiratory care departments have made new methods of record keeping necessary, from the standpoint of patient care and because of legal requirements. Standard VII of the JCAH Standards for Respiratory Care Services states that "reports of all respiratory care services provided to the patient shall be made part of the patient's medical record."[1] This Standard, and its interpretation, makes old systems of record keeping, where the therapist was not allowed access to the patient's chart and merely checked off that a specified task had been done, not only obsolete but also inadequate. The documentation required by the Standard includes reference to *at least* the "type of therapy, dates and times of administration, specifications of the prescription, [and] effects of therapy, including any adverse reactions."

Today the process of correctly communicating the condition and status of the patient, as well as fully describing the procedures rendered, is as much a legal and ethical requirement of quality patient care as is actually performing the procedure. Accurate, informative, basic record-keeping systems are practical, cost-effective, and available to any department, regardless of size. The only limitation is the lack of innovative department administration in developing these systems.

One of the first steps toward development of a modern record-keeping system is the establishment of a departmental *task list* that should cover all areas of departmental activity. Once the goals and objectives are decided on, development of a means of achieving them is the next logical step. How is it to be done and what is to be done? A task list partially answers these questions. If the identified tasks are satisfactorily completed, then a department can be said to be meeting its goals. If there are inappropriate or incomplete tasks, or ones that are counterproductive, then the goals and objectives of the department are not being met. These tasks vary to a great extent from department to department; a list of possible activities is given on p. 142.

The record-keeping system, which forms much of the data base from which the department operates, rests solely on the information collected at the bedside. This information is not only crucial to the coordinated care of the patient, but also to department planning. Methods of getting this information to the department may range from a carbon copy to a computer terminal. Each department must develop a system that meets its own needs.

Facts on what is actually being done to the patient and the patient's reaction are crucial; therefore, each therapist should be provided with a list of the required information (observation lists or parameter checks) that is easy to handle and can be rapidly, but accurately, filled out. Of primary importance is that the list be restricted to *factual* information such as the treatment performed, pulse rate, tidal volume, and medication administered. Subjective opinions are best eliminated. Other therapist observations may be included in the data, but factual information gives the most accurate picture of a patient's progress and the quality of care. Given on p. 143 is a list of the data that might be considered. Obviously, only the parameters of pertinence determined in one's own department and individualized to the patient should be recorded.

From the activities list and parameter checklist, a *qualitative* overview of departmental function can be ascertained. The next step involves collecting and analyzing the frequency with which such functions are performed in order to derive a *quantitative* basis for departmental function (statistical analysis) that, in turn, will serve as departmental historian (retrospective analysis), prophet, and planner (prospective analysis). Such statistical analyses should consider that some departmental activities are "invisible" (*i.e.*, they are real and necessary functions of the department, the charges for which are divided among the "visible" functions of the department) (see below).

OXYGEN THERAPY

Visible (generally seen and appreciated, if not understood, by the patient)

1. Equipment: masks, cannulas, tubing, flowmeters
2. Oxygen
3. Solutions or medications used
4. Nurse or therapist when directly administering therapy

Invisible (generally not seen by the patient but vital to the process)

1. Director's time: medical, technical
2. Supervisor's time
3. Report time
4. Equipment repair, maintenance, and sterilization (*see* Chap. 7)
5. Oxygen storage and transport (*see* Chap. 15).
6. In-service and other education
7. Clerical and billing time
8. Charting
9. Hospital-determined indirect expenses
   a. Plant operation (heat, air conditioning, lights, telephone, grounds, security, dietary, housekeeping)
   b. Plant depreciation
   c. Administrative and personnel costs
   d. Noncollectible billing

Analysis of these activities and their assigned charges comprises the basis for periodic departmental statistical reports, some suggested components of which are listed on p. 144.

Before quality-control information is obtained from the basic record collection, each department must determine what "quality" should be for that specific institution. Certainly the quality of patient care would be ideal if therapist performance were uniform across the country, regardless of the size of an institution.[15] However, taking data from one institution and trying to apply it to another will not take into account important factors such as physical plant layout, size of staff, patient type and load, methods of therapy, and other factors unique to each institution. One of the chief controlling factors will be cost-effectiveness, since what may be financially practical for one institution may be financially impossible for another. If, however, administrators and personnel are motivated and innovative, the basic data can be used in ways limited only by the ingenuity and capabilities of the people using the system.

DEPARTMENTAL ACTIVITY LIST

1. Aerosol therapy
   - Nebulizer treatment
   - USN treatment
   - Isolette
   - Pediatric tent
   - O_2 hood
   - Intermittent nebulizer treatment
2. Airway care
   - Suctioning*
   - Intubation*
   - Extubation*
   - Tracheotomy care*
3. Bronchoscopy assistance
4. Calibration of devices
5. Chest physiotherapy
   - Percussion, vibration, and positioning
   - Breathing exercises
   - Breathing retraining
6. Clinical visits
7. Generation of progress notes*
8. CO_2 production measurements*
9. Carbogen treatment
10 CPAP*
11. Resuscitation
12. Education and training
    - Preoperative patient training
    - Rehabilitation training
13. Continuing education*
    - Rounds
    - Chest conferences
    - Pulmonary conferences
    - Instructor activity
    - Inservice education activities
14. Equipment change
15. Equipment check*
16. Equipment cleaning (general)*
17. Equipment repair*
18. Equipment setup
19. Establishment of patient goals and objectives*
20. Use of resuscitators (hand)*
21. Home visits
22. Humidity therapy
    - Isolette
    - O_2 hood
23. IPPB with or without USN
24. Observation*
    - Patient
    - Student
    - Special procedure
25. Oxygen therapy
    - Isolette
    - Pediatric tent
    - O_2 hood
    - Cannula
    - Nonrebreathing mask
    - Partial rebreathing mask
    - Air entrainment mask
    - Simple mask
    - Face tent
26. Longitudinal patient assessment*
27. Portable O_2
    - O_2 walker
    - O_2 cylinder
28. Quality control functions*
29. Respirator adjustment*
30. Social service evaluation
31. Spirometry
    - Bedside, prebronchodilator or postbronchodilator
32. Sputum induction
33. Transportation of patient*
34. Endotracheal and tracheotomy tube changes
35. Ventilator management
36. Weaning*
37. Blood gas sampling
38. Body plethysmography
39. Closing volume studies
40. Blood gas analysis
41. Exercise testing
42. Isoflow/volume study
43. Lung compliance study
44. Nitrogen washout
45. P_{50}
46. Scholandering of gases

*Possible nonchargeable items (*see* text).

CLINICAL OBSERVATIONS OF POSSIBLE IMPORTANCE

1. Patient name
2. Patient number
3. Patient room number
4. Date of therapy
5. Mode of therapy (oxygen, aerosol, IPPB)
6. Patient interface (mask, trach tube, mouthpiece)
7. Mode of breathing (spontaneous, assist, control, IMV)
8. Therapist time spent
9. Patient time spent
10. Reason therapy not done
11. Timer number
12. Timer reading
13. Patient condition
14. Patient attitude
15. Patient body weight (kg)
16. Patient position during therapy
17. Total fluid intake (previous 8 hr)
18. Total fluid output (previous 8 hr)
19. Tracheostomy tube size
20. Inflation hold
21. Inspired gas temperature
22. Mechanical flow rate
23. Peak patient inspiratory flow rate
24. Peak patient expiratory flow rate
25. Lost volume (gas compressibility and leakage)
26. Description of cough
27. Description of sputum
28. Auscultation of breath sounds
29. Pretherapy pulse
30. Pretherapy respiratory rate
31. Pulse during therapy
32. Respiratory rate during therapy
33. Tidal volume during therapy
34. Posttherapy pulse
35. Posttherapy respiratory rate
36. Blood pressure
37. Arterial mean pressure (when available)
38. Patient temperature
39. CVP (when available)
40. Pulmonary wedge pressure (when available)
41. Urine output
42. Cardiac output
43. Vital capacity
44. Patient inspiratory effort
45. Patient expiratory effort
46. $P_{E_{CO_2}}$
47. Ventilator rate
48. Spontaneous patient tidal volume
49. Total expired minute volume
50. Mechanical dead space
51. Mechanical sighs/hr
52. Inspiratory time
53. Expiratory time
54. I/E ratio
55. $F_{I_{O_2}}$
56. Cuff volume and pressure
57. Peak machine pressure
58. Static machine pressure
59. PEEP/CPAP pressure
60. Static compliance
61. Type of medication
62. Strength of medication
63. Quantity of medication
64. Site of activity (*e.g.,* left radial artery for arterial blood sampling)
65. Indication of adverse patient reaction
66. Number of incentive spirometer breaths
67. *p*H
68. Pa_{CO_2}
69. $P_{A_{O_2}}$
70. Pa_{O_2}
71. O_2 content
72. A-a gradient
73. Base excess
74. HCO_3
75. V_D/V_T
76. O_2 uptake
77. A-V O_2 difference
78. $P\bar{v}_{O_2}$
79. % shunt
80. Hemoglobin concentration
81. Narrative comment: Description of therapy beyond standard observations

A THEORETICAL DEPARTMENTAL STATISTICS LIST

Income

1. Number of treatments (by modality)
2. Number of patients receiving treatments (by modality)
3. Units of care* (by modality)
4. Charges per patient:
    a. by modality
    b. by disease category
    c. by location (*e.g.,* RICU, pulmonary unit, rehabilitation program)
5. Departmental income (by modality)
6. Total gross charges per period
7. Net departmental revenue
8. Gross and net revenue divided by total number of staff
9. Gross revenue per patient
10. Gross revenue per modality
11. Gross revenue divided by number of procedures = gross revenue per procedure

Costs

1. Total personnel salaries
2. Equipment and supplies
3. Direct and indirect overhead
4. Total costs divided by number of treatments* = costs per task

Work Load

1. Total time per individual procedure = average time per procedure
2. Total time per individual therapist
3. Total time per individual patient
4. Total number of procedures per individual patient
5. Total number of tasks*
6. Total of individual tasks*
7. Total tasks per total staff = average individual task performance

*Procedures, tasks, and units of care are all indices of work done, but the terms are not synonymous. For example, an IPPB treatment with bronchodilator aerosol may be thought of as 1 procedure, 5 separate tasks, and 3 units of work. In the same scale, oxygen therapy may be 1 procedure, 3 separate tasks, and 0.5 unit of work. The scaling of work varies from department to department. A procedure comprises variable numbers of tasks; units of work usually reflect the *time* required to perform a task or series of tasks. Thus an IPPB treatment in a cooperative patient may take 15 minutes (*e.g.,* 3 units of work); in an uncooperative patient, a whole hour may be required (12 units of work).

FINANCES AND BUDGETING

This section on the economic aspects of departmental administration is primarily concerned with budget preparation and cost control as they relate to the respiratory care department. Since, however, there is a close correlation between departmental budgets and the overall hospital budget, it is important to be aware of the basic objectives of the hospital, which incorporate planning, forecasting, and controlling activities.

To make a budget functional, the department must not only be aware of, but also must comply with, the institution's basic goals and long-term plans for meeting those goals. Although the budget, by itself, cannot set standards of patient care, the act of budgeting forces the department to think in terms of quality as well as quantity functions, and sharpens the decision-making process. The process of budgeting thus tends to force the total organization to make plans for the most effective use of available resources. It also helps to coordinate activities between various departments.

A budget manual, as well as a budget calendar, should be made available to department heads and others responsible for detailed parts of the budget. Because oral instructions can prove unsatisfactory, the manual should clearly outline procedures for budget preparation, including review and revision procedures, the periods covered, and the procedures for approval. It should also include the scope and purpose of the budgetary program; the authority, duties, and responsibilities of section heads for the preparation, review, revision, and approval of the budget; and a checklist relating to budgetary policy, scope, and contents.

Three main types of budgets can be prepared for various purposes.

1. The *appropriation budget,* which is commonly associated with government agencies, anticipates a specific level of spending for a forecast level of activity in a certain period. The major flaw of this type of budget is its inflexibility and the lack of built-in controls necessary to provide efficient use of the committed resources. In situations where departmental activity is variable from period to period, working within the constraints of an appropriation budget may be difficult.
2. The *forecast budget,* which may be used either for capital plans or for continuing operational

programs, is based on best estimates of departmental activity. Although not as inflexible as the appropriation budget, the forecast budget loses some of its value if the actual level of activity deviates significantly from the planned level of activity and its administration does not respond promptly to the changing needs of the department.

3. The *flexible budget* is built on the premise that certain costs will vary from the level of activity and that other costs will remain relatively fixed over a wide range of activity. Although the flexible budget requires fairly elaborate data collection and processing procedures, it is management's most efficient way of controlling costs while retaining flexibility once the fiscal year is underway.

Although budgetary periods vary from one hospital to another, most institutions use short-term operating budgets that cover a 1-year period as a basis for planning. Projections are generally made for 1-month segments within the budgetary year, with shorter time intervals being required for certain special projections.

Other budgetary approaches have been used. The *13-month budget*, for example, provides equal-length intervals of 28 days, since comparison between months is sometimes difficult when the budget is prepared on a monthly basis with a varying number of days in each month. This method provides for only 364 days of the year; therefore, provision must be made to pick up the extra day (or days during leap year). The *rolling quarter budget* was developed because of the need for regular reviews and involves detailed estimates for the next operating quarter, with less detailed estimates provided for the remaining three quarters of the 12-month period. Since estimates are less reliable the further they project into the future, regular budgetary reviews are necessary so that indicated adjustments may be made to prevent the budget from losing its significance.

Before establishing a budgetary system, the institution, in cooperation with the various departments, should define objectives and long-term goals and analyze the current situation in terms of these objectives. Broadly, these objectives should define the geographic area to be served and the types of services to be provided, reflecting in the process current economic and demographic trends in the area. Long-term goals, which are based on these objectives, help the hospital administration develop an orderly growth pattern that will meet future requirements for physical facilities and services. This type of planning also aids the administration in anticipating major capital needs far enough in advance to institute a program for securing capital funds.

With the translation of plans into financial terms, an obvious need arises for a suitable accounting system framework within which the budget can be built. The people given authority for the operation of the system should have the responsibility for incurring various costs and should accept accountability for fulfilling their share of the overall plan within the guidelines developed in the formulation of policy.

Statistical data should be made available before each new budgetary period, which usually occurs once every year. Knowledge of past performance, trends in types of patients served, new programs, changing composition of the medical staff, economic factors in the community, and demographic trends and changes in the area provide a reasonable starting point for projecting what is likely to happen in the near future.

These trends should be noted not only before budget renewal, but also after it as well. It is important to be continually aware of the implications of the budget on an up-to-date basis. A formal budget-reporting program must therefore be implemented by the accounting department. Normally these reports will be issued monthly, with more frequent reports during unusual circumstances. Proper use of periodic reports will simplify accurate projections of the department's financial position at any future date in the budgetary year and, more important, at year's end.

ORGANIZATION OF THE BUDGETARY PROGRAM

Key people and groups who play necessary roles in the budgetary process are the *governing board*, which establishes goals and policies and gives final approval to the budget; the *administrator*, who is ultimately responsible for the formulation and execution of the budget and who uses the budget to evaluate the performance of various organizational elements; the *department heads*, who should develop a budget for their own areas of operation within the framework of the broad policies and plans set forth by higher authority; the *controller* (or chief financial executive), who should develop procedural details, forms, and schedules, provide past statistical and dollar data for operating personnel, coordinate the review and revision of budget estimates, develop the final documents for submission to the governing board, and develop periodic budget performance reports and variance analysis; and the *budget committee*, which is usually headed by the controller but might include the administrator, the controller, and one or more department heads. Medical staff representatives and the governing board serve in an advisory capacity.

The budget committee, which acts primarily in an advisory capacity during the preparation of the budget, reviews the budgetary estimates in terms of plans established and coordinates various portions from interacting areas once sub-budgets have been prepared. The committee will also recommend revisions or changes as inconsistencies occur, as well as appoint an appeals board when major differences of opinion arise over the scope of the plans.

Budgetary Coordination and Timing

The participation of department heads in the preparation of the budget is absolutely necessary. Such participation stimulates more efficient management and promotes cost-consciousness throughout the department. Before preparing their detailed budgetary estimates, however, such individual department heads should be supplied with historical data (both dollar and statistical) by the director of the department or by the budget director (or controller) of the hospital. The budget director is usually responsible for the coordination of all budgetary activities, including processing and summarizing the detailed estimates into the master budget documents. Working through his office in the early developmental stages of budgeting has its advantages.

All departmental expense budgets should be submitted to the administration for review and coordination. After agreement has been reached between department heads and administration on necessary alterations and revisions, the accounting department is responsible for preparing the formal expense-budget document.

After completing the expense, revenue, and capital budgets, the treasurer or controller can compile the cash budget. If, based on estimates contained in the operating and capital budgets, the cash budget reflects cash-balance deficiencies, adjustments in other departmental budgets or other means of generating cash should be determined by the administration. An overall budget-plan summary, including a brief narrative report, a condensed income statement, a summary of capital requirements, and an analysis of available cash, should be submitted to the governing board for discussion and approval. Detailed estimates should be available to the controller so that he can answer any questions raised by the board. Condensed information about significant factors considered in preparing forecasts of anticipated activity and estimates of the impact on hospital services finances focuses emphasis and attention on essentials, thereby expediting consideration of important matters.[2]

THE PROCESS OF DEVELOPING CHARGES

No single facet of departmental management is subject to more variables than the process of charge-setting. When a therapist is asked, "Why do you charge $10 per IPPB treatment?" he may answer: "Because I was told to," (by whom?) or, "Because X, Y, and Z Hospitals nearby do," (why?) or, more commonly, "Because that's what it costs to keep us in the black." (But does it?) In these days of push–pull inflation, there is a more rational approach.

The cost of a procedure may be divided into four portions: indirect costs; salary; other direct costs; and an appropriate and necessary profit margin. In the interest of brevity, various parameters of a typical charge-setting operation are outlined below in terms of the above-mentioned four variables.

Let

1 = indirect costs

1A = number of procedures (*e.g.*, IPPB) done per year

1B = 1A ÷ total number of procedures done by the department per year

1C = total indirect costs for the department per year

$$1D = \frac{1C}{1A} = \text{indirect costs per "costed procedure"}$$

2 = salary costs

2A = salary *per minute* per full-time equivalent (FTE). Here the salary must include base wage and benefits (FICA, sick leave, vacations and holidays, health and life insurance, retirement and pension plans, and workmen's compensation). The total of these benefits is often between 20% and 30% of the base wage, a point that may surprise some administrators

2B = direct time the therapist spends performing the procedure with the patient

2C = ancillary time spent in the "invisible part"

of the procedure (e.g., administrative time, medical director's time, equipment sterilization, maintenance and repair, and clerical and billing time). This may be one third of the actual personnel *time* it takes to perform a procedure

2D = (1B + 2C) = total time spent performing procedure

2E = (2A × 2D) = total salary cost per "costed procedure"

3 = other direct costs

3A = 1A

3B = 1B

3C = total *direct* costs for the department per year *minus* salary costs

$$3D = \frac{3C}{3A} \times 3B = \text{direct nonsalary cost per "costed procedure"}$$

4 = profit margin. This term is often misunderstood, particularly in nonprofit hospitals. It is the charge in excess of costs that must be made to support the non-income-generating centers of the hospital, to purchase new and replace old equipment, and the like.

For example, let us calculate the charge for a routine IPPB treatment, with bronchodilator, given the following information on the above parameters.

Step 1 (indirect costs):

1A = 36,000; 1B = 0.5; IC = $150,000

$$ID = \frac{\$150{,}000}{36{,}000} \times 0.5 = \$2.08:$$

Step 2 (salary costs):

2A = $0.12/min.; 2B = 20 min.

2C = 10 min.; 2D = 30 min.

2E = ($0.12/min. × 30 min.) = $3.60.

Step 3 (other direct costs):

3A = 36,000; 3B = 0.5; 3C = $100,000

$$3D = \frac{\$100{,}000}{36{,}000} \times 0.5 = \$1.39.$$

Step 4 (profit margin): This will vary from institution to institution and from procedure to procedure. Here, let it equal 30% of the other costs:

4 = 0.3 (1D + 2E + 3D) = $2.09.

Step 5 (total charge = sum of steps 1–4)

$2.08 + $3.60 + $1.39 + $2.09 = $9.16.

USE OF COMPUTERS IN RESPIRATORY CARE

The trend toward computer use in hospitals makes it possible for respiratory care departments to create highly sophisticated record-keeping systems. In fact, a hospital or department with computer capability can record, as a permanent part of patients' medical records, a daily summary of each patient's therapy, including all patient data collected at the time of each procedure, as well as any pertinent comments by the therapists. The sheer volume of data used in such programs as the Systematized Hospital Uniform Reporting (SHUR) sponsored by the AART is difficult to implement without the use of a computer. What is true for the use of computers in departmental record keeping is equally, if not more, pertinent in recording charges, as discussed above.

Established respiratory care services, as well as those undergoing rehabilitation, will have to consider the practically inevitable impact that computerization will have on respiratory therapy during the 1980s and beyond. We will mention in the Physical Facilities section of this chapter that facilities planning for new departments or expanding existing departments may have to accommodate some form of computer system. The physical location of computer hardware in the department and in intensive care areas should be well thought out to promote ease of use and maximum convenience.

The specter of computerization raises far more complex questions than merely the placement of terminals. Obviously the type of operations and functions to be handled by the computer should be planned and agreed on by all concerned well in advance of the system's installation. Ideally, the computer's applications to the department should be agreed on in advance of the actual purchase of the system. This frequently does not happen when the respiratory care service applications are a subset of a much larger, hospital-wide computer application. If the system will be dedicated solely to the respiratory care service, then tailoring to the individual needs of the department may be more feasible.

The question of whether to acquire a so-called microcomputer or minicomputer or to time-share on a hospital-wide mainframe system will be answered in part by an examination of the anticipated computer uses. Microcomputers (including some of the popular and readily available "personal computers") may have many applications in a respiratory care service for dedicated functions such as tracking statistics, attendance records, and blood gas analysis and pulmonary function testing. Hemodynamic and blood gas calculations and interpretations can be readily performed on a microcomputer. It should be expected that respiratory therapy software of increasing quantity, quality, and ingenuity will become available over the next few years. Much of that software will probably be developed, or at least suggested, by respiratory therapists using personal microcomputers in their departments. It has even been suggested that the installation of a consumer-oriented microcomputer in respiratory care departments is desirable for training and developing *computer-literate* respiratory therapy practitioners.

Microcomputers and mainframe systems represent a much larger investment as far as purchase price and operating cost. However, they may serve many users simultaneously through a system of remote terminals and printers. These larger systems require a correspondingly larger number of users or a substantial amount of actual computing time in order to be economical. It is likely that a respiratory care service would be one of many using departments rather than being the sole user of such systems. The fact that monitoring systems for collecting and filing physiological data are frequently based on a minicomputer-type central processor and storage method might suggest that such an existing system could handle certain additional respiratory therapy data. This approach may, in certain circumstances, be preferable to the acquisition of a dedicated microcomputer.

In those departments in which the acquisition of any type of conventional computer system is unlikely, the possibility of purchasing either a sophisticated programmable calculator or one of the recently introduced brands of "hand-held computer" should be considered. These units are inexpensive ($300–500) and easy to use, although there is little available software at present; users will have to develop their own programs for their specific applications. But this limitation, as in the case of the microcomputer, is bound to pass as more and more users develop programs that will eventually be shared in the scientific journals or offered for sale in the software marketplace. In concert with the increased availability of software for the programmable calculators and hand-held computers, the availability of low-cost printers, plotters, and mass storage peripherals for these devices will enhance their attractiveness and usefulness. Arguably, their relatively low price can enable the acquisition of multiple units (one for each critical care area, for example) instead of one larger and centrally located microcomputer system.

Regardless of the type of computer equipment that may exist in any respiratory care service at present, it can be anticipated that a substantial number of respiratory therapy departments will either acquire their own computer equipment or tie into a hospital-wide system throughout this decade and beyond. Thus the need arises for at least one person within these departments to develop skills related to "computerization" generally and the department's actual computer equipment specifically. Although the respiratory therapy profession is only at the threshold of its "computer age," it is likely that a person will be required in computerized departments for coordinating computer activities, developing and overseeing program and software implementation, training respiratory therapy practitioners, and coordinating cooperative programs between respiratory care, biomedical engineering, and computer and information service departments.

THE AUDIT PROCESS AND QUALITY CONTROL

Standards for good-quality patient care can be rendered ineffective without an organized method for determining whether these standards are being met. Indeed, since the Darling decision in 1965 (*see* Chap. 5), an increasing body of law speaks to the issue of hospital responsibility for patient care. The Medicare and Medicaid enactments of 1966 (Titles 18 and 19) mandated utilization review of patient hospitalizations covered by that legislation. In 1968, the Supreme Court of Massachusetts held that local standards of care were no longer acceptable benchmarks of quality care in any particular area, given that national standards were readily accessible through participation in the printed media, conferences, and other types of postgraduate education. To be "up-to-date" in Bedford, Massachusetts, one would need to be "up-to-date" in Boston!

Respiratory care departments must establish mechanisms for evaluation and selfassessment of the quality of patient care they deliver. Departmental self-surveillance activities aimed at evaluating performance in the delivery of patient care are part of a hospital-wide quality-assurance program (QAP). The term "quality assurance" has been used to indicate

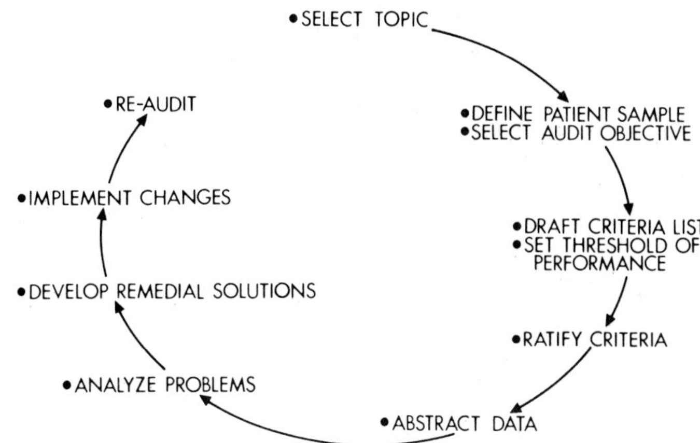

Fig. 6-5. Diagrammatic representation of the audit program process as suggested by the California Medical Association and the California Hospital Association (the "California model").

that programs developed on these bases will accomplish more than simple surveillance or assessment of care provided within an impatient facility; it implies that the department will make a further commitment to bring about change by appropriate corrective action if suboptimal levels of care are identified; it can, therefore, *assure* the patient community it serves that the care is of the highest quality and that it is cost-effective.[3]

Hospital boards and physicians generally, despite the historical precedents cited, have been somewhat complacent about the yield and cost-effectiveness of the audit procedure. Readers, however, should not be deterred; *for good or ill, the audit procedure is here to stay, in one form or another, for years to come.* Several *forms* of audit have been proposed, some by the JCAH, others by hospital associations or state medical societies. Whichever audit vehicle is chosen is probably of little account. What *is* important is that some QAP exist and be operative in every department.

The basic objectives of a respiratory care department QAP are to identify, analyze, and correct departmental areas of suboptimal care through the use of retrospective, concurrent, or prospective evaluation mechanisms; to comply with the requirements of regulatory agencies, health insurers, consumer groups, and so forth;* to reduce departmental and institutional exposure to risk of legal actions for malpractice, negligence, and so forth; and to provide a management tool for assessing and developing departmental patient care policies and procedures.

*Examples include the Social Security amendments of 1972 (PL 92-603) and the pertinent JCAH standards (Quality of Professional Services [supplemental standard], March 1975).

The two main types of QAP are departmental audit and utilization review, which are discussed in detail in the following section.

AUDIT QUALITY CONTROL

This section discusses the selection of audit topics, the definition of patient or procedure samples, and the selection of audit objectives; lists some examples of objectives for audit topics, demonstrating the development of a draft criteria list; and describes some methods for verifying and clarifying criteria, including methods of ratifying criteria, threshold for action levels and organizing analysis, and action planning (Fig. 6-5).

Selecting an Audit Topic

An audit topic should demonstrate that high-quality care is provided to a significant group of patients, identify problems in the pattern of patient care, and initiate remedial action. Appropriate topics might include an admission or discharge diagnosis (e.g., bronchial asthma), a specific diagnostic procedure (e.g., arterial blood gas analysis), a surgical procedure (e.g., tracheostomy), a physical finding (e.g., abnormal breath sounds) or a symptom (e.g., dyspnea), or a treatment modality or procedure (e.g., IPPB).

Criteria for the topic selection include a high occurrence rate, the fact that treatment significantly alters the health of the patient, and a specific interest on the part of the hospital or department in what is thought to be a problem area. Generally, only topics known to be amenable to proper medical intervention should be selected.

EXAMPLES OF SPECIFIC OBJECTIVES WITHIN AUDIT TOPICS*

Topic: Tracheostomy
Objective: To improve the quality of tracheostomy care.

Topic: Arterial blood gases
Objective: To improve the management of turnaround time from time requested, drawn, and report-charted.

Topic: Chronic obstructive pulmonary disease
Objective: To increase the accuracy of diagnosis at the time of admission.

*Note that audit objectives are simply narrower aspects of the topic.

The audit committee (those persons assigned the responsibility for doing the audit) should make the final topic selection to ensure that they are comfortable with the topic and can identify with it. Interest and enthusiasm for the audit are very important. Much of the information needed for the audit can be supplied by statistics by the respiratory care department itself.

Defining the Patient Sample

Many variables may be important when selecting a homogeneous patient population to make up the audit sample, such as age, sex, mode of treatment, primary or associated diagnosis, and anything that might apply to a particular institution. A statistically significant number of patients for the audit (probably randomly selected) should be studied. The most homogeneous population possible should be identified *before* setting audit criteria because the standards of care may vary with different groups of patients.

Some important considerations in defining a homogeneous population include mode of treatment, severity of illness, condition at admission (conscious, unconscious), terminal/salvageable, and the social and psychological resources of the patient or family.

Setting Audit Objectives

An *audit objective* is a critical aspect of an audit topic that serves as a focus for development of criteria (see below). Without clear objectives and criteria, the audit could lead to either a long laundry list of detailed criteria for care or a few criteria that are too general to uncover real problems. The critical aspects of care within a topic can usually be covered by doing two or three audits on that topic, using different objectives each time.

Developing a Draft Criteria List

The draft criteria list comprises four to eight clear sentences that are used as unique and essential indicators relative to the objective of the audit. The audit topic may be limited to process or outcome criteria or may include both. The criteria list should be developed by a small, multidisciplinary group of health professionals involved in the care of the patients to be reviewed in the audit. The following basic steps should be followed in order to complete the development of the draft list.

1. Using the nominal group process of "brainstorming," the group should list ideas for criteria, discuss the priority of these possible criteria, and select the most important for the draft criteria list. These criteria should be simple enough so that *no physician or therapist decision-making* is necessary by those who will abstract the information.
2. Using standard procedures for verifying and clarifying criteria, the draft criteria are refined. The group may rely on the medical records department member for assistance.
3. The group should review the topic, objective, and patient sample and modify them, if necessary, in relation to the draft criteria.
4. The group should set threshold for action levels (see below) for each criterion.
5. The group should develop a draft of a criteria list for presentation to all practitioners whose care will be audited (see Table 6–2). The presentation (ratification) will include
   A. the audit topic;
   B. the objective for this topic;
   C. a well-defined patient sample;
   D. four to eight clear draft criteria that are indicators of the critical aspects of care;
   E. threshold for action levels for each criterion, indicating the minimum degree to which the group feels the criterion should be met;
   F. a statement that "all charts that do not meet the criteria will be reviewed by appropriate committee members."

Table 6-2. A Completed Audit: Arterial Blood Gas Sampling*

CRITERIA (I)	THRESHOLD FOR ACTION (II) %	ACTUAL PERFORMANCE (III) %
1. Patient will exhibit at least one of the following signs before the first arterial blood gas (ABG): **a.** chest pain. **b.** abnormal respiratory pattern. **c.** cyanosis or dusky skin. **d.** abnormal breath sounds.	90	80
2. Each ABG drawn shall have the following recorded: **a.** pulse rate. **e.** oxygen % or liters/min. **b.** respiratory rate. **f.** sampling site. **c.** temperature. **g.** patient position. **d.** mode (how breathing?).	95	90
3. A written order requesting the ABG before blood is drawn.	98	75
4. Every order requesting that a repeat ABG be drawn shall be complied with, except when a written statement notifying the physician or nurse that **a.** patient is not available. **b.** patient refused. **c.** problem with the vessel arose.	100	96
5. If sampling is complicated by prolonged bleeding, hematoma during the procedure, or an arterial line complication, a statement about the complication, what was done for the patient, and that the physician or nurse was notified must be recorded.	100	NA (no complication occurred)
6. If a repeat ABG was drawn, the previous sample must be abnormal, or patient will have exhibited the signs listed under criterion 1 after the previous ABG.		
Note: All charts that do not meet the criteria will be reviewed by appropriate committee members.		
Plan: Letters to supervisors regarding remedial action taken.		
Action: Letter sent on (date).		
Reaudit: 6 months.		

*Items that appear in columns I and II have been ratified by the staff before beginning the audit. Performance, or outcome, appears in column III. This audit demonstrates satisfactory arterial blood gas sampling technique involving an inpatient population (excluding NICU). Its objective is to improve the management of arterial blood gas sampling.

Methods for Verifying and Clarifying Criteria (R-U-M-B-A)

Relevant. Each criterion must be specifically related to the objective of the audit and be stated as clearly and concisely as possible.

For example, each arterial blood gas (ABG) drawn shall have the following recorded:

a. heart rate;
b. site drawn;
c. respiratory rate;
d. FI_{O_2} or liter flow of oxygen.

Understandable. Each criterion must be clear and specific; it must be worded explicitly as a complete statement to eliminate any possible misinterpretation.

Example: A patient receiving oxygen therapy should have initial blood gas determinations that demonstrate hypoxemia; for example, $Pa_{O_2} \leq 60$ mm Hg.

Measurable. Each criterion should include the time frame and frequency of the activity or the specific range of test data expected.

Example: A respiratory therapist must be involved in performing tracheostomy care within 8 hours of the tracheostomy or admission.

Behavioral. Each criterion should be an indicator of the activity of a specific group of practitioners or patients in order to identify what or whose behavior should be changed.

Example: A respiratory therapist must be involved in performing tracheostomy care within 8 hours of the tracheostomy or admission.

Achievable. Each criterion should be realistic, given the present state of the art, the local patient population, and the department staff's capabilities.

Example: Mortality from pneumonia may be expected to be higher in a small rural facility serving a population that is largely comprised of elderly patients.

Threshold for Action Level

The threshold for action is the minimum percentage of charts or instances that should meet a criterion to indicate an expected performance pattern. Actual performance below that threshold level obligates the group to recommend action to modify (improve) the performance pattern. The threshold for action does not need to be 100% (perfection) but rather a level the ratification group accepts as an acceptable level of care.

The reason for carefully setting a threshold for action level are

1. to state how often the criterion must be met to assure that a high quality of care has been achieved for this sample of patients;
2. to look for obstacles affecting group performance;
3. to have an objective means of determining when action must be taken to improve patient care;
4. to indicate the value of the criterion to those doing the audit. If the threshold for action level is set below 95%, the group should reconsider whether this criterion is an indicator of *critical* care;
5. to commit the group to examine why a criterion's actual performance level is lower than its threshold for action level.

To determine the threshold for action for each criterion, the following questions should be asked:

1. Is the language of the criterion specific and consistent with the level of compliance chosen?
2. Assuming that 100 patients with the same discharge diagnosis were to be reviewed, could you be assured of quality performance if 98, 95, or 90 patients' records document that the criterion had been met?
3. Conversely, if fewer than 98%, 95%, or 90% of the records contained no such documentation, would you be concerned about the quality of patient care?
4. What does the medical literature (or the Professional Activities Study/Medical Audit Program or California Health Data Corporation statistics) reveal to be the norm for this group of patients?
5. If the data indicate this threshold was met or exceeded, would you be willing to defend the quality of patient care in your department?
6. Conversely, if the data indicate this threshold was *not* met, would you be willing to defend the quality of patient care in your department?

Ratification of Criteria

The single, most important segment of criteria development is criteria ratification. Each member of the staff whose performance will be affected by the audit should be presented with the draft objectives, criteria, and threshold for action levels. Substantive changes in the audit may appropriately derive from their feedback. The audit committee must be willing to compromise on some threshold for action levels and to give up some criteria or to add new ones. The strength of this process is uniform commitment by the staff to the audit procedure *and its implications.*

Data Abstraction

Data abstraction is usually performed by medical record department personnel, although it could just as readily (but probably not as efficiently) be performed in the respiratory care or nursing department. Charts that fail to meet criteria are then sent to the audit committee for review.

Problem Analysis and Action Planning

Who Should Be Involved? The following are people who might be included in a well-structured analysis and action planning committee:

1. Those *working on the audit*
2. Those genuinely *interested* in the problem
3. Those actually *affected* by the problem
4. Those generally *knowledgeable* about all aspects of the problem
5. Those in a position to *make decisions about policy* in the problem area
6. Those in a position to *implement policy* to attempt to alleviate the problem

Optimum Analysis and Action Groups. The following criteria are important to the development of well-coordinated optimum analysis and action groups:

1. Between four and seven members
2. People having worked on problem-solving together
3. At least two people who have assumed leadership roles (one person who is task-oriented; the other group/process-oriented)
4. No hidden agendas on the part of the members
5. Ability to approach a problem objectively
6. Willingness to commit time and effort to these problems

Planning and Reporting System

Whether the problem-solving committee comprises the same people who initiated the audit or is assembled specifically to work on the problems revealed in the audit, a designated member should report the status of their efforts at regular intervals to the audit committee. Regular reporting is essential to remind the audit committee that the audit cycle has not been completed and to keep the departmental management and the medical director informed of audit activities during the completion of the cycle. It might be necessary to involve the audit committee if unresolvable problems arise. There is a need to have an efficient *coordinator* who keeps careful minutes, schedules meetings, and monitors the committee's fact-finding efforts. Such documentation is essential evidence of a thorough audit program.

Reporting of Results

The results of an audit can be reported at departmental meetings. Problem analysis, the procedure used to analyze performance gaps discovered during an audit, as well as remedial action taken to correct any deficiencies discovered, should also be reported. Letters must be sent to the supervisory and administrative staff and to the governing body, informing them of the efforts of those involved in the audit and of the improvement in patient care that was followed. Significant or unique audit findings and accomplishments might be presented in the medical literature.[4]

The Re-audit

The final step of the cycle is the periodic reaudit. The frequency of this process depends on the severity and magnitude of the problems found during the initial audit. Many experts feel that even in the best hospitals, QAP audits will reveal far more problems with *process* (systems) than with poor practice standards or *outcome*. Accordingly, the responsibility for correcting systems problems very frequently will fall on departmental administrators, who are encouraged to learn from their medical colleagues the problems and the benefits of auditing, a new tool of management.

UTILIZATION REVIEW

The nation's medical insurance groups are placing pressure on hospitals and physicians to resort to respiratory services only for patients who need them. A recent Congressional Office of Technology Assessment study reported that much of the use of respiratory services has occurred without sufficient scientific evidence demonstrating that it brings about measureable improvement in the patient's physical condition.

To combat this, medical insurance groups in cooperation with professional medical associations such as the American College of Physicians and the American Academy of Pediatrics have drawn guidelines for hospitals to control the ordering of respiratory services to patients. If respiratory care services do not voluntarily respond to these guidelines, health insurance companies will begin to halt payment in the near

Table 6-3. Classification of the Clinical Status of Patients with Respiratory Disease

LEVEL OF CARE	APPROXIMATE LENGTH OF STAY
I. Life support: early recognition of cardiorespiratory failure and initiation of emergency care toward life support	Short as possible in transit to level II
II. A. Intensive or critical respiratory care directed toward reversing cardiopulmonary failure threatening life	3 days
B. Subintensive care directed toward stabilization of cardiopulmonary condition	5 days
III. Continuing acute or subacute respiratory (general ward) care	1 to 2 weeks
IV. Chronic or rehabilitation respiratory care (skilled-nursing facility level [SNF])	7 to 10 weeks
V. Extended respiratory management, including home care and outpatient rehabilitation, directed toward prevention of recurrent respiratory failure and stabilization of chronic lung disease	Variable
VI. Symptomatic treatment of progressive chronic lung disease, preterminal outpatient	Indefinitely

future. Documentation of a respiratory service need should always accompany a physician's order. One answer to federal demands to reduce the cost of respiratory services while improving the quality of respiratory care is to prepare protocols for nursing and respiratory care personnel to carry out physician's orders while providing information for the medical staff.[13]

At present, many general hospitals are well equipped to deal with acute, severe respiratory problems; however, the present health care system does not provide adequate resources to support patients with lesser degrees of pulmonary disability. Such patients are cared for in acute-care hospitals, which is wasteful of money and personnel and creates dilemmas of both ethics and utilization.

A logical classification of the clinical status of patients with respiratory disease is presented in Table 6-3.

Patients in levels I, II, and III are appropriately treated in well-equipped and adequately staffed general hospitals. The early phases of convalescence are also appropriately managed in such hospitals. Those patients convalescing rapidly will be discharged to their homes.

In many instances, when a patient's convalescent phase is prolonged, the acute care hospital is an economically wasteful facility. For such level IV patients, a less intensive facility that can provide continued supportive care would be desirable. When patients have convalesced to a stable functional level, they may either return to normal health or enter level V. Depending on the level of permanent disability, patients in levels V or VI will be discharged to return home or may require indefinite care in the support facility. Some will simply require assistance in the routines of daily living, whereas others will require supportive respiratory care and rehabilitation. Many patients will require both types of service. A small number of patients with stable, severe, chronic respiratory failure may require continuous ventilator support.

Patients in this latter setting will not require the intensive monitoring and active nursing care of the general hospital. Facilities for patients in levels IV, V, and VI must provide resources for, and personnel skilled in, patient education, the use of respiratory therapy equipment, chest physiotherapy, occupational therapy, and general physical therapy. A limited number of personnel skilled in cardiopulmonary resuscitation, maintenance of a patent airway, and the administration of oral, parenteral, and nebulized medication must be available; however, staff/patient ratios should be much lower than those of a general hospital.

Those responsible for the care of patients with respiratory disease are seriously troubled by the current lack of facilities in other than general hospitals that can provide acceptable care for patients in levels I, II, and III. This is of particular concern because, in some instances, private and government insurance programs will not cover the cost of convalescent care in acute care facilities.

The problem is not merely a lack of facilities. Were such facilities available, it is doubtful that sufficient numbers of skilled personnel would be available to staff them.

Table 6-4. Charting Responsibilities of the Physician, Nurse, and Respiratory Therapist to Satisfy Utilization Review Requirements*

PHYSICIAN'S RESPONSIBILITY	RESPIRATORY CARE AND NURSING DEPARTMENT RESPONSIBILITY
1. Admitting diagnosis, history and physical examination	**1.** Accession notes
2. Daily progress notes reflecting **A.** patient status **B.** response to therapy **C.** response to laboratory and x-ray findings **D.** plans for discharge **E.** justification of transfer (*e.g.,* ICU ward, rehabilitation visit, home) **F.** justification for longer than usual stay	**2.** Problem list including justification for modalities to be used **3.** Daily progress notes reflecting patient status and response to therapy **4.** Correlation of patient status with pulmonary function and arterial blood gas abnormalities **5.** Automatic "stop therapy" orders where indicated (*e.g.,* O_2, IPPB) **6.** Charting of complications of therapy as well as benefits **7.** Avoidance of needless duplication of tests or duplication of services

*This table is not meant to be a comprehensive review of everything normally documented by these workers.

Utilization review is concerned with type and quality of care as surely as is the audit process. It also is concerned with *location* of care, as was discussed above, although the options of intelligent and humane transfer of patients from level III to level IV and higher categories are at present limited.

Review teams must be satisfied that a patient's stay is medically indicated. Table 6-4 illustrates some parameters used in evaluating the need for continuing hospitalization in a patient with respiratory disease. These parameters *must be documented* in the patient's chart, and not just in the general knowledge of the care team.

TOPICS FREQUENTLY EXAMINED IN UTILIZATION REVIEW

1. Patients receiving respiratory therapy services should have a pulmonary diagnosis noted in the chart. History, physical, laboratory, and x-ray data should support the presence of pulmonary problems, and these should be evidenced in the initial workup, progress notes, and discharge summary.
2. Patients at prolonged bed rest or with restricted chest motion or postoperative patients can justifiably be given respiratory therapy, especially if there is a history of smoking, chronic pulmonary disease, or congestive heart failure.
3. Most patients receiving oxygen therapy should have initial blood gas determinations that demonstrate hypoxemia (e.g., $P_{O_2} \leq 60$ mm Hg) and should have follow-up blood gases if oxygen therapy is continued.
4. In many cases, the justification for respiratory therapy services will be obvious from the admission history, physical examination, and laboratory work; however, when a question does exist, the reason respiratory therapy services are needed should be documented in the progress notes (e.g., ineffective cough, tenacious or excessive secretions, atelectasis, pulmonary embolism, paroxysmal cough, wheezing, or dyspnea).
5. Respiratory stop orders should be instituted at least every 5 days, and physicians should reorder therapy as indicated by the clinical condition.
6. Progress notes and respiratory care flow sheets should contain an assessment of the patient's response to respiratory therapy. An accurate record-keeping system is legally, ethically, and morally crucial to the operation of a respiratory care department. Accurate documentation is not only required for the auditing process and for third-party payer reimbursement but

also is critical to quality patient care. Inadequate and inaccurate record keeping can predispose a patient to possibly lethal care, can place in jeopardy the physician who is legally responsible for the patient's care, and can set up the next therapist for involvement in continuing dangerous treatment. Documentation is as important as performing the therapy itself.

7. Charge slips should include itemization of *all* treatments given daily, with justification appearing in the chart as described above. Therapists and administrative personnel share the responsibility for ensuring that a basic minimum of accurate, factual data be recorded for the treatment of each patient. The data should be shared with, and explained to, other members of the health care team in a spirit of cooperation that results in improved patient care. The critical and primary function of the departmental record-keeping system, however, must be to focus on bedside data collection.
8. Finally, both audits and utilization reviews, according to the JCAH, are preferably done on the most frequently seen disease states and on the most commonly employed respiratory care modalities.

PHYSICAL FACILITIES

In nearly all cases, the physical facilities of both the hospital and the respiratory care service will greatly influence the overall organization of the respiratory care department. Major factors such as services offered, equipment inventory, and personnel selection and deployment may be mediated, at least in part, by the prevailing of planned physical facilities.

An extreme example of this assertion is found in a number of municipal hospitals that comprise old buildings that lack piped medical gas systems. Although the respiratory care departments in these facilities strive for excellence, clearly a multitude of concessions must be made on account of the physical plant. Certain types of therapies may not be available because of the lack of piped medical gases. Something as basic as a Venturi oxygen mask with aerosol entrainment provided by a nebulizer driven by compressed air may not be available because of the cost and inconvenience of providing compressed air cylinders at the bedside. Indeed, the mere ability to provide oxygen at any given bedside may require cylinders, special equipment, and a unique division of labor among the department's employees. Fortunately, as hospital planners and architects endeavor to design new hospitals and rehabilitate older ones, comprehensive medical gas installations in all appropriate areas are becoming commonplace. Nevertheless, some managers and practitioners must accept the eventuality of contemporizing departmental organization within already existing facilities that have little likelihood of renovation.

Some practitioners and managers are more fortunate and can expect to become involved in the rehabilitation and redesign of their respiratory care service physical facilities within the next few years. Sometimes this rehabilitation accompanies the reconstruction of an area, the addition of a "new wing" or the expansion of an intensive care unit. If a substantial amount of respiratory care activities are planned for the rehabilitated or expanded area, then thought should be given to relocating the respiratory care service to that area if its current facilities are inadequate or its location relatively inaccessible. Occasionally, the opportunity arises for a practitioner or manager to become involved in the building of a respiratory care department from the ground up in a new hospital or in an existing hospital that has no such department. In any event, those persons responsible for planning the new department or its renovation should remember that an institution never completes the funding of a *poorly planned* respiratory care department. Since successful facility planning depends on the attention to details consistent with the department's philosophy of operation, it is unfortunate when a planner accepts the job but is unwilling or unable to cope with details. The therapist who is going to direct the department must be very interested in details of planning. *The Respiratory Care Service Functional Programming Worksheet,* published by the U.S. Department of Health, Education, and Welfare, is recommended as a guide for developing a comprehensive approach before the initiation of a building project.[17]

Planning should go through various steps before reaching the drawing board stage, and the input of an appropriate respiratory therapy practitioner or manager should be available at all stages. At an early stage of planning, answers to some of the following *basic questions* should be sought:

1. What is the total number of staff?
2. What are the types of functions and services that the department will be providing?

3. Will the department perform its own equipment cleaning and sterilization, or will this be done by the Central Sterile Supply?
4. Will the respiratory care department be responsible for performing blood gas analyses and maintaining the instruments, or will this be done by any other department? How many blood gas instruments will be needed? Will they be remotely located in satellite laboratories or centrally operated in a main blood gas laboratory?
5. Will the department perform its own equipment repairs and maintenance, or will this be handled by another department or a contracted service?
6. Is a Central Sterile Supply exchange cart system available for providing basic respiratory therapy disposable supplies to all patient units, or will the department have to maintain its own supplies?
7. Is the department to be centralized or decentralized with respect to facilities?
8. Will the department need satellite space and storage areas in or near various parts of the hospital, including the critical care units?
9. Is the hospital planning any additional expansion?
10. What is the 10-year projected growth?

The checklist on p. 158 from the first edition of this book can be readily adapted to tracking the progress of new and rehabilitated respiratory care services at any stage of the planning process.

CONTINUING EDUCATION

Despite current financial constraints on manpower utilization, the interpretation of JCAH Standard II of 1983 states that a respiratory care department is responsible for "the development of programs for the orientation and inservice education of technical and supportive respiratory care personnel."[1] AART standards for continuing education are equally broad and nondefinitive.

The fact that the JCAH and AART have created guidelines rather than regulations has too often been misinterpreted. Continuing education can easily deteriorate into change-of-shift classroom lectures on subjects that have little relevance to the very real problems facing therapists, and which are characterized by boredom and lack of progress. As the need for the improvement of the quality of patient care increases, the very process by which that quality can be achieved moves horizontally or descends in direct proportion to the lack of high-quality continuing education.

If continuing education is ever to play the crucial role it should in improving patient care, those responsible for continuing education must accept the fact that it is a vital part of the operation of a respiratory care department. Basic goals must be set within each institution, since any continuing education program should seek change and improvement. The program should help therapists to become better educated to do a better job by making them aware of changes in procedures, concepts, and equipment. It should also help therapists to understand their job better by making them aware of changes in policy and their own individual roles in patient care. Continuing education must be education for productivity, not education for its own sake.

Determining the needs of each individual department is the first step in designing a productive continuing education program. There are several ways by which such needs can be identified. Bringing in outside experts or resources has been one common method; however, this has met primarily a philosophical rather than a practical need. All too often, outsiders enter the continuing education program with preconceived ideas of what should be taught and do not really analyze or try to understand the problems and needs of each individual department. It is "canned education" based on educational theory rather than practical need.

"More attention is being given now to building in-house capabilities rather than depending on outside experts or resources."[8] Therapists are beginning to assume the role of educators. Certainly an involved therapist employed by a respiratory care department is closer to the needs and problems of that department than an outside expert would be. The therapist–educator, in addition, is answerable to management, which is also concerned with defining and meeting the needs of that department. A director of continuing education, whether his is a full-time job or one of several responsibilities, cannot simply set up a classroom situation, teach a subject, and then leave, content that the job has been done. The in-house director's job is not completed until change and improvement have been effected.

Closely allied with the general educational needs of the department is the need for emphasis on specific areas. One method, the "critical incident analysis,"

1. Will the main base of operation of the respiratory care service have
   - A. administrative/work center only, or
   - B. both of the above plus the pulmonary function laboratory and the treatment center for outpatients?
2. In a centralized, consolidated respiratory care base of operations, which of the following functional spaces will need to be provided?
   - A. reception and patient waiting area
   - B. staff conference space
   - C. staff locker and toilet spaces
   - D. public/patient toilet spaces
   - E. classroom for patient, personnel, or student demonstration and instruction
   - F. bed treatment space
   - G. ambulatory treatment cubicles and lounge/chair spaces
   - H. pulmonary testing laboratory
   - I. blood-gas analysis laboratory
   - J. soiled equipment, cleanup, preparation, packaging, and sterilizing space
   - K. equipment maintenance and repair space
   - L. ready-to-use equipment storage and dispatch space
   - M. gas cylinder storage closet
   - N. supply file storage space
   - O. medical director's office
   - P. technical director's office
   - Q. supervisors' offices
   - R. therapists'/technicians' offices
   - S. staff conference office
   - T. waiting area
   - U. secretaries' space
3. What are basic requirements for the patient reception/waiting area?
   - A. number of seating spaces?
   - B. number of wheelchair patients to be accommodated?
   - C. number of stretcher cases to be accommodated?
4. What are basic requirements for the staff conference space?
   - A. number to be seated for staff conferences?
   - B. storage cabinets?
5. What are basic requirements for multipurpose educational classroom space?
   - A. number of patients at one time?
   - B. number of personnel/students at one time?
   - C. counter with sink?
   - D. x-ray view boxes?
   - E. piped oxygen, vacuum, compressed air?
   - F. closet or shelves for anatomical models and audiovisual aids?
6. What will be the requirements for bed treatment space?
   - A. number of beds?
   - B. separate or cubicled spaces?
   - C. work counter with sink?
   - D. supply closets?
7. What will be the basic requirements for ambulant-patient treatment space?
   - A. approximate dimensions?
   - B. number of patients at one time?
   - C. treatment counter with angled seating?
   - D. counter stalls for each patient?
   - E. piped oxygen and compressed air to each patient treatment counter space?
   - F. counter inset tissue dispenser and undercounter soiled tissue receptacle at each patient treatment space?
   - G. armchairs, reclining lounge chairs, and postural drainage chairs in open treatment space with piped oxygen and compressed air at each location?
   - H. number of each type?

8. What will be the basic requirements for a medication preparation and storage station?
   - **A.** location *vis-à-vis* treatment areas?
   - **B.** modular medication station with sink and locked cabinets?
9. Will space for exercise tolerance equipment be required?
   - **A.** as part of pulmonary function testing space?
   - **B.** in treatment area?
   - **C.** treadmill?
   - **D.** other exercise equipment to be accommodated?
   - **E.** piped oxygen outlets?
10. What will be the basic requirements for the pulmonary function testing laboratory?
    - **A.** approximate dimensions?
    - **B.** piped oxygen, vacuum, compressed air?
    - **C.** counter with sink?
    - **D.** x-ray view boxes?
    - **E.** counter with sink for blood gas analyses?
    - **F.** storage shelves, cabinets, and closets for equipment and accessories?
11. What will be the basic requirements for the soiled (used) equipment receiving and decontamination space?
    - **A.** approximate dimensions?
    - **B.** equipment disassembly counter with deep double sinks?
    - **C.** disinfection immersion tanks? dimensions?
    - **D.** separate from cleanup preparation area?
    - **E.** negative air exhaust?
    - **F.** wet-room wall and floor finishes?
    - **G.** wall or overhead drip racks?
12. What will be the basic requirements for the equipment cleanup, assembly, packaging, and sterilizing space?
    - **A.** approximate dimensions?
    - **B.** counter with deep double sinks?
    - **C.** ultrasonic glassware/instrument cleaner?
    - **D.** equipment assembly/packaging counter?
    - **E.** parts storage cabinets and closets?
    - **F.** supply storage cabinets and closets?
    - **G.** steam autoclave? type and dimensions?
    - **H.** ethylene oxide sterilizer and aerator? type and dimensions?
    - **I.** any need for recourse to, or joint use of, sterilizing services and equipment in central services?
    - **J.** heat sealer?
    - **K.** tube dryer?
    - **L.** cabinets, shelving, closets, and floor space for storage and holding ready-to-use equipment and accessories?
13. What will be the basic requirements for the equipment maintenance and repair space?
    - **A.** part of, or separate from, cleanup preparation space?
    - **B.** approximate dimensions?
    - **C.** work counter/bench?
    - **D.** carpenter's tool cabinet?
    - **E.** parts storage cabinets and closets?
    - **F.** oxygen and compressed air supply?
14. What are basic requirements for the storage of gas cylinders?
    - **A.** number and sizes of cylinders to be stored?
    - **B.** types of gases to be stored?
    - **C.** closed, 1-hour fire-rated space?
    - **D.** dry, well-ventilated space remote from ignition sources and readily combustible materials?
    - **E.** self-closing door?

(continued)

15. Will there be a need for a janitorial closet within the respiratory care base of operations, or will the equipment decontamination space be used for this purpose?
16. Will all door openings be 44 inches clear?
17. Will electrically powered respiratory equipment from which a current could flow to the patient's body through direct electrical connection or through moist breathing circuits be checked routinely by an approved shock-hazard detecting device to ensure protection of the patient against possible current leakage?
18. Will minimum requirements of the most current versions of the life-protection and safety codes and standards of the National Fire Protection Association, National Board of Fire Underwriters, National Safety Council, U.S. Standards Institutes, National Bureau of Standards, Building Officials' Council of America, and American Society of Heating and Air Conditioning Engineers be adhered to in design of all structural and mechanical elements and services of all functional components of the respiratory care unit?
19. Will Hill–Burton's latest version of *Minimum Requirements of Construction and Equipment for Hospital and Medical Facilities* (DHEW Publ. No. [HRA] 74–4000) represent minimum requirements for mechanical services of the respiratory care unit?
20. Other than the following components, will any others, require special ambient air conditions or air handling within the respiratory base of operations?
    A. receiving and decontaminations space? negative air pressure?
    B. toilet spaces? negative air pressure?
    C. janitorial space? negative air pressure?
21. Will special filtration equipment to provide bioclean air be installed in the air supply system to, or at, the air input outlets in any of the patient pulmonary testing or treatment spaces?
22. Will any patient rooms on selected nursing units be equipped with special filtration equipment to provide bioclean ambient air?
    A. patient spaces in ICU/CCU?
    B. rooms or grouping of rooms on selected nursing units?
23. In what spaces and in what numbers will oxygen air and vacuum be required?
    A. decontamination?
    B. cleanup and preparation?
    C. treatment beds?
    D. treatment cubicles?
    E. pulmonary function testing?
    F. classroom?
    G. exercise space?
    H. blood gas laboratory?
    I. equipment maintenance and repair?
24. Which functional components of the respiratory care center need to be on standby electrical power?
    A. monitoring equipment?
    B. computers?
    C. other life-support devices?
25. Will any patient spaces on nursing units designated for care of pulmonary patients need to be on standby emergency electrical power?
    A. selected patient spaces or rooms on general-care nursing units to which respiratory care patients will be assigned?
    B. entire bed complement or any pulmonary/chest disease nursing unit that is set up as such?
26. Will any component spaces of the respiratory care center call for distinctive lighting fixtures or lighting intensities?
27. In what component spaces of the respiratory care center will 110/220 volt duplex receptacles be required?

28. What spaces will require wall-mounted clocks?
    A. waiting spaces?
    B. all treatment spaces?
    C. all work spaces?
    D. pulmonary function testing?
    E. classroom?
    F. staff conference?
    G. RICU?
29. What spaces of the respiratory care center will require wall-mounted two-light x-ray film illuminators?
    A. medical director's office?
    B. technical director's office?
    C. pulmonary function testing?
    D. staff conference room?
    E. classroom?
30. What spaces of the respiratory care center will require flush-mounted or wall-hung storage and supply cabinets and open adjustable shelving? (For each such space indicate whether cabinets are to have solid or glass doors, are to be over or under work counters; indicate approximate dimensions. For open shelving, indicate depth, number of shelves or linear feet of shelving required.)
31. What offices, classrooms, or conference space of the unit will require built-in bookcases and tack/chalk boards? (Indicate linear feet of book shelving required for respective spaces and dimensions of tack/chalk boards.)
32. Where should recessed drinking fountains be located in the waiting area of the respiratory care center?
33. Will all lavatories and work sinks be equipped with wrist or elbow controls and gooseneck nonsplash faucets?
34. What spaces will require lavatories?
    A. all testing and treatment spaces?
    B. classroom?
    C. medical director's office?
    D. staff conference room?
    E. elsewhere?
35. What spaces of the respiratory care center will require work counters? (Indicate whether with or without sinks; type of sinks and whether cabinets, shelving, and open space are required below; approximate length; laminated or stainless steel surface.)
36. Will the decontamination immersion tanks or counter sinks in the soiled equipment receiving/decontamination space have dimensions and attachments calling for special fabrication? (If so, detail dimensions and describe fully.)
37. Will a prefabricated, modular medication unit incorporating closed, locked storage, sink, and work surface be used for drug additive preparation in the treatment space?
    A. preferred location?
    B. special plumbing or electrical services, or both, required?
    C. 4 feet wide? 6 feet wide?
    D. other dimensions or features?
38. Will a modular, prefabricated nourishment station or a conventional kitchenette module incorporating sink, work counter, hot plate, refrigerator, and storage cabinets be installed for convenience of the staff?
    A. in what location?
    B. special plumbing and electrical services required?
39. If an ultrasonic glassware/instrument cleaner is to be used in the cleanup preparation room,
    A. what will be its dimensions?
    B. will it be counter-mounted or freestanding?
    C. what special electric and plumbing services will be required?

(continued)

40. What makes and models of sterilizing equipment will be used?
    A. steam autoclave?
    B. pasteurizer?
    C. ethylene oxide sterilizer?
    D. aeration cabinet?
    E. any of the above counter-mounted?
    F. special electric or plumbing services required for any of the above?
41. At what points in the respiratory care base of operations will telephones be required?
    A. wall-mounted?
    B. desk?
    C. public phone in waiting area?
42. Will the respiratory care center be tied into the hospital's cardiac arrest alert system? Where will annunciators be located?
43. Which spaces in the respiratory care center will be linked to the hospital's general paging and piped-music system?
    A. waiting area?
    B. treatment spaces?
    C. work areas?
    D. conference classroom spaces?
44. Will the respiratory care unit be tied into the hospital's pneumatic tube system?
    A. receptionist/secretarial desk terminal?
    B. any other terminals?
45. Will there be any need for an internal audio or audiovisual intercom system within the respiratory care base of operations? (If so, between which functional components?)
46. Will external functional activities be tied in to respiratory care center by
    A. audiovisual intercom?
    B. direct writing intercom?
    C. pneumatic tube system?
    D. mechanical conveyors?
    E. messenger/transport/patient escort systems?
47. Who will be responsible for transporting or escorting patients (bed-bound, stretcher, wheelchair, ambulant, outpatients or referred extramural patients) to and from the respiratory care center?
    A. respiratory care personnel?
    B. nursing department personnel?
    C. a hospital-wide patient escort transportation service?
48. Will acoustical ceilings be used throughout the entire respiratory care base of operations?
    A. composition material?
    B. aluminum pan?
49. In what areas of the respiratory care unit will carpeting be used?
50. In the interest of creating a tranquil, noninstitutional environment, will consideration be given to using wood-grain veneers or other wall coverings in components of the respiratory care center to be used by patients?
51. If the hospital is not fully air-conditioned, will the respiratory care unit be independently air-conditioned?
52. Will general illumination throughout the respiratory care base of operations be subdued indirect lighting to promote a relaxed feeling and supplemented selectively by auxiliary lighting, where needed, for special examinations, equipment inspections, and the like?

has been described by Robert F. Mager in his book *Goal Analysis*.[9] This method utilizes information gleaned from reports on procedures that have not been done correctly or well enough and have led to undesirable consequences. For example, an increase in nosocomial infections during an 8-month period on a neurosurgical unit may be due to poor suctioning or equipment-handling technique. Once this has been determined through the analysis, the next step for continuing educators would be to design a program of instruction on aseptic/sterile techniques.

A respiratory care audit is another means of identifying deficiencies in quality of care delivered. Once the audit has identified deficiencies resulting from lack of information or skills training, continuing education courses may be designed to correct these deficiencies.

The concept of *shared services* can only serve to strengthen the continuing education process. In an area where there are several hospitals or schools, each could contribute to hiring a full-time director of continuing education who would be closely involved, as an employee, with all the institutions and their needs. Smaller, outlying hospitals could also be involved because, while small departments can certainly have good continuing education programs, they often do not have access to the sophisticated equipment and resources of a larger hospital. The possibilities for a meaningful continuing education program that is financially within easy reach are unlimited through the shared services concept.

Shared services need not be limited only to other respiratory care departments. Other departments within the institution, such as nursing, physical therapy, the clinical laboratory, or radiology, may have established continuing education programs that could meet the needs of respiratory therapists. Then, too, respiratory therapy continuing education need not be limited to respiratory therapists. Nursing service and physical therapy would likely benefit from certain programs such as chest examination and respiratory drug pharmacology. Although the primary emphasis of any departmental continuing education is based on the particular needs of that department, it is not an isolated function of any one department.

It is part of the function of continuing education to provide therapists within each given institution with the tools they need to evaluate their own performance. Moving away from task-oriented toward interactive problem solving helps the therapist to achieve the dynamic capability of forming personal guidelines for each patient–therapist relationship. The therapist needs to know not only which knobs to set where, but also how the patient should be responding and what the therapist can, and cannot, do to help that patient psychologically as well as physiologically. Supervisory personnel are a vital part of the process of productive continuing education because a supervisor educates continually. It is the job of supervisors to inquire, observe, offer alternatives and assistance, encourage, teach, and effect change.

Management, which has an obligation and a vested interest in the program, stays involved in continuing education by being aware of the department's needs. The director must keep the supervisors up-to-date on policy and procedure changes and must encourage, assist, and try to motivate them, as well as give them the same kind of tools and guidelines for performance and personal involvement that the supervisor is expected to provide for the therapist. Continuing education for productivity is one of the most important tools of management.

An involved medical director can and should play an important role in continuing education.[18] Weekly rounds and conferences where therapists and all members of the health care team can discuss patient problems and ask pertinent questions are invaluable additions to any continuing education program. This is one way of helping the therapist to move away from the task-oriented to the situation-coping environment that leads to improved patient care. A concerned physician can provide an overview of care and conditions from a diagnostic as well as therapeutic view-point. From this, the therapist can see and define his own personal involvement in the total picture of patient care.

The specific teaching methods used by a department to accomplish change and improvement must be determined by each in-service director, keeping in mind that education for the sake of education is not the goal; rather, it is education for the improvement of individual performance and improvement of the quality of patient care that is desired. "Core-group" teaching, "hands-on" learning, relevant classroom activities, conferences, audiovisual media, individual study modules, and interactive problem solving (role playing) are all useful components of an effective program of continuing education. Whatever the method, however, there is a common requirement for any method to assure quality education, and that is the use of behavioral (instructional) objectives[11] and appropriate testing measurements.[10]

The use of behavioral objectives not only identifies the expected outcome or proposed changes in the participant's behavior, but also necessitates the organization of the instructor's thoughts, which, in turn, must yield a more organized and effective presentation. Behavioral objectives not only provide direction for the teaching/learning process, but also provide both the teacher and student with a basis for objectively evaluating the teaching done and the learning accomplished through the course.[5] With written instructional objectives available for any course taught, it follows then that the next step would be to evaluate the material to see *if what is being taught is being learned, and if what is being learned is being used.*

Four specific evaluation processes will be discussed briefly. The first, pretesting and posttesting, is a technique widely used and variably accepted at present. If both the pretests and posttests are essentially the same and there is a noticeable improvement in the posttest score, then it follows that this improvement was probably due to appropriate instruction. Statistical measurements obtained by means of "Fisher's table of t" have been used to identify the success of training programs.[14] In this method, pretest and posttest scores are evaluated by statistical methods, and the results will indicate if the difference in pretest and posttest scores was the result of the instructional process or merely due to chance.

Improved posttest behavior does not *directly* correlate with improved patient care, although such an association is frequently made. Long-term behavioral and attitudinal changes are much more difficult to evaluate, if indeed such tools are available to measure these changes.

Retrospective department audit, as described earlier, provides yet another method to evaluate the effectiveness, or lack of it, in continuing education programs. If, for example, respiratory therapists had received training in arterial blood gas sampling and a respiratory care audit on arterial blood gas sampling revealed persistent deficiencies related to this procedure, then it might well be concluded that the continuing education instruction had not been effective. Although this example suggests that instruction was not effective, most audits, hopefully, will more often reveal the appropriateness and effectiveness of continuing education instruction.

The final, but certainly not any less important, method is the first-hand observation of respiratory therapists and technicians in the course of patient care. By observing what is actually being done, it will be possible to determine if what is being taught is what is being done. If so, then the effort devoted to continuing education will be justified; if not, instruction must be reevaluated and educational programs designed that will meet the department's objectives.

REFERENCES

1. Accreditation Manual for Hospitals (From H-101), 2nd ed. Chicago, Hospital Accreditation Program, 1973
2. American Hospital Association: Budgeting Procedures, Financial Management Series, 1971, p 7
3. American Hospital Association (AHA): Quality Assurance Program for Medical Care in the Hospital. Chicago, AHA, 1974, sect 12, p 2
4. California Medical Association and California Hospital Association: Education-Patient Care Audit Workshop Program. San Francisco, 1975
5. Continuing education: How to do it. Respir Care *21*:244, 1976
6. Dale E: Organization, 2nd ed, p 104. New York, American Management Associations, 1967
7. Dinsmore FW: Developing Tomorrow's Managers Today. New York, Amacom, 1975, p 2
8. Lippitt GL: Training in the world today. Training 5:48, 1975
9. Mager RF: Goal Analysis, p 8. Belmont, California, Fearon Publishers, 1972
10. Measuring Instructional Intent. Belmont, California, Fearon Publishers, 1973
11. Preparing Instructional Objectives, 2nd ed. Belmont, California, Fearon Publishers, 1975
12. Newman WH: Administrative Action, 2nd ed, pp 128–236. Englewood Cliffs, Prentice–Hall, 1963
13. Nielsen–Tietsort J et al: Respiratory care protocol: An approach to in-hospital respiratory therapy. Respir Care 26:430, 1981
14. Novack SR: Scientific "proof" that your training program works: How to develop statistical evidence your management will buy. Training 13(3), March 1976
15. Skalnik B: IPPB: A question of quality. Respir Care 6(6):81, 1976
16. Townsend R: Up the Organization, p 134. New York, Alfred A. Knopf, 1970
17. U.S. Department of Health, Education, and Welfare: The Respiratory Care Services Functional Programming Worksheet (HRS)74–4004. Washington DC, DHEW, 1972
18. Yanda RL: In-service and other education, In Yanda RL (ed): The Management of Respiratory Care Services. New York, Projects in Health, 1976

BIBLIOGRAPHY

Dale E: Organization. New York, American Management Associations, 1967

Dinsmore FW: Developing Tomorrow's Managers Today. New York, Amacom, 1975

Drucker P: Technology, Management, and Society. New York, Harper & Row, 1970

FitzGerald JM et al: Fundamentals of Systems Analysis, New York, Wiley, 1973

Herkimer AG Jr: Understanding Hospital Financial Management. Germantown, Maryland, Aspen Systems Corp., 1978

Joint Commission on Accreditation of Hospitals: Accreditation Manual for Hospitals. Chicago, JCAH, 1976

McGregor D: The Human Side of Enterprise. New York, McGraw–Hill, 1960
Mager RF: Measuring Instructional Intent, or "Got a Match?" Belmont, California, Fearon Publishers, 1973
Maier NRF: Psychology in Industrial Organizations, 4th ed. Boston, Houghton Mifflin, 1973
McLaughlin AJ: Organization and Management for Respiratory Therapists. St. Louis, CV Mosby, 1979
Miller WF: Guidelines for organization and function of hospital respiratory care services. Chest 78:79, 1980
Newman WH: Administrative Action, 2nd ed. Englewood Cliffs, Prentice–Hall, 1963
Preparing Instructional Objectives, 2nd ed. Belmont, California, Fearon Publishers, 1975
Rakich JS et al: Managing Health Care Organizations. Philadelphia, WB Saunders, 1977
Townsend R: Up the Organization. New York, Alfred A. Knopf, 1970
Yanda RL: The Management of Respiratory Care Services. New York, Projects in Health, 1976

In the modern world of health care, where audit is an integral part of quality assurance, the following references may be helpful:

Eddy L et al: Multidisciplinary retrospective patient care audit. Am J Nursing 75:961, 1975
Gonnella JS et al: The staging concept: An approach to the assessment of outcome of ambulatory care. Med Care 14:13, 1976
Rosenberg C (moderator): The professional responsibility for the quality of health care (panel discussion at the 1975 Annual Health Conference of the New York Academy of Medicine). Bull NY Acad Med 52(1):86, 1976

7

Equipment Evaluation, Maintenance, and Quality Control

Charles B. Spearman • Howard G. Sanders, Jr.

Most current respiratory therapy modalities involve the use of some piece of equipment. Preventive maintenance and quality control must be provided to assure optimum equipment performance and to prevent equipment malfunction. Many of these devices are life-supportive in nature, and their proper operation is critical.

The interpretation of Standard IV of the Joint Commission on Accreditation of Hospitals, pertinent to respiratory care services, states that policy statements of the department must contain reference to "examination, maintenance and performance (of) all respiratory care equipment." This statement helps establish an operational precedent for these responsibilities, as do the following statements from the Occupational Safety and Health Act (OSHA).

1. The hospital has the responsibility of furnishing effective equipment and for its inspection as to proper functioning.
2. The hospital must provide the most current safety additions to any piece of equipment in use, or must replace it.

The Compressed Gas Association (CGA) and the National Fire Protection Association (NFPA) provide safety suggestions concerning respiratory care equipment. Another group, the Association for the Advancement of Medical Instrumentation (AAMI), provides guidelines concerning the qualifications of personnel involved in equipment maintenance and describes how such qualifications may be acquired. The Food and Drug Administration (FDA), has recently been given considerable authority to regulate devices as well as drugs. Under this legislation, device manufacturers must register with the government, keep records, and report defects involving their products.

None of the groups specify exactly how such equipment care and testing should be provided or documented. The purpose of this chapter is to provide some guidelines from which a hospital can draw when deciding on the best methods of providing proper maintenance and quality control of its respiratory therapy equipment. It is *not* our intention to supply a complete evaluation and maintenance protocol; rather, we shall introduce the topic and discuss information based on our experiences and that of others. Our approach is to discuss briefly considerations for equipment evaluation, then to describe five basic options for a maintenance program followed by some considerations for equipment used in the home. We recognize the obvious overlaps and the possibility of combining these five options.

EVALUATION OF EQUIPMENT PERFORMANCE

As modern technology's influence on the allied health professions increases, a greater number of devices will be available each year. Each respiratory therapy department must have appropriate expertise and methods available to it for evaluating which types and brands of equipment to purchase. For some hospitals this may entail purchasing substantial amounts of test equipment, provision of physical space, and hiring of additional personnel to participate in this process. This equipment, space, and staff may very well be combined into an in-house maintenance program. Smaller hospitals may be able only to survey larger institutions for recommendations and input. It would be appropriate for larger, teaching-oriented institutions to feel a moral obligation to provide such information to surrounding, smaller community hospitals.

Although it is always desirable to use the "best" equipment for therapy, the risk of poor performance of new and perhaps untested equipment without proper evaluation must also be considered. Purchasing new or replacement equipment should be an orderly undertaking. Spiraling costs of health care dictate that equipment purchases be monitored carefully. The following is a minimum list of primary considerations in making a new purchase.

1. The equipment should provide a needed function and one not available from existing equipment. It is not appropriate to purchase equipment for common use that has been used only in a few research projects and that is not yet universally accepted as current.
2. The equipment should "fit in" well with the existing equipment. For example, a device that operates by compressed air should obviously have ample sources of this gas available.
3. Flexibility of the device should be considered. It may be appropriate for adaptations or retrofits to take place later. In electric monitoring equipment, for example, modules may need to be switched to meet existing situations and upgraded from simple to more complex systems without discarding the original components.
4. The manufacturer should allow a trial period for its equipment to be used in the hospital, or at least supply names of hospitals where the equipment is being used.
5. Consideration of the manufacturer's experience in the business is also important. A new product may have been hurried into production without proper clinical and laboratory testing and thus provide poor performance.
6. The ease of, and time involved in, training personnel to use the new equipment should be considered.
7. Some manufacturers provide training, such as audiovisual aids and seminars. If so, these should be obtained for user orientation.
8. The equipment should be inspected to see whether the device has been manufactured for hospital use, meeting all the safety requirements of the various agencies.
9. It should be determined whether the equipment can be performance-checked with the existing maintenance facilities or whether other new testing equipment will be needed.
10. Information from the manufacturer, such as service bulletins and parts inventory, can be helpful. Some parts may need to be purchased along with the device to provide greater efficiency during its use.
11. The purchase of various types or brands of equipment that perform similar functions can compound problems of parts inventory and personnel training. In some situations, however, such as in teaching hospitals, a variety of equipment may be desirable and even mandatory.
12. The ecological impact of the device should be considered. Is the product disposable? How is it ultimately disposed of? How much storage space is required? What is its energy consumption?
13. The unit should be compatible with current cleaning and sterilizing systems. Small parts that can be lost, broken, or misassembled during operation and cleaning should be noted.
14. The matter of durability is important but usually difficult to determine without experience with the equipment. However, a good inspection may reveal fragile appendages, poor shock mounts, sloppy alignment screws, uncalibrated adjustment knobs, and so forth.
15. An advantageous economical comparison with similar equipment can be made.
16. If the equipment requires a major capital expenditure, a look into the economics of leasing may be appropriate. An advantage of leasing is that no large initial investment is made

Table 7-1. Function Parameters to be Checked and Alterations and Repairs Commonly Made by Clinical, Cleaning, and Maintenance Personnel

EQUIPMENT	CHECKS BY CLINICAL OR CLEANING PERSONNEL, OR BOTH	ADDITIONAL CHECKS BY MAINTENANCE PERSONNEL
Flowmeters	Leaks Flow valve Foreign matter in Thorpe tube Structural defects	Clean internally Replace faulty parts Check accuracy of flow
Regulators	Manometer zero when not pressurized Inlet and outlet threads Missing manometer lens Leaks	Clean internally Replace faulty parts Check outlet pressure precisely Check safety valves
Compressors	Excess noise Water discharge Outlet pressure if obtainable Cleanliness of visible parts Filters Electrical line cord	All electrical components Electrical leaks Internal filters Shock mounts Internal pneumatic connections Flow capabilities against pressure
Air/O_2 mixers	Relation of O_2 setting and O_2 concentration obtained from outlet Leaks Functioning alarms and bypass systems Integrity of pneumatic hoses	Check inlet filters Precise O_2 calibration Pneumatic hoses Clean and replace faulty parts Pressure and flow capabilities
O_2 analyzers	Meter zero Meter span against air and O_2 Battery check Drying agents Alarm system Reaction time	Precise calibration (may include internal adjustments) Battery inspection and test Inspection of all internal parts (*e.g.,* circuit boards, tubing, meters)
Gas-powered resuscitators	Leaks Valve operation Pressure regulating mechanism Pneumatic hose	Inlet filters Pressure output Flow output Clean internally and replace faulty parts
Manual resuscitator bags	Leaks Valve action Pressure pop-off if used Structural damage	Replace faulty parts Pressure testing for bag and valve integrity
Respirometers	Structural damage Volume with volume standard Zeroing of meter Water accumulation Battery check if it applies	Battery check Clean and adjust Electrical service if it applies
Pneumatic nebulizers	Leaks Structural damage Aerosol generation O_2 mixing function where it applies	Repair structural damage Aerosol volume output Check O-ring seals and filters Test of heater function
Ultrasonic nebulizers	Aerosol generation Height of geyser Fan noise Fan filter Water leaks Structural damage	Electrical leak test Aerosol volume output Frequency check

(continued)

Table 7-1. Function Parameters to be Checked and Alterations and Repairs Commonly Made by Clinical, Cleaning, and Maintenance Personnel *(continued)*

EQUIPMENT	CHECKS BY CLINICAL OR CLEANING PERSONNEL, OR BOTH	ADDITIONAL CHECKS BY MAINTENANCE PERSONNEL
Humidifiers	Water and air leaks Heater function Structural damage Integrity of internal valves and diffuser if used Air temperature	Humidity output Precision leak test Repair structural damage Electrical leak test of heater if used Calibration of heater Test of heater function
Ventilators	Pressure Flow Leak test PEEP Inspiratory hold operation Sensitivity Volume delivered Alarm systems Pneumatic hoses Structural damage Rate Sigh rate and volume Pop-off and pressure limits All visible filters Compressor noise Circuitry competence O_2 concentration	Electrical leak test Precision dynamic testing and calibration of all ventilator functions using a lung analog and recording functions for future reference, such as flow, volume, and pressure Observation or replacement of all internal filters
Alarms	Visual alarms Audio alarms Delay timer Check of calibration	Battery check Electrical leak test Precision calibration

in equipment that may be obsolete fairly soon. Thus the immediate outlay of money is smaller. If this equipment has a very limited use period and is available for lease during these times, leasing may be more economical.

17. Whenever possible, a full performance evaluation should be completed before purchase in all clinical situations where the device may be used.
18. The warranty and its application to the equipment in relation to its use and maintenance must be considered. With some equipment, departmental maintenance procedures may surpass the warranty itself, or, alternatively, their use may endanger the viability of the warranty.

Whenever possible, newly purchased equipment should be thoroughly inspected and tested to ensure proper working order before clinical use. It can be determined not only whether a unit meets factory specifications, but also whether it meets a given clinical facility's requirements. Devices may be purchased that have factory specifications that differ from those the hospital sets as its own standards. It is important that each type of device be given a range of acceptable specifications appropriate for the use of that unit in that particular environment.

Performance evaluation of current equipment obviously begins with day-to-day use in the clinical setting. Ideally, technicians and therapists are trained to use equipment at their disposal, not only in the theoretical therapeutic value and potential dangers of treatment being provided, but also in the proper operation and use of the equipment involved. In the procedure manual for each device, a concise section on troubleshooting should be included.

Table 7-1 lists some general categories of equipment common to respiratory therapy departments, with suggestions of items to be considered when per-

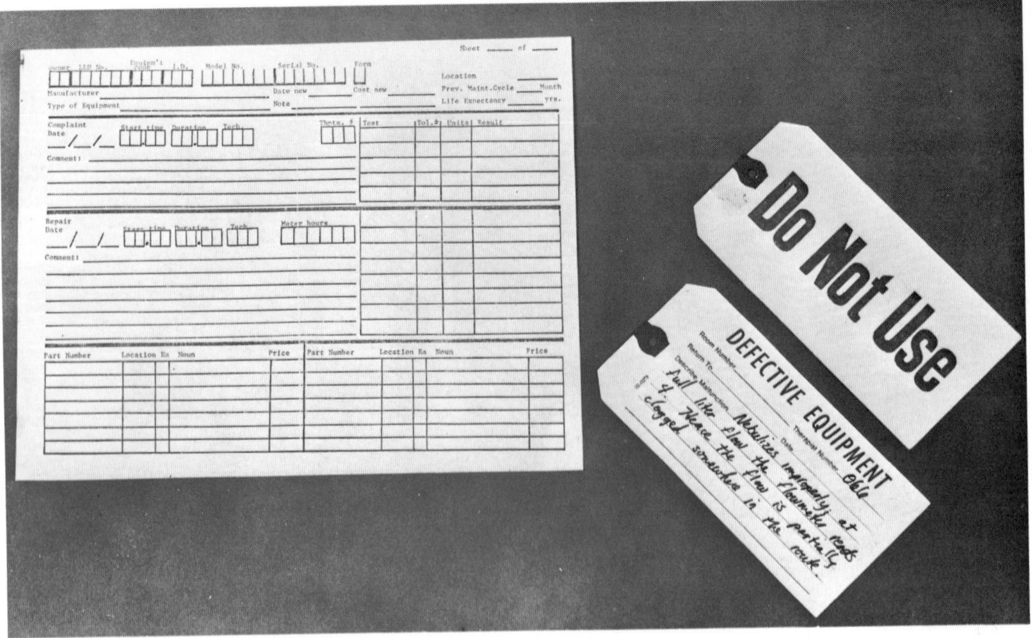

Fig. 7-1. History and data sheet and tags used to identify broken or malfunctioning equipment. Note space provided on the tag for a description of the irregular behavior of the device.

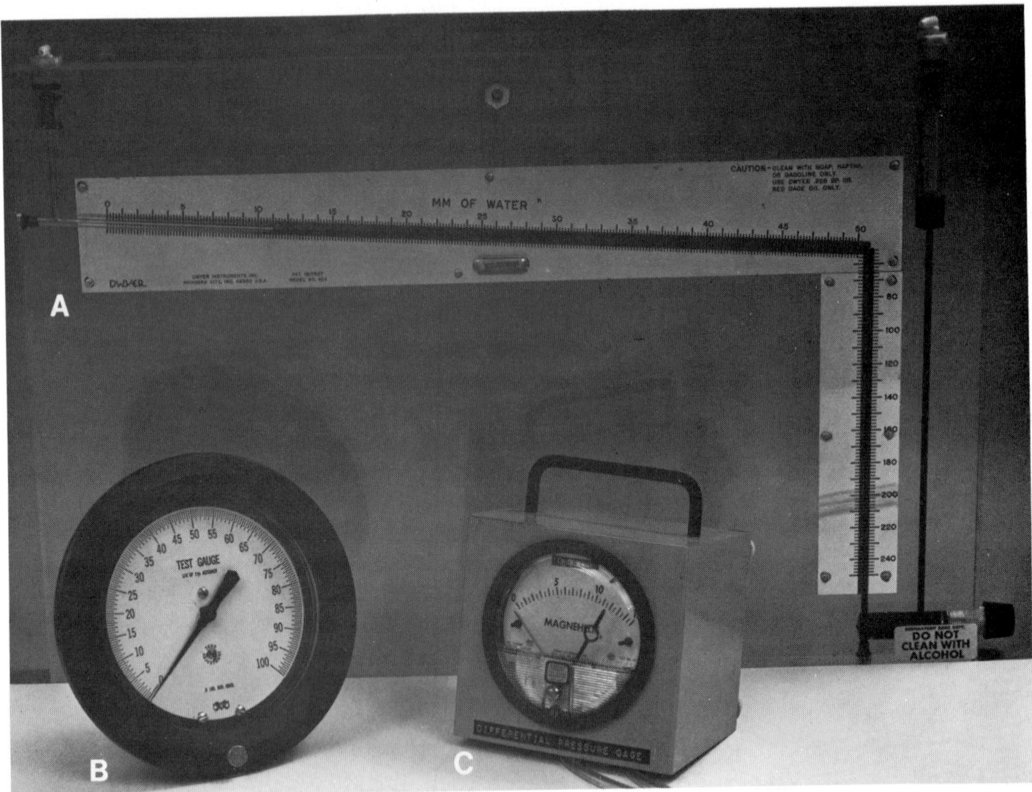

Fig. 7-2. Devices for pressure standards. *A* is an oil-filled column calibrated from 0 to 240 mm H_2O to be used for static measurements of relatively low-pressure systems. *B* is used when measuring higher pressures and is calibrated in pounds per square inch gauge (psig). Its accuracy claims are within 0.25%. *C* can be used for measuring differential pressures where small pressure gradients exist or for low-pressure systems compared to atmospheric pressure.

sonnel are evaluating device operation. The tasks of clinical personnel and cleaning personnel have been combined in the interest of space, but these groups may be separate in many hospitals. In most instances the procedures used by the maintenance personnel will include those performed by the clinical group as well as more sophisticated measuring, recording, and repairing.

When clinical personnel suspect that a unit is malfunctioning or represents a potential hazard, they should have it removed from the clinical setting and tagged with a DO NOT USE sign (Fig. 7-1). A brief description of the problem, including the evaluation steps used by the clinician, should accompany the device to the maintenance facility. If the defective equipment has actually been in use and the difficulty has been recorded on the patient's record, then the immediate solution (such as a statement that the device has been replaced by a normally functioning unit) should also be recorded there.

A system of test devices to compare equipment function must be devised. These "standards" will vary in their sophistication, absolute accuracy, and cost for each institution according to the size and the type of maintenance facilities being used. Generally it is desirable for measuring devices used as standards to have an accuracy of about ±1% or better or to provide an accuracy of ten times greater than the device being tested. Many such devices, however, are expensive and highly impractical for some institutions. Often factory specifications and check-out procedures do not call for such accuracy.

In the following section some devices commonly used as testing devices for respiratory therapy equipment are discussed. This overview will *not* attempt to describe the principles of how these items function or procedures for their use. Whole textbooks have been dedicated to these purposes, and the interested reader is referred to the bibliography at the end of this chapter for further study. Examples of testing devices that have been used in standardization are shown in Figures 7-2 through 7-14, including devices for measuring pressure, flow, volume, temperature, and electrical safety.

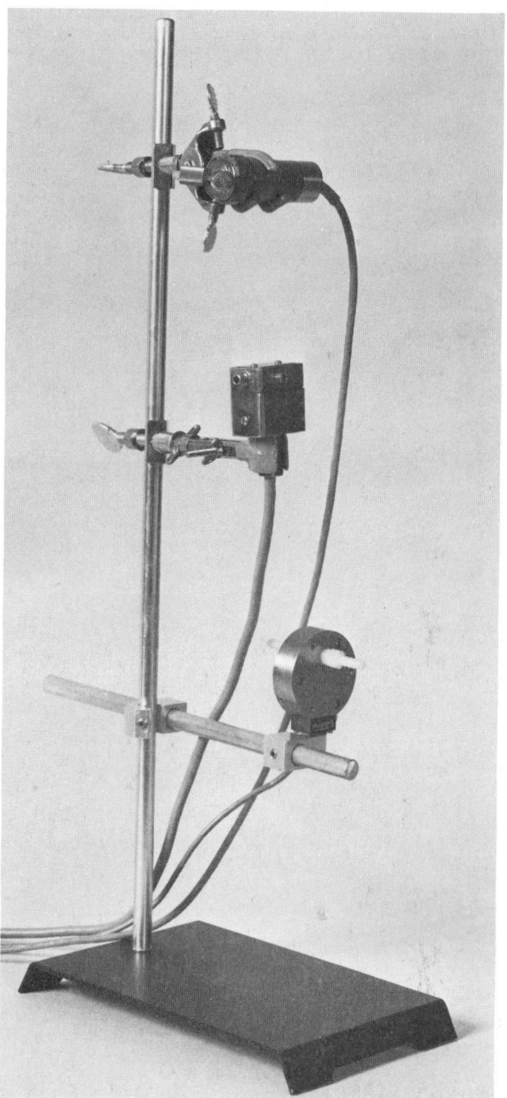

Fig. 7-3. Examples of electrical pressure transducers. These must be connected to appropriate amplifiers and display units and provide accurate measurements of pressures under either dynamic or static conditions. Calibration of these units generally depends on comparison with other devices, such as those shown in Figure 7-2.

PRESSURE STANDARDS

A wide range of gas pressures from a few centimeters of water (cm H_2O) to over 2000 pounds per square inch (psi) are used in various respiratory therapy equipment. Figure 7-2(A) illustrates a test device calibrated in millimeters of water (mm H_2O) that is used for calibrating low-presure manometers. This unit can be very accurate when used for static measurement comparisons but does not measure pressures that fluctuate abruptly, such as with ventilators. Electrical pressure transducers such as those shown in Figure 7-3 can provide accurate, dynamic pressure measurements when coupled with appropriate amplifiers and records, but they also require that a static pressure standard be used for their own calibration. Gauges such as those shown in Figure 7-4 can be used for

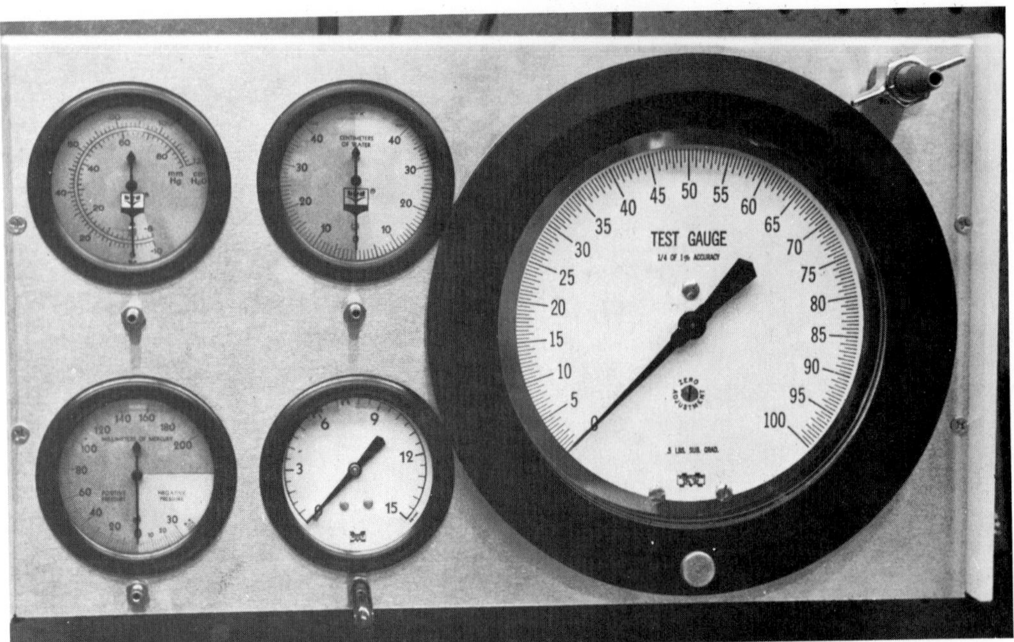

Fig. 7-4. Examples of pressure manometers mounted into a portable carrying case for sample measurements in cm H_2O, mm Hg, and psig values.

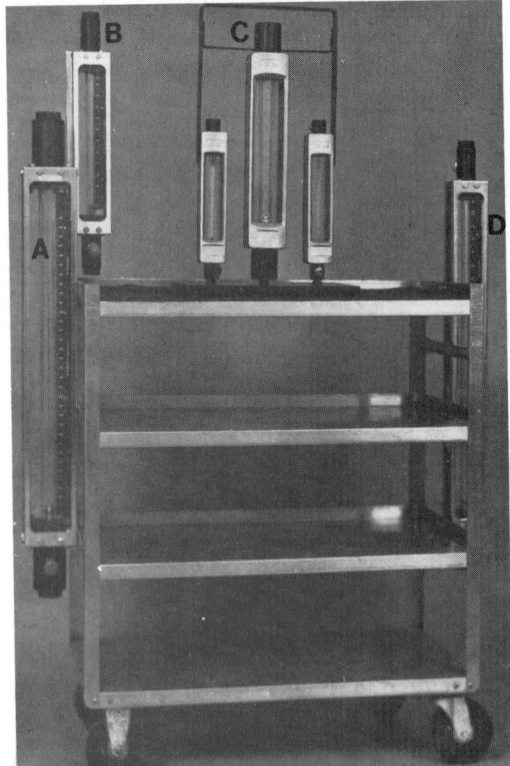

Fig. 7-5. Thorpe tube-type flowmeter standardization devices. *A, B,* and *D* are custom-built units calibrated for 735 mm Hg atmospheric pressure and for air measurement. Flows of more than 600 liter/min can be measured accurately by the larger unit. *C* is a set of three flowmeters calibrated at 760 mm Hg (sea level) atmospheric pressure, for use with oxygen.

measuring pressures in psi, mm Hg, and cm H_2O. Many of the pressure-sensing devices are position-dependent and should be used on a level surface.

These are only a few examples of devices commonly used for pressure testing. Others are available as well, some of which have accuracy specifications traceable to the National Bureau of Standards. However, these units can be very expensive and often unnecessary for most clinical applications.

FLOW STANDARDS

Figure 7-5 shows large Thorpe-tube-type flowmeters. These units can be used to check constant or slowly changing flow rates and are often used to calibrate other flow-measuring devices such as those in Figure 7-6. Since these flowmeters are calibrated for a specific gas composition and at a certain barometric pressure (such as pure oxygen at 760 mm Hg), corrections for their readings may have to be applied when other gases, at different barometric pressures, are used. These devices can also be built to order, as was the case for three of those in Figure 7-5. They were calibrated for air at a barometric pressure of 735 mm Hg. Any restriction to the outflow of these flowmeters that causes a pressure higher than the calibration pressure will result in an inaccurate (low) reading. (These are *not* pressure-compensated flowmeters.)

The accuracy of these flowmeters can be checked periodically by collecting gases from them in a large-volume collecting device, such as a Tissot-type water

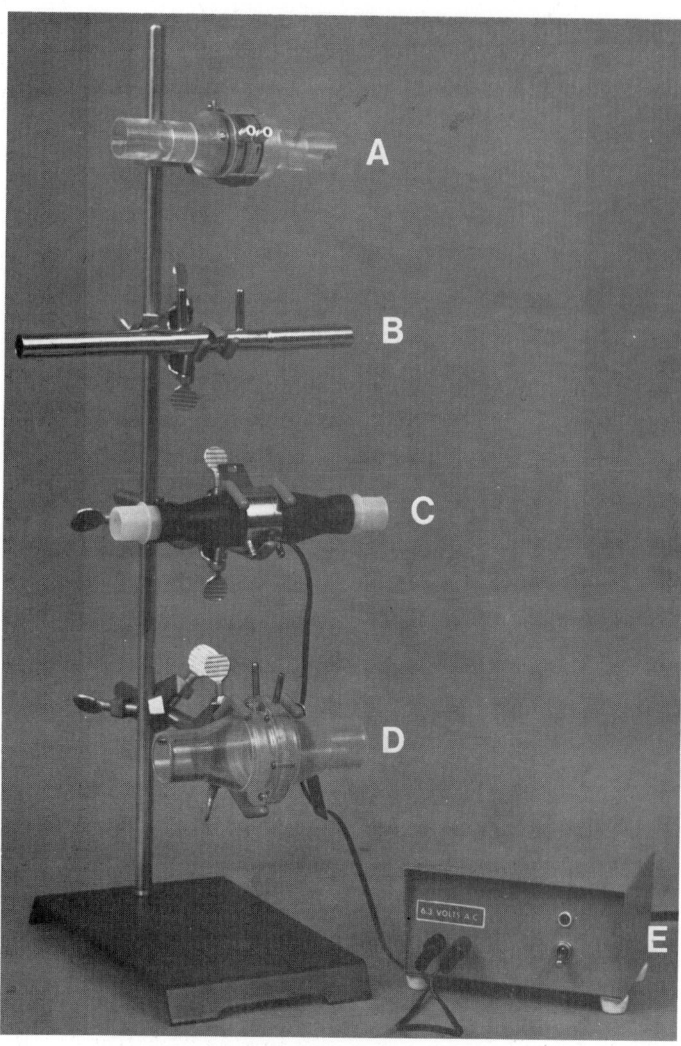

Fig. 7-6. Pressure-differential pneumotachometers for flow measurement. *A* = Pitot tube unit; *B* = fixed orifice type; *C* = heated metal mesh type; *D* = screen type; *E* = heater module used for the *C*-type pneumotachometer. When these devices are used in a pressure-changing environment, such as in line with mechanical ventilators, their accuracy may become compromised similar to that of a backpressure uncompensated Thorpe tube flowmeter.

sealed spirometer, while timing the collection period. Correction curves for using these flowmeters with different gases can be made in the same manner and are especially useful when evaluating equipment with more than one gas, such as air and oxygen.

Figure 7-6 illustrates differential pressure measuring devices. By measuring the difference in pressure across a known resistance during gas movement, flow rates can be calculated and displayed using the appropriate electronic amplifiers, recorders, and so forth (Figs. 7-7 and 7-8). The screen, heated mesh, fixed orifice, and Pitot tube pneumotachometers are all sensitive to gas density and internal pressures, and are therefore most accurate when used with a constant gas composition and internal (reference) pressure (usually atmospheric) against which they have been calibrated. Although their absolute accuracy may not be greater than ±10% when used under changing internal pressures and gas compositions, they have still been recommended for use in evaluating positive pressure ventilators. The flow-rate wave forms produced by one ventilator compared to another under similar conditions may provide useful information in addition to the absolute accuracy of the recordings themselves. These pneumotachometers can provide an accurate means for documenting flow rates if the same gas composition and pressure used for calibration are used for making measurements. Each brand and type should have an accuracy and flow range recommended by its manufacturer to which the user can refer. The signal produced by these units is proportional to flow and can be electrically manipulated (by an integrator) to provide another signal that is proportional to volume.

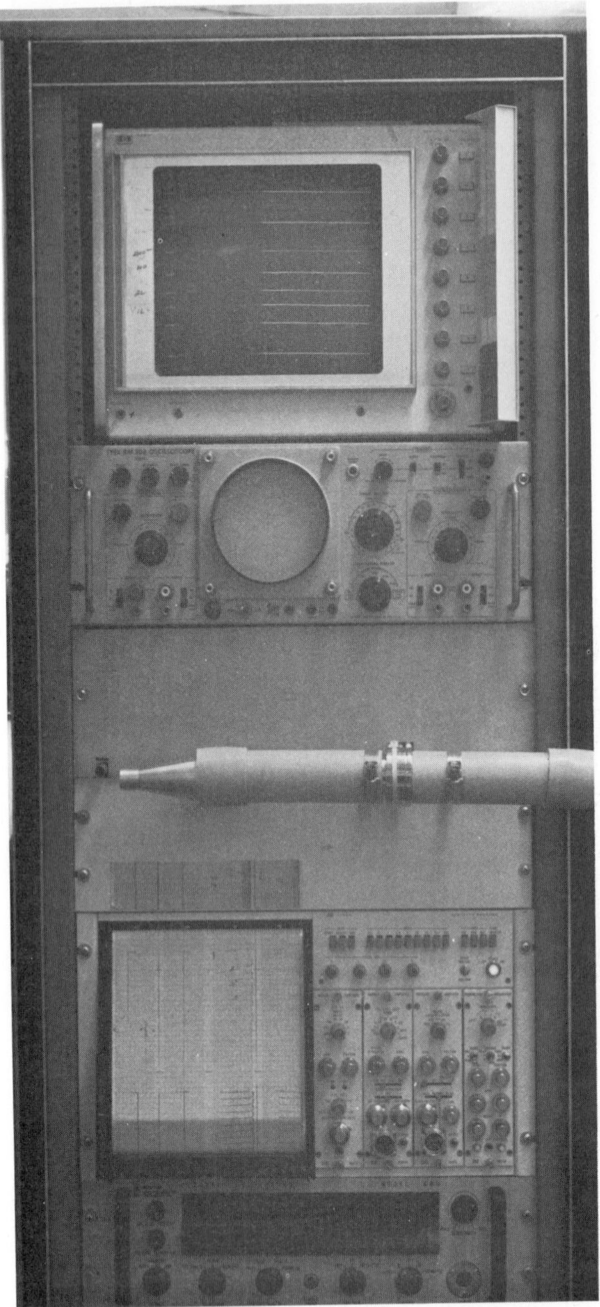

Fig. 7-7. Example of a modular system for various amplifiers and oscilloscopes and a strip recorder for measuring and documenting equipment function.

VOLUME STANDARDS

Probably the most commonly used volume standard in respiratory therapy is the water-sealed spirometer (Fig. 7-9). Water-sealed spirometers tend to be reliable and accurate and can provide a permanent record tracing, if necessary. The volume displacement required to raise the spirometer's bell a specific distance is commonly called a "bell factor." This factor varies with spirometers of differing sizes and must be known for accurate measurements. Temperature and pressure corrections may be needed in some situations, but

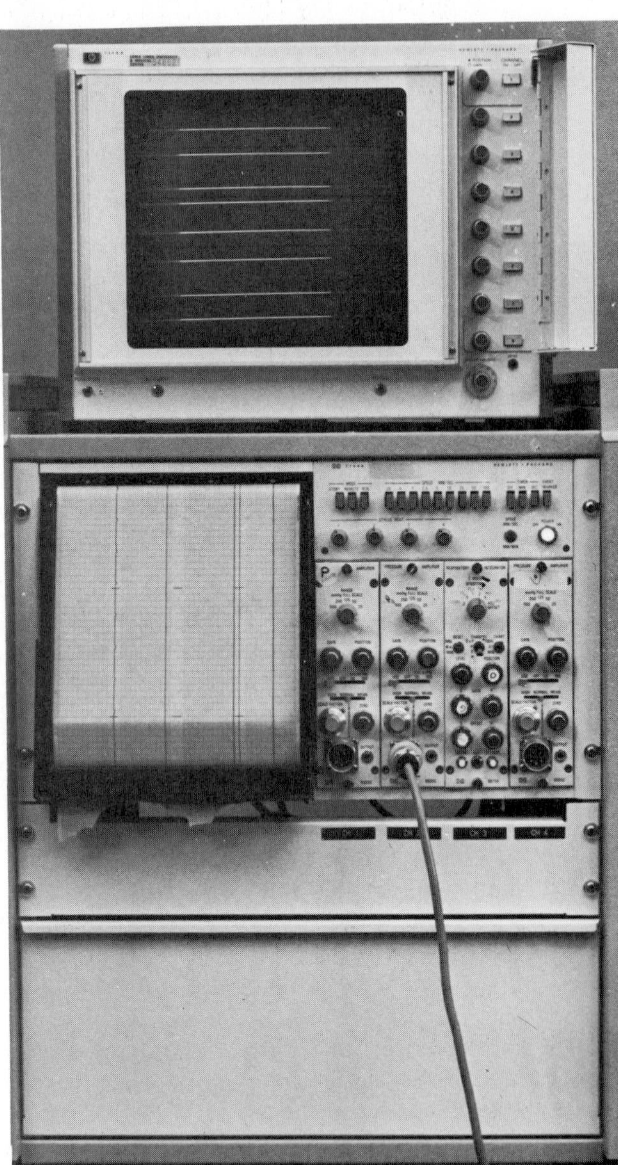

Fig. 7-8. Example of a portable four-channel amplifier and strip chart recorder with an accompanying eight-channel oscilloscope. This unit is set up to measure two pressure parameters: a flow (pressure-differential signal) tracing; and a volume signal, which is integrated from the flow channel. The system can be used in the laboratory or at the bedside.

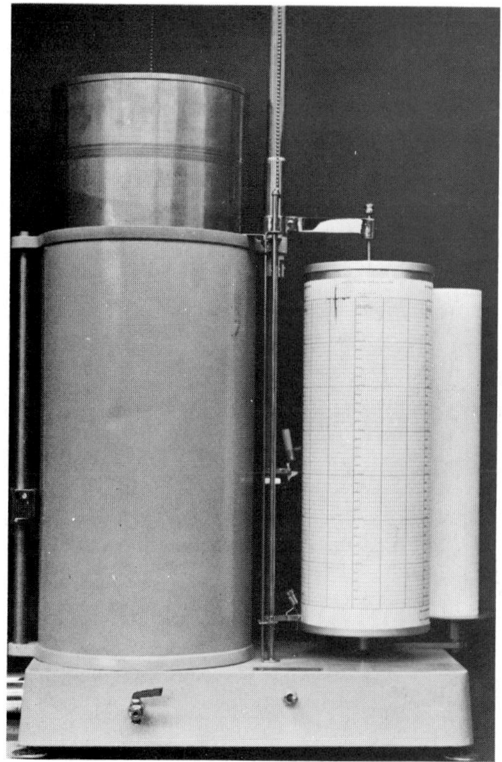

Fig. 7-9. A Collins 13.5-liter water-seal spirometer. This device is one of the most commonly used "volume standards" in respiratory care.

generally they are not needed when evaluating *therapeutic* devices at ambient conditions.

These spirometers can also be used to evaluate flow-metering devices under constant flow conditions. The graphic record of volume as opposed to time can be compared to the flow displayed on the metering device. If necessary, a correction graph can be made over a range of flows as well as with different gases such as air and oxygen.

Another type of volume standard is shown in Figure 7-10. Although generally quite accurate and simple to use, these syringes, must be used carefully when the flow rate at which the volume is expelled is crucial—that is, these devices are usually manually operated, and if the preset volume is expelled through a device that is flow-dependent (such as a rotary vane respirometer) to check its volume-measuring accuracy, care must be used to ensure that the proper flow ranges are not exceeded. Because this is difficult to accomplish, some manufacturers of volume-measuring devices do not recommend the use of these syringes.

Although not a volume standard *per se*, the efficiency of using a calibrated test lung analogue is worth mentioning (Fig. 7-11). This device can be very helpful in simulating patient resistance and compliance factors during mechanical ventilator evaluation. "Delivered' volumes can be read on the appropriate scale and checked against more precise volume standards.

TEMPERATURE STANDARDS

Figures 7-12 and 7-13 show three temperature monitors that can be used. Two are electronic, and the other is a standard mercury-filled glass tube. The most economical would be a high-quality mercury thermometer; however, some of the newer electronic types are easier to use and can be adapted to a recorder. If the electronic temperature-sensing device is used primarily, it should be checked periodically with another temperature standard, such as the mercury thermometer.

ELECTRICAL SAFETY STANDARDS

Electrical safety can be achieved by diligent inspection of all electrical components and the use of testing equipment (Fig. 7-14). The hazard detector in this group is of prime importance and is used for detecting electrical leaks with the attendant potential for serious electrical shock. Even new equipment should be hazard-tested before being used clinically.

Fig. 7-10. Calibrated "super syringe." Generally available from 500-ml to 5-liter sizes, these syringes provide a very accurate source for volume standardization, particularly in devices that are flow independent.

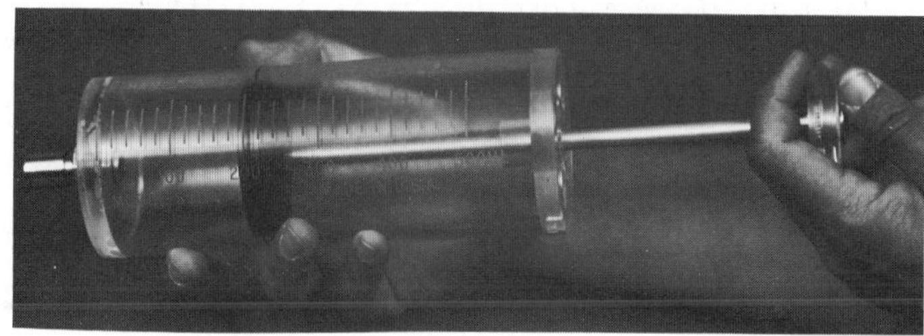

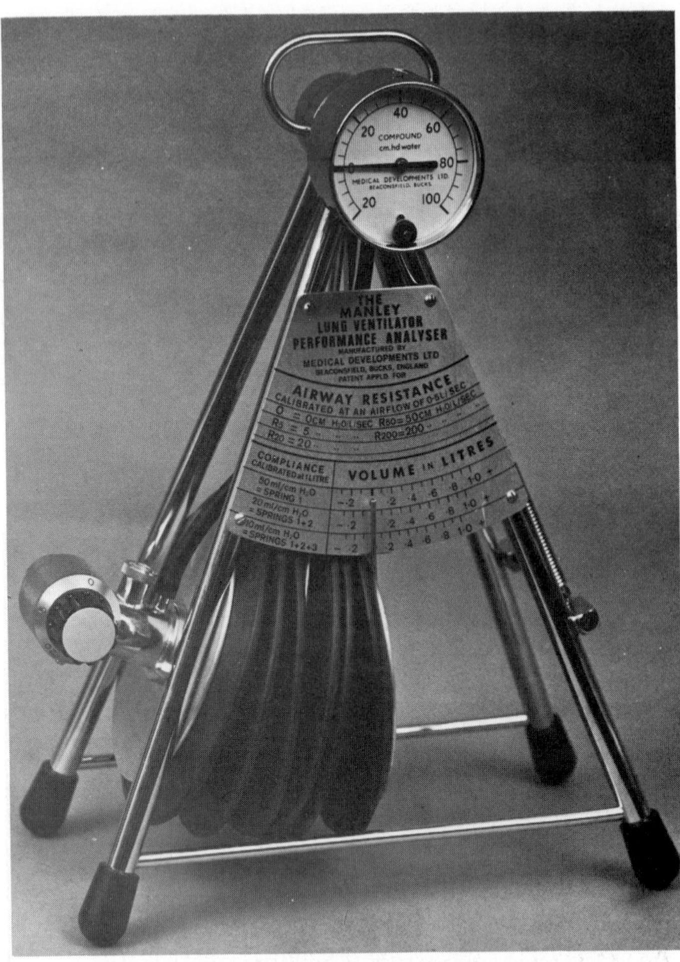

Fig. 7-11. Lung analogue for use with mechanical ventilators can simulate changing patient conditions by altering compliance and resistance values.

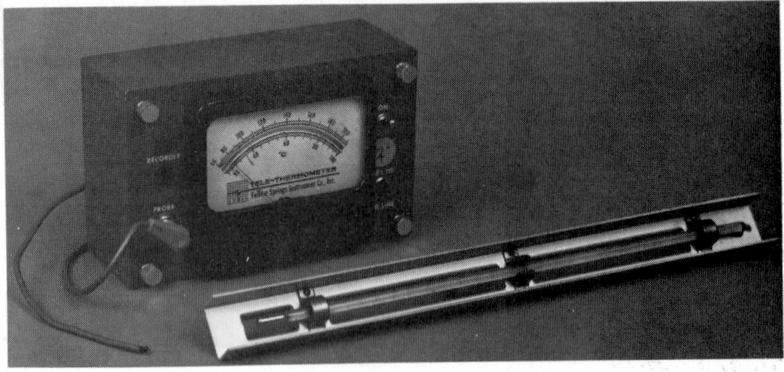

Fig. 7-12. Electrical and mercury thermometers.

SPACE

To perform efficient equipment evaluation, one needs adequate space (i.e., space for testing equipment, storage of maintenance manuals, performance records, and several large pieces of equipment at the same time). The Joint Commission on Accreditation of Hospitals has stated that "space, facilities, and equipment for the service shall be appropriate for the effective and timely care of the patient." The interpretation of this standard states that "the respiratory care service shall be provided with adequate, conveniently located space for specified work areas for cleaning, sterilizing, and repairing equipment." Equipment evaluations performed in a closet or hallway cannot be expected to provide accurate information and probably are better left to an outside contractor.

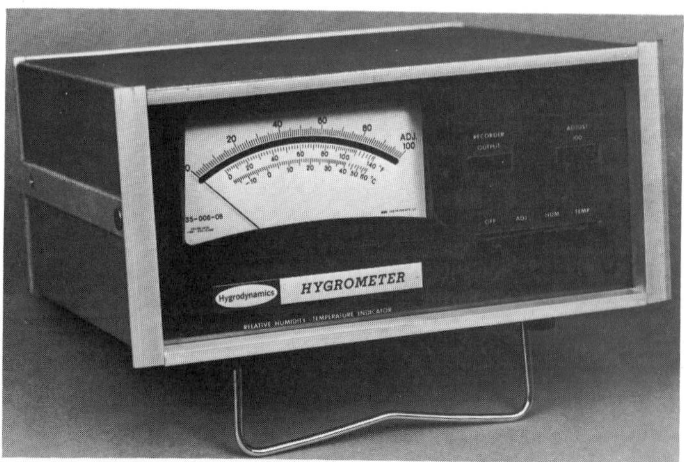

Fig. 7-13. Electrical hygrometer for measuring relative humidity and accurate temperatures on an analog meter or a recording device.

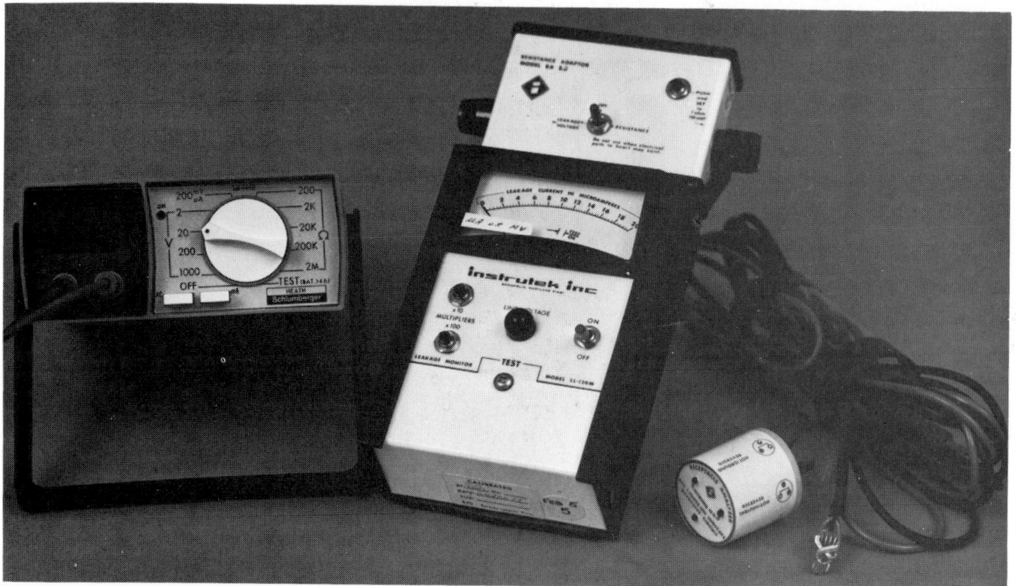

Fig. 7-14. Electrical leakage detectors and receptacle ground tester. The ground tester tests the correctness of wiring of the electrical receptacle.

AVAILABLE OPTIONS FOR MAINTENANCE PROGRAMS

RETURN TO THE MANUFACTURER OR DEALER

Probably the most frequently used option for repairing respiratory therapy equipment has been to ship the device to its manufacturer or to a factory-authorized dealer. It is highly unlikely that a modern department of respiratory therapy could use such a means for preventive maintenance and repair of all the equipment being used. Rather, the large variety of types and brands of devices will usually dictate that some other option be chosen for much or all of the equipment care.

"Down time," or the length of time a device is not available for use, is a primary consideration for any maintenance program. In this case the down time includes packing and shipping the device, the maintenance itself, and the return shipping. To predict the length of time the service will take is usually difficult. Many manufacturers and their dealers have not provided such estimates in the past and are reluctant to make such a commitment. Because the down time may be prolonged, a larger inventory of equipment may be needed.

Obviously, the locality of the repair service can be a major influence as to the usefulness of this option. If the equipment in question is manufactured and serviced within the hospital's local area, this type of servicing program may be most appropriate. In this case not only may an estimate of down time be feasible, but also replacement or loan equipment may be available as well.

The hospital must maintain records of maintenance and repair data. Therefore one deciding factor should be whether the manufacturer or dealer is willing to supply this information. Often a device is returned to the hospital after repair work has been completed with no accompanying reports or records, a clearly unacceptable practice.

Size and initial cost of the items will often be deciding factors for choosing to return certain equipment to the manufacturer. For example, oxygen flowmeters generally require only simple, inexpensive maintenance and may not require the time and costs of shipping. Other large, initially expensive equipment, such as mass spectrometers, body plethysmographs, and the like, also may not lend themselves to the rigors of shipping. In these cases it may be appropriate for a factory representative or an authorized dealer to provide service at the hospital itself. Some manufacturers offer a mobile service unit for maintenance and repair of their equipment on a contractual basis. However, these services are few, may cover only a small area, and are generally restricted to the company's own products.

Warranties may also influence equipment maintenance. Some ventilators on the market may be allowed to be sold only where a dealer and factory-trained personnel are available for specific periodic maintenance. The actual service available, however, may vary from dealer to dealer. The hospital may, in fact, wish to seek a dealer other than a local one if the facilities and services provided warrant it. Warranties themselves differ from one item to the next, and it is sometimes appropriate for a hospital with adequate facilities to provide its own service when the warranty is unsatisfactory or not applicable to the situation.

Certain elements of equipment function, accuracy, and safety *must* be provided by the hospital itself, and it is simply not feasible for a modern respiratory therapy department to depend solely on the manufacturer or dealer to provide all such preventive maintenance checks.

HOSPITAL ENGINEERING DEPARTMENT

Whether it is called medical electronics, biomedical maintenance, or, as it will be referred to here, the engineering department, such a facility may provide a good maintenance program for respiratory therapy equipment. This department has the advantages of being in-house and of having personnel with backgrounds in mechanical or electronic engineering; it may also have established some communication with manufacturers. This department will already be acquainted with various safety standards and regulations as well as with the data collecting systems used by the hospital. Cooperation between respiratory therapy and engineering departments will obviously be of primary importance if such a program is to be successful.

A serious commitment must be made by the engineering department to provide adequate and timely service to the respiratory therapy department. Ideally, personnel from both units should meet and discuss how the equipment is used, emphasizing critical life-support devices, how repair and maintenance procedures will be accomplished, what standards of performance are necessary, and what special training for personnel is available and needed. A records system must be established and should include mechanisms to obtain the documentation required by third-party payers in order that the services may be recompensed. The equipment inventory and history records should be available to both departments at any time.

Because devices will certainly have to be taken out of service periodically for performance checks, a system must be established for replacement of such needed equipment. Someone from the respiratory therapy department must be responsible for establishing and maintaining an adequate exchange system so that a crisis situation does not occur because of lack of operating equipment.

Although the engineering department may be responsible for maintaining the equipment for respiratory care, this does not void the respiratory therapy department's responsibilities for such devices. In fact, a greater effort may be needed to ensure that the engineering department realized the use and proper function of the devices involved. Most engineering departments are primarily set up to service electronic equipment and may not be familiar with many of the mechanical pneumatic devices that respiratory therapy uses. Therefore the staff involved may require reeducation, much of which the various manufacturers may provide. It may be appropriate for the respiratory therapy department to supply qualified personnel to the engineering department for design or implementation of specific procedures. The vast amounts and diversity of types of equipment used by respiratory therapy will likely cause the engineering department to require substantial additional space for work areas, inventory, and supplies compared to the area needed for other duties.

Once again an ongoing liaison is mandatory if such a joint effort is to realize success.

RESPIRATORY THERAPY DEPARTMENT PROGRAM

For optimum control of procedures, policies, performance standards, record–data collection, and equipment use, the equipment maintenance and quality control program ideally should be located *within* the respiratory therapy department. However, with such a venture come large amounts of responsibility, high initial costs, substantially increased physical space and inventory requirements, new personnel, and new in-service considerations.

Obviously, strong administrative support is vital for such a program. In some hospitals it may indeed be difficult to establish justifiable need for a complete maintenance facility that provides services primarily for one department, when there already may be another facility (such as engineering) that supplies maintenance for the rest of the institution's equipment. Such justification will depend on the size of the department involved and on the numbers and variety of equipment used. Once an in-house program is started, whether under respiratory therapy, engineering, or both, the administrative staff must be made aware of the substantial economic and spatial commitment.

The parts' inventory can be very large, particularly for teaching hospitals that require a wide variety of equipment. Experience will likely be the best teacher for knowing which replacement parts to carry for each device. In some areas where communication between the respiratory therapy department and a competent local dealer has been established, it may be possible for most of the inventory to be kept by the dealer. In this case the dealer must be ready to supply, upon demand, the needed items.

Measurement standards, as have been discussed previously, must be decided on by the department. Their cost-effectiveness can be enhanced if they are used for evaluation of new or prototype equipment and for research as well as for the maintenance program itself.

Once again the personnel involved in the actual maintenance and repair of the equipment must be qualified to provide such services adequately. Their initial training and subsequent continuing education should be formally documented. Respiratory therapy technicians and therapists who have been trained in patient care procedures may or may not be able to fulfill the maintenance technician's duties. Those who have training or experience in both respiratory care and mechanical or electrical engineering are ideal for such positions. Regardless of the person's qualifications, it is vital that he be acutely aware of the nature of the equipment and its use in patient care and of the immense responsibility of his position. In-service orientation sessions can, and should, be provided for these workers on technical and practical changes in the field and in the changing patient-care needs of the hospital.

Once such a department is committed to supplying its own quality-control program, physical space will be a primary concern. The space must be adequate to provide room for test equipment, work benches, inventory shelves, and drawers. In some hospitals, small, closetlike spaces have been used, only to frustrate the technicians attempting to provide care for equipment that can scarcely fit through the door. The space available can influence not only the quality of equipment care, but also the safety of the procedures themselves. Adequate wiring, lighting, and ventilation are a must. Many of the tools used will be common types, popular for pilfering. Therefore the space should have locking doors or at least locking cabinets for storage. Figures 7-15 through 7-17 show examples of work benches and inventory storage.

It may be feasible for larger institutions that have a working interdepartmental maintenance program to provide services for the small hospitals of the area. This may be economical and practical. The increased number and variety of procedures may warrant full-time rather than part-time staff, thus making better use of the relatively expensive test equipment purchased. The increased amount of data gathered should also aid the department in future equipment-purchasing choices.

Quality of equipment performance must be defined and documented for each device. Often the manufacturer's data will supply needed procedural information and acceptable specifications. However, each hospital's use of, and demands on, the devices will vary. The department must decide whether the man-

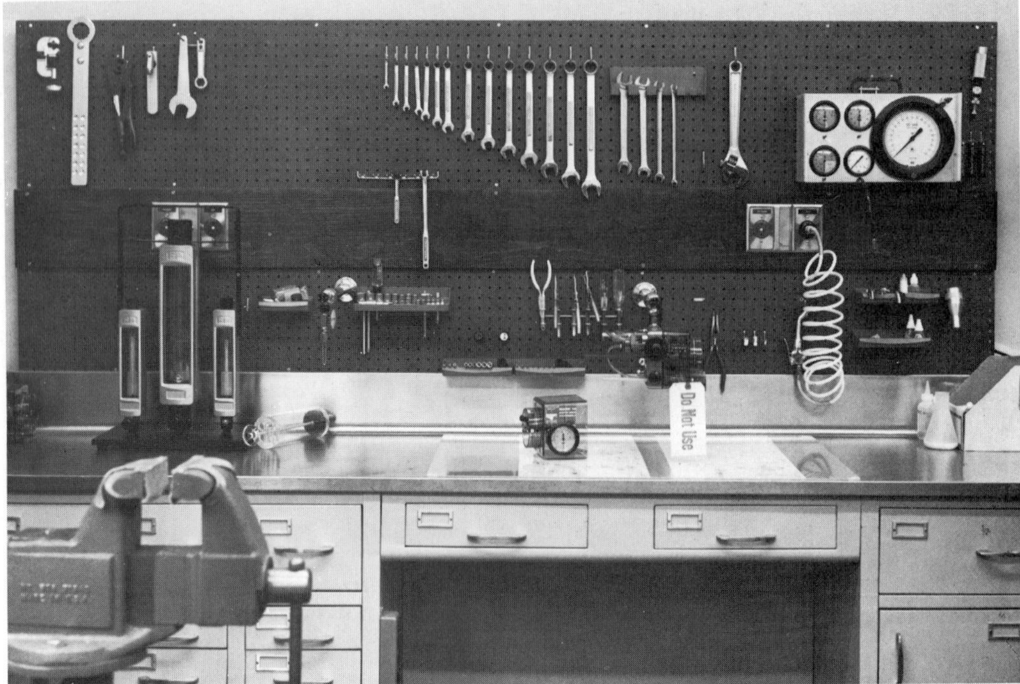

Fig. 7-15. Pneumatic work bench. The compressed gas outlets, pressure and flow standards, and tools shown here require adequate space for storage as well as working area for promoting quality equipment evaluation and maintenance.

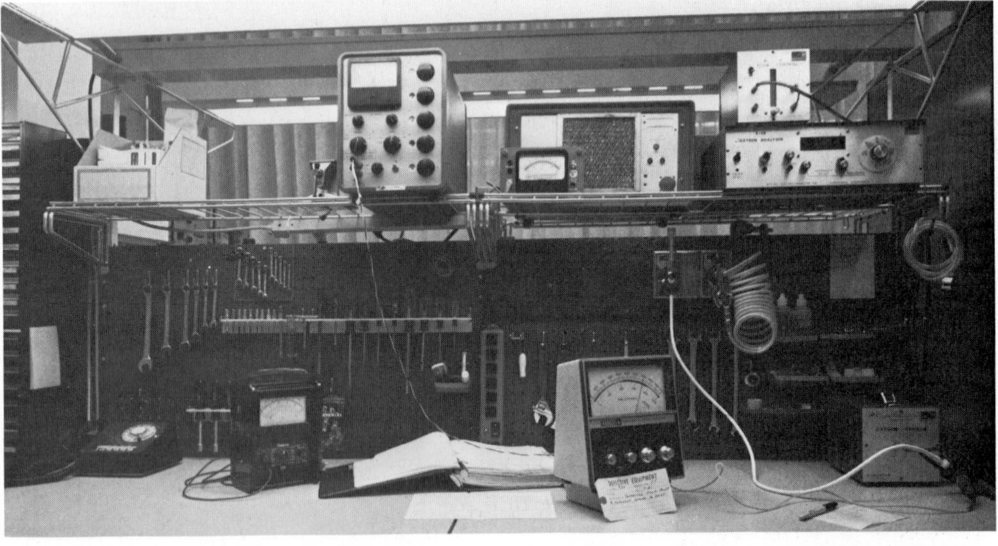

Fig. 7-16. Electrical work bench. This example again emphasizes the space requirements needed for maintaining equipment common to hospitals. Electrical safety, temperature, and oxygen measurement standards are readily available to the work bench. Note the small drawers on the extreme left for storing needed replacement parts.

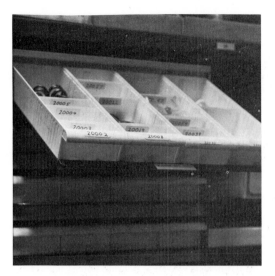

Fig. 7-17. Numerous small parts must be available to maintenance personnel. Drawers such as these provide a good storage system.

ufacturer's specifications are acceptable for each piece of equipment. If they are not, then the procedure used for testing and calibration should specify the new expectations. Quality is obviously a nebulous term that lends itself poorly to definitions and categorization. Whatever level of controls are placed on the maintenance programs, documentation as to the procedure and specifications used is extremely important.

Some equipment may not be serviced within the respiratory therapy department without voiding the warranty. For certain, devices may be of little or no consequence if the warranty itself is less than optimal. If warranty service is required and the device leaves the maintenance area to be sent to the manufacturer or dealer, then that process should be duly documented. If possible, the manufacturer should be asked to supply information on any repairs required so that those procedures may be entered into the operational history record for that device.

The more cooperation between the equipment manufacturers and the respiratory therapy department, the better. The departmental maintenance system can make or break such needed communications. Appropriate feedback from respiratory therapy departments to the manufacturer about repair records, parts availability, and performance specifications can add much-needed input to future equipment design and planning. If prototype investigations are done, the manufacturers must be aware of and consider basic patient-care needs. The respiratory therapy department should make every attempt to coordinate the evaluations and clinical trials so as to provide the most complete and accurate data possible to the manufacturer. The maintenance facility should be the starting place for such a trial because there the unit can be initially inspected and evaluated for safety and performance.

The hospital is, of course, legally responsible for the proper working order of its equipment, regardless of who provides the maintenance services. Documentation of adequate procedures, policies, and continuing education of personnel is a key factor in defending the adequacy of any such service.

CONTRACT SERVICES

Another option whereby respiratory therapy departments may obtain equipment maintenance and repair is the use of a local company that offers such a program of equipment maintenance and repair on a contractual basis. This situation should not be confused with service companies that provide an entire respiratory therapy "department," including equipment and personnel. Such a company may provide normal maintenance of specified equipment for some predetermined dollar amount, generally excluding the cost of parts, on a periodic basis. Items delineated in the contract usually include types of equipment, an identification system, minimum time between evaluations, evaluation procedures, records data, responsibilities of the hospital and company, and minimum costs.

Damaged equipment is repaired at an additional cost beyond the maintenance fee. Rates of the repair costs can often be estimated either at the time the contract is agreed on or just before the repair procedure. As experience is gained for each type of equipment, an estimated repair cost may be included as a guide to the total cost of such a service.

Contract services have several potentially desirable features.

1. A minimum cost for maintenance can be predetermined.
2. The costs of needed inventory of parts, measuring devices, physical space, and personnel are the company's responsibilities.
3. Repair and maintenance warranties beyond the manufacturer's own can be part of the contract.

4. Definitive information on down time and costs of repair for various pieces of equipment can be made available to the hospital without the hospital doing its own accumulating of raw data.
5. The contracting company shares in the legal responsibilities for the equipment's functional operation.
6. If the service company provides similar services to other hospitals in the area, it is reasonable to expect that their technicians may become familiar with certain equipment sooner than the technicians of a hospital-based program because of the increased exposure.

The reliability and stability of the contract service are obviously important concerns. Practical considerations include such problems as down time for equipment, cooperation between the two institutions, availability of emergency service and backup for life-support equipment, and the respiratory therapy department's input to the company's maintenance procedures and quality control systems.

Down Time

Down time for normal maintenance for major equipment such as ventilators, ultrasonic nebulizers, and spirometers can be shortened if the service company begins its rotation of items by exchanging the units temporarily with working units provided by the company. This may not be needed in every case, but the hospital should consider this procedure when the system is developed.

If the company is not immediately local, much of the down time may be due to travel. The ideal situation for both the company and the hospital seems to be a mobile service. A step-van (Fig. 7-18) or similar vehicle can be equipped with relatively large amounts of testing equipment and parts inventory. Electrical power can be supplied to the carrier by the hospital. The availability of the mobile unit on the hospital

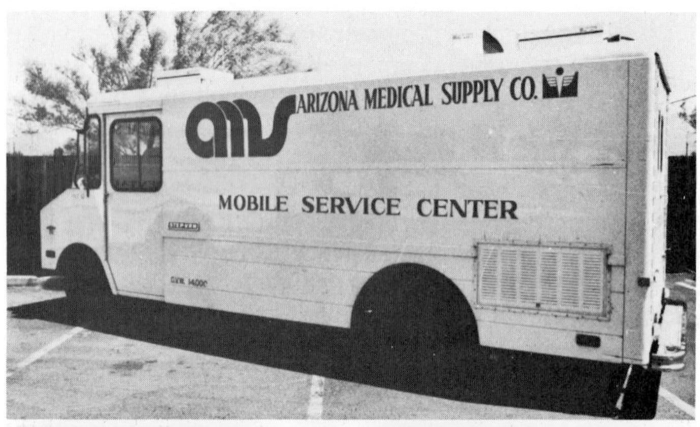

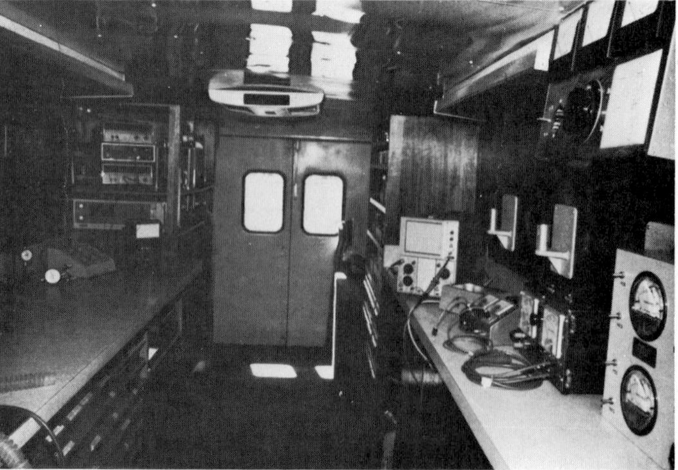

Fig. 7-18. A mobile maintenance vehicle, showing both the external and internal features. Various testing devices, tools, and replacement part inventory can be available in such a unit when properly arranged.

grounds can minimize travel time and help facilitate adequate equipment rotation.

Cooperation

Beyond the limits of the responsibility of both parties as written in the contract lie all the practical, everyday considerations of its implementation. Someone in the respiratory therapy department who understands its general operations must be responsible for the coordination of the maintenance and repair service. Whether this person actively transfers the equipment from the clinical setting is for the individual parties to decide. Obviously someone who is aware of the nature of patient care must be actively involved in the removal and return of the equipment in question.

Emergency Service

If a company is responsible for normal maintenance and repair, then the same company should provide reasonable services for emergency repair or temporary replacement of certain life-support equipment. The importance of such a backup procedure should be established by preplanning in the initial contract negotiations, and not after a crisis situation. This can be a critical problem for small hospitals with only limited amounts of life-support devices (such as ventilators and, blood gas analysis devices), which the contract service can usually readily supply. When equipment replacement is necessary, the company should be expected to supply similar equipment that does not require extra training of personnel by the hospital. The company will most likely charge for this service in rental fees or by other mechanisms as agreed on in advance by both parties.

Respiratory Therapy Department Input

It is just as important for the respiratory therapy service to be aware of the procedures used by the contract company as it is for hospital management to be aware of the procedures used by a hospital-based program. From the beginning of such a program and periodically thereafter, the procedures used by the company should be reviewed briefly. The service company should be receptive to the specific needs of each hospital, and there need to be provisions for procedural change even in the middle of an ongoing contract. Determinations of minimum quality will differ between institutions of varying sizes and financial structures. The versatile company should be prepared to offer individual adjustments to its basic contract at reasonable costs.

Both the maintenance procedures and the personnel actually performing them should be available for scrutiny. Qualifications for such personnel must be equal to or greater than those for technicians who would perform the same duties were the service hospital-based. The contract service should follow the guidelines of the various agencies mentioned earlier in this chapter, if service is to be rendered acceptably. The company should be expected to provide documentation of its personnel's qualifications and continuing education to the respiratory therapy department or other agencies that influence the hospital's accreditation procedures.

Reliability and Stability of the Contract Company

Determination of the reliability of a company may be difficult to establish until after a program has begun. However, some estimations can be made subjectively through past experience with the company by either the hospital concerned or by questioning other hospitals in the area and the local Better Business Bureau. If the hospital is not sure of the type of service to be provided, a probationary period may be stipulated in the contract. During formation of the contract, which may require considerable time, cooperation between the institutions will be established. Some insight may be gained during this time by the responsiveness to suggestions and contractual rewrites made by the company.

COMBINATION PROGRAMS

The diversity of size and variety of responsibilities assumed by various respiratory therapy departments dictate that some combination of the foregoing options will likely prove optimal in many situations. A variety of factors can influence the type of combination program that is appropriate. The size and location of the institution and the sophistication of the equipment used will have an influence. If a hospital is in an area where an adequate contract service can be provided, then it may be appropriate for much of the maintenance to be provided through such a service. If specific manufacturers or their authorized dealers are nearby, some equipment maintenance may be delivered by them. When the size of the hospital is such that reasonably comprehensive in-house maintenance is already being provided for most of the other departments, then some respiratory therapy equipment may also be taken care of there. If the respiratory care services are large enough to warrant the sophisticated testing equipment, trained personnel, and physical space required to provide a nearly complete in-house maintenance program, then other smaller hospitals in the area may very well arrange to have some of their own equipment maintained by that program as well.

The following are examples of combination programs that have been divided into categories relative to hospital size. These are only illustrative examples and not recommendations *per se*.

Fewer Than 100 Beds

Some type of respiratory care is likely to be provided by all small hospitals. Small institutions may encounter the most difficulty in establishing a maintenance program because of financial problems and geographical location. They are not exempt, however, from the moral and ethical obligation to provide adequately functioning equipment for patient care.

For some of the equipment (flowmeters, humidifiers, pneumatic nebulizers), someone in the hospital itself, either in the respiratory therapy department, if one exists, or perhaps in the general maintenance area, could be responsible for upkeep. The clinical staff should be acquainted at least with routine calibration and troubleshooting procedures for the devices they use. Larger equipment, such as ventilators and electronic devices, could be serviced by a contract service periodically, if, in fact, one is available. Here the mobile service has a definite advantage. If contract maintenance service is not available, then perhaps a larger institution within reasonable distance may provide the service.

New equipment under warranty and sophisticated apparatus, such as volume ventilators and monitoring systems, may have to be checked and maintained periodically by the manufacturer or authorized dealer. It may well be appropriate for certain smaller institutions to limit their respiratory care equipment to simple intermediate-care devices, particularly if a transport mechanisms is or can be available so that critically ill patients may be taken to a facility that offers more comprehensive services.

Renting or leasing certain equipment during time of need can also be a valid approach for smaller hospitals. Particularly when various devices are being serviced, the small hospital must be conscious of alternative equipment availability.

Between 100 and 300 Beds

The range of respiratory care within a hospital of intermediate size will vary greatly and depend on many factors. A teaching institution may provide more acute care facilities, for example, than a community hospital of the same size. Here the hospital might have at least one person to coordinate the equipment maintenance programs. One option would be that all flowmeters, humidifiers, nebulizers, and ventilators be maintained within the respiratory therapy department itself, while all primarily electrical equipment be maintained by the engineering group. Sophisticated electric-pneumatic ventilators, monitors, pulmonary function apparatus, and the like could be serviced by the manufacturer or a contract service.

Again some facilities of substantial size with sophisticated maintenance capabilities may provide some relief to the smaller hospitals.

More Than 300 Beds

In a large hospital the evaluation and quality control of respiratory-care-related devices may fall completely within the hospital itself. If a combined program were used, an option would be for the respiratory care department to manage and supply nearly all required care to pneumatic, pneumatic-electric, and simple electric devices, while the engineering department would service sophisticated electronic equipment. On a job per job basis, the institution could supply service to smaller facilities in the area or a mobile service, as previously discussed.

MAINTENANCE OF RESPIRATORY THERAPY HOME-CARE EQUIPMENT

The daily care of home equipment ideally starts with a hospital-based training program. If the patient is hospitalized a training period should be initiated with the same equipment the patient will use at home. These training sessions should include disassembly and assembly of the equipment and some means of evaluating the performance of the device by the patient. If the proficiency of the patient is inadequate near the time of dismissal from the hospital, an extra effort must be applied by the staff at this point. The patient's spouse or some other family member or friend should be taught how to use and clean the equipment.

Regardless of the type of device used in the home, the clinical staff who train patients for home therapy must also provide complete and explicit information on the cleaning and care of the devices.

CLEANING PROCEDURES

Most therapeutic modalities used at home use liquids either for aerosolization or for simple addition of water vapor to dry medical gases. These liquids may provide a medium for microorganism growth and the potential for infecting or reinfecting the patient during use (*see* Chap. 19). While absolute sterilization of equipment between treatments is ideal, it is not practical or even necessary in the home. However, a step-by-step procedure for disassembling, cleaning, disinfecting, drying, reassembling, and storing the equipment on a scheduled basis should be provided. Regardless of the solutions used or recommended, a primary consideration should be the frequency of the cleaning procedure. Aerosol-producing units provide a greater potential for contamination than do simple humidifying devices, and therefore their cleaning should be more frequent. Again the manufacturer may provide information that can serve as a guideline.

Individual patient needs should be considered when establishing the cleaning procedure. For example, one patient may be able to use only soaking solutions with minimum scrubbing because of physical disability. Another patient may have an automatic dishwasher that provides very hot water and a drying cycle that may be ideal for the equipment being used.

PERFORMANCE CHECKS

Each device used by the patient should be accompanied by a written description for its normal operation as well as some simple performance checks. The list should include the steps for each treatment and periodic checks.

When investigating operation and performance standards for a given piece of equipment, the manufacturer should be the first place to look for information. Most pieces of home equipment, when purchased new, have an operator's manual, some of which may provide performance criteria (*see* Fig. 7-19 and the appendix to this chapter). If the operator's manual does not provide needed information, a service manual can often be obtained from the manufacturer. The evaluation of the performance of home

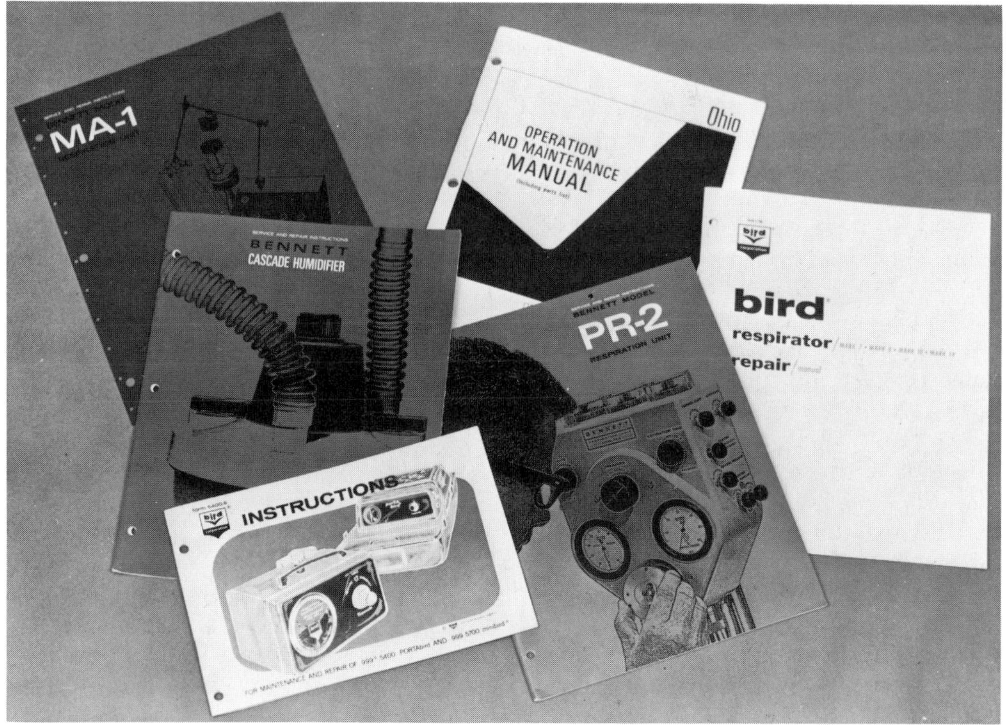

Fig. 7-19. Examples of various operation manuals. A variety of such information should be available from manufacturers for their respective equipment.

therapy equipment need not be an elaborate, complicated procedure; in fact, it should not be. Some very simple means of evaluation should be devised for the home patient so that he can be warned of malfunctioning equipment. Periodically, home therapy equipment should be taken into a more sophisticated testing area and given a complete evaluation for possible electrical leaks, compressor malfunction, ultrasonic frequency variances, flaws in flow and pressure capabilities, total aerosol output of ultrasonic nebulizers, and so forth. Most of these tests are difficult to perform in the home, and, ideally, if this requires some time, the maintenance facility should provide an alternate piece of equipment while the equipment is being evaluated and, if necessary, repaired.

It has been our experience that much of this maintenance and performance evaluation can be done while the patient is in the hospital, even though it may be before the scheduled evaluation time. The equipment is then checked and ready to perform when the patient is discharged. A retraining session for the use and care of the equipment may also be appropriate at this time.

Figure 7-20 shows a few examples of various types of home care equipment. One simple device to determine the pressure capabilities of the machine in the field is an aneroid manometer. This manometer should be calibrated so that it can be used as a "standard" for checking other manometers.

Another performance-evaluating device is a simple tube with a fixed orifice that can be attached to a positive-pressure generating device. By monitoring the pressure behind the fixed orifice, both pressure and flow capabilities of the device can be evaluated. A predetermined amount of minimum pressure acceptable is determined on more elaborate flow and pressure devices. This aneroid manometer and tube with a fixed orifice (Fig. 7-21), along with some instructions, can provide a simple means for the patient to check the performance of his equipment in his home.

Other variables that can be inspected in the home by the patient or the visiting therapist include electrical components such as the cord and switches on the equipment. Visual inspection for insulation breaks and cracked casings and feeling for excessive warmth of the unit are simple, yet important, methods of problem detection. Dirty filters (Fig. 7-22) are also a frequent source of difficulty. Compressors are often used for home respiratory therapy, and excessive noise or discharge of particles from the cooling vents can indicate oncoming failure of these devices. Many of these units are not intended for continuous use, and this consideration should be conveyed to the patient.

When aerosol-generating devices such as ultrasonic nebulizers are used, some subjective visual inspection of the aerosol produced can be helpful. With experience the patient will know how dense the aerosol should appear and whether the mist output is intermittent or continuous. If an air blower is used to deliver the mist, it can be evaluated by observing the horizontal distance over which the aerosol is propelled. Again, deviations from the typical operation of these devices may be indications for them to be taken to a maintenance facility for further evaluation.

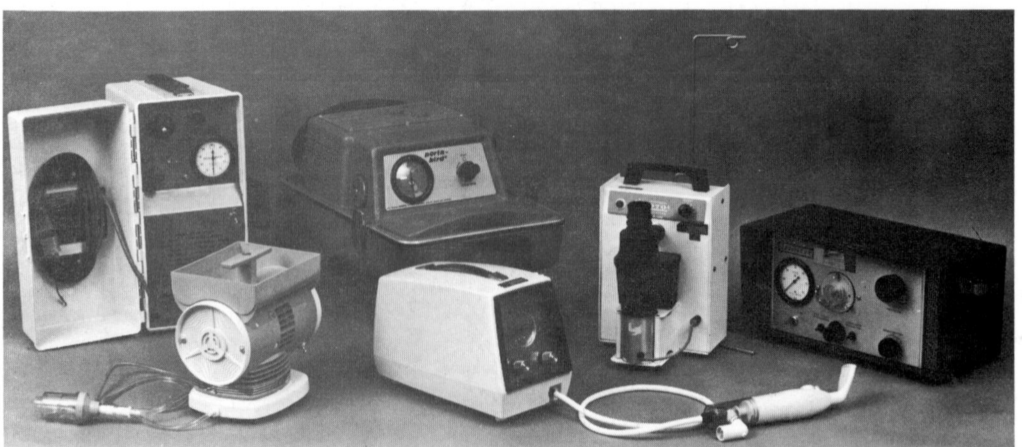

Fig. 7-20. Various devices often used for inhalation of aerosols for respiratory therapy in the home. Care of these devices is discussed in the text.

MAINTENANCE SCHEDULE

Devices used in the home should be routinely checked by a maintenance facility, just as they should be in the hospital. A predetermined schedule for these checks should be given to the patient during his initial training in the use of the device. The time intervals between maintenance checks should be individually determined, depending on the type of equipment and the patient's use of the device.

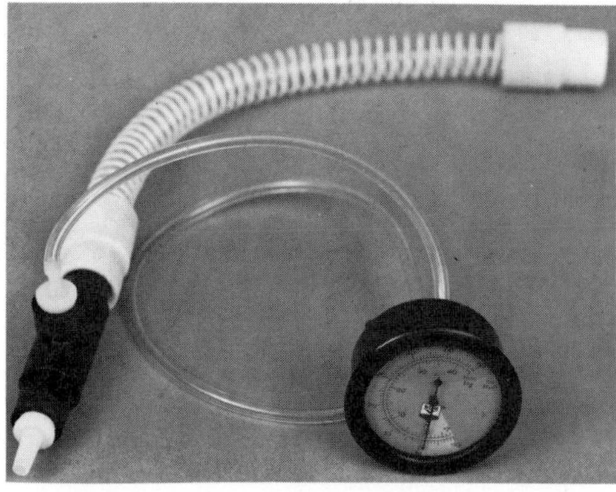

Fig. 7-21. A simple, portable testing device. This system can estimate adequacy of a general flow range in some devices by measuring the pressure exerted against a known resistance (*see* text).

SUMMARY

The need for ongoing equipment evaluation, maintenance, and quality control of respiratory care equipment is obvious. The type of program designed to accomplish this at an optimal level will be different for each institution, depending on its size, type of care provided, financial capability, and a multitude of other factors. Of the five separate options for programs offered here, no one option is likely to suit an institution's total needs; some combination of these options is likely to be more appropriate. It is the obligation of institutions to analyze their individual capabilities and to develop a complete program of equipment care.

APPENDIX

The following is a selected group of manufacturers involved with devices commonly used for equipment evaluation, maintenance, and quality control from which the reader may obtain further information. The inclusion of a manufacturer does not indicate any endorsement by the authors or the publishers.

Fig. 7-22. Portable positive-pressure device in need of cleaning. Many such devices use air filters, which should be checked and changed periodically. The difference in the appearance of the clean filters held in the hand compared to those still in the unit indicates a need for replacement.

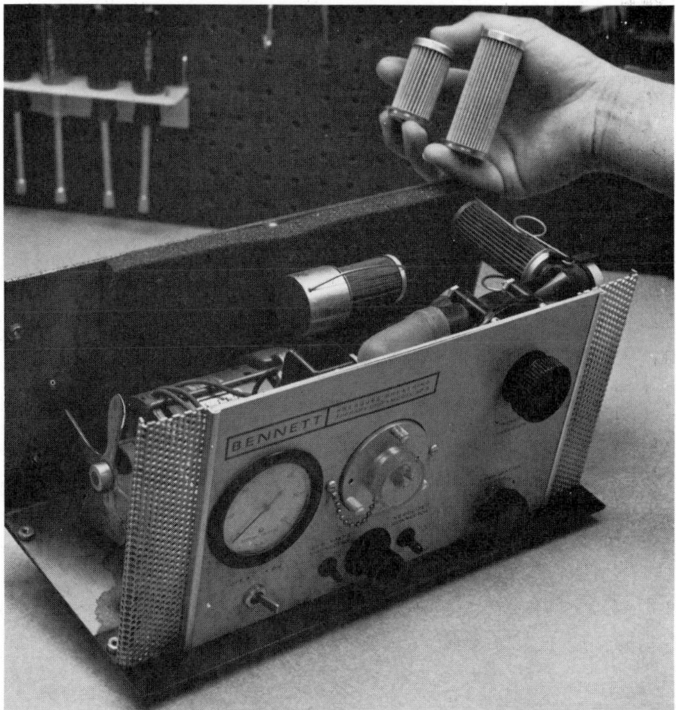

Primary Medical Gas Systems

Air Compressors

Chemetron Medical Division
Allied Health-Care Products, Inc.
1720 Sublette
St Louis, MO 63110

Dryair Inc.
P. O. Box 11149
Nashville, TN 37211

ITT Pneumotive
P. O. Box 4748
4601 Central Avenue
Monroe, LA 71203

Ohio Medical Products, Division of Airco
3030 Airco Drive
P. O. Box 7550
Madison, WI 53707

General Medical Gas Delivery Systems

Chemetron Medical Division
Allied Healthcare Products Inc.
1720 Sublette
St Louis, Mo 63110

Ohio Medical Products
3030 Airco Drive
P. O. Box 7550
Madison, WI 53707

Oxequip's Health Industries
12601 South Springfield
Chicago, IL 60658

Puritan–Bennett Corporation
13th and Oak
Kansas City, MO 64106

Pneumatic valves, pressure regulating devices, and other related equipment

Bay Corporation
25700 First Street
Westlake, OH 44145

Gould Incorporated
Valve and Fittings Division
6300 West Howard Street
Chicago, IL 60648

Ohio Medical Products
3030 Airco Drive
P. O. Box 7550
Madison, WI 53707

Puritan–Bennett Corporation
13th and Oak
Kansas City, MO 64106

Western Enterprises
33672 Pin Oak Parkway
Avon Lake, OH 44012

Gas Analysis Equipment

Applied Electrochemistry, Inc.
735 North Pastoria Avenue
Sunnyvale, CA 94086

Beckman Instruments, Inc.
2500 Harbor Blvd.
Fullerton, CA 92634

Boehringer Laboratories, Inc.
P. O. Box 337
Wynnewood, PA 19096

Erich Jaeger Inc.
P. O. Box 5465
Rockford, IL 61125

Perkin–Elmer
2771 North Garey
Pomona, CA 91767

P. K. Morgan Instruments Inc.
17 Millpond off Harkaway Road
North Andover, MA 01845

Gas Pressure Devices

Dwyer Precision Inc.
P. O. Box 51182
266 North 20th Street
Jacksonville Beach, FL 32250

Gould Incorporated Medical Products Division
SRL Medical
2676 Indian Ripple Road
Dayton, OH 45440

Hewlett-Packard Company
175 Wyman Street
Waltham, MA 02254

Meriam Instrument Company
10920 Madison Avenue
Cleveland, OH 44102

MKS Instruments Inc.
34 Third Avenue
Burlington, MA 01803

Setra Systems Inc.
One Strathmore Road
Natick, MA 01760

Validyne Engineering Corporation
8626 Wilbur Avenue
Northridge, CA 91324

Wallace and Tiernan
Division Pennwalt Corporation
25 Main Street
Belleville, NJ 07109

Gas Flow Devices

Brooks Manufacturing Corporation
3147-53 Emerald Street
Philadelphia, PA 19134

Dynasciences
Township Road
Blue Bell, PA 19422

Fischer and Porter
Warminster, PA 18974

Hans Rudolph Inc.
7200 Wyandotte
Kansas City, MO 64114

Hewlett–Packard Company
175 Wyman Street
Waltham, MA 02254

Meriam Instrument Company
10920 Madison Avenue
Cleveland, OH 44102

Wallace and Tierman, Division of Pennwalt Corporation
25 Main Street
Belleville, NJ 07109

Gas Volume Devices

Fiske/Med-Science Park
600 Wheeler Road
Burlington, MA 01803

Hans Rudolph Inc.
7200 Wyandotte
Kansas City, MO 64114

Jones Medical Instrument Company
200 Windsor Drive
Oak Brook, IL 60521

Timeter Instrument Corporation
2501 Oregon Pike
Lancaster, PA 17601

Vacumed Inc.
2261 Palma Drive
Ventura, CA 93003

Warren E. Collins, Inc.
220 Wood Road
Braintree, MA 02184

Temperature Measurement Devices

American Scientific Products, General Offices
1430 Waukegan Road
McGraw Park, IL 60085

Yellow Springs Instruments Company
Box 279
Yellow Springs, OH 45387

Electrical Safety Devices

Bio Tek Instruments Inc.
One Mill Street
Burlington, VT 05482

Dynatech Nevada Inc.
2000 Arrowhead Drive
P. O. Box 1925
Carson City, NV 89701

Instrutek Corporation
401 North Broad Street
Philadelphia, PA 19108

Timeter Instruments Corporation
2501 Oregon Pike
Lancaster, PA 17601

Ohmic Instruments Corporation
2501 Oregon Pike
Lancaster, PA 17601

Humidity and Aerosol Devices

American Scientific Products, General Offices
1430 Waukegan Road
McGraw Park, IL 60085

Climet Instrument Company
Box 151
Redlands, CA 92373

Miac/Razco, Pacific Scientific Instruments Division
141 Jefferson Drive
Menlo Park, CA 94025

Hygrodynamics
949 Selim Road
Silver Springs, MD 20910

Lung Analogues

Bear Medical Systems Inc.
9335 Douglas Drive
Riverside, CA 92503

Dixie USA Inc.
P. O. Box 13060
Houston, TX 77219

Electronic Amplifier and Recording Equipment

Beckman Instruments Inc.
Electronic Instruments Division
3900 River Road
Schiller Park, IL 60176

Gould Inc. Medical Products
Division of SRL Medical
2676 Indian Ripple Road
Dayton, OH 45440

Hewlett–Packard Company
175 Wyman Street
Waltham, MA 02254

Validyne Engineering Corporation
8626 Wilbur Avenue
Northridge, CA 91324

BIBLIOGRAPHY

General

Bancroft ML et al: Health device legislation: An overview of the law and its impact on respiratory care. Respir Care 23:1179, 1978

Crane FA: To lease or purchase. J Am Hosp Assoc 45:89, 1971

Gish GB: The hospital as part of a community of equipment needs. Respir Care 20:922, 1975

Gross R: Keeping mechanical ventilators dependable. Respir Care 20:942, 1975

Health Devices Sourcebook: A Directory of Medical Devices and Manufacturers. Plymouth Meeting, PA, ECRI, 1981

Judge D: Leasing: A way to use equipment without buying it. Mod Hosp 117:123, 1971

Kernaghan SG: Financing the purchase of respiratory care equipment. Respir Care 20:934, 1975.

Nobel JJ: Guidelines for equipment purchasing control. Respir Care 20:929, 1975

Nobel JJ: The future of medical devices and how to avoid the worst of it. Respir Care 20:945, 1975

Oslick T: Equipment needs of a hospital's respiratory therapy program. Respir Care 20:925, 1975

Phillips DF: Leasing comes of age. J Am Hosp Assoc 46:126, 1972

Saposnick AB: Maintenance and repair of gas, humidity, and aerosol equipment. Respir Care 20:938, 1975

Shapiro AG et al: JCAH standards: Learn to use the tool. J Am Hosp Assoc 48:100, 1974

Thomas Register of American Manufacturers and Thomas Register Catalog File. New York, Thomas Publishing, 1982

1982 Buyer's guide. Respir Care 26:1283, 1981

Measuring Devices and Standards

Cook AM et al: Therapeutic Medical Devices: Application and Design. Englewood Cliffs, NJ, Prentice–Hall, 1982

Cromwell L et al: Medical Instrumentation for Health Care. Englewood Cliffs, NJ, Prentice–Hall, 1976

Cromwell L et al: Biomedical Instrumentation and Measurements, 2nd ed. Englewood Cliffs, NJ, Prentice–Hall, 1980

DeMarre DA et al: Bioelectric Measurements. Englewood Cliffs, NJ, Prentice–Hall, 1983

Norton HN: Sensor and Analyzer Handbook. Englewood Cliffs, NJ, Prentice–Hall, 1982

Pacela AF: The Guide to Biochemical Standards, 8th ed. Brea, CA, Quest Publishing, 1981–1982

Sykes MD et al: Principles of Clinical Measurement, 2nd ed. Oxford, Blackwell Scientific Publications, 1981

8

The Economics of Respiratory Care

Thomas J. DeKornfeld

Since the first edition of *Respiratory Care* has been published, the economic aspects of health care delivery have come under increasing scrutiny. Even before 1976, the immense escalation of medical costs and the increasing concern expressed about the quality of medical care and the cost–benefit ratio of complex and expensive medical services made it mandatory that the economic aspects of respiratory care be examined in some detail.

There are two segments in the health care system that are currently under heavy fire from all directions, including by the federal government, state governments, consumer groups, and even some within the health care industry. These two segments are the hospitals and the physicians. In the view of most critics, these two segments are jointly and individually responsible for health costs having risen much more sharply than the *consumer price index* or other economic indicators.

The assumptions basic to this discussion are that respiratory care services are generally beneficial; that patients, indeed, require at least some of these services at least some of the time, and that both the administrative and therapeutic decision-making process and the actual delivery of care are a professional responsibility for which adequate compensation must be provided.

It would be naive to assume that the regulation of the $200 billion health care industry—which approximates 10% of the *gross national product*—is a simple matter or that such a giant organization, operated by fallible and occasionally dishonest and rapacious people, will be free of extraordinary difficulties. Nevertheless, it is clearly our mandate to approach not only the scientific but also the economic aspects of health care with the utmost seriousness and with a profound commitment to do the best possible job, in the best possible way, *and* at the lowest possible cost.

In recent years the scientific basis of respiratory care has been questioned, and this very legitimate concern has had profound effects on the practice of the specialty. Certain techniques and procedures have almost disappeared, whereas others have proliferated but in turn have been challenged by newer observations. It is a rather fundamental tenet that there should be a *reasonable cost–benefit ratio* for all activities in which a service is rendered for financial or other compensation. While it would be tempting to delve into the intricacies of cost–benefit ratios, it is deemed more prudent to keep this chapter, as much as possible, on a factual basis and to consider the economic aspects of respiratory care from a purely fiscal point of view, assuming that there is a reasonable cost–benefit ratio in respiratory care activities. This consideration could take a variety of forms, and there are many ways in which economic problems can be presented. In order to approach this often neglected area in an orderly fashion, we need first to discuss the general fiscal principles that govern the hospital as a "business" organization. This discussion must include the general financial management of the hospital, with particular reference to the ever-increasing influence of governmental agencies that have become the dominant factors in financing health care and that affect profoundly the economic climate in which the hospital and all its components must operate. Since most respiratory therapy personnel devote most of their time and efforts to patients in the hospital, it behooves them and all other hospital-based health professionals to have a good understanding of the ways in which hospitals operate not only from the professional but also from the financial point of view.

On this basis, this chapter discusses [1] the general financial management of hospitals; [2] the cost of respiratory services to the patient; [3] the cost of maintaining a respiratory therapy department for the hospital, including the option of contract services; [4] the economics of medical direction; [5] the cost of education in respiratory care; and [6] budget preparation. These discussions will examine current practices but will also include some speculations on the future economic development of the health care industry, with special reference to respiratory care. This chapter will reflect some of my economic prejudices. I believe that access to quality health care is a fundamental human right and that the financing of these rights is a societal responsibility.

GENERAL FINANCIAL MANAGEMENT OF HOSPITALS

"A well managed hospital operation is generally not the result of individual genius or effort. Rather, it is the product of the efforts and intellects of a group of individuals organized to function in concert."[3] No organizational structure fits all the different types of hospitals, but three basic elements must be present for sound financial management.

1. An *organizational table* that not only delineates the lines of authority and which is sufficiently flexible to allow for expansion and for change, but which also delineates the roles and authority of all administrative personnel.
2. *Written accounting and operating practices* are important because a complex organization with significant turnover in personnel must have precise procedure manuals available for training new personnel and for assuring a strict adherence to agreed upon procedures and practices. These operational manuals are very similar to the well-known departmental policy and procedure manuals and usually suffer from the same weaknesses.
3. *Quality personnel* are obviously an important component. The success or failure of financial management of a major institution such as a hospital depends largely on the quality of the personnel entrusted with the financial operations and on the ability of the operational and fiscal management people to cooperate intelligently and well. Quality of performance must be maintained at all levels of operation—from those who set policy, to those who have to enforce it, and to those who have to implement it.

The role of the financial management team is to balance the hospital's budget—that is, to attain a level of income that will, ideally, be equal to or exceed the cost of operating the hospital. In principle, this same type of process is performed by every economic unit of the nation, whether it be an individual, a family, an industrial organization such as General Motors, or, indeed, the state and federal governments. The hospital performs a number of functions and provides a number of services that generate revenue, and its expenses must be covered by that revenue. Parenthetically, it should be stated that while corporations generally are in business for money, most hospitals are "not for profit" organizations. This does not mean that they are not allowed to show a profit at the end of the year but simply that nonprofit hospitals do not have to pay taxes on their income and that whatever excess of income they generate has to be used for the benefit of the hospital, and cannot accrue to any individual or group of individuals.

The sources of revenue available to hospitals—other than federal, state, or municipal hospitals that are largely or entirely tax supported—are primarily generated from patients. Most hospitals have some additional sources of revenue such as private donations, bequests, fund drives, or interest on cash reserves, but most hospitals rely almost entirely on patient revenue. In the past, most patients paid their own bills, but in recent years most of the hospitals' income has been obtained from "third-party payers." The third party is an insurance organization that may be a private insurance company, a prepaid health maintenance organization (HMO), or a tax-supported government organization such as Medicare and Medicaid. The changes in the distribution of hospital charges between 1974 and 1983 in a large academic health center in the midwest are noted below.

	1974	1983
Blue Cross	40%	33%
Medicare–Medicaid	30%	40%
Private Insurance Carriers	15%	15%
Patients	15%	12%

This distribution represents gross billing and does not mean that these four payer groups paid identical amounts for specific services rendered. In fact, Blue Cross and the federally supported Medicare–Medicaid program pay only the cost of the services rendered on a very carefully negotiated basis, and frequently pay less than the true cost of the service. The private insurance carriers pay at least a cost-plus premium for the so-called covered services, whereas the patient who pays his own bill and has no insurance, does not have the bargaining power of the third party payers and must make up the difference between the cost of operating the hospital and the revenues generated from the third-party payers. This is an inequitable situation, but the third-party payers distinguish sharply between what they consider reimbursable costs and the true costs of operating the hospital. Needless to say, the reimbursable costs are always less than the true costs, and thus the hospital has to make up this deficit either from patients who pay their own bill or from some outside source.[2,7]

Although it is beyond the scope of this chapter to discuss the fine details of the complex calculations that serve as the basis for negotiations between hospitals and the government "Medi-plans," it may be of interest to give a broad outline because an increasing number of nongovernment plans, for example, Blue Cross, follow the same system, and because an appreciation of this problem may make it easier to understand the very real fiscal constraints under which hospitals are forced to operate.

Basically, Medicare, Medicaid, and Blue Cross do not compensate hospitals on the basis of individual patient bills but rather on the basis of "reasonable" bulk costs. This means that if it costs "x" dollars to operate the hospital and if 10% of patients are covered by Medicare, then Medicare will pay 10% of "x," assuming that the costs that make up "x" are deemed "reasonable" by Medicare. Obviously this system has two major weaknesses from the hospitals' perspective: The payments are retrospective, and the definition of what is "reasonable" is subject to arbitrary interpretation. The fact that payments are retrospective produces significant cash-flow problems, because there is always an appreciable lag-time between the reimbursement received by the hospital and the hospital's obligation to meet its expenses in a timely fashion.

The second problem for the hospital ensues from the interpretation of "reasonableness." A cost that may be considered reasonable one year may be considered unreasonable the next year, and, indeed, entire services may be arbitrarily considered unreasonable after the hospital has already provided that service. For instance, the "routine" preoperative chest x-ray that was a reasonable, reimbursable expense some years ago has recently been declared nonreimbursable.

From the viewpoint of the individual consumer and society as a whole, this form of retrospective reimbursement is disadvantageous because it holds little, if any, inducement for cost containment. In fact, it was precisely this type of financing that not only allowed the enormous expansion in services and costs during the socially conscious and economically prosperous 1960s and early 1970s but which actually encouraged it.

More recently, when a major inflationary period was followed by a very severe depression, increased unemployment and serious economic difficulties, the magic word has become "cost containment." The voluntary cost containment urged by the President of the United States and by all sections of the public and private sector has only been partially successful in slowing the inflationary spiral of health care costs. The use of the states' regulatory powers to control the charges reimbursed by the Medi-plans was doomed to failure because it was contrary to the basic principles of retrospective reimbursement and because astute hospital financial managers were able to reallocate expenses from the highly visible "containment" areas to less obvious "noncontainment" and fully reimbursed areas.

Since the "retrospective reimbursement" was an obvious and dramatic failure, the federal government, in the spring of 1983, issued two sets of regulations: One was the result of legislative action, whereas the other was issued under the regulatory power of the Department of Health and Human Services (HHS).

The Tax Equity and Fiscal Responsibility Act of 1982 (TEFRA) affects primarily the hospital-based physicians and those engaged in the practice of laboratory medicine. Its primary target was the pathologists, but TEFRA will also have effects on pulmonary physicians and anesthesiologists in charge of pulmonary function and blood gas laboratories.

The compensation for these laboratory determinations will be strictly regulated, and physician compensation will be based entirely on the demonstrable and justifiable professional expense associated with the determination.

Other parts of the TEFRA regulations affect the reimbursement of hospital outpatient visits and some other hospital based functions of all physicians.

At present TEFRA regulations pertain only to Medicare patients, but it is generally recognized that it will be only a short time before the same reimbursement scheme will be applied to Medicaid patients and to all patients covered by Blue Cross/Blue Shield contracts. Whether the private insurance companies will follow suit is uncertain at present but is certainly highly likely.

It is estimated that the implementation of TEFRA in October 1983 will lead to a 40% reduction in reimbursement for the affected areas and to a saving for the government of hundreds of millions of dollars.

The impact on the general practice of medicine will probably be moderate. The major impact will be on those who derived most of their income from mechanized laboratory services. Thus, indirectly, respiratory therapy may be affected, since removal of the profit motive will undoubtedly lead to a decrease in laboratory use.

The second type of regulation issued by HHS is much more significant and is referred to as Diagnosis Related Grouping (DRG). The DRG system, tested quite successfully in New Jersey, is an almost pure, prospective payment system. When fully implemented in 1986–1987, the hospitals will be paid a predetermined amount for each patient falling into one of 467 diagnostic subgroups. The amount of dollars paid for each patient will at first be determined on the basis of regional averages, but within 3 years only national averages will be used. Under DRGs the hospital will know, in advance, that if it cares for 20 patients with staphylococcal pneumonia, it will be paid 20 times X dollars. Some room will be allowed for maneuvering for the exceptional case, but basically both the payer and the payee will have limits set on the number of health dollars that changes hands within one fiscal year.

This form of prospective, cost-per-case, reimbursement system will definitely be a major factor in changing the present health care delivery system. The impact on hospital fiscal management and on physician and other health care provider behavior will be profound. The hospital will have to increase the productivity of all of its resources. Staffing patterns will have to be adjusted and capital expenditures and new programs scrutinized very strictly. Efficiency will have to be increased and waste of all kinds curtailed. In other words, hospitals will have to focus on the bottom line as does any other business, rather than relying on their ability to manipulate cost reports as they did for the old-fashioned retrospective reimbursement.

Since hospitals will quickly become cost conscious, physician behavior will also have to change. Admissions will have to be limited to the really necessary ones; hospital stay will have to be shortened as much as is consistent with good care, and the use of laboratory, x-ray, and all ancillary services will have to be limited to those that are essential. No longer will it be permissible to order unnecessary studies or use therapeutic modalities of doubtful or unproven merit.

If this system is really fully implemented, it is likely to affect respiratory care quite significantly. Positions will be eliminated; salary levels will be investigated and either reduced or held steady; capital and commodity budgets will be sharply curtailed, and the educational functions of the "nonteaching" hospitals will be significantly curtailed. To put it into the vernacular, it will be an entirely new ballgame.

Just as TEFRA, the DRG system pertains only to Medicare patients initially, although it is a foregone conclusion that it it will be only a short time before it is extended to most, if not all, patients.

One additional change, already introduced in California and, with some modifications, in New York and Massachusetts is the so called preferred provider system. Under this system the third-party payers negotiate for the least expensive hospital and physician services and contract with those who offer the best terms. This approach, besides leading to a massive shakeout of uncompetitive hospitals and physician groups, will limit the free choice of the patient and is being fought vigorously on this basis.

All these developments are too recent to enable me to predict with any precision the effects they are going to have. It is my conviction, however, that if implemented properly and not sabotaged by greed and narrow-minded reactionaryism, these developments will result in a better world for all of us.

Regardless of how much the hospital can recover from third-party payers, it is important that the method whereby costs are allocated be discussed because this is the basis of all third-party reimbursement and because it has direct bearing on the charges made by the respiratory therapy department.

As a general principle of the cost analysis program, the hospital must identify the different units of the organization that can be designated as cost centers and that either generate income or generate only expenses. Among the former are respiratory therapy, radiology, clinical laboratories, the operating rooms, and the "daily charge" or "room charge." Among the latter are medical records, laundry, maintenance, housekeeping, administration, and trash removal. Once all the cost centers are identified and divided into general cost centers that cost money and final cost centers that generate income, the cost of the general centers must be distributed among the income-producing final cost centers. The simplest method of distribution is "direct apportionment," where the costs are distributed to the final cost centers on some arbitrary basis, such as percentage of total income generated, square footage of space used, number of employees, and so forth. This system is simple but unfair, since it does not consider the varying levels of demands made on the general cost centers by the final cost centers or the services rendered by one general cost center to another. Most hospitals use more equitable methods of assigning costs to the final cost centers, including the "step down" method, the "double apportionment" method, and the "multiple apportionment" or "algebraic" method. The last method is considered the most satisfactory but is complex and usually requires a computer. (For a detailed discussion of these methods, *see* Reference 3.)

Once the costs have been allocated to the final cost centers, these centers must generate the income to cover the costs of the entire hospital operation. This is done by setting the charges and rates at a level that generates a total revenue equal to, or slightly in excess of, the total hospital cost. Several ways are discussed below in which rates and charges can be determined very rationally and in reasonable approximation to the real cost of the service plus the appropriate indirect cost to compensate for the non-income-producing cost centers and for other financial obligations of the hospital (Fig. 8-1).

METHODS OF DETERMINING RATES AND CHARGES

Weighted Procedure Rate Method

The weighted procedure rate method (*see* Tables 8-1, 8-2) uses a relative value guide for individual services performed, taking into account such factors as time, cost of equipment, and type of personnel performing task. This system is suitable for certain respiratory therapy procedures, and the dollar value assigned to each unit within the relative value guide can be changed easily to conform to the changing total economic costs of the unit. The weighted procedure rate method is also suitable for determining daily rates and for the different rates of private, semiprivate, and ward facilities.

Hourly Rate Charges Method

The hourly rate method (*see* Table 8-3) is particularly suitable for operating rooms, anesthesia, physical therapy, and respiratory therapy, where the primary cost of the unit is time spent with the patient and where additional charges can be made for materials, equipment, and the like.

Surcharge Rate Method

The surcharge rate method (*see* Table 8-4) is suitable for determining charges in cost centers that deal primarily in "goods," such as the pharmacy, where drugs are dispensed to patients with a "mark up" over the hospital's cost of the drug. The percentage increase in the "cost" of drugs will be the same as the percentage increase in cost assigned to the pharmacy, as related to the true cost of the pharmacy.

Regardless of the system whereby costs are ultimately allocated to the final cost centers, the hospital bill that the patient receives has two major items. The first one is the "daily rate," which represents the hospital's hotel–restaurant function and which also includes the general costs from which all patients benefit similarly. Such costs include nursing services, food services, laundry, and the administrative costs of the hospital. These various charges may vary according to the level of care and the nurse–patient ratio. Thus the daily charges will be substantially higher in intensive care areas, less in intermediate or stepdown areas, and even less in general care areas.

Unfortunately, a rigorous accounting of these costs and a proportional assignment of the costs of the general cost centers to the final cost centers represented by the "daily charge" would produce a daily charge figure far higher than the currently charged rates and would cause considerable reaction among the public, for whom the daily rate is the most visible and most readily identifiable component of the hospital bill. For this reason, and largely on a regional hospital consensus basis, the daily charges are kept at a level that the public is likely to accept despite the fact that the daily charges are insufficient to compensate the hospital for the real costs of this area of the hospital's operation.

To compensate for the deficit created by the cost of daily care and the charges made for it, the hospital must distribute this deficit to the other final cost centers equitably. This means that the special services any patient receives and which can be identified with great precision will be assigned costs in excess of the true cost of the service, even including the originally prorated costs of the non-income-producing cost centers. Thus, respiratory therapy services, laboratory, x-ray, operating rooms, pharmacy, and other departments will have their costs inflated to allow the daily rates to remain within reasonable and societally acceptable bounds. In fact, the daily rates in most hospitals reflect an actual loss that is then made up by the individual patient services listed above.

Although this system is used almost universally and has gained acceptance by third-party payers, it is inequitable because, under this system, the sickest patient who requires the most individual services will pay a disproportionate cost of the total hospital operation. Conversely the patient admitted to the hospital for minor diagnostic studies or for a "rest cure" and whose hospital bill consists primarily of "daily charges" pays less than his proper share of the operating expenses of the hospital.

A strange yet little noted and poorly appreciated corollary of patient costs is the patient's lack of input into the economic decision-making process. One of the characteristics of a free economy is a competitive-

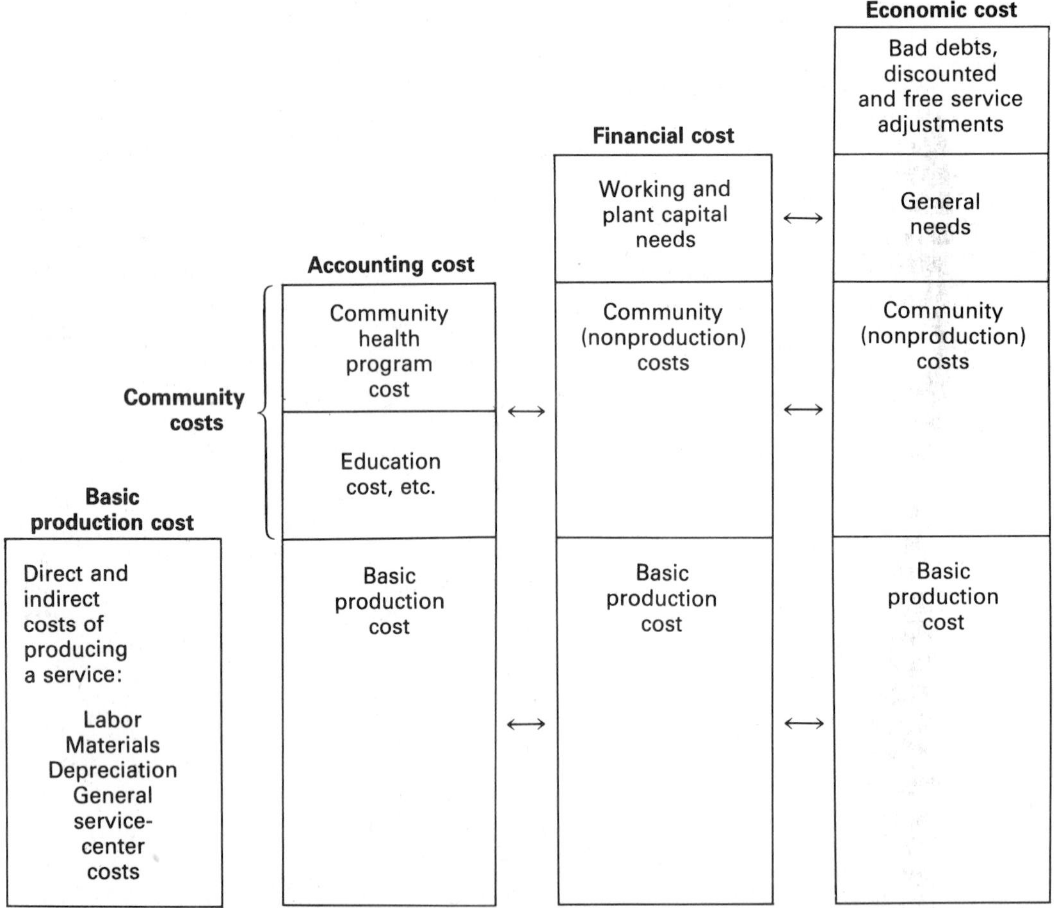

Fig. 8-1. Rate-setting in theory. The graphic relationships shown are purely illustrative; they are not meant to reflect the relative sizes of the various cost premiums. (Adapted, with permission, from Berman HJ et al: The Financial Management of Hospitals, 4th ed. Ann Arbor, Health Administration Press, 1979)

Table 8-1. Weighted Procedure Rate Method: Laboratory Charges

ASSUMPTIONS

- Accounting costs for the laboratory = $150,000
- Financial and economic costs for the laboratory = a 20% addition, or $30,000*
- Total economic cost for the laboratory (financial requirements) = $180,000
- Weighted units computation (example represents only a sample of all tests performed):

Amylase, blood	2,000	2.5†	5,000
Bleeding time	2,500	1.9	4,750
Hematocrit	3,800	0.8	3,040
Platelet count	3,900	1.0	3,900
Uric acid	1,500	1.5	2,250
Total weighted units (all tests)			120,000

CALCULATION STEPS

- Total economic cost ÷ total weighted units = charged/weighted unit:
  $180,000 ÷ 120,000 = $1.50
- Charge/weighted unit × unit value of test = charge/test:
  $1.50 × 2.5 = $3.75 charge/amylase, blood test
  $1.50 × 1.9 = $2.85 charge/bleeding time test
  $1.50 × 0.8 = $1.20 charge/hematocrit test
  $1.50 × 1.0 = $1.50 charge/platelet count test
  $1.50 × 1.5 = $2.25 charge/uric acid test

(Adapted, with permission, from Berman HJ et al: The Financial Management of Hospitals, 4th ed. Ann Arbor, Health Administration Press, 1979)

*Premium for economic and financial costs should be based on historical accounting data (bad debt and free service element), subjective estimates, and policy decisions.

†These weighting factors are used only for purposes of illustration. Individual hospitals should select weighting factors on the basis of their own unique physical plants, processing techniques, capital–labor mix, and so forth.

ness among the providers of services of all kinds, and, indeed, rigorous federal legislation dating back three quarters of a century penalizes all attempts to eliminate this competitive element from all but a few public services. In addition, consumers seeking nonhealth services generally have the opportunity of "shopping around" and of obtaining the best value for their money. In most instances, such a consumer not only has advance information about the cost of the services required but also at least some method of assessing the quality of the product he is buying. In health care, there is a distinct lack of these options. Although patients generally have a free choice of physicians and may have a choice of hospitals, they are rarely informed in advance of the total cost of the services they will need and have no control over the costs they will incur during any hospitalization. Many patients assume that their "insurance" will cover all hospital and medical expenses only to find at the time of discharge that they owe the hospital a substantial sum of money for services that their insurance policy did not cover and which, sometimes, they do not even recall having received.

Worse yet is the fact that while the patient has some choice of physicians and may have a choice of hospital, he has no choice of the individual health care providers in the hospital and depends entirely for the quality of care he receives on chance and the general internal quality control that the hospital chooses to exercise over its own personnel. Although this issue may not appear to be an "economic" one, it clearly falls into this broad category. Quality service is obviously a part of the economic package of health care, and, of two patients who may have the same hospital bill, one may have bought a Cadillac while the other ends up with an Edsel.

It is vital for the improvement of health care in this country that the patients have a clear understanding about the services they receive, that they understand the economics of health care, and that they may be certain that if they pay for a Cadillac they, indeed, receive a Cadillac. This last issue is one of quality control in the entire range of medical and hospital services. Organized medicine, third-party payers, and federal regulation will hopefully find a way to assure quality care.

At the time of this writing (summer 1983), there is considerable pressure from both the federal government and consumer groups to encourage competitive advertisement from physicians and health care facilities. Generally, this is commendable, but its eventual outcome is not clear and appears to still be being fought by organized medicine and the health care industry. The advantage of competitive advertising in the health care field is that it will give the consumer an opportunity to compare prices, but the potential disadvantages are that unscrupulous advertisers may entice the unsophisticated public to select services on the basis of cost alone. This, in turn, will inevitably lead to potentially dangerous and shoddy practices that may cause untold harm before being recognized and corrected.

Courts have found that professional advertising is permissible provided that it is not "misleading."

Table 8-2. Weighted Procedure Rate Method: In-Patient Unit Charges

ASSUMPTIONS

	Private Room	*Semiprivate Room*	*Ward*	*Total*
• Type of facility				
Expected patient days	2,000	6,000	2,000	10,000
Facility unit value	2	1.5	1	
Total weighted units	4,000	9,000	2,000	15,000

• Costs
  Accounting, financial; and economic costs that are to be allocated on the basis of patient days = \$350,000
  Accounting, financial, and economic costs that are to be allocated on the basis of unit value = \$150,000

CALCULATION STEPS

• Costs to be allocated on the basis of patient days ÷ patient days = patient day charge factor:
  \$350,000 ÷ 10,000 = \$35
• Costs to be allocated on the basis of unit values ÷ total weighted units = unit value charge factor:
  \$150,000 ÷ 15,000 = \$10
• Unit value charge factor × unit value of facility = unit value charge factor/facility:
  \$10 × 2.0 = \$20 unit value charge factor/private room bed
  \$10 × 1.5 = \$15 unit value charge factor/semiprivate room bed
  \$10 × 1.0 = \$10 unit value charge factor/ward bed
• Patient day charge factor + unit value charge factor/facility = charge/in-patient unit:
  \$35 + \$20 = \$55 charge/private room bed
  \$35 + \$15 = \$50 charge/semiprivate room bed
  \$35 + \$10 = \$45 charge/ward bed

EXPLANATION

• Certain cost elements, such as nursing, dietary, medical records, and working capital needs, are mostly applied uniformly to all patients. Thus they should be allocated on the basis of patient days. Based on accounting data (budgets), the hospital should determine the total amount of costs that should be allocated on a patient-day basis. This cost should then be divided by total patient days to determine cost per day.
• Those cost elements that cannot be allocated uniformly should be distributed on a weighted-value basis. The mechanics of this distribution are basically the same as those depicted in the outline on laboratory charges. Cost elements that fall into this category include bad debts, plant capital needs, depreciation, housekeeping, and plant operations.
• As the final step, the charges, as determined in the two above steps, should be combined to produce charge per type of facility.

(Adapted, with permission, from Berman HJ et al: The Financial Management of Hospitals, 4th ed. Ann Arbor, Health Administration Press, 1979)

Recently a number of physicians have advertised their services. It is too early to evaluate the effects of this move.

COST OF RESPIRATORY SERVICES TO THE PATIENT

Respiratory therapy services encompass a wide scope of procedures. Manipulations may range from the placement of a room humidifier or the administration of oxygen to the most sophisticated, continuous respirator care.

The methodology whereby the cost of these services can be determined has been detailed above, and generally one of these methods is followed in calculating the cost of the individual procedures. This represents a change in hospital accounting procedures, which has been demanded by the emergence of the third-party payers as a major force in the financial management of hospitals.

Table 8-3. Hourly Rates

ASSUMPTIONS

- Accounting costs for the operating room = $100,000
- Financial and economic costs for the operating room = 30% addition, or $30,000
- Total economic costs for the operating room = $130,000
- Expected hours of use = 2,000
- Average number of personnel per operation = 4

CALCULATION STEPS

- Total economic cost ÷ hours of use = rate/hour: $130,000 ÷ 2,000 = $65 charge/hour
- Hours of use × typical number of personnel = man-hours of use (2,000 × 4) = 8,000 man-hours
- Total economic cost ÷ man-hours of use = rate/man-hour: $130,000 ÷ 8,000 = $16.25 charge/man-hours

(Adapted with permission, from Berman HJ et al: The Financial Management of Hospitals, 4th ed. Ann Arbor, Health Administration Press, 1979)

Traditionally, fees for respiratory therapy services were set either by the hospital administration alone or by the administration and the respiratory therapy department jointly. Fees were set at a level generally corresponding to similar services in other hospitals in the area and were usually high enough to generate considerable revenues to the hospital. In fact, the charges usually had very little relation to the actual costs of the service rendered and were frequently determined on the principle of "whatever the traffic will bear." The respiratory therapy department was often viewed as one of the most consistent and generous income producers of the hospital, and hospital administrators learned to expect that it would subsidize the non-income-producing divisions of the hospital.

Unfortunately, setting the charges for a procedure, whether done on a true cost basis or even if padded to reflect the added costs of a share of the primary cost centers, does not indicate whether the procedures performed were appropriate.

The enthusiastic salesmanship of respiratory therapists combined with the sincere desire of physicians to find a therapeutic modality for a large number of patients for whom there was little else to offer led to abuses of many respiratory therapy procedures. The apparent temporary benefits of IPPB and the theoretical considerations that suggest IPPB may be of benefit in a large number of patients with respiratory and other ailments led to the use of this treatment modality in literally tens of thousands of patients when there was little or no valid medical indication for its use.

Chapter 23 in *Respiratory Care* discusses the problems of IPPB in detail, and thus my chapter is obviously not the site for a discussion of the merits of this procedure. Nevertheless, the therapeutic value of IPPB does indeed become a proper subject for economic concern if it were eventually demonstrated that this basic component of respiratory care and major contributor to departmental revenues rests on dubious scientific grounds.

Blood gas determinations and pulmonary function studies also lend themselves to considerable abuse. Nobody questions the significant contributions that these studies *can* make to the diagnostic and therapeutic decision-making process; yet in many instances these procedures are ordered unnecessarily, performed unreliably, and interpreted incorrectly, at considerable cost to the patient and of benefit only to the hospital. If we exclude from consideration those (hopefully exceptional) stituations in which procedures are ordered for profit alone, these aspects of respiratory care become a proper subject for controlled scientific study and improved and expanded continued education.

Table 8-4. Pharmacy Charges

ASSUMPTIONS

- Accounting cost for pharmacy = $50,000
- Financial and economic cost for pharmacy = a 20% addition, or $10,000
- Total economic cost for pharmacy = $60,000
- Cost of drugs billed to patients = $45,000

CALCULATION STEPS

- Total economic cost − cost of drugs billed to patients = total surcharge: $60,000 − $45,000 = $15,000
- Total surcharge ÷ cost of drugs billed to a patient = percentage mark-up: $15,000 ÷ $45,000 = 33.3%
- Percentage mark-up × cost of drugs* = surcharge 33.3% × $12 = $4
- Surcharge + cost of drugs = charge/drugs: $4 + $12 = $16 charge

(Adapted, with permission, from Berman HJ et al: The Financial Management of Hospitals, 4th ed. Ann Arbor, Health Administration Press, 1979)

*Assumed drug cost for a particular prescription.

SERVICE	CHARGE (in dollars) 1975	1983
Continuous Respiratory Care		
1st day (or part thereof)	75.00	250.00
Each additional day (or part thereof)	50.00	230.00
1st day in recovery room	40.00	
IPPB Apparatus [with or Without Ultrasonic Nebulization (USN)]		
1st day (or part thereof)	10.00	13.00
Each additional day (or part thereof)	6.00	8.00
IPPB supervised treatment (without USN)	3.00	8.00
IPPB and ultrasonic supervised treatment	7.00	18.00
ULTRASONIC NEBULIZER SUPERVISED TREATMENTS		
Sputum Induction		
1st treatment	10.00	15.00
Each additional treatment	4.00	10.00
MANUAL VENTILATION EQUIPMENT—available at bedside		
1st day	5.00	10.00
Each additional day (or part thereof)	3.00	9.00
O_2 TENTS OR CROUPETTES		
1st day (or part thereof)	30.00	55.00
Each additional day (or part thereof)	20.00	37.00
Standby	5.00	7.00
AEROSOL EQUIPMENT		
1st day (or part thereof)	15.00	33.00
Each additional day (or part thereof)	10.00	27.00
Standby	5.00	11.00
CONTINUOUS ULTRASONIC NEBULIZATION		
1st day (or part thereof)	25.00	36.00
Each additional day (or part thereof)	20.00	30.00
O_2 MASK, CATHETERS, CANNULA, OR AUXILIARY O_2		
1st day (or part thereof)	15.00	33.00
Each additional day (or part thereof)	10.00	27.00
Standby	5.00	11.00
COMPRESSED GASES (per day or fraction thereof)		
Compressor (Dia pump) (motor)	5.00	19.00
ROOM HUMIDIFIER		
1st day (or part thereof)	5.00	NA
Each additional day (or part thereof)	2.00	NA

As the educational level of respiratory therapists has improved, and particularly as more physicians become better informed about the uses and limitations of respiratory care, a more rational approach to utilization can be expected. This educational process is the joint responsibility of the schools of respiratory therapy and of the medical organizations that are primarily concerned with the training and utilization of respiratory therapy services. The main thrust in the general improvement of hospital utilization and in the rational and justified use of diagnostic and therapeutic treatment modalities will, hopefully, derive from the internal and external audit procedures mandated by Title XI of the Social Security Act, the so-called Professional Standards Review (PSRO) amendment.[8]

Increasingly more sophisticated equipment, and better and more expensive human and mechanical monitoring of life-support systems, will necessarily increase the cost of respiratory care. It is essential, therefore, that the cost of respiratory care services be determined on a rational time/cost-plus basis. Respiratory care charges can and should be lowered where overcharging is taking place, and every effort must be made to use only those services that can be justified on a medical basis.

Without any attempt to justify their reasonableness, I compare (on p. 200) the charges made for all respiratory therapy services in a large midwestern hosital in March 1975 and in July 1983.

COST OF RESPIRATORY CARE SERVICES TO THE HOSPITAL

The general principles whereby cost accounting of respiratory therapy can be achieved must determine the actual costs the hospital incurs when it establishes and maintains a respiratory therapy department. Basically, the hospital's costs for a respiratory therapy department comprise salary, capital equipment, commodity equipment, and space.

SALARY BUDGET

By far the major item is the salary budget, which accounts for nearly two thirds of the usual department budget. The salary ranges for respiratory therapy technologists vary widely from area to area but are generally higher than those of other health care professionals with similar or even higher educational backgrounds. The reason for this discrepancy is that the demands for trained respiratory technologists have increased much more rapidly than could be met by the training programs. In addition, respiratory therapy technologists have, as described earlier, produced substantial revenues and have thus been in a favorable bargaining position.

The shortage of qualified technologists produced another anomalous situation. Hospitals with more rigid salary structures—for example, state university hospitals, Veterans Administration hospitals, and county and city hospitals—have found it impossible to compete with private hospitals where salary changes could be made as rapidly and frequently as necessary. This has created an income differential between these institutions similar to the academic versus private practice income situation for physicians. Many of the leaders in respiratory therapy, working in teaching hospitals, have been forced to make considerable financial sacrifices to stay in a "teaching hospital" or under more intensive and more stimulating medical direction. This is unfortunate because it has forced some excellent therapists to take jobs in hospitals in which their skills and knowledge could not be appreciated, and it has placed many others in the position of accepting a lower salary in order to work in an "academic" environment. Both organized respiratory therapy and patients owe much to these young men and women who work in leadership positions in public hospitals.

Salary ranges vary widely, as already indicated. They are highest in major cities on the east and west coasts and tend to be lower in the middle west and south. The scale for registered staff therapists is reported to range from $10,000 to $18,000, whereas chief therapists command salaries in some areas as high as $30,000 to $50,000. Nonregistered school graduates or certified technicians earn proportionately less, and their income ranges are reported from $7,000 to $16,000.

The list below compares 1974–1975 and 1980–1981 ranges in an academic health center in the midwest.

TITLE	SALARY RANGE (in dollars) 1974–1975	1982–1983
Chief respiratory therapist	13,600–19,700	30,000–45,000
Assistant chief	11,700–17,000	25,000–35,000
Clinical supervisors*	10,700–15,500	20,000–28,000
Therapists	7,060–10,240	18,000–24,000
Technicians	6,720– 9,840	11,000–18,000

*Clinical supervisors must be registered therapists.

In examining the changes in salary ranges, we find that they barely keep up with the inflationary decrease in purchasing power. The true value of the increased salary expressed in terms of "real dollars"—that is, the amount of goods and services this amount of dollars can purchase—may well be at or below the comparable value of the 1975 salaries. Admittedly the "cost of living index" is not a good measure of true purchasing power because few of us buy homes or cars with any regularity. Nevertheless wage and salary administrators and department managers must give serious attention to the threatened erosion of the true income, and thus the living standard of respiratory care personnel.

There is some indication that the rate of increase in salaries paid to respiratory therapy technologists is beginning to slow and, in some instances, even stabilize. The biggest reason for this is the increasing number of school graduate respiratory technologists. The almost alarming proliferation of schools and the concomitant increase in graduates markedly weakens the bargaining position of the individual respiratory technologist and strengthens the hand of the hospital and wage administrators, especially where a surplus of trained technologists exists.

Before abandoning the area of salaries as the major cost item in the operation of a respiratory therapy department, we must remember that the salary paid to the recipient is only part of the total salary cost. Every "salary" agreement also includes a significant financial commitment on the part of the employer, which is in addition to the actual salary and which is known as the "fringe benefit package." This term includes all the noncash benefits that employees receive and comprises such items as vacation and sick time, retirement benefits, social security, and health, accident, and life insurance. In determining the cost of the salary package that the hospital has to provide to maintain a respiratory therapy department, a sum of about 15% to 20% must be added to the cash salary actually paid to employees. In both industrial and health settings one of the major causes of increased costs was the astronomical escalation of the fringe benefit package.

Because salary policies generally tend to follow the patterns established by the major collective bargaining agreements between industry and organized labor, it is becoming increasingly obvious that those members of the health care system who currently do not participate in collective bargaining have already benefited from the negotiated salary and fringe benefits agreements between employers and organized employees. Probably within the next decade, all hospital employees and other health care providers will have their incomes determined by agreement reached at the bargaining table between "management" (administration) and a small negotiating team representing a job-family, a specialty, or even the entire medical, nursing, and technologic group. Although it is contrary to the so-called American system of free enterprise, in the not-too-distant future professional incomes may be regulated by the state or federal government, with limits being set for the maximum professional compensation dependent on such variables as specialty qualifications, patient load, and seniority. From the broader perspective of national good rather than the narrow view of individual benefit, I view such developments as professional collective bargaining, quality control of performance, and reasonable income limitations with considerable equanimity.

CAPITAL BUDGET

The second major item in the cost of maintaining a respiratory therapy department is the capital budget. This item reflects the cost of purchasing all major respiratory therapy equipment as well as other major items of equipment necessary to the functioning of a department without actually being of a specific technical nature. Thus the capital budget includes not only those items of respiratory care that cost in excess of a specified sum (usually $500), but also office equipment, furniture, cleaning and sterilization equipment, calculators, computer hardware, and the like.

The capital equipment budget of every department should be based on the services the department is expected to render, and the 1982 JCAH Standard IV states that "The respiratory care department/service shall have equipment and facilities to assure safe, effective and timely provision of respiratory care services to patients." Thus every hospital that maintains a respiratory therapy service must have the equipment needed to perform the functions of the department specified in the procedure and policy manual.

Even if the hospital has no facilities or intentions to engage in long-range management of difficult respiratory patients, no hospital can claim to be a modern health care facility if it does not have at least one or two IPPB machines. One of these, at least, must have the appropriate ancillary equipment so that apneic patients may be ventilated with adequate humidification at least long enough for emergency measures to be taken and arrangements made to transfer the patient to the nearest hospital that has the human and mechanical resources to deal with extended respiratory care.

This purpose can be achieved with the least expensive "pressure cycled" ventilators that have adequate humidifiers. While, theoretically, a "volume ventilator" has obvious advantages and should be considered in the capital budget planning of every hospital, the actual purchase of such expensive equipment can be justifiably postponed until more pressing needs are met or until the hospital has reached the level of sophistication that makes the appropriate use of such equipment a reasonable and proper part of patient care. I believe that the most expensive equipment is not necessarily the best and that one of the most important considerations in purchasing respirators is the availability of fast, efficient service by the manufacturer. Thus, in different parts of the country, the choice of equipment may be made purely on the basis of the local service organization's efficiency. This consideration is too often neglected. While sales organizations are uniformly efficient and even aggressive, service organizations vary enormously from manufacturer to manufacturer, and the makers of fine equipment have deservedly bad reputations for rapidly losing interest in their customers once the sale has been consummated.

There is also considerable difference in the complexity of respirators; although some units can be serviced and even repaired by properly trained respiratory therapy technologists, others require expert repair facilities or return to the factory. This may cause delays of weeks and even months, during which time the hospital may be without its only suitable piece of equipment for even short-term emergency respirator care.

In considering the cost of capital equipment, the hospital's accounting department must consider the depreciation of this equipment. The construction of the capital budget must use one of the standard schemes for depreciation allowance, for example, the "straight line" or one of the "accelerated depreciation" methods. For details of these methods, the reader is referred to Berman and Weeks.[3]

COMMODITY BUDGET

The commodity budget includes the multitude of equipment less than $500 in unit cost and also the necessary "administrative" equipment without which a department cannot function. The former includes drugs, masks, catheters, and all other minor pieces of equipment, whereas the latter comprises such items as record forms, accounting forms, stationary, mailing, and telephone costs, and the like.

The size of the commodity budget depends entirely on the level of services rendered by the department, the number of procedures performed, and the total number of patients cared for. It is the least amenable to economies and has suffered recently from the rapidly increasing costs of minor equipment which, in the aggregate, represents a significant sum of money. The tendency toward using disposable equipment has also significantly increased the commodity budget and has undoubtedly contributed to the increased total cost of respiratory care.

Disposable equipment has evident advantages. It is convenient to use, may be sterile when purchased, and eliminates the need for expensive, time- and space-consuming sterilizing and packaging procedures. On the other hand, it is expensive to purchase, requires extensive storage facilities, and usually does not totally eliminate the need for cleaning and sterilizing space and personnel. In addition, the enormous proliferation in the use of disposable equipment begins to present a significant problem in disposal because, with few exceptions, "disposable" respiratory care equipment is not biodegradable and cannot usually even be disposed of by incineration. Although this may appear to be a relatively minor concern for the individual hospital, it does begin to present a national problem for which no adequate solution has been suggested at present.

SPACE

The last major economic consideration is the matter of space. Although this is a significant item and a major problem for all hospitals, the value placed on space is difficult to quantitate with precision and varies widely among institutions.

Traditionally, the respiratory therapy department has been located in an area originally designed for some other purpose, and these areas were adapted, more or less, adequately for the purposes of housing the "new" department. By a curious coincidence, this space seems to have been located, with few exceptions, in the basement of the hospital, far from vertical transportation, supported with inadequate utilities, and, not infrequently, infested with vermin. It is gratifying to see that JCAH Standard IV addresses itself specifically to the problem of space and facilities. Hopefully this standard, combined with the increased use of respiratory care services, will physically remove the department from the nether regions and place it in areas more suitable to its role in patient care.

A curious anomaly of hospital space must be mentioned. The hospital itself represents a very major capital investment, but one that differs substantially from almost any other type of major building project. The initial cost of acquiring the land, erecting the structure, and providing the original equipment is not borne either by the people who operate the hospital and provide the patient services or by the consumer of these services. Hospitals are usually built with major donations, local fund drives, or public funds such as revenue bonds, tax funds, and federal contributions under the Hill–Burton Act.

With respect to the physical plant, the only expense the patients contribute to directly is the debt retirement and the general use and depreciation of facilities and equipment (indirect overhead), which has been referred to elsewhere in this chapter and which is illustrated as a cost item in Figure 8-1.

CONTRACT SERVICES

The only method whereby a hospital can unify the cost of the entire respiratory care service is to contract for the services of a commercial respiratory care organization. A number of these, around the country, are prepared to offer complete packages comprising staff, equipment, and medical direction. The usual arrangement is that for a given consideration, the commercial service company provides trained personnel, all appropriate equipment, and even a medical director. The financial arrangement may be a negotiated but fixed sum or may be a percentage of the revenues generated by the respiratory therapy service. The company may rent space from the hospital, or space may be part of the hospital's commitment.

Although this arrangement has some obvious advantages to the hospital, it is generally unsatisfactory unless some conditions are rigidly adhered to. Since the contract service company is a business venture, it naturally makes every effort to make its operation as profitable as circumstances allow. There are a number of instances within my personal knowledge where the staff provided was of a low level of competence, where the equipment was less than ideal, and where medical direction was provided from a distance.

It is convenient for the hospital to avoid the necessary growing pains involved in establishing a department with all that implies, but the hospital still must not abdicate its responsibilities to its patients, and it must maintain control over the quality of care rendered to the patients regardless of whether the service is performed by its own employees or by a contract service. Thus, use of a contract service organization is acceptable only when the hospital, through its administration and professional staff organization, maintains control over the activities of the service company. This means that the hospital must be able to specify the qualifications of the therapists and maintain the right of rejection of therapists who personally or professionally do not measure up to the standards expected from a good respiratory care department. Second, the hospital must have some control over the equipment used by the service company and make sure that this equipment is appropriate to the particular needs of that hospital. Finally, but most importantly, an absentee medical director is totally unacceptable, and is indeed contrary to the JCAH "Standards." Therefore, even if a service company provides technologists and equipment, the medical direction must be provided by a member of the hospital staff who is always available for consultation and for all the other duties that the medical director of respiratory therapy must perform.[1,4]

COMPENSATION OF THE MEDICAL DIRECTOR*

The problem of compensating physicians is becoming increasingly complex. Until relatively recently, most physicians outside government service were compensated directly or indirectly by the patients to whom a specific service was rendered. Physicians working entirely or partially in a hospital setting were expected to contribute some of their time to "administrative" and "educational" activities in the hospital. Administrative activities included service on hospital committees, whereas educational activities were largely limited to a few lectures or seminars in the framework of required or voluntary, continuing, or in-service staff education. An exception was provided by faculty members of medical schools, who were expected to make significant time commitments to education at all levels and who participated actively in the education of allied medical professionals as part of their full-time commitment, without additional compensation for this activity.

*Parts of this section have been published in *Hospital Medical Staff*[5] and are reprinted here by permission of the publisher, the American Hospital Association.

In recent years, the development of professional associations in the allied medical specialties, the requirements of the national certifying bodies in these specialties, the requirements of the JCAH, and the efforts of the National Association of Medical Directors of Respiratory Care have established the position of Medical Director of Respiratory Therapy as a requirement for recognition and accreditation. Under these rules the medical director has become a responsible functionary in the hospital structure with significant responsibilities and duties requiring substantial commitments of time and effort. Thus the traditional methods of physician compensation on a "fee-for-service" basis are no longer adequate to ensure competent and concerned performance of the medical directorship of an allied medical service in the hospital.

The alternative methods of compensation for the physician who functions as medical director of an allied medical specialty are particularly pertinent to respiratory therapy but may also be appropriate for other allied medical specialties where a medical director is required by the professional organization or the JCAH.

There are three methods whereby a medical director of respiratory therapy can be compensated adequately for his or her important role in administrating the respiratory therapy department, teaching the respiratory therapists, and serving as a resource person to the hospital staff in respiratory care.

1. The full-time salaried physician in a government hospital (Armed Forces, Veterans Administration, Public Health Services) or in an academic health center may fill this role as a regular assignment or appointment and devote his entire professional activities to this important area.
2. A physician may engage in a full-time contract relationship with the hospital to provide a complete respiratory care package. In this instance, the physician employs the technical staff, purchases and owns the respiratory care equipment, rents space and other facilities from the hospital, and engages to provide all services under appropriate supervision that the patients in that particular hospital may require. Under this arrangement, the physician as an individual or as professional corporation bills the patients or the third-party payers for services rendered and collects the fees so generated.

   This is a somewhat rare arrangement but in several instances it seems to function satisfactorily and the patients are provided with excellent respiratory care by well-trained technologists under competent, full-time medical supervision using good equipment. The major disadvantage of this scheme is that it totally depends on the integrity of the medical director and that it is prone to abuse, particularly if the medical director is in the position of ordering treatments, and thus may be tempted to increase services even though the patients may not require them. In addition, under these circumstances, the hospital or the medical staff organization has little, if any, control over respiratory therapy personnel or equipment and techniques used.

   In some instances a single physician has functioned in this capacity and, under these arrangements, in a group of hospitals. This is clearly undesirable because medical direction cannot be optimally provided simultaneously in two or more hospitals, and patient care is bound to suffer. If at all acceptable, this type of contract service must be limited to a single institution, and the medical director must be a regular member of the hospital staff with all the requirements and qualifications that a hospital staff appointment ordinarily entails.
3. In all other arrangements, technical personnel are employed by the hospital, and equipment and space is provided by the hospital. Under these conditions, the medical director assumes responsibility for managing the department and for educating the technologists and is compensated by the hospital for these activities. He receives no direct compensation from patients for services rendered by the department and receives professional fees only from his own private patients or on a consultation basis from patients for whom his services are requested by other physicians on the hospital staff.

The hospital's contribution to the medical director's income serves only to enable him to devote time to administrative and educational activities. The amount of this compensation may be based on a percentage of the total income generated by the respiratory therapy department, may be based on straight time, or may be a fixed sum negotiated in advance between the medical director and the hospital.

Under a percentage arrangement, the medical director usually receives 5% to 20% of the gross income of the department. This is not uncommon and involves relatively little bookkeeping. Nevertheless, it is a situation that may be abused and which leaves the medical director potentially vulnerable, particularly if he has the opportunity to exert any control over the amount and type of respiratory care services provided to patients in that particular hospital. Although most medical directors would function ethically even under a percentage arrangement, I consider it undesirable because of its abuse potential and because income purported to be for managing and teaching is not proportional to the time spent by the medical director in these activities.

A more appropriate form of compensation is provided on a straight-time basis. Under this scheme, the medical director is paid by the hospital on an hourly basis only for the time actually spent in managing or teaching. It is a cumbersome method that requires careful bookkeeping and which has the additional disadvantage that neither the medical director nor the hospital can accurately predict the amount of total compensation that the medical director will receive.

The most satisfactory and ethically sound arrangement involves a fixed, negotiated sum that the hospital agrees to pay to the medical director for assuming complete administrative and educational control over the respiratory therapy department. The sum agreed on naturally will bear a direct relationship to the estimated time involvement of the medical director but removes the stigma of hourly employment and places the relation between the medical director and the hospital on a sound and respectable professional basis. This agreement should be for a limited time and should be revised annually if the size and complexity of the administrative and educational activities increase or decrease.

If the medical director is also responsible for a significant amount of teaching of students from a college or a university, then this educational institution should also compensate the medical director for time so spent. It is unreasonable to expect that the cost of clinical education of students should be borne by patients of the affiliated hospital.

In summary, the medical director must be a competent, concerned physician who is prepared to devote time and effort to the administration and education of the respiratory therapy department and its personnel. For this time and effort he must be compensated proportionally to the time and effort expended, and every precaution must be taken to avoid any arrangement that may lead to abuse or criticism on ethical or professional grounds.

COST OF EDUCATION IN RESPIRATORY THERAPY

Chapter 2 discusses in detail the current philosophy and mechanics of education of respiratory therapy technologists, but an area that will be considered in this chapter is the cost of clinical education currently being borne almost entirely by the hospital.

Clinical education may be divided into two phases: the "in service" education of the employees of the hospital, and the cost of providing clinical instruction to students enrolled in a formal school of respiratory therapy. In-service education is clearly a hospital responsibility and again comprises two major parts. The first is the orientation and basic instruction of new employees who have received no formal training in respiratory therapy and who wish to enter the field through "on-the-job training" (OJT). A fairly rigid educational program must be designed to provide this OJT, which implies that the permanent staff and particularly the technical director have to devote considerable time to the indoctrination of new employees. Since time, at least in this context, is money, OJT adds considerably to the indirect costs of the department. In larger departments, one of the more senior and experienced members of the department may be specifically assigned to provide this training, and thus it becomes a direct cost that the hospital assumes and which must be identified and considered in budget planning for the department.

The new Standards of the JCAH that became effective on January 1, 1982, address themselves to, among other matters, the training of respiratory care personnel. Standard II states that "Personnel shall be prepared for their responsibilities in the provision of respiratory care services through appropriate training and education programs." It seems that *all* respiratory therapy personnel must be "qualified"—that is, have some degree of formal education with specified educational and behavioral objectives and with some assurance of competence. If this interpretation of Standard II is correct, the entry skill level into respiratory care will be raised, and there will be little, if any, need for OJT. This will significantly decrease the educational costs in the departments provided that the cost of educating *bona fide* students is borne by the educational institution, as suggested below.

The second phase of in-service education is the continuing education and skill improvement of the regular employees. This phase is assuming an increasingly important role in maintaining the department at a high level of efficiency and is also essential in adapting to the requirements of rapidly changing technology. It is only through this continuing education process that employees can achieve rational career mobility and progress through the various hospital rank and salary levels on a sound basis rather than on the traditional and obsolete basis of pure seniority.

Continuing education includes both a program of educational activities within the department and the opportunity to attend local, regional, or even national educational meetings, seminars, and workshops. Every good hospital must provide these opportunities for its employees, although the cost in large departments may be considerable.

An entirely different economic problem is the cost of the clinical education of students from accredited educational institutions. This remains an unsolved problem, or, more precisely, the solution is an unsatisfactory one. In fact, the educational institution, while it collects tuition from its students and usually receives additional revenues per student from the state or federal government, pays little or nothing for the clinical phases of the education and expects the affiliated hospitals to provide this by donating their space and the time of their full-time employees. Thus, indirectly, the patients pay for the clinical education of students from whom they may not receive any direct benefit.

This system, while obviously appealing to the school, is unfair to patients and should not be permitted to continue. Several solutions are possible. One is for the school to contribute appropriately to the salary of one or more hospital employees charged with the clinical teaching and supervision of the students. Another method is for the school to send its own clinical instructors with the students into the clinical facility so that the regular employees do not have to devote any time to the students and are free to do the work for which they were employed and for which the hospital pays them. Both of these approaches, while having advantages and disadvantages, have proved successful in a number of institutions, and the method chosen depends largely on local circumstances. The important fact to recognize is that the clinical phases of education are not different from the basic classroom instruction and that the entire cost of the total educational experience should be underwritten either by the student or, ideally, by society, and should not become part of the hidden costs of hospitalization.

Unfortunately, the clinical phase of education is expensive because it requires a very low instructor–student ratio and because some clinical education must be provided by highly paid professionals. Thus, schools claim that they cannot afford to compensate the hospital for these educational services. This argument is a specious one, and the schools must adjust their economic planning as rapidly as possible to encompass the entirety of the educational process. This will probably have to be done through legislative appropriation in public institutions, but legislatures appear to be more receptive to this approach than they have been in the past.

In private educational institutions, program budgeting will have to recognize the cost of clinical education, and those schools and colleges that cannot or will not adapt to the financial requirements of clinical education will have to draw the obvious conclusions and discontinue this type of educational activity.

BUDGET PLANNING

The elements of financial management discussed above must all be incorporated into the budget planning process. This process is a prospective assessment of the revenues and costs of the operation of the respiratory therapy department as one part of the hospital which in turn has to construct its own budget for the forthcoming fiscal year. The principles of preparing a budget are relatively simple, and the budget planning process for the department and the hospital is quite similar. Nevertheless, some differences are important and need to be discussed.

Generally, the budgetary process can be defined as making an educated guess on income and expenses based on previous experience, and predictable changes anticipated during the budget year. With rare exceptions, budgets are prepared for a 12-month period which is referred to as the fiscal year. This may start any time during the calendar year, but the two most common starting dates for the fiscal year are January 1 or July 1. Some institutions, for reasons of convenience, may follow a different fiscal year pattern.

The first step in the budget planning process is estimating known expenditures during the upcoming fiscal year. These expenditures include salaries, capital and commodity requirements, and other known expense items. Allowance must be made for salary increases that are to be granted during the fiscal year and for cost increases caused by inflation, expanded services, new commitments, and other factors.

To balance this projected budget, probable revenues must be estimated based on past performance and on estimated changes in services to be rendered during the next fiscal year. If the estimated income is less than the known expenditures, the charges must be adjusted or the planned expenditures decreased. If the department generates income in excess of expenses, this overage (profit) is absorbed into the general funds of the hospital and is used to defray the costs of the non-income-producing areas of the hospital, according to one of the methods described earlier in this chapter.

The main difference in the budget process between the department and the hospital is that the department does not have to consider daily, weekly, or monthly income–expense balances or the current debt to asset ratio of the hospital, and can rely on the hospital to cover temporary differences between income and expenditures. In other words, the department generates income by rendering services for which the hospital bills the patient or the third-party payers. In return for this, the hospital pays the salaries, buys the equipment, and provides the physical facilities in which the department functions.

In theory, at least, the hospital as a major organization comprising a number of units operates in the same way. In practice, however, the hospital assumes a fixed commitment to its employees and to the vendors who furnish equipment and supplies. Payrolls have to be met regularly on a weekly, biweekly, or monthly basis, and the vendors must be paid within a specified time after delivery of the goods that the hospital has ordered. To be able to meet its obligations, the hospital must have funds at hand. These funds originate from the payment of bills the hospital presents to patients and to third-party payers. Unfortunately, the lag time between billing and collecting is considerable and indeed both patients and third-party payers may take weeks or months before they compensate the hospital for services rendered. In view of this, the hospital must maintain a sufficient cash reserve to meet its obligations while waiting to collect the charges made. The money owed to the hospital is referred to as "accounts receivable," and some of these accounts receivable may never be collected, since some patients cannot or will not pay their bills and some third-party payers may pay only what they consider "allowable charges." These may, in fact, be less than the cost of the services rendered.

Obviously therefore, the financial management of the hospital and the budget planning for the entire institution is a complex juggling act. There must always be enough money on hand to meet current obligations. There must always, hopefully, be enough continuous cash income so that the cash reserves may be kept at a minimum. There has to be some contingency plan to meet sudden major expenses for which the cash reserves may be insufficient. If the hospital has to borrow money to pay its bills, it has to pay interest on this loan, and the keeping of large cash reserves also represents a "loss" since the money, so held, is nonproductive. Further, the hospital cannot charge interest on the accounts receivable and thus is squeezed between fixed obligations, uncertain income, escalating costs, the high price of borrowed money, and inability to exert significant economies by reducing the number of employees or eliminating non-income-producing, but essential, services.

"A hospital's budget exists and is only meaningful within the context of the institution's corporate plan."[3] Every hospital administrator should remember this statement.

The financial planning that culminates in the formulation of the budget must be made subservient to the overall purposes of the institution and its many operational subdivisions. Unless this principle is accepted and adhered to, the budget process becomes an oppressive management tool. Policy decisions will be based on fiscal considerations rather than fiscal decisions being made in order to achieve the policy aims of the institution.

Clearly it is difficult to orchestrate the frequently divergent views of programmatic and fiscal planning. Budgeting is a fiscal function that has as its primary purpose the translation of management plans into the realization of dollars and cents. In this process a number of factors must be considered: the need to inspect closely the entire operation of the institution; to examine the cost–benefit ratios of procedures, departments, and divisions; to review retrospectively the accomplishments of the past budgeting period, and to recommit the institution to the needs and demands of the internal and external community it serves.

In the past, the budget construction was a relatively simple process in which the revenue centers took the previous budget period allocations as given and estimated the incremental needs for the next budget period, with reference to increases in costs and with relatively little reference to evaluation of performance and to the changing relative importance of the different components of the cost centers. This system was simple and rapid but made few, if any, allowances toward the overall purposes of the institution and did not really serve as a significant management tool.

A significant change in budgeting technology and philosophy was created by the introduction of "zero based budgeting."[5] This technique, which has proved its value in both industrial and governmental settings, assumes that every cost center must submit a full justification for any continued funding, must offer a series of alternatives, and, generally, that no funding will be provided unless it can be shown on a comparative basis that the request is not only meritorious on its own but also that it is more meritorious than requests emanating from other cost centers.

As far as the process is concerned, there are two major components. At the operational level the department heads must prepare a description and an evaluation of all the activities existing and proposed within their departments. At the management level these so-called decision packages are rank ordered based on various objective (cost–benefit) and subjective considerations.

A disadvantage of the zero-based budgeting process is the amount of hard work it imposes on the lower-level and middle-level managers. It also, by itself, may lead to a number of rather arbitrary decisions and must therefore be supplemented by another budgeting technique known as "program budgeting." Program budgeting serves to evaluate alternative programs trying to accomplish the same purpose but by different routes. Ideally program budgeting and zero-base budgeting should be used to support and to complement each other.

It would take us far beyond the scope of this chapter to enter into the many intricate financial management procedures whereby a hospital can "keep its head above the water" and avoid the obviously unsatisfactory option of declaring bankruptcy and closing its doors. It is hoped that the reader will have a better understanding of the financial problems that continuously confront hospital management, will be more concerned with exercising careful planning and rigid economies, and will be less impatient when management responds with exasperating slowness to demands that seem so simple, so modest, and so obviously desirable from the viewpoint of the individual or of the department making them.

SUMMARY

This chapter presents an overview of the financial aspects of respiratory care. The hospital's general financial management is briefly outlined, and then these principles are applied specifically to the costs and revenues of respiratory care. The role and compensation of the medical director are detailed at length, and several fiscally sound and ethically correct solutions are offered.

Although there are various ways in which the current high costs of respiratory care services can be curtailed or even reduced, by far the most important considerations are improved education of medical and technological personnel, a more intelligent and appropriate use of human and mechanical resources, and, most important, a careful and thoughtful internal or external audit that requires that all procedures performed by the respiratory therapy department be medically justified, properly performed, regularly evaluated, and promptly discontinued when further respiratory care can no longer be justified on the basis of sound therapeutic management.

It is both likely and desirable that the initial steps in the regionalization of medical care and the sharing of medical facilities will progress. There is also a strong suggestion that some form of national health insurance may replace, or at least significantly modify, the current fragmented method of paying for medical services, and it is very probable that this national health insurance scheme will have profound effects not only on hospital services but also on the practice and method of compensation of professional services. A major step in this direction is represented by TEFRA and the DRG concepts discussed earlier.

It is hoped that a better, more rational, and more equitable system can and will be developed that will make health services available to all who require them at a reasonable individual cost and of a high standard of quality in which all health care providers can take justifiable pride.

GLOSSARY

Since financial management uses a highly specialized vocabulary, the following brief glossary may assist the reader.

ACCELERATED DEPRECIATION—Depreciation methods that write-off the cost of an asset at a faster rate than the write-off under the straight line method. The two principal methods of accelerated depreciation are sum-of-years digits and double declining balance.

ACCOUNTING—The art of recording, classifying, and summarizing in a significant manner, and in terms of money, transactions that are at least partly of a financial character and interpreting the results thereof.

ALGEBRAIC METHOD—A cost-finding technique that involves the simultaneous distribution of general service cost-center costs to both general service and final cost centers.

CAPITAL BUDGETING—The process of planning expenditures on assets whose returns are expected to extend 1 year.

COST—The monetary valuation applied to an asset or service that has been obtained by an expenditure of cash or by a commitment to make a future expenditure.

COST-BASED REIMBURSEMENT—The reimbursement approach generally used by third-party payers. Under this approach, the third party pays the hospital for the care received by covered patients at cost; with the expense elements included and excluded from cost determined by the third party.

COST CENTER—A unit, department, or other administrative subdivision of the hospital.

COST CENTER, GENERAL SERVICE—One of the above units that does not generate income.

COST CENTER, FINAL—An income generating unit or division of the hospital to which the costs of the general service cost centers are allocated.

COST FINDING—The process of apportioning or allocating the costs of the non-revenue-producing cost centers on the basis of the statistical data that measure the amount of service rendered by each center to the other centers.

DIAGNOSIS RELATED GROUPS (DRG's)

DIRECT DISTRIBUTION—A cost-finding technique that involves the distribution of general service cost-center costs directly to final cost centers.

DOUBLE DISTRIBUTION—Cost-finding technique that involves the distribution of general service cost-center cost first to the appropriate general service centers and then to final cost centers.

FINANCIAL STRUCTURE—The entire right-hand side of the balance sheet, the way in which a firm is financed.

INTERNAL CONTROL—The plan of organization of all the coordinate methods and measures adopted within a business to safeguard its assets, check the accuracy and reliability of its accounting data, promote operating efficiency, and encourage a chance to prescribe managerial policies.

RELATIVE VALUE UNITS—Index number assgned to various procedures based on the relative amount of labor, supplies, and capital needed to perform the procedure.

RESPONSIBILITY ACCOUNTING—An accounting system that accumulates and communicates historical and projected monetary and statistical data relating to revenues and controllable expenses, classified according to the organizational units that produce the revenues and are responsible for incurring the expenses.

STEP DOWN—A cost-finding technique that involves a single distribution of general service cost centers to both general service and final cost centers.

TAX EQUITY AND FISCAL RESPONSIBILITY ACT (TEFRA)

THIRD-PARTY PAYERS—An agency such as Blue Cross or Medicare Program that contracts with hospitals and patients to pay for the care of covered patients.

REFERENCES

1. American Thoracic Society statement: Inhalation therapy contract services. Am Rev Respir Dis 105:652, 1972
2. Anderson OW: Blue Cross Since 1929. Accountability and Public Trust. Cambridge, MA, Ballinger, 1975
3. Berman HJ et al: The Financial Management of Hospitals, 4th ed. Ann Arbor, Health Administration Press, 1979
4. Burton GG: Letter: Inhalation therapy contract services. Am Rev Respir Dis 107:308, 1973
5. DeKornfeld TJ: Respiratory care: Compensating the medical director. Hosp Med Staff 4:12, 1975
6. Pyrrh PA: Zero Base Budgeting. New York, John Wiley & Sons, 1973
7. Stevens R et al: Welfare Medicine in America: A Case Study of Medicaid. New York, The Free Press, 1974
8. U.S. Code—Congressional and Administrative News. Washington, DC, U.S. Government Printing Office, Oct 30, 1972

BIBLIOGRAPHY

Berki SE: *Hospital Economics.* Lexington, MA, Lexington Brooks, D.C. Heath & Co, 1975. A standard textbook with excellent bibliography. for the more sophisticated student interested in the general economic problems of hospitals.

Berman HJ et al: *The Financial Management of Hospitals.* 4th ed. Ann Arbor, Health Administration Press, 1979. The primary reference text for this chapter. It is very clear, understandable introduction to the basic money management from hospital administration's point of view.

Hay LE: *Budgeting and Cost Analysis for Hospital Management.* Bloomington, IN, Pressler Publications, 1963. An in-depth study for advanced study, particularly on budgeting.

Hiss D: *An Economic Analysis of Health Insurance with Special Reference to Blue Cross.* Lafayette, IN, Purdue University Press, 1971. This small monograph uses the Blue Cross Plan as a model and compares it with government and commercial insurance plans. An "optional insurance plan" is developed and tested against a number of economic and political assumptions. For those interested in the theory of health insurance.

Hospital Financial Management. Oak Brook, IL, *Journal of the Hospital Financial Management Association.* The leading journal dealing with hospital economic matters. A must for all professionals in the health finance area.

O'Donnell PJ: *A Consideration of Third Party Cost Reimbursement and its Influence on the Price of Patient Care in Hospital.* Cincinnati, Xavier University, 1970. A historical review and analysis of cost reimbursement. The effects, advantages, and disadvantages of this system and examined and alternative methods of reimbursement are discussed.

Silvers JB et al: *Financial Management of Health Institutions.* Flushing, NY, Spectrum Publications, 1974. Includes many case histories of financial management problems with separate chapters on opportunities for case analysis. A useful and interesting work using a refreshing approach to problem solving.

Section Two

THE RATIONAL, SCIENTIFIC BASIS OF RESPIRATORY THERAPY TECHNIQUES

9

Respiratory Gas Exchange Mechanisms

George G. Burton

The main function of the lung is to expose approximately equal flows of air and blood to each other over a large interface area, so that efficient respiratory gas exchange may occur. Although the lung has secondary functions, such as the storage of a small amount of blood, filtration, metabolic capabilities, and the biosynthesis of certain compounds, its main function is that of gas exchange. The respiratory care team is specifically concerned with the distribution and magnitude of pulmonary ventilation, although respiratory care techniques may directly or indirectly influence other physiologic processes in the lung, such as the flow and distribution of blood.

The gas exchange process is composed of several intertwined mechanisms, any or all of which can be affected by disease processes, causing them to fail to function at any given time. It is the task of the bedside clinician, nurse, or therapist to try to decide quickly the cause of the patient's *symptoms* and then to move forward to *treatment* in a rapid, although well-considered, way.

SYMPTOM–PATHOLOGY RELATIONSHIPS

Figure 9-1 illustrates a hypothetical, yet practical, relationship between increasing pulmonary pathology and symptomatology. This relationship is often not understood by students until they have been in the field of respiratory care for many months. What is implied is that the lung demonstrates little, if any, visible alteration in its efficiency when first involved by a disease process. Thus the effects of cigarette smoking, industrial exposure, or air pollution go on for years without any significant recognized disability on the part of the patient. Several years ago a young athlete, who previously had one entire lung removed (for cavitary pulmonary tuberculosis), went on to win an international tennis meet in Mexico City, more than 7500 feet above sea level. This is an extreme example of just how much loss of respiratory functional reserve can occur before disability becomes apparent.

Further, the most common symptoms of pulmonary disease—shortness of breath and cough—are often shrugged off by victims of pulmonary disease as the expected effects of our polluted environment, their own cigarette smoking, obesity, or age. This is a real tragedy and one that makes early diagnosis of pulmonary disease difficult, without application of some of the pulmonary function tests described in Chapters 10 and 11. The message of the left side of Figure 9-1 is that considerable lung damage can occur without clinically visible impairment of the gas exchange mechanism. The liver is another organ that functions in much the same way. It can be extensively involved with metastatic carcinoma or cirrhosis before signs of liver failure develop.

The right side of Figure 9-1 tells a different story. When the structure–function relationships of the lung are severely disturbed, as in advanced emphysema or pulmonary fibrosis, small amounts of *additional* damage, such as airways edema, small pneumothoraces, pleural effusions, or small areas of pneumonia, will clearly produce severe disability, progressing to respiratory failure. Treatment of these "small" complications or exacerbations may reverse the process to the extent that the patient, although disabled, can return once again to a fairly functional state. The attainment and the maintenance of an activity state conso-

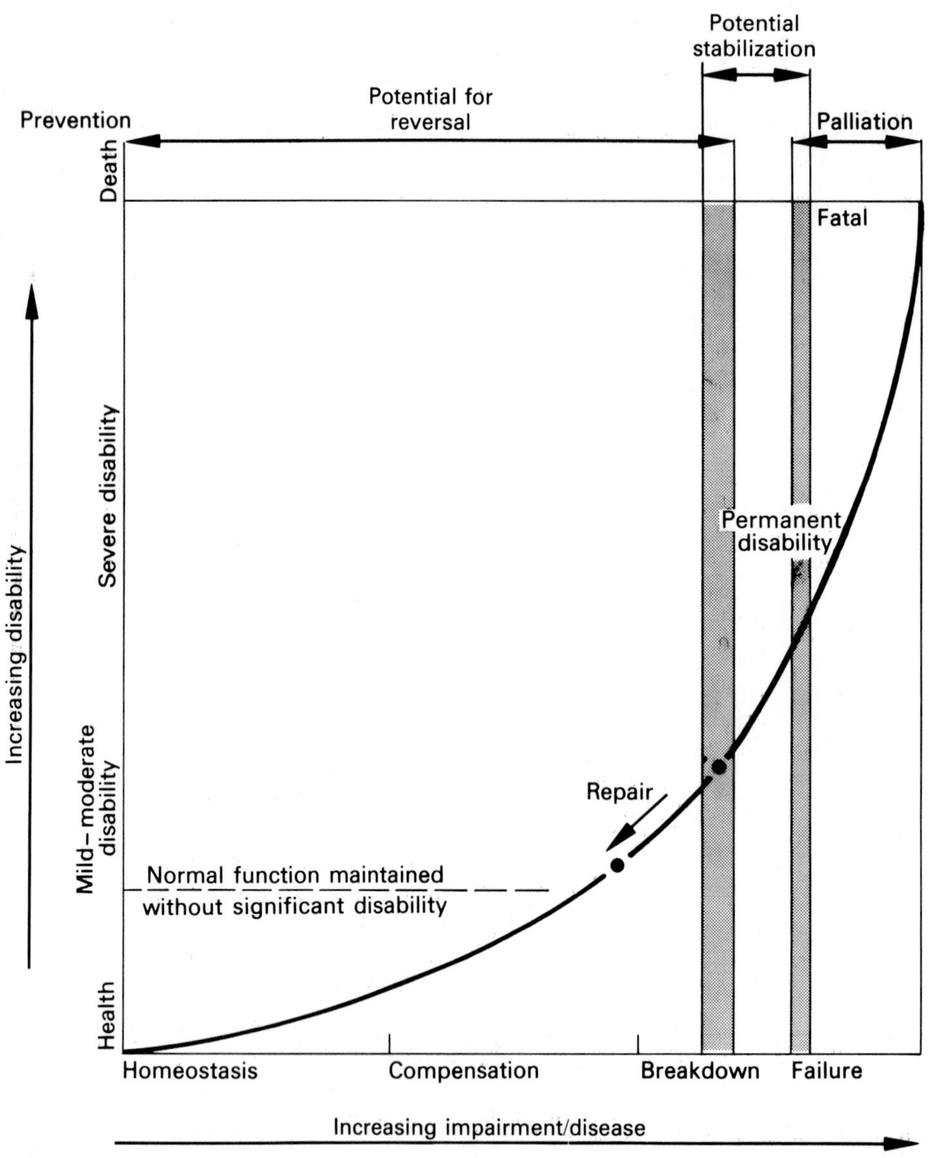

Fig. 9-1. Early in the course of progressive pulmonary disease, symptoms are scarcely noted by the patient because of the enormous physiologic functional reserve of the lung (*see* text). With more advanced disease, small exacerbations or complications cause successively more disability. (Adapted from Hatch TF: Changing objectives in occupational health. Am Ind Hyg Assoc J 23:1, 1962)

nant with the degree of the patient's pulmonary disability are the goals of most pulmonary rehabilitation programs.

With even more advanced disease, small exacerbations or complications cause successively more disability, and supportive or palliative care may be all one has to offer the patient.

Students would do well to consider the implications of this disability–impairment scale at every turn in their contact with patients. In its simplest interpretation, considerable disease involvement produces few symptoms in the early stages, but late in the course of pulmonary disease the reverse is true.

THE GAS EXCHANGE PROCESS

Oxygen and carbon dioxide move between the external air and the metabolizing cells by the processes of bulk gas flow and simple diffusion, from areas of high to low partial pressure, much as a stream runs downhill through a series of channels and over waterfalls. The success of this process, which depends on adequately matched flows of air and blood as well as membrane diffusion processes, can be gauged with a large degree of accuracy by measuring the P_{O_2} and P_{CO_2} of arterial blood.

Figure 9-2 is a model of the total respiratory gas exchange mechanism as an engineer might envision it. The *external gas exchanger* comprises two parallel pumps, one for air and one for blood, in series with two sets of parallel conducting tubes (the tracheobronchial tree and the pulmonary arterial circulation) and an interface where air and blood so transported come into close contact (the alveolar–capillary membrane).

The *internal gas exchanger* distributes oxygenated blood to the tissues and removes carbon dioxide and other metabolic end-products from them. It comprises the left ventricle and systemic arteries, capillaries, and veins containing hemoglobin. The internal gas exchanger is in series with the *external, cellular,*

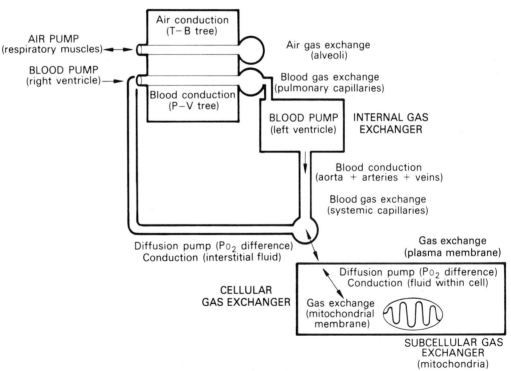

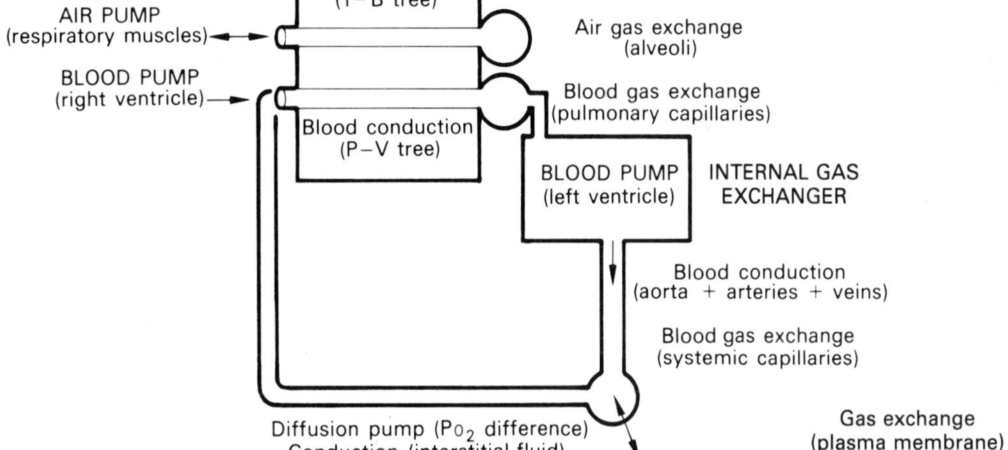

Fig. 9-2. A model of the respiratory gas exchange mechanisms. T-B tree = tracheobronchial tree (airways); P-V tree = pulmonary vascular tree (pulmonary arterial system). (Modified from Gee JBL, Robin ED: Disorders of Respiratory Gas Transport and Metabolism. Scientific Clinician, Vol 1, Unit 2. New York, McGraw-Hill, 1966)

Table 9-1. Clinical Application of Gas Exchanger Model

EXCHANGER COMPONENT	SITE OF ABNORMALITY	EXAMPLES OF DISEASES AFFECTING	BEDSIDE FINDINGS
EXTERNAL			
Air pump	Control of ventilation	Respiratory-depressant drugs, CO_2 narcosis, carotid body excision, sleep apnea	Hypopnea or apnea
	Neuromuscular	Cervical spine injury, poliomyelitis, myasthenia gravis	Hypopnea or apnea; may observe diaphragmatic or chest wall weakness
	Chest wall	Trauma, pleurisy, pleural effusion, kyphoscoliosis, obesity	Restricted chest wall expansion
	Parenchymal	Pulmonary fibrosis, congestive heart failure, respiratory distress syndrome	Shallow rapid breathing, rales
Blood pump	Right ventricle	Infarction (rare) Failure of, secondary to pulmonary hypertension	Elevated CVP RV gallop, $P_2 > A_2$
Tracheobronchial tree	Airways	Foreign bodies, sputum, bronchospasm, external compression, tumor	Wheezes, rales, sputum production
Terminal respiratory unit	Respiratory bronchioles and alveoli	Emphysema	Decreased breath sounds, expiratory prolongation
		Pulmonary (alveolar) edema	Moist rales, LV gallop
Pulmonary vascular tree	Pulmonary arteries and capillaries	Pulmonary emboli, hypoxia-induced pulmonary vasoconstriction, essential pulmonary hypertension	Signs of cor pulmonale
	Pulmonary venous system	Pulmonary venous hypertension	Signs of left ventricular failure
Air–blood interface	Alveolar–capillary membrane	Pulmonary edema, hyaline membrane disease, pulmonary fibrosis, adult respiratory distress syndrome	Tachypnea, rales (x-ray and DL_{CO} much more sensitive)
INTERNAL			
Blood conduction	Arteries and capillary lumen	Atherosclerosis (*e.g.,* coronary artery disease, emboli, extravascular pressure producing ischemia—plaster casts)	Asymmetrical or absent pulses, arrhythmias, etc.
	Hemoglobin	Anemia, hemoglobinopathies, carbon monoxide poisoning	Pallor in anemia, rubor in carbon monoxide poisoning

and *subcellular gas exchangers*. In the last-named compartment, molecular oxygen enters into substrate oxidation by acting as a terminal electron acceptor. For instance, in the metabolism of glucose,

$$C_6H_{12}O_6 + O_2 \rightarrow 6\ CO_2 + 6\ H_2O + \text{energy}.$$

This type of reaction requires an intracellular P_{O_2} of less than 5 torr and is responsible for about 70% of the total oxygen consumption. The other 30% is accounted for by various biosynthetic processes outside mitochondria.

Implied, but not shown in Figure 9-2, is the concept that *all* pumps and tubes must be functioning simultaneously and continuously and, in the case of the blood circulation, *hemoglobin* must be contained as the biochemical transport vehicle for oxygen. Of most importance is the understanding that, in engineering terms, the gas exchange mechanism is a "go–no go" system; that is, if one part of the system fails, even though the others are temporarily functioning adequately, the overall function of the system will be impaired.

In trained athletes the system just described can produce maximal rates of oxygen consumption 10 to 15 times that at rest (oxygen consumption equal to nearly 4 liters/min at sea level). One of the most disabling effects of heart and lung disease is the decreased maximal rate of oxygen transport and thus of the capacity to work and exercise.[4]

Table 9-1 is a modification of Figure 9-2, wherein the exchanger components, some disease processes that affect them, and physical findings at the bedside are outlined. Its application in the prompt institution of rational therapy will hopefully be apparent to the reader, who will, for instance, ask the appropriate questions to determine which gas exchanger components are involved when faced with a dyspneic patient. Disorders of cellular and subcellular gas transport, such as cyanide poisoning, are rare and are not discussed here.

EMBRYOLOGY AND GROWTH OF THE LUNG

The primordia of the lung arise from the primitive pharynx and differentiate into discernible structures by about the 4th week of gestation. The epithelial lining of the airways arises from primitive endoderm; the pleurae arise from the mesoderm. By the 16th week of gestation, the bronchial tree has developed 20 generations of branches (*i.e.*, to and including the terminal bronchioles). The fetal lung is not used as an organ of gas exchange. During gestation the lung serves as one of the main sources of amniotic fluid and surfactant. Its airless alveoli quickly expand during the first few breaths of life (see Fig. 9-3).

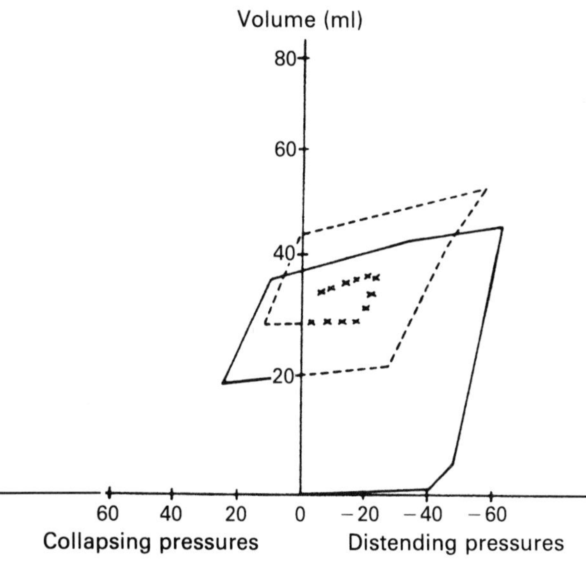

Fig. 9-3 Schematic representation of volume–pressure relationships in the lungs of newborn infants during the first (—), second (---), and third (XXX) breaths. (Avery ME: In pursuit of understanding the first breath. Am Rev Respir Dis 100:295, 1969)

At birth one has the normal complement of airways down to the terminal bronchioles, which lengthen and enlarge up to about 8 years of age. The respiratory bronchioles, alveolar ducts, and alveoli increase in number until about age 8 and in size throughout adulthood. The average alveolar diameter is around 50 μm* between ages 1 and 2 and about 200 μm at age 70. By way of comparison, in emphysema the alveoli are enlarged to more than 225 μm in diameter. In the adult the right lung weighs about 600 g and the left 550 g, with considerable variation because of the weight of blood and extravascular fluid that they may contain.

The mean pulmonary artery pressure *in utero* is slightly greater than the aortic pressure, and right-to-left shunting occurs through the patent ductus arteriosus and foramen ovale.

SUBDIVISIONS OF LUNG

The right lung has three lobes: upper, middle, and lower. The left lung has two: upper and lower. Anal-

*A micron is 1/1000 of a millimeter.

ogous to the right middle lobe on the left is an anterior, dependent portion of the upper lobe called the lingula. These lobes are further divided into segments as described in Figure 9-4. (Another useful illustration of the bronchopulmonary segments is found in Chapter 26.) These segments lend themselves to *en bloc* removal at surgery because each segment has its own airway and arterial and venous circulation, which makes intersegmental dissection possible. Knowledge of the location is of further importance in applying intelligent chest physical therapy, particularly during percussion–vibration and postural drainage proce-

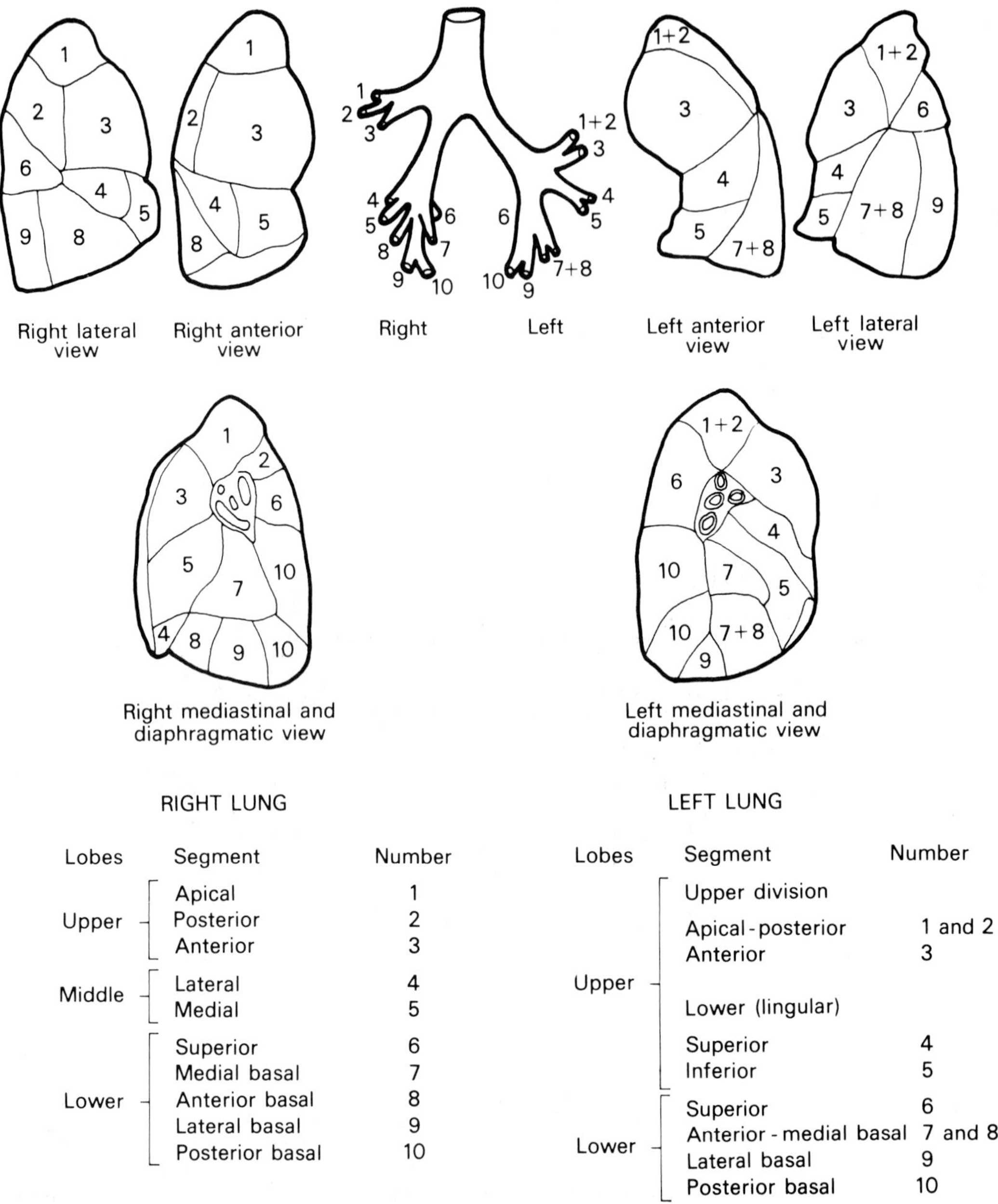

RIGHT LUNG

Lobes	Segment	Number
Upper	Apical	1
	Posterior	2
	Anterior	3
Middle	Lateral	4
	Medial	5
Lower	Superior	6
	Medial basal	7
	Anterior basal	8
	Lateral basal	9
	Posterior basal	10

LEFT LUNG

Lobes	Segment	Number
Upper	Upper division	
	Apical-posterior	1 and 2
	Anterior	3
	Lower (lingular)	
	Superior	4
	Inferior	5
Lower	Superior	6
	Anterior-medial basal	7 and 8
	Lateral basal	9
	Posterior basal	10

Fig. 9-4. Pulmonary lobes and segments. The diagram views the lungs in lateral, anterior, and mediastinal diaphragmatic projections. The numbered airways correspond to the bronchopulmonary segments.

dures (*see* Chap. 26), in the localization and interpretation of abnormalities in the chest x-ray (*see* Chap. 14), and finally in the accurate localization of physical findings in the chest (see Chap. 13).

THE ALVEOLAR–CAPILLARY UNIT

The alveolar–capillary unit shown in Figure 9-5 is the fundamental unit of gas exchange. Basically it is composed of a polygonal-shaped alveolus about 150 μm in diameter with a rich investment of pulmonary capillaries. About 300,000,000 such units are in the adult human lung.[1] The membrane separating capillary blood from this air-conditioning space is between 0.01 and 0.5 μm in width. Although *potentially* highly permeable, except in disease states the alveolar–capillary membrane is relatively impermeable to the liquid constituents of blood, although some flow of these constituents to and from the pulmonary lymphatics does occur at all times. The alveolar–capillary membrane has a total area of between 50 and 100 m^2, depending on body size, and is extremely well suited to its function of gas exchange.

Approximately equal flows of air and blood must present themselves to the alveolar–capillary units for effective gas exchange to occur. Optimally there is good but variable "matching" of air and blood flows to the lung; a ventilated but nonperfused alveolus, or a perfused but nonventilated alveolus, is totally without function as a gas exchange participant ("wasted ventilation" or "right-to-left shunt," respectively). Thickening of the alveolar–capillary membrane, as in interstitial pulmonary edema, also reduces the efficiency of gas transport. If the thickening is severe enough, a shuntlike effect develops, and no oxygenation of venous blood occurs in the units thus affected.

Function of the alveolar–capillary unit is also ensured if the respiratory pump moves air down the branching airways by bulk flow and distally to the terminal bronchioles by intraluminal gas diffusion; only if the alveolar–capillary membrane is of such character as to allow effective diffusion of gases; *and*

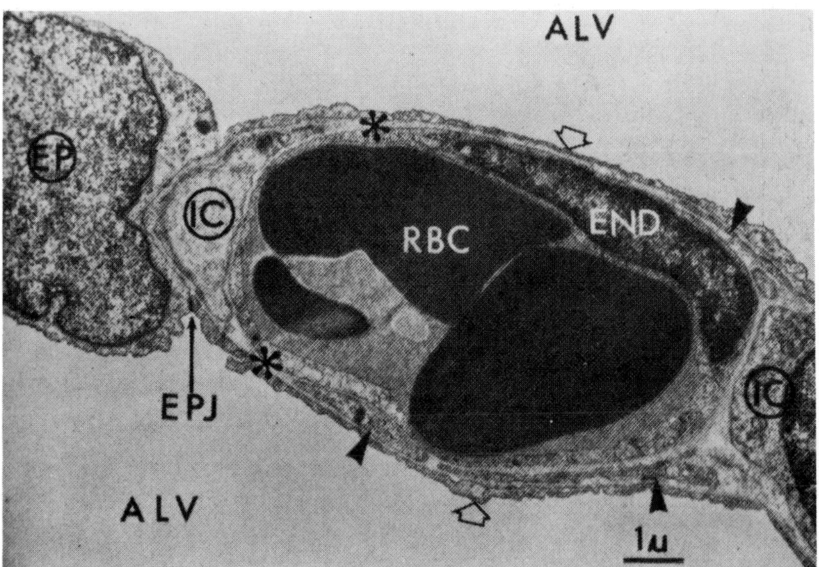

Fig. 9-5. Portion of an interalveolar septum lined by thin cytoplasmic processes (*open arrows*) of type I pneumonocytes *(EP)* (X 10,000 before reproduction). A junction *(EPJ)* between two epithelial cells is shown on the left side. A capillary, lined by endothelium *(END)* and containing three red cells *(RBC)*, occupies the central portion of the septum. The interstitium contains interstitial cells *(IC)* and processes of fibroblasts *(solid arrows)*. Between the endothelium and epithelium, the interstitial space is very narrow. In some areas (*) the interstitium is represented only by fused epithelial and endothelial membranes, thus reducing the space between air and blood to a layer 10 nm thick. (Fishman AP, Pietra GG: Handling of bioactive materials by the lung. N Engl J Med 291:884, 1974. Reprinted by permission from the *New England Journal of Medicine*)

only if the right heart output is distributed through open pulmonary vessels to the pulmonary capillary bed. I shall now discuss each of these gas transport mechanisms in more detail.

THE THORAX AS AN AIR PUMP

The chest wall and diaphragm function as a pump with variable frequency and variable displacement. The components of this pump are the bony thorax (thoracic spine, ribs, scapulae, clavicles, sternum) and respiratory muscles. The primary muscle of inspiration during tidal breathing is the diaphragm. Although the ribs are raised by contraction of the internal intercostals, contraction of both sets of these muscles provides rigidity to the intercostal spaces. With exercise and in disease states associated with increased work of breathing, the accessory muscles of breathing, including the intercostals, the scalenii, sternocleidomastoids, trapezii, and rhomboids, are involved.

The ribs articulate on the thoracic spine in such a way as to elevate and widen the thorax during inspiration (so-called bucket handle action), whereas the diaphragm flattens in the process of contracting, further enlarging the thoracic cavity.

The diaphragm is a fibromuscular separation between the chest and the abdomen, comprising three muscular portions: the sternal, the costal, and the vertebral. The central portion of the diaphragm is made up of tendinous tissue and at the periphery, skeletal muscle, which attaches to the chest wall. The diaphragm may function voluntarily (e.g., during a deep inspiration) or may function involuntarily during normal breathing. The diaphragm is innervated by the phrenic nerve arising from spinal cord roots C-3, C-4, and C-5, with components of lesser importance coming from the lower thoracic nerves. A corollary of diaphragmatic contraction is an increased transabdominal pressure gradient. Thus, during normal breathing, there is synchronous interaction between the rib cage, diaphragm, and, to a lesser extent, the abdominal musculature. Current data suggest that the diaphragm, *acting alone*, is the "prime mover" of normal resting ventilation[3] and that other muscular movements may be secondary.

The thoracic cavity (pleural space) is essentially a closed, potential space delineated by the visceral and parietal pleural margins. With enlargement during inspiration, the intrapleural pressure falls, and a pressure gradient develops between the mouth (atmospheric pressure) and the alveoli (subatmospheric pressure). This pressure gradient during tidal breathing is between −3 and −5 cm H_2O and is enough to ensure tidal volumes of between 300 and 750 cc of air per breath, provided that airflow resistance is not exceedingly high.

Expiration during quiet breathing is a passive procedure that requires no muscular contraction unless airway resistance or pulmonary compliance is abnormal. Expiration is normally achieved by recoil of the lung parenchyma and chest wall. The abdominal muscles are the major effectors of active expiration. During forced expiration or with deep rapid breathing, as occurs during exercise, the abdominal muscles contract, causing depression of the lower thoracic cage and *positive* intraabdominal and intrapleural pressure. Such events also occur during coughing, sneezing, and the performance of the Valsalva maneuver.

The muscular work of the respiratory air pump is so small as to consume less than 5% of the total oxygen consumption of the body at rest and 30% during severe exercise, when the minute volume is 70 liters/min. The oxygen cost of breathing increases markedly when the airway resistance is high or the compliance of the lung is low. If, in addition, the ventilation is "wasted" on underperfused areas of the lung, then the normally efficient breathing process becomes very inefficient indeed.

AIRWAYS AND AIRFLOW

UPPER AIRWAY

Air is delivered to the lungs through the nose and nasopharynx and then through the branching airways, where about 23 to 25 divisional generations later it reaches the alveoli. The nose, pharynx, hypopharynx, and larynx are the great "air conditioners" of the airway. Air is warmed and humidified, soluble noxious gases absorbed into the fluid lining the walls, and particles greater than 50 μm in diameter removed in these intricate passages. Nearly one third of patients with chronic obstructive pulmonary disease have associated upper airway disease (see Table 9-2).

As the airways divide, each generation becomes narrower, shorter, and more numerous than its predecessor. Table 9-3 classifies these airways by name, generation number, mean diameter, and structure. During inspiration the airways widen and elongate slightly. During expiration they become slightly narrowed. This expiratory reduction in diameter (particularly in the terminal, relatively unsupported airways) is profound in pulmonary emphysema. Bronchi

Table 9-2. Association Between Upper Airway Diseases and Chronic Obstructive Lung Diseases

LUNG DISEASE	COMMONLY ASSOCIATED UPPER AIRWAY CONDITIONS
Bronchial asthma	Allergic rhinitis, nasal polyposis, sinusitis
Chronic bronchitis	Sinusitis, recurrent tonsillitis
Bronchiectasis	Sinusitis (Kartagener's syndrome with situs inversus)
Emphysema	Elevated nasal airway resistance (mechanism unknown)

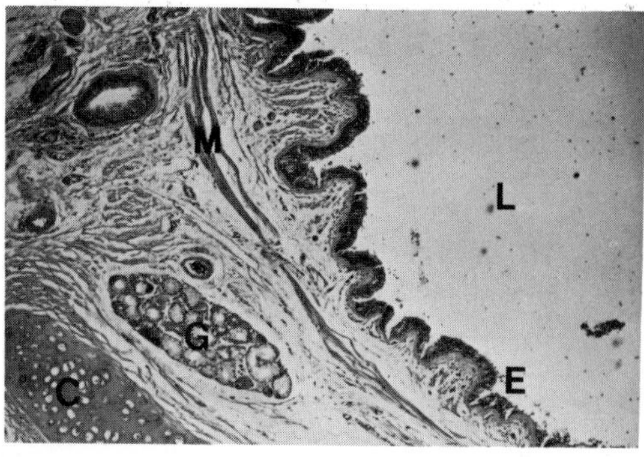

Fig. 9-6. Cross-sectional view of cartilaginous central airway. L = lumen; E = epithelial surface; M = smooth muscle; G = submucous gland; C = cartilage

of between 0.6 and 0.7 mm in diameter supply the so-called primary lobule, which is the smallest subdivision of lung recognized on gross dissection by its limiting septa, sometimes outlined with anthracotic pigment.

Proceeding distally into the lung the airways can be classified longitudinally into cartilaginous airways, the trachea and bronchi (see Fig. 9-6); the membranous airways, the bronchioles; and finally the gas exchange or respiratory airways themselves, the respiratory bronchioles, alveolar ducts, alveolar sacs, and alveoli.

CENTRAL AIRWAYS

The proximal or conducting airways are well supported by a U-shaped cartilaginous ring. The noncartilaginous portion is located posteriorly. The sole function of the proximal airways is to conduct gas by bulk flow from the mouth and nose to the distal airways. Distally, at or near the level of the lobar bronchi, the cartilaginous rings are replaced by a circumferential structure of cartilage plates, which irregularly encircle the airway. These rings and plates are interconnected by a strong fibrous layer within which is a circularly arranged smooth muscle investment. The bronchial smooth muscle is innervated by the vagus nerve, stimulation of which causes airway constriction. Smooth muscle in the upper airway can also narrow under direct stimulation. The role of the autonomic nervous system in maintaining normal airway caliber is discussed elsewhere (see Chap. 20).

The surface of the cartilaginous airways is lined with pseudostratified columnar ciliated epithelium (see Fig. 9-7A), interspersed by clear cells that secrete thick viscid mucus—the goblet cells. Deep to the cartilaginous rings and plates are nests of mucous glands that connect with the airway lumen by means of

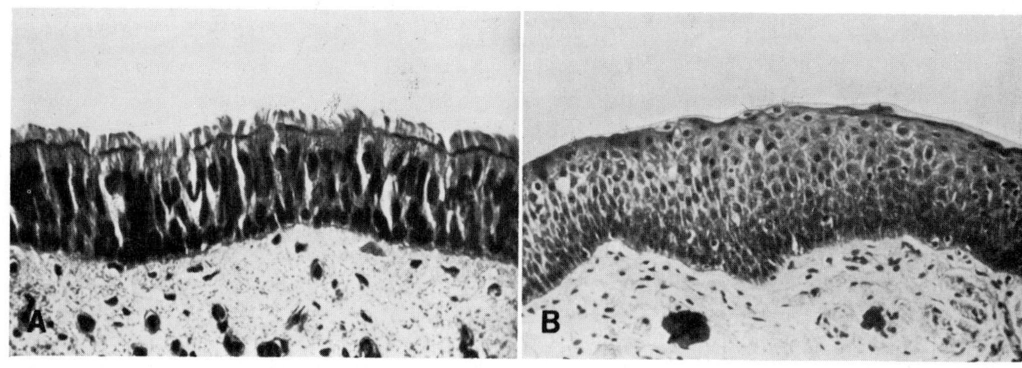

Fig. 9-7. Normal pseudostratified columnar ciliated epithelium *(A)* is contrasted with that seen in chronic bronchitis *(B)*. Note the replacement of the normal ciliated epithelium by metaplastic squamous cells *(B)*.

Table 9-3. Description of the Human Airways*

STRUCTURE	NO. UNITS	GENERATION	MEAN DIAMETER mm	AREA SUPPLIED	CARTILAGE	SMOOTH MUSCLE	EPITHELIUM	NUTRIENT CIRCULATION
CONDUCTIVE ZONE								
Mouth, nasopharynx, oropharynx	1	0		Both lungs				
Trachea	1	I	18	Both lungs	U-shaped	Closes open end of cartilage		
Bronchus	2	II	13	One lung			Columnar ciliated	
Lobar bronchi	4→5	II→III	7→5	Lobes				Bronchial circulation
Segmental bronchi	18	III	4	Segments	Irregular helical-shaped			
Smaller bronchi	32 ↓ 2,000	III	3→1	Secondary lobules		Helical bands		
TRANSITIONAL AND RESPIRATORY ZONE								
Bronchioles Terminal bronchioles	4,000 ↓ 65,000	IV→XIV	1→0.5				Cuboidal	
Respiratory bronchioles	130,000 ↓ 500,000	XV→XX	0.5	Primary lobules	Absent	Muscle bands between alveoli	Cuboidal to flattened cuboidal	
Alveolar ducts	1,000,000 ↓ 4,000,000	XXI→XXII	0.3	Alveoli		Thin bands in alveolar septa	Alveolar epithelium	Pulmonary circulation
Alveolar sacs	8,000,000	XXIII	0.3					

*The first 16 generations make up the conductive zone, whose sole purpose is to transport gases to and from the distal transitional and respiratory zone. Distal to the alveolar sacs are the alveoli themselves (*see* text). (Data modified from Weibel ER: Morphometry of the Human Lung. New York, Springer-Verlag, 1963)

ducts. These glands secrete a mixture of thick and thin mucus and may be made to secrete their products by vagal stimulation. Both the submucous glands and cartilage gradually disappear distally in the region of the membranous airways.

The surface of the epithelial cells is coated by a thin, complex layer of mucus secreted by the glands just described. This mucus blanket is propelled toward the pharynx by the cilia at a rate of about 1000 strokes per minute. Adverse conditions such as cigarette smoking, drying of the airways, alcoholism, and hypoxia interfere with ciliary action and may suppress it altogether. Ciliary function may be overwhelmed by an excessive thickness of the overlying mucus coat (e.g., during exacerbations of asthma or chronic bronchitis). Ciliated epithelium's ability to regenerate after damage is not known. At biopsy or autopsy in patients with chronic bronchitis, one often sees replacement of the ciliated epithelium with squamous metaplasia, as shown in Figure 9-7B. The only way secretions can pass such damaged areas is by mist flow (flow that produces shearing forces) induced by coughing, postural drainage, or suctioning.

The cartilaginous airways comprise a large part of the *anatomical dead space*, that portion of the airways containing no alveoli and thus taking no direct part in gas exchange. The volume of this space is about 150 ml, averaging about 1 ml per pound of body weight in the normally proportioned adult. (A very obese person will have a smaller anatomical dead space in relation to body weight, whereas a thin person will have a larger one.) Its entire function, as mentioned above, is to channel inspired air into the gas-exchanging regions of the lung. The blood supply of these airways is through the *bronchial circulation*, which arises from the aorta. A large portion of the venous drainage from this circulation returns to the left heart, thus contributing to the normal anatomic shunt.

Pressure required to move air through the conducting (central) airways is very small (on the order of 2.0 cm H_2O/liter/sec). The normal lung beyond it, as already stated, is easily distensible, requiring a pressure of less than 3.0 cm H_2O to achieve a tidal volume of 500 ml. The total cross-sectional area of the conducting airways, however, is small (less than 200 cm^2), and thus, because airway resistance is inversely proportional to the total cross-sectional area, these airways form more than 80% of the total airway resistance in humans.[5]

In the central (cartilaginous) airways, particles 2 to 10 μm in diameter impinge at the bifurcations by *impaction* or settle onto their surfaces by *sedimentation*. Such particles are usually transported out of the airways to the pharynx by the mucociliary escalator just described, where they are then swallowed or expectorated. Smaller particles and relatively insoluble gases are not efficiently removed by solution, impaction or sedimentation, and penetrate deeper into the lung.

TRANSITIONAL AIRWAY

At the level of the terminal bronchiole, the cartilaginous supports of the airway disappear and are replaced by an increasingly prominent investment of smooth muscle and connective tissue that contains elastic fibers. The cartilaginous airways thus end in the terminal bronchioles, which have a diameter of about 0.6 mm. No secretory glands are found in bronchioles distal to the terminal bronchioles, although goblet cells persist. The mucosa is now composed of low, ciliated columnar cells that become more cuboidal as one approaches the distal terminal bronchiole. In bronchitis the number of goblet and inflammatory cells in the bronchioles may markedly increase. Again the blood supply to these airways is from the bronchial arterial system.

The transition from cartilaginous to membranous airways is gradual. The bronchioles contribute considerably less to the anatomic dead space and airflow resistance than do the cartilaginous bronchi. Clearance of material in this part of the lung is by movement of a coating of fluid derived from the liquid film that lines the surface of the terminal respiratory units, secretions from the mucous glands, and the goblet cells.

RESPIRATORY AIRWAY

The lung distal to the terminal bronchiole has been variously called the terminal respiratory unit (TRU), acinus, or secondary lobule. It comprises the respiratory bronchiole and its subdivisions. Five to ten acini constitute the primary pulmonary lobule. There are about 100,000 TRUs in humans, which in turn subserve some 300,000,000 alveoli.

The respiratory bronchioles demonstrate occasional alveoli budding from their walls. This is the start of the so-called respiratory zone of the airway.

Within the acinus, or secondary lobule, the respiratory bronchioles are continuous with the terminal bronchioles. They are less than 0.5 mm in diameter and are supported solely by the connective tissue framework of the lung. The smooth muscle investment so prominent in the proximal membranous airways now becomes less clearly defined, and the epithelial mucosa becomes entirely monolayered. Only occasional cilia are seen but no goblet cells. So-called Clara cells, believed to secrete serous fluid, are interspersed here with a low cuboidal epithelium.

The gas exchange airways distal to the terminal bronchioles are supplied by the *pulmonary circulation* rather than the systemic. The distance from the terminal bronchiole (where bulk gas flow ceases) to the alveolar–capillary membrane is at most 5 mm, yet the respiratory zone makes up most of the resting lung volume (about 2500 ml).

INTERAIRWAY AND INTRAALVEOLAR COMMUNICATIONS

Various types of airway intercommunications are important in the pathophysiology of emphysema and in the spread of alveolar disease. The interlobular septa are not clearly defined in the central portions of the lung, and extension of disease through these communications may explain the more rapid spread of alveolar lesions such as bronchopneumonia. The alveolar pores of Kohn and the accessory bronchiolar communications (channels of Lambert) are largely responsible for the collateral movement of air throughout the lung. When obstruction occurs proximal to these pores and channels, a shunt would occur in perfused areas distal thereto unless some physiological allowance was made.

The alveolar pores of Kohn[2] are smoothly rounded and occasionally reinforced by a ring of elastic tissue (*see* Fig. 9-8). Several workers have shown an increase in the size and number of pores with increasing age corresponding to the enlargement of the air spaces. With advancing age the pores of Kohn show a predilection for the lung borders, especially in the apices of the upper and lower lobes. They are frequently identified in patches near the hila and also near the larger bronchi and blood vessels.

The bronchiolar channels, described by Lambert in 1955, are connections between the bronchioles and adjacent alveoli. These channels are lined with cuboidal epithelium and are one of the prime sites for deposits of anthracotic pigment. As many as five of these connections have been observed in a single terminal bronchiole.

ALVEOLAR CYTOARCHITECTURE

As seen in Figure 9-5, the alveolar–capillary unit comprises several types of cells. Knowledge on the me-

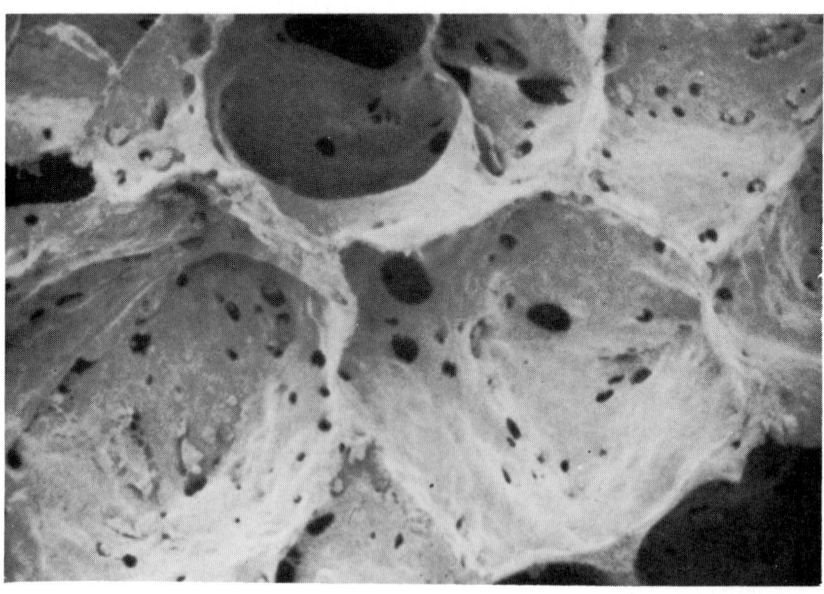

Fig. 9-8. Scanning electron micrograph showing an alveolar duct surrounded by alveoli. Note the holes in the alveolar walls (pores of Kohn) and the rough cells lining some of the alveoli (alveolar macrophages). (Courtesy of C. E. Cross, M.D., University of California at Davis)

Table 9-4. Alveolar Cell Types, Their Function, and Known Metabolic Profile

CELL TYPE	FUNCTION	ENERGY REQUIREMENT	SUBSTRATES
I	Structural support, gas transfer	Low	Glucose
II (granular pneumocytes)	Surfactant production	Probably high	Glucose, fatty acids, lipids, amino acids
Alveolar macrophages	Scavenger/phagocyte	High	Glucose
Endothelial cells	Gas transfer	High	Biogenic amines, adenine nucleotides, prostaglandins (?), polypeptide hormones, lipids

tabolism and function of these cells is increasing (see Table 9-4). The thin, type 1 epithelial cells are known to have a relatively rapid turnover, to be oxygen sensitive, and to be involved early in oxygen toxicity. Their thin extensive cytoplasmic extensions allow them to facilitate gas exchange. The fatter, type II "corner" cells are fewer in number, have fewer organelles in the cytoplasm, and are involved in the production of surfactant. The importance of this material will be discussed later.

Large cells with wrinkled cytoplasmic surfaces are also scattered around the alveoli. These cells are the *alveolar macrophages*, the scavengers of the alveoli. They are thought to originate in bone marrow and are exfoliated regularly from the alveoli, then swept up and out of the lung by the mucociliary escalator. The metabolism of alveolar cells has been widely studied because of these cells' relative accessibility by bronchoalveolar lavage.

The alveolar–capillary is lined with thin *endothelial cells*, which recently have been demonstrated to have intracellular junctions through which can pass particles with a molecular weight of up to 60,000 daltons (e.g., albumin) in acute pulmonary edema or nearly 500,000 in the adult respiratory distress syndrome (ARDS).

The interstitium of the lung contains tropocollagen, collagen, and fibrous and elastic connective tissue. Under inflammatory conditions, migratory white blood cells (PMNs) and histiocytes may be seen. At the junction of the respiratory bronchioles and the alveolar ducts, aggregations of lymphocytes may be seen that with recruited PMNs confer on the lung an important immediate local response to microorganisms and allergens.

AIRWAYS: A SUMMARY

The airways can be considered as a series of branching, ever narrower and shorter tubes exerting *(per tube)* increasing resistance but, in the aggregate, less and less of the total airway resistance. These airways extend first through a conductive zone with no alveoli, then into a transitional zone beginning at the terminal bronchiole, and finally end in the respiratory zone (respiratory bronchioles, alveolar ducts, and alveolar sacs). As the airways branch, the total cross-sectional area of the airways increases from about 110 cm^2 at the level of the terminal bronchioles to 50 to 100 m^2 of alveolar surface. *Note that the unitage of these measurements rises from square centimeters to square meters.*

The volume of the conductive zone makes up the *anatomic dead space*. Some of the alveolated airways and alveoli distal to the conductive zone have relative hypoperfusion with respect to their ventilation. In a normal upright person the volume of these airways and alveoli is negligible, and the anatomic and so-called physiologic dead spaces are roughly synonymous. In disease processes, however, there may be many poorly perfused alveoli, resulting in a *physiologic dead space* that may be considerably larger than the anatomic dead space.

SURFACTANT AND THE ROLE OF SURFACE-ACTIVE FORCES IN THE LUNG

The pulmonary circulation is one of relatively low resistance and high compliance. Studies using radioxenon as a tracer have clearly shown preferential distribution of blood flow to *dependent* lung zones, no matter whether the subject is in the erect, supine, or lateral decubitus position. Accordingly, the dependent lung zones are relatively engorged with blood (and, accordingly, have more blood flow per unit lung volume) compared to the nondependent areas. Studies using techniques wherein living tissue is rapidly frozen have shown that alveoli in the dependent portions of the lung are smaller than their nondependent neighbors.

Were it not for the presence of surfactant, such small alveoli and the smaller airways would tend to collapse, especially during expiration when their size normally becomes smaller. Surfactant is thought to be produced by the type II alveolar cell. It is a phospholipid composed mainly of dipalmitoyl lecithin; its production depends on an adequate blood supply to the lung parenchyma. The effect of this material is to reduce surface tension as the radius of the alveoli and the small airways decreases. The importance of this material will be appreciated by a consideration of the law of LaPlace, wherein the pressure (P) inside a spherical structure with radius (r) is related to surface tension (T), or $P = 2T/r$. For a given surface tension the pressure required to keep a sphere from collapsing will be greater as the radius decreases. In the alveoli, of course, at end-expiration the normal alveolar pressure is essentially atmospheric; in small alveoli the reduction in radius becomes critical, and surface tension would rise to critical (collapsing) levels. Surfactant reduces the value of T and allows the alveoli and small airways to remain open at low transpulmonary pressures.

A reduction in surfactant promotes alveolar instability and atelectasis. Depletion of surfactant may occur after repeated bronchial lavage, in drowning victims, after open-heart surgery where membrane oxygenation is used, after exposure to high concentrations of oxygen, in oxidant air-pollution-induced toxicity, and in the neonatal and adult respiratory distress syndromes. An excess of surfactant is thought to be present in the relatively rare condition known as pulmonary alveolar proteinosis. The exact nature of the removal and fate of surfactant is unclear at present.

PULMONARY ARTERIAL AND BRONCHIAL CIRCULATION

PULMONARY CIRCULATION

The lung must participate in acid–base homeostasis as well as provide respiratory gas exchange; thus the respiratory processes are clearly interlocked with circulatory processes in addition to electrolyte and water balance, temperature control, and metabolism. The lung, through alveolar ventilation, excretes the major portion of the acid load of the body by eliminating CO_2, which, although excreted as a gas, exists transiently as a potent but highly dissociable acid (H_2CO_3) in the body.

The right ventricle delivers the entire cardiac output to the pulmonary arterial circulation. The right ventricle may be described as a variable displacement, variable frequency blood pump that produces a pulsatile flow. By special techniques this pulsatile flow may be demonstrated even in the fine pulmonary capillaries. The output of the right ventricle varies from about 5 liters at rest to more than 20 liters/min. during severe exercise.

The usual two-dimensional view of the pulmonary capillary is unfair; in fact, the lung can be thought of as "an emulsion of blood in air" separated only by the fine and delicate alveolar–capillary membrane. At any time the volume of blood in the pulmonary capillaries (Vc) is between 75 and 150 ml, which increases by about 100 ml during peak exercise, presumably by vascular "recruitment" or opening of normally closed or underperfused capillaries.

The average time in which blood resides in alveolar capillaries and is exposed to alveolar air is less than 1 second. During exercise this residence time is shortened considerably. When gas exchange between alveolar and incoming fresh air is incomplete or alveolar–capillary thickening prolongs transmembrane diffusion time, ventilation–perfusion mismatch occurs, and saturation of capillary blood with oxygen is incomplete. These relationships worsen further during exercise.

The main pulmonary artery divides at the hilus into a left and right pulmonary artery. These further subdivide, in general paralleling the divisions of the airways, down to about the level of the terminal bronchiole (see Fig. 9-9). Unlike the diminishing stiffness of the walls of the branching airway, the pulmonary circulation tends to *gain* stiffness as it branches. The proximal pulmonary arteries make up what is known as the "capacitance" portion of the lesser (pulmonary) circulation. Here the vessel walls largely comprise elastic tissue and resemble the aorta and larger systemic blood vessels.

In the normal adult human lung, pulmonary blood vessels 0.1 to 1.0 mm in diameter have media consisting of smooth muscle fibers bounded by internal and external elastic laminae. These vessels and the pulmonary capillary network compose the "resistance" portion of the pulmonary circulation. The walls of the muscular pulmonary arteries lie close to the bronchioles, respiratory bronchioles, and alveolar ducts. When the blood vessels become less than 0.1 mm in size (the level of the terminal bronchioles), the walls of the pulmonary arterioles are composed largely of smooth muscle, which may contract under various stimuli, most notably hypoxemia and acidosis.

Finally, at the level of the *pulmonary arterioles* (< 0.1 mm in diameter), the muscular layer gradually disappears until the vessel wall contains only the endothelium and an elastic lamina. These vessels directly supply the alveolar ducts and alveoli, ending in the pulmonary capillaries.

Generally the pulmonary arterial circulation should be thought of as one with high compliance, where vascular resistance is less than one fifth that of the systemic circulation. A mean pulmonary arterial pressure of less than 12 mm Hg at rest and 15 mm Hg during exercise propels the entire cardiac output through the pulmonary circulation. The function of this circulation is to distribute the entire cardiac output over the nearly 100 m^2 surface area of the alveolar–capillary membrane.

A knowledge of normal cardiac chamber and vascular pressures is essential in understanding many of the pathologic conditions that will be discussed in later chapters. Figure 9-10 illustrates these relationships. The right ventricular pressure is 25/0 mm Hg. Cardiac output from this circulation drains into the left atrium, which has a mean pressure of about 5 mm Hg. Stevens has described a rational approach wherein the etiology of acute respiratory failure can be separated into pulmonary, cardiac, or combined cardiopulmonary causes by measurement of these chamber and vascular pressures, using the Swan–Ganz catheter.[7]

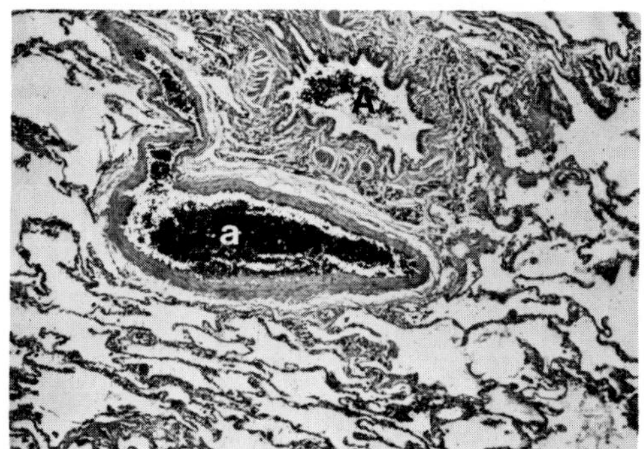

Fig. 9-9. The pulmonary arterial circulation closely follows the arborizing, branching airway. This photomicrograph demonstrates this relationship. A = airway; a = pulmonary arterial segment

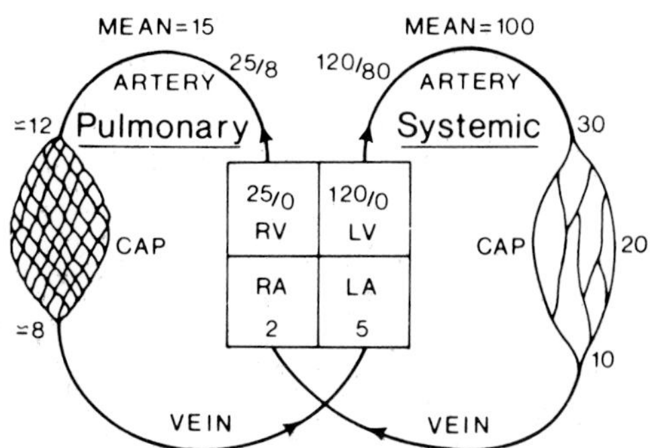

Fig. 9-10. Heart chamber and vascular pressures in the greater *(systemic)* and lesser *(pulmonary)* circulations. To a certain extent, particularly in the lung, these pressures are modified by hydrostatic differences. Figures are in mm Hg. (West JB: Respiratory Physiology: The Essentials. Baltimore, Williams and Wilkins, 1974)

MATCHING OF AIRFLOW AND BLOOD FLOW

Gas exchange does not occur optimally if ventilation ($\dot{V}$) and perfusion ($\dot{Q}$) are not adequately matched. As mentioned earlier, blood flow per unit lung volume is greatest in the dependent portions of the lung, largely because of the generally passive-resistant nature of the pulmonary arterial circulation and the unopposed, gravity-dependent flow of blood to dependent areas. Ventilation is also greater in dependent lung areas, largely owing to the geometry of the lung and the fact that greater distending forces (negative intrathoracic pressure) can be generated when there is the closest pleural approximation. $\dot{V}/\dot{Q}$ ratios are highest in the nondependent parts of the lung, about unity in midlung (*i.e.*, at about the level of the third and fourth ribs in the upright position), and lowest in the dependent portions of the lung.

Figure 9-11 shows three schematized units in which abnormal $\dot{V}/\dot{Q}$ relationships are compared to normal. Since abnormalities of ventilation–perfusion ratios cause most of the abnormalities found in var-

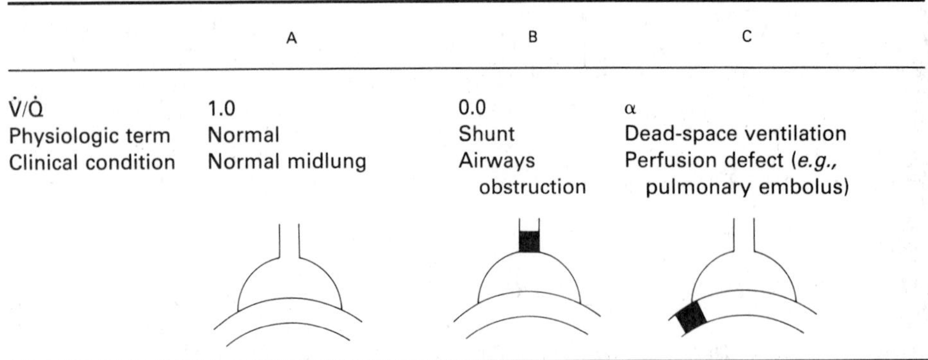

A
B
C
V̇/Q̇
Physiologic term
Clinical condition
1.0
Normal
Normal midlung
0.0
Shunt
Airways obstruction
α
Dead-space ventilation
Perfusion defect (e.g., pulmonary embolus)

Fig. 9-11. Ventilation–perfusion relationships in normal and diseased lungs. Areas resembling *C* occur at the apices of normal lung, which are underperfused with respect to ventilation, and resemble *B* at the bases, where the converse occurs.

ious disease states, it behooves the student to consider each disease in terms of the question, What is the ventilation–perfusion abnormality here? Only if he understands this will he understand what therapy is indicated and the limitations of his therapy on the disease state in question. A classic treatise on this important topic has been prepared by West.[9]

Ventilation–perfusion inequality is by far the most common cause of hypoxemia, caused by relative or absolute shunt, dead space ventilation, or both. If total alveolar ventilation is normal, overventilated alveoli can compensate for underventilated alveoli as far as maintaining CO_2 homeostasis (CO_2 content) but cannot make up for the oxygen deficit in underventilated alveoli because of the difference in the solubility (dissociation) curves of the two gases.

PULMONARY VENOUS SYSTEM

Like the arteries, the pulmonary veins initially are in proximity to the bronchi. At the very periphery of the lung the veins move away from the bronchi and pass between the lobules, whereas the arteries and bronchi travel together down into the center of the lobules. The pulmonary veins possess thinner walls than do the arteries, arriving to a less developed muscular layer at all stages of life. Current work has shown that the pulmonary arterioles arborize into a system of pulmonary capillaries that encase the interdigitating alveoli much as a lace napkin might lie over the top of an open umbrella. The diameter of the pulmonary capillaries is about 10 μm, just enough for red blood cells to pass through end to end. This meshwork of pulmonary capillaries rejoins to form the pulmonary venules, which subsequently drain into the pulmonary veins and the left atrium.

THE BRONCHIAL CIRCULATION

The bronchial circulation originates from the aorta and nourishes the entire tracheobronchial tree down to the terminal bronchioles. The respiratory bronchioles, alveolar ducts, and alveoli normally receive oxygenation and metabolic substrates from the pulmonary arterial circulation. At the junction of the terminal bronchi and respiratory bronchioles there is a rich anastomosis between capillaries supplied by both bronchial and pulmonary arteries.

The bronchial circulation is hypertrophied in bronchiectasis and to a lesser extent in chronic bronchitis. In these conditions rupture of these vessels into the terminal respiratory units can occur, with resultant hemoptysis. Most venous drainage is into the left atrium, contributing to the normal anatomical shunt.

CONTROL OF RESPIRATION

The arterial pH, P_{O_2} and P_{CO_2} respond to changing metabolic demands with a fidelity that is relatively unparalleled in nature.[8] At sea level maximum oxygen transport capacity and aerobic exercise capacity are limited not by ventilation but by the maximal cardiac output that can be achieved during exercise. The lungs themselves become a significant impediment to oxygen transport and begin to impose a limit on exercise capacity in all the disease states discussed in Section Three of *Respiratory Care*.

The complex neural and humoral mechanisms whereby alveolar ventilation is regulated are now only beginning to be understood. The literature on respiratory control is exceedingly complex, and the interested reader should refer to the bibliography and to Chapter 34 for additional information.

NEURAL CONTROL OF RESPIRATION

Attempts to understand respiratory rate and periodicity have caused us to reinterpret studies wherein various portions of the brain or brain stem were transected or electrically stimulated. When the upper cervical spinal cord is severed, voluntary and rhythmic contraction of the main respiratory muscles is not possible. Breathing is the only automatic function subserved entirely by skeletal muscle. In contrast the heart continues to pump blood when completely denervated.

The respiratory system is under both voluntary and involuntary control. The behavioral or voluntary centers are located in the motor cortex of the forebrain and the limbic cerebral area. Efferent fibers descend through the corticospinal and rubrospinal tracts in the dorsal and lateral spinal cord. Certain conscious acts, such as speaking, response to anxiety or fear, voluntary hyperventilation, and breath-holding, interfere with the rhythmic respiratory pattern and are mediated by means of these pathways. The metabolic or automatic system has its origins in as yet not completely localized portions of the lower pons and medulla (*i.e.*, in the brain stem). The afferents (inputs) for this system come from peripheral chemoreceptors, the glossopharyngeal and vagus nerve, and various proprioceptors. The efferents (outputs) involve the phrenic nerve, which innervates the diaphragm, and nerve cells in the ventral and lateral columns of the upper thoracic spinal cord, which innervate the intercostal muscles. Mitchell and Berger, in their recent review, admit that despite more than a century of study, the nature of the cellular organization of those parts of the brain stem (pons and medulla) responsible for respiratory rhythmicity "still remains one of the mysteries of neuro- and respiratory physiology."[6] This important reference deserves more than the short overview presented here and should be read.

To complicate matters further, the way in which the voluntary and involuntary pathways is integrated in the spinal cord is still debatable, although the location of the tracts themselves is well known. The effect of lesions in the cerebral cortex, midbrain, brain stem, and spinal cord on respiratory rate, depth, and periodicity is discussed in Chapter 34.

HUMORAL CONTROL OF RESPIRATION

Chemoreceptors are located in the carotid and aortic bodies and in the medulla. There structures are responsible for the basic chemical control of respiration and function as chemical regulators, adjusting the level of ventilation to maintain the arterial P_{CO_2} as constant as possible, combating the effects of increased (H^+) end elevating the arterial O_2 when this is necessary.

Carotid and Aortic Bodies (Peripheral Chemoreceptors)

Peripheral chemoreceptors are stimulated to a certain degree by elevation of arterial P_{CO_2} or, as in metabolic acidosis, elevation of (H^+), but more effectively by a fall in the oxygen tension of arterial blood. Carotid bodies are found at the bifurcation of the common carotid arteries, and their afferents to the medulla pass via the glossopharyngeal nerve (IX). The aortic bodies are located near the arch of the aorta, with afferents conveyed via the vagus nerve (X). When these structures are denervated in animals, the ventilatory response to hypoxemia is severely blunted. In humans the aortic bodies respond readily to hypoxemia with an afferent discharge, but the carotid bodies are essentially nonfunctional, except in rare instances. The hyperpnea of CO_2 inhalation is depressed only slightly by denervation of the aortic and carotid bodies. When increased P_{CO_2} or H^+ is combined with hypoxemia, however, a considerable increase in ventilation occurs when these centers are intact.

Medullary Chemoreceptors

Chemosensitive areas responsive to changes in P_{CO_2} and H^+ exist in the medulla. These medullary centers are influenced primarily by the (H^+) of cerebrospinal fluid (CSF) which, unlike blood, has no rapidly responsive effective buffer system, so that changes in P_{CO_2} produce maximal changes in (H^+); for example, CSF protein is low compared to nerve proteins, and the concentration of HCO_{3-} is lower and less responsive to changes in arterial P_{CO_2} than in peripheral blood. The medullary centers respond more slowly to abrupt changes in P_{CO_2} (5–10 min) than do the peripheral chemoreceptors, which respond in seconds.

Figure 9-12 summarizes current thinking on the interaction of peripheral and central chemoreceptors in the cortical control of ventilation.

Other (Nonchemical) Influences

Nonchemical influences include the voluntary or behavioral system just duscussed, joint proprioceptors, and stretch receptors that inhibit inspiration, located in the smooth muscle of the airways. In association with this last-mentioned group, deflation receptors

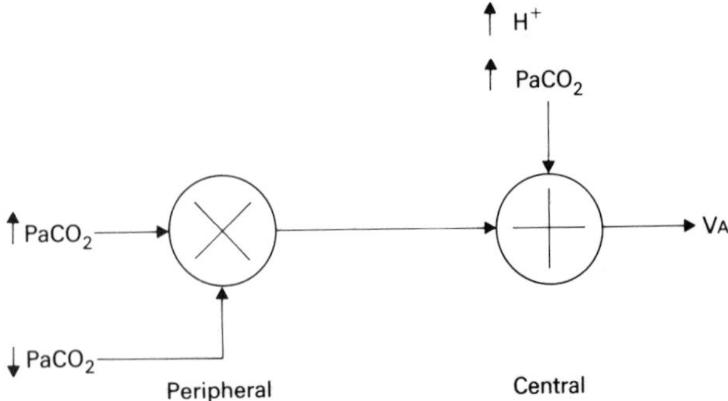

Fig. 9-12. Peripheral and central chemoreceptor and ventilatory control. Note that the effects of hypoxemia and hypercapnia on peripheral chemoreceptors are multiplicative. Carbon dioxide and $[H^+]$ stimulate central chemoreceptors in a fashion additive to the peripheral afferent input. (Modified from Cunningham DJC: Integrated Aspects of the Regulation of Breathing: A Personal View. MTP International Review of Science, Physiology Series One, Vol 2. Baltimore, University Park Press, 1974)

exist that stimulate inflation; collectively, these form the *Hering–Breuer reflexes*.

In summary, the sites or mechanics by which respiratory rhythmicity occurs have still not been completely identified or illustrated, but the search continues.

REFERENCES

1. Angus EE, Thurlbeck WM: Number of alveoli in the human lung. J Appl Physiol 32:483, 1972
2. Cordingley JL: The pores of Kohn. Thorax 27:433, 1972
3. Goldman MD, Mead J: Mechanical interaction between the diaphragm and rib cage. J Appl Physiol 35:197, 1973
4. Johnson RL: The lung as an organ of oxygen transport. Basics of RD, 2(1), 1973
5. Macklem PT, Mead J: Resistance of central and peripheral airways measured by a retrograde catheter. J Appl Physiol 22:395, 1967
6. Mitchell RA, Berger AJ: Neural regulation of respiration. Am Rev Respir Dis III:206, 1975
7. Stevens PM: Assessment of acute respiratory failure: Cardiac versus pulmonary causes. Chest 67:1, 1975
8. Wasserman K, Burton GG, Van Kessel AL: Interactions of physiologic mechanisms during exercise. J Appl Physiol 22:71, 1967
9. West JB: Ventilation/Bloodflow and Gas Exchange, 2nd ed. Oxford, Blackwell Scientific Publications, 1970

BIBLIOGRAPHY

The Gas Exchange Process

Johnson RL: The lung as an organ of oxygen transport. Basics of RD 2(1), 1973 (published by the American Thoracic Society). An excellent description of the circumstances by which the lungs, whose function at sea level is usually not rate-limiting in exercise, may be so when derangements in alveolar ventilation or pulmonary diffusion occur.

Wasserman K, Whipp BJ: Exercise physiology in health and disease. Am Rev Respir Dis 112:219, 1975. This classic "state of the art" discussion, though tedious reading in spots, will be particularly helpful to the reader who has access to an exercise physiology laboratory, which can be used to advantage in localization of defects in the respiratory–cardiovascular gas transport chain.

Embryology and Growth of the Lung

Not previously much considered in the purview of respiratory care, the development of neonatal respiratory therapy as a subspecialty promises that future generations of workers will need to know more regarding these topics than they do presently. Herewith are a few selected references.

Avery ME: The Lung and Its Disorders in the Newborn Infant. 3rd ed. Philadelphia, WB Saunders, 1975. Chapters 1 through 4 are pertinent to this section.

de Leuck AVS, Porter R (eds.): Ciba Foundation Symposium: Growth and Development of the Lung. Boston, Little, Brown & Co., 1967

Dunnill MS: Postnatal growth of the lung. Thorax 17:329, 1962

Scarpelli EM (ed): Pulmonary Physiology of the Fetus, Newborn, and Child. Philadelphia, Lea & Febiger, 1975

The Thorax as an Air Pump

Peters RM: The Mechanical Basis of Respiration: An Approach to Respiratory Pathophysiology. Boston, Little, Brown & Co, 1975. Chapters 1, 4, and 9 are concise expressions of complex topics.

Functional Anatomy

Nagaishi C: Functional Anatomy and Histology of the Lung. Baltimore, University Park Press, 1972. A definitive, beautifully illustrated treatise, well worth including in any departmental library.

10

Routine Pulmonary Function Tests

John E. Hodgkin

Evaluation of pulmonary function can be of significant benefit for various reasons (*see* the list below). One of the most common reasons for performing pulmonary function tests is to determine the cause of dyspnea in the patient who complains of shortness of breath. Selected tests are helpful in differentiating dyspnea of cardiac origin from that of pulmonary origin. Before diagnosing psychogenic dyspnea, one must determine that pulmonary function is indeed normal.

Preoperative evaluation of patients with lung disease will help to determine the risk of surgery and postoperative cardiorespiratory failure. Pulmonary function testing may aid in outlining an appropriate preoperative respiratory care program, improving the patient's chances of undergoing surgery without complication.[2]

The cause of polycythemia (an elevated hemoglobin and red cell mass) is often obscure. Polycythemia secondary to hypoxemia may be detected by arterial blood gas analysis. Patients with polycythemia rubra vera or secondary polycythemia owing to erythropoietin-secreting tumors usually have normal arterial blood oxygen levels and normal pulmonary function.

Pulmonary disease may be detected by specific pulmonary function tests before the onset of signs or symptoms of a respiratory disorder. The early detection of pulmonary disease may help the physician to outline a corrective program (e.g., convincing the patient to stop smoking) that may prevent progression or allow for reversal of the disease (e.g., bronchitis).

Serial pulmonary function testing gives objective data on the course of a pulmonary disorder. This information can help the physician to determine whether a specific therapeutic regimen is beneficial.

Patients are frequently referred for evaluation to determine whether their pulmonary disorder is severe enough to warrant disability. The physician may be asked to determine whether the patient's occupation has caused or significantly aggravated the underlying pulmonary disease. Medicolegal considerations are often involved in this request for evaluation. It is often only with a combination of pulmonary function studies that a patient's pulmonary status can be determined objectively.

Various pulmonary function tests are available. This chapter will discuss spirometry and total lung capacity determination, the most common pulmonary function tests used. The reader is referred to Appendix A for the specific methods involved in performing the tests and for predicted normal values. Examples of abnormal pulmonary function data are also presented in Appendix A at the end of this book.

VALUE OF PULMONARY FUNCTION TESTS

1. Distinguishing cause of dyspnea
2. Evaluating potential risk of surgery
3. Differentiating primary from secondary polycythemia
4. Detecting pulmonary disease early
5. Objectively measuring effect of therapy
6. Evaluation of disability for medicolegal reasons
7. Evaluating effect of occupation on pulmonary function

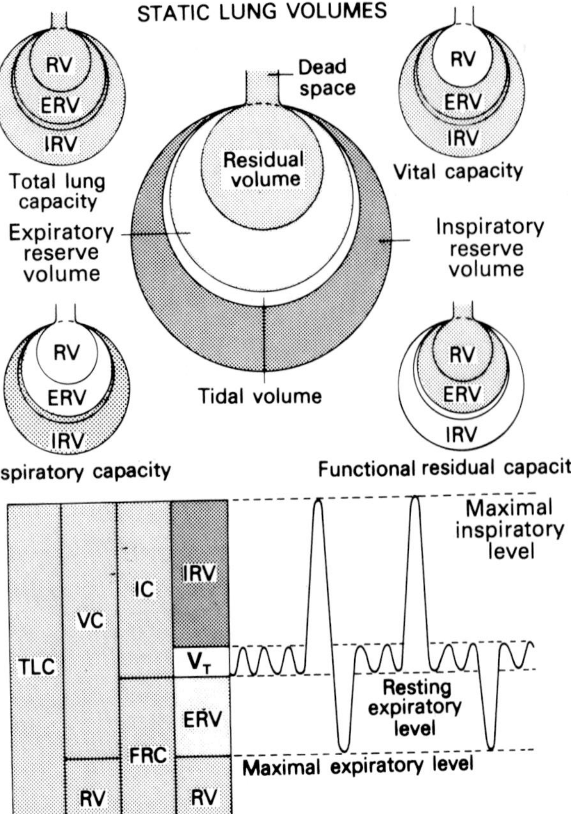

Fig. 10-1. Division of total lung capacity into lung volumes and lung capacities. In the small diagrams surrounding the large central one, the shaded areas outline the *volumes* that comprise the various lung *capacities.* (Adapted from Comroe JH Jr *et al*: The Lung: Clinical Physiology and Pulmonary Function Tests, 2nd ed. Chicago, Year Book Medical Publishers, 1962)

SPIROMETRY

LUNG VOLUMES

There are four standard lung volumes. A grouping of these lung volumes together results in four standard lung capacities (Fig. 10-1). The volume of air inhaled or exhaled with routine breathing is known as the *tidal volume* (V_T). The maximum amount of air that can be inhaled, starting at the top of a tidal volume breath, is known as the *inspiratory reserve volume* (IRV). The maximum volume of air which can be exhaled from the resting expiratory level (after the tidal volume has been exhaled) is known as the *expiratory reserve volume* (ERV). The air left inside the chest after a maximal exhalation is known as the *residual volume* (RV).

The maximum volume of air that can be inhaled from the resting expiratory level (*i.e.*, the sum of the tidal volume and inspiratory reserve volume) is known as the *inspiratory capacity* (IC). That volume of air inside the thoracic cage at the resting expiratory level is called the *functional residual capacity* (FRC) (*i.e.*, the sum of the ERV and RV).

The maximum volume of air that can be exhaled after a maximal inspiration is known as the *expiratory vital capacity* (EVC). The total volume of air that can be inhaled after a maximal expiration is known as the *inspiratory vital capacity* (IVC). These measurements may be made from a slow inhalation or exhalation (*slow vital capacity* [SVC]) or may be done as a maximal flow rate maneuver. The volume of air exhaled at a maximal rate after a complete inspiration is known as a *forced vital capacity* (FVC). The volume of gas in the chest after maximal inspiration is known as the *total lung capacity* (TLC) (i.e., the sum of the four lung volumes).

The residual volume *cannot* be determined with routine spirometry. Therefore, those lung capacities that include the residual volume (FRC and TLC) are also not obtainable with spirometry. The determination of these measurements will be discussed later in this chapter.

FLOW RATES

Determination of flow measurements is crucial in detecting obstructive airway disease. Flow is equal to a change in volume divided by time:

$$\dot{V} = \frac{\Delta V}{t}.$$

Flow rates are generally determined during forced inspiratory or forced expiratory maneuvers. The most common flow rates used are those determined during an FVC. The volume of air exhaled during the first second of an FVC is known as the *forced expiratory volume in 1 second* (FEV_1) (see Fig. 10-2). The volume exhaled during the first half second is the $FEV_{0.5}$ and that exhaled during the first 3 seconds is the FEV_3.

The flow rate between 200 ml and 1200 ml of the FVC is known as the *forced expiratory flow between 200 ml and 1200 ml* ($FEF_{200-1200}$) (see Fig. 10-2). The flow rate between 25% and 75% of the vital capacity, originally called the *maximal midexpiratory flow* (MMF), is known as the *forced expiratory flow between 25% and 75% of the vital capacity* ($FEF_{25\%-75\%}$) (see Fig. 10-2). The peak flow that can be achieved during the FVC is known as the *peak expiratory flow* (PEF). This cannot be detected by usual spirometry and must be determined either by flow-volume loop analysis (see Chap. 11) or with the use of a peak flowmeter.

The FEV_1 may be presented as *FEV_1/observed FVC* (FEV_1/FVC%), providing additional information in differentiating obstructive from restrictive pulmonary disease. Normally, one should be able to exhale about 75% of the forced vital capacity in the first second, decreasing slightly with age. Additionally, one should be able to exhale 95% or more of the FVC in the first 3 seconds. Presentation in this fashion is more valuable than looking at the FEV_1 or FEV_3 alone (see section on Interpretation of Routine Pulmonary Function Tests).

The first 25% of an FVC maneuver is *effort-dependent*. The last 75% of the FVC, however, is relatively *effort-independent* (e.g., most patients can be coaxed to deliver enough effort to reach the maximal flow point at those lung volumes. (Greater effort does not result in higher flow rates.) Theoretically, therefore, flow rates that are predominantly located in the lower 75% of the vital capacity are advantageous for purposes of interpretation in that they are relatively effort-independent. Since the $FEF_{25\%-75\%}$ lies in this portion of the FVC, it is theoretically a better measurement than the other expiratory flow values.

MAXIMAL VOLUNTARY VENTILATION

The maximum volume of air that can be breathed in or out in 1 minute is known as the *maximal voluntary ventilation* (MVV). This test was formerly called the *maximal breathing capacity* (MBC). However, MVV is the preferable term, since the measurement may not represent the maximal capacity but rather only the best that the patient will voluntarily perform. The measurement is usually made by having the subject breathe air in and out maximally for 10 to 15 seconds. One then calculates the volume that would be inhaled or exhaled over a 1-minute period if this level of performance could be maintained for the full 60 seconds.

When interpreting the results of this test, one must remember that the maneuver is very effort-dependent; it is generally not a very helpful test. Normal is considered to be equal to or greater than 80% of predicted. Some use the product of $FEV_{1.0} \times 30$ or $FEV_{0.75} \times 40$ as a way of estimating a patient's MVV.

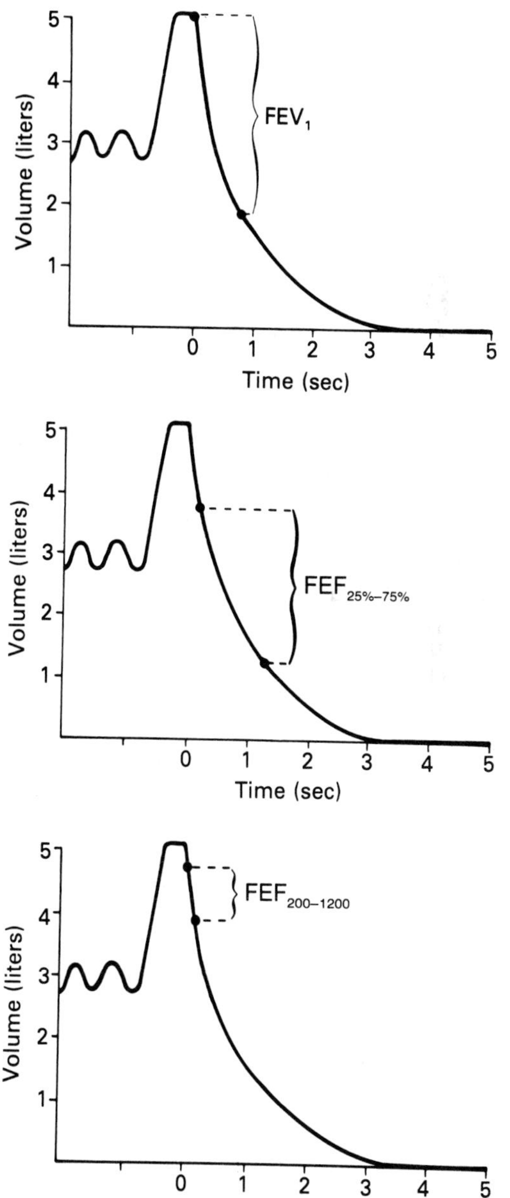

Fig 10-2. Determination of flow rate measurements from a normal spirometric tracing

DETERMINATION OF TOTAL LUNG CAPACITY

As already noted, RV, FRC, and TLC cannot be measured with routine spirometry. There are three methods available for determining these values (see Appendix A at the end of this book for a detailed discussion of the methodology of the tests).

GAS ANALYSIS TECHNIQUES

RV, FRC, and TLC may be estimated by analyzing relatively insoluble gases that can be breathed using either an open-circuit or closed-circuit method. Relatively insoluble gases are necessary because they will not leave the alveolar gas readily to dissolve in lung tissue or blood.

Nitrogen Washout Open-Circuit Method

The subject begins to breathe 100% oxygen at the end of a tidal volume exhalation. The amount of gas in the chest at the start of the test, then, is equivalent to the FRC. The unknown volume of gas in the patient's lungs at the start of the test contains about 80% nitrogen. As the subject breathes 100% oxygen, all exhaled gas is collected. By knowing the volume of gas exhaled during the study and the fraction of nitrogen in this gas, the volume of nitrogen in the lungs at the start of the test can easily be calculated. Since this represents 80% of the starting FRC, FRC can be calculated. Minor corrections need to be made for the small amount of nitrogen present in "100%" oxygen that passes from the blood and lung tissue into the alveolus during the washout study.

Using the determined functional residual capacity, RV and TLC can be calculated as follows.

$$\text{FRC} - \text{ERV} = \text{RV}$$
$$\text{RV} + \text{VC} = \text{TLC}$$

Helium Dilution Closed-Circuit Equilibration Method

The study starts with a known amount of helium in a bellows or bag-spirometer system. The starting concentration of helium in the lungs is zero. The subject rebreathes helium from the bag-spirometer system until equilibration between the lungs and bag-spirometer system is reached. By knowing the new concentration of helium in the system, along with the starting volume of gas and helium fraction in the bag-spirometer system, the starting lung volume (*i.e.*, FRC) can be readily calculated. The helium dilution and nitrogen washout methods are essentially equivalent with regard to accurate determination of RV, FRC, and TLC.

The major disadvantage of the gas analysis methods for determining lung volumes is that alveolar gas may be trapped in the lungs of patients with obstructive airway diseases. Therefore, all of the nitrogen may not wash out during the short time that the test is performed, or the alveolar gas may not reach true equilibration for helium concentration with the bag-spirometer system. The standard length of time for the nitrogen washout test is 7 minutes; however, to wash out all of the nitrogen from the alveoli completely may take 20 to 30 minutes in patients with significant obstructive airway disease. Therefore, lung volumes determined in the usual manner using these methods may grossly underestimate FRC, RV, and TLC if the tests are not continued until all of the gas is adequately washed out of the alveoli, or equilibrated with the closed system, depending on the technique used. This underestimation of lung volumes, however, does not occur with the other two methods of lung volume determination to be described.

BODY PLETHYSMOGRAPH METHOD

The subject to be studied may be placed within a body plethysmograph (body box) (Fig. 10-3) to determine

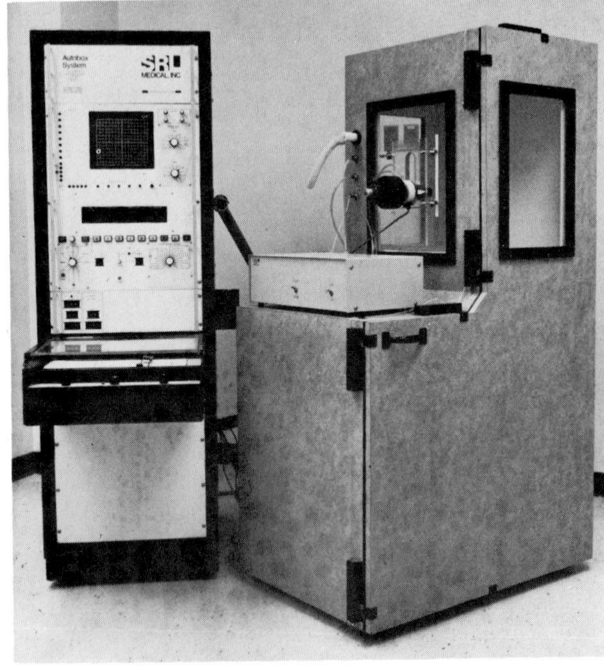

Fig. 10-3. Example of a flow-type body plethysmograph

accurate thoracic gas volume measurements. Body plethysmographs are of three types: variable-pressure, in which the patient breathes air from within the box, and a pressure transducer is used to calculate changes in lung volume; variable-volume, in which the patient breaths air through a tube from outside the box, and a spirometer is used to measure changes in thoracic gas volume; and flow, where a pneumotachograph is used instead of a spirometer to measure the change in lung volume. Variable-pressure boxes are used more commonly because they are easier to keep accurately calibrated.

The principle of measurement of thoracic gas volume in the body plethysmograph is based on *Boyle's law:*

$$P_1V_1 = P_2V_2.$$

With the patient sitting inside the box, at end expiration, a shutter can be occluded in the patient's mouthpiece-airway system, and the patient continues to breathe against this obstruction using a suck–blow maneuver.

The starting alveolar pressure (P_1), new alveolar pressure (P_2), and change in alveolar volume can be measured. Using these data, the starting unknown FRC volume (V_1) can be determined. This method is not only much more rapid than the other methods, but also gives accurate thoracic gas volume measurements in the presence of obstructive airway disease. The major drawback to the method is the considerable cost involved in purchasing a body plethysmograph.

CHEST ROENTGENOGRAM METHOD

The arithmetical calculation of lung volume from posteroanterior (PA) and lateral chest roentgenograms taken at total lung capacity can be readily used to determine thoracic gas volumes (Fig. 10-4). There is excellent correlation between the plethysmographic and radiologic determinations of total lung capacity not only in normal subjects, but also in patients with obstructive airway diseases.[1] The major advantage of this method is that it is accurate and yet economically feasible in any pulmonary function laboratory.

INTERPRETATION OF ROUTINE PULMONARY FUNCTION TESTS

Abnormal spirograms tend to have one of two patterns: obstructive or restrictive. Occasionally one will find combined obstructive and restrictive pulmonary

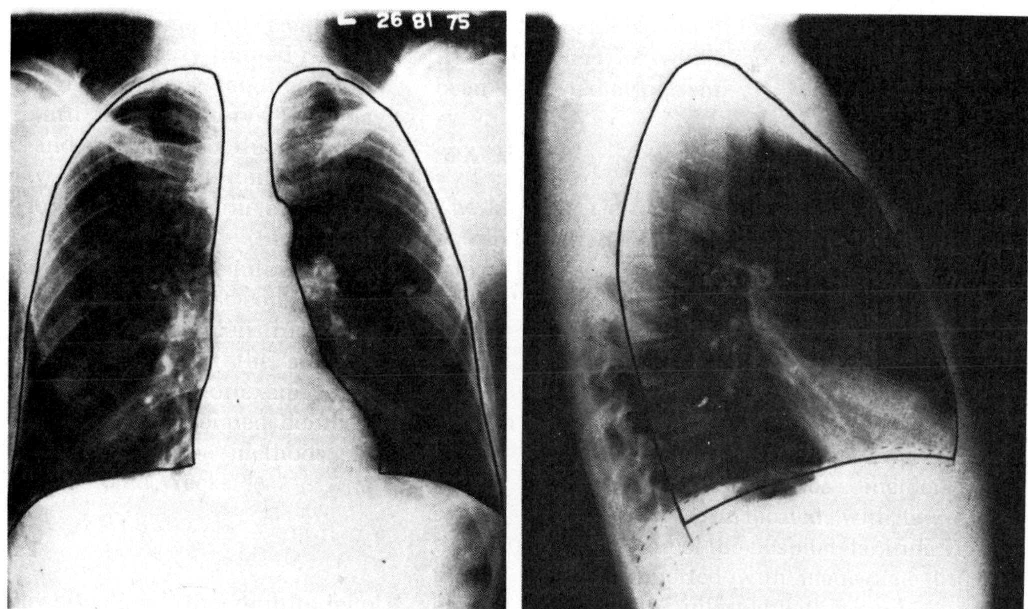

Fig. 10-4. Determination of total lung capacity using the chest roentgenogram method. The areas outlined in the posterior–anterior and lateral chest films are measured by planimetry and simple calculations made to determine the total lung capacity. (Harris TR, Pratt PC, and Kilburn KH: Total lung capacity measured by roentgenograms. Am J Med 50:756, 1971)

disease (*see* Table 10-1 for a classification of obstructive and restrictive pulmonary disorders).

Lung volume and flow-rate measurements are generally accepted as normal if they are between 80% and 120% of the predicted normal. It is now recognized, however, that normal patients may fall below 80% of predicted normal and would thus be incorrectly labeled as having pulmonary disease. Therefore, some laboratories use the statistical measure of standard deviation to help define the normal population. If one, for example, used the mean predicted normal minus 1.65 times the standard deviation value, 95% of the population would lie above this value.

If one wants to avoid labeling the normal person as abnormal (e.g., on life-insurance examinations), using "normal" predicted values that take standard deviation into account would result in fewer false positives. Data are now being gathered to help define appropriate standard deviations for pulmonary function test data, which hopefully will better delineate between normal and abnormal pulmonary function test values.

Table 10-1. Types of Pulmonary Disease

I. *Obstructive Pulmonary Disease*
  1. Emphysema
  2. Chronic bronchitis
  3. Bronchial asthma
  4. Bronchiectasis
  5. Cystic fibrosis
  6. Tracheobronchomalacia

II. *Restrictive Pulmonary Disease*
  A. Intrapulmonic
    1. Interstitial fibrosis
    2. Pulmonary edema
    3. Pneumonia
    4. Vascular congestion
    5. Adult respiratory distress syndrome
    6. Pneumoconioses
    7. Sarcoidosis
  B. Extrapulmonic
    1. Thoracic
      a. Kyphoscoliosis
      b. Multiple rib fractures
      c. Rheumatoid spondylitis
      d. Thoracic surgery
      e. Pleural effusion
      f. Pneumothorax or hemothorax, or both
    2. Abdominal
      a. Abdominal surgery
      b. Ascites
      c. Peritonitis
      d. Severe obesity
    3. Neuromuscular defects
      a. Poliomyelitis
      b. Guillain–Barré syndrome
      c. Myasthenia gravis
      d. Tetanus
      e. Drugs (*e.g.,* curare, kanamycin)
    4. Respiratory center depression
      a. Narcotics
      b. Barbiturates
      c. Anesthesia

OBSTRUCTIVE PATTERN

The VC is usually normal in mild obstructive airway disease. With severe obstruction to air flow, air trapping occurs, and the VC becomes reduced. If a slow VC or inspiratory VC (two-stage VC) is significantly larger (e.g., 300 ml greater) than the FVC, air trapping during the forced expiratory maneuver may be present.

The FEV_1 may be normal in early obstructive airway disease. However, the FEV_1/observed FVC is usually reduced, making the latter determination a more sensitive indicator of obstruction to air flow than the FEV_1 alone. The $FEF_{25\%-75\%}$ is one of the most sensitive spirographically determined expiratory flow measurements for detecting early obstructive airway disease.[3]

The MVV is often normal in the presence of early obstructive airway disease but is reduced in moderate to severe impairment to air flow. A classic pattern for air trapping is often detected on the spirographic tracing during an MVV maneuver in patients with significant obstructive airway disease (Fig. 10-5).

The TLC is normal to increased in obstructive airway disease. A markedly increased TLC in the stable patient (e.g., greater than 130% of predicted) suggests the presence of emphysema. The RV normally makes up about 35% of the TLC, increasing with age. The RV/TLC ratio (RV/TLC%) is often normal in early obstructive airway disease but increased in moderate to severe disease. Other lung volumes such as ERV, IRV, and V_T are quite variable and usually of little value in determining the pattern of pulmonary impairment. An isolated reduction in ERV is commonly seen in centripetal obesity but may simply be secondary to decreased effort during the terminal phase of exhalation.

Inhalation of a bronchodilator is commonly used to determine whether reversible airways obstruction is present. Generally, one should see at least a 15% improvement in flow rates or lung volumes to say that there is bronchodilator-induced improvement. At times, one will miss improvement in the postbronchodilator spirogram unless flow measurements at identical absolute lung volumes are compared (*i.e.*, by use of a body plethysmograph). For example, $\dot{V}$ max 50% may be quite similar in pre-bronchodilator and postbronchodilator spirograms where the FVC is significantly larger after bronchodilator inhalation, whereas flow at the 50% point of the prebronchodilator VC may be significantly higher at that same lung volume point on the postbronchodilator spirogram.

A definite improvement in flow rates or lung volumes after bronchodilator inhalation suggests the presence of bronchial asthma, although pulmonary function sometimes improves acutely in those with chronic bronchitis. A failure to improve dramatically after bronchodilator inhalation on spirometry does not rule out benefit from the chronic administration of bronchodilators.

In some laboratories, inhalation of irritants or allergens is used to detect the presence of reactive airways disease. Bronchospasm induced by mecholyl or histamine inhalation is characteristic of bronchial asthma. Inhalation of a specific allergen, with a resultant reduction in pulmonary function, may aid in the diagnosis of certain pulmonary disorders. An example would be bronchospasm induced by *Aspergillus* antigen inhalation in a patient with allergic bronchopulmonary aspergillosis. Laboratory personnel should be adequately prepared to treat severe bronchospasm that may occur in patients exposed to this type of provocation testing.

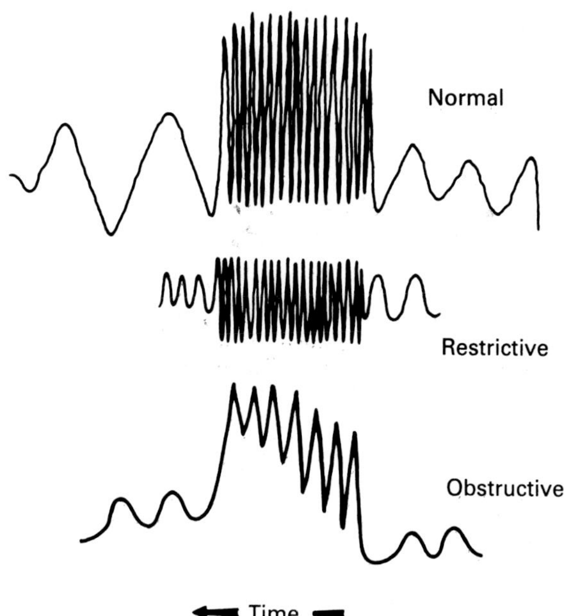

Fig. 10-5. Spirographic tracings showing maximal voluntary ventilation maneuvers. Normal is compared with restrictive disease and obstructive airway disease.

RESTRICTIVE PATTERN

All lung volumes and capacities are reduced in classic restrictive disease. The flow rates may be reduced, normal, or increased. The reduction in flow rate, if present, would be proportional to the reduction in VC. Expiratory flow rates that are more reduced than the reduction in VC would suggest the presence of concomitant obstructive airway disease. Although the FEV_1 and FVC are classically reduced, the FEV_1/observed FVC is normal in pure restrictive disease. This helps to differentiate the reduced FEV_1 of obstructive disease from that of restrictive disease.

The MVV may be normal to reduced. The RV/TLC ratio will be normal in pure restrictive disease.

COMBINED OBSTRUCTIVE AND RESTRICTIVE PATTERN

Patients may, and occasionally do, have more than one cardiopulmonary disorder, which may result in a combined obstructive and restrictive pulmonary function abnormality. Examples of this would be cases of emphysema (obstructive) with mild congestive heart failure (restrictive), or tracheal stenosis (obstructive) with concomitant obesity (restrictive). The VC is reduced in combined obstructive and restrictive disease. The flow rates are reduced disproportionately to the reduction in VC. The FEV_1/observed FVC will be reduced. The MVV may be normal to decreased.

A common error is to assume that a reduced FVC indicates the presence of restrictive pulmonary disease. The VC may be reduced solely because of air trapping from obstructive airway disease. To be certain that restrictive disease is present, in association with a reduced VC and reduced FEV_1/observed FVC, one should demonstrate that a reduced TLC is present. Serial changes in the TLC might be helpful. For instance, the TLC in a patient with emphysema may change from supernormal to normal as a concomitant restrictive process is developing. The RV/TLC ratio will be increased in the presence of combined obstructive and restrictive disease.

Table 10-2 summarizes the patterns of function-testing abnormalities in obstructive, restrictive, and combined obstructive and restrictive pulmonary disease.

Table 10-2. Patterns of Pulmonary Function Abnormality

FUNCTION	NORMAL* (%)	OBSTRUCTIVE	RESTRICTIVE	COMBINED
FVC	≥80	N to ↓	↓	↓
FEV_1	≥80	N to ↓	↓	↓
FEV_1/FVC%	≥75	↓	N to ↑	↓
$FEF_{25\%-75\%}$	≥80	↓	↑, N, or ↓	↓
TLC	80–120	N to ↑	↓	↓
RV/TLC%	25–40	↑	N	↑

*Normal (N) values represent the percentage of predicted value except for FEV_1/FVC% and RV/TLC%, which are absolute percentages.

PULMONARY FUNCTION TESTING IN CHILDREN

The evaluation of pulmonary function in infants and children presents unique challenges. Routine equipment often needs to be modified because of the smaller subjects. Children may not be fully cooperative, and the ability of the pulmonary laboratory technician to achieve maximal patient performance may be tested to the ultimate.

The incidence of significant respiratory disorders in neonates and small children in which pulmonary function testing would be helpful is, fortunately, relatively small. During this age period, the pulmonary status is generally evaluated by a careful history and physical examination. Chest roentgenography and arterial blood gas analysis are helpful supplemental aids that do not require an extraordinarily complex set-up and where patient cooperation is not as vital.

An in-depth discussion of the technology and a presentation of normal standards are beyond the scope of this chapter. The student particularly interested in this topic is referred to other source material now available.[4]

SUMMARY

Pulmonary function equipment must be carefully calibrated to ensure accuracy of the data obtained. Also crucial to the collection of interpretable data is the presence of a well-trained pulmonary laboratory technician. Unless the person directing the performance of the test coaxes the patient to achieve maximal performance and learns to accept only valid efforts, the results achieved are often uninterpretable. The correct performance of simple pulmonary function maneuvers, however, will give valuable data that are essential in evaluating pulmonary status properly.

REFERENCES

1. Harris TR, Pratt PC, Kilburn KH: Total lung capacity measured by roentgenograms. Am J Med 50:756, 1971
2. Hodgkin JE, Dines DE, Didier EP: Preoperative evaluation of the patient with pulmonary disease. Mayo Clin Proc 48:114, 1973
3. McFadden ER Jr, Linden DA: A reduction in maximum midexpiratory flow rate: A spirographic manifestation of small airway disease. Am J Med 52:725, 1972
4. Polgar G, Promadhat V: Pulmonary Function Testing in Children: Techniques and Standards. Philadelphia, WB Saunders, 1971

BIBLIOGRAPHY

Spirometry

Bartlett RG Jr, Brubach H, Specht H: Some factors determining the maximum breathing capacity. J Appl Physiol 12:247, 1958

Bates DV, Macklem PT, Christie RV: Respiratory Function in Disease, 2nd ed. Philadelphia, WB Saunders, 1971

Comroe JH Jr et al: The Lung: Clinical Physiology and Pulmonary Function Tests, 2nd ed. Chicago, Year Book Medical Publishers, 1962

Dawson A: Reproducibility of spirometric measurements in normal subjects. Am Rev Respir Dis 93:264, 1966

Leuallen EC, Fowler WS: Maximal midexpiratory flow. Am Rev Tuberc 72:783, 1955

Petty TL: Pulmonary Diagnostic Techniques. Philadelphia, Lea & Febiger, 1975

Pulmonary terms and symbols: A report of the ACCP–ATS Joint Committee on Pulmonary Nomenclature. Chest 67:583, 1975

Determination of Total Lung Capacity

Bates DV, Macklem PT, Christie RV: Respiratory Function in Disease, 2nd ed. Philadelphia, WB Saunders, 1971

Bedell GN et al: Plethysmographic determination of the volume of gas trapped in the lungs. J Clin Invest 35:664, 1956

Comroe JH Jr, Botelho SY, DuBois AB: Design of a body plethysmograph for studying cardiopulmonary physiology. J Appl Physiol 14:439, 1959

Comroe JH Jr et al: The Lung: Clinical Physiology and Pulmonary Function Tests, 2nd ed. Chicago, Year Book Medical Publishers, 1962

Curtis JK, Emmanuel D, Rasmussen HK: Improved apparatus for determining the functional residual capacity of the lung by the open circuit method. Am J Med 18:531, 1955

Gildenhorn HL, Hallett WY: An evaluation of radiological methods for the determination of lung volume. Radiology 84:754, 1965

Hale FC, Cohen AA, Hemingway A: Reliability of the estimation of functional residual capacity in the emphysematous patient. Am Rev Respir Dis 87:820, 1963

Harris TR, Pratt PC, Kilburn KH: Total lung capacity measured by roentgenograms. Am J Med 50:756, 1971

Loyd HM, String ST, DuBois AB: Radiographic and plethysmographic determination of total lung capacity. Radiology 86:7, 1966

Mead J: Volume displacement body plethysmograph for respiratory measurements in human subjects. J Appl Physiol 15:736, 1960

Meneely GR, Kaltreider NL: The volume of the lung determined by helium dilution. Description of the method and comparison with other procedures. J Clin Invest 28:129, 1949

Ruppel G: Manual of Pulmonary Function Testing. St Louis, CV Mosby, 1975

Skoogh BE, Rizell F: High frequency volume displacement body plethysmograph. Scand J Clin Lab Invest 31:419, 1973

Weiner RS, Cooper P: Measurement of functional residual capacity. A comparison of two closed-circuit helium-dilution methods. Am Rev Tuberc 74:729, 1956

Interpretation of Routine Pulmonary Function Tests

Bates DV, Macklem PT, Christie RV: Respiratory Function in Disease, 2nd ed. Philadelphia, WB Saunders, 1971

Cherniack RM: Pulmonary Function Testing. Philadelphia, WB Saunders, 1977

Comroe JH Jr et al: The Lung: Clinical Physiology and Pulmonary Function Tests, 2nd ed. Chicago, Year Book Medical Publishers, 1962

Hodgkin JE et al: Chronic obstructive airway diseases: Current concepts in diagnosis and comprehensive care. JAMA 232:1243, 1975

Pulmonary Function Testing in Children

Bernstein L et al: Pulmonary function in children. I. Determination of norms. J Allergy 30:514, 1959

Bjure I: Spirometric studies in normal subjects. IV. Ventilatory capacities in healthy children 7 to 17 years of age. Acta Paediatr 52:232, 1963

Cherniack RM: Ventilatory function in normal children. Can Med Assoc J 87:80, 1962

Chu JS et al: Lung compliance and lung volume measured concurrently in normal full term and premature infants. Pediatrics 34:525, 1964

Cook CD et al: Studies of respiratory physiology in the newborn infant. I. Observations on normal premature and full-term infants. J Clin Invest 34:975, 1955

Cook CD et al: Studies of respiratory physiology in the newborn infant. J Clin Invest 36:440, 1957

Cook CD, Motoyama EK: Respiratory physiology in infants and children. In Smith RM: Anesthesia for Infants and Children. St Louis CV Mosby, 1968

Giammona ST, Daly WJ: Pulmonary diffusing capacity in normal children, ages 4 to 13. Am J Dis Child 110:144, 1965

Morse M, Cassels DE: Cardiopulmonary Data for Children and Young Adults. Springfield, IL, Charles C Thomas, 1962

Nelson NM: Neonatal pulmonary function. Pediatr Clin North Am 13:769, 1966

11

Specialized Pulmonary Function Tests

John E. Hodgkin

Most patients who present with respiratory symptoms can be adequately evaluated with routine spirometry and lung volume studies. However, it is often beneficial to obtain one or more of the specialized tests to be described in this chapter.

In patients who will not provide maximal effort during spirometry, certain other tests that are effort-independent can provide the physician with valuable data. When medicolegal aspects are involved, tests can be performed that do not allow the patient to alter voluntarily the results in order to appear disabled.

Routine spirometry may show a pulmonary impairment, but often only with more specific tests can a precise diagnosis be made. The spirogram is not a very sensitive way of detecting early lung disease, so the physician may desire to order other tests to detect disease at an earlier stage.

A description of the methods for performing these specialized tests, along with tables of normal values, are provided in Appendix A at the end of this book.

DIFFUSING CAPACITY

Many tests have been proposed for determining the ability of gases to diffuse across the alveolar–capillary membrane. The components of this membrane are depicted in Figure 11-1. The most common gas used for determining diffusing capacity is carbon monoxide, which is inhaled in very low concentration (e.g., 0.2%). The ability of carbon monoxide to move from the alveolus to the capillary is diminished in patients with interstitial lung diseases. Those interstitial pulmonary disorders resulting in a reduced diffusing capacity have classically been grouped together into the "alveolar–capillary block syndrome." However, factors other than thickening of the alveolar–capillary membrane can also result in reduced diffusing capacity as measured by carbon monoxide inhalation.

Other factors that affect "diffusing capacity" include loss of alveolar–capillary membrane surface area; abnormalities of alveolar ventilation; lung perfusion; ventilation/perfusion matching; red blood cell mass and the red cell membrane; and affinity of hemoglobin for carbon monoxide. Some workers have separated the pulmonary diffusing capacity into three parts: the membrane component (D_M); the red blood cell and hemoglobin component; and the pulmonary capillary blood volume (V_C). The methods commonly used, however, make no attempt to separate these component parts.[6]

The technique most widely used is the "*single-breath method.*" The patient inhales a gas mixture containing a low concentration of carbon monoxide, then holds his breath for about 10 seconds before exhaling. The diffusing capacity can be calculated by determining the amount of carbon monoxide that has moved from the alveolar gas into the blood.

The other major technique used is the *steady-state method*. Numerous steady-state techniques have been developed with suggested advantages for each of the methods. With this technique the patient breathes a known mixture of gas containing a low concentration of carbon monoxide. When the alveolar carbon monoxide level reaches a plateau, certain measurements are made. Most of the variations in technique relate to the method for determining alveolar carbon monoxide (PA_{CO}) The alveolar carbon monoxide level can be calculated from [1] inspired P_{CO} and determination of dead space using PA_{CO_2}; [2] assuming that end tidal P_{CO} and PA_{CO} are equal; and [3] assuming the dead space volume and subsequent calculation of PA_{CO}. The steady-state method may be performed either at rest or with exercise. Some believe that exercise makes the steady-state method more reliable and reproducible because the increased cardiac output of exercise distributes blood throughout the pulmonary capillary bed more evenly than at rest; accordingly, spurious reductions in Vc because of regional underperfusion are minimized.

Although a reduction in diffusing capacity for carbon monoxide may correctly be interpreted as suggesting the presence of a thickened alveolar–capillary membrane owing to interstitial lung disease, in most patients with interstitial lung diseases the development of hypoxemia is secondary to ventilation/perfusion mismatch rather than to the presence of a true diffusion block due to thickening of the alveolar–capillary membrane.[4]

Despite these limitations the diffusing capacity test is one of the most sensitive indicators of early interstitial lung disease. For example, the diffusing

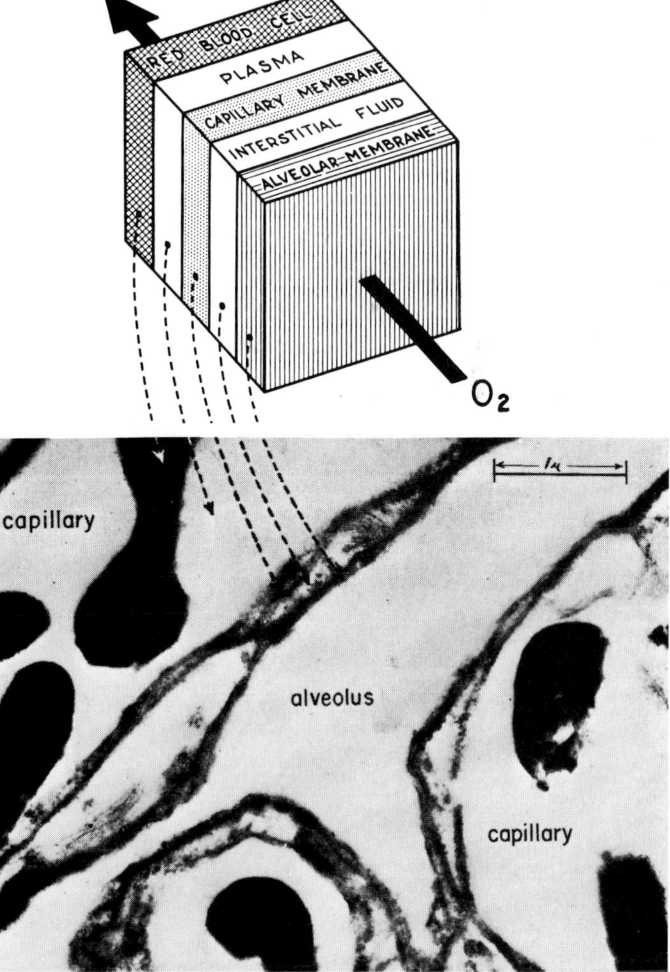

Fig. 11-1. Diagrammatic representation of the alveolar–capillary membrane and an electron micrograph of lung parenchyma. (Comroe JH Jr *et al:* The Lung; Clinical Physiology and Pulmonary Function Tests, 2nd ed. Chicago, Year Book Medical Publishers, 1962)

capacity may be significantly reduced in pulmonary sarcoidosis, whereas the chest roentgenogram, lung volume studies, and resting arterial blood gases are still within normal limits.

In addition to assisting in the early diagnosis of pulmonary disorders, the diffusing capacity is one of the best tests to follow for determining response to specific therapy. A deteriorating diffusing capacity in a patient with sarcoidosis or interstitial pneumonitis–fibrosis would suggest a poor response to the therapy initiated.

One of the proposed ways to diagnose anatomic emphysema is to demonstrate the presence of a significantly reduced diffusing capacity[14] (e.g., less than 50% of predicted) in the presence of chronic obstructive airway disease. The reduced diffusing capacity in this situation largely is due to loss of alveolar–capillary membrane.

The diffusing capacity for the lung is reported in milliliters of carbon monoxide that diffuse per minute across the alveolar–capillary membrane per millimeter of mercury difference in the partial pressure of carbon monoxide between the alveolus and the capillary:

$$DL_{CO} = \text{CO ml/min/mm Hg CO.}$$

VENTILATION INDICES

The respiratory rate *(frequency)* is the variable of pulmonary function most frequently measured at the bedside. However, more important than the number of breaths per minute is the patient's *minute ventilation.* Minute ventilation = tidal volume × respiratory rate (frequency).

$$\dot{V}E = f \times VT$$

Even more crucial than knowing the minute ventilation, however, is determining the *alveolar ventilation.* Alveolar ventilation is inversely porportional to Pa_{CO_2} and is calculated as follows:

$$\dot{V}A = f(VT - VD),$$

where the dead space (VD) is obtained from the modified Bohr equation

$$VD/VT = \frac{Pa_{CO_2} - P\bar{E}_{CO_2}}{Pa_{CO_2}}.$$

The physiologic dead space to tidal volume ratio is most important in the clinical setting.

It is often important to estimate the *dead space to tidal volume ratio* (VD/VT). The *anatomical dead space* includes those airways not perfused by the pulmonary capillaries (*i.e.*, trachea, bronchi, and bronchioles). However, in disease states, alveoli themselves may not be perfused. Nonperfused alveoli constitute the *alveolar dead space* and represent an inconsequential volume in normal humans. The anatomical dead space plus the volume of alveolar dead space equals the *physiologic dead space.*

The method for determining VD/VT requires the collection of exhaled gas and an arterial blood sample (*see* Appendix D, Fig. D-1). Although the minute ventilation may be constant, the alveolar ventilation may vary significantly depending on the VD/VT ratio (Fig. 11-2). Normally, the VD/VT ratio is about 0.35; however, it increases gradually with age.

UNIFORMITY OF VENTILATION

Uniformity of ventilation is a critical factor in determining the ability of gas exchange to take place. Several tests are available for evaluating this factor.

Single-Breath Nitrogen Test

The single-breath nitrogen test is performed by having the patient exhale maximally, followed by an inhalation of 100% oxygen up to total lung capacity. By then measuring nitrogen concentration and plotting this versus lung volume during the subsequent exhaled slow vital capacity, a single-breath nitrogen curve can be developed (Fig. 11-3).

Four phases of the single-breath nitrogen curve have been described. Phase I represents exhalation of dead space gas that contains only 100% oxygen; phase II represents a mixture of dead space and alveolar gas; phase III represents the alveolar plateau owing to exhalation of mixed alveolar gas; and phase IV represents the "closing volume," which will be discussed later. If areas of lung are not emptying uniformly, the alveolar plateau (phase III) will be steeper than normal. The percentage of nitrogen increasing by more than 1.5 on the alveolar plateau between the 750-ml exhaled point and the 1250-ml exhaled point suggests the presence of significant nonuniform ventilation.

Nitrogen Washout Test

The nitrogen washout test for determining lung volumes has been discussed in Chapter 10. During the nitrogen washout study, while the patient is breathing 100% oxygen, the concentration of nitrogen in each exhaled breath should drop exponentially. If the pa-

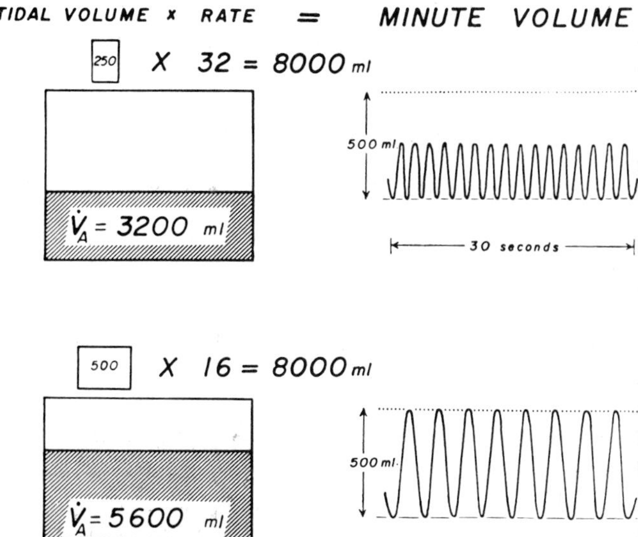

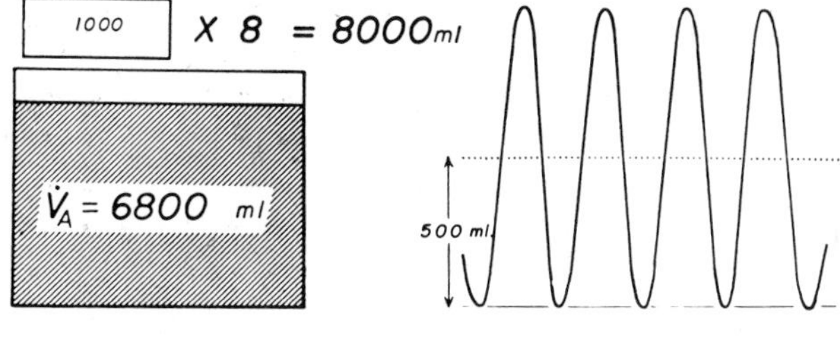

Fig. 11-2. Diagrammatic representation of the effect of a varying VD/VT ratio on alveolar ventilation. Note that the minute ventilation is identical in all three examples. However, the alveolar ventilation varies markedly as the tidal volume and VD/VT ratio vary. T.V. = tidal volume; D.S. = dead space volume. Dead space ventilation (V̇DS) is indicated by the unshaded portion of the boxes. (Comroe JH Jr *et al:* The Lung: Clinical Physiology and Pulmonary Function Tests, 2nd ed. Chicago, Year Book Medical Publishers, 1962)

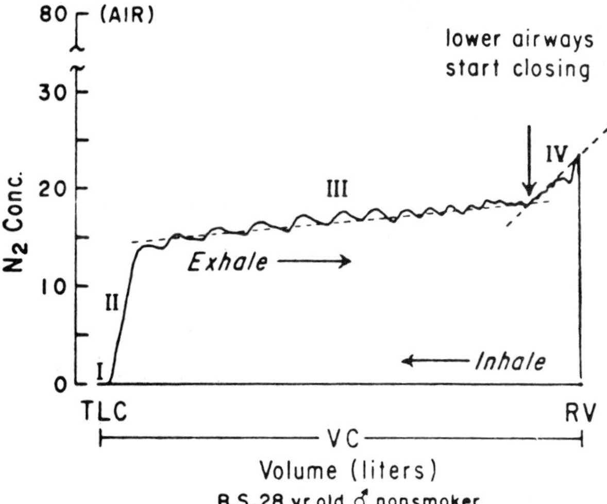

Fig. 11-3. Single-breath nitrogen test showing the four phases of the single-breath nitrogen curve. (Buist AS, Van Fleet DL, Ross BB: A comparison of conventional spirometric tests and the test of closing volume in an emphysema screening center. Am Rev Respir Dis 107:744, 1973)

tient is breathing slowly and regularly, a nitrogen plateau should also be developed at the end of each exhaled breath. Both the presence of peak nitrogen concentrations higher than on previous breaths and the loss of the flat nitrogen plateau indicate the presence of nonuniform ventilation (Fig. 11-4).

At the end of the 7-minute nitrogen washout study the subject exhales maximally, and the nitrogen concentration of this final exhaled breath is reported as the *nitrogen index*. There should be less than 2.5% nitrogen present during this last exhaled breath. A nitrogen index of 2.5% or greater again suggests the presence of significant nonuniform ventilation. The breath-by-breath analysis during nitrogen washout is significantly more sensitive than either the slope of phase III of the single-breath nitrogen study or the nitrogen index in detecting the presence of nonuniform ventilation.

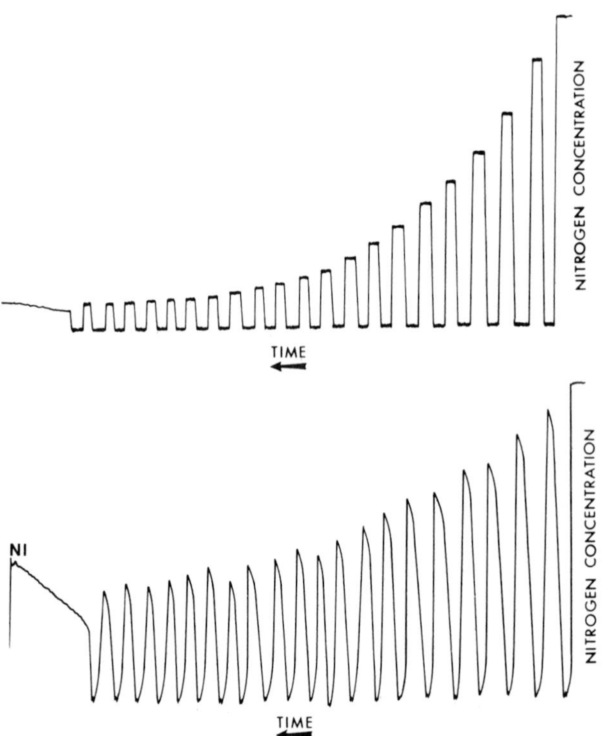

Fig. 11-4. Nitrogen washout tracings. The upper pattern is that seen normally. Note that each breath has less exhaled nitrogen than the previous breath and that there is a nitrogen plateau at the end of each exhaled tidal volume. In the lower tracing the pattern of obstructive airway diseases is depicted. Note the presence of spikes or irregular height as well as the increased nitrogen index, NI (the nitrogen content of the last exhaled breath), indicative of the presence of nonuniform ventilation

Helium Mixing Time

With the closed-circuit helium dilution method for determining lung volume (discussed in Chapter 10), an estimate of the presence of nonuniform ventilation can also be obtained. If the "helium mixing time" (the time required to reach a helium plateau during the study) is prolonged, the presence of nonuniform ventilation is suggested. A helium mixing efficiency index can be calculated by determining the number of breaths taken to reach 90% of the final equilibrium value.

FLOW-VOLUME LOOP ANALYSIS

If during forced inspiratory and forced expiratory vital capacity maneuvers, one plots flow versus lung volume, a flow-volume curve is developed (Fig. 11-5). There are several advantages to evaluating forced vital capacities in this manner.

1. Evidence is accumulating that analysis of flow at lung volumes in the lower portion of the vital capacity provides more sensitive indicators of small airway obstruction than usual spirographic analysis.[13] For example, flow at 50% of the vital capacity ($\dot{V}max_{50\%}$) and at 75% of the vital capacity ($\dot{V}max_{75\%}$) will be reduced earlier in the development of obstructive pulmonary disease than will values such as the forced expiratory volume in 1 second (FEV_1). Flattening of the slope (e.g., between $\dot{V}max_{50\%}$ and $\dot{V}max_{75\%}$) may also be more sensitive in detecting obstructive airway disease than are the usual spirographic data.
2. One can easily determine peak expiratory flow (PEF) and peak inspiratory flow (PIF) from flow-volume loop analysis, whereas these measurements cannot be made on the usual spirogram.
3. Lesions that produce large airway obstruction, such as bilateral vocal cord paralysis, tracheal stricture, and tracheal tumors, may be detected by flow-volume loop analysis when they would not be suspected from the routine spirogram.[12] A variable extrathoracic large airway obstruction (such as laryngeal carcinoma) produces a plateau on the inspiratory flow-volume loop, whereas a variable intrathoracic large airway obstruction (such as a tracheal carcinoid tumor) produces a plateau on the

forced expiratory flow-volume loop. A fixed large airway obstruction (tracheal stricture) will produce plateaus on both the inspiratory and expiratory loops. Various flow-volume loops are shown in Figure 11-6.

4. The comparison of flow-volume curves performed with the subject breathing room air with those with the subject breathing a helium–oxygen mixture (80% helium and 20% oxygen) has been promoted for detecting small airway obstruction (Fig. 11-7). The test is based on the fact that turbulent flow (as seen in larger airways) is density-dependent. The inhalation of the helium–oxygen mixture, which is a lower density than room air, results in higher flows in the normal person at volumes greater than 10% of the vital capacity. Laminar flow, as seen in smaller airways, depends on gas viscosity rather than on density. With the development of small airway disease, a larger percentage of the airway resistance occurs in the smaller airways. As a result, the flow-enhancing effect of the less dense helium–oxygen gas mixture will disappear at

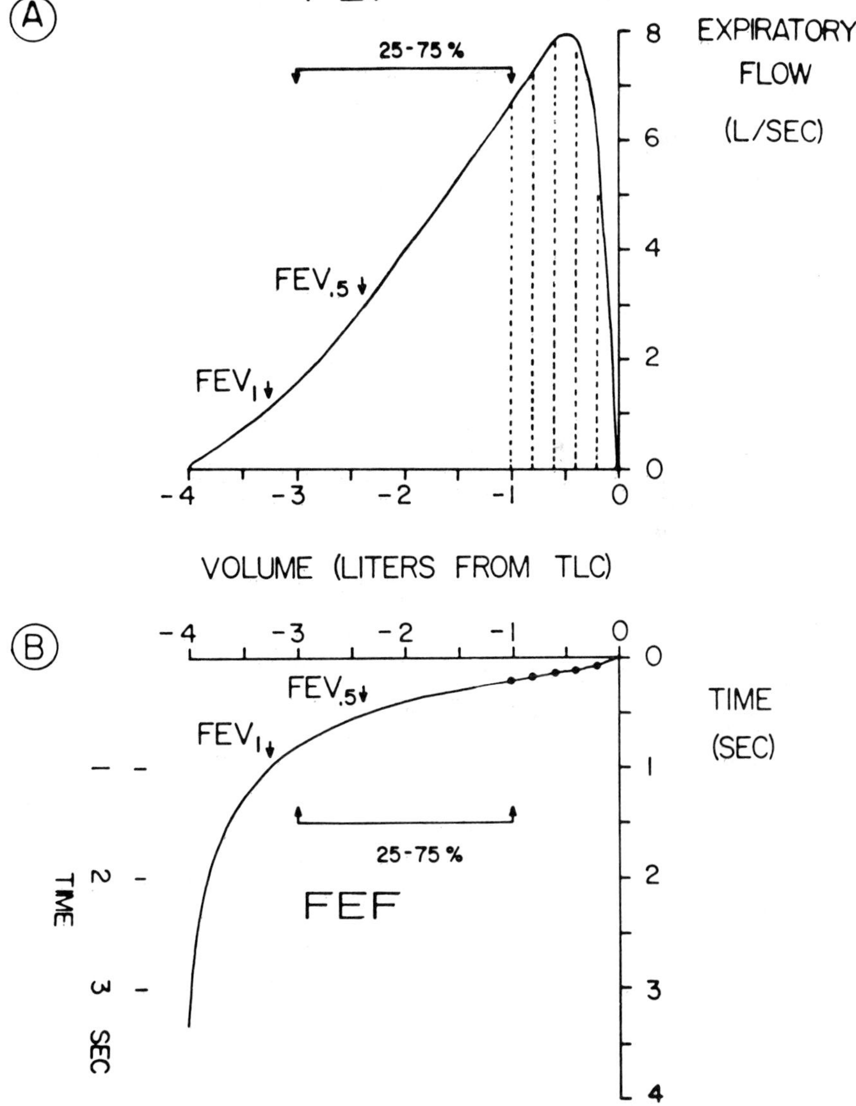

Fig. 11-5. Comparison of a routine spirometric tracing and an expiratory flow-volume loop display. The vertical dashed lines in A indicate instantaneous flow rates that correspond to exhaled volumes in spirometric tracing B. (Modified from Hyatt RE: Dynamic lung volumes. In Fenn WO, Rahn H (eds). Handbook of Physiology, Sect. 3, Respiration, Vol II. Washington DC, American Physiological Society, 1964)

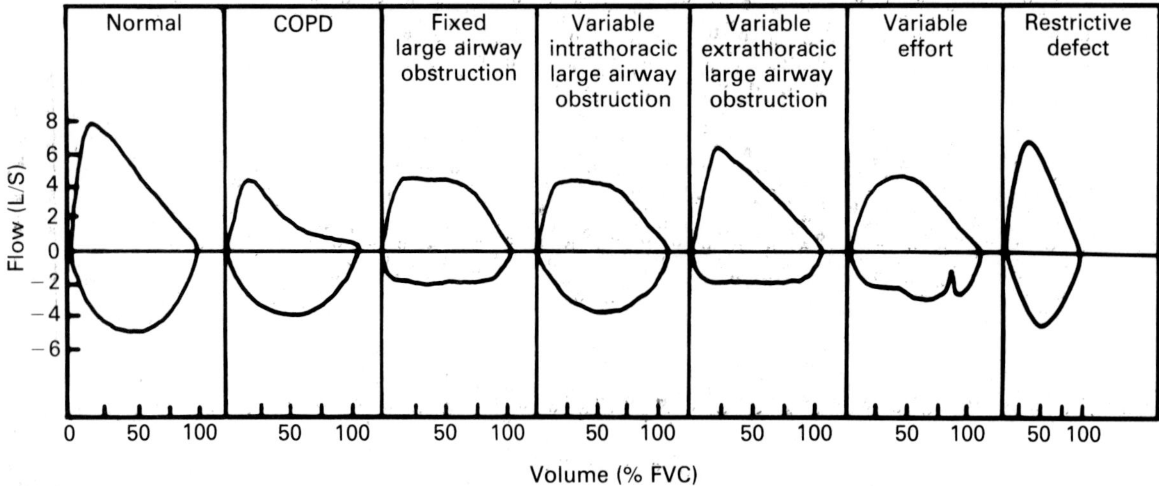

Fig. 11-6. Characteristic flow-volume loops from various lesions. The TLC is to the left of each panel. (Lauer J: Computer methods in spirometry: Diagnosis and flow-volume curve analysis. Unpublished thesis, Loma Linda University Graduate School, Loma Linda, California, 1973)

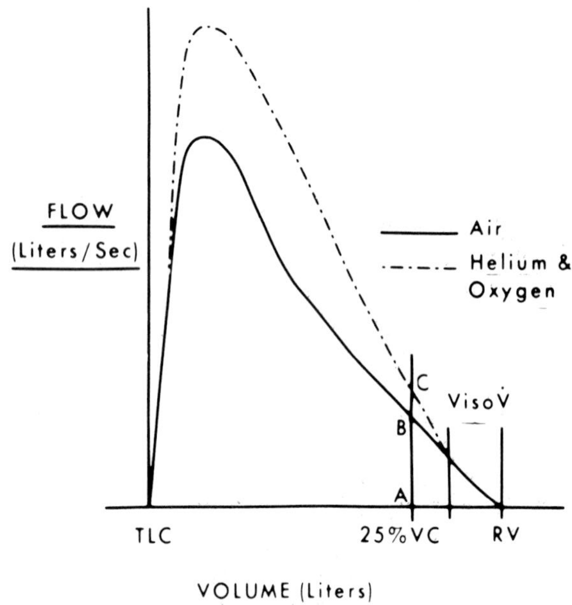

Fig. 11-7. Maximal expiratory flow-volume curves breathing air and He + O_2. The response to He + O_2 is expressed as the percentage of increase in flow compared to flow in air at 25% of VC (*i.e.*, BC/AB × 100 = $\Delta\dot{V}_{25}$). The point where flows breathing air and He + O_2 are the same is identified, and Viso$\dot{V}$ is measured from this point to RV. (Hutcheon M et al: Am Rev Respir Dis 110:458, 1974)

lung volumes well above 10% of the vital capacity. The lung volume at which the flows on the two curves becomes identical is known as the "*volume of isoflow*" (Viso$\dot{V}$). With small airway narrowing, the Viso$\dot{V}$ increases. One can also compare the difference in maximal flows on the curves after 50% or 75% of the VC has been exhaled (referred to respectively as the $\Delta\dot{V}max_{50\%}$ and $\Delta\dot{V}max_{75\%}$). A narrowing of the difference in maximal flows between the two curves when measured at these isovolume points suggests the presence of obstructive disease in the small airways. This test is considered to be more sensitive in detecting abnormality in the small airways than are the usual spirometric measurements.[9]

Normal flow-volume loop data, corrected for age, body size, sex, and smoking habits, are now being collected in many centers. With these data in hand, hopefully more precise criteria can be established for flow-volume loop analysis.

MECHANICS OF BREATHING

COMPLIANCE

The stiffness or elasticity of the respiratory system is expressed as its compliance. This measurement is normally made under static conditions and is reflected as the change in volume produced by a unit pressure change:

$$C = \frac{\Delta V}{\Delta P}.$$

The respiratory system must be separated into two portions when considering compliance; the lung itself and the chest wall. The compliance of the chest wall is further divided into that of the bony thorax and that of the diaphragm–abdominal wall system.

Pressure volume (PV) curves can be developed under static conditions by measuring the pressure developed at each lung volume over the VC. The pressure measured for developing the PV curve for the total respiratory system is the transrespiratory system pressure (*i.e.*, alveolar pressure minus atmospheric pressure [pressure at the body surface]):

$$P_{RS} = P_{alv} - P_{bs}.$$

The pressure used to develop the PV curve of the lung itself is the transpulmonary pressure (*i.e.*, alveolar pressure minus pleural pressure):

$$P_L = P_{alv} - P_{pl}.$$

In developing the chest-wall PV curve the trans-chest-wall pressure is used (*i.e.*, atmospheric pressure minus pleural pressure):

$$P_W = P_{bs} - P_{pl}.$$

Pleural pressure is estimated by measuring intrathoracic pressure, using an esophageal balloon. That intrapleural and esophageal pressures are equivalent is assumed.

The PV curves for the chest wall, lung, and total respiratory system are depicted in Figure 11-8.

Alveolar pressure is equivalent to oral pressure (pressure at the airway opening) if the airway between the mouth and the alveolus is open and there is no air flow (*i.e.*, the measurement is made under static conditions):

$$P_{alv} = P_{ao}.$$

Compliance is normally calculated from that portion of the PV curve in the 1-liter range above the end-resting tidal volume point (*i.e.*, that lung volume achieved after exhalation of the tidal volume). For example, for the calculation of lung compliance,

$$C_L = \frac{\Delta V}{\Delta P_L}.$$

If the change in lung volume above the end-resting tidal volume point is 1 liter, and the change in transpulmonary pressure over this 1-liter volume is 5 cm of water, then

$$C_L = \frac{1 \text{ liter}}{5 \text{ cm } H_2O};$$

$$C_L = 0.2 \text{ liters/cm } H_2O.$$

The normal static compliance for the lung and the chest wall systems is the same (*i.e.*, 0.2 liters/cm H_2O). The compliances of the total respiratory system, lung, and chest wall are related in a reciprocal fashion:

$$\frac{1}{C_{RS}} = \frac{1}{C_L} + \frac{1}{C_W}.$$

Therefore normal C_{RS} = 0.1 liter/cm H_2O.

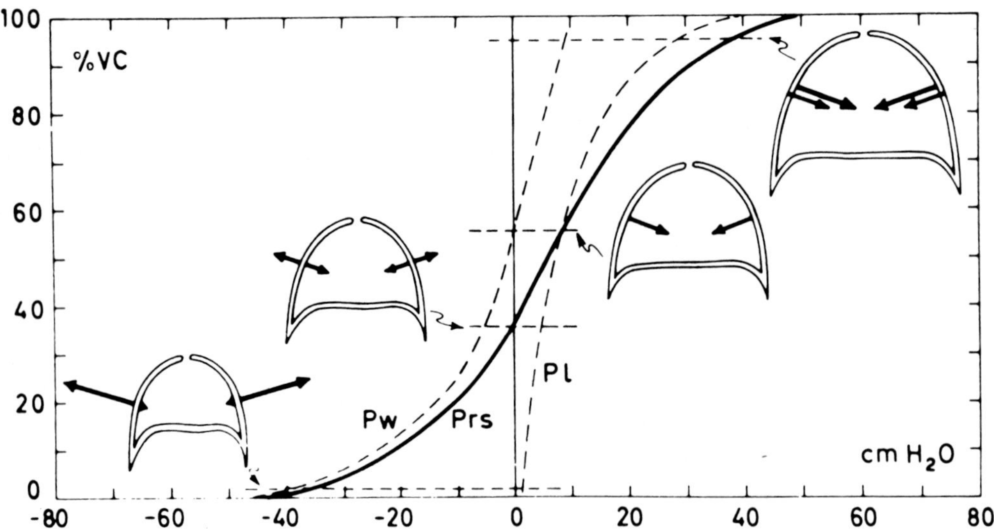

Fig. 11-8. Pressure-volume curves for the chest wall, lung, and total respiratory system. Pw = transchest-wall pressure; Prs = transrespiratory system pressure; PL = transpulmonary pressure. The static forces of the lung and chest wall are pictured (not to scale) by the arrows in the schematic diagrams. (Agostoni E, Mead J: Statics of the respiratory system. In Fenn WO, Rahn H (eds): Handbook of Physiology, Sect 3, Respiration, Vol 1 (Chap 13). Washington DC, American Physiological Society, 1964)

Elastance and compliance are related in a reciprocal fashion:

$$E_L = \frac{1}{C_L}.$$

A decrease in the stiffness of the lung is represented by a decreased elastance and an increased compliance. An abnormally high lung compliance in a stable patient with obstructive pulmonary disease indicates the presence of anatomic emphysema. Lung compliance is generally normal in chronic bronchitis and bronchial asthma. Lung compliance may be increased or decreased in an acute attack of asthma. A decrease in lung compliance suggests the presence of interstitial or alveolar pulmonary disease such as pulmonary fibrosis, sarcoidosis, and pulmonary edema (Fig. 11-9).

Compliance is related directly to lung volume, and thus is meaningless unless related to the patient's lung volume. For example, the compliance of a newborn lung is almost the same as the compliance of an adult lung when expressed as liter/cm H_2O/liter of lung volume. When the difference in lung volume is not taken into account, the neonate's lung compliance is about 0.006 liters/cm H_2O, whereas the adult's lung compliance is about 0.2 liters/cm H_2O. Therefore it is helpful to divide lung compliance by the lung volume at which the measurement is made, a value known as *specific compliance:*

Specific compliance

$$= \frac{C_L}{V_L \text{ at which compliance is measured}}.$$

Chest wall compliance may be decreased in patients who have kyphoscoliosis, ankylosing spondylitis, prominent obesity, severe pectus excavatum, and neuromuscular disorders associated with spasticity of the muscles. A reduced compliance of the lung or chest wall results in an increased work of breathing since the pressure required to produce a volume change is increased.

Compliances of the chest wall and total respiratory system are not routinely measured because they are affected by skeletal muscle contraction. Therefore, unless the muscles are totally relaxed, the measurements are invalid. Lung compliance, on the other hand, can be determined readily, even if the subject is not relaxed.

During quiet tidal volume breathing the change in transpulmonary pressure (PL) between the beginning and end of a tidal volume breath can be used as

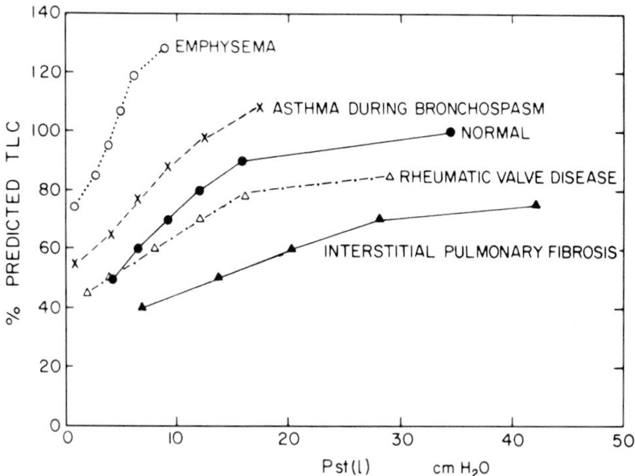

Fig. 11-9. Pressure–volume curves for the lung with examples of both obstructive airway diseases and interstitial lung diseases. (Bates DV, Macklem PT, Christie RV: Respiratory Function in Disease, 2nd ed. Philadelphia, WB Saunders, 1971)

the ΔP for the denominator in the equation, with the tidal volume being the ΔV:

$$\text{Cdyn} = \frac{V_T}{\Delta P_L}.$$

When compliance is measured in this manner, it is known as *dynamic compliance* (Cdyn). Normally, dynamic compliance of the lung is equal to static compliance (Cst). However, with obstructive airway disease, dynamic compliance decreases when compared to static compliance. In early obstructive airway disease, one can demonstrate a decreasing CL_{dyn} with increasing respiratory rate (Fig. 11-10). This is known as *frequency dependence of compliance* (*i.e.*, decreasing dynamic compliance with increasing respiratory frequency).

The presence of frequency dependence of compliance is one of the most sensitive indicators of small airway obstruction and is often abnormal in the presence of a normal spirogram. However, the measurement of transpulmonary pressure to determine the ΔP requires the use of an esophageal balloon, which is somewhat invasive. Proper collection of data also involves very accurate calibration of equipment. These factors make it a poor mass-screening test for the early detection of obstructive airway disease.

It is often valuable, with a patient who requires respirator support, to follow an estimate of lung stiffness known as *effective compliance*. The usual way of determining this measurement is to divide the tidal volume delivered by the peak inspiratory pressure required to deliver the volume. It is often mistakenly assumed that "compliance," when determined this way, is a reliable indicator of lung stiffness. However, the peak pressure required to deliver the tidal volume is influenced by factors in addition to lung compliance: airway resistance and chest-wall compliance. Also the peak pressure increases, without any change in airway diameter or respiratory system stiffness, if the tidal volume or the inspiratory flow rate is increased. Therefore, since this value is not solely an estimate of lung compliance, it is now known as *effective compliance, dynamic*.

If one applies an inspiratory hold, after the tidal volume has been delivered, either by using a prolonged inspiratory plateau or by occluding the exhalation line, one can obtain a measurement of the "static" pressure required to hold the lung at this inspired tidal volume point. By dividing the tidal volume by this new static pressure, a value known as *effective compliance, static* is obtained. This allows one to determine respiratory system compliance changes accurately, since airway resistance is now eliminated as a factor. Changes in respiratory system stiffness may still be due to factors other than lung compliance (e.g., changes in chest wall compliance secondary to muscle spasm or abdominal distention).

RESISTANCE

For air to flow down a tube, there must be a difference in pressure between the two ends of the system known as the "driving pressure." Resistance is defined as the pressure differential, or driving pressure, required to produce a unit flow:

$$R = \frac{\text{driving pressure}}{\dot{V}}.$$

Resistance is measured under dynamic conditions while air flow is occurring. *Pulmonary resistance* (RL) can be separated into *airway resistance* (Raw) and *lung tissue (viscous) resistance* (Rti):

$$R_L = \text{Raw} + \text{Rti}$$

Total respiratory system resistance is equal to pulmonary resistance plus *chest wall resistance*.

$$\text{Rrs} = R_L + \text{Rw}$$

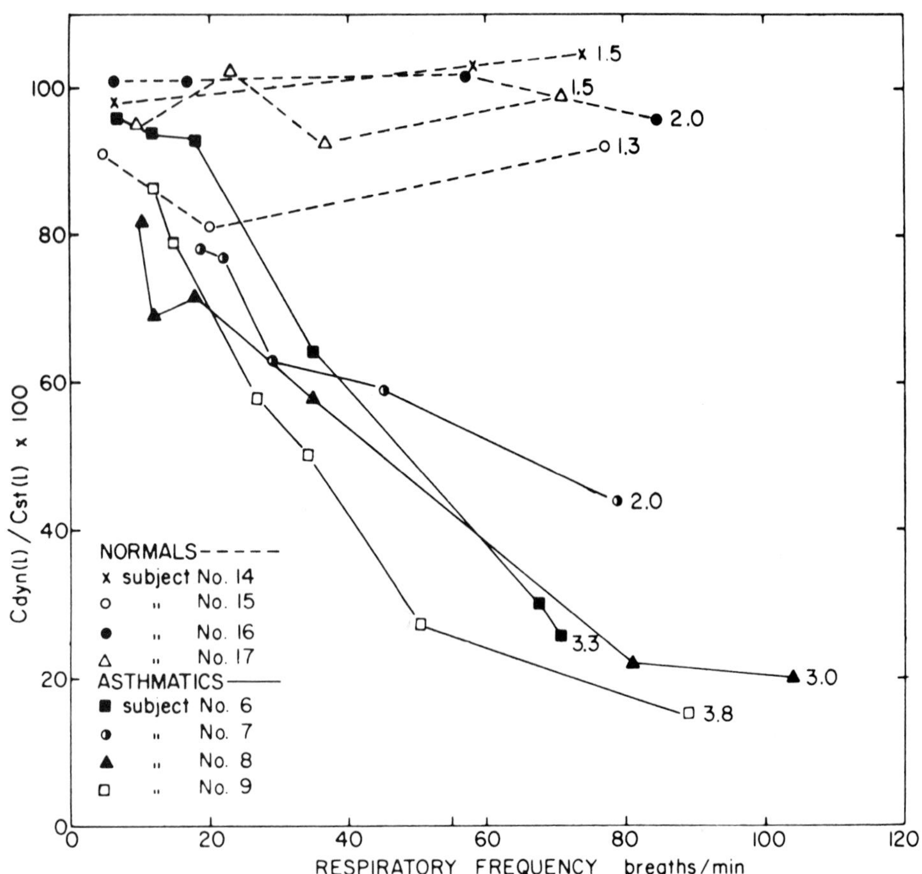

Fig. 11-10. Dynamic compliance, Cdyn(L), is seen to decrease with increasing breathing frequency in asthmatic patients but not in normal subjects. (Woolcock AJ, Vincent NJ, Macklem PT: Frequency dependence of compliance as a test for obstruction in the small airways. J Clin Invest 48:1097, 1969)

Chest wall resistance and lung tissue resistance are relatively minor. Lung tissue resistance may be increased by interstitial lung disease such as sarcoidosis, but is rarely a limiting factor to breathing.

Airway resistance is the major factor in determining the work of breathing due to resistance, accounting for about 80% of the total respiratory system resistance. The small airways (< 2 mm diameter) are responsible for only about 10% of the airway resistance, and these may be narrowed without any significant change in airway resistance.[8]

Airway resistance is equal to the driving pressure across the airway (pressure at the airway opening minus alveolar pressure) divided by flow:

$$\text{Raw} = \frac{\text{Pao} - \text{Palv}}{\dot{\text{V}}}.$$

Since pressure at the airway opening, or mouth pressure, is essentially the same as atmospheric pressure, one needs only to measure alveolar pressure and air flow.

$$\text{Raw} = \frac{\text{Palv}}{\dot{\text{V}}}.$$

Pulmonary resistance is equal to the driving pressure across the airway and lung tissue divided by flow:

$$\text{R}_\text{L} = \frac{\text{Pao} - \text{Ppl}^*}{\dot{\text{V}}}.$$

*The changes in pleural pressure during flow are responsible for overcoming lung elasticity, not just airway and lung tissue resistance. If one subtracts from the total transpulmonary pressure that which is required to overcome elastic recoil, then the remaining pressure is that needed to overcome pulmonary resistance.

Airway resistance is the measurement of pulmonary mechanics most commonly used in pulmonary function laboratories. This technique requires the use of a body plethysmograph. While the patient "pants" through a flow meter, changes in alveolar pressure are detected by changes in body box pressure. Airway resistance can be rapidly calculated by this technique. Normal values for airway resistance are 0.5 to 1.5 cm H_2O/liter/sec.

Pulmonary resistance may be measured by noting changes in transpulmonary pressure required to produce flow. This technique is more invasive because an esophageal balloon to measure transpulmonary pressure changes is required.

Total respiratory system resistance may be measured while the patient breathes quietly on an oscillator system in which forced oscillations are generated at or near a resonant frequency of the lung. The basis for the technique is that factors of compliance are eliminated so that only the flow-resistive pressure is being measured. An advantage to this method is that no esophageal balloon or body plethysmograph is required.[5]

The relation between airway resistance and lung volume is hyperbolic, with the reduction in resistance as lung volume increases due to an increased diameter of the airways. Some physiologists prefer to express airway resistance in an inverse relation, a factor known as *conductance* (Gaw), since changes in conductance with lung volume changes are linear.

$$\text{Gaw} = \frac{1}{\text{Raw}}$$

When conductance is divided by the lung volume at which the airway resistance is measured, the value is known as *specific conductance* (SGaw):

$$\text{SGaw} = \frac{\text{Gaw}}{V_L \text{ at which Raw measured}}.$$

The reciprocal of specific conductance is *specific airway resistance* (SRaw):

$$\text{SRaw} = \frac{1}{\text{SGaw}}.$$

An increase in airway resistance is typical for obstructive airway diseases including asthma, chronic bronchitis, and emphysema. The increased work of breathing in obstructive airway diseases is due to an increase in resistance to air flow, particularly during expiration.

CLOSING VOLUME

A modification of the single-breath nitrogen test, known as the "closing volume," evaluates phase IV of the single-breath nitrogen test (*see* Fig. 11-3). In most normal subjects the nitrogen concentration increases abruptly toward the end of the expiratory vital capacity maneuver during the single-breath nitrogen test.

The explanation for this increase in nitrogen concentration is as follows: the patient exhales maximally, and then 100% oxygen is inhaled to the maximum lung volume achievable. During the initial part of this inhalation, the first gas to enter the alveoli is the dead-space gas containing about 79% nitrogen. This gas preferentially goes to the apices of the lung, partially filling the alveoli. As the inhalation continues, the gas, now composed of 100% oxygen, completes the filling of the alveoli at the apices, but the major portion goes to the alveoli at the bases of the lung. A differential nitrogen concentration is thus established: The gas in the apices has a higher nitrogen concentration than that in the bases. As the subject exhales, and the diaphragm ascends, a point is reached where the small airways just above the diaphragm tend to close, limiting air flow from these areas. The air flow now comes from the upper lung fields, where the alveolar gas has a higher nitrogen concentration, thus resulting in a sudden increase in the nitrogen concentration toward the end of exhalation (phase IV).

The volume above residual volume where this increase in nitrogen concentration occurs is known as the "closing volume." The closing volume plus the residual volume is known as the "closing capacity" (Fig. 11-11). In early small airway obstruction the closing volume and closing capacity increase (*i.e.*, because of narrowing of the lumen of the airways, they "close" at a higher lung volume during exhalation). This is generally presented as the CV/VC ratio or the CC/TLC ratio. These variables of pulmonary function may be increased, indicating the presence of small airway obstructive disease, in the presence of a normal spirogram.[3] There is some evidence that the CC/TLC ratio is more sensitive than the CV/VC ratio in detecting obstructive airway disease.

Only a nitrogen meter and a method for determining lung volumes are needed for performing this test, which is not invasive. Although this procedure has been widely used for screening purposes in patients with potential obstructive pulmonary disease, its value and precise role have yet to be determined.

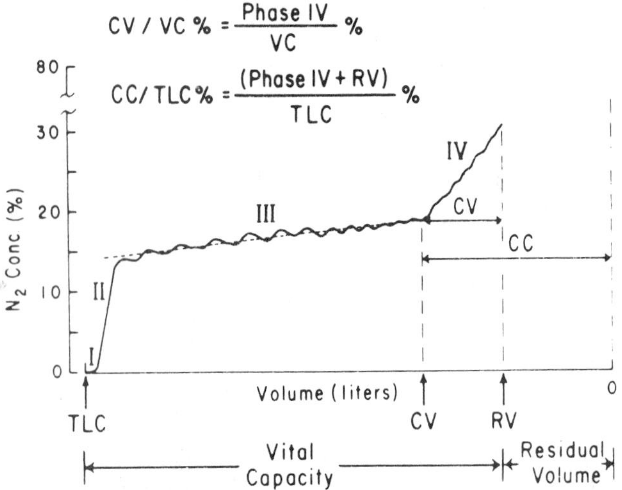

Fig. 11-11. Use of the single-breath nitrogen test to determine closing volume and closing capacity. (Buist AS, Ross BB: Quantitative analysis of the alveolar plateau in the diagnosis of early airway obstruction. Am Rev Respir Dis 108:1078, 1973

MAXIMAL RESPIRATORY PRESSURES

The maximal respiratory pressures that can be generated on inspiration and on expiration are excellent indicators of restrictive lung disease due to neuromuscular problems. These pressures may be markedly decreased in the presence of normal lung volumes and normal arterial blood gases. Pulmonary disability owing to such diseases as myasthenia gravis, Guillain–Barré syndrome, hypothyroidism, and amyotrophic lateral sclerosis may be best detected by the measurement of maximal respiratory pressure. An instrument known as a "bugle," developed at the Mayo Clinic, makes the testing of maximal respiratory pressures easily attainable (Fig. 11-12).[2]

SUSTAINED VENTILATORY CAPACITY

The maximal voluntary ventilation (MVV) has been used to measure a patient's ability to hyperventilate over a short period of time (see Chap. 10). Maximal respiratory pressures can be measured, as described above, to evaluate respiratory muscle strength. More recently, practitioners in rehabilitation medicine have become interested in determining respiratory muscle endurance, for example, the ability to hyperventilate for a sustained period.[11]

A system can be established that allows for eucapnic hyperventilation so that one can measure the "sustained ventilatory capacity." Such measurements have demonstrated the ability to enhance respiratory muscle endurance, and thus exercise performance, through specific training programs.[16]

VENTILATION/PERFUSION LUNG SCANS

Radioactive techniques have been developed that allow both qualitative and quantitative comparison of ventilation and lung perfusion. Inhalation of xenon, with radioactive scanning to determine the location of the inhaled xenon, and venous injection of radioactive materials such as xenon, technetium, and radioactive iodinated serum albumin allow for determination of the location of pulmonary ventilation and perfusion.

Uneven distribution of ventilation with air trapping can be readily detected by xenon inhalation. In patients with chronic obstructive pulmonary disorders, matching ventilation and perfusion defects throughout the lungs are typical. Pulmonary arterial obstruction (e.g., due to pulmonary embolism or tumor) can be detected as a perfusion defect. The $\dot{V}/\dot{Q}$ scan is perhaps most useful in diagnosing pulmonary emboli. A perfusion defect in an area of lung that has normal ventilation is highly suggestive of a pulmonary embolus (Fig. 11-13).

Ventilation/perfusion lung scans have replaced bronchospirometry in the differential evaluation of lung function. Quantification of the relative amount of ventilation or perfusion contributed by an area of lung can easily be determined. For example, postoperative lung function following a pneumonectomy may be accurately predicted by doing preoperative lung scans.[15] If 40% of the total lung perfusion is present in the left lung in a patient who is to undergo a left pneumonectomy for bronchogenic carcinoma, the predicted postoperative FEV_1 will be the preoperative FEV_1 times 0.6. This technique can be helpful in predicting the risk of pneumonectomy in a patient with pulmonary disease. For example, performing a pneumonectomy would be very risky if the predicted postoperative FEV_1 is less than 0.8 liters, since postoperative cardiorespiratory failure in such a patient occurs frequently.[7]

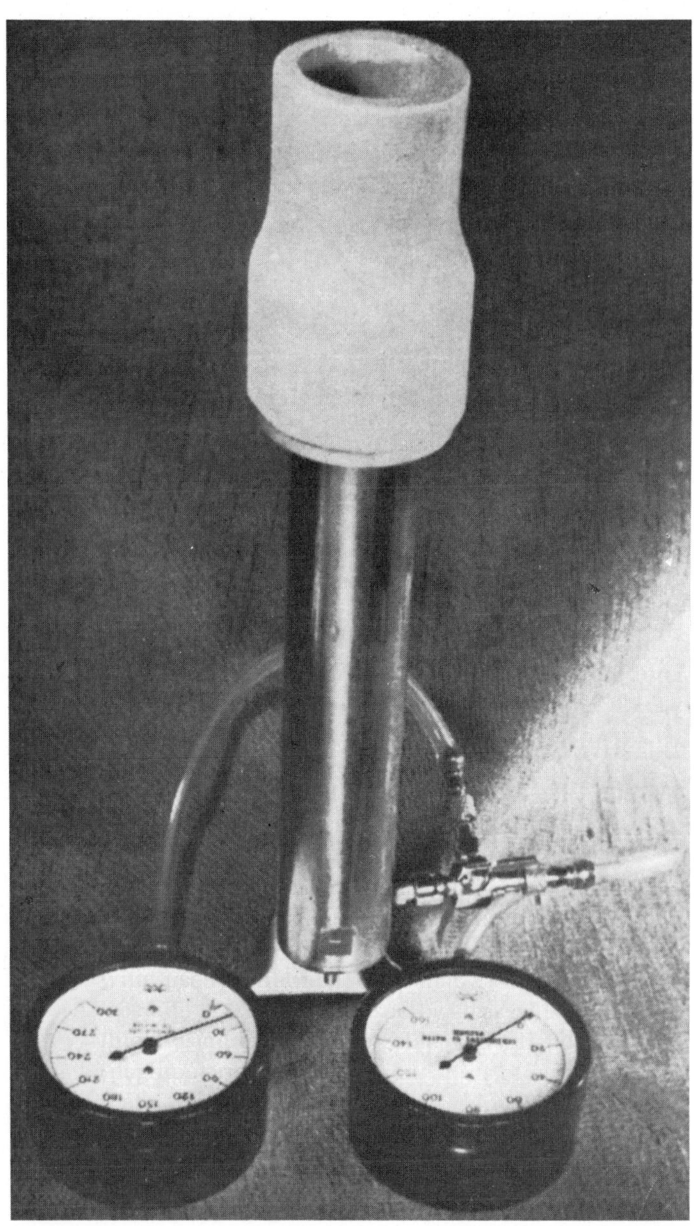

Fig. 11-12. This "bugle" is useful in determining maximal respiratory pressures. (Black LF, Hyatt RE: Maximal respiratory pressures: Normal values and relationship to age and sex. Am Rev Respir Dis 99:696, 1969)

EXERCISE TESTING

Exercise testing, measuring pulmonary as well as cardiac parameters, was previously confined to the research laboratory but has now become clinically relevant. Reasons for evaluating a person's exercise capability[1] include [1] to test fitness for work and vigorous sports; [2] to evaluate the functional status of the cardiovascular or pulmonary systems in health and disease, including the determination of present status, the prediction of the likelihood of developing cardiovascular disease, and the prognosis if the disease is already present; [3] to evaluate the effect of preventive, therapeutic, and rehabilitation programs, including the effects of medication, surgery, diet, and physical conditioning; and [4] to collect information helpful in outlining an exercise training program (*i.e.*, the "exercise prescription").

In the clinical arena the most common reason for performing exercise testing is to attempt to determine if coronary artery disease is present. Exercise testing, followed by an organized exercise training program, however, is becoming increasingly useful in the patient with pulmonary disease as well.

The major role for exercise testing in patients with chronic obstructive lung disease is to evaluate the patient before outlining a regular exercise schedule. Objective evidence of improved physical condition can be readily demonstrated in patients with chronic bronchitis and emphysema if they follow a program faithfully (see Chap. 27).

Generally the best overall indicator of cardiopulmonary health and physical fitness is a person's maximum oxygen uptake ($\dot{V}O_{2max}$). However, in some patients with cardiac or respiratory disease, it may be risky to perform "maximal" exercise; thus various submaximal exercise test regimens have been developed. From such data one can calculate the patient's presumed $\dot{V}O_{2max}$ on the basis of predictive formulas, or nomograms.[1]

One should have the appropriate equipment available for quality exercise testing. The indications and contraindications for testing, as well as the indications for stopping the test procedure, should be well known to any laboratory offering these tests. For a thorough review of exercise physiology and indications for and techniques of exercise testing, one should consult the literature.[1,10,17]

SLEEP STUDIES

An increasing awareness of episodes of hypoventilation and periodic apnea during sleep is developing. Complaints such as excessive daytime sleepiness, ir-

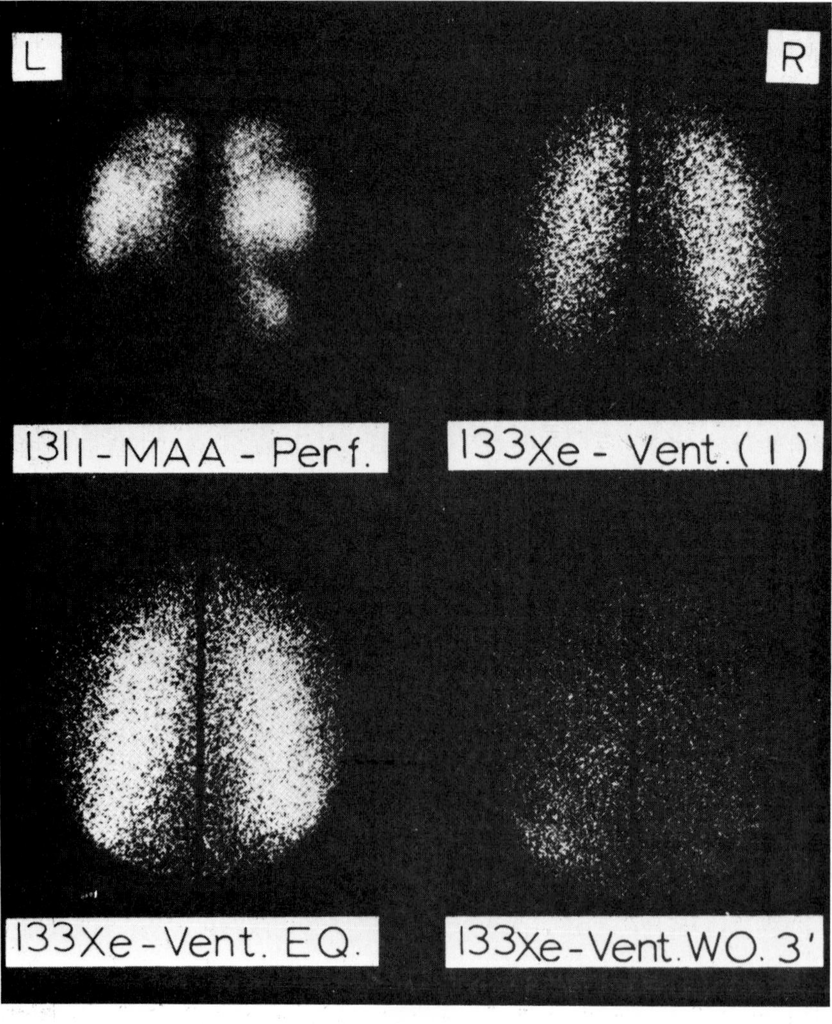

Fig. 11-13. Posterior view $\dot{V}/\dot{Q}$ scans in a patient with pulmonary embolism and a negative chest roentgenogram. Note multiple defects on a perfusion scan *(upper left)* with homogenous ventilation of these nonperfused zones (*upper right,* first breath; *lower left,* equilibrium). Modest delay in washout from small zones of left lower lobe *(lower right)* is seen, (Moser KM: Clinical applications of ventilation/perfusion scintiphotography. In Baum GL (ed) Textbook of Pulmonary Diseases, 2nd ed. Boston, Little, Brown, 1974)

ritability, and findings of unexplained polycythemia and cor pulmonale may be due to "sleep apnea." See Appendix C for a discussion of the methodology of sleep studies.

CONTROL OF VENTILATION

The factors that stimulate the ventilatory drive include hypoxemia, hypercapnia, and acidosis. Some patients partially or completely loose the ability to respond to these ventilatory stimuli. Although both the carotid bodies and the medullary chemoreceptor can respond to hypercapnia and acidosis, only the carotid bodies sense hypoxemia. A discussion of the methodology for testing ventilatory control is also provided in Appendix A.

SUMMARY

A proper use of the specialized pulmonary function tests discussed in this chapter will often help to clarify the diagnosis in a patient who presents with confusing signs and symptoms. These tests provide a valuable supplement to a careful history and physical examination in detecting and delineating respiratory diseases. Serial pulmonary function tests often help the physician and allied health personnel to follow objectively the course of a pulmonary disorder.

REFERENCES

1. Anderson KL et al: Fundamentals of Exercise Testing. Geneva, World Health Organization, 1971
2. Black LF, Hyatt RE: Maximal respiratory pressures: normal values and relationship to age and sex. Am Rev Respir Dis 99:696, 1969
3. Buist AS, Van Fleet DL, Ross BB: A comparison of conventional spirometric tests and the test of closing volume in an emphysema screening center. Am Rev Respir Dis 107:735, 1973
4. Finley JN, Swenson EW, Comroe JH Jr: The cause of arterial hypoxemia at rest in patients with 'alveolar-capillary block syndrome.' J Clin Invest 41:618, 1962
5. Fisher AB, DuBois AB, Hyde RW: Evaluation of the forced oscillation technique for the determination of resistance to breathing. J Clin Invest 47:2045, 1968
6. Forster RE: Diffusion of gases. In Fenn WO, and Rahn H (eds): Handbook of Physiology: Respiration I. Baltimore, Williams & Wilkins, 1964
7. Hodgkin JE: Evaluation before thoracotomy. West J Med 122:104, 1975
8. Hogg JC, Macklem PT, Thurlbeck WM: Site and nature of airway obstruction in chronic obstructive lung disease. N Engl J Med 278:1353, 1968
9. Hutcheon M et al: Volume of isoflow: A new test in detection of mild abnormalities of lung mechanics. Am Rev Respir Dis 110:458, 1974
10. Jones NL, Campbell EJ: Clinical Exercise Testing, 2nd ed. Philadelphia, WB Saunders, 1982
11. Keens TG et al: Ventilatory muscle endurance training in normal subjects and patients with cystic fibrosis. Am Rev Respir Dis 116:853, 1977
12. Miller RD, Hyatt RE: Obstructing lesions of the larynx and trachea: Clinical and physiologic characteristics. Mayo Clin Proc 44:145, 1969
13. Morris JF, Koski A, Breese JD: Normal values and evaluation of forced expiratory flow. Am Rev Respir Dis 111:755, 1975
14. Murray J et al: Early diagnosis of chronic obstructive lung disease. University of California, San Francisco (specialty conferences). Calif Med 116:37, 1972
15. Olsen GN, Block AJ, Tobias JA: Prediction of post-pneumonectomy pulmonary function using quantitative macroaggregate lung scanning. Chest 66:13, 1974
16. Sonne LJ, Davis JA: Increased exercise performance in patients with severe COPD following inspiratory resistive training. Chest 81:436, 1982
17. Wasserman K, Whipp BJ: Exercise physiology in health and disease, Am Rev Respir Dis 112:219, 1975

BIBLIOGRAPHY

General

Bates, DV, Macklem PT, Christie RV: Respiratory Function in Disease, 2nd ed. Philadelphia, WB Saunders, 1971

Cherniak RM: Pulmonary Function Testing. Philadelphia, WB Saunders, 1977

Comroe JH Jr et al: The Lung: Clinical Physiology and Pulmonary Function Tests, 2nd ed. Chicago, Year Book Medical Publishers, 1962

Fishman AP: Assessment of Pulmonary Function. New York, McGraw–Hill, 1980

West JB: Respiratory Physiology: The Essentials. Baltimore, Williams & Wilkins, 1974

Diffusing Capacity

Filley GF et al: Pulmonary gas transport. A mathematical model of the lung. Am Rev Respir Dis 98:480, 1968

Forster RE: Diffusion of gases. In Fenn WO, Rahn H (eds): Handbook of Physiology, Sect 3: Respiration, Vol. 1. Washington DC, American Physiological Society, 1964

Forster RE: Exchange of gases between alveolar air and pulmonary capillary blood: Pulmonary diffusing capacity. Physiol Rev 37:391, 1957

Krogh M: The diffusion of gases through the lungs of man. J Physiol 49:271, 1915

McNeill RS, Rankin J, Forster RE: The diffusing capacity of the pulmonary membrane and the pulmonary capillary blood volume in cardiopulmonary disease. Clin Sci 17:465, 1958

Murray J et al: Early diagnosis of chronic obstructive lung disease: University of California, San Francisco (specialty conferences). Calif Med 116:37, 1972

Ogilvie CM et al: A standardized breath holding technique for the clinical measurement of the diffusing capacity of the lung for carbon monoxide. J Clin Invest 36:1, 1957

Wagner PD, West JB: Effects of diffusion impairment on O_2 and CO_2 time courses in pulmonary capillaries. J Appl Physiol 33:62, 1972

Ventilation Indices

Becklake MR, Goldman HI: The influence of pulmonary dead space on lung mixing indices: S Afr J Med Sci 19:21, 1954

Bouhuys A, Lundin G: Distribution of inspired gas in lungs. Physiol Rev 39:731, 1959

Buist AS, Ross BB: Quantitative analysis of the alveolar plateau in the diagnosis of early airway obstruction. Am Rev Respir Dis 108:1078, 1973

Comroe JH Jr, Fowler WS: Lung function studies. VI. Detection of uneven alveolar ventilation during a single breath of oxygen; a new test of pulmonary disease. Am J Med 10:408, 1951

Fowler WS: Intrapulmonary distribution of inspired gas. Physiol Rev 32:1, 1952

Otis AB et al: Mechanical factors in distribution of pulmonary ventilation. J Appl Physiol 8:427, 1956

Rossier PH, Bühlmann A: The respiratory dead space. Physiol Rev 35:860, 1955

Flow-Volume Loop Analysis

Dosman J et al: The use of a helium-oxygen mixture during maximum expiratory flow to demonstrate obstruction in small airways in smokers. J Clin Invest 55:1090, 1975

Fry DL, Hyatt RE: Pulmonary mechanics: A unified analysis of the relationship between pressure, volume, and gas flow in the lungs of normal and diseased human subjects. Am J Med 29:672, 1960

Hutcheon M et al: Volume of isoflow: A new test in detection of mild abnormalities of lung mechanics. Am Rev Respir Dis 110:458, 1974

Hyatt RE, Black LF: The flow-volume curve: A current perspective. Am Rev Respir Dis 107:191, 1973

Hyatt RE, Schilder DP, Fry DL: Relationship between maximum expiratory flow and degree of lung inflation. J Appl Physiol 13:331, 1958

Miller RD, Hyatt RE: Obstructing lesions of the larynx and trachea: Clinical and physiologic characteristics. Mayo Clin Proc 44:145, 1969

Takishima T et al: Flow-volume curves during quiet breathing, maximum voluntary ventilation, and forced vital capacities in patients with obstructive lung disease. Scand J Respir Dis 48:384, 1967

Mechanics of Breathing

Campbell EJM, Agostoni E, Newsom–Davis Jr: The Respiratory Muscles: Mechanics and Neural Control. Philadelphia, WB Saunders, 1970

DuBois AB, Botelho SY, Comroe JH Jr: A new method for measuring airway resistance in man using a body plethysmograph: values in normal subjects and in patients with respiratory disease. J Clin Invest 35:327, 1956

Fisher AB, DuBois AB, Hyde RW: Evaluation of the forced oscillation technique for the determination of resistance to breathing. J Clin Invest 47:2045, 1968

Mead J: Mechanical properties of lungs. Physiol Rev 41:281, 1961

Rah H et al: The pressure-volume diagram of the thorax and lung. Am J Physiol 146:161, 1946

Schilder DP, Hyatt RE, Fry DL: An improved balloon system for measuring intraesophageal pressure. J Appl Physiol 14:1057, 1959

Vincent NJ et al: Factors influencing pulmonary resistance. J Appl Physiol 29:236, 1970

Woolcock AJ, Vincent NJ, Macklem PT: Frequency dependence of compliance as a test for obstruction in small airways. J Clin Invest 48:1079, 1969

Closing Volume

Buist AS, Ross BB: Predicted values for closing volumes using a modified single breath nitrogen test. Am Rev Respir Dis 107:744, 1973

Buist AS, Ross BB: Quantitative analysis of the alveolar plateau in the diagnosis of early airway obstruction. Am Rev Respir Dis 108:1078, 1973

Buist AS, Van Fleet DL, Ross BB: A comparison of conventional spirometric tests and the test of closing volume in an emphysema screening center. Am Rev Respir Dis 107:735, 1973

Hyatt RE, Rodarte JR: "Closing volume," one man's noise—other men's experiment. Mayo Clin Proc 50:17, 1975

McCarthy DS et al: Measurement of "closing volume" as a simple and sensitive test for early detection of small airway disease. Am J Med 52:747, 1972

Maximal Respiratory Pressures

Black LF, Hyatt RE: Maximal respiratory pressure: Normal values and relationship to age and sex. Am Rev Respir Dis 99:696, 1969

Black LF, Hyatt RE: Maximal static respiratory pressures in generalized neuromuscular disease. Am Rev Respir Dis 103:641, 1971

Byrd RB, Hyatt RE: Maximal respiratory pressures in chronic obstructive lung disease. Am Rev Respir Dis 98:848, 1968

Sustained Ventilatory Capacity

Belman MJ, Mittman C: Ventilatory muscle training improves exercise capacity in chronic obstructive pulmonary disease patients. Am Rev Respir Dis 121:273, 1980

Keens TG et al: Ventilatory muscle endurance training in normal subjects and patients with cystic firbrosis. Am Rev Respir Dis 116:853, 1977

Sonne LJ, Davis JA: Increased exercise performance in patients with severe COPD following inspiratory resistive training. Chest 81:436, 1982

Ventilation/Perfusion Lung Scans

Bates DV, Ball WC Jr, Bryan AC: Use of xenon^{133} in studying the ventilation and perfusion of the lung. Dynamic Clinical Studies With Radioisotopes. U.S. Atomic Energy Commission, 1964

Hodgkin JE: Evaluation before thoracotomy. West J Med 122:104, 1975

Moser KM: Clinical applications of ventilation/perfusion scintiphotography. In Baum GL (ed): Textbook of Pulmonary Diseases, 2nd ed. Boston, Little, Brown & Co, 1974

Moser KM et al: Correlation of lung photoscans with pulmonary angiography in pulmonary embolism. Am J Cardiol 18:810, 1966

Olsen GN, Block AJ, Tobias JA: Prediction of post-pneumonectomy pulmonary function using quantitative macroaggregate lung scanning. Chest 66:13, 1974

Sabiston DC Jr, Wagner HN Jr: The diagnosis of pulmonary embolism by radioisotope scanning. Ann Surg 160:575, 1964

West JB: Pulmonary function studies with radioactive gases. Annu Rev Med 18:459, 1967

Exercise Testing

Andersen KL et al: Fundamentals of Exercise Testing. Geneva, World Health Organization, 1971
Jones NL, Campbell EJ: Clinical Exercise Testing, 2nd ed. Philadelphia, WB Saunders, 1982

Sleep Studies

Block AJ et al: Sleep apnea, hypopnea, and oxygen desaturation in normal subjects. N Engl J Med 300:513, 1979
Guilleminault C, Tilkian A, Dement WC: The sleep apnea syndromes. Ann Rev Med 27:465, 1976
Phillipson EA: Regulation of breathing during sleep. Am Rev Respir Dis (Suppl)115:217, 1977

Control of Ventilation

Kelsen SG, Fishman AP: Clinical assessment of the regulation of ventilation. In Fishman AP (ed): Assessment of Pulmonary Function. New York, McGraw–Hill, 1980
Severinghaus JW: Proposed standard determination of ventilatory responses to hypoxia and hypercapnia in man. Chest (Suppl)70:129, 1976
Whitelow WA, Derenne J, Milic–Emili J: Occlusion pressure as a measure of respiratory center output in conscious man. Respir Physiol 23:181, 1974

12

Blood Gas Analysis and Acid–Base Physiology

John E. Hodgkin • Clarence A. Collier

The evaluation of oxygenation and acid–base status in critically ill patients is crucial to their proper management. Treating patients in acute respiratory failure without examining arterial blood gas values is akin to treating patients in diabetic coma without utilizing blood glucose values. Arterial samples for analysis must be obtained because peripheral venous samples may be grossly misleading with regard to adequacy of oxygenation and acid–base balance. It is impossible to properly manage patients who require assisted ventilation without using arterial blood gas data.

The proper technique for performing arterial punctures can be easily learned by respiratory therapists and nurses, so that physicians need not be available to obtain samples. Proper maintenance of equipment with accurate calibration and performance of quality control is essential, however, to assure valid results.

ARTERIAL PUNCTURE

Arterial blood samples may be drawn from multiple sites. Samples are most commonly obtained from the radial artery, brachial artery, or femoral artery. It is important to consider the availability of collateral circulation when selecting a site for arterial puncture. Both the radial and brachial arteries normally have excellent collateral blood flow; however, there is a marked lack of collateral flow if the femoral artery becomes obstructed in the area just below the inguinal ligament. Since radial artery puncture is relatively safe and the radial artery is the most easily accessible site for drawing arterial blood, this site is preferable.

The Allen test as originally described involves occluding the radial artery at the wrist for 3 minutes and noting if there is any change in color of the palmar epithelium.[2] If no change in color occurs, circulation is sufficient through the ulnar artery. Next, the ulnar artery is occluded for 3 minutes, with the color of the hand again being noted. Blanching of the hand would suggest radial artery occlusion. A modification of this test is used commonly today.[8] After the patient has made a fist to force blood from the hand, pressure is applied to compress both the ulnar and radial arteries. When the hand is relaxed, the palm and fingers are blanched. Obstructing pressure is then removed from the ulnar artery while the radial artery remains compressed. If the ulnar artery is patent, the hand should quickly become flushed within 10 to 15 seconds. If this does not occur, radial artery puncture should be avoided in that wrist. Once adequate collateral circulation has been demonstrated, the patient is prepared for puncture of the radial artery.

The patient's arm should be positioned comfortably, using a rolled or folded towel to hyperextend the radial or brachial site. The skin surface should be cleansed thoroughly (e.g., with 70% isopropyl alcohol) before the arterial puncture.

Using a disposable 3-ml syringe with a 25-gauge, ⅝ inch long needle, 0.8 ml to 1.0 ml of 2% xylocaine can be injected around the artery to achieve surface and subcutaneous anesthesia, provided the patient gives no history of allergy to local anesthesia. The use of a local anesthetic is not essential in many cases but may relieve apprehensiveness or be helpful in reducing arterial vasospasm if difficulty in obtaining an arterial sample is anticipated.

About 1 ml of heparin (sodium heparin with a concentration of 1000 units/ml) should be drawn into a 5-ml or 10-ml glass syringe, using a 21-gauge, 1-inch short-bevel needle. Once the syringe has been lubricated with heparin, all excess heparin should be expelled. For the arterial puncture, plastic syringes may be used; however, the barrel on a glass syringe slides much more readily while the sample is being obtained, making it easier for blood to flow into the syringe under its own pressure. Newer designs in disposable plastic syringes have minimized their disadvantages.

The syringe should be held much as one holds a pencil, with the needle bevel facing cephalad; the skin should be punctured at approximately a 45° angle. The position of the artery should be determined using the fingers of the opposite hand.

The needle is then advanced slowly through the skin into the subcutaneous tissue. If the needle is advanced too rapidly, it may pass through the artery without blood being obtained. As soon as the needle enters the artery, blood will readily fill the syringe. With the needle in the artery a pulsation should be visualized. If no pulsation is present, one should suspect that the needle is in a vein rather than in an artery.

About 3 ml to 4 ml of blood should be obtained. When the needle is withdrawn, a folded 4- × 4-inch gauze should be placed over the site and pressure applied for about 5 minutes (longer if the patient is anticoagulated or has a bleeding disorder). If any bleeding occurs at the end of this time, pressure should be maintained until no further bleeding occurs. A protective gauze strip can be placed around the wrist and an elastic bandage then placed *part way* around the wrist to continue pressure on the puncture site.

Any air bubbles in the syringe should be expelled immediately from the sample. The syringe should then be capped, placed in a cup of crushed ice, and delivered immediately to the blood gas laboratory for proper analysis.

The reader is referred to Appendix B for methods of blood gas measurement.

MEASUREMENTS OF OXYGENATION

Numerous factors can be evaluated to determine whether tissue oxygenation is adequate. Each of these measurements yields information helpful in managing the patient properly. A thorough understanding of the significance of each of these factors, as well as a knowledge of their limitations, is critical.

OXYGEN TENSION

The partial pressure of oxygen, created by the random collision of molecules of the gas, may be readily measured. This tension may be measured in inspired gas ($P_{I_{O_2}}$), arterial blood ($P_{a_{O_2}}$), venous blood ($P_{\bar{v}_{O_2}}$), and capillary blood ($P_{c_{O_2}}$). Formulas for calculating $P_{I_{O_2}}$ are given below.

1. Dry gas formula:

$$P_{I_{O_2}} = P_B \times F_{I_{O_2}},$$

where P_B = barometric pressure and $F_{I_{O_2}}$ = the fractional concentration of inspired oxygen. At sea level the $P_{I_{O_2}}$ for room air (i.e., 21% oxygen) would be

$$P_{I_{O_2}} = 760 \text{ mm Hg} \times 0.21 = 159 \text{ mm Hg}.$$

2. Humidified gas formula:

$$P_{I_{O_2}} = (P_B - \text{water vapor pressure}) \times F_{I_{O_2}}.$$

For room air at sea level,

$$P_{I_{O_2}} = (760 \text{ mm Hg} - 47 \text{ mm Hg}) \times 0.21$$
$$= 149 \text{ mm Hg in humidified room air with a normal water vapor pressure.}$$

The $P_{a_{O_2}}$ is a measure of the partial pressure of oxygen dissolved in the plasma of arterial blood and may be reported in either mm Hg or torr.* The $P_{a_{O_2}}$ is

*The units mm Hg and torr may be used interchangeably when referring to partial pressure of gases within the earth's atmosphere; the difference between the two is so small as to be negligible.

the most important determinant of the amount of oxygen that binds to hemoglobin (see below).

The alveolar oxygen tension (PA_{O_2}) may be calculated from the alveolar air equation as follows:

$$PA_{O_2} = PI_{O_2} - \frac{PA_{CO_2}}{R} + \left[PA_{CO_2} \times FI_{O_2} \times \frac{1 - R}{R}\right]$$

This is valid if there is no CO_2 in the inspired gas. R represents the ratio of CO_2 production to O_2 uptake. Since the term in square brackets is a small correction factor (2 mm Hg when $FI_{O_2} = 0.21$, $PA_{CO_2} = 40$ mm Hg, and $R = 0.8$), and Pa_{CO_2} is assumed to be equivalent to PA_{CO_2}, many reduce the formula to the following.

$$PA_{O_2} = PI_{O_2} - \frac{Pa_{CO_2}}{R}.$$

If R = 0.8, then this becomes

$$Pa_{O_2} = PI_{O_2} - Pa_{CO_2} \times 1.25^*$$

Others present the alveolar air equation as follows (assuming PA_{CO_2} is equal to Pa_{CO_2}).

$$PA_{O_2} = PI_{O_2} - Pa_{CO_2}\left[\frac{1}{R} - FI_{O_2} \times \frac{1 - R}{R}\right]$$

This can be rewritten as

$$PA_{O_2} = PI_{O_2} - Pa_{CO_2}\left[FI_{O_2} + \frac{1 - FI_{O_2}}{R}\right].$$

Assuming an R of 0.8, while the patient breathes room air, the equation simplifies to

$$PA_{O_2} = PI_{O_2} - Pa_{CO_2} \times 1.20.^*$$

PI_{O_2} may be calculated using the gas formulas above and Pa_{CO_2} measured directly.

Calculation of alveolar P_{O_2} allows one to determine the *alveolar–arterial oxygen difference* [P(A-a)O_2]. The Pa_{O_2} "normally" decreases with age as a result of increasing ventilation/perfusion imbalance with normal aging.

The normal Pa_{O_2} for a person breathing room air may be predicted using the following formulas.

Predicted Pa_{O_2} (ages 14–84, supine)[14]

$$= 103.5 - (0.42 \times \text{age}) \pm 4.$$

*This factor changes slightly with changes in FI_{O_2}.

Table 12-1. Normal, Supine, Pa_{O_2}, and P(A-a)O_2 Values (Sea Level)

AGE *yr*	Pa_{O_2} *mm Hg*	P(A-a)O_2 *mm Hg*
20	96–104	<5
30	92–100	<9
40	88–96	<13
50	84–92	<17
60	79–87	<22
70	75–83	<26
80	71–79	<30
90	66–74	<35

This was the formula from Sorbini's data, at 500-m elevation. When the data are corrected for a barometric pressure of 760 mm Hg, the formula for predicting the normal Pa_{O_2} at sea level becomes

$$109 - (0.43 \times \text{age}) \pm 4.$$

The predicted Pa_{O_2}, according to Mellemgaard, (ages 15–75, seated)[10]

$$= 104.2 - (0.27 \times \text{age}) \pm 6.$$

Table 12-1 gives examples of age-predicted Pa_{O_2}. Since the Pa_{O_2} decreases with age, then the alveolar–arterial oxygen difference increases with age. It is invalid to assume that the standard normal Pa_{O_2} is 80 to 100 mm Hg and the normal P(A-a)O_2 is 10 to 15 mm Hg, since these "normal" values do not take age into account. From the above formulas, it should also be recognized that the Pa_{O_2} is usually lower when the patient is supine than when upright.

It is sometimes useful to determine the a/A O_2 ratio (Pa_{O_2}/PA_{O_2}).[7] Whereas the P(A-a)O_2 varies as the FI_{O_2} is changed, the a/A O_2 ratio remains relatively stable. One can, therefore, use the a/A O_2 ratio as an index to the status of lung function when the oxygen concentration being delivered to the patient is altered (see Equations and "Rules of Thumb" for Management of Patients in Appendix D for examples of using the a/A O_2 ratio).

OXYGEN SATURATION

Oxygen saturation is a measurement of the amount of oxygen bound to hemoglobin compared to hemoglobin's maximum capability for binding oxygen.

$$O_2 \text{ saturation} = \frac{\text{ml } O_2 \text{ bound to hemoglobin} \times 100}{\text{maximum ml } O_2 \text{ hemoglobin is capable of binding}}$$

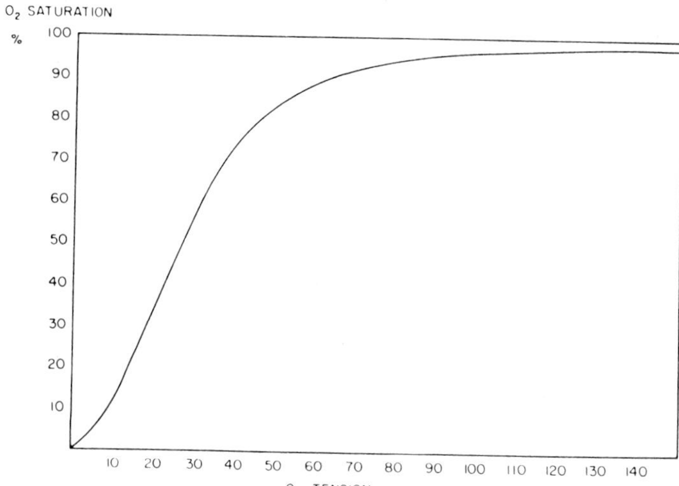

Fig. 12-1. Oxyhemoglobin dissociation curve, showing relationships between P_{O_2} and O_2 saturation. (Bates DV, Macklem PT, Christie RV: Respiratory Function in Disease, 2nd ed. Philadelphia, WB Saunders, 1971)

The O_2 saturation is expressed as a percentage, with normal being equal to or greater than 96%.*

The characteristic relation between P_{O_2} and O_2 saturation is known as the oxygen dissociation curve (Fig. 12-1). This relationship is described by an S-shaped curve. At higher oxygen tensions the curve is relatively flat, whereas at lower oxygen tensions the curve becomes quite steep.

The flat part of the oxyhemoglobin dissociation curve is an advantage in the lung, where, despite significant drops in alveolar oxygen tension, the hemoglobin in the pulmonary capillaries will bind oxygen almost to full capacity. For example, the PA_{O_2}, and thus the Pa_{O_2}, may drop significantly because of obstructive airway disease; however, unless the Pa_{O_2} is below about 60 mm Hg, the O_2 saturation in the blood that leaves the pulmonary capillary will be almost normal.

The steep portion of the curve is an advantage at the tissue level, where small decrements in P_{O_2} result in a rapid release of oxygen by hemoglobin, characterized by a rapidly decreasing O_2 saturation. In other words, as oxygen tension drops at the tissue site, the hemoglobin molecule readily releases oxygen to make it available for tissue use. The Pa_{O_2} is a more sensitive indicator of mild hypoxemia than is O_2 saturation, since the upper portion of the curve is relatively flat.

*The O_2 saturation may be somewhat lower, normally, as the Pa_{O_2} decreases below 80 mm Hg with aging. For example, for a Pa_{O_2} of 70 mm Hg, the normal O_2 saturation at a normal pH would be about 93%.

P_{50} MEASUREMENT

It has been recognized for many years that multiple factors may shift the position of the oxygen dissociation curve. As a general rule those factors that shift the curve to the right are an advantage to the patient, since a rightward shift indicates a reduced affinity of hemoglobin for oxygen, resulting in an increased release of oxygen to the tissues. A shift to the left indicates that hemoglobin's affinity for oxygen is increased, so that hemoglobin does not release oxygen normally at the tissue site.

The P_{50} measurement is a way of expressing the position of the oxygen dissociation curve and is defined as the P_{O_2} at 50% saturation and at a pH of 7.40, P_{CO_2} of 40 mm Hg, and temperature of 37°C. Normally, the P_{50} is about 26.5 mm Hg. An increased P_{50} (e.g., P_{50} of 30 mm Hg) would indicate that the oxygen dissociation curve is shifted to the right (Fig. 12-2).

Factors known to shift the curve to the right include chronic hypoxemia, acidosis, hypercapnia, and fever. Alkalemia, hypocapnia, and hypothermia shift the curve to the left. Changes in pH, P_{CO_2}, and temperature affect hemoglobin's affinity for oxygen but will not affect the P_{50} measurement, if, as is standard, the P_{50} is determined with the blood at a normal pH, P_{CO_2}, and temperature. Some do calculate the P_{50} at the patient's temperature, P_{CO_2}, and pH that exist in the blood sample (*in vivo* P_{50}).

The importance of *2,3-diphosphoglycerate* (2,3-DPG), a red-cell phosphate enzyme affecting hemoglobin's affinity for oxygen, is well recognized. If the level of 2,3-DPG increases in the red blood cell, hemoglobin's affinity for oxygen is decreased, thus making more oxygen available to the tissue. This is a com-

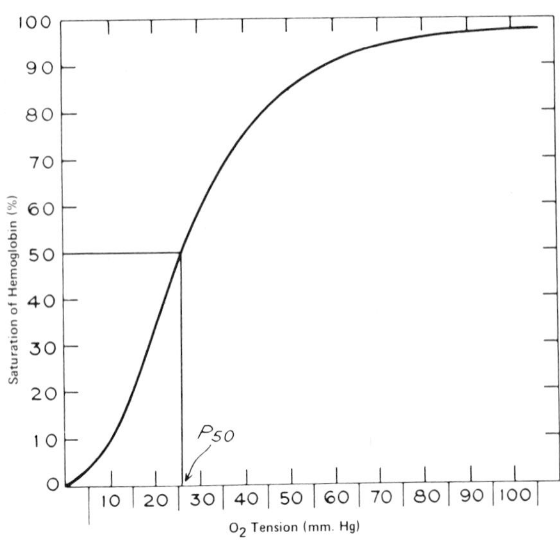

Fig. 12-2. Oxyhemoglobin dissociation curve depicting the P_{50} (P_{O_2} at 50% O_2 saturation). The P_{50} is normally approximately 26.5 mm Hg (Comroe JH Jr: Physiology of Respiration. Chicago, Year Book Medical Publishers, 1974. Data of Severinghaus JW: J Appl Phys 21:1108, 1966)

pensatory mechanism by which tissue oxygenation can be aided in the face of hypoxemia. Hypoxia results in an increased 2,3-DPG level in the red blood cell, thus increasing oxygen release from hemoglobin. This is one of the methods by which humans adapt to the hypoxia of high altitude.

Pyruvic kinase deficiency and thyrotoxicosis also result in an increased 2,3-DPG level, decreasing hemoglobin's affinity for oxygen. A decrease in 2,3-DPG levels, such as occurs in hexokinase deficiency and myxedema, results in a shift of the oxygen dissociation curve to the left (*i.e.*, decreased P_{50}).

Blood preserved in acid citrate dextrose (ACD) loses most of its red cell 2,3-DPG within several days, whereas blood preserved in citrate phosphate dextrose (CPD) maintains its 2,3-DPG levels for weeks.[12] Thus ACD-preserved blood more than several days old when transfused raises the hemoglobin level and oxygen-carrying capability; however, the hemoglobin in these red cells does not release oxygen to the tissues normally for the first 18 to 24 hours after infusion.

Certain congenital hemoglobinopathies also result in a shift of the oxygen dissociation curve. For example, hemoglobin Kansas shifts the curve to the right, resulting in improved oxygen release to the tissues. On the other hand, hemoglobin Rainier shifts the curve to the left, resulting in impaired oxygen release. Patients with hemoglobins that shift the curve to the right may present with anemia, whereas patients with hemoglobins resulting in a decreased P_{50} may present with polycythemia. When carbon monoxide binds to hemoglobin (carboxyhemoglobin), the curve is also shifted to the left.

Fetal hemoglobin (hemoglobin F) results in a curve that is markedly shifted to the left. It helps the fetus to obtain oxygen from the mother during intrauterine life. However, fetal hemoglobin rapidly disappears after birth; otherwise oxygen release from hemoglobin to the tissues would be grossly impaired. Table 12-2 provides a list of factors that shift the oxygen dissociation curve.

The P_{50} can be calculated from blood gases and O_2 saturation from a single sample of blood, without tonometry, with results within 2 mm Hg of standard P_{50} measurements when the O_2 saturation in the sample is between 20% and 90%.[1,6]

OXYGEN CONTENT

The O_2 content, although often not reported by the laboratory, is really more important than the Pa_{O_2} or O_2 saturation, since it is a quantitative measure of the amount of oxygen present in the blood. It is reported as "ml of oxygen per 100 ml of whole blood" or as "volumes percent." There are two components to the oxygen content.

1. The amount of oxygen dissolved in plasma: $P_{O_2} \times 0.003$ = ml O_2 dissolved per 100 ml whole blood
2. The amount of oxygen bound to hemoglobin: Hemoglobin G% × 1.39* × O_2 saturation = ml O_2 bound to hemoglobin

Calculation of the normal O_2 content for arterial blood with a Pa_{O_2} of 100 mm Hg, a hemoglobin of 15

*The factor 1.34 has been used for many years; however, current data suggest that 1.39 is more valid.[9]

Table 12-2. Factors that Shift the Oxygen Dissociation Curve

TO THE LEFT	TO THE RIGHT
Alkalosis	Acidosis
Hypocapnia	Hypercapnia
↓ 2,3-DPG	Fever
Hexokinase deficiency	↑ 2,3-DPG
Myxedema	Pyruvic kinase deficiency
ACD-preserved bank blood	Thyrotoxicosis
Certain congenital hemoglobinopathies (*e.g.*, hemoglobin Rainier)	Hypoxia
Fetal hemoglobin	Anemia
Carboxyhemoglobin	Certain congenital hemoglobinopathies (*e.g.*, hemoglobin Kansas)

G%, and an oxygen saturation of 98% would be as follows.

1. The amount of oxygen dissolved in the plasma:
   $100 \times 0.003 = 0.3$ ml O_2 per 100 ml blood
2. 15 G% $\times$ 1.39 $\times$ 0.98 = 20.4 ml O_2 bound to hemoglobin per 100 ml blood:
   O_2 content = 0.3 + 20.4 = 20.7 ml O_2 per 100 ml whole blood

Normally the tissues as a whole extract only about 25% of the oxygen carried in the arterial blood. The normal venous O_2 content is about 15 ml O_2/100 ml blood. One of the mechanisms by which tissues cope with hypoxemia or with increased oxygen demand is to increase the amount of oxygen extracted from the blood. However, some tissues have less capability for increasing extraction than others. The heart normally extracts 60% to 70% of the O_2 in the coronary arterial blood. The skeletal muscles extract about 40% of the O_2 available to them at rest, the brain 30%, and the kidneys 6%. During maximal exercise only about 25% of the oxygen content of arterial blood returns to the heart (*i.e.*, mixed venous O_2 content is about 5 ml O_2/100 ml blood).

Measurements of O_2 content are particularly important in the conditions described below.

Anemia

An anemic patient may have a normal Pa_{O_2} and O_2 saturation and be suffering from tissue hypoxia because of the reduced oxygen carrying capacity resulting from severe anemia.

Carbon Monoxide Poisoning

Carbon monoxide binds to hemoglobin with an affinity 210 times greater than that of oxygen. In this situation the Pa_{O_2} may be relatively normal, yet the patient would suffer from tissue hypoxia because of the reduced O_2 saturation and O_2 content. If the O_2 saturation is calculated (using a "normal" oxygen dissociation curve) from a measured Pa_{O_2}, both the reported O_2 saturation and O_2 content values will be incorrect in a patient with carbon monoxide poisoning. As mentioned earlier, carboxyhemoglobin also results in a leftward shift of the oxygen dissociation curve, which further contributes to tissue hypoxia.

Methemoglobinemia and Sulfhemoglobinemia

As mentioned earlier, abnormal types of hemoglobin result in an inability of hemoglobin to bind oxygen. Again the Pa_{O_2} may be relatively normal, and yet the patient will have significant tissue hypoxia because of the reduced O_2 saturation and O_2 content. Here also, unless the O_2 saturation is measured directly, one will calculate a falsely high O_2 content.

Figure 12-3 is a diagrammatic representation of the effect of shifts of the oxygen dissociation curve on O_2 content and the amount of oxygen available to the tissues. A reduced P_{50} results in an increased O_2 content in the venous blood, indicating that less oxygen has been released to the tissue.

MIXED VENOUS P_{O_2} ($P\bar{v}_{O_2}$)

Of equal importance to the O_2 content in terms of oxygen delivery to the tissues is the cardiac output.

$$O_2 \text{ delivery} = O_2 \text{ content} \times \text{cardiac output}$$

An arterial blood sample can provide data with regard to the Pa_{O_2}, O_2 saturation, P_{50}, and O_2 content. It does *not*, however, provide information on cardiac output, effectiveness of tissue perfusion, and quantity of oxygen being extracted by the tissues.

The measurement of P_{O_2} in a blood sample taken from the pulmonary artery ($P\bar{v}_{O_2}$) gives perhaps the best overall indicator of the adequacy of tissue oxygenation. At rest the normal $P\bar{v}_{O_2}$ is 35 to 40 torr. A value less then 35 torr in a critically ill patient suggests that oxygen extraction is increased and tissue oxygen delivery may be inadequate. One must then look at the multiple factors involved in oxygenation to determine the cause for the tissue hypoxia. An arterial–venous O_2 content difference greater than 5 vol %

would similarly suggest that delivery of oxygen to the tissues may be inadequate. Measurement of P_{O_2} in a peripheral venous sample provides information relating only to the adequacy of oxygenation in the tissue being drained by that particular venous system. Measurement of P_{O_2} in a sample obtained through a central venous catheter in the superior vena cava may also give misleading information since, in critically ill patients, the P_{O_2} in blood samples from this area tends to be somewhat higher than the true mixed venous P_{O_2} ($P\bar{v}_{O_2}$) of blood taken from the pulmonary artery.[11]

Blood may be easily sampled from the pulmonary artery through a flotation-type, balloon-tipped catheter such as a Swan–Ganz catheter. This type of catheter is frequently used in the care of critically ill patients so that left ventricular function may be carefully monitored with "wedge pressure" measurements. Cardiac output may also be measured with the use of these catheters, using dye dilution or thermal dilution techniques.

In patients with the adult respiratory distress syndrome (see Chap. 36), the implementation of positive end-expiratory pressure (PEEP) along with mechanical ventilation can be life-saving; however, PEEP can occasionally reduce cardiac output. In such patients the introduction of PEEP might result in actual worsening of tissue oxygen delivery. If the Pa_{O_2} improves with the introduction of PEEP but the $P\bar{v}_{O_2}$ decreases, worsening of tissue oxygenation has occurred because of reduced cardiac output. The optimal level of PEEP ("best PEEP") may be chosen by selecting the amount of PEEP that results in the highest $P\bar{v}_{O_2}$.[15] The $P\bar{v}_{O_2}$ can also be very helpful in determining the amount of supplemental oxygen needed (i.e., the FI_{O_2} needed to provide satisfactory oxygenation of the tissues). One should remember that the $P\bar{v}_{O_2}$ represents a sample of blood from all perfused organs of the body. Some organs may be hypoxic despite a normal $P\bar{v}_{O_2}$.

Finally, if tissue metabolism is markedly reduced, as occurs in cyanide poisoning (which inhibits cytochrome oxidase), the difference between arterial and venous O_2 content and P_{O_2} narrows, even though severe cellular hypoxia is present.

CAUSES OF HYPOXEMIA

The measurement of Pa_{O_2} is commonly used to determine whether hypoxemia is present. However, hypoxemia properly refers to low O_2 concentration in the blood. Arterial O_2 content may be normal despite a reduced Pa_{O_2} if the hemoglobin is increased. On the other hand, the O_2 content may be significantly reduced from anemia despite a normal Pa_{O_2}. *Hypoxemia and tissue hypoxia are not the same thing;* tissue hypoxia may be present despite a normal arterial O_2 content.

An obvious cause for reduced arterial oxygen tension is a decreased PI_{O_2}. This is most commonly related to living at high altitude. When patients with pulmonary disease are discharged from a hospital located at low altitude (e.g., sea level) and return to their homes at a higher altitude (e.g., 5000-ft elevation), their arterial P_{O_2} may drop significantly. This must be kept in mind when determining whether supplemental oxygen will be needed for the patient at discharge. Furthermore, the PI_{O_2} in pressurized aircraft is equivalent to that found at approximately 5000 to 8000-ft elevations, and this must be taken into account should the patient plan to travel in airplanes.

If one eliminates altitude there are basically four causes for hypoxemia, discussed below.

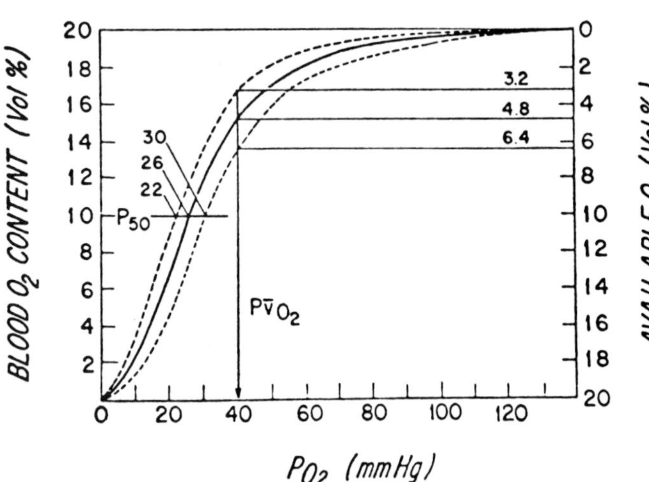

Fig. 12-3. Effect of shifts of the O_2 dissociation curve on O_2 content and the amount of oxygen available to the tissues. The isopleths represent different P_{50} values, ranging from 22 to 30 mm Hg. A reduced P_{50} is associated with an increased O_2 content in the venous blood, indicating that less oxygen has been released to the tissue (low A-V O_2 difference). (Snider GL: Clinical Interpretations of Blood Gases. Audiographic Series, Vol 1. American College of Chest Physicians)

Overall Hypoventilation

The minute ventilation may be decreased as a result of a reduction in tidal volume, slowing of respiratory rate, or both. Alveolar ventilation drops as a result of the decreased minute ventilation, resulting in hypoxemia. The differential diagnosis of factors that produce hypoventilation includes respiratory center depression owing to drug overdose, effect of anesthesia during the early postoperative period, excessive postoperative analgesia, the Pickwickian syndrome, thoracic deformities such as kyphoscoliosis and rheumatoid spondylitis, and neuromuscular disturbances.

Ventilation/Perfusion ($\dot{V}/\dot{Q}$) Mismatch

$\dot{V}/\dot{Q}$ mismatch is the most common cause of hypoxemia. When units of lung are underventilated with respect to their perfusion (low $\dot{V}/\dot{Q}$), the pulmonary capillary blood that leaves these units is underoxygenated, and hypoxemia results. Examples include bronchospasm, mucoid obstruction of the airway with resultant atelectasis, obstruction of airways associated with chronic bronchitis, and emphysema, pneumonia, and pulmonary edema. High $\dot{V}/\dot{Q}$ units do not directly cause hypoxemia, since the blood perfusing these units becomes well oxygenated.

Diffusion Defect

The alveolar–capillary membrane may occasionally be thickened to the extent that diffusion is reduced enough to result in hypoxemia. This is unusual, however, since normally at rest the hemoglobin in the pulmonary capillary is fully saturated by the time the blood is one third of the way past the alveolus. The alveolar–capillary membrane can be widened significantly without resting hypoxemia occurring. In most interstitial lung diseases (e.g., sarcoidosis, pulmonary fibrosis, and interstitial pneumonitis), hypoxemia is due to $\dot{V}/\dot{Q}$ mismatch rather than to diffusion defect. It is therefore a misnomer to refer to these diseases as "alveolar–capillary block syndrome."

Shunt

Anatomic right-to-left shunts such as the tetralogy of Fallot and pulmonary arteriovenous fistulas result in hypoxemia. Physiologic shunts that are correctable with proper respiratory care also cause hypoxemia; for example, in lobar atelectasis resulting from a mucus plug obstruction, if the collapsed area of lung continues to be perfused, this functions as a shunt (*i.e.*, the blood does not come in contact with normally ventilated alveoli).

With proper evaluation the cause of a patient's hypoxemia may be determined. The $P(A-a)O_2$ is normal in the presence of overall hypoventilation and high altitude and is increased in the other three causes of hypoxemia: $\dot{V}/\dot{Q}$ mismatch, diffusion defect, and shunt. A "rule of thumb" that works reasonably well for determining the cause of hypoxemia in adult patients is to note the *sum of the* Pa_{O_2} *and* Pa_{CO_2}. If, on room air, the sum is between 110 and 130 mm Hg, the cause of the hypoxemia is overall hypoventilation. If the sum is less than 110 mm Hg on room air or on supplemental O_2, the cause is $\dot{V}/\dot{Q}$ mismatch, diffusion defect, or shunt. If the sum is more than 130 mm Hg and the laboratory report states that the patient was on room air, one should suspect an error: Either the patient was on supplemental oxygen or an error was made in either the Pa_{O_2} or Pa_{CO_2} measurements. These are general observations that apply to most adults and can be helpful if one has difficulty in clinically evaluating the cause of an abnormal $P(A\text{-}a)O_2$.

With the use of the $P(A\text{-}a)O_2$ or the sum of the Pa_{O_2} and Pa_{CO_2}, one can differentiate hypoxemia owing to overall hypoventilation from other causes of hypoxemia. One must then look at other tests to differentiate $\dot{V}/\dot{Q}$ disturbance, diffusion defect, and shunt. Such measurements as the nitrogen washout, single breath nitrogen test, and helium dilution tests give evidence for the presence of $\dot{V}/\dot{Q}$ mismatch and nonuniform ventilation. Comparison of pulmonary ventilation and perfusion lung scans can give a semiquantitative analysis of $\dot{V}/\dot{Q}$ matching over the lung fields.

The carbon monoxide diffusing capacity test can evaluate the patient for the presence of a diffusion defect. The diffusing capacity is one of the most sensitive indicators of the presence of interstitial lung disease.

The presence of a shunt can be detected by placing the patient on 100% oxygen. The patient breathes 100% O_2 for about 20 minutes, and then an arterial sample is obtained. For a patient at sea level, there is about a 5% shunt for every 100 torr the Pa_{O_2} is below 550 to 600 torr. This "rule of thumb" works reasonably well down to a Pa_{O_2} of 100 torr. One should remember that everyone normally has about a 2% to 4% "physiologic" shunt. Unfortunately, the administration of 100% oxygen to detect a shunt in patients with diseased lungs has a major drawback: When alveoli that are supplied by partially obstructed airways are filled with a high percentage of oxygen, they are prone to collapse. Alveoli that normally contain a large

Table 12-3. Determination of the Causes of Hypoxemia

	$P(A\text{-}a)O_2$	$P_{O_2} + P_{CO_2}$ *mm Hg*
Overall hypoventilation	Normal	110–130 on room air
$\dot{V}/\dot{Q}$ mismatch* Diffusion defect† Shunt‡	Increased (in all three)	<110 on room air or on oxygen

*$\dot{V}/\dot{Q}$ lung scans are useful in demonstrating mismatching.
†Use diffusing capacity test ($D_{L_{CO}}$).
‡Detect by placing patient on 100% O_2.

amount of nitrogen resist collapse because nitrogen is not significantly absorbed by the blood perfusing the alveolus; however, when this nitrogen is replaced by oxygen, which is readily absorbed by the blood that comes in contact with the alveolus, the alveolus can rapidly collapse, resulting in a shunt. Therefore, administration of 100% oxygen in diseased patients may indeed produce a significant physiologic shunt. In patients with hypoxemia resulting from overall hypoventilation, $\dot{V}/\dot{Q}$ mismatch and diffusion defect, inhalation of 100% oxygen will correct the hypoxemia—that is, the Pa_{O_2} should reach the level expected for normal subjects inhaling 100% oxygen.

Table 12-3 summarizes the laboratory clues to the various causes of hypoxemia.

EVALUATION OF ACID–BASE STATUS

USUAL MEASUREMENTS

Evaluating certain variables is necessary to determine accurately acid–base status of patients. One cannot look at any one acid–base measurement but must look at a combination of factors to arrive at a proper interpretation before appropriate treatment is initiated.

pH Measurement

The measurement most commonly used to reflect the hydrogen concentration of the blood is the pH.

$$pH = \log \frac{1}{[H^+]}$$

Normally, the arterial blood pH is in the range of 7.35 to 7.45.

Acidemia is present if the pH is less than 7.35, and *alkalemia* is present if the pH is greater than 7.45.* The presence of a normal pH does not rule out an acid–base disturbance.

Carbon Dioxide Tension (P_{CO_2}) Measurement

The partial pressure of CO_2, created by CO_2 molecules dissolved in the plasma, may be readily measured. The Pa_{CO_2} is normally in the range of 35 to 45 mm Hg.

The lungs are the major organ for excretion of acid, eliminating about 13,000 mEq/day of volatile acid, the CO_2 of H_2CO_3, whereas the kidneys excrete about 60 to 80 mEq/day of nonvolatile acids.

The Pa_{CO_2} represents the respiratory component of an acid–base disturbance. It is the product of the following relationships.

$$F_{A_{CO_2}} = \frac{CO_2 \text{ production } (\dot{V}CO_2)}{\text{alveolar ventilation } (\dot{V}A)}$$

Therefore,

$$Pa_{CO_2} = \frac{0.863 \times \dot{V}CO_2}{\dot{V}A}$$

0.863 corrects for the fact that $\dot{V}A$ is reported in liters/min (BTPS), $\dot{V}CO_2$ is reported in ml/min (STPD), and $F_{A_{CO_2}}$ is converted to PA_{CO_2}. (Pa_{CO_2} is substituted for PA_{CO_2} since they are believed to be equivalent.)

By definition, *alveolar hypoventilation* is present if the Pa_{CO_2} is greater than 45 mm Hg. *Alveolar hyperventilation* is indicated by a Pa_{CO_2} less than 35 mm Hg. A high-minute volume is not synonymous with alveolar hyperventilation; for example, in severe chronic obstructive airway diseases an elevated Pa_{CO_2} may be present despite the presence of an increased minute ventilation when most of the increased ventilation is dead space ventilation due to a high dead space to tidal volume ratio.

Plasma Bicarbonate (HCO_3^-) Measurement

Bicarbonate is normally in equilibrium in plasma, in red cells, and in other body cells in the following relationship.

$$CO_2 + H_2O \overset{\dagger}{\rightleftharpoons} H_2CO_3 \rightleftharpoons H^+ + HCO_3^-$$

*The terms acidosis and alkalosis refer to the total body acid–base status, which may or may not be mirrored in the arterial blood pH.

†This reaction is increased 13,000-fold by the presence of carbonic anhydrase in the red cell and in the kidney. However, this enzyme is not present in the plasma.

Normally, the arterial plasma bicarbonate is in the range of 22 to 26 mEq/liter (or mM/liter). Usually the plasma bicarbonate measured on a chemistry panel is similar to that calculated from the pH and P_{CO_2} measured in the blood gas laboratory, but occasionally there is a sizeable discrepancy. Which value is the correct one?

Whereas arterial blood samples are usually kept anaerobic and cool and are analyzed soon after withdrawal, clinical laboratory samples are usually venous, may not be anaerobic, and often are analyzed hours after the sample has been obtained. In AutoAnalyzers used in most clinical chemistry laboratories, the CO_2 that evolved when the plasma is acidified is measured. There may be a loss of CO_2 while the plasma is in the sample cups. In addition, because this method assumes a normal pH, there may be some errors in bicarbonate determination in patients with an abnormal pH. Usually if we trust the accuracy of the P_{CO_2} and pH, we should accept the calculated plasma bicarbonate. If the P_{CO_2} and pH measurements in the blood gas laboratory are accurate, then the calculated plasma bicarbonate from the blood gas laboratory should be accepted as valid if there is a significant discrepancy between that value and the one reported by the clinical laboratory.

Although the plasma bicarbonate is usually referred to as the metabolic component of an acid–base disturbance, there is a small respiratory component to the plasma bicarbonate. If one acutely hypoventilates, resulting in an increased CO_2 tension, the equilibrium reaction shifts to the right, resulting in a slight, instantaneous increase in plasma bicarbonate.

$$\uparrow CO_2 + H_2O \rightarrow H_2CO_3 \rightarrow H^+ + HCO_3^-$$

Therefore, the plasma bicarbonate does not only represent the renal-regulated or metabolic component, but also is slightly affected by acute changes in alveolar ventilation.

BUFFER SYSTEMS

Buffers are substances that minimize the change in the concentration of hydrogen ion (or pH) in a solution when hydrogen or hydroxyl ions are added or removed. A buffer system is a mixture of a weak acid and its conjugate base. Most of the hydrogen ions added to this mixture combine with the base, and most of the H^+ removed from the mixture by adding base are replaced from the acid of the acid–base pair. Several buffer systems operate in the blood to minimize the wide fluctuations of pH that might occur if respiratory or metabolic aberrations were present.

BUFFER VALUE

The buffer value of a buffer system is the amount of acid that must be added to change the pH of the buffer system by one pH unit. The usual dimensions are mM/liter/pH unit or a slyke (abbreviated sl) in honor of D.D. Van Slyke.[16] The buffer value of most buffer systems is greatest when the acid–base pair is present in equal concentrations, and this condition exists when the pH is equal to the pK of the acid–base pair. The exception to this is the bicarbonate–carbonic acid buffer system that buffers equally well at all values of pH. The maximum buffer value of most buffers is 0.575 × buffer concentration in mM/liter. The buffer value of the bicarbonate–carbonic acid system is 2.3 × bicarbonate concentration in mM/liter regardless of pH.

Bicarbonate/Carbonic Acid (HCO_3^-/H_2CO_3) System

The bicarbonate/carbonic acid system is the most important buffer system of the body. It is quantitatively a more powerful buffer than other buffers and buffers equally well at all ranges of pH. This unique property is due to the volatility of CO_2. It also functions as an effective buffer because of the ability of the lungs to regulate CO_2 and of the kidneys to regulate plasma bicarbonate. The relationship of pH to the HCO_3^-/H_2CO_3 system is represented by the equation

$$pH = pK + \log \frac{(\text{salt})}{(\text{acid})};$$

$$pH = pK + \log \frac{(HCO_3^-)}{(H_2CO_3)}.$$

This equation is not useful as it stands because there is no simple way to measure H_2CO_3. The plasma H_2CO_3 is proportional to the free CO_2, which in turn is equal to (P_{CO_2} × 0.03). The *Henderson–Hasselbalch equation* can then be written

$$pH = 6.1 + \log \frac{(HCO_3^-)}{(Pa_{CO_2} \times 0.03)}$$

Therefore the pH is a function of the relation of HCO_3^- to Pa_{CO_2} in the following fashion:

$$pH \sim \frac{HCO_3^-}{Pa_{CO_2}} \sim \frac{\text{metabolic component}}{\text{respiratory component}}.$$

PROTEIN BUFFERS (Pr^-/HPr)

Quantitatively, hemoglobin is the most important "chemical buffer" in whole blood. Plasma proteins are the most important "chemical buffers" in plasma, but, quantitatively, plasma proteins are less important than hemoglobin.

PHOSPHATE ($HPO_4^=$/$H_2PO_4^-$) BUFFER SYSTEM

The phosphate buffer system is relatively unimportant quantitatively as a blood buffer system. Phosphate is a very important intracellular buffer.

There is an interrelationship between the bicarbonate/carbonic acid buffer system and the other body buffers.

$$CO_2 + H_2O \rightleftharpoons H_2CO_3 \rightleftharpoons H^+ + HCO_3^-$$
$$+$$
$$BUF^-$$
$$\upharpoonleft\downharpoonright$$
$$HBUF$$

Each of the three buffer systems of blood acts to minimize the effect of excess hydrogen or hydroxyl ions, but only the nonbicarbonate buffers (Hb, plasma proteins, and phosphate) buffer the effect of a rising or falling P_{CO_2}. This effect is expected because the P_{CO_2} is part of the bicarbonate-CO_2 system.

"*IN VITRO*" and "*IN VIVO*" BUFFER SYSTEMS

The effectiveness of a buffer system is proportional to its concentration. Most of the nonbicarbonate buffers of the extracellular fluid (ECF) are concentrated in the blood compartment, but the P_{CO_2} and bicarbonate are rather evenly distributed to the interstitial fluid as well as to the blood plasma. Since in an adult the ECF volume is about three times the blood volume, the effective concentration and hence buffering power of nonbicarbonate buffers in the entire ECF is only about one third of that in the blood. It is these considerations that cause the arterial blood taken from a living subject to react differently than the same blood in a test tube when subjected to changes of P_{CO_2}.

MEASUREMENTS TO EVALUATE THE METABOLIC COMPONENT

The respiratory component of acid–base balance is evaluated by measurement of the P_{CO_2}. No excess or deficit of fixed acid or base will influence this evaluation. Measures of the metabolic component will be discussed below.

PLASMA BICARBONATE

Plasma bicarbonate should always be calculated from the measured P_{CO_2} and pH. This can be done quickly using the nomogram of Figure 12-4. A line connecting the P_{CO_2} and pH is extended to the HCO_3^- line. We noted earlier that the plasma bicarbonate is affected to a small degree by respiratory changes. Many experienced physicians simply make a qualitative mental correction of the bicarbonate for the respiratory effect. The effect is never greater than about 4 mEq/liter of HCO_3^-. There are a number of indirect calculations to quantitate the respiratory correction. They can all be calculated by using a nomogram, but the best one can be calculated in one's head at the bedside if the laboratory has not calculated it for him (*see* discussion on Extracellular Fluid Base Excess).

IN VITRO CORRECTIONS

These calculations are all based on the buffering power of whole blood in the test tube. Whole blood has a nonbicarbonate buffer value of 30 mEq/liter [H^+] per pH unit or slykes (sl),[16] which means that it would take 30 mEq/liter of [H^+] added in the form of carbonic acid to change the pH 1 unit.

STANDARD BICARBONATE

The standard bicarbonate has been defined as the "plasma bicarbonate" concentration when the blood has been equilibrated at a P_{CO_2} of 40 mm Hg, a temperature of 37°C, and the hemoglobin is 100% saturated with oxygen. This measurement theoretically allows one to look at the "metabolic component" of a plasma bicarbonate, eliminating the "respiratory component." For example, in *acute* respiratory failure, with a Pa_{CO_2} of 85 mm Hg, the plasma bicarbonate may be slightly increased; however, the "standard bicarbonate" would still be normal. The acute elevation in plasma bicarbonate as a result of the hypercapnia is due to an increased "respiratory" component rather than to a "metabolic" increase in bicarbonate. The normal standard bicarbonate is 22 to 26 mEq/liter. A graphic solution for standard bicarbonate is shown in the example in Figure 12-5. The standard bicarbonate works best to correct for the respiratory component of bicarbonate only when there is little or no metabolic component. This limits its usefulness.

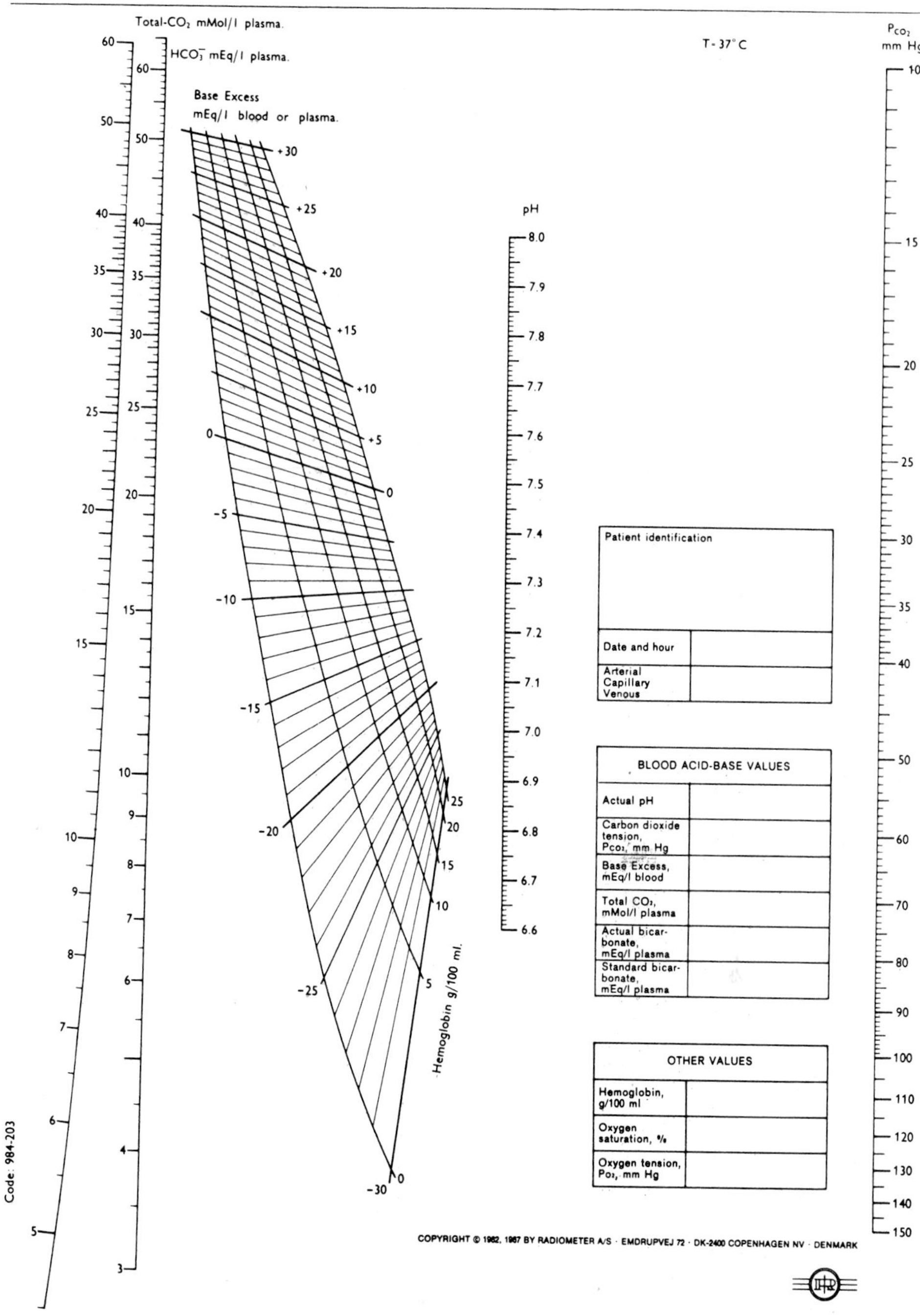

Fig. 12-4. Siggaard–Andersen alignment nomogram for determination of base excess, total CO_2, actual bicarbonate, standard bicarbonate, T_{40} bicarbonate, and BE_{ECF}. *See* Appendix B for methods of calculation. (Reproduced by permission of O. Siggaard–Andersen and Radiometer A/S, Copenhagen, 1963)

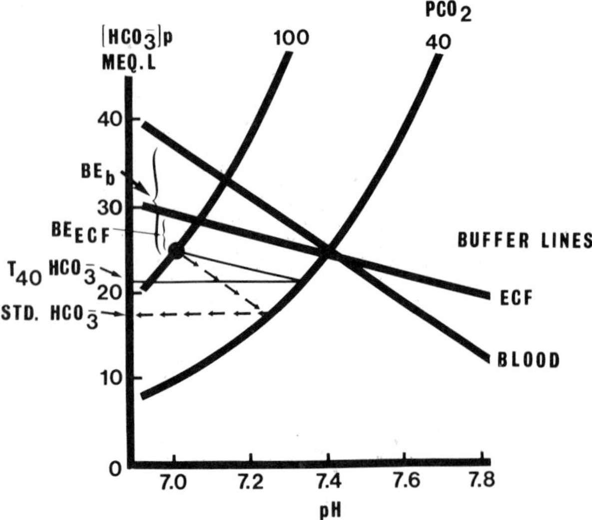

Fig. 12-5. In this graph, the $[HCO_3^-]$ of the plasma is plotted against the pH. The CO_2 isopleths are curved lines. The buffer lines represent the nonbicarbonate buffer value of ECF and blood, respectively. The buffer lines represent the average pathway for pure respiratory (P_{CO_2}) changes in the respective compartments. The slope of the lines is the buffer value of about 10 for ECF and about 30 for blood. The slope is $\Delta HCO_3^- / \Delta pH$, whereas buffer value was defined in the text as ΔH^+ added/ Δ pH. The ΔHCO_3^- is stoichometrically identical to the ΔH^+ added for CO_2 as shown by the equation

$$CO_2 + H_2O \rightleftharpoons H_2CO_3 \rightleftharpoons H^+ + HCO_3^-.$$

Most of the H^+ is buffered by the nonbicarbonate buffers, but the $[HCO_3^-]$ remains as a quantitative marker of the $[H^+]$ added.
The solid point • represents a patient with acute respiratory failure and a mild metabolic acidosis caused by lactic acidemia due to hypoxia.
Measured values are

$$P_{CO_2} = 100 \quad pH = 7.01.$$

Calculated values are

$$(HCO_3^-)p = 24;$$
$$BE_{ECF} = -5;\ BE_b = -12;$$
$$T_{40} = 21;\ STD\ HCO_3 = 17.$$

The BE_{ECF} or BE_b can be determined graphically from the deviation of the patient point from the ECF or blood buffer lines, respectively. Because of inhomogeneities within the compartments, the values obtained in this way are larger than the true values obtained from Figure 12-4. The BE_b correction factor = 1 − 0.0143 Hb (g/dl). The BE_{ECF} correction is very small and can be ignored.

The T_{40} HCO_3^- and standard HCO_3^- may be determined by extending a line from the patient point parallel to the ECF or blood buffer lines, respectively. The HCO_3^- level at the point of intersection with the P_{CO_2} = 40 line is the desired value.

BUFFER BASE

The buffer base includes the total concentration of anions in the blood available to buffer hydrogen chemically or by elimination of CO_2. The buffer base thus includes bicarbonate, hemoglobin, plasma proteins, and phosphates. The normal buffer base, with a hemoglobin of 15 G%, is 48 mEq/liter.

In pure respiratory acid–base disturbances, the "buffer base" theoretically should remain normal. For example, in acute hypercapnia,

$$\uparrow CO_2 + H_2O \rightarrow H_2CO_3 \rightarrow H^+ + HCO_3^-$$
$$+$$
$$BUF^-$$
$$\downarrow$$
$$HBUF.$$

BUF^- includes protein and phosphate buffers. An increased Pa_{CO_2} results not only in an increased hydrogen ion, but also in an *increased plasma bicarbonate* (HCO_3^-). The interaction with the other buffer systems, however, results in an equal *reduction in the nonbicarbonate buffers* (BUF^-). Since the "buffer base" comprises bicarbonate *and* the other buffers, the total "buffer base" should remain normal in the presence of a pure respiratory acid–base disorder. However, *in vitro* and *in vivo* changes in buffer base in response to changes in Pa_{CO_2} are different, as will be described. There is no direct simple way to estimate accurately the total buffer base of the blood, but changes in buffer base are easy to describe in terms of base excess.

BASE EXCESS OF BLOOD

Base excess of blood (BE_b) is another way of reflecting an increase or decrease in the buffer base. Normally, the BE_b is −2 to +2 mEq/liter. A BE_b greater than +2 means that acid has been removed or base has been added, and a BE_b (base deficit) less than −2 means that acid has been added or base removed. The BE_b represents the amount of fixed acid needed to titrate the blood to bring the pH to 7.4 *after* the blood has been equilibrated to a P_{CO_2} of 40 mm Hg. "Fixed acid" refers to any volatile acid other than carbonic acid. A negative BE_b would require titration with a base. The BE_b is represented graphically in Figure 12-5 and can be calculated accurately from Figure 12-4.

This is an elegant way to quantitate the metabolic component of the blood, but unfortunately it is an *in vitro* measure. The BE_b will not change if CO_2 is added to blood *in vitro*, but if CO_2 is added to a living patient the BE_b will decrease, as shown in Figure 12-6. Therefore, this test is of limited usefulness.

IN VIVO CORRECTIONS

In vivo corrections are better than the *in vitro* calculations because they represent the state of the entire extracellular fluid, not just the blood. The T_{40} *bicarbonate* and the *base excess of the ECF* (BE_{ECF}) are available *in vivo* measurements and are calculated essentially the same way as the standard bicarbonate and BE_b, but the buffer value of the ECF is used instead of that of blood. An acute elevation of Pa_{CO_2} owing to alveolar hypoventilation does result in an increase in plasma bicarbonate and a decrease in the other buffers; however, because the capillary wall is permeable to bicarbonate but not to the principal nonbicarbonate buffers (*i.e.*, proteins), some of the bicarbonate formed in response to acute hypercapnia diffuses through the capillary wall into the interstitial fluid. The bicarbonate formed as a direct result of the buffer response to acute hypercapnia is distributed throughout the extracellular fluid space; thus the increase in blood bicarbonate is only about one third that which would be seen in an *in vitro* system with a single volume of distribution. Therefore, the increase in plasma bicarbonate *in vivo* in response to acute CO_2 retention is less than would occur in a setting *in vitro*, making standard bicarbonate an unreliable indicator of the "metabolic" component of the plasma bicarbonate in acute hypercapnia. Since the reduction in nonbicarbonate buffers is the same but the increase in plasma bicarbonate is less than would occur *in vitro*, the total blood buffer base or blood base excess may, in fact, decrease in association with acute hypercapnia. In this situation, the decrease in blood buffer base or blood base excess would not then represent a superimposed metabolic disturbance (e.g., metabolic acidosis), but would be related only to the *in vivo* response to acute CO_2 retention.

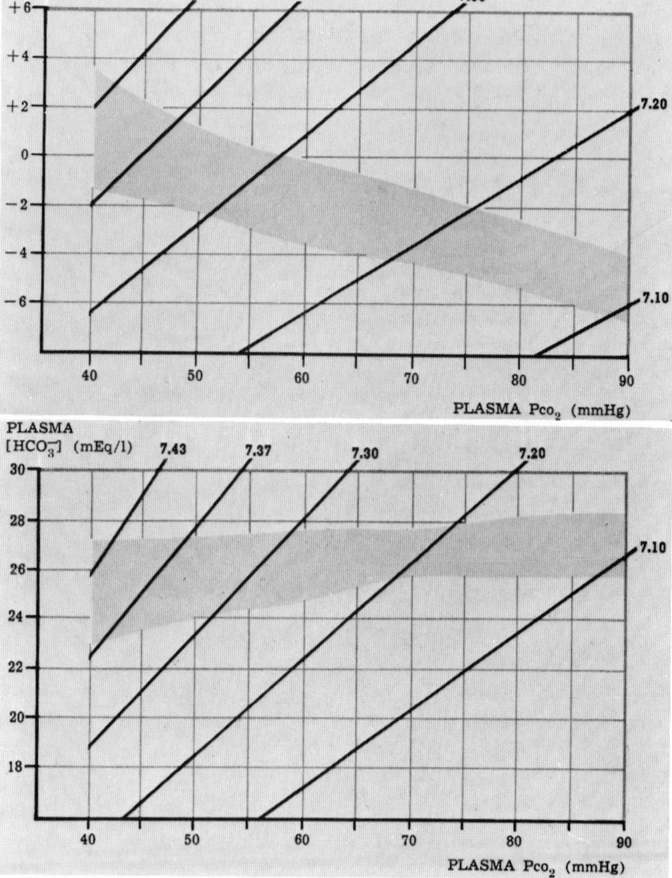

Fig. 12-6. Ninety-five percent confidence-limit bands for acute CO_2 retention. Note that the blood base excess does drop below −2 with acute CO_2 retention even though there has been no change in "metabolic component." (Winters RW et al: Acid–Base Physiology in Medicine, 2nd ed. Cleveland, The London CO, 1969)

Superficially, it appears that the pathway of acute hypocapnia is the same for *in vitro* blood as for a living subject. The effect of acute hypocapnia on *in vitro* blood is exactly what would be predicted by extrapolation from hypercapnia experiments. In the living subject, however, very frequently a true superimposed metabolic acidosis occurs which is due to a lactic acidosis. The lactic acidosis may be produced by a reduced blood flow to some tissues caused by hypocapnia and alkalemia or by reduced excretion or reduced metabolism of lactate due to the same causes. The T_{40} bicarbonate and BE_{ECF} measures reveal the presence of this metabolic acidosis, but the *in vitro* measures do not show it.

T_{40} BICARBONATE

Since it was recognized that, with acute hypercapnia, the increase in plasma bicarbonate that occurs *in vivo* is less than that which occurs *in vitro*, and therefore that *in vitro* nomograms used to calculate standard bicarbonate might be invalid, a new calculation known as the T_{40} bicarbonate was developed.[3] A method of calculating it graphically is shown in Figure 12-5. It can also be calculated accurately from Figure 12-4. A bedside estimation can be done by assuming that an acute increase in Pa_{CO_2} of about 15 mm Hg will increase the plasma bicarbonate by about 1 mEq/liter. The change in plasma bicarbonate expected to occur with acute CO_2 retention would be

$$\Delta HCO_3^- = \frac{\text{observed } Pa_{CO_2} - 40}{15}.$$

The T_{40} bicarbonate is equal to the observed plasma bicarbonate minus the ΔHCO_3^- expected to occur secondary to the acute CO_2 elevation. For example, if the Pa_{CO_2} equals 85 mm Hg, then

$$\Delta HCO_3^- = \frac{85 - 40}{15} = 3 \text{ mEq/liter}.$$

If the observed plasma HCO_3^- = 28 mEq/liter, then

$$T_{40} \text{ bicarbonate} = 28 - 3 = 25 \text{ mEq/liter}.$$

Therefore, in this example, the slightly elevated bicarbonate was due to acute CO_2 retention and did not indicate increased "metabolic bicarbonate."

Since changes in plasma bicarbonate with acute CO_2 retention are different *in vivo* than *in vitro*, T_{40} bicarbonate is a more reliable measure than is standard bicarbonate in patients with acute hypercapnia.

In acute hypocapnia, T_{40} bicarbonate is also more reliable than standard bicarbonate because it will detect the concomitant lactic acidosis when the standard bicarbonate will be normal, misdiagnosing the condition.

Use of the ratio of 15:1 (P_{CO_2}: plasma bicarbonate) for estimating T_{40} bicarbonate, useful in acute hypercapnia, is unreliable in acute CO_2 reduction. A more precise method for estimating T_{40} bicarbonate must be used for Pa_{CO_2} values below 35 mm Hg.[4] A ratio of 5:1 (P_{CO_2}:plasma bicarbonate) to estimate changes in plasma bicarbonate secondary to acute hypocapnia is quite reliable when the Pa_{CO_2} is less than 35 mm Hg. The T_{40} bicarbonate becomes more inaccurate when a large metabolic component is also present.

Base Excess of ECF (BE_{ECF})

The BE_{ECF} is easy to calculate accurately even at the bedside and is a measure of the metabolic component of the entire ECF provided the patient has been in a quasi-steady-state for about 10 minutes. It can be defined as the "titratable basicity" of the ECF. In other words, it represents the amount of fixed base or acid that would have to be added to the ECF to bring the pH to 7.4 *after* the P_{CO_2} has been brought to 40 mm Hg.[5,13]

The calculation is shown graphically in Figure 12-5. The BE_{ECF} is the deviation from the ECF buffer line. The BE_{ECF} can also be calculated from Figure 12-4, but a quite accurate bedside calculation is

$$BE_{ECF} = \Delta\, HCO_3^- + 10\, \Delta\, pH,$$

where

$$\Delta\, HCO_3^- = \text{actual } HCO_3^- - 24$$

and

$$\Delta\, pH = \text{actual } pH - 7.4.$$

The 10 is the approximate slope of the ECF buffer line in mEq HCO_3^-/liter/pH unit. (The slope depends on the hemoglobin concentration of the blood and on the ratio of blood volume to ECF volume.) A slope of 11.6 was obtained in a group of normal subjects. The value of 10 makes the calculation easier.

COMPARISON OF *IN VITRO* AND *IN VIVO* MEASURES

Using the following set of numbers from an arterial blood analysis, compare the *in vitro* and *in vivo* measures.

		Normal Values
pH	= 7.14	7.35–7.45
Pa_{CO_2}	= 85 mm Hg	35–45 mm Hg
Plasma HCO_3^-	= 28 mEq/liter	22–26 mEq/liter
Standard HCO_3^-	= 21 mEq/liter	22–26 mEq/liter
T_{40} HCO_3^-	= 25 mEq/liter	22–26 mEq/liter
BB_b	= 44 mEq/liter	46–50 mEq/liter
BE_b	= −4 mEq/liter	−2 to +2 mEq/liter
BE_{ECF}	= 1.4 mEq/liter	−2 to +2 mEq/liter

BE_{ECF} is derived as follows.

$$\begin{aligned} BE_{ECF} &= (\Delta\ HCO_3^-) + 10\ (\Delta\ pH) \\ &= (28 - 24) + 10\ (7.14\text{–}7.40) \\ &= (4) + 10\ (-0.26) \\ &= 4 - 2.6 \\ &= 1.4\ \text{mEq/liter} \end{aligned}$$

The plasma HCO_3^- is slightly elevated; however, the T_{40} HCO_3^- and the BE_{ECF} are normal, which indicates that the increased plasma HCO_3^- is of "respiratory" origin, from the hypercapnia, rather than of "metabolic" origin. The reduced standard bicarbonate, BE_b and BB_b are inaccurate because they are derived from *in vitro* observations that are different from *in vivo* observations in acute hypercapnia. The reduced blood buffer base and BE_b result from the leakage of HCO_3^- from the blood into the perivascular tissues, which occurs *in vivo* with acute hypercapnia. The normal BE_{ECF} accurately indicates that this is a pure respiratory acidosis, with a normal metabolic component.

A study of Figure 12-5 reveals the following relationships between BE_b and BE_{ECF} and standard bicarbonate and T_{40} bicarbonate:

$$\begin{aligned} &\text{Below pH 7.4, } BE_b < BE_{ECF}; \\ &\text{Above pH 7.4, } BE_b > BE_{ECF}; \\ &\text{Above } P_{CO_2} \text{ 40 mm Hg, standard } HCO_3^- < T_{40}\ HCO_3^-; \\ &\text{Below } P_{CO_2} \text{ 40 mm Hg, standard } HCO_3^- > T_{40}\ HCO_3^-. \end{aligned}$$

BE_{ECF} is the only test of the four that is indicative of the metabolic component under all circumstances. The reasons for the superiority of the BE_{ECF} are twofold: First, the BE_{ECF} uses an *in vivo* buffer value to compute the metabolic component. Hence, the value of BE_{ECF} is realistic and can be directly applied to living subjects. Second, the BE_{ECF} is a measure of the amount of strong base that needs to be added or removed to make the pH 7.4 *after* the P_{CO_2} has been made 40 mm Hg. The T_{40} bicarbonate is an *in vivo* measure but suffers from the fact that with a marked metabolic component, especially a severe metabolic acidosis, the intersection of the *in vivo* buffer line with the P_{CO_2} 40 line will occur at an abnormal pH. This will produce values for T_{40} bicarbonate that are qualitatively correct but not quantitatively correct.

The one drawback of the BE_{ECF} calculation is that it assumes a Blood/ECF volume ratio of 1:3. In conditions of severe overhydration or underhydration and with a newborn or very young child, this assumption is incorrect. In pediatric disease, it is probably better to look at the plasma bicarbonate and not to correct it for a respiratory component. This has the effect of assuming that the effective nonbicarbonate buffer value of the fluid compartments is zero. This undoubtedly is not true, but it probably is very low.

Table 12-4 shows a comparison of plasma HCO_3^-.

Table 12-4. Comparison of *in vitro* and *in vivo* Measures of Metabolic Component

	pH	Pa_{CO_2}	PLASMA HCO_3	BE_{ECF}	T_{40} HCO_3	BE_b	STANDARD HCO_3
Acute hypercapnia	↓↓	↑	↑	N	N	↓	↓
Chronic hypercapnia	↓	↑	↑↑	↑↑	↑↑	↑	↑
Metabolic acidosis	↓↓	↓	↓↓	↓↓	↓	↓↓↓	↓↓↓
Metabolic alkalosis	↑	↑	↑	↑	↑	↑↑	↑↑
Acute hypocapnia	↑↑	↓	↓↓	↓	↓	N	N
Chronic hypocapnia	↑	↓	↓↓↓	↓↓↓	↓↓↓	↓↓↓	↓↓↓
Mixed respiratory and metabolic acidosis	↓	↑	N or ↓	↓	↓	↓↓	↓↓
Mixed respiratory and metabolic alkalosis	↑	↓	N or ↑	↑	↑	↑↑	↑↑

T_{40} HCO_3^-, BE_{ECF}, standard HCO_3^-, and BE_b in typical clinical disorders. The plasma HCO_3^- gives values that might be misinterpreted in respiratory abnormalities with or without a primary metabolic component. The T_{40} HCO_3^- may be misleading in severe acidosis. The standard HCO_3^- and BE_b have the greatest potential of misinterpretation qualitatively and quantitatively. The BE_{ECF} may be misleading in small children or marked fluid imbalance but otherwise is based on the most sound physiological grounds. All tests will give qualitatively correct results in very severe acid–base imbalances of any kind, but in the less severe cases the *in vitro* tests and, to a lesser extent, the plasma HCO_3^- and the T_{40} HCO_3^- may be misinterpreted.

TRANSPORT OF CO_2

Carbon dioxide can be transported to the lungs from the tissues in six forms (Fig. 12-7). When CO_2 enters the plasma, it may [1] remain dissolved in plasma, [2] become bound to plasma proteins to form carbamino compounds, or [3] join with water to form carbonic acid and then hydrogen ion and bicarbonate. However, most CO_2 enters the red blood cells, where it again may [1] be present as dissolved CO_2, [2] become bound to hemoglobin to form carbamino compounds, or [3] join with water to form carbonic acid and then hydrogen ion and bicarbonate.

The reaction

$$CO_2 + H_2O \rightarrow H_2CO_3 \rightarrow H^+ + HCO_3^-$$

is catalyzed by carbonic anhydrase present in the red blood cell but not in plasma. Because of this mechanism for rapid conversion of CO_2, most tissue-generated CO_2 enters the red blood cell and is converted to H^+ and HCO_3^-.

Since the red blood cell membrane is impermeable to protein anions but permeable to such diffus-

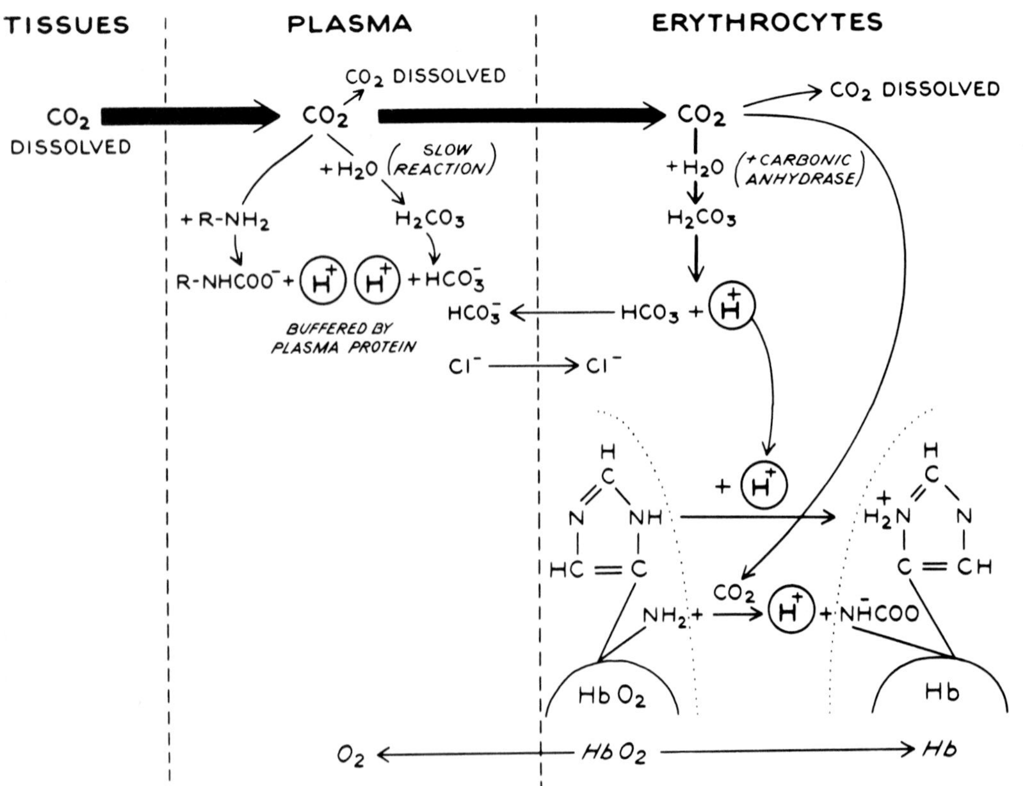

Fig. 12-7. Carbon dioxide transport in blood. About 70% to 80% of CO_2 is transported as HCO_3^- in the plasma, 10% is carried as carbamino compounds both inside and outside the cell, and about 7% as dissolved CO_2. The reverse of these reactions occurs when the blood reaches the lungs, allowing for rapid elimination of CO_2 (Comroe JH Jr: Physiology of Respiration. Chicago, Year Book Medical Publishers, 1974. Redrawn from Davenport H: The ABC of Acid–Base Chemistry, 5th ed. Chicago, University of Chicago Press, 1969).

ible anions as Cl^- and HCO_3^-, the diffusible anions will distribute themselves unequally on the two sides of the red blood cell membrane. As oxygenated blood reaches the tissues, oxyhemoglobin begins to lose its oxygen. Because reduced hemoglobin is a weaker acid than is oxyhemoglobin, the hemoglobin anion concentration decreases as oxygen is given up to the tissues. Since the intracellular cation, K^+, remains relatively constant, HCO_3^- and Cl^- move from the plasma into the cells to reestablish the anionic equilibrium. As CO_2 enters the red blood cell from the tissues, the H^+ ion formed is buffered by the hemoglobin, resulting in a further decrease in the total hemoglobin anion. Because this addition of CO_2 to the red cell also results in HCO_3^- production, a portion of this HCO_3^- diffuses out into the plasma. The amount of HCO_3^- that diffuses from the red cell into the plasma is less than would have occurred if the hemoglobin anion concentration had remained unchanged. In other words, if CO_2 is being added to the red blood cell at the same time that hemoglobin is releasing oxygen to the tissues, less HCO_3^- diffuses out of the cell than would have were there no change in the hemoglobin anion concentration. The anion concentrations for both Cl^- and HCO_3^- are higher in red blood cells in venous blood than in those in arterial blood. Since there are more osmotically active particles inside red cells in venous blood, water diffuses into the cells, resulting in swelling. This phenomenon of Cl^- moving from the plasma into the red cells at the same time as CO_2 is taken up by the red cells might more properly be called an "anionic shift" rather than the "chloride shift," as it is commonly termed.

About 60% to 90% of the CO_2 is transported from the tissues to the lung in the form of HCO_3^-, with most of this having been formed in red cells but transferred out to the plasma for transport. Some 10% to 20% of the CO_2 is transported as carbamino compounds, with less than 10% being transported as dissolved CO_2.

REGULATION OF HYDROGEN ION AND BICARBONATE IN THE KIDNEY

The regulation of plasma bicarbonate is predominantly carried out by the kidney. Although the lungs can vary the CO_2 level in the blood within minutes, it takes hours to days for the kidney to change the

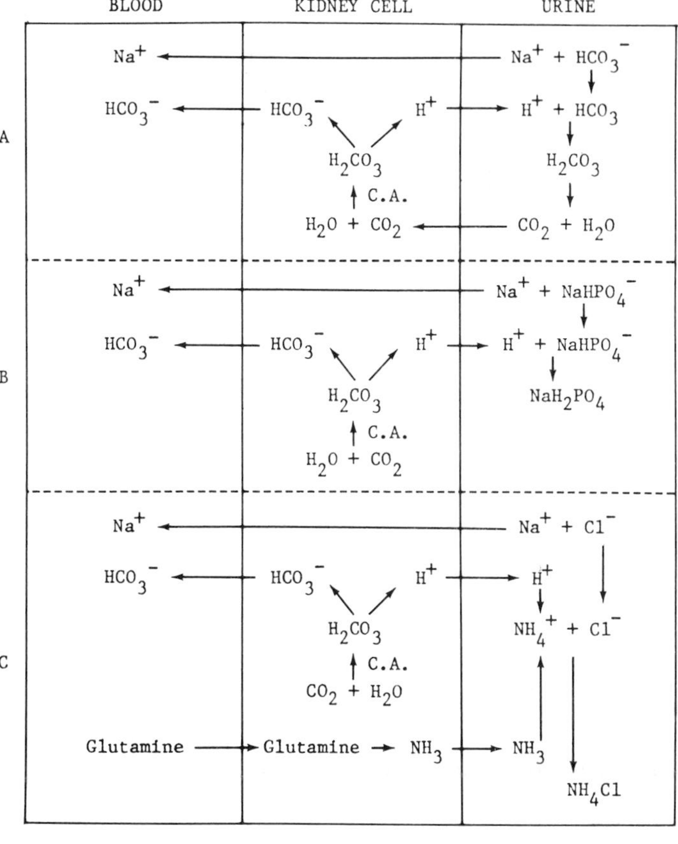

Fig. 12-8. Mechanisms for reabsorption of sodium from the urine into the blood (take place in the distal convoluted tubule and collecting duct system). Mechanism A depicts the usual mechanism for reabsorption of bicarbonate from the glomerular filtrate. In mechanism B, H^+ is excreted in the form of "titratable acid." In mechanism C, the glutamine mechanism, H^+ is excreted in the form of NH_4Cl. C.A. = carbonic anhydrase.

bicarbonate level in the plasma. The reabsorption of sodium from the urine by the kidney cell and its return to blood is accompanied by the regeneration of bicarbonate (Fig. 12-8). Normally, about 90% of the bicarbonate filtered through the glomerulus is returned from the renal tubule to the blood by the reabsorption (reclamation) mechanism depicted in Figure 12-8 (Mechanism A). Normally, about two thirds of the acid excreted in the urine is in the form of ammonium chloride (e.g., via the glutamine mechanism), and one third is in the form of titratable acid (e.g., NaH_2PO_4).

If respiratory acidosis due to hypercapnia (elevated Pa_{CO_2} occurs, the kidney attempts to compensate for this by regenerating extra bicarbonate. On the other hand, when respiratory alkalosis due to hypocapnia (a decreased Pa_{CO_2}) occurs, the kidney reduces the amount of bicarbonate regenerated, resulting in increased hydrogen ion in the plasma, in an attempt to compensate for the alkalosis. Carbonic anhydrase is also present in the kidney cell, resulting in acceleration of the reaction $CO_2 + H_2O \rightleftharpoons H_2CO_3$.

CAUSES OF ACID–BASE IMBALANCE/ ACID–BASE DISORDERS

RESPIRATORY ACIDOSIS

Respiratory acidosis is caused by hydrogen ion accumulation as a result of hypercapnia.

$$\uparrow CO_2 + H_2O \rightarrow H_2CO_3 \rightarrow H^+ + HCO_3^-$$
$$+$$
$$BUF^-$$
$$\downarrow$$
$$HBUF$$

The increased P_{CO_2} results in increased hydrogen ion concentration and acidosis. The plasma HCO_3^- is increased slightly as a result of hypercapnia. Although decreases in buffer base of the blood, and hence in BE_b, occur, the buffer base of the ECF and BE_{ECF} is unchanged.

Respiratory acidosis may be due to overall hypoventilation associated with respiratory center depression and neuromuscular disturbances in the presence of normal lungs, or may indicate respiratory failure associated with chronic obstructive airway diseases (e.g., emphysema and chronic bronchitis). Other disorders such as severe pulmonary edema due to left ventricular failure and significant pulmonary embolism may also result in respiratory acidosis.

RESPIRATORY ALKALOSIS

Hypocapnia (decreased Pa_{CO_2} due to hyperventilation) results in a loss of hydrogen ion.

$$\downarrow CO_2 + H_2O \leftarrow H_2CO_3 \leftarrow H^+ + HCO_3^-$$
$$+$$
$$BUF^-$$
$$\uparrow$$
$$HBUF$$

Although plasma bicarbonate decreases slightly in this reaction, the other buffers increase. Many patients with hypocapnia show no change in BE_{ECF}, as would be theoretically predicted. The few patients who show a mild lactic acidosis have a negative BE_{ECF} but a normal BE_b. Respiratory alkalosis is commonly associated with neurogenic hyperventilation, interstitial lung diseases, pulmonary embolism, asthma, hyperventilation syndrome, and severe hypoxemia.

METABOLIC ACIDOSIS

Metabolic acidosis may occur due to the increased metabolic formation of acids by the body (e.g., diabetic ketoacidosis and lactic acidosis), reduction in excretion of acids by the kidney (e.g., acidosis associated with renal failure), or the exogenous addition of acids to the bloodstream (e.g., ammonium chloride and hydrochloric acid).

$$CO_2 + H_2O \leftarrow H_2CO_3 \leftarrow \uparrow H^+ + HCO_3^-$$
$$+$$
$$BUF^-$$
$$\downarrow$$
$$HBUF$$

This primary increase in hydrogen ion results in both a reduction in plasma HCO_3^- and BUF^-, resulting in a reduction in buffer base and base excess of blood and of the ECF.

Metabolic acidosis may also result from a loss of plasma bicarbonate (e.g., diarrhea, excessive loss associated with an ileostomy, and excess renal loss [renal tubular acidosis]), or from the exogenous administration of acetazolamide (Diamox), a carbonic anhydrase inhibitor that blocks the regeneration of bicarbonate in the kidney.

$$CO_2 + H_2O \rightarrow H_2CO_3 \rightarrow H^+ + \downarrow HCO_3^-$$
$$+$$
$$BUF^-$$
$$\downarrow$$
$$HBUF$$

A loss of plasma bicarbonate results in increased hydrogen ion formation. Both HCO_3^- and BUF^- are reduced, resulting in a reduction in buffer base and base excess of both blood and ECF. The BE_b will show a greater deficit than the true deficit of the ECF as shown by the BE_{ECF}.

In patients with metabolic acidosis, evaluating the *"anion gap"* can be a clue to the presence and cause of the acid–base disturbance. Normally, the difference between the major plasma cation sodium and the sum of the major plasma anions chloride and bicarbonate is about 10 to 15 mEq/liter. For example,

Cation	Anions
Na^+ = 140 mEq/liter	Cl^- = 100 mEq/liter
	HCO_3^- = 25 mEq/liter
Total = 140 mEq/liter	Total = 125 mEq/liter

If the difference is greater than 15, the "anion gap" is increased. This suggests the presence of other circulating anions, as would be seen with diabetic ketoacidosis, lactic acidosis, uremic acidosis, and the ingestion of methanol, paraldehyde, ethylene glycol, and salicylates. If metabolic acidosis is due to the simple addition of H^+—for example, from HCl or NH_4Cl—or the loss of HCO_3^-—for example, from diarrhea or acetazolamide administration, the "anion gap" is normal.

Bicarbonate therapy should be considered for severe metabolic acidosis. If bicarbonate therapy is desirable, arterial blood gas results can be used as a guideline to therapy.

The total deficit in buffer base of the ECF compartment is easily calculated by multiplying BE_{ECF} by the ECF volume. If we assume that the ECF volume is 24% of the body weight in kg, the equation is

$$\text{Deficit in } BE_{ECF} = 0.24 \times \text{wt (kg)} \times BE_{ECF}.$$

For instance, if the weight is 70 kg and $BE_{ECF} = -10$ mEq/liter, then

$$\text{Deficit in } BE_{ECF} = 0.24 \times 70 \times (-10) = -168 \text{ mEq}.$$

If the acidosis affected only the ECF compartment in the above example, 168 mEq of bicarbonate would completely correct the metabolic deficit of the ECF, and if the P_{CO_2} were 40 mm Hg, the pH would be 7.40. Of course, the acidosis will not only involve the ECF compartment but also include the intracellular fluid (ICF) compartment. However, there is no guide as to what the ICF deficit is. Experience has shown that the total body deficit may be two to four times the ECF deficit and has been observed as high as eight times the ECF deficit. If there are continuing losses of bicarbonate, these must also be replaced.

If one wanted to return the pH back to 7.40 (assuming the P_{CO_2} remained constant) then about one half of the calculated deficit in BE_{ECF} would be infused intravenously, a blood gas would be drawn in about 20 minutes, the new BE_{ECF} would be calculated, and about one half of the new deficit would again be given intravenously. This approach would be continued until the desired pH is achieved.

In diabetic ketoacidosis with a pH below 7.1, it may be desirable to give enough bicarbonate to raise the pH to at least 7.1. This objective will require only comparatively small amounts of bicarbonate.

Principles of bicarbonate therapy in lactic acidosis are similar to those in ketoacidosis. There is evidence that vigorous bicarbonate therapy may make lactic acidosis worse.

METABOLIC ALKALOSIS

The loss of hydrogen ion by nasogastric suction or excessive diuretic and steroid therapy results in metabolic alkalosis.

$$CO_2 + H_2O \rightarrow H_2CO_3 \rightarrow \downarrow H^+ + HCO_3^-$$
$$+$$
$$BUF^-$$
$$\uparrow$$
$$HBUF$$

Both plasma bicarbonate and BUF^- are increased, resulting in an increase in buffer base and base excess of both blood and ECF.

Hypokalemia can cause and perpetuate metabolic alkalosis. Since sodium reabsorption in the distal convoluted tubule and collecting duct system can be accomplished by excretion of either an H^+ or K^+ ion into the urine in exchange for the Na^+, a deficit of potassium means that H^+ is used mainly for this sodium reclamation, resulting in continuous HCO_3^- regeneration (Figure 12-8).

An increased plasma bicarbonate associated with injudicious use of exogenous intravenous or oral bicarbonate may also result in metabolic alkalosis.

$$CO_2 + H_2O \leftarrow H_2CO_3 \leftarrow H^+ + \uparrow HCO_3^-$$
$$+$$
$$BUF^-$$
$$\uparrow$$
$$HBUF$$

The increased HCO_3^- is associated with an increased BUF^-, resulting in an increase in the buffer base and base excess of both blood and ECF. The BE_b will show a greater excess than the true excess of the ECF, as shown by the BE_{ECF}. Table 12-5 provides a list of acid–base disturbances.

INTERPRETATION OF ACID–BASE DISORDERS

In attempting to properly interpret acid–base disorders, one must remember the basic relationship implied in the Henderson–Hasselbalch equation:

$$pH \sim \frac{HCO_3^-}{P_{CO_2}} \sim \frac{\text{metabolic component}}{\text{respiratory component}}.$$

Two of the three factors in this relationship must be known to evaluate accurately the acid–base disturbance. When interpreting acid–base data, one should look at the pH to determine whether acidemia or alkalemia is present, remembering that a normal pH does not rule out an acid–base disorder.

Whether the respiratory component is normal or abnormal may be determined by looking at the Pa_{CO_2}. One must then decide whether the observed Pa_{CO_2} would explain the observed pH.

Whether the metabolic component is abnormal may be determined by looking at the plasma bicarbonate. There is, however, a small respiratory component to the plasma bicarbonate, so that the BE_{ECF} more accurately reflects the metabolic component of the plasma bicarbonate.

One should also decide whether "compensation" is present. If a primary respiratory acidosis has occurred, for example, within hours the intracellular buffers will contribute to an increase of plasma bicarbonate and BE_{ECF}. This is brought about by H^+ entering the cell in exchange for K^+. Also within hours the kidney will begin to alter the plasma bicarbonate in an attempt to compensate for the respiratory disturbance. The kidney response is slow, *requiring 72 hours* or more for maximal effect. If a primary metabolic disorder occurs, within minutes the lung will begin to compensate for the metabolic disorder by altering alveolar ventilation to change the Pa_{CO_2}. *It may take up to 12 hours for the lung to compensate maximally*. In the past the presence or absence of compensation has been categorized as follows.

1. *Uncompensated*. The presence of an abnormal pH due to deviation of one component with the other component still within normal limits (e.g., presence of metabolic acidosis with a Pa_{CO_2} still within the normal range).
2. *Partially compensated*. Deviation of one component with the other component changing appropriately to compensate for the acid–base disorder. However, the pH is still abnormal.
3. *Completely compensated*. Deviation of one component with an appropriate change of the other component so that the pH has been restored to normal (i.e., between 7.35 and 7.45).

It is now well recognized that with a major deviation from normal of one component, it is not pos-

Table 12-5. Causes of Acid–Base Disturbances

RESPIRATORY ACIDOSIS

- Overall hypoventilation
  - Pickwickian syndrome
  - Drug overdose
  - Head injury
  - Neuromuscular disturbance (*e.g.*, myasthenia gravis)
  - Kyphoscoliosis
- Chronic obstructive lung disease
- Pulmonary edema, severe

RESPIRATORY ALKALOSIS

- Neurogenic hyperventilation
- Interstitial lung diseases
- Pulmonary embolism
- Acute asthma
- Hyperventilation syndrome

METABOLIC ACIDOSIS

- Increased metabolic formation of acids
  - Diabetic ketoacidosis
  - Uremic acidosis
  - Lactic acidosis
- Exogenous addition of acids
  - Ammonium chloride
  - Hydrochloric acid
- Loss of bicarbonate
  - Diarrhea
  - Ileostomy loss
  - Renal tubular acidosis
- Exogenous administration of Diamox

METABOLIC ALKALOSIS

- Loss of hydrogen ion
  - Nasogastric suction
  - Persistent vomiting
  - Diuretic therapy
  - Steroid therapy
- Exogenous bicarbonate

Siggaard-Andersen Acid-Base Chart

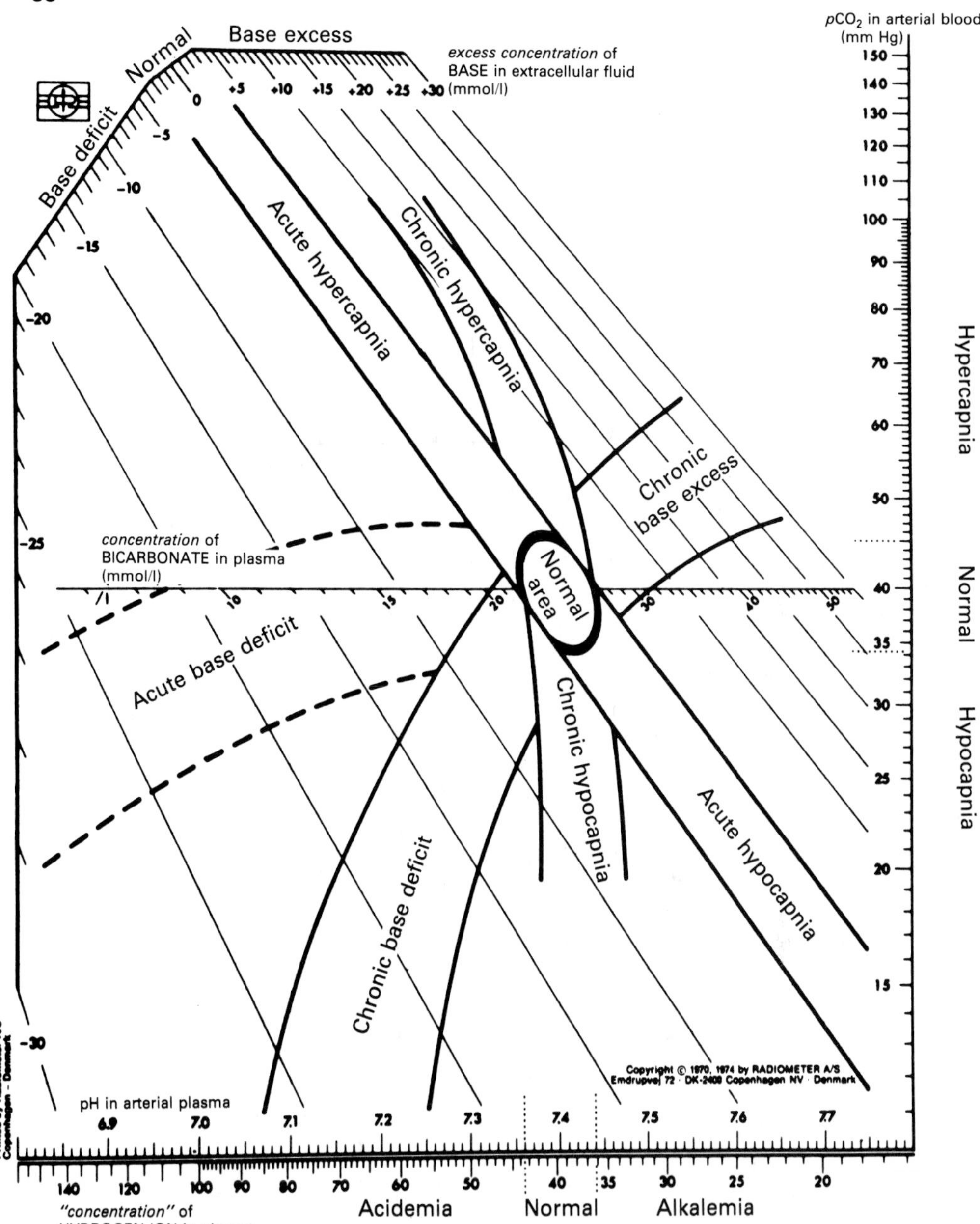

Fig. 12-9. Depiction of 95% confidence-limit bands by Siggaard–Andersen. (Reproduced by permission of O. Siggaard–Andersen and Radiometer A/S, Copenhagen, 1971). Note that extracellular fluid base excess is depicted on this "*in vivo*" nomogram.[13] The BE_{ECF} remains normal with acute hypercapnia, whereas the blood base excess, depicted in Figure 12-6, decreases.

sible for the other component to restore the pH to normal; for example, with severe diabetic ketoacidosis, it is impossible for the lung to increase alveolar ventilation sufficiently to reduce Pa_{CO_2} to the extent where pH would be restored to normal. Also, in the presence of severe chronic respiratory failure, the normal kidney may not be able to regenerate enough bicarbonate to return the pH to the normal range.

Since physiologic compensatory mechanisms are unable to compensate fully (*i.e.*, return the pH to normal) for major deviations in acid–base status, it has become apparent that determining the extent to which one could maximally return the pH toward normal would be more appropriate. Studies in animals and in humans have helped to determine the degree of compensation that can be expected for any given disturbance.

One way of evaluating the compensation is to consider the acid–base data from such studies. In a group of 100 subjects, the results are distributed in a bell-shaped curve. It has become accepted to compare a patient's acid–base data to the middle 95% of the curve, recognizing that 2.5% of the subjects' data will be above and 2.5% below the mid-95% of subjects. These data have been developed into "95% confidence-limit bands" that aid in the proper interpretation of various acid–base disturbances. These bands have been developed for both acute and chronic acid–base disturbances. In the presence of *acute* hypercapnia, for example, one can determine the appropriate pH, plasma bicarbonate, and BE_{ECF} for any given Pa_{CO_2} (Figs. 12-6 and 12-9). In the presence of *chronic* hypercapnia, one can determine the expected pH to be achieved for a certain level of Pa_{CO_2} (Fig. 12-9); for example, in chronic hypercapnia associated with a Pa_{CO_2} of 85 mm Hg and a pH of 7.38, under the old acid–base terminology this would be interpreted as a completely compensated respiratory acidosis. Examination of this point on Figure 12-9 reveals, however that it lies considerably to the right of the 95% confidence band for chronic hypercapnia, indicating that the level of plasma bicarbonate and BE_{ECF} is inappropriately high for this Pa_{CO_2} and that the patient has a chronic respiratory acidosis with a superimposed metabolic alkalosis.

The proper terminology for compensation using 95% confidence-limit bands would express the compensation as "maximal" or "less than maximal" (*see* Fig. 12-9 for further examples of 95% confidence-limit bands). It is impossible to interpret acid–base disorders accurately and completely without a knowledge of [1] the duration of the acid–base disturbance (observation of serial arterial blood gases are often helpful in this respect) and [2] the patient's clinical condition (*i.e.*, whether disorders are present that could lead to respiratory or metabolic acid–base disturbances).

Occasionally one will have a "combined" or "mixed" acid–base disturbance; for example, if changes in both the P_{CO_2} and plasma bicarbonate would result in acidosis, the patient would have a combined respiratory and metabolic acidosis. Mixed respiratory and metabolic alkalosis may also occur. (*See* Appendix E for further examples of the proper interpretation of arterial blood gas data; also *see* Equations and Rules of Thumb for Management of Patients in Appendix D for useful guidelines relating to oxygenation and acid–base disorders.

SUMMARY

A proper understanding of arterial blood gas data is crucial to the proper management of critically ill patients. Interventions based on blood gas data can be made in management that will result in a reduced morbidity and mortality.

REFERENCES

1. Aberman A, Cavanilles JM, Weil MH et al: Blood P_{50} calculated from a single measurement of pH, PO_2, and SO_2. J Appl Physiol 38:171, 1975
2. Allen EV: Thromboangiitis obliterans: Methods of diagnosis of chronic occlusive arterial lesions distal to the wrist with illustrative cases. Am J Med Sci 178:237, 1929
3. Armstrong BW, Mohler JG, Jung RC et al: The in vivo carbon dioxide titration curve. Lancet 1:759, 1966
4. Armstrong BW: Rapid changes in $PaCO_2$ and HCO_3. Respir Care 21:808, 1976
5. Collier CR: Oxygen affinity of human blood in presence of carbon monoxide. J Appl Physiol 40:487, 1976
6. Collier CR, Hackney JD, Mohler JG: Use of extracellular base excess in diagnosis of acid–base disorders: A conceptual approach. Chest 61:6S, 1972
7. Gilbert F, Keighley JF: The arterial/alveolar oxygen tension ratio: An index of gas exchange applicable to varying inspired oxygen concentrations. Am Rev Respir Dis 109:142, 1974
8. Greenhow DE: Incorrect performance of Allen's test—ulnar artery flow erroneously presumed inadequate. Anesthesiology 37:356, 1974
9. Kelman GR: Computer program for the production of O_2–CO_2 diagrams. Respir Physiol 4:260, 1968
10. Mellemgaard K: The alveolar–arterial oxygen difference: Its size and components in normal man. Acta Physiol Scand 67:10, 1966
11. Scheinman MM, Brown MA, Rapaport E: Critical assessment of use of central venous oxygen saturation as a mirror

of mixed venous oxygen in severely ill cardiac patients. Circulation 40:165, 1965
12. Shafer AW, Tague LL, Welch MH et al: 2,3-Diphosphoglycerate in red cells stored in acid–citrate–dextrose and citrate–phosphate–dextrose: Implications regarding delivery of oxygen. J Lab Clin Med 77:430, 1971
13. Siggaard–Andersen O: An acid–base chart for arterial blood with normal and pathophysiological reference areas. Scand J Clin Lab Invest 27:239, 1971
14. Sorbini CA, Grassi V, Solinas E: Arterial oxygen tension in relation to age in healthy subjects. Respiration 25:3, 1968
15. Suter PM, Fairley HB, Isenberg MD: Optimum end-expiratory airway pressure in patients in acute pulmonary failure. N Engl J Med 292:284, 1975
16. Woodbury CW: Body acid–base state and its regulation. In Ruch TC, Patton HD (eds): Physiology and Biophysics, Circulation, Respiration and Fluid Balance, 20th ed, pp 480–524. Philadelphia, WB Saunders, 1974

BIBLIOGRAPHY

General

Comroe JH Jr: Physiology of Respiration, 2nd ed. Chicago, Year Book Medical Publishers, 1974

Jones NL: Blood Gases and Acid-Base Physiology. New York, Brian C Decker, 1980

Mohler JG, Collier CR, Brandt W et al: Blood gases. In Clausen JL (ed): Pulmonary Function Testing: Guidelines and Controversies. New York, Academic Press, 1982

Shapiro BA, Harrison RA, Walton JR: Clinical Application of Blood Gases, 3rd ed. Chicago, Year Book Medical Publishers, 1982

West JB: Respiratory Physiology: The Essentials. Baltimore, Williams & Wilkins, 1974

Winters RW, Engel KE, Dell RB: Acid–Base Physiology in Medicine: A Self-Instruction Program, 2nd ed. Cleveland, The London Co (Copenhagen, Radiometer A/S), 1969

Woodbury CW: Body acid–base state and its regulation. In Ruch TC, Patton HD (eds): Physiology and Biophysics, Circulation, Respiration and Fluid Balance, 20th ed, pp 480–524. Philadelphia, WB Saunders, 1974

Oxygenation

Bunn HF, Jandl JH: Control of hemoglobin function within the red cell. N Engl J Med 282:1414, 1970

Finch CA, Lenfant C: Oxygen transport in man. N Engl J Med 286:407, 1972

Jones NL: Blood Gases and Acid-Base Physiology. New York, Brian C Decker, 1980

Kelman GR: Computer program for the production of O_2–CO_2 diagrams. Respir Physiol 4:260, 1968

Klocke RA: Oxygen transport and 2,3-diphosphoglycerate (DPG). Chest 62:79S, 1972

Mansell A, Bryan C, Levison H: Airway closure in children. J Appl Physiol 33:711, 1972

Mellemgaard K: The alveolar–arterial oxygen difference: Its size and components in normal man. Acta Physiol Scand 67:10, 1966

Mohler JG, Collier CR, Brandt W et al: Blood gases. In Clausen JL (ed): Pulmonary Function Testing: Guidelines and Controversies. New York, Academic Press, 1982

Sorbini CA, Grassi V, Solinas E: Arterial oxygen tension in relation to age in healthy subjects. Respiration 25:3, 1968

Acid–Base Balance

Albert MS, Dell RB, Winters RW: Quantitative displacement of acid–base equilibrium in metabolic acidosis. Ann Intern Med 66:312, 1967

Arbus GS et al: Characterization and clinical application of the "significance band" for acute respiratory alkalosis. N Engl J Med 280:117, 1969

Astrup P et al: The acid–base metabolism: A new approach. Lancet 278:1035, 1960

Bia M, Thier SO: Mixed acid base disturbances: A clinical approach. Med Clin N Am 65:347, 1981

Brackett NC Jr, Cohen JJ, Schwartz WB: Carbon dioxide titration curve of normal man: Effect of increasing degrees of acute hypercapnia on acid–base equilibrium. N Engl J Med 272:6, 1965

Cohen JJ, Schwartz WB: Evaluation of acid–base equilibrium in pulmonary insufficiency: An approach to a diagnostic dilemma. Am J Med 41:163, 1966

Jones NL: Blood Gases and Acid–Base Physiology. New York, Brian C Decker, 1980

Kildeberg P: Respiratory compensation in metabolic alkalosis. Acta Med Scand 174:515, 1963

McCurdy DK: Mixed metabolic and respiratory acid–base disturbances: Diagnosis and treatment. Chest 62:35S, 1972

Mohler JG, Collier CR, Brandt W et al: Blood gases. In Clausen JL (ed): Pulmonary Function Testing: Guidelines and Controversies. New York, Academic Press, 1982

Rastegar A, Thier SO: Physiologic consequences and bodily adaptions to hyper- and hypocapnia. Chest 62:28S, 1972

Schwartz WB, Brackett NC Jr, Cohen JJ: Response of extracellular hydrogen ion concentration to graded degrees of chronic hypercapnia: Physiologic limits of defense of pH. J Clin Invest 44:291, 1965

Shapiro BA: Clinical Application of Blood Gases. Chicago, Year Book Medical Publishers, 1973

Winters RW: Studies of acid–base disturbances. Pediatrics 39:700, 1967

Woodbury CW: Body acid–base state and its regulation. In Ruch TC, Patton HD (eds): Physiology and Biophysics, Circulation, Respiration and Fluid Balance, 20th ed, pp 480–524. Philadelphia, WB Saunders, 1974

13

Practical Physical Diagnosis in Respiratory Care

George G. Burton

No matter how thorough the admitting physician's history-taking and physical examination may be, subsequent interrogation and reevaluation of the respiratory patient is often rewarding. The patient may add to, retract, or amend information he gave the physician during the rush of admission procedures; these bits of social or historical data may be more important than much of the information already on the hospital chart.

Repeat chest physical examinations are also key to the evaluation of patients undergoing respiratory care procedures. Under vigorous therapy, chest physical findings may change and be the first clue to alterations in the disease process. New complications (e.g., wheezes where normal breath sounds were previously heard) or early signs of improvement (e.g., rales developing in the resolution stage of pneumonia) may appear. The repeated interview and limited cardiopulmonary examination thus serves several important purposes.

1. It provides essential information vital to accurate differential diagnosis
2. It "double checks" the often harried work of the initial examination
3. It allows the allied health worker to assess longitudinally the psychologic and sociologic, as well as the physiologic, impact of the illness (and treatment) on the patient
4. It creates and maintains patient–therapist rapport in a way that no simple respiratory therapy treatment can do

The Joint Commission on Hospital Accreditation has indicated that therapists and nurses should record physical findings before, during, and after therapy as part of the permanent patient record in order that the results of treatment can be judged objectively (Standard III, Interpretation). In situations where a patient does not demonstrate improvement in physical findings or in his symptoms of shortness of breath or sputum production, respiratory therapy treatment modalities should not be continued for days or weeks without change. Third-party payers may simply refuse to reimburse the hospital for such unmonitored "treatments." Accordingly, in addition to concern about blood gas measurements, spirometric improvement, and other variables, it becomes imperative for the aggressive respiratory care worker to learn how to interview and examine a patient at the bedside and to interpret these findings in the light of the patient's condition.

BRIEF RESPIRATORY HISTORY

Clarification of the patient's complaint is usually the first step in the successful interview. In the patient with cardiopulmonary disease, these complaints are usually cough and dyspnea.

COUGH

Coughing is not normal, except very occasionally. The incidence of cough increases rapidly among smokers and those with various diseases. Of itself cough is a nonspecific but important finding. In a recent study, however, 86% of patients with chronic, persistent cough were *specifically* diagnosed.[1] Questions to be asked about cough should reassure the therapist that he is dealing with more than the "tickle in the throat" associated with postnasal drainage or with hysteria.

Questions about cough should consider the volume and character of the expectorated secretions (*see* Chap. 19), which may indicate the nature of the disease process to some extent. The patient's own description of the site where the cough originates should not go unnoted.

Finally, definitive treatment of cough may be simple or complex. Its precise nature is predicated on first determining its *precise* cause, and then embarking on disease-specific rational therapy.

SHORTNESS OF BREATH (DYSPNEA)

The most common of respiratory symptoms is also the most misleading. Is the patient *claiming* dyspnea when he really *means* fatigue, weakness, hyperventilation, or chest discomfort (e.g., "tightness in the chest" or, more commonly, "congestion")? The careful questioner must ascertain the difference. Similarly, questions on exertional dyspnea must be carefully phrased. I have been chagrined to find that a patient who would admit to *no* shortness of breath on exertion later admitted that he did not, could not, or would not exert (e.g., because of arthritis in the hip joint, leg cramps, or just plain laziness).

The degree of dyspnea should be assessed first. The American Medical Association has devised a rating scale for respiratory impairment that is useful in the initial and longitudinal evaluation of dyspnea (see Table 13-1). Use of this scale is valuable in disability determinations and in respiratory rehabilitation programs and gives at least a *roughly* quantifiable idea of the patient's respiratory limitations.[2] Within the framework of these guidelines, one can view dyspnea as an imbalance between the patient's need to, and *ability* to, breathe. (A corollary of this concept implies that relief of dyspnea may be achieved in two general ways: by reducing the *need* for ventilation, for example, by weight loss, exercise conditioning, reduction of fever, or work modification techniques; and by enhancing the ability to breathe, for example, by improving ventilation–perfusion relationships in the lung.)

Next should follow questions that probe such areas as the precipitating (and relieving) factors of dyspnea, such as duration, temporal factors, positional factors, and daytime–nighttime variation. Episodic shortness of breath that wakes one from sleep is called paroxysmal nocturnal dyspnea. Patients with severe heart or lung disease may need to sit up or have the head of the bed elevated to breathe comfortably (orthopnea). Both these symptoms suggest congestive heart failure, but they often occur in other conditions as well.

In evaluating possible causes of dyspnea, one must be wary of accepting the patient's own idea of

Table 13-1. Severity of Dyspnea in Evaluating Permanent Impairment*

CLASS I	CLASS II	CLASS III	CLASS IV	CLASS V
Dyspnea only on severe exertion ("appropriate" dyspnea)	Can keep pace with person of same age and body build on the level without breathlessness, but not on hills or stairs	Can walk a mile at own pace without dyspnea, but cannot keep pace on the level with a normal person	Dyspnea present after walking about 100 yards on the level, or upon climbing one flight of stairs	Dyspnea on even less activity, or even at rest

*(Modified from Committee on Rating of Mental and Physical Impairment: Guides to the evaluation of permanent impairment—the respiratory system. JAMA *194*:919, 1965)

his diagnosis as the actual truth. Many patients believe, or have been told, that they have emphysema when in fact they do not. Many patients are convinced that their dyspnea results from "*only* my emphysema" when indeed the dyspnea is due to an associated pneumonia. Although it is important to ascertain how the patient assesses his own situation, it is the physician, nurse, or therapist who must make the correct diagnosis. Particularly misleading are complaints of "tuberculosis" (on the basis of a positive tuberculin skin test), "emphysema" (on the basis of increased anteroposterior diameter of the chest), "asthma" (anything that wheezes), and "pneumonia" (cough with fever, but no roentgenogram). Despite all the foregoing potential pitfalls, the careful history and physical examination remain the cornerstones of the clinical evaluation; they attain more significance when performed repeatedly, as in the course of a hospitalization or in a protracted pulmonary rehabilitation program.

PHYSICAL EXAMINATION

VIEW FROM THE DOOR

The examiner is well advised to resist the temptation to rely on the stethoscope as the primary diagnostic tool of his trade. A moment's reflection on the implications of the scene as viewed at the entrance to the patient's room may predict, with surprising accuracy, what will be heard during auscultation. The stethoscope is the *last*, not the first, tool to use in examination of the chest.

Attendant Garb

The respiratory care worker who sees the patient's physician and other attendants dressed in isolation gowns, caps, masks, and gloves can narrow the diagnostic possibilities from several hundred down to a relative handful: tuberculosis; *Pseudomonas sp.* infection; staphylococcal infection; depressed immune status of the patient (reverse isolation); and hepatitis.

Care must be taken that such infections do not spread to other patients by means of contaminated equipment, clothing, or unwashed hands. This problem is discussed in Chapter 19.

Graphic Sheet

A glance to see whether the patient is febrile will usually separate the diagnostic possibilities into infectious and noninfectious categories. The most common causes of fever in respiratory disease patients are pneumonia, tuberculosis, severe *acute* bronchitis, and atelectasis.

Although the temperature (particularly if taken rectally) and the pulse rate are usually reliable indicators of patient condition, the respiratory *rate* often is not. If one observes one's colleagues attempting to count the respiratory rate in spontaneously breathing patients, the reasons for this will become instantly apparent. In adults the normal breathing frequency ranges from 8 to 10 breaths per minute when the person is asleep to 20 to 30 breaths per minute when the patient is having an arterial puncture, is apprehensive, or is in pain. Which number, then, is charted? Certainly at times the patient will hold his breath or hardly seem to breathe at all, whereas at other times he may hyperventilate. With all this in mind, it is a wonder that the old "R" part of the "TPR" survived as long as it has. The science of pneumotachography, as used in sleep apnea studies, may soon ameliorate this problem in critically ill patients.

However, a *change* in respiratory rate is important. For example, consider the patient who has been breathing 10 to 12 times per minute day after day, shift after shift, who then suddenly doubles or triples his respiratory rate, accompanied by fever, cough, or increased sputum production. This *is* important and usually indicates the presence of hypoxemia, perhaps secondary to atelectasis, or one of the infectious processes already mentioned.

Breathing Patterns and Position

The supine, bedsheet-covered patient who breathes 8 to 15 times per minute with a tidal volume of 300 to 500 cc may tempt one to call a STAT while still standing at the entrance to the patient's room. Such breathing, although delivering perfectly adequate alveolar ventilation, may be accompanied by hardly any *visible* muscular activity!

The normal patient demonstrates no *position dependence* for ease of breathing: Respiration is comfortable while prone, supine, or in either lateral decubitus position. The normal patient may occasionally take a deep sigh and change position, but these movements are casual and not associated with any visible effort.

Patients with unilateral lung disease may be more comfortable lying on the "good" side (e.g., patients with pleurisy or fractured ribs), but this is not a constant finding. Patients with severe airways obstruction assume the arms-braced, sitting-up "emphysematous habitus" (Fig. 13-1). In this position the accessory muscles of respiration elevate and expand the thoracic cage across the fixed shoulder girdle, and gravity assists the downward motion of the diaphragm.

Normal breathing, as mentioned above, is easily performed regardless of position, is rhythmic, and is not associated with visible muscular effort. The length of expiration is slightly longer than inspiration (I:E ratio of 3 to 3:5). In obstructive pulmonary disease, the respiratory rate may be slow or normal, but expiration is prolonged. Breathing is usually rapid and shallow in restrictive pulmonary disease (e.g., interstitial fibrosis, pleural effusion, or congestive heart failure).

When the work of breathing increases, either from increased airways resistance, from decreased pulmonary compliance, or during moderate to severe exercise, the accessory muscles of respiration become involved. There is much more tossing of head, neck, arms, shoulders, and chest cage, and clearly to even the casual observer the ease of normal breathing is no longer present. Abnormal breathing patterns are detailed in Chapter 34.

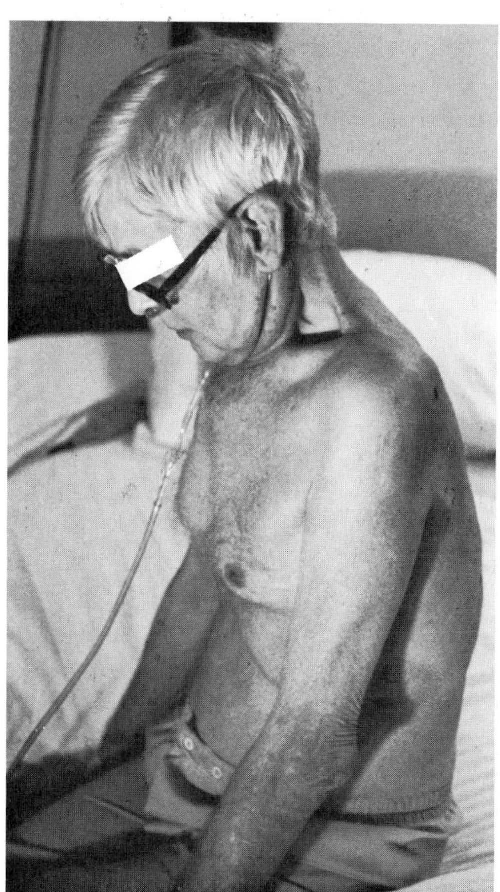

Fig. 13-1. The typical "emphysematous habitus." the patient sits with arms braced on bed or table to stabilize the insertions of the accessory muscles of respiration and thus aid in the work of breathing.

Sounds of Breathing

From the door the normal, spontaneously breathing patient may snore, occasionally cough, or audibly sigh, but generally is quiet. Audible wheezing, stridor, or gurgling respirations are signs of upper airway obstruction that require prompt attention. Suctioning, repositioning of the patient, or insertion of an oropharyngeal airway may be indicated. The *loudest* sounds are made by abnormalities in the *larger* (upper) airways. The stridor of childhood croup (allergic tracheobronchitis) is a good example. *Continuous snoring* during sleep may be the earliest symptom of sleep apnea, discussed in detail in Appendix C.

Equipment in Use

The patient on oxygen therapy *presumably* would be hypoxemic without oxygen supplementation; the patient on a respirator would hypoventilate without it; the patient using an ultrasonic nebulizer probably has thick, tenacious secretions; the patient taking bronchodilator medication from a nebulizer or an IPPB device presumably has one of several obstructive pulmonary diseases. The patient using a postural drainage board has either a lung abscess, bronchiectasis, or cystic fibrosis. All this seems clear. It is surprising how rarely the peripheral vision of the respiratory care worker encompasses these well-known devices and incorporates their presence into his diagnostic thinking process.

Sputum

The patient with hypertension gets his blood pressure measured and charted; the obese patient is weighed and the results are charted. The patient with arrhythmias is placed on a monitor with a trend recorder. What can be observed about the patient with respiratory disease? The answer is his *sputum*. Better medical centers now ask patients to expectorate all sputum into bedside containers. These containers are preferably made of clear plastic and should be examined by the respiratory team at frequent intervals. Notable variables are [1] volume/time period, [2] consistency and viscosity, [3] purulence or lack of it, and [4] presence or absence of blood. In hospitalized pa-

Table 13-2. Disease States Associated with Abnormal Gross Appearance of the Sputum*

TYPE OF SPUTUM	LUNG ABSCESS	ACUTE BRONCHITIS	CHRONIC BRONCHITIS	PNEUMONIA	PULMONARY EDEMA	BRONCHIECTASIS	TUBERCULOSIS	LUNG CANCER	PULMONARY INFARCTION	BRONCHIAL ASTHMA	CYSTIC FIBROSIS	ASPIRATION PNEUMONIA
Mucoid (white or clear)			X							X		
Mucopurulent		X	X								X	
Purulent (yellow or green)	X	X		X		X						X
Fetid	X					X					X	X
Bloody		X		X	X	X	X	X	X			
Frothy, sometimes pink					X							

*The most characteristic sputum appearance, consistency, and odor are listed.

tients with respiratory disease, the volume, color, and consistency of the sputum expectorated should be charted at the end of each shift.

The diagnostic implications of gross sputum examination are seen in Table 13-2. Chapter 19 further outlines the importance of the gross and microscopic examination of the sputum. Particularly viscous, adherent sputum is seen in asthma, bronchitis, and cystic fibrosis. If the container must be violently agitated to dislodge a bit of sputum from the side of the jar, one can be assured that the patient *also* has had difficulty in removing such secretions. Systemic hydration or humidification of inspirated air, or ultrasonic nebulization of fluids, may be indicated. Suctioning or postural drainage may be needed as well.

Purulent green or yellow sputum is seen in bronchitis, pneumonia, lung abscesses, cystic fibrosis, and bronchietasis. In bronchietasis excessively large amounts of thick, tenacious sputum are commonly expectorated, unless the patient lives in areas of very low ambient humidity.

Sputum that contains bright red blood is seen most typically in carcinoma of the lung, tuberculosis, and bronchiectasis. Bleeding from the upper airway, particularly the posterior nasopharynx and periodontal tissues, must be excluded before beginning an unnecessary, extensive workup. Darker blood ("rusty sputum") is expectorated in several types of pneumonia and is classical in pneumococcal and *Klebsiella* pneumonia.

Clear mucoid sputum occurs characteristically in bronchial asthma. Tiny threads of mucopolysaccharide that represent casts of the small airways (Curschmann's spirals) may be seen clinging to the side of the sputum jar in some cases.

In acute alveolar pulmonary edema, the sputum is thin, frothy, and sometimes blood-tinged. The same pink color in expectorated sputum is sometimes seen in patients using isoetharine (Bronkosol) and other bronchodilators.

Particularly foul-smelling, fetid sputum indicates chronic suppurative lung abscesses or bronchiectasis. Sputum that contains anaerobic organisms and *Pseudomonas sp.* has a particularly putrid odor.

Markings on the Chest

Although some physicians will use a felt-tipped pen to outline various physical findings (such as diaphragmatic excursion) on a patient's chest, this is not really common. If a patient's skin is covered with reddish-purple markings that outline the central mediastinum, he most likely has carcinoma of the lung or another malignant disease that involves the mediastinum. A lead "mantle" fits outside these marked-off areas to prevent radiation pneumonitis from the effects of radiotherapy.

INSPECTION OF THE CHEST

The "view from the door" completed, one now approaches the patient for the formal examination. The interval interview may be accomplished during this period. If possible, ask the patient to disrobe completely to the waist and examine him while he sits on the side of the bed or in a chair. This step should not be performed hastily.

Inspection is the first formal step in the chest examination, followed in order by palpation, percussion, and auscultation.

CHEST CONFIGURATION

In infancy the chest is more or less circular when viewed from the head down. With the coming of puberty the chest increases in its lateral diameter so that the anteroposterior diameter of the chest is much less than its lateral dimension. With advancing age the chest may increase slightly in anteroposterior diameter. In patients with severe obstructive pulmonary disease, the anteroposterior diameter of the chest is markedly increased (the so-called barrel chest deformity). This may occur in severe childhood asthma as well as in emphysema.

Unilateral hyperexpansion of the chest is seen in rare conditions such as agenesis of the contralateral lung or congenital hemiatrophy. *Apparent* hyperexpansion may be seen in the contralateral lung in patients with pneumothorax, fibrothorax, or massive atelectasis in the affected lung. In short, the normal chest should be symmetrical. Sternal deformities, pectus excavatum (sternal depression), or pectus carinatum (sternal outward bowing) usually produce no severe physiologic sequelae.

Deformities of the spine, however, are often responsible for severe pulmonary disability. Spinal curvature is seen in kyphosis, scoliosis, arthritis, and spinal tuberculosis. In ankylosing spondylitis, loss of the normal thoracic and lumbosacral curves results in a straight, immobile spinal column (so-called poker spine). In such patients, limitation of chest expansion eventually may occur, with loss of lung volume and cor pulmonale being the end results.

Abdominal protuberance from centripetal obesity or lax abdominal musculature must be looked for, preferably with the patient both standing and lying supine. Obesity predisposes the patient to hypoventilation and atelectasis in the basilar portions of the lung. Severe obesity associated with overall alveolar hypoventilation, reduced CO_2 responsiveness, and cor pulmonale is called the "pickwickian syndrome."

Scars

Scars of past surgeries or trauma on the neck and chest wall are often so well healed as to be overlooked. Their discovery will often bring out important, previously overlooked bits of historical information (e.g., that the patient had lung cancer or tuberculosis or that his hoarseness is from recurrent laryngeal nerve palsy secondary to thyroid disease).

Breast Examination

Examination of the breasts is not pertinent to ferreting out the causes of cough or dyspnea. Surgical absence of the female breast should be noted and may explain later findings if breast carcinoma metastatic to lung has occurred. Male nurses and therapists need not palpate or examine the female breast in most instances, and then only when accompanied by another female or physician in the room. This seemingly minor point has been the root cause of some narrowly averted lawsuits.

Reduced or Absent Hemithorax Movement

Reduced or absent movement of one hemithorax may indicate pain in that area from fractured ribs or pleural disease; diminished diaphragmatic excursion; or a unilateral pneumothorax. It may also indicate accidental intubation of one mainstem bronchus (usually the right). Symmetry of motion of the chest is as critical as symmetry of shape.

Localization of Findings

Good practice requires that abnormal findings be localized as precisely as possible. Vertical imaginary lines drawn through the sternum, spine, midclavicle, midscapula, and down from the anterior, middle, and posterior axillary folds are of historical interest but of limited usefulness. Some of these imaginary lines are illustrated in Figure 13-2. Although helpful in rough localization of findings in the vertical plane, they require one to record cumbersome comments (e.g., "rales were heard 3.0 cm medial to the right midscapular line 30 cm from the top of the shoulder").

Of considerably more use is knowledge of lobar and segmental topographical anatomy and reporting of physical findings with comments such as "wheezes were heard in the anterior segment of the right upper lobe." Figure 13-3 illustrates the approximate location of the lobes of the right lung in the right anterior oblique projection. Figure 13-4 illustrates the topographical correlates of the upper and lower lobes in the anterior oblique projection of the left chest. The posterolateral extent of the lower lobes must be emphasized. Almost the whole posterior chest, from midscapula to diaphragm, is composed of these lobes.

Anteriorly the upper and middle lobes lie under the right chest; on the left side the upper lobe and its dependent portion, the lingula, occupy most of the anterior chest.

The horizontal fissure, which separates the right upper from the right middle lobe, underlies the fourth anterior rib, in line with the nipple in males. On the left the lingular segment of the uper lobe is in a position analogous to the right middle lobe.

Segmental anatomy is described in detail in Chapter 26; the topographical relationships are illustrated in Figure 13-5. The reader is encouraged to practice his skills in precise anatomical localization of physical findings using these illustrations as guidelines.

PERCUSSION

Chest percussion as a physical diagnosis technique is usually vastly overrated; it is underrated as a *therapeutic* technique in patients with retained secretions. That caveat aside, even expert percussion of the chest can rarely localize lesions smaller than 4 to 5 cm in diameter. Thus, it is relatively *useless* in the localization of segmental infiltrates or "coin" lesions. The technique is useful, however, in defining the extent of larger lesions such as lobar pneumonias, pleural effusions, motion of the diaphragm on deep inspiration, and heart and liver size.

Percussion should be performed with the patient sitting or standing, since compression of the chest by body weight makes percussion in the prone or lateral decubitus position misleading at best.

Percussion is performed in two ways: by direct firm tapping of the patient's chest with the flexed fingertip *(immediate percussion)* (Fig. 13-6A); or by tapping over the distal portion of the interposed third finger *(mediate percussion)* (Fig. 13-6B). Immediate percussion is excellent for gross localization of the abnormalities listed above; mediate percussion is best for more precise localization. These techniques can be practiced by attempting to localize the studs in a convenient wall. One should note a dull, nonresonant

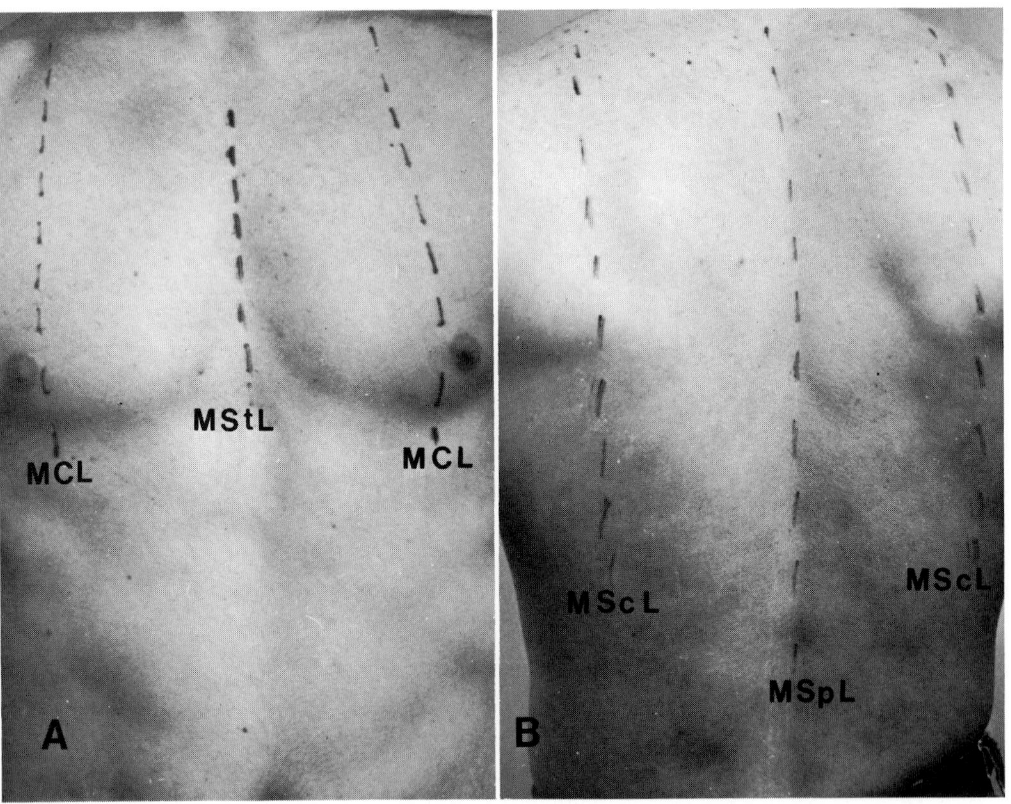

Fig. 13-2. Vertical imaginary lines used in the localization of chest physical findings. *(A)* Anterior chest. *(B)* Posterior chest. MCL = midclavicular line; MStL = midsternal line; MScL = midscapulae line; MSpL = midspinous line.

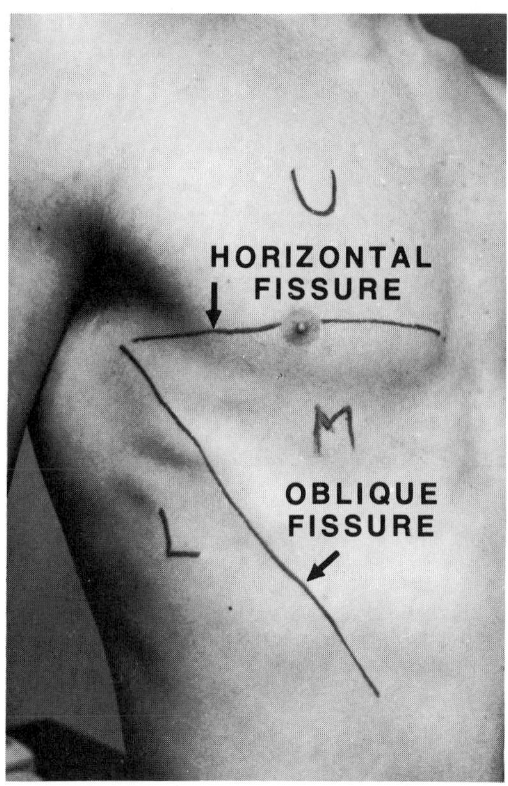

Fig. 13-3. Approximate location of the lobes of the right lung, seen in the lateral anterior oblique position. Posteriorly the superior segment of the lower lobe extends to approximately midscapula. U = upper lobe; M = middle lobe; L = lower lobe.

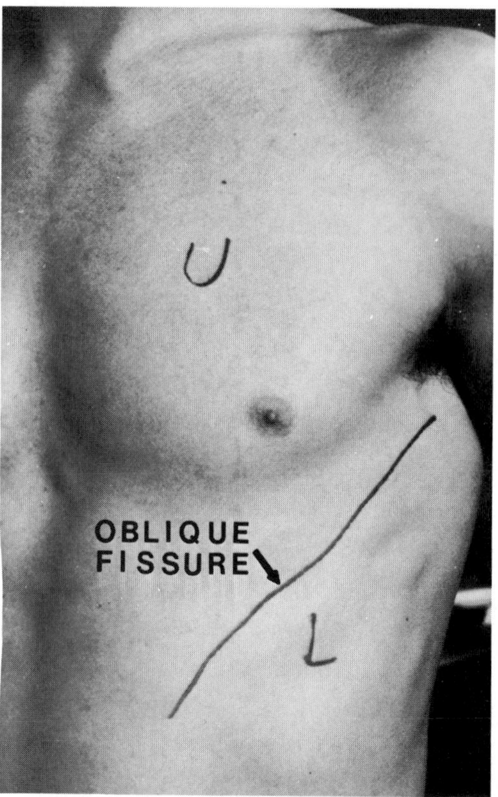

Fig. 13-4. Approximate location of the lobes of the left lung, in the lateral anterior oblique position. The anterior, dependent portion of the left upper lobe above the oblique fissure is known as the lingula and is in a position analogous to the right middle lobe.

sound over the denser wooden stud compared to the resonant, air-containing, hollow wall between the studs.

A resonant sound is heard over a normal, air-containing lung. Hyperresonance (tympany) may be heard in conditions that cause pulmonary air trapping or in patients with pneumothorax. Dullness or flatness should be percussed over the heart and liver. The areas of resonance at the lung apices (Kronig's isthmuses) should be identified by mediate percussion (Fig. 13-7). Asymmetry of the absolute width of these areas is more significant than their actual width. Dullness or flatness in the area of Kronig's isthmuses may indicate apical consolidation, as in carcinoma or tuberculosis.

Probably the most important contribution chest percussion makes to the physical examination is that of determining the extent of diaphragmatic excursion. Normally the diaphragms descend between 4 to 6 cm on deep inspiration. Descent of the diaphragm is normally equal on both sides of the chest (Fig. 13-8). If excursion of the lung on one side is prevented by diaphragmatic paralysis, adhesions, or masked by a pleural effusion, the difference in height of the resonance-dullness border will be apparent.

Dullness or flatness to percussion is produced by consolidation of the lung parenchyma or fluid interposed between the chest wall and lung. Such conditions include pleural effusion or thickening, carcinoma, pneumonia, emphysema, and tuberculosis.

AUSCULTATION

Since the early 1800s, when Laënnec first described the stethoscope, the great temptation of entering students has been to take out this device, lay it on the patient's chest, and say, "Ah ha! I hear wheezes" (or rales or rhonchi), to write these findings down, and to think of the examination as complete. This is not

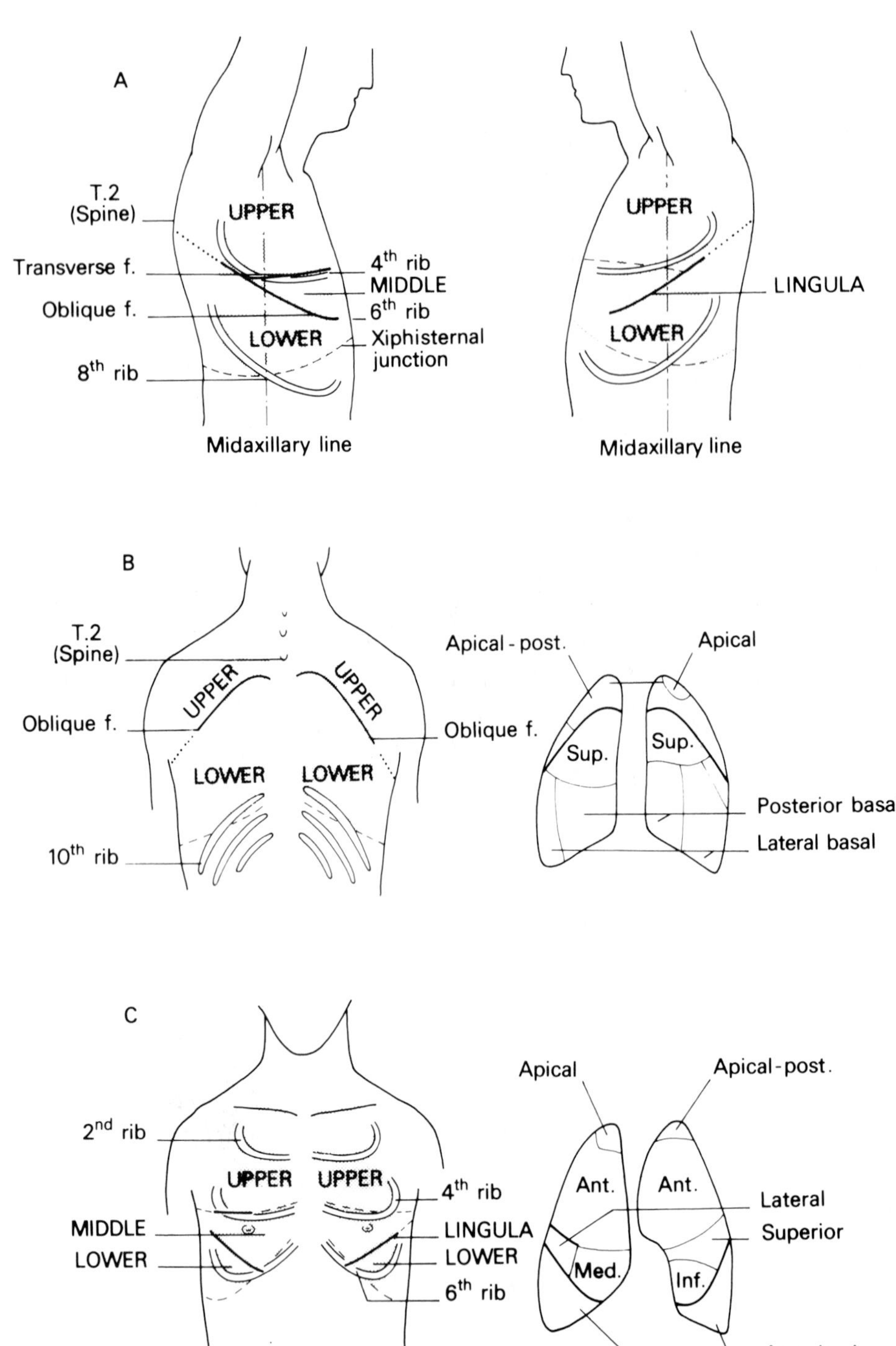

Fig. 13-5. Topographical relationships with respect to the pulmonary segments. *(A)* Lateral; *(B)* posterior; and *(C)* anterior projections.

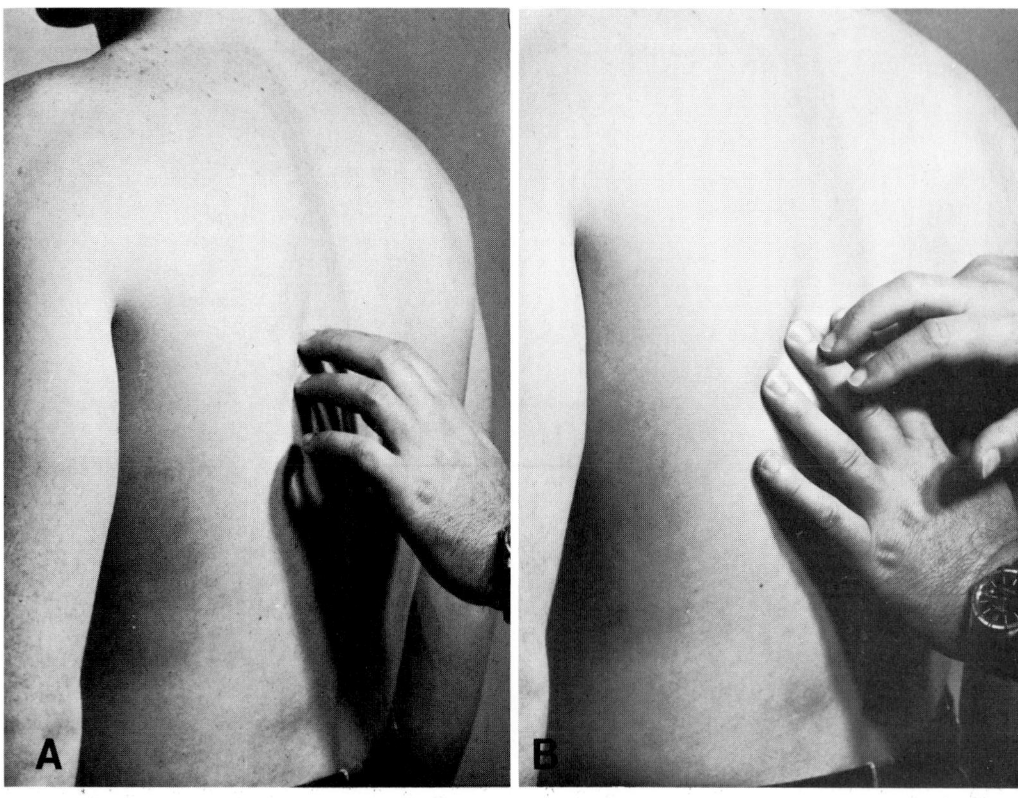

Fig. 13-6. Immediate *(A)* and mediate *(B)* chest percussion technique.

always the case, despite the importance of auscultation as an examination technique.

The vocabulary of chest auscultation is confusing, although a Joint Committee of the American College of Chest Physicians and the American Thoracic Society has attempted to standardize many of the terms and symbols in use for pulmonary disease and function.[3] Their report has recently been updated.[4] The Joint Committee has suggested that breath sounds be described only as normal, decreased in intensity, or bronchial, and that only fine crackles (fine rales), coarse crackles (coarse rales), wheezes (sibilant rhonchi), and rhonchi (sonorous rhonchi) be listed as acceptable terms for adventitious sounds. Although I agree with the Joint Commission, I believe that other terms are still sufficiently common to warrant discussion in this chapter.

Normal breath sounds have a higher frequency (100–>1000 Hz) than do normal heart sounds and murmurs (60–400 cps), are generally of less intensity, and are lower pitched. In addition, breath sounds may change from moment to moment: a patient with rhonchi at one time may be absolutely "clear" to auscultation the next, after bronchodilator therapy. Finally, since audible breath sounds are generated only by air-

Fig. 13-7. Krönig's isthmuses (areas of relative resonance above the lung apices). Loss of resonance or unequal width of the two isthmuses may indicate disease in the upper lobes.

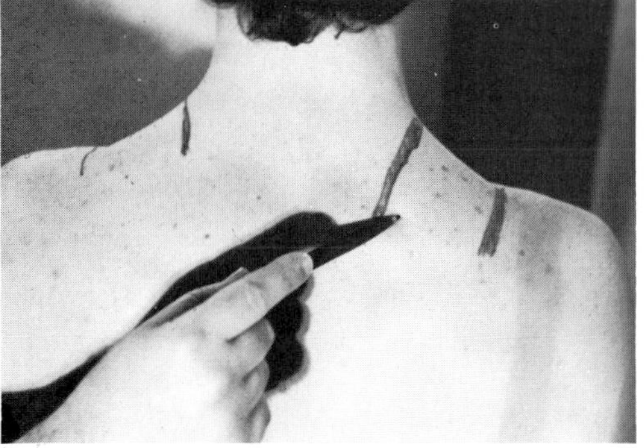

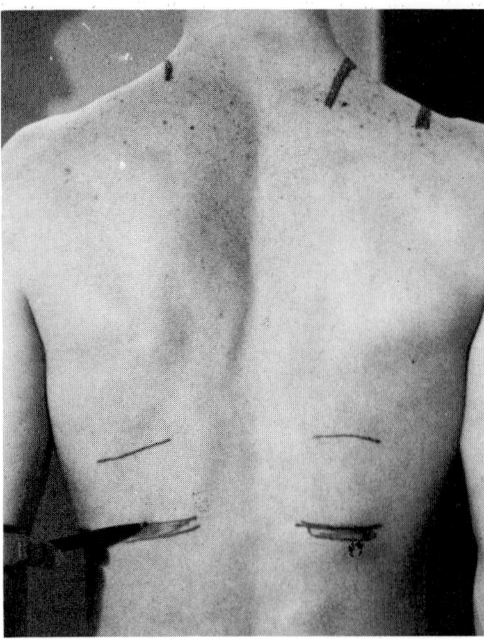

Fig. 13-8. Posterior view of the thorax illustrating the normal diaphragmatic excursion between inspiration *(lower horizontal lines)* and expiration *(upper horizontal lines)*. Percussion resonance is appreciated above the diaphragm and flatness below.

flow velocities greater than those achieved during tidal breathing, the patient's ability to sustain hyperventilation limits the amount of time that can be spent in auscultation. These factors combine to make recording of breath sounds for teaching purposes difficult. With these problems in mind, the beginner will be well advised to practice listening to the various normal breath sounds on willing roommates, spouses, or, better yet, children, whose thin chest walls greatly facilitate the examination. Finding patients with "pure" abnormal breath sounds is somewhat difficult (e.g., crackles and wheezes frequently occur simultaneously). Knowledge of "pure" findings in specific patients should be shared with one's colleagues so that all may benefit.

Absolute quiet is necessary for thorough examination of the chest with the stethoscope. Relatives should be asked to leave the room; television sets, radios, and running water should be turned off; the doorway to the hall should be closed; and all machines that make sounds should, if possible, be disconnected. In nonintubated, hypopneic, or apneic patients, good breath sounds may be induced by having an assistant ventilate the patient with a manual resuscitation bag.

The earpieces of the stethoscope should conform to the size and shape of the examiner's external auditory canal. If possible, the patient should sit errect with the back muscles relaxed so that all lobes can be auscultated. The chest should be completely exposed: Clothing that rubs against the stethoscope tubing introduces artifacts difficult to distinguish from some types of abnormal breath sounds.

The binaural stethoscope is the basic tool for auscultation. The diaphragm of the stethoscope filters out most low-pitched sounds. Since most breath sounds are relatively high-pitched, the diaphragm is used almost exclusively in the chest examination. It should be pressed firmly against the chest wall to screen out extraneous sounds.

Extraneous, nonpulmonary sounds may confuse the beginner. These sounds arise from the examiner's breathing on the stethoscope tubing, from sounds produced by muscles, tendons, and joints of the chest wall, and from hair on the patient's chest. This last-mentioned problem, if excessive, can be solved by moistening the skin or, in extreme cases, by shaving the area to be examined.

The bell of the stethoscope is valuable when listening for lower-pitched sounds, such as diastolic heart murmurs. It is also helpful in examining children and in thin or debilitated patients, where it can be applied over the intercostal muscles between their protuberant ribs.

Table 13-3 is a composite, diagrammatic representation of *normal* breath sounds. In the diagrams of the right side of the table, the inspiratory phase of respiration is represented by an upward stroke and expiration, by a downward stroke. The pitch, amplitude, length (on a 1–5 scale), and distinctive characteristics of each of the various sounds are outlined. The length of each line is determined by the amount of time that part of the respiratory cycle is heard. The thickness of the line represents the amplitude or loudness of each part of the breath sound. The angle the upward or downward strokes make with the horizontal is a schematic representation of the pitch of the breath sound—the greater the angle, the higher the pitch. The part of the chest where the individual breath sounds are characteristically heard is described below; heard elsewhere (*see* below), the sounds may be *abnormal*.

NORMAL BREATH SOUNDS

Normal Vesicular (Alveolar) Breathing

These sounds can be heard best over most of the chest, except directly over the trachea and central bronchi.

Their intensity is related directly to inspiratory flow rate. The site of generation of these sounds is unclear: Although they are called vesicular (the Latin word for "small vessels") or alveolar breath sounds, as far as is currently known no real air *flow*, and thus no sound, occurs in the alveoli themselves. Accordingly these sounds must arise in airway units larger than alveoli (presumably in the lobar or segmental bronchi).[5]

The vesicular breath sound has been described as "crisp," "breezy," and "like the sighing of wind." None of these terms is entirely descriptive. The inspiratory component is louder, slightly higher-pitched, and longer than the expiratory phase. There is no pause between the phases.

Normal vesicular sounds are accentuated in children and other people with thin chest walls. They are diminished in conditions such as emphysema, pleural effusion, and pleural thickening and are absent in pneumothorax. Like other breath sounds, they are greatly accentuated by deep breathing.

Tracheal and Bronchial Breathing

Over the intrathoracic trachea and major bronchi a different breath sound is heard. It is loud, harsh, and has a "tubular quality." Here the expiratory phase is often longer and louder than the inspiratory phase. Sounds that originate in the larger airways (*i.e.*, the trachea and main bronchi) are generally louder and of a lower pitch (400–800 Hz versus 1000–2000 Hz) than those that originate in the smaller bronchi. There is often a short pause between the inspiratory and expiratory phases.

Bronchovesicular Breath Sounds

As the name suggests, bronchovesicular breath sounds are a combination of the two sounds just described. They are heard best over the central airway (around the sternum and in the intrascapular area). Bronchovesicular breathing is sometimes also heard over the anterior and apical segment of the right upper lobe, where large bronchi are relatively close to the chest wall.

They are more muffled than bronchial breath sounds. Inspiration and expiration are roughly equal in length, and there is no pause between inspiration and expiration. Inspiration and expiration are of similar intensity.

In disease of the lungs, bronchial or bronchovesicular breath sounds are heard in areas other than those described above. Any process that causes the normally air-filled alveoli and small airways to be consolidated or fluid-filled results in bronchial breath sounds if the bronchial tree is open to airflow. Bronchovesicular breath sounds will be heard in areas of partial consolidation. Over pleural effusions, distant bronchial breathing may be heard.

Table 13-3. Normal Breath Sounds

TYPE	LOCATION WHERE TYPICALLY HEARD	PITCH	AMPLITUDE (LOUDNESS)	INSPIRATION: EXPIRATION RATIO	DESCRIPTION	GRAPHIC ILLUSTRATION
Vesicular	Over most of chest except major airways	Low	Moderate	3:1	"Breezy" (sound of wind in trees)	
Tracheal	Over trachea	Very high	Very great	5:6	Loud, harsh "tubular"	
Bronchial	Over major central airways	High	Great	2:3	Hollow tubular	
Broncho-vesicular	Over major central airways	Medium	Moderately great	1:1	"Breezy," tubular, "tent-shaped"	

ABNORMAL BREATH SOUNDS

Absent and Diminished Breath Sounds

Breath sounds will appear to be *absent* when the patient is not breathing, when the stethoscope is being used improperly, or when the patient has a pneumothorax, severe emphysema, an underlying pleural effusion, pleural thickening, or is severely obese. *Diminished* or variable-intensity breath sounds are diagnostic hallmarks of emphysema.[6]

Rhonchi and Wheezing

Rhonchi (see Table 13-4) are low-pitched, continuous sounds with a dominant frequency of 200 Hz or less. They have been described as a "snoring" or "gurgling" sound. Such sounds are often associated with diseases in which sputum production is characteristic, for example, bronchitis, resolving pneumonia, asthma. A bit of sputum vibrating in the airway may produce these sounds, which are often modified, or even eliminated, by coughing.

Wheezes (see Table 13-4) are high-pitched, continuous sounds that often increase in pitch and decrease in intensity toward the end of a forced expiration. Their dominant frequency is 400 Hz or more. Although often occurring in asthma, wheezes are also associated with other conditions, such as emphysema, congestive heart failure (with or without frank pulmonary edema), partial obstruction of an airway by a foreign body or tumor, the carcinoid syndrome.

Forgacs has postulated that both rhonchi and wheezes may arise from constricted, or semiobstructed, airways, where (by virtue of Bernoulli's principle) the velocity of gas flow increases at the point of constriction.[5] As higher intrathoracic pressures are generated, the airway orifice may become even narrower. At some point of narrowing, a "critical lumenal size" may be reached, and turbulent airflow across it may then produce either rhonchi or wheezes.

Stridor

Crouplike breath sounds are usually loud enough to be heard without a stethoscope. Their presence indicates large (upper) airway obstruction, as in laryngotracheobronchitis (childhood croup), foreign body aspiration, laryngeal tumors, or tracheomalacia. They are usually loudest on inspiration.

Table 13-4. Adventitious Sounds*

ACOUSTIC CHARACTERISTICS	TIME-EXPANDED WAVEFORM	RECOMMENDED TERM	ACCP† REPORT	CURRENT BRITISH USAGE	OTHER TERMS	SOME COMMON CLINICAL ASSOCIATIONS
Discontinuous, interrupted, explosive sounds—loud, duration of about 10 msec. Low in pitch: initial deflection width* averaging 1.5 msec.		Coarse crackle	Rale	Crackle	Bubbling rales, coarse crepitations	Pulmonary edema, resolving pneumonia
Discontinuous, interrupted, explosive sounds—less loud than above and of shorter duration. They average less than 5 msec in duration and are lower in pitch.		Fine crackle	Rale	Crackle	Fine crepitations	Interstitial fibrosis
Continuous sounds—longer than 250 msec, high-pitched dominant frequency of 400 Hz or more; a hissing sound.		Wheeze	Sibilant rhonchus	High-pitched wheeze	Sibilant rale, muscial rale	Airway narrowing
Continuous sounds—longer than 250 msec, low-pitched, dominant frequency about 200 Hz or less; a snoring sound.		Rhonchus	Sonorous rhonchus	Low-pitched wheeze		Sputum production

*(ATS News, Winter 1981. Modified and reprinted with permission)
†ACCP = American College of Chest Physicians.

Amphoric or Cavernous Breath Sounds

Amphoric sounds are best heard in expiration and occur over cavitary lesions that communicate with open airways. The sound is classic and will not be missed once one has heard it. It resembles the noise made by blowing across the mouth of an empty bottle. It may also be heard over a pneumothorax.

Metamorphosing or Variable Breath Sounds

Normally one should expect to hear reasonably constant breath sounds in any given area of lung, as described previously. When secretions intermittently occlude the airway, hybrid sounds that change from vesicular to tubular, or from bronchovesicular to asthmatic, may occur in midcycle, caused by the bronchus suddenly opening or closing in response to foreign material. Pedunculated tumors of the airway, such as bronchial adenomas, may produce this finding when the patient changes position from side to side.

Crackles or Rales

The rale (French rale = rattle) was first heard through a stethoscope by Laënnec, although originally described 2000 years earlier by Hippocrates, who mentioned it in cases of pneumonia and pleural empyema.

Crackles are low- to medium-pitched, discontinuous, interrupted, "explosive" sounds that are often quite loud. The origin of these sounds is still widely debated. Current theory holds that the coarse crackles of fulminant pulmonary edema are caused by rupture of fluid films and bubbles in the airway filled by edema fluid. Forgacs believes that the crackles of *interstitial* pulmonary edema and interstitial fibrosis result from the sudden release of energy stored in the lung after delayed opening of airways that had closed, perhaps prematurely, at the end of the previous expiration.[5] These rales usually occur predominantly in inspiration.

Many types of adjectives describe the various types of rales. The classification of rales seems to be constantly changing and varies from author to author. Modifying terms such as "wet," "dry," "atelectatic," "bubbling," "crepitant," and "Velcro" are all used to describe rales in various textbooks and journals.

Pleural Friction Rubs

When the visceral and parietal pleurae are inflamed and adherent, as in pleurisy, a characteristic loud, grating, discontinuous sound is heard, often described as that of "creaky shoe leather." Such sounds are often heard exactly where a patient complains of chest-wall discomfort; if so, the diagnosis of pleurisy is confirmed. Many conditions cause pleurisy: tuberculosis, pulmonary infarction, pneumonia, and both primary and metastatic carcinoma. One must not confuse the sounds made by chest hair and the movement of bones, joints, and muscles (chest wall crepitations) with true pleural friction rubs.

BEDSIDE ASSESSMENT OF PULMONARY FUNCTION

We have reviewed the importance of observing the ease with which the patient breathes, the position in which he chooses to do so, and the various sounds heard with and without the stethoscope. One further helpful maneuver is to assess the time required for all sounds to cease in the chest during the expiratory portion of a forced vital capacity maneuver. This *forced vital capacity time* should not exceed more than 3 seconds. Prolonged expiration greater than 5 seconds in duration indicates the presence of airway obstruction. Wheezing may accompany the prolonged expiration. Such patients will not be able to blow out a match held more than 3 to 5 inches from their mouths without pursing their lips (positive "*match test*").

SUMMARY

Table 13-5 summarizes the typical physical findings in the common, most important pulmonary diseases. Not mentioned previously is the finding of fremitus (vibration) abnormalities. Generally, consolidated or partially consolidated areas of lung that communicate with the larynx by means of open airways vibrate more vigorously than normal. This finding is particularly striking over a resolving pneumonia, where the spoken "one-two-three" or "ninety-nine" may be appreciated as increased vibration on the lateral aspect of the examining hand (tactile fremitus; see Fig. 13-9) or as exceptionally clear transmission of the normally muffled spoken word through the stethoscope (increased vocal fremitus, egophony, or, in the extreme, whispered pectoriloquy).

Chest physical diagnosis is not difficult if approached systematically, not neglecting the peripheral assessment detailed in this chapter—"the view from the door." To be helpful, it must be repeated

Table 13-5. Summary of Typical Physical Signs in the More Common Respiratory Diseases

PATHOLOGICAL PROCESS	MOVEMENT OF CHEST WALL	PERCUSSION NOTE	BREATH SOUNDS	ADVENTITIOUS SOUNDS AND ACCOMPANIMENTS
Consolidation: as in lobar pneumonia, extensive pulmonary infarction, or pneumonic tuberculosis	May be reduced on side affected	Dull	High-pitched, bronchial	Fine rales early; coarse rales later
Diffuse lobular pneumonia	Often symmetrically diminished	May be impaired	Usually harsh vesicular with prolonged expiration	Rhonchi and coarse rales
Pulmonary cavitation (typical signs present only when cavity is large and in communication with bronchus)	Normal or slightly reduced on side affected	Impaired	"Amphoric" or bronchial	Coarse rales
Atelectasis: from obstruction of major bronchus by secretions, carcinoma, foreign body or tuberculous lymph nodes	Reduced on side affected	Dull	Diminished or absent if complete; high-pitched bronchial otherwise	Usually rales appear after deep breath or cough
Bronchiectasis	Normal	Slightly impaired	Low-pitched bronchial	Coarse or sibilant rales
Pleural effusion or empyema	Reduced or absent (depending on size) on side affected	Dull to absent	Diminished or absent (occasionally high-pitched bronchial)	Pleural rub in some cases
Pneumothorax	Reduced or absent (depending on size) on side affected	Normal or hyperresonant	Diminished or absent (occasionally faint high-pitched bronchial)	High-pitched rales when fluid present
Bronchitis (acute or chronic)	Normal	Normal	Vesicular with prolonged expiration	Rhonchi, usually with some coarse rales
Bronchial asthma	Normal or symmetrically diminished	Normal or hyperresonant	Vesicular with prolonged expiration	Rhonchi, mainly expiratory and high-pitched (wheezes)
Diffuse pulmonary emphysema	Symmetrically diminished *en bloc* motion	Usually hyperresonant	Diminished vesicular with prolonged expiration	Rhonchi and coarse rales from associated bronchitis
Diffuse pulmonary fibrosis and other forms of interstitial lung disease	Symmetrically diminished	Normal	Harsh vesicular with prolonged expiration	Coarse crepitations uninfluenced by coughing
Pulmonary edema	Normal or increased	Normal	Bronchial if interstitial: vesicular if alveolar-filling	Moist rales

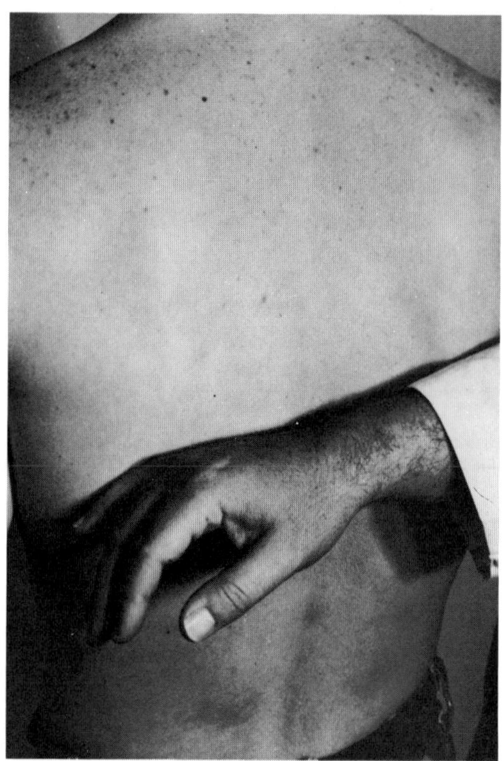

Fig. 13-9. Checking for tactile fremitus. The lateral edge of the examiner's hand is held against the patient's chest wall. Normal vocal sounds are transmitted through the chest wall and appreciated only as faint vibrations.

frequently. As in all procedures, practice makes perfect.

REFERENCES

1. Ad Hoc Committee on Pulmonary Nomenclature (ATS): Updated nomenclature for membership reaction, p 8. ATS News, Winter 1981
2. Committee on Rating of Mental and Physical Impairment: Guides to the evaluation of permanent impairment—the respiratory system. JAMA 194:919, 1965
3. Forgacs P: The functional basis of pulmonary sounds. Chest 73:399, 1978
4. Irwin RS, Corras WM, Prather MR: Chronic persistent cough in the adult: The spectrum and frequency of causes and successful outcome of specific therapy. Am Rev Respir Dis 123:413, 1981
5. Ploysongsang Y, Pare JAP, Macklem PT: Lung sounds in patients with emphysema. Am Rev Respir Dis 124:45, 1981
6. Pulmonary terms and symbols: A report of the ACCP/ATS Joint Committee on Pulmonary Nomenclature. Chest 67:583, 1975

BIBLIOGRAPHY

Barbee RA, Kettel LJ, Burrows B: The medical history in evaluation of patients with pulmonary diseases. Basics of RD 2, No. 4, 1974

Loudon RG: Cough: A symptom and a sign. Basics of RD 9, No. 4, 1981

Murphy RLH, Holford SK: Lung sounds. Basics of RD 8, No. 4, 1980. (This article is reprinted in Respir Care 25:763, 1980.)

14

Roentgenographic Patterns of Worsening Pulmonary Function

Glen A. Lillington

The analysis and interpretation of chest roentgenograms is a science that can scarcely be encompassed within a single chapter with a limited number of illustrations. This presentation will therefore not attempt to summarize a body of knowledge to which large and learned tomes have been devoted but will be directed toward three goals.

1. To acquaint paramedical readers with the terminology and some of the basic concepts peculiar to radiologic techniques of information gathering.
2. To demonstrate some of the "typical" radiologic patterns of abnormality, particularly those that occur in the seriously ill patient and are associated with deterioration of pulmonary function.
3. To emphasize that radiologic analysis may be critically important in some instances but seriously misleading in others. The stethoscope is not only a more convenient diagnostic tool than radiologic examination, but also, at times, more sensitive and occasionally more precise.

SOME BASIC PRINCIPLES IN CHEST ROENTGENOGRAPHY

Roentgenographic visualization of body structures depends on *contrast*. As the roentgenographic beam passes through the tissues to register on the radiographic film, differential absorption of the beam by different tissues occurs. The greater the "radiodensity" of the tissue, the greater the absorption of the beam, and the image of the tissue or organ will be relatively white (radiopaque). Less dense tissues are radiolucent and appear blacker on the film.

Chest roentgenography is made possible by the relative radiolucency (blackness) of the air-filled alveoli, which provide contrast to (and outline) the denser tissues such as bone, intrapulmonary vessels, and mediastinal structures, which are solid or fluid filled.

Because calcium has the greatest radio-opacity of any endogenous material, calcified structures are usually easily detected on the roentgenogram. Certain exogenous substances (tin, iodine, barium), which may appear in the thorax, have a "metallic density" similar to calcium. Body fluids and most tissues have a lesser degree of radio-opacity, usually referred to as "water density" or "tissue density." The degree of radio-opacity also depends on the *thickness* of tissue through which the beam has penetrated. The heart, which is large, will appear more opaque than the much smaller right or left pulmonary artery.

In most lung diseases, the "air density" of the affected area of lung is replaced (or displaced) by the "water density" of the disease process, resulting in the appearance of *increased radio-opacity*. Such abnormalities are commonly referred to as "shadows," and the size, shape, distribution, location, and homogeneity of such shadows provide clues to the radiologist in predicting the possible nature of the abnormality.

Certain thoracic diseases result in *increased radiolucency* if the air–tissue ratio in the affected area is increased. This is most commonly due to loss of lung tissue (emphysema, bullae, cavities), hyperinflation (asthma or a check-valve bronchial obstruction), or a collection of air in an abnormal location (pneumothorax or pneumomediastinum).

VALUE AND LIMITATIONS OF CHEST ROENTGENOGRAPHY

The chest roentgenogram is an extremely sensitive *detector* of certain abnormalities in the lungs. Commonly one encounters patients in whom routine chest roentgenography has revealed evidence of disease despite no symptoms or signs on physical examination. In addition to the detection of disease, the chest roentgenogram displays the *pattern* of abnormality, which provides valuable clues to determining the cause of the disorder. At times the roentgenographic pattern in itself is specifically diagnostic. More commonly the abnormal pattern suggests a limited number of diagnostic possibilities, which must then be further investigated by other techniques. *Serial chest roentgenograms taken at appropriate intervals provide a dynamic portrait of the disease process, information that has diagnostic value and prognostic implications and allows one to monitor the effectiveness of therapy.*

To interpret chest roentgenograms properly, one must be constantly aware of the *limitations* of the technique. In patients with bronchial asthma or chronic bronchitis, the chest roentgenogram may appear entirely normal even when the disease is severe. Emphysema may cause little change in the chest roentgenogram until an advanced stage has been reached. Primary lung cancer (bronchogenic carcinoma) usually cannot be detected by roentgenography until the tumor mass has reached a size of 1 cm in diameter, at which time the tumor may have already been present for 10 years or longer. Relatively large lesions may be virtually undetectable on the chest roentgenogram if they are located in the "blind" areas where the lung tissue is obscured by neighboring solid organs (heart, great vessels, or diaphragm).

Respiratory insufficiency may result from extrapulmonary abnormalities, including overdosage of sedative drugs leading to respiratory center depression, trauma to the brain and spinal cord, and neuromuscular disorders such as poliomyelitis and myasthenia gravis. These disorders of the "ventilatory pump" may occur in the presence of normal lung parenchyma, and the chest roentgenogram may appear completely normal unless complications occur.

Conversely, moderate or even extensive abnormalities on the chest roentgenogram are not always accompanied by severe symptoms or marked abnormalities in pulmonary function. This dichotomy between radiologic appearance and pathophysiologic reality tends to occur most commonly in sarcoidosis, pneumoconiosis, and histiocytosis X.

NORMAL CHEST ROENTGENOGRAM

The standard (routine) chest roentgenographic study comprises two views, both obtained with the subject in the upright position: a film obtained in the posteroanterior projection (the PA film); and a lateral projection, either right or left (the lateral film). The exposures should be made with respiration suspended in the full inspiratory position, with the subject properly positioned so that there is no rotation in either frontal or lateral projection, and with appropriate exposure techniques to enhance contrast without underpenetration or overpenetration.

When the patient is seriously ill, many or all of these ideal circumstances may be unattainable. The physician may often be asked to interpret a supine anteroposterior (AP) film (with no lateral view), badly overpenetrated, taken on a subject who was rotated and was in a state of submaximal inspiration and breathing at the time of exposure. Such films can yield valuable diagnostic information provided the reader is fully aware of the many apparent but spurious abnormalities on such films, which are related solely to the suboptimal technique. Conversely, the radiologic appearance of actual disease that is present may be significantly modified by the suboptimal technique.

In situations where the patient must have an AP film while intubated, the respiratory care worker can assist the x-ray technician by inflating the patient's lungs before the film exposure, either with a resuscitation valve or bag or with the inspiratory hold or "sigh" control of the ventilator.

NORMAL RADIOLOGIC ANATOMY

A full description of the normal radiologic anatomy of the thorax is beyond the scope of this chapter, and the reader is referred to the classic descriptions in the standard texts (*see* the Bibliography). Some pertinent data are included in the following description of the techniques of inspecting the radiographic film.

INSPECTION OF THE PA CHEST FILM

It is a self-evident truth that an abnormality cannot be interpreted that has not first been detected.* Many factors are operative in the unavoidable observer error that occurs in radiology,[4] but failures in perception can be reduced by following a standard and specific pattern in which the different components of the chest roentgenogram are systemically inspected during the interpretative process. The precise order in which one studies the various structures is less important than the consistency with which one applies the method (*see* Fig. 14-1).

The *extrathoracic soft tissues* should be inspected briefly. If the patient is female, the breast shadows should be checked. Absence of one breast will result in relative hypertranslucency over the lower lung on the affected side. Large breasts cause considerable haziness over the lower lung fields that can be confused with pneumonia or pulmonary congestion. Nipple shadows may be mistaken for solitary nodules. The presence of subcutaneous emphysema may be apparent in the neck or lateral chest wall.

The *bony thorax* is inspected, including ribs, spine, manubrium, and scapulae. A cervical rib is present in 1% to 2% of normal persons. Rib fractures and lytic lesions of bone should be sought. Scapulae that overlie the lung may be confused with pleural lesions. The presence of kyphosis or scoliosis makes interpretation of the chest roentgenogram more difficult.

The proper *positioning* of the patient is verified by comparing the relationship of the medial ends of the clavicles to the midline. Slight degrees of rotation may create a spurious appearance of tracheal deviation, cardiac displacement, or cardiomegaly.

The diaphragms should have a normal rounded contour with clear costophrenic angles. The right diaphragm is usually 2 cm higher than the left, and normally the dome is at the level of the anterior end of the sixth rib. Unilateral or bilateral elevation of the diaphragm should be noted.

The *mediastinal contour* should be inspected for shifting of the mediastinum from the midline position, cardiomegaly, abnormalities in position or size of the large vessel shadow, mediastinal widening, and the presence of air or calcium within the mediastinum.

The *hilar areas* are inspected with particular attention to changes in size or position of one hilum or both hila. The left hilum is usually about 2 cm higher than the right. Untoward displacement of the hilum strongly suggests possible volume loss of a lobe of the lung on that side.

The *vascular pattern* in the lungs is assessed, tracing the vessels from the hilum to the periphery. The vascular shadows should progressively diminish in size as one scans outward from the hila. Minor increases or decreases in vascularity are difficult to detect. Changes in the vascular pattern may be localized or generalized.

The *lung fields* are then inspected for localized areas of increased or decreased translucency. The

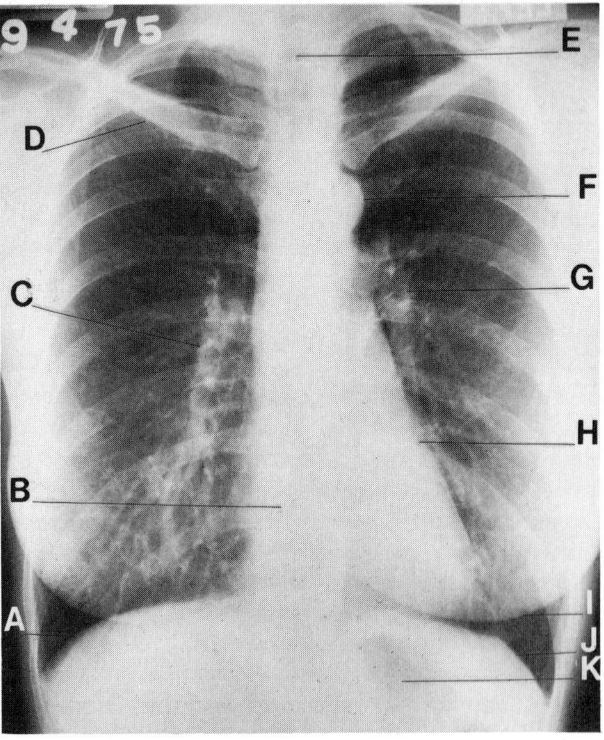

Fig. 14-1. Posteroanterior chest roentgenogram of a young woman. *(A)* Right hemidiaphragm, convex upward with a clear costophrenic angle; *(B)* thoracic spine; *(C)* right hilum (the hilar opacity is mainly due to pulmonary arteries); *(D)* right clavicle; *(E)* midline lucency due to intratracheal air; *(F)* aortic knob (this becomes more prominent in older persons); *(G)* left hilum, usually situated higher than the right hilum; *(H)* left heart border; *(I)* inferior margin of left breast; *(J)* left hemidiaphragm usually a little lower than the right; *(K)* gas bubble within stomach.

*One is reminded of the recipe for hasenpfeffer (rabbit stew), which begins "First, you must catch one big rabbit."

lung fields should be covered systematically, comparing one side with the other.

The *lateral chest roentgenogram* (Fig. 14-2) is inspected similarly. As the two lungs are superimposed in this projection, the interpretation is somewhat more difficult. Mediastinal lesions and at times intrapulmonary lesions may be seen in the lateral projection in cases in which the PA roentgenogram appeared normal.

AP SUPINE CHEST FILM

As previously noted, the AP supine (or semierect) chest roentgenogram has inherent disadvantages that must be recognized if erroneous interpretations are to be minimized. The fact that the film was exposed with this technique is usually indicated in some fashion, on the film itself or on the requisition. Radiologic clues that the projection was AP include high clavi-

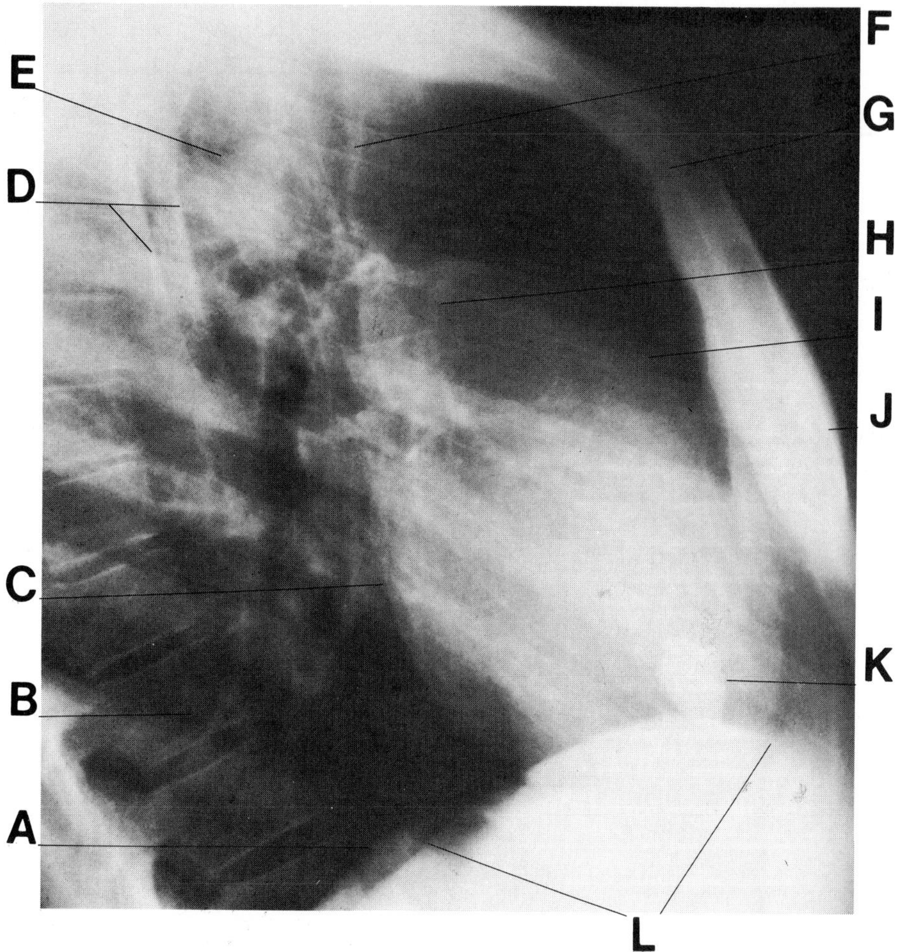

Fig. 14-2. Chest roentgenogram, right lateral projection. *(A)* Left hemidiaphragm, the laterality of which can be determined because the gastric air bubble can be seen beneath it; *(B)* thoracic spine (the intervertebral disc spaces are shown clearly); *(C)* posterior wall of the heart; *(D)* scapulae; *(E)* upper margin of the aortic arch; *(F)* anterior wall of the trachea (posterior to this is the tracheal air lucency); *(G)* sternum. The manubriosternal joint is visible; *(H)* right hilum, anterior to the left hilum in the lateral projection; *(I)* anterior border of the heart; *(J)* breast shadows; *(K)* rounded opacity owing to the presence of a small benign tumor (fibrous mesothelioma) within the oblique fissure on the right (this, of course, is not a normal structure); *(L)* right hemidiaphragm.

cles and transverse course of ribs (because the path of the roentgen beam often has a cephalad angulation) and the tendency of the scapulae to overlie the lung fields.

Assessment of heart size is difficult because the magnification effect on the heart and the elevation of the diaphragms often create an erroneous impression of cardiomegaly. The position-induced diaphragmatic elevation and the frequent failure of the patient to perform a maximal inspiration result in basilar haziness, suggesting pulmonary congestion or pleural effusion.

SPECIAL RADIOLOGIC TECHNIQUES

Special techniques are available to enhance the value of the radiologic examination. Although some of these are not particularly pertinent to the subsequent discussion, the most important techniques will be included here and discussed briefly.

CHANGES IN THE POSITION OF THE PATIENT

In addition to the standard PA and lateral projections, other views are sometimes helpful. *Oblique* projections aid in localizing lesions and at times provide evidence of disease that was not apparent on the the standard films. The *apical lordotic* projection allows an improved view of the apical and subapical areas of the lungs (Fig. 14-3) and is particularly helpful in identifying tuberculous disease. The *lateral decubitus* film is usually obtained with the affected side dependent and is particularly valuable in detecting the presence of small pleural effusions and in demonstrating that some large opacities seen on standard roentgen-

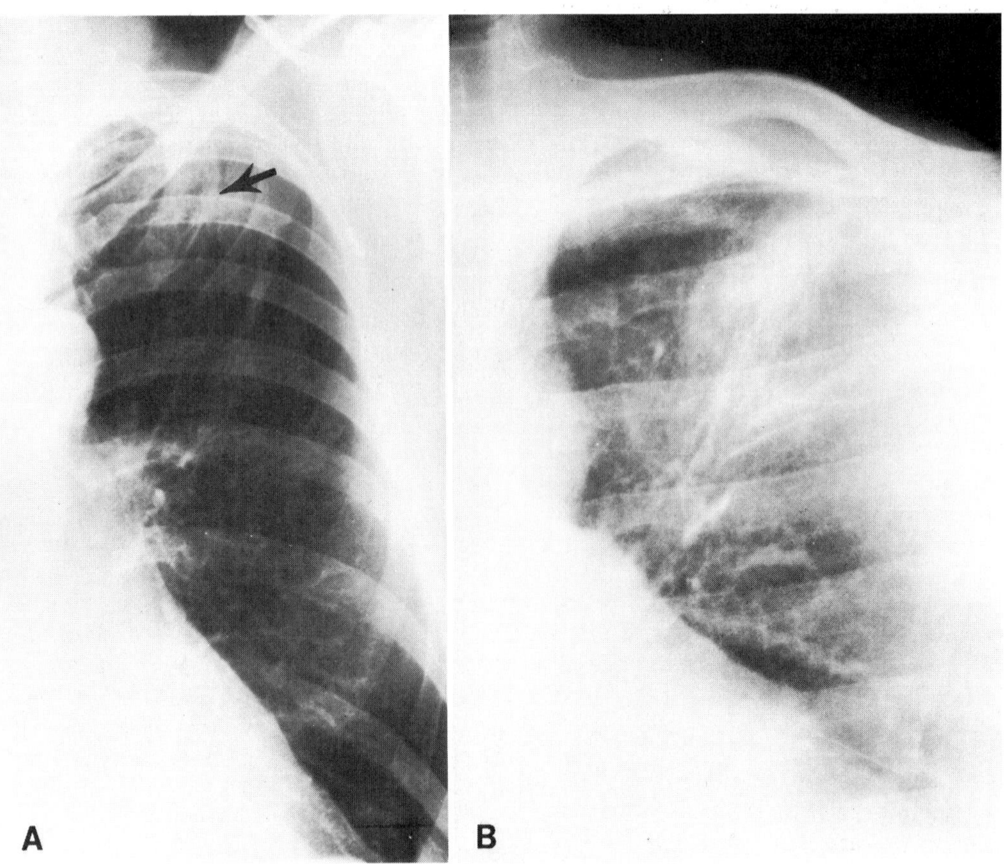

Fig. 14-3. Apical lordotic projection film. *(A)* Posteroanterior chest film showing poorly defined consolidation *(arrow)* in the upper left lung behind the clavicle and first rib. *(B)* Apical lordotic view clearly shows large ovoid mass in left upper lung. Final diagnosis was bronchogenic carcinoma.

ograms are caused by free pleural fluid and not by parenchymal consolidation. This projection will also shift fluid levels within pulmonary cavities, which at times has some diagnostic usefulness.

The *end-expiratory* PA chest roentgenogram does not, strictly speaking, involve a change in the position of the patient but is included here for convenience. This provides an objective measurement of diaphragmatic excursions when compared with the standard end-inspiratory chest roentgenogram and is valuable in detecting localized air trapping within the lung and in identifying a small pneumothorax. If a mediastinal shift is present (such as in a tension pneumothorax), a change in the degree of shift may occur between inspiration and expiration, which is useful in determining which hemithorax is the abnormal one: The mediastinum appears to move toward the normal side on expiration.

CHANGES IN RADIOLOGIC CONTRAST

On occasion it is useful to alter the technical factors affecting exposure and radiation density to produce an overpenetrated film that delineates certain abnormalities more clearly. This is never a substitute for the standard chest roentgenogram. Similarly, the use of the Potter–Bucky diaphragm improves the clarity with which structures of certain lesions, particularly cavities, can be seen.

DIAGNOSTIC PNEUMOTHORAX AND PNEUMOPERITONEUM

The injection of gas into the peritoneal cavity (diagnostic pneumoperitoneum) is useful in elucidating disease processes in or around the diaphragm. Air is occasionally injected into a pleural cavity (diagnostic pneumothorax) to delineate certain pleural lesions more clearly.

TOMOGRAPHY

Body-section roentgenography (tomography, planigraphy, laminography, stratigraphy) facilitates the study of intrathoracic lesions obscured in standard chest roentgenograms by the opacities of overlying structures. Tomograms essentially consist of a series of roentgenographic sections that are "cut" (focused) at different depths. Each film shows a sharp image of the structures in that plane, with blurring of the images anterior and posterior to that plane. Tomograms are usually obtained in the PA projection but can be obtained in other projections under special circumstances. Tomograms are particularly helpful in establishing the presence or absence of a disease process in cases in which standard chest roentgenograms do not show the lesion clearly. The size and shape of the lesion, the sharpness of its margins, the presence of cavitation and calcification, and the surrounding vascular patterns are well demonstrated by tomography (Fig. 14-4). In addition, the patency of the tracheobronchial tree is often well shown by this technique.

BRONCHOGRAPHY

Bronchography utilizes the instillation of a radio-opaque substance into the tracheobronchial tree. The medium adheres to the bronchial mucosa and allows radiologic visualization of the bronchi (Fig. 14-5). The standard bronchographic medium contains iodine, although barium has been used occasionally, and in the future inhalation of tantalum dust may well be the ideal technique. Bronchograms clearly show narrowing, dilatation, or obstruction of the bronchi. Bronchography causes some discomfort to the patient and increases hypoxemia and airway resistance, which involves an element of risk to the patient with diminished pulmonary function. The main contraindication to bronchography is allergy to the local anesthetic or to the bronchographic medium.

ANGIOGRAPHY

Angiography is the injection of a radio-opaque medium into the pulmonary vascular tree to outline the size, patency, and pattern of the blood vessels. In the investigation of pulmonary diseases, injections of angiographic media into appropriate areas may be used to opacify one or more of the following: the leg veins, the inferior vena cava, the superior vena cava and its tributaries, the cardiac chambers, the pulmonary trunk and pulmonary arteries, the pulmonary veins, the aorta and its branches in the thorax or abdomen, and the bronchial arteries. Angiographic study of the pulmonary arteries is probably the most commonly used of these procedures. It is extremely valuable in diagnosing pulmonary embolism (see Chap. 33) but has other uses as well.

FLUOROSCOPY

Fluoroscopy is related to standard chest roentgenography as the motion picture is related to still pictures. It provides a dynamic picture of the thorax and its contents during inspiration and expiration and throughout the cardiac cycle. The usefulness of chest fluoroscopy has increased in recent years with the advent of the image-intensifier fluoroscope and the use of cinefluoroscopy to provide a permanent recording of the abnormalities visualized. Fluoroscopy is less sensitive than standard roentgenograms in detecting certain pulmonary lesions; it is therefore an adjunct to standard chest roentgenograms, not a substitute for them. In addition, fluoroscopic examination entails a much greater radiation exposure than standard chest roentgenograms.

Fluoroscopy provides valuable information about the motion of the diaphragms and mediastinum and detects the presence of air trapping. The relative expansion of the two lungs during inspiration is well shown. Mediastinal lesions can be better defined in terms of location and movement during breathing and swallowing. It is difficult, however, to differentiate the pulsatile expansion of a vascular mediastinal mass

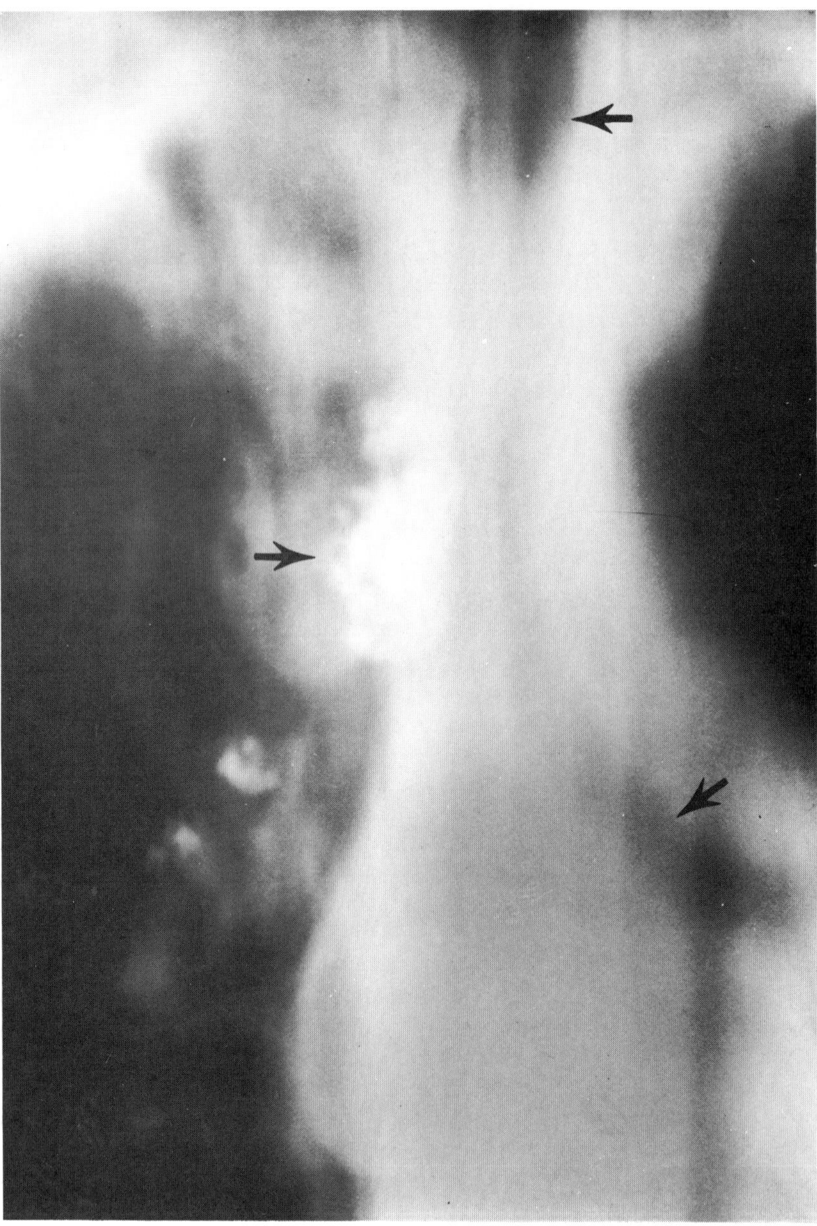

Fig. 14-4. Tomographic cut in the posteroanterior projection at 12 cm from the posterior thoracic wall. Tracheal air lucency is seen *(upper arrow).* A calcified mass of benign lymph nodes occupies the angle above the right main bronchus *(middle arrow).* Smaller calcified nodes are seen in the lower right hilum. Air in the left main bronchus is seen *(lower arrow).* (Lillington GA, Jamplis RW: A Diagnostic Approach to Chest Diseases, 2nd ed. Baltimore, Williams & Wilkins, 1977).

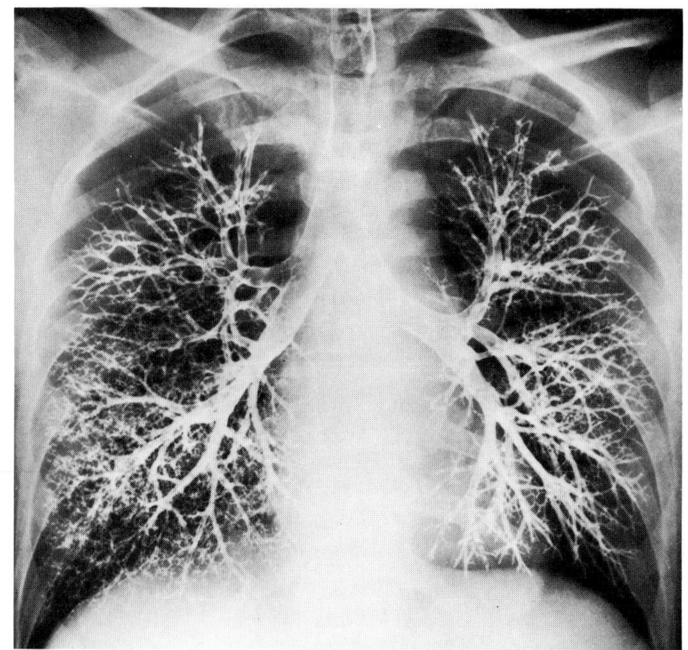

Fig. 14-5. Normal bilateral bronchogram (posteroanterior view). Note the progressive diminution of airway caliber moving from the carina peripherally. The opaque medium coats the inner walls of the bronchial tree.

from the transmitted movement of a nonvascular mass adjacent to a large arterial vessel. In most instances barium is swallowed during fluoroscopy to detect abnormalities and displacements of the esophagus.

RADIOLOGICAL ESTIMATION OF PULMONARY FUNCTION

Numerous attempts have been made to use roentgenographic techniques for estimating the various functions measured by standard pulmonary function tests. The standard fluoroscopic methods obviously provide some information about the total expansibility of the lungs and the relative volume contributions of the two sides, but quantitation is extremely difficult. The specialized techniques of *roentgen kymography* and *roentgen densitometry* have shown a fairly good correlation with spirometric measurements of vital capacity and flow rates and have an advantage in that regional variations in these parameters are detectable. These methods have not found wide acceptance.

Total lung capacity can be measured fairly accurately from the standard end-inspiratory PA and lateral chest roentgenograms. The method is tedious, however, and is not commonly used (see Chap. 10).[5]

THE THORACIC CT SCAN

The computed tomographic (CT) scan, also known as the computer-assisted tomographic (CAT) scan, is a relatively new technique but one that has already had a major impact on the practice of pulmonary medicine. The method provides cross-sectional (transverse) tomographs of the body structures at multiple levels (Fig. 14-6).

The CT scan is a supplement to, and not a replacement for, conventional chest radiography. It is particularly helpful in detecting the presence and determining the size, shape, location, and radiodensity of mediastinal masses. In the lungs, it helps differentiate pleural from parenchymal masses, detects pulmonary nodules and subpleural lesions not visible on standard films or tomograms, and clearly shows lesions in the bones and thoracic wall. The full usefulness of the thoracic CT scans is still being determined.

With more modern scanning devices, it is possible to perform the examination on "critically ill" patients receiving controlled ventilation.

PULMONARY VENTILATION AND PERFUSION SCINTISCANS

Although pulmonary scintiscanning is not, strictly speaking, a roentgenologic technique, its diagnostic usefulness is worth considering. With pulmonary scintiscans the radiation emitted from various *radioisotopes* introduced into the lungs is measured, rather than the radiations emitted by the *roentgen tube* and transmitted through the lungs, as in standard roentgenography.

Pulmonary scintiscans measure the volume and spatial distribution of either ventilation or perfusion in the lungs. The standard lung *perfusion* scintiscan utilizes albumin particles that are tagged or labeled with radioactive iodine. This material is injected intravenously, and during its passage through the lungs some of the albumin particles impact in the small pulmonary capillaries. A scanning device is then passed over the thorax, and the pattern of gamma radiation is recorded as an index of the distribution and volume of perfusion in the lungs. Subsequently, radioactive technetium has been used for perfusion scans and, more recently, radioactive xenon dissolved in saline.

Similarly, both the distribution pattern and the volume of *ventilation* within the lungs are measured by scanning the thorax while the patient takes one or several breaths of gas that contains radioactive xenon.

The scanning or recording devices now used are all variations on the Anger scintiscan camera. These devices allow a complete recording of the emitted radiation in any projection within 10 to 15 seconds. Ideally, separate scans are taken in the anterior and the posterior projections and both lateral projections.

The diagnostic usefulness of ventilation and perfusion scintiscans lies in the fact that a number of pulmonary diseases will give rise to abnormalities in either ventilation or perfusion, or both. Although the pattern that emerges is not entirely specific for any single process, it does delineate the abnormality in physiology that can then be correlated with clinical and roentgenographic information to provide markedly increased diagnostic precision.

Pulmonary scintiscanning is used most commonly in detecting *pulmonary embolism*. The lodgement of an embolus within a lobar or segmental pulmonary artery is followed by a marked decrease or complete absence of perfusion in the involved area. Ventilation to the area, however, is usually fairly well maintained at least for the first 24 to 48 hours. Ventilation/perfusion scans taken within the first 48 hours will then show a highly characteristic pattern of diminished or absent perfusion with normal ventilation (*see* Chap. 33). This is called a "nonmatching" defect. If the embolized area eventually undergoes infarction, ventilation will also decrease or disappear in the region of the perfusion defect. This type of combined or "matching" ventilation/perfusion defect is not specific for pulmonary infarction, however, but may be seen with other conditions, including pneumonia, asthma, emphysema, atelectasis, and bronchogenic carcinoma.

Ventilation/perfusion scintiscans are also useful in studying cases of *bullous emphysema*, particularly in selecting those patients who can be expected to benefit from surgical resection. The technique also has some usefulness in other pulmonary parenchymal and vascular conditions.

RADIOLOGIC PATTERNS OF DIFFUSE LUNG DISEASE

The development of multiple areas of increased opacification, widely distributed throughout both lungs, is a relatively common clinical problem. Such patients commonly have serious deterioration of pulmonary function and form a major component of intensive care units' population.

A large number of diseases (well over 100) can cause diffuse pulmonary opacification. Differential diagnosis is aided by the fact that there are four basic radiologic patterns of diffuse lung disease: the alveolar-filling pattern, the interstitial pattern, the vascular pattern, and the bronchial pattern.

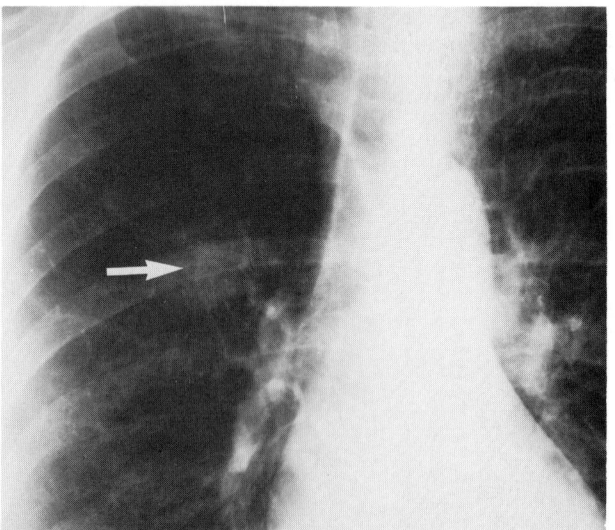

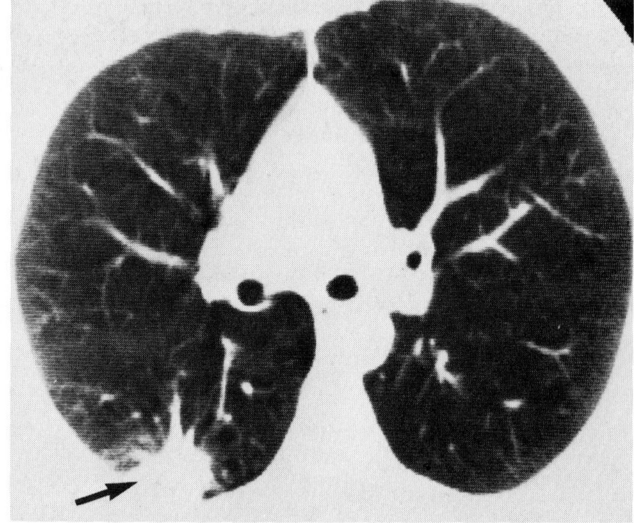

Fig. 14-6. Thoracic CT scan. *(Left)* The standard chest film shows a poorly demarcated mass *(arrow)* in the right lung. It was not clearly identified in the lateral projection. *(Right)* CT scan shows the mass *(arrow)* in the right lung adjacent to the posterior chest wall. This view is a transverse section just below the level of the carina, with the orientation as if the patient is lying supine and the observer is looking up toward the head.

THE ALVEOLAR-FILLING PATTERN

Filling of the alveolar spaces with fluid or solid tissue presents a fairly characteristic roentgenographic appearance that can be recognized in most cases, particularly when diffuse involvement is present. Alveolar-filling lesions are soft, fluffy, and poorly demarcated. The individual lesions are 0.5 cm to 1 cm in diameter but frequently coalesce to form larger, irregular, poorly demarcated lesions that may be several centimeters in diameter. The normal vascular pattern becomes blurred or even obliterated, as the alveolar opacification reduces the contrast between the air density of the lung and the water density of the vessels. A peripheral ("bat's wing") distribution is often seen when an alveolar-filling process diffusely involves the lungs (Fig. 14-7). Another diagnostically important manifestation of alveolar-filling disease is the "air bronchogram." The consolidated alveoli around the bronchi and bronchioles outline the hyperlucent air within the bronchial tree, revealing a characteristic arborizing pattern (Fig. 14-8). Diffuse alveolar filling may also show a "ground-glass" appearance.

Diffuse alveolar-filling disease may be acute or chronic. The most common cause of *acute* disease is pulmonary edema, either cardiogenic or noncardiogenic. Other causes include certain viral pneumonias (particularly influenza and cytomegalovirus), pneumocystis infection, shock lung, fat embolism, and intraalveolar hemorrhage. These conditions cannot be distinguished from one another based on radiologic appearances. Generally, the defect in pulmonary function is proportional to the magnitude of the radiologic abnormality. In many instances, impaired oxygen transfer is severe enough to warrant the use of the term adult respiratory distress syndrome (ARDS).

Chronic diffuse alveolar-filling disease may be due to pulmonary alveolar proteinosis, desquamative interstitial pneumonitis, alveolar microlithiasis, alveolar cell carcinoma, and (rarely) sarcoidosis and lymphoma. Bronchogenic spread of tuberculosis or fungal disease may have this appearance, although the distribution is usually less symmetrical.

INTERSTITIAL PATTERN

Interstitial tissue comprises the alveolar walls, the intralobular vessels and interlobar septa, and the connective tissue framework that surrounds the pulmonary arteries, veins, and bronchial tree. Consolidation resulting from disease primarily involving interstitial tissues has certain characteristics that often allow recognition of the roentgenogram pattern. Interstitial dis-

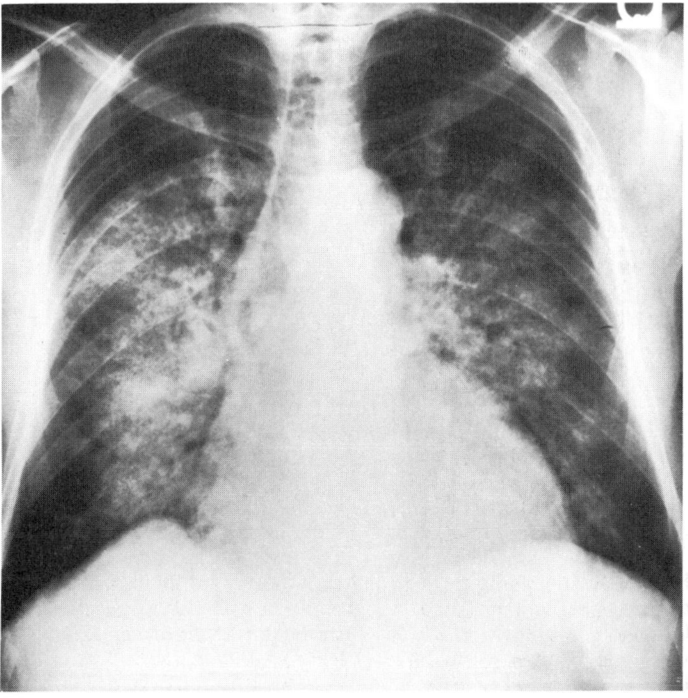

Fig. 14-7. Bilateral perihilar distribution of pulmonary edema (the "bat-wing" or "butterfly" distribution). The soft, fluffy, poorly circumscribed and confluent alveolar lesions are seen clearly. This appearance occurs in both cardiogenic and noncardiogenic pulmonary edemas and sometimes with other types of alveolar disease. In this case the patient had renal failure, and the edema was caused by fluid overload.

ease typically shows a branching linear pattern with multiple thin strands radiating toward the periphery of the lung, often intersecting to form a reticular network. This phenomenon is primarily due to thickening of the interlobular septa and may be caused by fibrosis, granuloma, lymphangitic carcinoma or interstitial edema. These linear streaks are called Kerley's lines and may be further differentiated into "A" lines (long linear streaks), "B" lines (short transverse streaks best seen at the periphery of the lower lung fields, Fig. 14-9A), and "C" lines (which form the diffuse reticular network; Fig. 14-9B).

The most characteristic feature of interstitial disease is "honeycombing," which consists of multiple rounded lucent areas, up to 1 cm in diameter, outlined by dense interstitial consolidations (Fig. 14-10). The air bronchogram effect is usually absent or not prominent in interstitial disease.

Many types of diffuse lung disease have both alveolar and interstitial components, with manifestations of both patterns radiologically. This is usually described as a "mixed" pattern.

Many diseases may give rise to diffuse interstitial disease. An important and common cause is diffuse pulmonary fibrosis, also known as fibrosing alveolitis and as "usual interstitial pneumonitis." This condition may be idiopathic or secondary to collagen-vascular diseases, certain fibrogenic drugs, asbestosis, excessive oxygen inhalation, or radiation. Other causes of diffuse interstitial disease of the reticular or honeycomb type include sarcoidosis, eosinophilic granuloma, lymphangitic carcinomatosis, lymphoma, and hypersensitivity pneumonitis from organic dust inhalation.

A variant form of the interstitial pattern is *miliary disease*, in which the chest roentgenogram shows a profusion of small nodules about 2 mm to 4 mm in diameter (Fig. 14-11). The prototype is miliary tuberculosis, but a diffuse fine nodularity of this type may also occur with fungal infections, sarcoidosis, certain pneumoconioses, metastatic tumors to lung, and varicella pneumonia. The distinction between the reticular and miliary patterns is often elusive, in which case the term "reticulonodular" disease may be used.

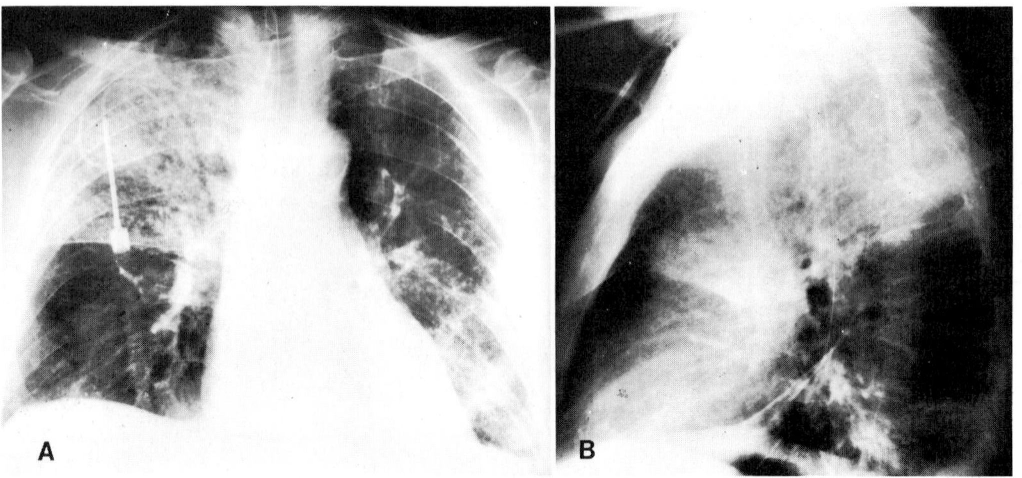

Fig. 14-8. Bacterial pneumonia, causing consolidation of the right upper lobe. This alveolar-filling process occupies the entire lobe, and a lucent "air bronchogram" can be seen within the consolidation, indicating that the opacity is alveolar and that the bronchus is patent. *(A)* Posteroanterior projection with the consolidation sharply limited inferiorly by the horizontal fissure. Overlying the right hemithorax is a catheter taped to the anterior chest wall which then passes down the right subclavian vein and superior vena cava. The tip is obscured within the mediastinal opacity. Patchy, confluent, poorly circumscribed opacities can also be seen in the lower left hemithorax. These are areas of bronchopneumonia. *(B)* Lateral projection. The sternum is to the left and the spine to the right. The pneumonic consolidation is sharply demarcated inferiorly by the horizontal fissure (anteriorly) and by the oblique fissure (posteriorly). Additional areas of bronchopneumonia can be seen above the left diaphragm posteriorly. The left diaphragm can be identified by the gastric air bubble.

The severity of impairment of pulmonary function correlates poorly with the severity of radiologic impairment in miliary disease. The critical task is to determine the etiology, particularly in infectious cases.

VASCULAR PATTERN

The pulmonary arteries and veins, as previously noted, form a somewhat indistinct branching pattern radiating peripherally from the hilum on the normal chest roentgenogram. Increases in the size of the pulmonary vessels cause an accentuation of this pattern, which superficially resembles interstitial disease. *Generalized* increases in vascularity may result from congenital heart disease with left-to-right shunts, polycythemia, and left heart failure. A striking feature of the last-mentioned disorder is increased prominence and loss of marginal sharpness of the vessels in the upper lung fields (Fig. 14-12).

A chest roentgenogram obtained while the lungs are in the end-expiratory position presents a spurious pattern of increased vascularity, particularly at the lung bases. *Localized* increases in vascularity are a common phenomenon in the redistribution of blood flow in patients with bullous emphysema.

Decreased vascularity may be focal, as in emphysema or pulmonary embolism, or diffuse, as in right to left shunts, pulmonic stenosis, and obstructive pulmonary hypertension. The central hilar vessels are often enlarged in obstructive pulmonary hypertension.

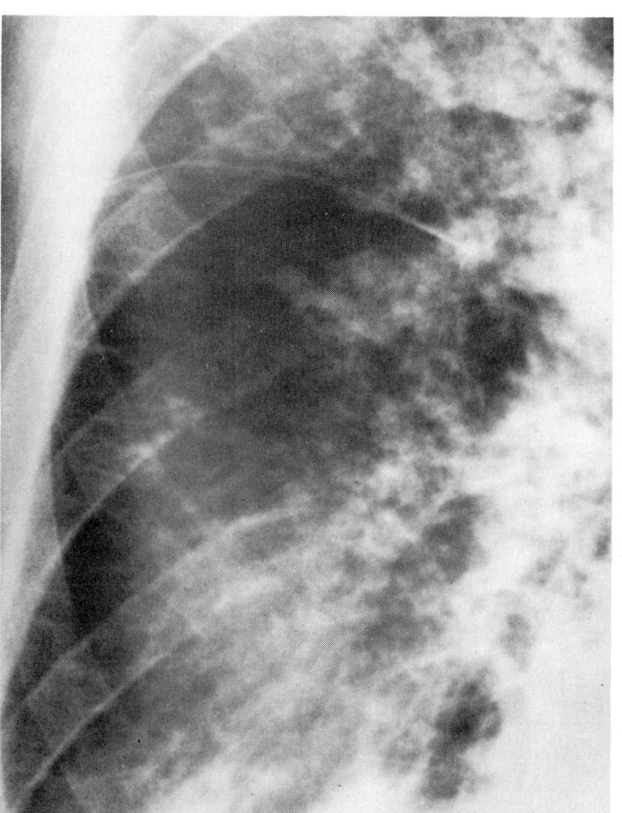

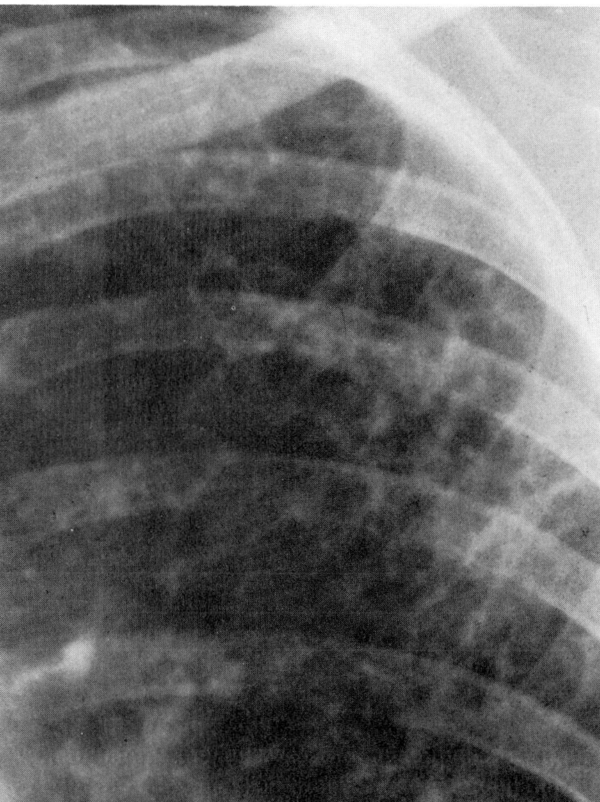

Fig. 14-9. *(Left)* Kerley B lines. These thin lines extend horizontally for 1 cm or 2 cm inward from the pleural surface and represent thickened interlobular septa. They result from pulmonary venous hypertension or pulmonary lymphatic obstruction and may, as in this case, provide an important clue to the presence of pulmonary edema of cardiogenic origin. *(Right)* Posteroanterior view showing upper left lung in a 32-year-old woman with biopsy-proven eosinophilic granuloma. A reticular pattern (also known as Kerley's C lines) is present. This pattern can occur in any type of interstitial lung disease.

THE BRONCHIAL PATTERN

Diffuse involvement of the bronchial tree by inflammatory disease may result in an irregular but diffuse pattern, often composed of linear streaks, branching in character. This can result from thickened bronchial walls (as in chronic bronchitis, asthma, bronchiectasis) or from peribronchial scarring (as in mucoviscidosis or allergic bronchopulmonary aspergillosis). In patients with chronic obstructive pulmonary disease, this appearance is often referred to as the "dirty lung"[7] and usually indicates that chronic bronchitis is a major component of the obstructive complex. The term "increased markings pattern" is also used.

PATTERNS OF LOCALIZED OPACIFICATION

Localized opacification refers to single or multiple areas of opacification that are "patchy" in distribution and usually associated with or surrounded by numerous small or large areas of lung that appear relatively normal. This can be subdivided into several types. Pulmonary *consolidation* implies a localized opacification due to filling of alveoli in the affected area with fluid, tissue, or exudate. The volume changes little, if at all, and the distribution is often lobar or segmental. An early radiologic sign is blurring of the normal vascular pattern in the consolidating area, with eventual complete loss of vessel outlines as the opacification increases. Even extensive consolidation is usually nonhomogeneous, giving a patchy radiologic appearance. Air bronchograms are typically present in nonobstructive consolidations.

Areas of consolidation may be single or multiple, unilateral or bilateral. Common causes include pneumonia (infectious or noninfectious), localized pulmonary edema, pulmonary contusion, localized alveolar cell carcinoma, and the early stage of pulmonary infarction.

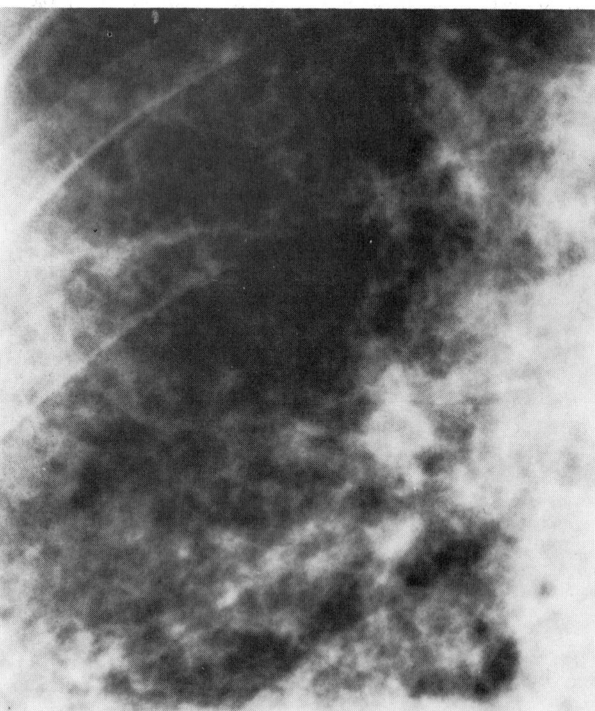

Fig. 14-10. Honeycomb lung in a patient with fibrosing alveolitis. The honeycomb cysts form dozens of rounded lucent areas, 5 mm to 10 mm in diameter, separated by opaque fibrous tissue.

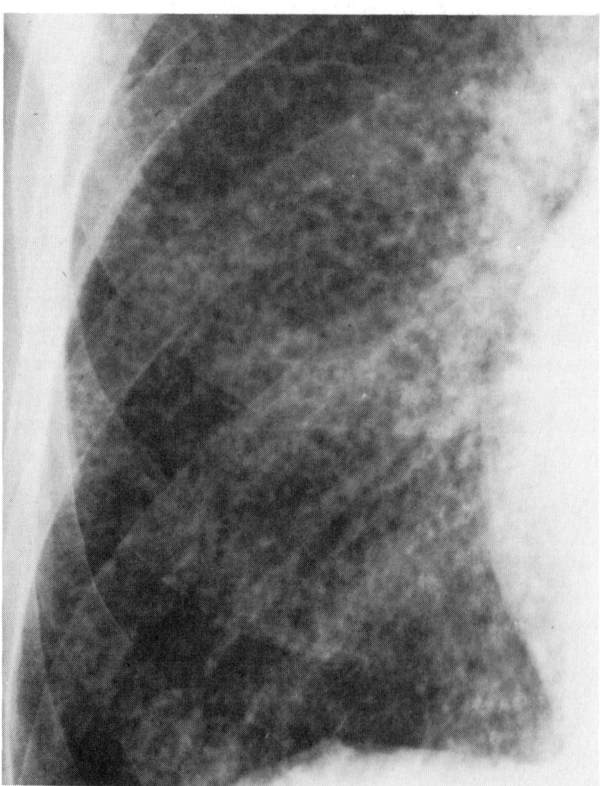

Fig. 14-11. Diffuse miliary nodules in a patient with disseminated coccidioidomycosis. The innumerable tiny nodules are well circumscribed and are 2 mm to 4 mm in diameter. A similar appearance occurs in miliary tuberculosis and is sometimes seen in other fungal diseases, sarcoidosis, coal-worker's pneumoconiosis, and metastatic tumors.

Atelectasis is an opacification due to loss of volume in a segment or lobe. When the collapse is due to obstruction of a bronchus with resorption of air in the lung distal to the obstruction, the opacification will be homogeneous in appearance. The vascular pattern is completely obliterated.

Pleural effusion creates a homogeneous opacification that will have a characteristic localization and appearance. Atypical appearance may result if pleural obliteration impairs the free flow of fluid in response to gravitational forces. A large pleural effusion may mask the radiologic features of accompanying consolidation or atelectasis. If the pleural effusion is not too large and the underlying lung is normal, one may detect a normal vascular pattern through the overlying pleural opacity, particularly if the film is a little overpenetrated.

A *replacement opacity*, also called a "destructive" lesion, is one in which the normal lung tissue in the affected area has been replaced by a disease process. In some instances, the normal tissue is pushed aside or compressed by a growing mass, whereas in other instances there has been tissue necrosis. Examples include nodules and masses, tuberculous and fungal infections, necrotizing pneumonias, undrained lung abscesses, and complete infarcts. Such lesions, single or multiple, tend to be homogeneous in density and often sharply circumscribed, although irregular, in shape.

PNEUMONIA

Pneumonia is an inflammatory consolidation of the lung, usually caused by an infection with microorganisms. Most pneumonias are acute in onset, bacterial in etiology, and alveolar-filling in their radiologic presentations. The opacification is usually nonhomogeneous.

BACTERIAL PNEUMONIAS

Bacterial pneumonias may result from a number of pathogenic microorganisms that may reach the lung through inhalation (commonly) or by hematogenous spread from an infection elsewhere (less commonly). Primary bacterial pneumonias caused by the pneumoccoccus *(Streptococcus pneumoniae)*, Friedlander's bacillus *(Klebsiella pneumoniae)*, and the staphylococcus are usually *lobar* or *segmental* in distribution (Fig. 14-13). Most commonly one lobe or segment is involved, although multiple areas of disease are sometimes seen particularly with staphylococcal pneumonia. These pneumonias are alveolar-filling in type, but if an entire lobe is involved the presence of an air bronchogram may be the most prominent indicator of the radiologic pattern. In many cases some of the small secondary lobules within the involved area are free of disease, and the soft fluffy lesions with irregular margins are then more apparent. Lobar bacterial pneumonias are usually primary in type and not a complication of underlying lung disease. Friedlander's pneumonia is particularly common in chronic alcoholics. Lobar pneumonias often have an acute onset with fever, cough, chest pain, dyspnea, and arterial hypoxemia. In occasional instances lobar consolidations may result from infection with tubercle bacilli or fungi.

Bacterial pneumonias caused by certain other microorganisms rarely show a lobar or segmental pattern and more commonly present as multiple, poorly circumscribed areas of alveolar consolidation that may involve one or both lungs. This pattern is often referred to as *bronchopneumonia*. Organisms that commonly present in this fashion include *Streptococcus, Hemophilus influenzae, Mycoplasma*, the coliform bacilli, *Pseudomonas, Proteus, Serratia*, and anaerobic bacteria. Staphylococcal pneumonias often show this pattern rather than a lobar or segmental consolidation, particularly if the route of infection is hematogenous. Bronchopneumonias are often secondary to some other predisposing process, including the use of immunosuppressive drugs, general debility, aspiration, endotracheal intubation, prolonged antibiotic use, and contaminated inhalation therapy equipment.

Necrosis may occur with bacterial pneumonias, particularly those caused by *Staphylococcus*, aerobic gram-negative bacilli, and anaerobic organisms. Drainage of the necrotic material results in the appearance of air-filled hyperlucent areas called cavities (Fig. 14-14). A cavity that changes rapidly in size (a pneumatocele) is a common complication in staphylococcal infections.

Bacterial pneumonias are commonly accompanied by parapneumonic pleural effusions. Occasionally frank empyema develops.

Certain bacterial pneumonias may appear to be nonbacterial because the organisms are rarely seen in sputum smears and are difficult to culture. These include *mycoplasma* pneumonia, one of the most common pneumonic diseases. Other examples are *psittacosis* (parrot fever) and *legionellosis* (Legionnaire's disease). Diagnosis is serologic or by lung biopsy. The radiologic pattern is usually bronchopneumonic.

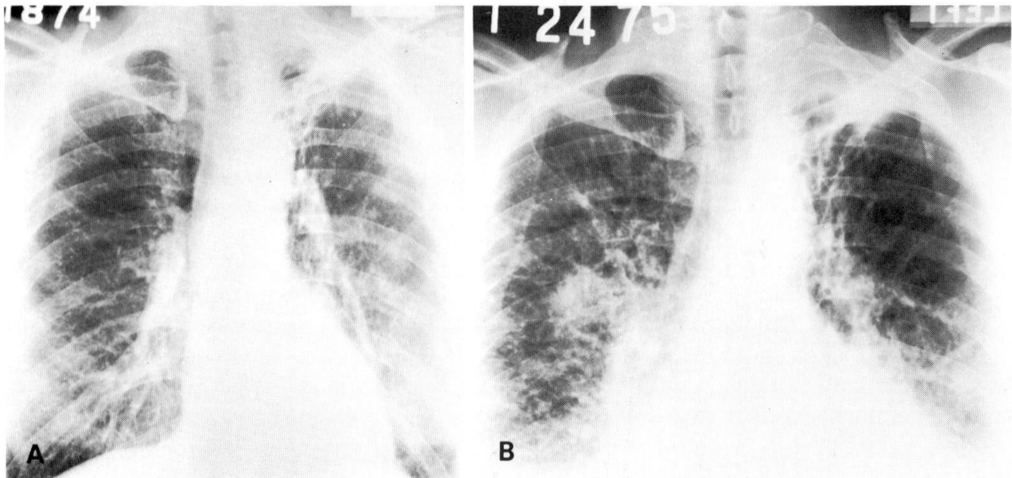

Fig. 14-12. Congestive heart failure. *(A)* Posteroanterior chest film at a time when cardiac function is normal. In the left hemithorax, apical scarring and elevation of the left hilum have resulted from previous active tuberculosis, with loss of volume in the left upper lobe during the healing process. *(B)* Two months later, this man has suffered an acute myocardial infarction and has developed congestive heart failure. The heart is enlarged. The hilar shadows are larger and have hazy margins. A diffuse reticular pattern is present, indicative of interstitial pulmonary edema, with frank alveolar fillings at the lung bases. The vascular shadows in the upper lungs are accentuated because of redistribution of blood flow.

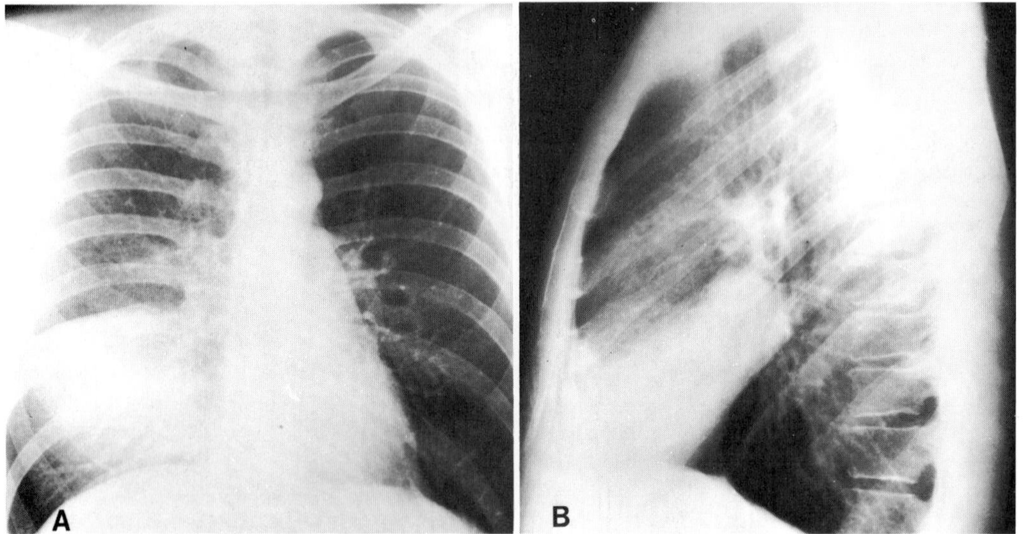

Fig. 14-13. Right middle lobe pneumonia. *(A)* Posteroanterior projection showing the consolidation with its characteristic triangular configuration. The upper border is limited by the horizontal fissure and the lateral border by the oblique fissure. Note that the costophrenic angle is clear and the right heart border is obliterated (the so-called silhouette sign). *(B)* Lateral view showing the roughly triangular opacity overlying the cardiac opacity. The upper margin of the consolidation is often more sharply outlined than in this case.

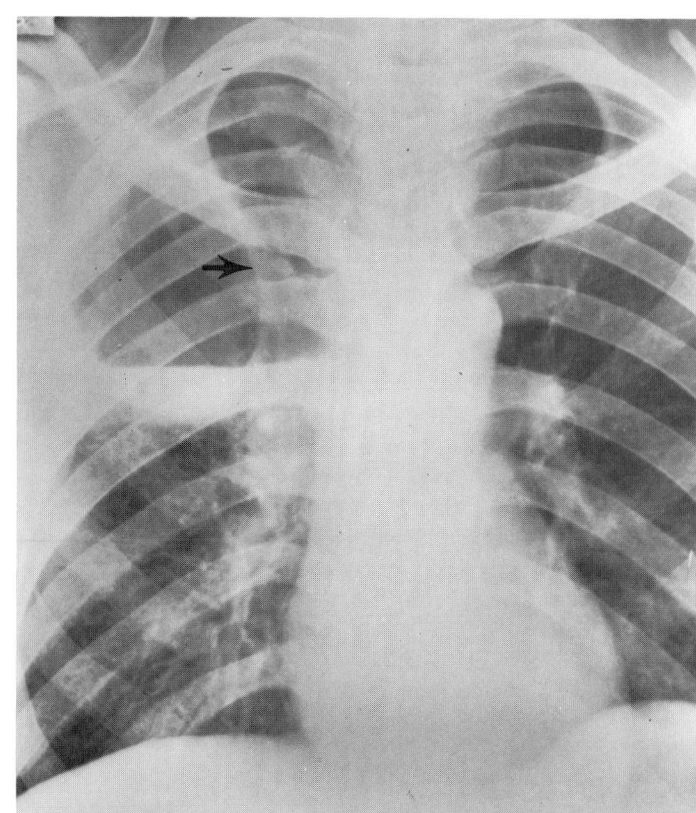

Fig. 14-14. Lung abscess. A large cavity is seen in the upper right lung, containing a small amount of opaque fluid. Note the horizontal air-fluid interface. The medial wall of the cavity is marked *(arrow)*. The superior wall is hidden by the clavicle and the lateral wall obscured by the ribs of the lateral chest wall.

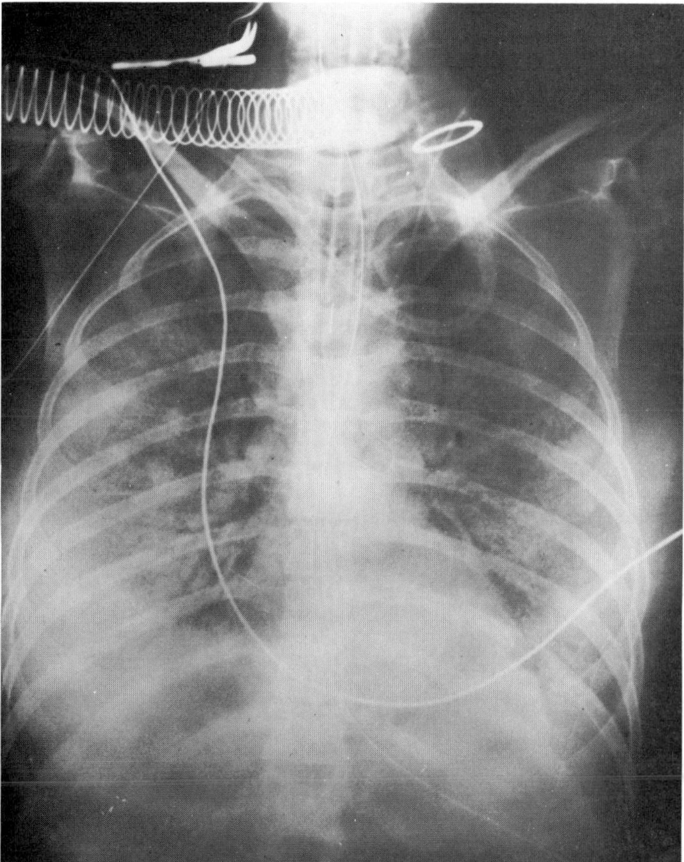

Fig. 14-15. Diffuse alveolar consolidation due to influenzal pneumonia. The diagnosis was proved by lung biopsy and by cultures.

VIRAL PNEUMONIAS

Viral pneumonias may present as a diffuse interstitial or alveolar-filling process. This is particularly common with influenzal (Fig. 14-15) and cytomegalovirus infections, which may be accompanied by severe hypoxemia and increased lung stiffness sufficient to qualify these diseases as examples of ARDS. Most viral pneumonias, however, present as a patchy bronchopneumonia, sometimes complicated by secondary bacterial infection. These illnesses may be only a temporary inconvenience to a previously healthy person, but can produce life-threatening respiratory insufficiency in the patient with chronic obstructive lung disease.

Viral pneumonia caused by measles or varicella may appear on the roentgenogram as miliary lesions or multiple nodules rather than as an alveolar-filling process.

TUBERCULOUS AND FUNGAL PNEUMONIAS

The tubercle bacillus and most fungi characteristically cause a chronic, slowly progressive, fairly well-localized destructive process that pathologically is often granulomatous in type. However, in the early primary stage of the infection, before the body develops resistance, single or multiple areas of pneumonia may occur with infection by the tubercle bacillus and certain fungi (*Coccidiodes* and *Histoplasma*). Other fungi may cause a pneumonic consolidation (sometimes rapidly spreading) if the host defenses have been compromised. Fungi that often behave in this fashion include *Cryptococcus*, *Phycomycetes*, *Candida*, and *Aspergillus*. Infection with *Phycomycetes* (a disease called mucormycosis) is most commonly seen in diabetic persons. *Candida* and *Aspergillus* superinfections often follow long-term antibiotic therapy and may occur after the use of immunosuppressive drugs.

Tuberculosis commonly presents as a chronic destructive granulomatous process in which consolidation, cavitation, fibrosis, and calcification are often present simultaneously. The apical and subapical areas of the lungs are most commonly involved (Fig. 14-16), and the disease is often bilateral. Quiescent "healed" tuberculosis may be converted to an active progressive disease by the use of adrenal corticosteroid drugs.

Certain fungal infections, particularly histoplasmosis and coccidioidomycosis, may demonstrate a similar clinical and radiographic pattern. Nocardiosis and actinomycosis usually behave similarly and are commonly included among the fungal diseases, even though the causative organisms (*Nocardia* and *Actinomyces*) are now classified as bacteria rather than fungi.

PARASITIC PNEUMONIAS

Pneumonias caused by parasitic infections are rarely seen in nontropical climates, with two exceptions. Amebic abscess of the liver may spread upward through the diaphragm to involve the right lower hemithorax, with roentgenographic changes indicative of pneumonic consolidation, pleural effusion, or pulmonary cavitation. Pneumonia caused by infection with *Pneumocystis carinii* presents as a diffuse alveolar-filling process and occurs almost exclusively in immunosuppressed patients.

NONINFECTIOUS PNEUMONIAS

On occasion, pneumonic consolidation may be related to physical or chemical irritation of the lung rather than to infection. The early stage of the reaction of the lung to radiation is pneumonic in type, although a diffuse interstitial fibrosis may eventually

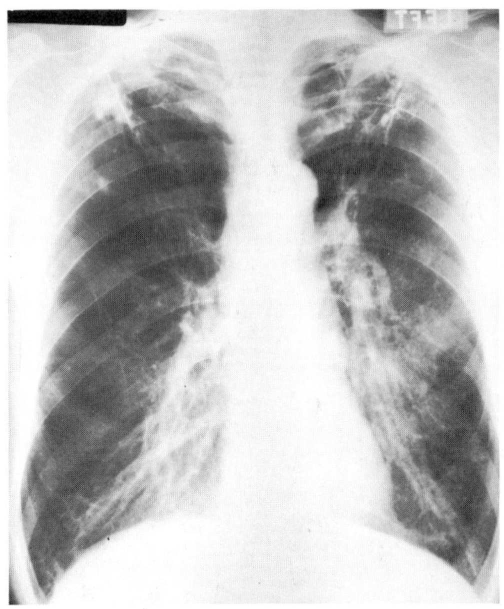

Fig. 14-16. Healed bilateral apical and subapical tuberculosis. The lesions are fibrotic and calcified; however, active tuberculous infection may be present in lesions that appear healed. This patient also has emphysema, which is apparent from the loss of lung markings in many areas of the lungs. Note the upward retraction of the left hilum due to fibrotic scarring and volume loss in the left upper lobe.

develop in the involved area. The inhalation of noxious fumes (nitrogen dioxide, chlorine, sulfur dioxide, phosgene) will cause a diffuse pneumonic process that is extremely acute and often fatal. Silo-filler's disease in an acute hemorrhagic pneumonitis of farmers from inhalation of nitrogen dioxide formed during the ensilage process.

The diffuse chemical pneumonia called *peptic* (or *aspiration*) *pneumonitis* is discussed under Diffuse Alveolar-Filling Processes.

Localized noninfectious pneumonias, solitary or multiple, may occur in systemic lupus erythematosus, aspiration of lipoid substances, and allergic alveolitis caused by inhalation of organic antigens.

SOLITARY AND MULTIPLE PULMONARY NODULES

A pulmonary nodule is a fairly well-circumscribed, roughly spherical, solid intrapulmonary lesion usually greater than 1 cm in diameter. A circumscribed lesion greater than 4 cm in diameter is usually designated a *mass* lesion rather than a nodule. Some nodules develop cavitation.

The *solitary nodule* is most commonly a healed or healing infectious granuloma that may result from tuberculosis, coccidioidomycosis, or histoplasmosis. Less commonly the solitary nodule is a lung tumor, either benign or malignant (primary or secondary). Other disease processes may occasionally present as a solitary nodule. If serial chest roentgenograms show that the nodule has not increased in size over 2 years or if it exhibits extensive calcification, it is safe to assume that the lesion is benign (Fig. 14-17).

Multiple nodules are usually due to intrapulmonary metastases from an extrapulmonary primary malignant lesion. Other causes include tuberculosis and fungal diseases, sarcoidosis, silicosis, and necrotizing granuloma. The appearance of multiple pulmonary nodules in an immunosuppressed host strongly suggests opportunistic infection with fungi.

A solitary nodule has little, if any, deleterious effect on pulmonary function. Its importance is related to possible malignancy. Multiple nodules, depending partly on number, size, distribution, and etiology, may reduce lung volumes, but blood gas values are often little affected.

ATELECTASIS AND LOSS OF VOLUME

Atelectasis is opacification of part, or all, of a lung due to loss of volume. Atelectasis may result from several different mechanisms; however, in common clinical usage the term atelectasis is applied to those losses of volume caused by bronchial obstruction or cicatrization (scar formation).

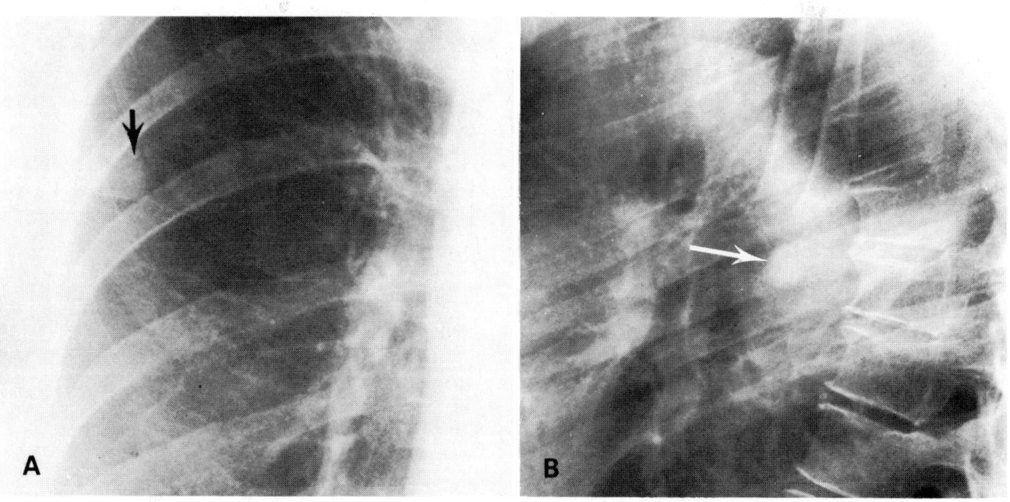

Fig. 14-17. Solitary pulmonary nodule due to coccidioidomycosis. *(A)* Posterolateral view of right hemithorax showing the 1.5-cm nodule situated far laterally *(arrow)* in the upper lung. *(B)* In the lateral view the nodule is clearly seen overlying the shadow of the lower aortic arch, halfway between the hilar opacity and the thoracic spine. The nodule is calcified. (Lillington GA, Jamplis RW: A Diagnostic Approach to Chest Diseases, 2nd ed. Baltimore, Williams & Wilkins, 1977).

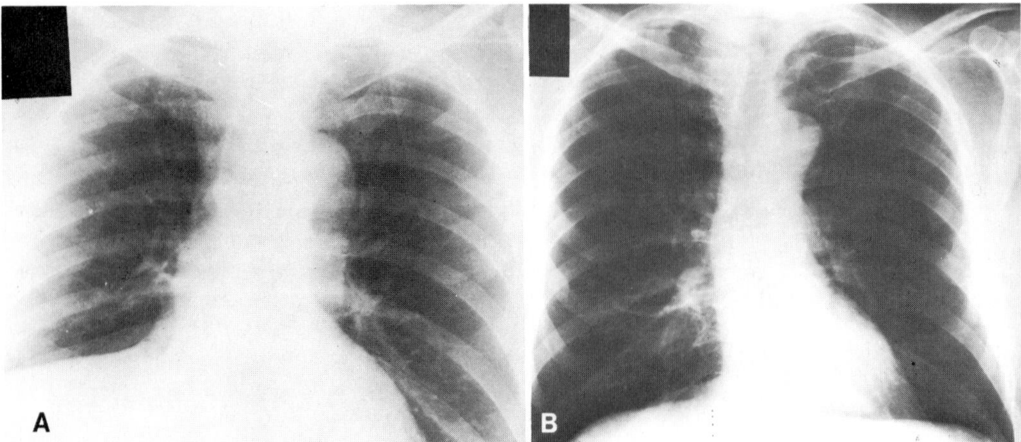

Fig. 14-18. Atelectasis of right lower lobe because of a mucus plug in an 18-year-old boy following intracranial surgery. *(A)* Posteroanterior chest film showing collapsed and airless right lower lobe simulating an elevated right hemidiaphragm. *(B)* Same patient 1 hour after bronchoscopic aspiration of the plug. The right lower lobe has reexpanded, and the diaphragm is now visible in its normal position.

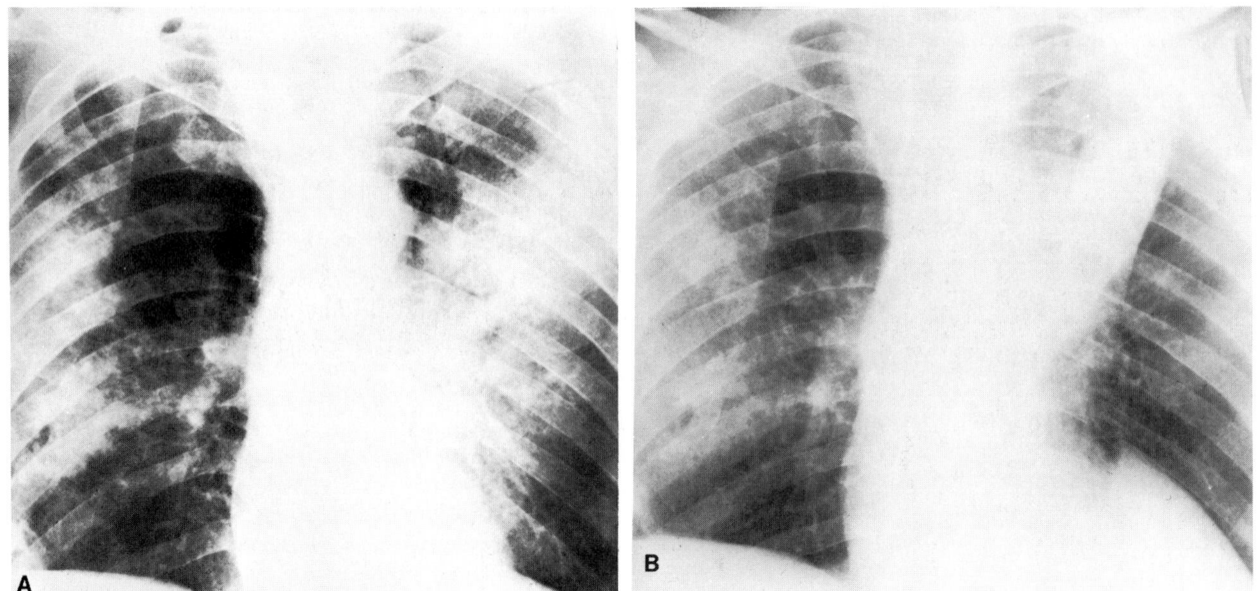

Fig. 14-19. Consolidation of left upper lobe followed by atelectasis. This is a case of active tuberculosis. *(A)* Posteroanterior projection showing a fairly dense alveolar consolidation in the left upper lobe with relative sparing of the apical segment but with involvement of the lingula. There is little loss of volume. On the right side are several areas of tuberculous bronchopneumonia, and there is a dense opacity due to pleural calcification above the lateral portion of the right hemidiaphragm. *(B)* Two weeks later. The left upper lobe bronchus has become occluded, and the left upper lobe is now atelectatic. It is smaller, denser, and now has a sharply demarcated lateral border. There is still some aeration within the apical segment. The left hemidiaphragm is now markedly elevated because of volume loss in the left lung.

BRONCHIAL OBSTRUCTION

Atelectasis may result from extrabronchial compression from tumors or enlarged lymph nodes, from endobronchial disease such as a bronchogenic carcinoma, bronchial adenoma, or inflammatory stricture, or from an intrabronchial mass such as an exogenous foreign body or a large mucus plug (Fig. 14-18). A movable intrabronchial mass may act as a "ball valve" that allows the air to be pumped out from the affected segment within minutes. More commonly air is slowly resorbed from the bronchioles and alveoli distal to the completely obstructed bronchus (Fig. 14-19).

CICATRIZATION ATELECTASIS

Cicatrization atelectasis occurs without bronchial obstruction. Rarely, it is a complication of organized pneumonia within a lobe. During the healing process scar tissue forms, and the contraction of the fibrous tissue causes loss of volume in the lobe. It is a common complication of chronic fibrocaseous tuberculosis, usually involving an upper lobe.

INDIRECT SIGNS OF ATELECTASIS

The secondary effects of collapse of a lobe are usually detectable on the chest roentgenogram and will indicate volume loss even if the opacification of the atelectatic segment is not clearly seen. These signs include elevation of the hemidiaphragm on the affected side, a decrease in size of the rib interspaces over the affected hemithorax, and in many instances a compensatory hyperinflation of the adjacent lobes or of the opposite lung. A shift of the hilum, either upward or downward, is sometimes detectable.

DIRECT SIGNS OF ATELECTASIS

The opacified collapsed segment, lobe, or lung usually has a characteristic appearance on the standard chest roentgenograms (Fig. 14-18).

DECREASED LUNG VOLUME OF OTHER TYPES

Decreased volumes of the entire lung occurs when the retractive force of the chest wall is impaired, allowing the elastic recoil of the lung to effect a decrease in volume. Common examples include hemidiaphragmatic paralysis (Fig. 14-20), multiple rib fractures with a flail chest, or air or fluid in the pleural space. In these cases the loss of volume is generalized, not localized, is partial and not complete, and the clinical and radiologic picture is dominated by the primary disturbance. Similarly the development of extensive scar tissue within a pleural space (fibrothorax) renders the affected hemithorax smaller and less expansile. Finally, an expanding lesion within the lung, such as a rapidly growing tumor, a lung abscess, or an expanding tension cyst, may cause some compression of the adjacent normal lung. Although loss of the volume of the lung is a feature of all these conditions, the term atelectasis is not used clinically in these circumstances.

BRONCHIAL OBSTRUCTION

Bronchial obstruction may have differing effects on the distal lung depending on the degree of obstruction and the rapidity with which it develops. Minor degrees of obstruction that have no major effect on airway dynamics will cause no roentgenologic changes. However, the presence of the localized obstruction may be apparent on stethoscopic auscultation over the

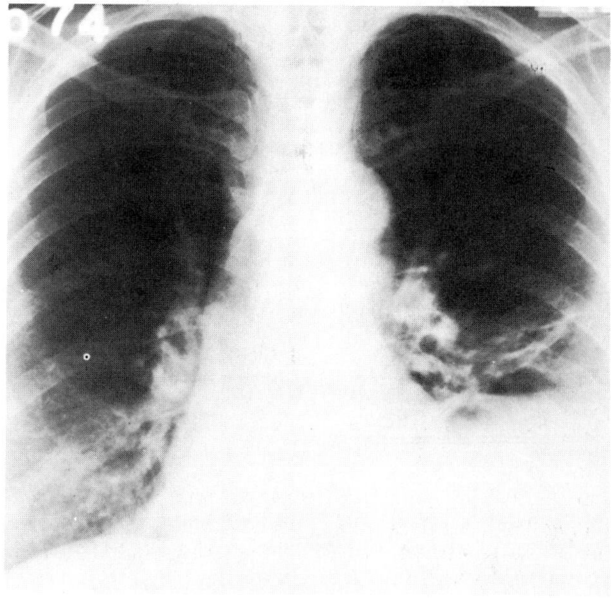

Fig. 14-20. Eventration of the left hemidiaphragm. The elevated hemidiaphragm showed paradoxical movement on sniffing. Usually the upper margin of the eventrated hemidiaphragm maintains a sharp convex contour. In this case a pulmonary infection has resulted in pleural adhesions between the diaphragm and the lung. Horizontal streaks of "discoid" atelectasis are seen. (Lillington GA, Jamplis RW: A Diagnostic Approach to Chest Diseases, 2nd ed. Baltimore, Williams & Wilkins, 1977).

affected area. A persistent localized wheeze may be noted if a partial obstruction is present.

An obstruction large enough to impair the clearance of mucoid secretions from the distal lung often results in pneumonia of the affected segment or lobe. This pneumonia will have the usual roentgenologic characteristics of a segmental or lobar alveolar-filling process and cannot be differentiated from nonobstructive pneumonias. If, however, the obstruction increases while the pneumonia is still present and eventually becomes complete, the affected segment or lobe becomes completely airless but will not shrink in volume because the alveoli are filled with inflammatory exudate. In such cases of *obstructive pneumonitis*

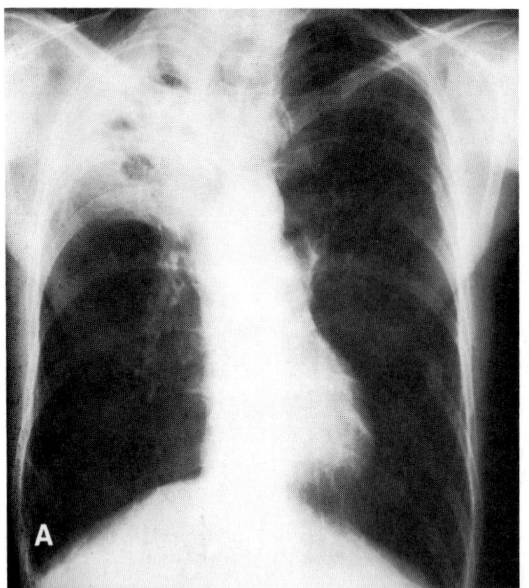

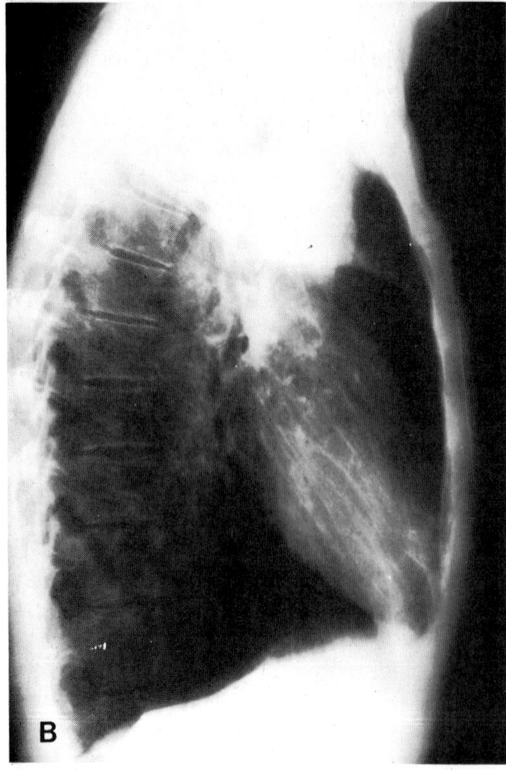

Fig. 14-21. Obstructive pneumonitis of right upper lobe because of bronchial occlusion by bronchogenic carcinoma. *(A)* On the posteroanterior (PA) view the lobe has lost some volume, as shown by the elevation of the horizontal fissure, which demarcates the consolidation inferiorly, but the fissure has not rotated to the diagonal position that would be expected if marked loss of volume were present. Cavitation is present within the lobe because of necrotizing pneumonitis. *(B)* Lateral view shows fissures elevated but retaining their normal angulation.

This man also has advanced pulmonary emphysema. In the PA view the lungs are hyperlucent because of hyperinflation and generalized destruction of lung parenchyma and vessels. The diaphragms are low and flat, and the small heart appears to be "hanging" in the mediastinum above the left hemidiaphragm. In the lateral view of diaphragms are flat and scalloped, and the sternodiaphragmatic angle is considerably greater than 90°. The retrosternal air shadow is large and so hyperlucent that it almost "cancels out" the consolidation in the anterior portion of the right upper lobe, immediately posterior to the sternum in the lateral view.

("drowned lung"), the air bronchogram will be absent, allowing one to infer the presence of bronchial obstruction as the cause of the homogeneous opacification of the lobe (Fig. 14-21). A complete bronchial obstruction that develops without secondary infection intervening will show the signs of *atelectasis* described previously.

An unusual but important manifestation of partial bronchial obstruction is *obstructive hyperinflation,* which occurs when the magnitude of the obstruction is such that it allows air to enter the lobe as the bronchus increases in size during inspiration but prevents egress of air as the bronchus decreases in size during expiration. The hyperinflated lobe or segment is hyperlucent and may cause some compression atelectasis of the adjoining or contralateral nonobstructed lung segments or lobes. Bronchography is sometimes used to confirm the presence and site of obstruction, and at times this technique provides some clues as to the etiology. In clinical practice bronchoscopic visualization and biopsy of the obstructing lesion are the most effective diagnostic tools.

PULMONARY CAVITIES AND CYSTS

A cavity is a hole within the lung parenchyma; it usually indicates that destruction of lung tissue has occurred, although sometimes it results from the evacuation of a congenital fluid-filled cyst. The terminology of cavitary lesions of the lung is confusing and somewhat inconsistent.

A *lung abscess* is a localized area of lung destruction caused by liquefaction necrosis, usually but not invariably due to pyogenic bacteria. A lung abscess may present with the roentgenographic appearance of a solid mass until the liquefied material drains into a bronchus. Subsequently the lung abscess appears as a thick-walled, round shadow containing air and often an air-fluid level (see Fig. 14-14). Lung abscess is most commonly due to aspiration of anaerobic organisms. Lung abscess may also develop as a complication of other necrotizing pneumonias, particularly staphylococcal or aerobic gram-negative bacterial infections. Obstruction of a bronchus may cause a necrotizing process in the distal lung that eventually forms an abscess. Hematogenous spread of infection to the lungs may result in multiple abscesses.

Cavitation occurs commonly in pulmonary *tuberculosis* and in *fungal infections* of the lungs. These cavities may have thick or thin walls. There are usually other lesions in neighboring portions of the lung as well.

Bullae are thin-walled, localized areas of emphysema. They vary in size but may be several centimeters in diameter in some cases. The wall of the bulla may not be roentgenographically visible or may present as one or more "hairline" shadows that form part of the wall but are not usually continuous around the entire air-containing structure (Fig. 14-22). Bullae may occur in otherwise normal lungs or may be a manifestation of diffuse obstructive emphysema. Secondary infection may occur, with the development of air-fluid levels, and the wall may then become thickened and more visible. A *pneumatocele* is a bulla that results from a check-valve obstruction of a bronchus and causes the bulla to increase rapidly in size. It occurs most commonly as a complication of staphylococcal pneumonia.

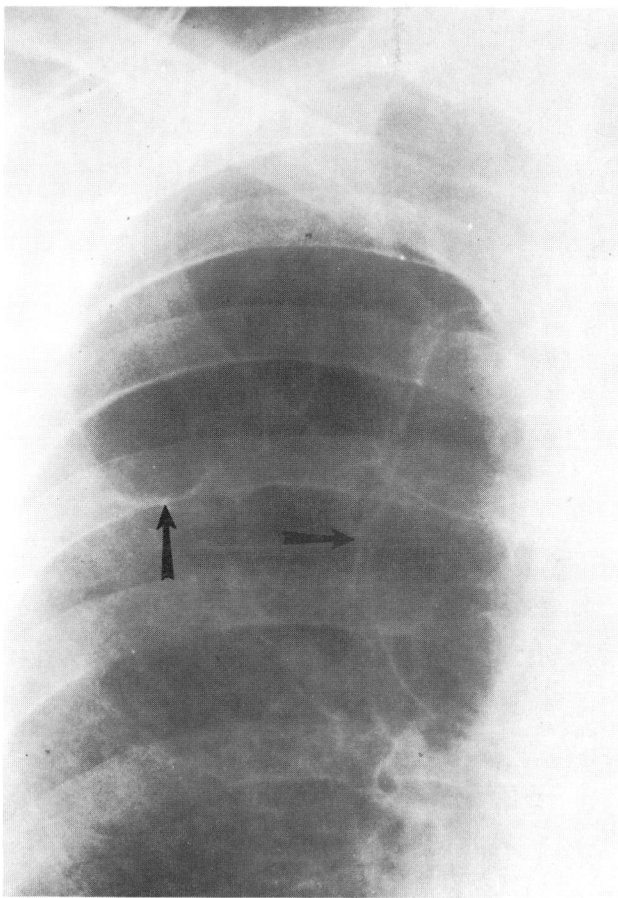

Fig. 14-22. Bullae in upper right lung. Thin, hairline shadows of the walls of the bullae are shown by arrows. Within the bullae there is little or no lung substance. This is a chest roentgenograph of a 76-year-old man with panacinar emphysema with bullous transformation.

Cavitation may occur within primary or secondary *neoplasms* of the lung, within *noninfectious granulomas*, and occasionally within an *infarcted* area secondary to pulmonary embolism. Hemorrhage, often life-threatening, may occur within cavitary lesions. A lung abscess may be a source of dissemination of infection throughout the body, resulting in septicemia or sometimes brain abscesses.

A *cyst* is a thin-walled cavity, usually congenital in origin. Many cysts are originally fluid-filled and contain air only if drainage of the contents has occurred.

DIFFUSE AIRWAY OBSTRUCTION

The diffuse obstructive airway diseases are a group of conditions characterized by generalized narrowing or partial obstruction of most of the bronchi and bronchioles in the lungs. Examples include asthma, chronic bronchitis, emphysema, and pulmonary cystic fibrosis (mucoviscidosis).

Diffuse obstructive airway disease leads to increased airway resistance, manifested physiologically by decreases in airflow rates. The increased airway resistance may be present during both inspiration and expiration, or during expiration alone.

Roentgenologic changes in diffuse obstructive airway diseases may be very obvious or fairly subtle. These changes, manifested in varying degrees by the different disease processes, include the following:

1. Hyperinflation—an increase in the total lung capacity as shown on standard end-inspiratory chest roentgenograms. The roentgenographic signs are depression and flattening of the diaphragms, a generalized increased translucency of the lung fields, and an increased size of the retrosternal air space as seen on the lateral projection.
2. Air trapping—a decreased ability to evacuate alveolar air during expiration. Detection of air trapping requires an end-expiratory roentgenogram to compare with the standard end-inspiratory roentgenogram. Fluoroscopic examination will supply similar information.
3. Diminution or loss of interstitial tissue and pulmonary vessels. The loss of interstitial tissue is most apparent if bullae are present; demonstration of diminution in vasculature may require "full chest" tomograms or angiography.
4. Increased lung markings. This occurs in some cases and is presumed to be caused by bronchial inflammation and peribronchial interstitial fibrosis. This appearance is often referred to as the "dirty lung."

ASTHMA

Asthma is an intermittent or reversible form of diffuse airway obstruction that often begins in childhood and is characterized by bronchospasm, swelling of the bronchial mucosa, and plugging of the airways with tenacious mucus. In about 50% of cases (extrinsic asthma), the disease is associated with atopic allergy; in the remainder (intrinsic asthma or asthmatic bronchitis), no definite allergic features can be identified, and the onset is often in middle age or later.

During symptom-free periods, a person's chest roentgenogram appears entirely normal in most instances. During an acute asthmatic attack the airway obstruction is manifested clinically by severe dyspnea and wheezing, and roentgenographically by reversible hyperinflation with some depression of the diaphragms and increased hypertranslucency. Destructive changes in the interstitial tissue do not occur, and the pulmonary vasculature is essentially normal. In short, an asthmatic attack may cause an acute deterioration of pulmonary function with relatively little radiographic change. In such cases the physical signs are diagnostic.

Complications of asthma may give rise to roentgenographic abnormalities.[6] Recurrent infections result in thickened bronchial walls and a "tram-line" appearance. Atelectasis may occur due to mucus plugs. Pneumomediastinum and pneumothorax may complicate asthma. Radiologic abnormalities in allergic bronchopulmonary aspergillosis include perihilar masses, consolidations, tram lines, nodules, and ring shadows.

CHRONIC BRONCHITIS

Chronic bronchitis is a chronic low-grade inflammation of the bronchi manifested by persistent cough and sputum production. Diffuse airway obstruction may be mild or severe. The chest roentgenogram is often normal but may show the pattern of "increased lung markings." In some instances there is a superimposed reversible or asthmatic component (chronic asthmatic bronchitis), and in these cases hyperinflation and air trapping may be noticeable. Unless complicated by emphysema, chronic bronchitis is not associated with destruction of interstitial tissue or loss of vasculature.

EMPHYSEMA

Emphysema is a destructive process in the pulmonary parenchyma, and the roentgenologic signs listed above (including loss of interstitial tissue and pulmonary vessels) are most marked in this condition (*see* Fig. 14-21). The diffuse airway obstruction is primarily expiratory due to collapse of the airways during expiration, and is manifested by exertional dyspnea. The presence of bullous disease may be very striking. In advanced cases hyperinflation is usually quite apparent, both on physical examination and by roentgenographic studies.

PNEUMOTHORAX AND MEDIASTINAL EMPHYSEMA

Pneumothorax is defined as the presence of air within the pleural cavity. Air may gain access to the pleural cavity through the chest wall, diaphragm, or mediastinum or from the lung through the visceral pleura. Pneumothorax may be traumatic, iatrogenic, or spontaneous.

TRAUMATIC PNEUMOTHORAX

Trauma may give rise to pneumothorax by several mechanisms, the most obvious being damage to the chest wall that allows atmospheric air to gain direct access to the pleural space. More commonly the underlying lung is lacerated, either from a penetrating foreign body or from injury to the lung by rib fracture. Another mechanism is traumatic fracture of a bronchus with resulting air leakage.

IATROGENIC PNEUMOTHORAX

Iatrogenic pneumothorax is now the most common form of this condition. Such pneumothoraces may be intentional (as in the induction of pneumothorax for diagnostic purposes), unavoidable (as in needle biopsy of the lung), or unintentional (which is the most common category). Iatrogenic pneumothorax usually results from perforation of the lung during various diagnostic or therapeutic procedures, including thoracentesis, liver biopsy, pericardiocentesis, intercostal nerve block, stellate ganglion block, transbronchial or percutaneous lung biopsy, attempted cannulation of a subclavian vein, and surgical procedures (such as tracheostomy) at the base of the neck. Procedures such as transtracheal needle aspiration and endoscopic injury of the thoracic esophagus may result in mediastinal emphysema, which subsequently ruptures into the pleural space. Pneumothorax as a complication of mechanical ventilation is discussed below.

SPONTANEOUS PNEUMOTHORAX

Spontaneous pneumothorax may occur as a complication of intrapulmonary or mediastinal disease processes. Most commonly it is seen in young people and is caused by rupture of a bleb at the apex of a lung. It is essentially a benign disorder that may, however, be recurrent and eventually require surgical correction (Fig. 14-23). Tuberculosis must be ruled out if the condition is recurrent. Pneumothorax resulting from intrapulmonary infectious diseases may be accompanied by empyema (*pyopneumothorax*).

Roentgenographic recognition of a pneumothorax depends on the loss of volume of the affected lung. A "hairline" linear shadow representing the visceral pleura may be seen, separated from the chest wall by the patternless hypertranslucency of the intrapleural air. A small pneumothorax may be difficult to detect on the standard end-inspiratory roentgenogram. The

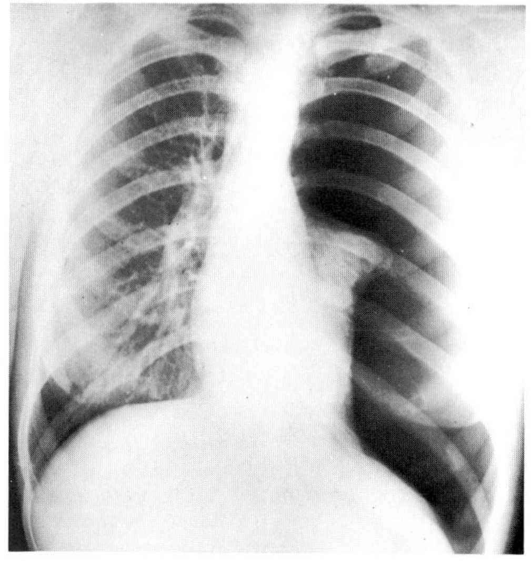

Fig. 14-23. Massive spontaneous pneumothorax in a young woman. The collapsed left lung forms a small opaque ball in the hilar area, whereas the rest of the hemithorax is filled with the patternless hypertranslucency of pleural air. Usually the lung does not collapse to this degree (*see* Fig. 14-24).

pneumothorax is always more obvious if films are taken in the end-expiratory position, and this is a very useful diagnostic maneuver in questionable cases.

With a small pneumothorax the air may be visible only in the apical and subapical areas. Pleural adhesions that prevent the retraction of portions of the lung may give rise to a loculated pneumothorax in which the intrapleural air is localized to one or more discrete areas instead of involving the entire pleural space (Fig. 14-24). The concomitant presence of blood, pus, chyle, or serous effusion is indicated if the air-fluid level is typical.

If a patient already has impaired pulmonary function, the development of a pneumothorax, even one that is small in degree, may cause serious respiratory difficulty, which can, however, be quickly relieved once the correct diagnosis has been established. Pneumothorax should be considered whenever there is an acute increase in dyspnea, particularly if unilateral chest pain is present.

MEDIASTINAL EMPHYSEMA

Mediastinal emphysema (pneumomediastinum) is the term applied to the presence of gas within the mediastinum. It is most common in newborn infants but may occur at any age. It may result from rupture of a major bronchus or the esophagus, or from the passage of air upward through the diaphragm or downward from the neck, but most commonly is secondary to rupture of alveoli and the subsequent dissection of air centrally along the bronchovascular sheaths into the mediastinum. This may occur as the result of trauma or from spontaneous rupture of alveoli (seen most often in asthmatic persons). It is a recognized complication of ventilator therapy, particularly with PEEP *(ventilator barotrauma).*

Roentgenographically, mediastinal emphysema is manifested by the presence within the mediastinum of one or more vertical linear hyperlucent streaks, most commonly appearing as an elevation of the mediastinal pleura from the underlying structures (Fig. 14-25). This is usually seen best on the left heart border. The roentgenographic changes are often subtle and frequently missed. The air may pass upward into the soft tissues of the neck and thoracic wall (subcutaneous emphysema), where it is easily visible on roentgenographic examination. Mediastinal emphysema often causes chest pain but usually has little deleterious effect on pulmonary function.

The artificial induction of a pneumomediastinum by injection of gas has been used as a diagnostic procedure in radiology, primarily for detecting enlarged mediastinal lymph nodes in cases of lung cancer.

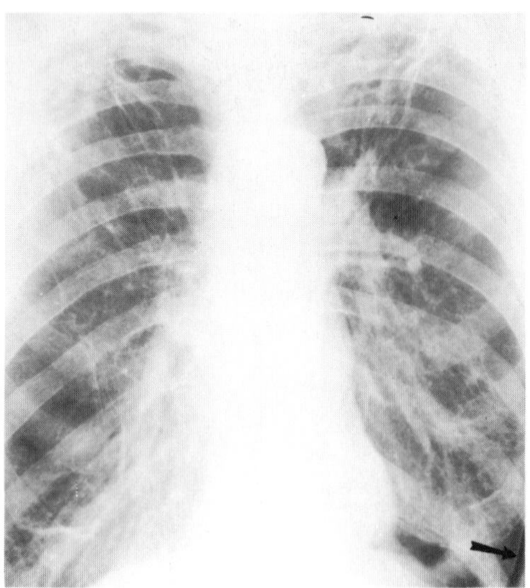

Fig. 14-24. Small loculated pneumothorax at the left base. Compare with Figure 14-16, which is of the same patient. Because of a ruptured emphysematous bleb after intermittent positive pressure breathing therapy, air has leaked into the pleural space *(arrow),* which is apparently bound by adhesions in most areas except the left base.

PLEURAL EFFUSIONS

A *pleural effusion* is fluid within the pleural space. This fluid may be blood (hemothorax), pus (empyema), chyle (chylothorax), or a relatively clear serous fluid, which may be a transudate or an exudate. The nature of the fluid cannot be determined by roentgenologic methods, and its identification depends on aspiration of the fluid with microscopic, bacteriologic, and chemical analysis.

A small pleural effusion appears roentgenographically as a haziness in the costophrenic angle or as complete obliteration of the angle. A larger effusion presents as a homogeneous opacity in the dependent portion of the thorax, with a poorly defined upper border that is generally concave and higher laterally along the chest wall (Fig. 14-26). The contour of the diaphragm is obliterated both in the upright PA and lateral projections. A very large pleural effusion causes complete opacification of the hemithorax with relatively less opacity at the top than at the bottom and often with evidence of mediastinal shift toward the normal lung.

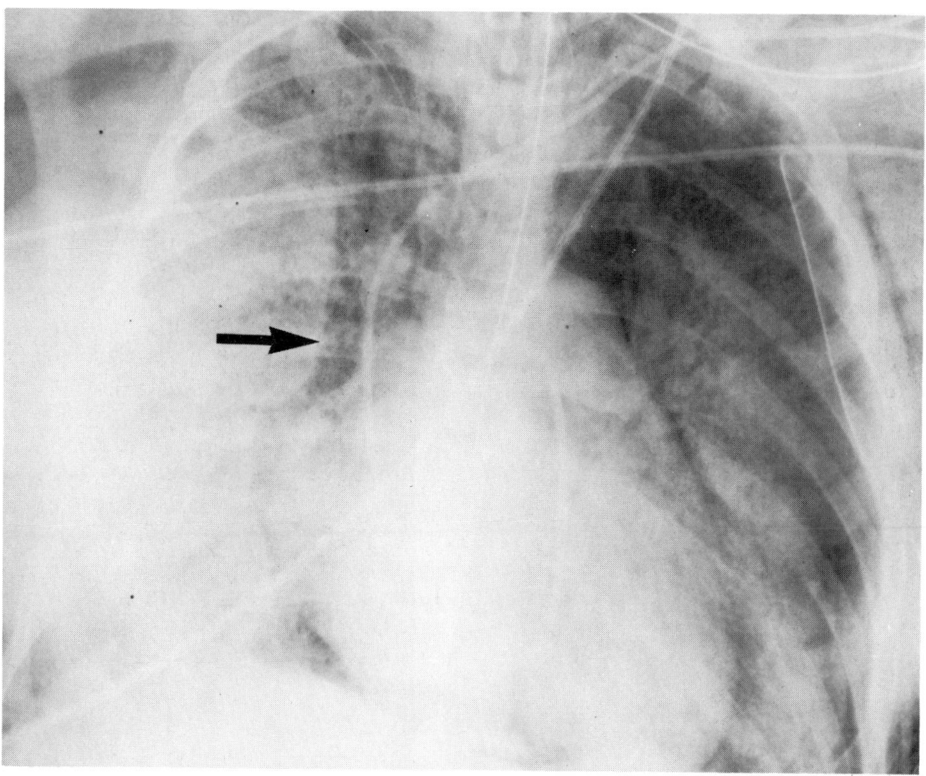

Fig. 14-25. Mediastinal emphysema. Posteroanterior film of a 16-year-old girl with acute respiratory distress syndrome and barotrauma. Note tracheostomy tube, Swan–Ganz catheter, and chest tube draining air from left pleural space. The mediastinal pleura *(arrow)* is lifted off by air. Subcutaneous air can be seen in the pectoralis muscles and in the lateral chest wall.

The appearances described above are obtained with the subject in the upright position and with a pleural space not bound down to any major degree by adhesions. If the exposure is made with the subject in the supine position, the pleural fluid layers out posteriorly, causing a diffuse haziness in the hemithorax. A *subpulmonic effusion* occurs between the lung and diaphragm and in the upright position simulates elevation of the diaphragm. An *interlobar effusion* collects within an interlobar fissure and resembles a mass lesion in the PA projection, but in the lateral view usually has a characteristic fusiform appearance. In all these cases a film taken in the lateral decubitus position will usually show movement of fluid to the most dependent portions of the hemithorax, establishing the true nature of the opacity (Fig. 14-27). A *transudative serous effusion* is identified by chemical studies of the fluid and results from changes in the hydrodynamic forces in the circulation. It may be regarded as a localized manifestation of a general tendency to form edema fluid. The most common cause is congestive heart failure. Other causes include cirrhosis and the nephrotic syndrome. In these condi-

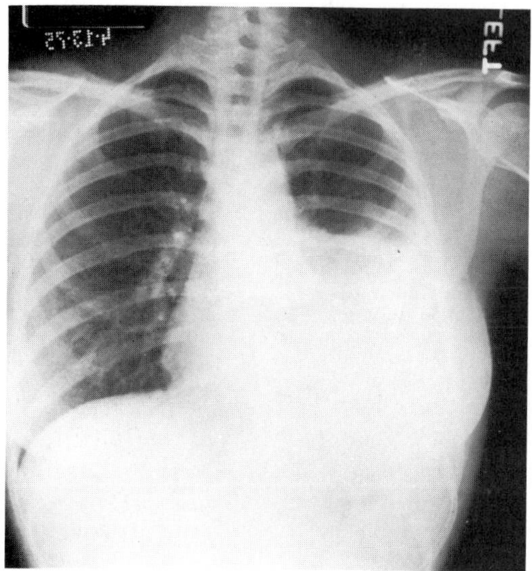

Fig. 14-26. Moderately large pleural effusion due to tuberculosis. There is a diffuse opacification in the lower half of the left hemithorax. The upper border of the opacity is concave upward. There is some shift of the heart to the right.

tions the effusion is often right-sided and associated with abdominal ascites, and the intrapleural fluid may result from the passage of ascitic fluid through diaphragmatic pores or lymphatics into the thorax.

Exudative serous effusions result from irritation of the pleural membranes, possibly due to inflammatory or malignant processes. Many inflammatory effusions are caused by an infection within the lung or mediastinum. An infection may also spread through the diaphragm to involve the pleural space; this occurs most commonly with subphrenic pyogenic abscess and with amebic infections of the liver.

Common causes of *inflammatory pleural exudates* include pneumonia, lung abscess, tuberculosis,

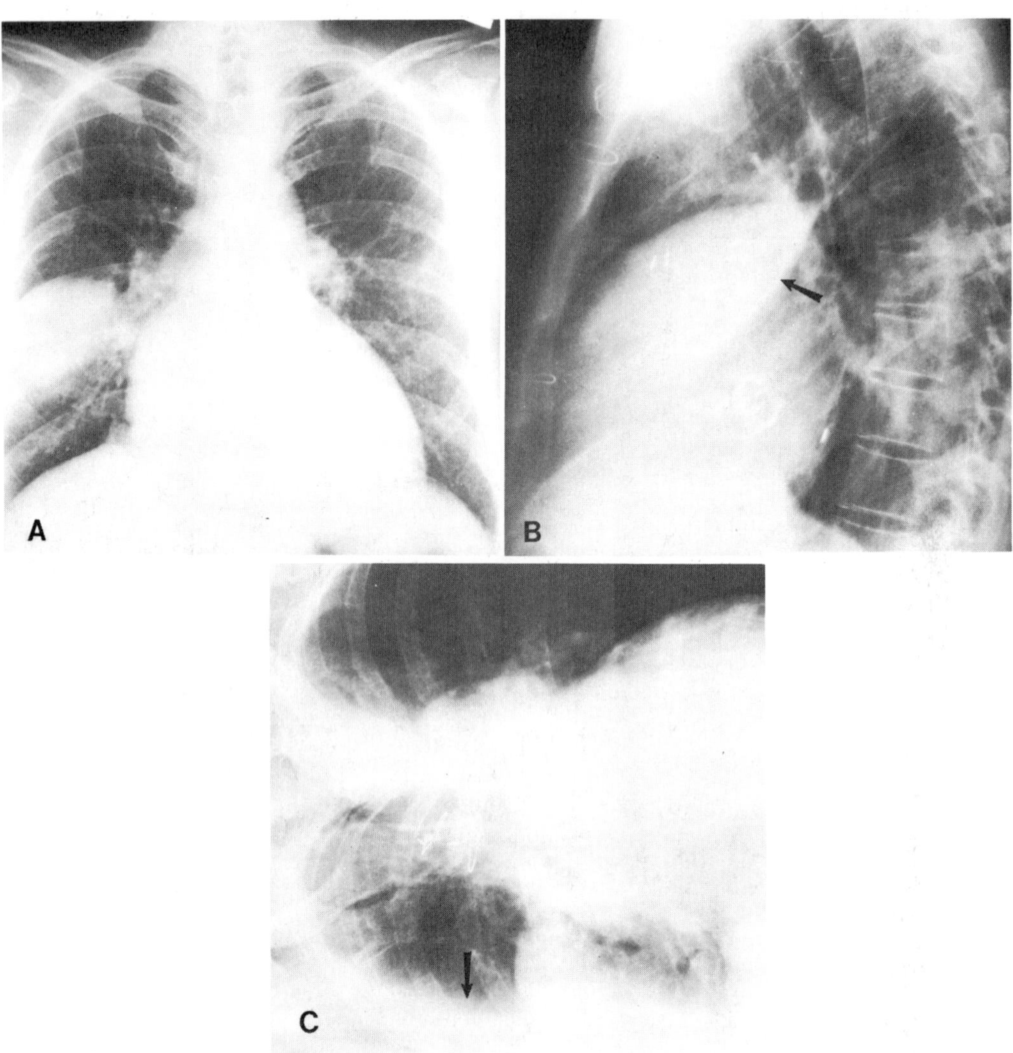

Fig. 14-27. Loculated interlobar effusion. *(A)* Posteroanterior chest film shows the fluid as a rounded opacity in the right hemithorax, resembling a tumor mass (pseudotumor). *(B)* Lateral film shows the characteristic fusiform appearance of interlobar effusion *(arrow)*, continuing upward as a thin diagonal line representing the upper portion of the oblique fissure. An artificial heart valve can be seen within the cardiac shadow, and surgical wires are seen encircling the sternum. *(C)* Right lateral decubitus film showing some passage of fluid out into the "lateral gutter," which is now the most dependent portion of the thorax.

fungal diseases, pulmonary infarction, acute pancreatitis, systemic lupus erythematosus, and the pleurisy of rheumatoid arthritis.

Malignant pleural effusions are most commonly caused by metastatic involvement of the pleura from a bronchogenic carcinoma or an extrapulmonary primary malignancy. Malignant effusions may occur with lymphomas. The most common primary malignant tumor of the pleural space is the diffuse pleural mesothelioma, often secondary to asbestos exposure.

EMPYEMA

Empyema is characterized by the presence of purulent pleural fluid and is usually caused by pneumonia or lung abscess. Other causes include tuberculosis, fungal disease, mediastinal abscess, and subphrenic abscess. Iatrogenic empyema may result from contamination of an uninfected pleural effusion by needles or drainage catheters passed into the pleural space. In almost all instances the infecting organism can be easily cultured from the aspirated empyema fluid.

The development of empyema is always a serious complication that requires prompt diagnosis and adequate mechanical drainage. Empyema should be considered whenever radiologic evidence of pleural effusion is present. Diagnosis depends on thoracentesis.

HEMOTHORAX

Hemothorax usually results from chest trauma, particularly rib fractures (Fig. 14-28) or from rupture of an intrathoracic aneurysm. It occurs occasionally with primary hemorrhagic disorders and anticoagulant drug use. The presence of a hemothorax often requires surgical intervention, either in the early stages to stop the hemorrhage or in the later stages to remove the resultant fibrin peel that may be encasing the lung and preventing adequate function on the affected side.

CHYLOTHORAX

Chylothorax is secondary to leakage of chyle from the thoracic duct and is usually caused by trauma or ma-

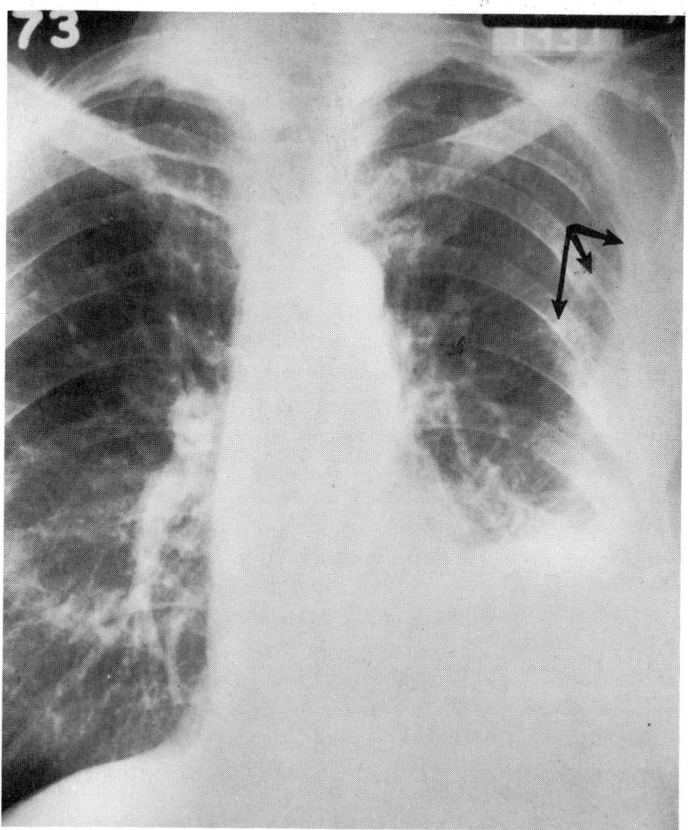

Fig. 14-28. Left hemothorax secondary to rib fractures *(arrows)*. The intrapleural opacity of the hemothorax cannot be differentiated radiologically from other types of pleural fluid.

lignant obstruction of the thoracic duct. The fluid usually has a characteristic milky appearance, but in questionable cases the true nature of the fluid must be determined by chemical studies. Chyliform and pseudochylous effusions resemble true chyle in some respects but can be differentiated chemically. These effusions are not due to leakage of chyle but result from the endogenous formation of lipids within a chronic, highly cellular exudative effusion or empyema.

Pleural effusion of any type will reduce pulmonary function to the extent that the intrapleural fluid volume reduces lung volume. In addition, pleuritic pain, when present, impairs the patient's ability to take a deep breath and to cough effectively, and the latter may lead to sputum retention.

DIAPHRAGMATIC ABNORMALITIES

The diaphragm is subject to relatively few primary diseases but is often affected by disease processes above or below it. *Bilateral depression* of the diaphragm is an important sign of hyperinflation and particularly indicates emphysema. *Bilateral elevation* of the diaphragm may result from obesity, ascites, painful breathing, or inability of the patient to take a deep breath. It is a common finding in obtunded patients lying in the supine position.

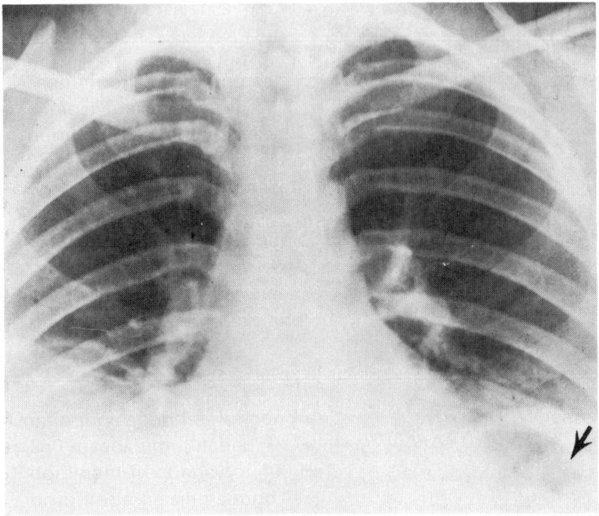

Fig. 14-29. Bilateral pulmonary emboli in a young woman. The elevated left hemidiaphragm is outlined by the gastric air bubble *(arrow)*. On the right, the diaphragm is also elevated but is not seen clearly. The thick, horizontal, curved linear opacity in the right third anterior interspace is discoid atelectasis (Fleischner's lines).

Unilateral elevation of the diaphragm may be an important sign of disease in or near the diaphragm and should never be ignored (Fig. 14-29). The most common cause of unilateral elevation of the diaphragm is an inflammatory or irritative process in the adjacent lung and visceral pleura. Such conditions include pulmonary embolism (with or without infarction), pneumonia, atelectasis, or pleurisy of any cause. Conditions of the diaphragm that cause unilateral elevation include paralysis owing to phrenic nerve dysfunction, and eventration, which is a loss of diaphragmatic muscle with thinning of the organ, probably congenital in origin (*see* Fig. 14-20). Conditions below the diaphragm causing its elevation include subphrenic abscess (usually secondary to abdominal surgery or perforation of an abdominal viscus) or a large cyst or hematoma in the upper abdomen. On occasion, gross enlargement of the liver may cause diaphragmatic elevation. In most cases of an elevated hemidiaphragm the respiratory excursions are reduced or may even be reversed (paradoxical movement). A diaphragmatic hernia may simulate unilateral elevation of the diaphragm. The recognition of an air-filled viscus within the hernia adds identification.

DIFFUSE ALVEOLAR-FILLING PROCESSES

The radiologic characteristics of alveolar-filling diseases have already been described. When the involvement is diffuse, involving multiple areas of both lungs, pulmonary function is usually markedly impaired. Clinically such patients are usually very dyspneic. Pulmonary function studies show the typical restrictive pattern with marked reduction in all lung volumes without evidence of obstructive airway disease. The lung is stiff and has a low compliance. The diffusing capacity is usually markedly reduced, and the arterial blood gases show severe hypoxemia associated with hypocapnia due to secondary hyperventilation. On occasion, widespread involvement of alveoli may be associated with carbon dioxide retention. The arterial hypoxemia may be very profound, and even high-flow oxygen supplementation may fail to raise the arterial oxygen tensions to levels that will alleviate the tissue hypoxia. The hypoxemia is primarily caused by shunting of blood within the lungs.

A diffuse alveolar-filling process frequently necessitates intubation and controlled mechanical ventilation, often with positive end-expiratory pressure.

Generally the severity of the physiologic abnormality is paralleled by the extensiveness of the radiologic findings, and deterioration or improvement in the radiologic picture is a useful index to the success of prevention or treatment. The nature of the substance that is filling the alveoli can rarely be determined from the radiologic characteristics of the abnormality. Differential diagnosis, upon which successful treatment is based, depends on the associated clinical features and, at times, the results of lung biopsy.

PULMONARY EDEMA

Acute pulmonary edema is the most common cause of acute alveolar filling (*see* Fig. 14-7). *Cardiogenic pulmonary edema* usually results from left ventricular failure (which may have various etiologic factors) or from pulmonary venous hypertension, most commonly seen in mitral valve disease (*see* Chap. 32). Cardiac enlargement is ordinarily present and provides the diagnostic clue. In patients with cardiogenic pulmonary edema the onset of frank alveolar filling may be preceded by enlargement and blurring of the hilar shadows, increased size of the upper lobe pulmonary veins owing to redistribution of blood flow, and a diffuse interstitial pattern accompanied by thickening of the interlobular septa (Kerley's B lines). Physical examination of the heart will usually reveal tachycardia and a gallop rhythm, and heart murmurs are often present. In the occasional case in which the diagnosis is in doubt, the demonstration of an elevated pulmonary wedge pressure on right heart catheterization will strongly suggest the cardiogenic origin of the disorder.

Noncardiogenic pulmonary edema may result from cerebral disorders, uremia, intravenous use of narcotic drugs such as heroin, transfusion reactions, excessive fluid intake (particularly by the intravenous route), near-drowning, and allergic reactions to drugs, among other causes. In these syndromes the heart is usually normal sized and the pulmonary wedge pressure is often normal. The diagnosis depends on a careful analysis of the history and surrounding clinical circumstances.

Pulmonary edema may result from prolonged exposure to elevated inspiratory tensions of *oxygen*. Because diffuse alveolar-filling diseases are among the most common indications for the use of high-inspired oxygen concentrations, the clinical recognition of oxygen toxicity is obviously difficult.

Unilateral pulmonary edema may occur if the patient has been lying for a prolonged time in a lateral decubitus position during the period when the edematous state developed. In rare instances unilateral pulmonary edema may occur in the underlying lung after rapid reexpansion of the lung during too rapid aspiration of a pneumothorax or pleural effusion.

ADULT RESPIRATORY DISTRESS SYNDROME AND RELATED CONDITIONS

A diffuse hemorrhagic intraalveolar exudation may occur after stress, including shock, severe trauma, septicemia, and intraabdominal catastrophes. The pulmonary abnormality usually begins 24 to 48 hours after the traumatic episode and is associated with severe dyspnea and profound hypoxemia. This syndrome is discussed in detail in Chapter 36. The profound physiologic disturbances that commonly occur in patients with diffuse alveolar disease are characterized by the term adult respiratory distress syndrome (ARDS).

Although the exact mechanisms through which the abnormality develops are not well understood, capillary wall injury with excessive leakiness appears to be a major factor. The diagnosis is usually made from the roentgenographic appearance of severe widespread alveolar opacification occurring in the clinical circumstances mentioned. Clinically the condition resembles acute pulmonary edema, and in many instances the use of massive amounts of intravenous fluids in treating the preceding shock state may be a major contributing factor to the development of ARDS. Once ARDS has developed, the pulmonary capillary wedge pressure is normal or low.

FAT EMBOLISM

Fat embolism is a similar posttraumatic syndrome that is considered to be secondary to embolization of fat globules into the pulmonary capillaries, followed by enzymatic breakdown of the fats with the release of fatty acids that irritate the lung. Presumably the fat globules originate from traumatized tissues. The condition occurs almost exclusively in people with bone fractures. Although the radiologic abnormalities are similar to those in shock lung, fat embolism has some special clinical characteristics that usually allow its identification, and it usually responds more readily to therapy.

VIRAL PNEUMONIAS

Diffuse pneumonitis caused by virus infection may result in a widespread alveolar-filling process and severe hypoxemia. Influenza and cytomegalovirus are the most commonly involved organisms.

INTRAALVEOLAR HEMORRHAGE

Widespread intraalveolar bleeding may result from spontaneous hemorrhagic states or from anticoagulant drug overdosage. In most instances, however, hemorrhages are manifestations of idiopathic pulmonary hemosiderosis, which occurs primarily in children and adolescents (perhaps as an immune response to milk), or Goodpasture's syndrome, which occurs primarily in young male adults and is caused by an immune disorder that affects the kidneys as well as the lungs. Clinical findings include the sudden appearance of a diffuse alveolar-filling process associated with a sudden fall in hemoglobin and usually hemoptysis. Recurrent attacks may lead to interstitial fibrosis.

ASPIRATION PNEUMONIA

The aspiration of small or large amounts of liquid or semisolid material into the lungs may cause bronchial obstruction or a pneumonic consolidation.[2,3] *Aspiration pneumonia* actually occurs in three forms. *Chemical* aspiration pneumonia (peptic pneumonitis, Mendelsohn's syndrome) is a diffuse alveolar-filling process that results from aspiration of gastric acids; it is frequently fatal. Predisposing causes include general anesthesia, comatose states, and nasogastric tubes or endotracheal tubes. The aspiration may be occult or follow gross emesis. The chest x-ray shows extensive alveolar filling (Fig. 14-30). *Bacterial* aspiration pneumonia is a localized consolidation of dependent portions of the lungs caused by repeated aspirations of small quantities of infected pharyngeal secretions; it is particularly common in alcoholics and in patients with poor oral hygiene, particularly if obtunded. Nasogastric tubes, endotracheal tubes, and swallowing difficulties are frequent predisposing causes. The infecting organisms are usually anaerobes or gram-negative aerobic bacilli; necrosis and abscess formation are common. *Lipoid pneumonia* (oil granuloma) results from the habitual use of mineral oil or oily nose drops and presents radiologically as a chronic consolidation simulating carcinoma. Oil substances are easily aspirated since the material may pass through the vocal cords without exciting the protective cough reflex.

CHRONIC ALVEOLAR-FILLING DISEASES

A number of diseases may be associated with persistent diffuse alveolar opacification, including sarcoidosis, infectious granulomas, alveolar cell carcinoma, and lymphoma. An unusual cause of chronic alveolar disease is pulmonary alveolar proteinosis. Most of these conditions require lung biopsy for diagnosis.

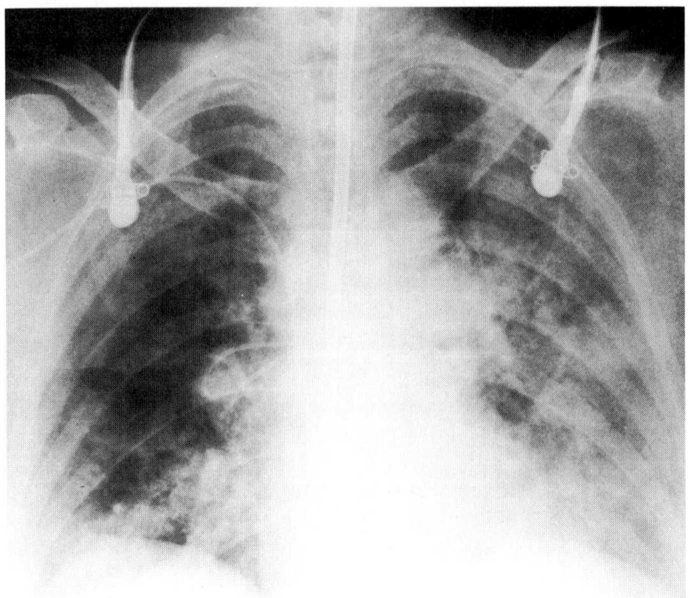

Fig. 14-30. Diffuse patchy alveolar opacification because of massive aspiration of gastric acid (peptic pneumonitis). In many cases, the distribution of the lesions is predominantly perihilar ("bat wing"). Diagnosis usually depends on the history of vomiting with aspiration because radiologic differentiation from other types of diffuse alveolar disease is usually impossible. This roentgenogram also shows artifacts peculiar to intensive care units: a midline tube passing down the esophagus for gastric decompression; two ECG leads; and a fine catheter inserted in the right arm that passes through the subclavian vein, superior vena cava, the right atrium and ventricle, the pulmonary trunk, and the right pulmonary artery.

DISSEMINATED INTERSTITIAL DISEASES

Diffusely disseminated diseases involving the interstitium of the lung are common. Although many criteria for the roentgenographic recognition of interstitial disease have been described, in many instances a definite differentiation of interstitial from alveolar-filling disease cannot be made with a great degree of confidence. The absence of an air bronchogram in a diffusely disseminated disease process suggests that the disease is interstitial in type. The most reliable signs are diffuse nodulation, linear streaks, and honeycombing, which refers to the appearance of multiple rounded lucent areas that are usually less than 1 cm in diameter (*see* Fig. 14-10).

Many of the diseases that may show a honeycomb-lung appearance are listed in Table 14-1. Alveolar processes such as ARDS and oxygen-induced pneumonitis may evolve into interstitial fibrosis. Conversely, the early stages of cardiogenic pulmonary edema produce an interstitial pattern before frank alveolar flooding with edema fluid occurs.

In most of these conditions, and particularly in the chronic ones, lung biopsy is needed to establish the diagnosis. In some instances the related clinical features will suggest the underlying etiology with considerable assurance. Physiologically, the diffuse interstitial diseases are characterized by small stiff lungs with a reduced diffusing capacity and hypoxemia, usually without carbon dioxide retention. In fact, hypocapnia is common, caused by secondary hyperventilation. The hypoxemia can usually be relieved by a moderate enrichment of inspired air with oxygen. Generally, the severity of the physiological abnormality is proportional to the extensiveness of the radiologic changes. There may, however, be gross disparity between clinical status and radiologic abnormalities in sarcoidosis, the patient usually appearing much better than his chest x-ray would indicate.

Table 14-1. Causes of Honeycomb Lung

- Fibrosing alveolitis ("usual interstitial pneumonitis")
  - Cryptogenic (idiopathic interstitial fibrosis)
  - Secondary
    - Collagen-vascular diseases
    - Fibrogenic drugs
    - ARDS
    - Oxygen toxicity
    - Tuberous sclerosis
    - Neurofibromatosis
- Desquamative alveolitis ("desquamative interstitial pneumonitis")
- Sarcoidosis
- Eosinophilic granuloma (histiocytosis X)
- Hypersensitivity pneumonitis
- Asbestosis
- Pulmonary hemosiderosis

PULMONARY EMBOLISM

The radiologic changes that accompany pulmonary embolism (*see* Chap. 33) are never distinctive, but they should suggest the diagnosis and indicate the need for more specific studies to identify positively the presence of the pulmonary embolus. In many instances pulmonary scintiscans will establish the diagnosis with high degree of assurance, and in other cases pulmonary angiography is needed. It is critically important to recognize the clinical and radiographic findings that will suggest the possibility of pulmonary embolism.

Massive pulmonary embolism is caused by the impaction of one or more large thrombi in the pulmonary outflow tract or main pulmonary arteries. Clinical features include the sudden onset of dyspnea, tachypnea, tachycardia, retrosternal chest pain, and in many cases a precipitous fall in blood pressure because of low cardiac output. If the patient survives long enough for appropriate diagnostic studies to be performed, the standard frontal projection chest roentgenogram will show relatively clear or even oligemic lung fields, usually with unilateral or bilateral increased hilar size, secondary to enlargement of the capacitance portion of the pulmonary arterial circulation. Pulmonary angiography is indicated in such circumstances and is almost invariably diagnostic.

Pulmonary emboli that involve one or more *medium-sized branches* of the pulmonary artery but do not cause infarction give rise to dyspnea and tachypnea, but pleuritic chest pain is unusual in these cases. The chest roentgenogram occasionally shows one or more oligemic, hyperlucent areas, but the common radiologic presentation is unilateral enlargement of the hilum or the lobar vessels, associated with elevation of the hemidiaphragm and the presence of discoid atelectasis (Fleischner's lines) (*see* Fig. 14-29). Discoid atelectasis appears as one or more transverse linear shadows, 1 mm to 3 mm in diameter and extending 2 cm to 4 cm in length, almost always horizontal in position and usually in the lower lung fields. The appearance of discoid atelectasis is not patho-

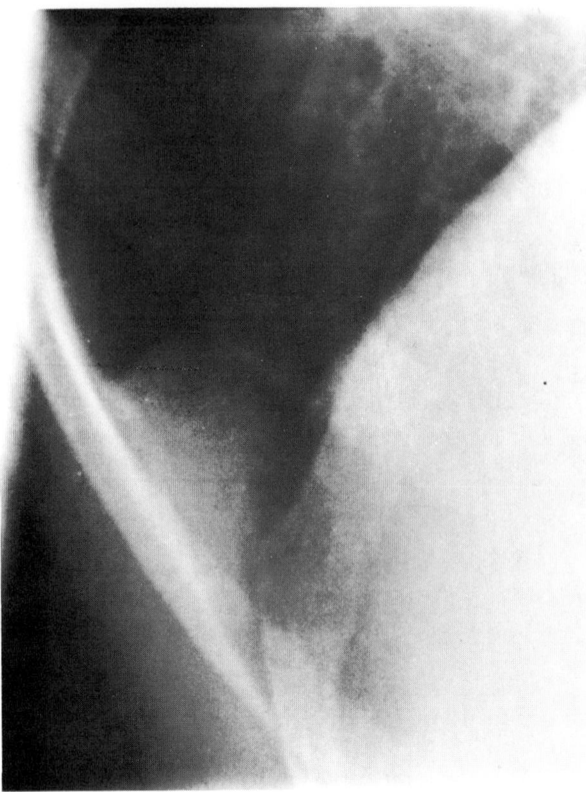

Fig. 14-31. Small pulmonary infarct seen in this magnified view of the right costophrenic angle. The infarct faces on the pleural surfaces adjacent to the costal chest wall and the diaphragm, and the convex free border is pointed toward the hilum. Unfortunately, the diagnosis here was obtained by surgical removal of the lesion, which was thought to be a tumor.

gnomonic of pulmonary embolism but should always suggest the diagnosis. It may also result from impaired motion of the hemidiaphragm and can occur with any condition that causes discomfort on breathing, including rib fractures, pleurisy, and upper abdominal surgery.

PULMONARY INFARCTION

Pulmonary infarction is ischemic necrosis of an area of lung distal to an embolus, occurring only in a small percentage of cases of embolism. Infarcts are often multiple and appear on the chest roentgenogram as one or more areas of consolidation, large or small, always abutting on a pleural surface (peripheral or interlobar) and often presenting a rounded contour on the margin facing the hilum (Fig. 14-31). Symptoms include dyspnea, tachypnea, pleuritic chest pain, and (often) hemoptysis. Pleural effusion is often present, and ipsilateral hilar enlargement with hemidiaphragmatic elevation is usually apparent. An infarct occasionally undergoes cavitation. Pulmonary scintiscanning is of limited usefulness, since an infarct will show a matching ventilation–perfusion defect similar to that occurring with any type of pulmonary consolidation. However, because emboli are commonly multiple, the scans may show one or more nonmatching defects in other nonconsolidated areas of lung that have been embolized but have not undergone infarction. Segmental pulmonary angiography is usually diagnostic. Recurrent showers of small pulmonary emboli may result in clinical and radiologic evidence of *chronic pulmonary hypertension*, with right ventricular enlargement, bilateral hilar enlargement, and clear or oligemic lung fields. Exertional dyspnea and exertional chest pain are often present. Differentiation from primary pulmonary hypertension is often difficult.

HILAR ENLARGEMENT

The hilum contains bronchi, lymph nodes, and blood vessels, but only the blood vessels are sufficiently large and radio-opaque to contribute to the normal hilar shadow. The increased size of the hilar shadow

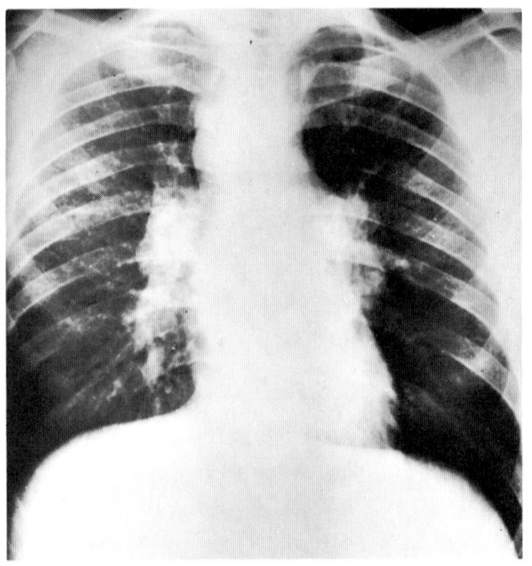

Fig. 14-32. Bilateral hilar adenopathy in sarcoidosis. The well-circumscribed, lobulated masses have been aptly described as having a "potato-node" appearance. Compare with the poorly demarcated hilar enlargement seen in Figure 14-12.

may be caused by vascular dilatation, enlargement of the lymph nodes because of disease, or development of a mass lesion, such as a bronchogenic carcinoma, within the hilum. The differentiation between lymphadenopathy and vessel enlargement as the cause of hilar enlargement can often be made on the standard chest roentgenogram and usually can be confirmed by tomographic or fluoroscopic studies. In occasional instances angiography is necessary.

Unilateral hilar enlargement of the *nonvascular* type may result from the development of an intrahilar mass lesion (tumor, bronchogenic cyst) or from the lymphadenopathy of tuberculosis, bronchogenic carcinoma, certain fungal diseases, and occasionally lymphoma. *Unilateral vascular enlargement* is most commonly caused by pulmonary embolism, but there are several rare causes, including pulmonary artery aneurysms and poststenotic dilatation due to pulmonic stenosis.

Bilateral hilar enlargement of the *nonvascular* type is most commonly caused by the lymphadenopathy of sarcoidosis (Fig. 14-32). Other causes include lymphoma, leukemia, some fungus infections, and certain pneumoconioses. Bilateral hilar enlargement caused by increased *vascular* shadows suggests pulmonary embolism, congestive heart failure (*see* Fig. 14-12), mitral stenosis, pulmonary arterial hypertension owing to chronic lung disease (cor pulmonale), and congenital heart diseases associated with a left-to-right shunt. In most instances the intrapulmonary arteries are also distended and prominent, although in massive central pulmonary embolism and in idiopathic pulmonary hypertension the lungs may appear oligemic.

IATROGENIC DISEASES OF THE LUNG

An iatrogenic disease is one caused by some action (or occasionally lack of action) of the physician. The rising incidence of iatrogenic disease has now become a major medical problem. These "diseases" are related to a progressive increase in invasive and potentially hazardous diagnostic procedures now used, and to the many toxic side-effects of the powerful drugs and complicated therapeutic procedures now available. Many iatrogenic diseases are unavoidable but predictable, and their prompt recognition depends on the physician's realization of their possible occurrence in certain clinical situations. The lungs are particularly susceptible to various iatrogenic diseases.

NOSOCOMIAL INFECTIONS

Pulmonary infections that have their onset after the patient has been admitted to the hospital may result from invasion by the indigenous pathogenic microbiologic flora of the hospital or may be a manifestation of infection by "saprophytic" organisms normally present in the body but which develop invasive potential because of reduced resistance in patients exposed to various diagnostic or therapeutic maneuvers. Predisposing factors include the use of broad-spectrum antibiotics or immunosuppressive drugs, invasive diagnostic or therapeutic procedures, swallowing difficulties allowing aspiration of food and infected pharyngeal secretions, tracheal intubation, and contaminated inhalation therapy equipment. Localization of the infection may be tracheobronchial, alveolar, or both.

Common infecting organisms include *Staphylococcus, Pseudomonas* and other aerobic gram-negative bacilli, anaerobic organisms, and bacteria and fungi normally of low pathogenicity, including *Aspergillus* and *Candida.* The roentgenographic features of nosocomial pneumonia are not characteristic except that the lesions are less likely to be lobar or segmental in distribution and commonly are multiple, bilateral, and poorly circumscribed (bronchopneumonia). Common complications include cavitation and pleural effusion or empyema.

POSTOPERATIVE PULMONARY COMPLICATIONS

Pulmonary complications are a major cause of morbidity and mortality after surgical procedures, and their incidence is greatly increased if preexisting pulmonary disease is present (*see* Chap. 37). Chronic obstructive airway diseases present the greatest hazard, since pulmonary function may already be borderline and the inability of the patient to generate an effective cough postoperatively predisposes to sputum retention. Surgical procedures on the thorax itself or on the upper abdomen are more likely to be followed by postoperative pulmonary complications than is surgery that involves other areas of the body.

Atelectasis

Atelectasis caused by obstruction of one or more bronchi by retained mucus plugs may occur during surgery or at any time in the postoperative period but usually appears within the first few days. Roentgenographic signs include changes indicating loss of volume and the opacity of the collapsed lobe or segment itself (see Fig. 14-18). The main contributing factor is the inability or unwillingness of the patient to cough effectively because of postoperative pain. In most instances postoperative atelectasis can be prevented by a vigorous program of pulmonary toilet both before and after surgery. Treatment for atelectasis is simple and effective provided the condition is recognized.

Postoperative Pulmonary Embolism

Postoperative pulmonary embolism may occur at any time in the postoperative period but most commonly appears several days after the surgical procedure. The radiologic signs of pulmonary embolism have already been reviewed. Predisposing factors include obesity, polycythemia, heart disease, malignancy, and orthopedic procedures to the limbs, particularly the treatment of hip fractures. In most instances clear-cut evidence of underlying thrombophlebitis will not be detectable on physical examination.

Postoperative Respiratory Insufficiency

Postoperative respiratory insufficiency has become increasingly common with the use of complicated surgical procedures on elderly or seriously ill patients. Chronic obstructive lung disease is the main predisposing factor. In many patients who develop respiratory insufficiency in the postoperative state, the chest roentgenogram shows no particular change from the preoperative film. The diagnosis primarily depends on arterial blood gas measurements. Prolonged, complicated surgical procedures associated with hypovolemic shock or sepsis may lead to the development of ARDS, in which case the chest roentgenogram reveals a diffuse patchy alveolar-filling process that develops 24 to 48 hours after the procedure.

DRUG-INDUCED DISEASES OF THE LUNGS

Certain drugs may have a direct *toxic* effect on the lungs. The prolonged use of high concentrations of oxygen in the inspired gas leads to hemorrhagic pulmonary edema, which is often not recognized because of the extensive radiographic abnormalities resulting from the underlying pulmonary disease that necessitated the oxygen therapy. *Allergic reactions* to drugs may cause pulmonary edema, asthmatic attacks, pulmonary vasculitis, or eosinophilic pneumonia. Certain drugs (bleomycin, busulfan, methotrexate, and several others) may cause a *diffuse interstitial pneumonitis* and *fibrosis*. Methysergide may cause *mediastinal fibrosis* with compression of the superior vena, the main bronchi, or the pulmonary veins. The prolonged use of adrenal corticosteroids often results in *mediastinal widening* due to fat deposits. The intravenous use of narcotic drugs such as heroin may result in noncardiogenic *pulmonary edema*.

FLUID OVERLOAD

Hospitalized patients, particularly those in intensive care units, commonly develop pulmonary edema from vascular overload with intravenous fluids. This possibility must be considered in any patient receiving intravenous fluids who develops a diffuse alveolar-filling process. The diagnosis can be confirmed in most instances by a careful study of intake/output data and serial body weights. The response to diuretic therapy is usually prompt and vigorous if renal function is adequate; in the presence of renal failure, even diminished oral fluid intake may cause pulmonary edema (see Fig. 14-7). In most cases, the pulmonary capillary wedge pressure is elevated.

COMPLICATIONS OF MECHANICAL VENTILATION

Mechanical ventilation is commonly used for maintaining life during episodes of respiratory insufficiency or respiratory failure. Certain hazards are, however, inherent in this form of therapy.[8]

Oxygen Toxicity

Oxygen toxicity has already been mentioned. The inspired oxygen concentration must be maintained at the lowest level that will yield an arterial oxygen tension of 60 to 80 mm Hg.

Endobronchial Infections

Bacterial colonization of the upper tracheobronchial tree is unavoidable when an endotracheal tube is in place, but the incidence and severity of secondary infections can be minimized by strict adherence to appropriate technique. Endobronchial infections are manifested by purulent bronchial secretions, often without any radiologic abnormality indicative of parenchymal pneumonia. Inadequate sterilization of inhalation therapy equipment may result in a serious or even fatal pulmonary infection that is often bilateral and sometimes necrotizing (associated with cavity formation).

Tube Misplacement

Displacement of the endotracheal tube into the right main bronchus usually results in the rapid development of atelectasis of the left lung. Atelectasis is easily recognized by stethoscopic examination, and a chest roentgenogram is confirmatory. This disorder can be avoided by radiographic monitoring of the tube placement and by routine stethoscopic examination of the lungs of the intubated patient at appropriate intervals.

Mediastinal and Subcutaneous Emphysemas

Mediastinal and subcutaneous emphysemas are infallible indices that air leakage is occurring (*see* Figs. 14-25, 14-33). If a tracheostomy has been performed, the leakage of air may be occurring from the tracheal incision or from the surgical site. More commonly, air in the tissues indicates that alveolar rupture has occurred, with dissection of the air centripetally along the bronchovascular bundles into the mediastinum and up into the subcutaneous tissues of the neck. This is commonly followed by the development of a *pneumothorax*, and the appearance of subcutaneous air should indicate the need for immediate chest radiographic examination. Other clinical signs that indicate a pneumothorax include tachycardia, shock, and decline of arterial blood gas values. The intubated and sedated patient cannot, of course, complain of chest pain or dyspnea. Roentgenographic recognition of a pneumothorax is simple if the collapse is massive, but the demonstration of a small amount of intrapleural air may require that the patient assume a somewhat upright position for the exposure of the film. The occurrence of interstitial emphysema and pneumothorax is surprisingly uncommon with intermittent positive pressure breathing but has a greatly increased incidence if PEEP is used.

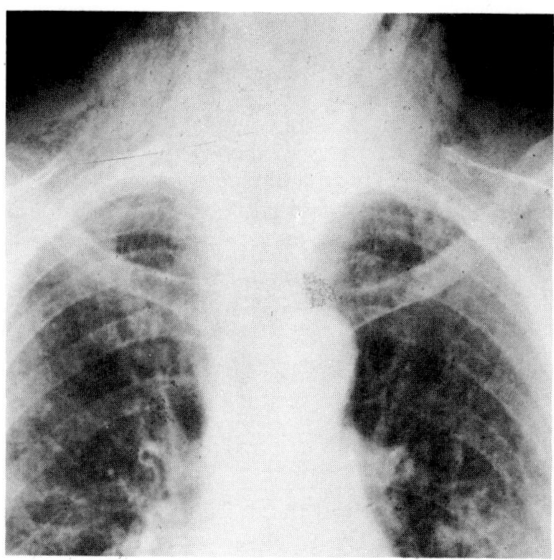

Fig. 14-33. Subcutaneous emphysema in the neck secondary to transtracheal aspiration for diagnostic purposes. Multiple linear lucencies represent air within subcutaneous fat and cervical muscles bundles. The patient has diffuse interstitial lung disease.

RADIATION PNEUMONITIS AND FIBROSIS

Radiation therapy in or near the lungs may result in acute radiation pneumonitis or chronic radiation fibrosis. *Radiation pneumonitis* appears within 1 or 2 months from the start of therapy and is manifested roentgenographically as a soft, fluffy alveolar process usually localized to the areas exposed to the radiation, although on occasion it may become generalized. *Radiation fibrosis* may be a sequela of radiation pneumonitis or may develop independently some months after radiation therapy has been completed. It is interstitial in its roentgenographic appearance and is characterized by its strict localization to the area of radiation exposure and its lack of segmental distribution. Secondary bronchiectasis within the involved area gives the infiltrate a nonhomogeneous character.

ENDOSCOPIC TRAUMA

Fiberoptic *bronchoscopy* is relatively atraumatic to the lung. Bronchoscopic biopsy of bronchial lesions may result in hemorrhage, more commonly with the larger-sized biopsies that are possible with the rigid bronchoscope. Bronchial bleeding may produce roentgenographic evidence of alveolar-filling consolidation in the affected lung area. Transbronchoscopic biopsies of peripheral lung may result in traumatic pneumothorax caused by penetration by the biopsy forceps of the visceral pleura (Fig. 14-34).

Esophageal endoscopic examination or bougienage may cause esophageal rupture, leading to acute mediastinitis. Roentgenographic findings include mediastinal widening, mediastinal emphysema, and often pneumothorax or hydropneumothorax. The esophageal perforation resulting from violent vomiting ("spontaneous" perforation of the esophagus) has identical radiologic characteristics.

OPPORTUNISTIC INFECTIONS

Opportunistic infections occur in patients with impaired host defenses. The "compromised host" may owe his vulnerability to his underlying disease (diabetes, impaired cellular or humoral immunity, splenectomy), to mechanical conduits (endotracheal tubes, intravenous catheters), or to the effects of drugs (adrenal steroids, cytotoxic drugs). The lungs are commonly the site of infection.

In the clinical and radiologic assessment of such patients, the roentgenographic abnormality is not necessarily caused by infection. It may be a manifestation of the primary underlying disease (particularly in lymphoma, leukemia, and metastatic carcinoma) and may result from an untoward reaction to treatment, such as alveolar hemorrhage due to platelet suppression, or interstitial fibrosis secondary to cytotoxic drugs.

The radiologic appearance of the lungs does provide some etiologic clues. Lobar and segmental consolidations suggest bacterial, fungal, or mycobacterial infections. Multiple nodules are often caused by fungal infection. Diffuse alveolar disease suggests pneumocystis or cytomegalovirus infection, alveolar hemorrhage, oxygen toxicity, or drug reactions. Diffuse interstitial disease in a compromised host may result from viral infection, lymphoma, or the chronic stage of drug reactions, radiation fibrosis, and oxygen-damaged lung. Miliary lesions suggest mycobacterial and fungal infection.

RADIOLOGY IN THE INTENSIVE CARE UNIT

Because patients in intensive care units tend to have life-threatening and rapidly changing pulmonary abnormalities, accurate interpretation is critically important, but the technical quality of the AP supine chest roentgenograms is necessarily suboptimal. Errors can arise from overinterpretation of abnormalities that may be spurious because of positional factors or differences in exposure on serial films. It has been wisely suggested that the interpreter of such roentgenograms attempt to provide answers to the following questions only.[1]

1. Is the film technically adequate?
2. Are there any rib fractures?
3. Are the endotrachael tube, gastric tube, and intravenous lines correctly positioned?
4. Is there pulmonary consolidation? One should determine if there is consolidation and whether it has changed on serial films. Attempts to predict etiology may be seriously misleading.
5. Is pleural fluid present?
6. Is atelectasis present?
7. Is a pneumothorax present?

The interpreter must constantly remember that pneumothoraces and pleural effusions often have atypical

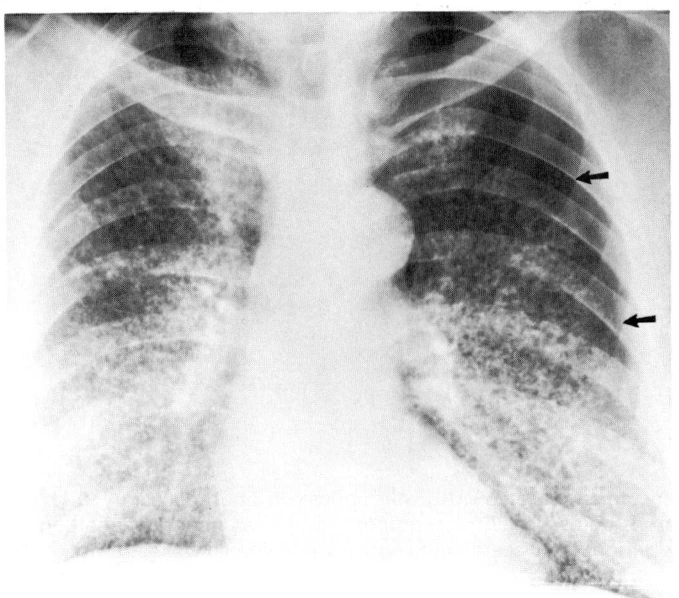

Fig. 14-34. Left pneumothorax because of perforation of the visceral pleura during transbronchial lung biopsy with the fiberoptic bronchoscope. This complication is rare if fluoroscopic guidance is used. The diagnosis of miliary tuberculosis was established by the biopsy. The lung edge is marked by arrows.

appearances on AP supine films and that penetration and contrast vary from film to film.

THORACIC TRAUMA

Thoracic trauma may result in various physiological and roentgenographic abnormalities in the thorax, the prompt recognition of which is imperative for successfully managing the patient. In most instances the fact that trauma to the thoracic cage has occurred is apparent from the history or from superficial inspection of the thorax; however, if an unconscious patient is brought to the hospital emergency room and inspection of the thorax reveals no obvious evidence of injury, traumatic lung damage may go unrecognized. Thoracic trauma must be suspected in all such cases and appropriate roentgenographic studies carried out. The mechanisms of production of thoracic trauma and the nature of the resulting lesions are extremely varied. I shall briefly indicate some of the more common abnormalities.

RIB FRACTURES

Rib fractures may result in various complications. One or two undisplaced rib fractures may have no deleterious effect other than pain. Special *rib films* may be needed to detect their presence. If the patient has chronic obstructive pulmonary disease, the cough suppression induced by the pain of the fractures may result in atelectasis or pneumonia. Multiple rib fractures will create an instability of the chest wall, known as *flail chest*, which may cause severe respiratory embarrassment. The modern treatment of flail chest with intubation and mechanical ventilation represents one of the more important advances in managing thoracic trauma. Flail chest is easily recognized on physical examination by the paradoxical movement of the traumatized chest wall and can be confirmed radiographically by inspiration and expiration films. Rib fractures may lacerate vessels and cause hemothorax (*see* Fig. 14-28) or may lacerate the lung and cause pneumothorax. The presence of air and fluid within the pleural space is manifested by the characteristic fluid level.

PENETRATING CHEST WOUNDS

Penetrating chest wounds cause pneumothorax both by entry of air through the chest wall wound and by leakage of air from the lacerated lung. Intrapleural hemorrhage is common, and chylothorax appears if the thoracic duct is injured. Intrapulmonary hemorrhage occurs along the pathway of the penetrating foreign body within the lung.

NONPENETRATING TRAUMA

Nonpenetrating trauma may result in the formation of an intrapulmonary hematoma (pulmonary contusion), which appears roentgenographically as a poorly circumscribed opaque consolidation without localization to segmental boundaries. The opacity appears within hours after the injury and clears spontaneously within 1 or 2 weeks. Occasionally closed-chest trauma may lacerate the lung internally to produce a cystlike hyperlucent space that may contain an air-fluid level because of intracavitary hemorrhage. Tracheobronchial rupture caused by nonpenetrating trauma results in pneumothorax, often accompanied by mediastinal and subcutaneous emphysema and frequently associated with fractures of the upper three ribs. Nonpenetrating trauma may cause hemothorax or chylothorax in some instances.

Mediastinal structures may be affected by nonpenetrating trauma. Traumatic pericarditis is often secondary to "steering wheel" injuries of the anterior chest. Traumatic rupture of the descending portion of the aortic arch may lead to formation of a false aneurysm, which presents on the chest roentgenogram as a left-sided mediastinal mass. Mediastinal hematoma resulting from traumatic injury of one or more small vessels causes generalized or diffuse mediastinal widening.

REFERENCES

1. Adams FG: A simplified approach to the reporting of intensive therapy unit chest radiographs. Clin Radiol 30:214, 1979
2. Bartlett JG: Anaerobic bacterial pneumonitis. Am Rev Resp Dis 119:19, 1979
3. Berkman YM: Aspiration and inhalation pneumonias. Semin Roentgenol 15:73, 1980
4. Fraser RG, Pare JAP: Perception in chest roentgenology. In Diagnosis of Diseases of the Chest, Vol I, 2nd ed. Philadelphia, WB Saunders, 1977
5. Miller RD, Offord KP: Roentgenologic determination of total lung capacity. Mayo Clin Proc 55:694, 1980
6. Palmer PES: Radiology of asthma. In Gershwin ME (ed): Bronchial Asthma. New York, Grune & Stratton, 1981
7. Thurlbeck WM et al: Chronic obstructive lung disease. A comparison between clinical roentgenologic, functional and morphologic criteria in chronic bronchitis, emphysema, asthma and bronchiectasis. Medicine 49:82, 1970
8. Zwillich CW et al: Complications of assisted ventilation. A prospective study of 354 consecutive episodes. Am J Med 57:161, 1974

BIBLIOGRAPHY

General Texts

Felson B: Chest Roentgenology. Philadelphia, WB Saunders, 1973

Felson B, Weinstein AS, Spitz HB: Principles of Chest Roentgenology: A Programmed Text. Philadelphia, WB Saunders, 1965

Fraser RG, Pare JAP: Roentgenologic signs in the diagnosis of chest disease. In Diagnosis of Diseases of the Chest, 2nd ed. Philadelphia, WB Saunders, 1977

Lillington GA, Jamplis RW: A Diagnostic Approach to Chest Diseases, 2nd ed. Baltimore, Williams & Wilkins, 1977

Simon GA: Principles of Chest X-ray Diagnosis, 4th ed. New York, Appleton–Century–Crofts, 1977

Pulmonary Scintiscans

Moser KM: Clinical applications of ventilation/perfusion scintiphotography. In Baum GL (ed): Textbook of Pulmonary Diseases, 2nd ed. Boston, Little, Brown & Co, 1974

Wagner HN: The use of radioisotopic techniques for the evaluation of patients with pulmonary disease. Am Rev Respir Dis 113:203, 1976

Thoracic CT Scans

Heitzman ER, Proto AV, Goldwin RL: The role of computerized tomography in the diagnosis of diseases of the thorax. JAMA 241:933, 1979

Mintzer RA: CT in the evaluation of pulmonary lesions. CRC Crit Rev Diagn Imaging 15:95, 1981

Radiologic Patterns

Heitzman ER: Pattern recognition in pulmonary radiology. In Heitzman ER (ed): The Lung: Radiologic–Pathologic Correlations. St Louis, CV Mosby, 1973

Itoh H et al: Radiologic–pathologic correlations of small lung nodules with special reference to peribronchiolar nodules. AJR 130:223, 1978

Infections

Genereux GP, Stilwell GA: The acute bacterial pneumonias. Semin Roentgenol 15:9, 1980

Janower ML, Weiss EB: Mycoplasmal, viral and rickettsial pneumonias. Semin Roentgenol 15:25, 1980

Palmer PES: Pulmonary tuberculosis—usual and unusual radiographic presentations. Semin Roentgenol 14:204, 1979

Diffuse Alveolar and Interstitial Disease

Carrington CB, Gaensler EA: Clinical–pathologic approach to diffuse infiltrative lung disease. In Thurlbeck WM (Ed): The Lung: Structure, Function and Disease. Baltimore, Williams & Wilkins, 1978

Felson B: The roentgen diagnosis of disseminated pulmonary alveolar diseases. Semin Radiol 2:3, 1967

Joffe N: The adult respiratory distress syndrome. AJR 122:719, 1974

Reed JC, Reeder WM: Honeycomb lung (interstitial fibrosis). JAMA 231:646, 1975

Pulmonary Embolism

Fleischner FG: Roentgenology of the pulmonary infarct. Semin Roentgenol 2:61, 1967

Lillington GA, Parsons GH: Acute pulmonary embolism. Hosp Med 16:11, 1980

Simon M: Plain film and angiographic aspects of pulmonary embolism. In Moser KM, Stein M (eds): Pulmonary Thromboembolism. Chicago, Year Book Medical Publishers, 1973

15

Manufacture, Storage, and Transport of Medical Gases

James M. Webb

OXYGEN

ATMOSPHERIC CONTENT

Oxygen is the third most abundant atom in the universe, with hydrogen and helium first and second, respectively, and carbon and nitrogen fourth and fifth, respectively. Oxygen composes only 0.09% of all atoms in the universe. At the earth's crust, however, where oxygen is the most abundant atom, it makes up about 54% of all atoms. There are about 37.7 Emoles* of oxygen in the atmosphere; 37.0 Emoles are in the form of molecular oxygen, and most of the rest is in the form of water vapor. In addition to molecular oxygen, the atmosphere contains a number of reactive gaseous species, including ozone. These other species are generally found at high altitudes or in smog.

Photosynthesis is the main producer and regulatory factor of oxygen in the atmosphere. The greatest amount of oxygen is produced on land by terrestrial photosynthesis (0.0073 Emoles per year). Approximately 0.0037 Emoles of oxygen per year are produced by oceanic photosynthesis, particularly close to land. The total production of oxygen for the earth is about 0.011 Emoles per year.

*One Emole represents 1×10^{18} moles, with a mole representing the gram molecular weight of the substance. For instance, a mole of free oxygen is 32 g, which corresponds to its molecular weight of 32.

Photosynthesis is the process whereby light energy from the sun converts carbon dioxide and water into glucose and oxygen. The chemical agent necessary for this transformation is chlorophyll. Chlorophyll is a pigment that traps energy. Interestingly, the enzyme system that catalyzes the production of energy-rich compounds is the same as the enzyme system that allows energy release from these compounds, in the presence of oxygen, in the animal body.

$$6\ CO_2 + 6\ H_2O \xrightarrow[\text{Radiant energy}]{\text{Chlorophyll}} C_6H_{12}O_6 + 6\ O_2$$

The rate of photosynthesis is primarily influenced by two factors: an increase in oxygen; and a decrease in carbon dioxide. Both factors decrease the rate of photosynthesis. Within the biosphere, the process of manufacturing oxygen is primarily the function of photosynthesis, and respiration is primarily the process by which oxygen is used. The end result of these two processes is a net production of oxygen that is practically zero. It takes about 3400 years for the oxygen in the air around the earth to be replaced.

The oxygen we breathe is necessary to support the metabolic process by which we convert carbohydrates, fats, and proteins into heat and energy. The amount of oxygen consumed by an average human being in a 24-hour period weighs about 2½ pounds,

1,000,000 CU. FT. OF DRY AIR CONTAINS	
781,400	CU. FT. NITROGEN
209,300	CU. FT. OXYGEN
9,300	CU. FT. ARGON
300	CU. FT. CARBON DIOXIDE
18	CU. FT. NEON
5	CU. FT. HELIUM
1	CU. FT. KRYPTON
1	CU. FT. HYDROCARBONS
.5	CU. FT. HYDROGEN
.08	CU. FT. XENON
.01	CU. FT. ACETYLENE

Fig. 15-1. Specific identifiable gases contained in 1,000,000 cu ft of dry air. (Courtesy of Union Carbide Corp., Linde Division)

which is roughly equal to the weight of the food that we consume in the same period of time. For our bodies to obtain this oxygen, we breathe about 500 cubic feet (15,000 qt) of air (Fig. 15-1).

LABORATORY METHODS

Until the early 1900s the manufacture of oxygen was primarily a laboratory experiment. In 1774, Joseph Priestley liberated the first pure oxygen on record by concentrating the sun's rays through a magnifying glass on mercuric oxide.[1]

Several other methods may be used for preparing oxygen in the laboratory setting. Heating potassium chlorate in the presence of manganese dioxide, which serves as a catalyst, is one method. Another is the electrolysis of water. By volume, water contains 2 parts hydrogen to 1 part oxygen (by weight water contains 1 part hydrogen to 8 parts oxygen). These elements can be split, leaving 1 part oxygen and 2 parts hydrogen. The difference between the volume and weight ratios can be explained by the fact that the atomic weight of oxygen is 16 times that of hydrogen.

The word "electrolysis" literally means "split by electricity." This is accomplished by passing an electric current through the water. Since water is a poor conductor of electricity, it is necessary to add a substance that will enable the electric current to pass through it. Generally a trace of mineral or sulfuric acid is added to the water to facilitate the conduction of the current through the water. As the current passes through the water, bubbles of gas appear near the two electrodes. Oxygen collects in the tube that contains the anode, and hydrogen collects in the tube that contains the cathode (Fig. 15-2). As explained earlier, for every milliliter of oxygen produced, 2 ml of hydrogen is produced.

Another method used for production of oxygen is the LeBrin process, by which oxygen is prepared from atmospheric air. This is an older process in which barium oxide (BaO) is heated to 500° C in air, producing barium peroxide. By raising the temperature of the barium peroxide to 800° C, oxygen and barium oxide will be liberated.

COMMERCIAL METHODS

Limited commercial production of oxygen began around the turn of the century in what was known as an "ozone generator." In this process fused sodium peroxide interacts with water. This method was both expensive and cumbersome and eventually gave way to the common technique of fractional distillation of liquefied air (sometimes referred to as the Joule–Kelvin method).[1]

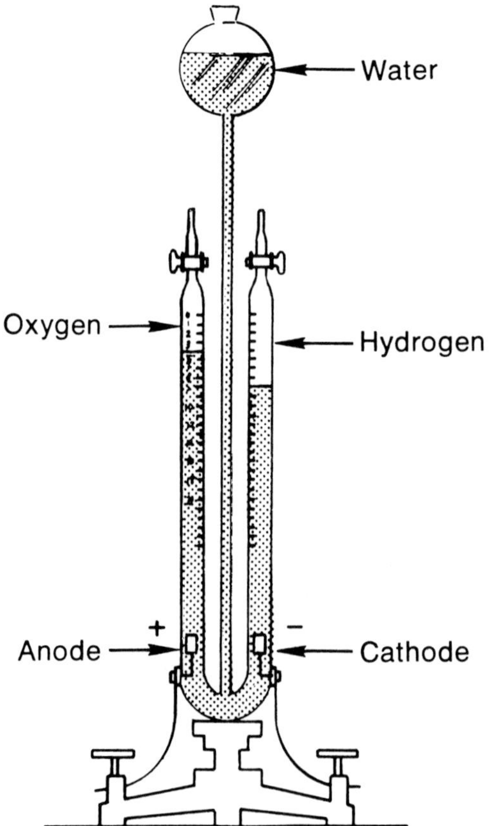

Fig. 15-2. Apparatus used for the electrolysis of water.

According to the Joule–Kelvin principle, when gases, under pressure, are released into a vacuum, the molecules tend to lose kinetic energy. The molecules withdraw from each other, and their cohesive attraction is lost in the vacuum. The loss in kinetic energy results in a decreased speed of the molecules, with a resultant lowering of the temperature, a necessary step for liquefaction of the air.

The complex process for the commercial preparation of oxygen can be divided into three stages: purification of the air; partial liquefaction of the air by refrigeration; and separation of oxygen from nitrogen by fractional distillation of the partially liquefied air. To start the process, air is compressed to about 1500 pounds per square inch gauge (psig) in a large compressor (Fig. 15-3). The initial increase in temperature caused by compression is reversed by a water-cooled heat exchanger. The air is then compressed further to approximately 2000 psig, after which it passes through an aftercooler and is delivered at room temperature to a countercurrent heat exchanger.

The purpose of the three-chamber countercurrent heat exchanger is to purify and to liquefy the compressed air partially through a refrigeration process. Using waste nitrogen as a cooling agent, the first chamber cools the air below the freezing point of water, condensing most of the water out of the air. The compressed air enters this chamber and is cooled to about −50°F, and leaves the chamber at about 32°F.

In the second chamber of the heat exchanger, the compressed air first enters a forecooler and is cooled to about −40°F by the evaporation of liquid ammonia. At this point, any water remaining in the air is frozen out. The partially purified air is then transferred to the third chamber of the heat exchanger, where it is cooled to about −265°F. At this stage of the process, the extremely cold air is still compressed at 200 psig and will not liquefy, since the critical pressure of air is about 530 psig. At any pressure above 530 psig, the meniscus, or curved upper surface of the column of liquid under pressure, disappears, and no separation between liquid and gas is evident; the air simply in-

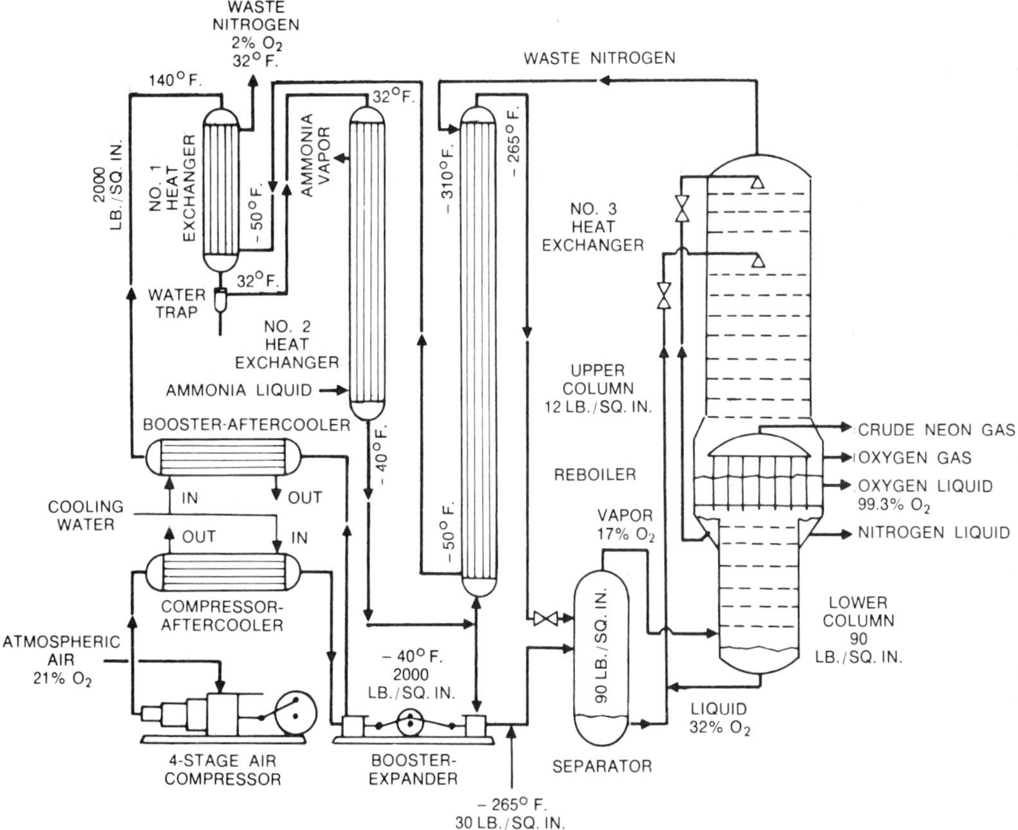

Fig. 15-3. Air separation plant for the production of liquid oxygen. (Courtesy of Union Carbide Corp., Linde Division)

creases in density as it is cooled. Therefore, the extremely cold air/fluid must be expanded to about 90 psig before it can be separated with a sizable fraction liquefied.

Still at −256°F but expanded to a much lower pressure, the air leaves the heat exchanger and passes into a separator, where liquid and vapor are separated. These are pumped in separate streams into the distillation column. The pressure of the liquid air is expanded further to about 12 psig as it enters the distillation column, where it is separated into its component gases.

In the distillation column the liquid passes over cylindrical shells containing perforated metal trays that are spaced at regular intervals. The liquid passes over the trays, whereas the gas rises through the perforations and bubbles through the liquid. The gas that passes through the liquid becomes progressively richer in nitrogen, whereas the liquid becomes richer in oxygen.

The entire process actually takes place in two phases. Air, in the form of vapor, enters the very bottom of the column, and nitrogen gas leaves through the top of the column, leaving 99.9% pure liquid oxygen.

The fractional distillation phenomenon can be explained through examination of the boiling points of various liquid gases. At one atmosphere, oxygen has a boiling point of −297.4°F, and nitrogen boils at −320°F. The rare gases contained in the liquid oxygen in its first impure state also have lower boiling points than does oxygen. Thus, by controlling the pressure, and therefore the temperature, within the two areas of the distillation column, the liquid nitrogen and other gases will evaporate faster, leaving pure liquid oxygen behind.

Two other methods of preparing oxygen for commercial use have been used on a limited basis: solid oxygen systems in which a solid chemical is converted to medically pure oxygen; and a unit that removes a portion of the nitrogen from room air by drawing it through a molecular sieve (see Chap. 18).

COMPRESSED AIR

At atmospheric temperature and pressure, air exists as a colorless, odorless, tasteless gas mixture. In air for human respiration ("respirable air"), the primary constituents are oxygen and nitrogen. Although other trace gases may be present and are considered useful in industry and for scientific purposes, it has never been determined that these trace gases serve any physiologic role in respiration.

Although nitrogen in the air does not serve any metabolic function, it aids in maintaining the inflation of the body cavities that are gas-filled, such as alveoli, sinus cavities, and the middle ear.

By increasing the forces acting upon it, air can be compressed. The percentage of oxygen in the air will remain the same; however, the partial pressure of the oxygen will increase. It is therefore critical to remember that even if the oxygen concentration is only 21% in a chamber filled with air under pressure, most materials that are combustible will ignite more readily and burn much more rapidly than they would if the air were at normal atmospheric pressure.

Since atmospheric air contains a large number of trace constituents, the Compressed Gas Association (CGA) has established a grading system for compressed air that limits the concentration of trace constituents for each specific grade. The oxygen concentration in all medically acceptable compressed air ranges from 19.5% to 23.5% oxygen, depending on the grade of air, with the balance being predominantly nitrogen. Grade J of the gas and grade B of the liquid are most commonly used for medical purposes.

Compressed air, when handled properly and with the same caution as any other compressed gas, has many important uses. In many instances it can be liquefied and purified. Aside from its medical applications, compressed air is used in aerospace technology, undersea exploration, navigation, and atomic energy projects. It is necessary for tunnel construction and is used by industry and firemen in self-contained breathing devices.

The most common method of producing compressed air for human respirators is by the compression of normal atmospheric air at the point of use, although it can be transported to that point or synthetically produced by combining already purified components. The process involves various types of compressors that take in ambient air and compress it to the desired working pressure. The choice of compressor depends on the volume of air required and the pressure at which the air is to be used. Usually, a rotary or centrifugal compressor is used when less than 150 psig is required. The coaxial screw-type compressor is adequate for pressures ranging from 150 to 300 psig. The piston or diaphragm-type compressor is suitable for a wide range of pressures. For most hospital use, the piston, rotary, or centrifugal compressor would generally be considered adequate. In hospital systems where the rate of consumption varies in the course of a day or week, an accumulator is recommended; it can be filled by the compressor and air withdrawn as needed.

Two processes are used in the manufacture of liquid air. In the *Linde process*, air under pressure enters a tube and is then allowed to reexpand to atmospheric pressure. According to the Joule–Thompson effect, as the air reexpands, it produces a cooling effect. By the continual influx and reexpansion of the compressed air, the chamber eventually reaches a temperature at which the air will liquefy. This liquid air is accumulated at the bottom of the container. In this process a pressure of 200 atm is necessary for liquefaction.

The second process for producing liquid air is the *Claude process*. In this process air is compressed and passes through an orifice into a cylinder head. The expanding gas in the cylinder head causes a piston to compress additional fresh air. In this process the cooling is obtained by the gas performing the external work of compressing a piston. Liquefaction is accomplished in a much shorter time and with a lower pressure (30 atm).

Several considerations are important in using compressors for human respiration. Proper lubrication and maintenance are essential to the efficient operation of the compressor. Compressors may be lubricated internally with water, or with water to which a small amount of soap or natural mineral oil has been added. The bearings and working parts of most compressors are lubricated, but the cylinder and compressor chamber are not. The use of plastic or other low-friction seals on the piston has eliminated the need for lubrication in these areas. In the diaphragm-type compressor, the chamber is separated from the lubricated portions of the compressor by a diaphragm. Therefore, the chamber is considered to be unlubricated.

The compressor must be properly maintained. A compressor that is allowed to overheat may produce undesirable odors or even carbon monoxide caused by decomposition of lubricants. The compressor intake should be located away from the contaminating exhaust of automobiles and the gasoline or diesel engine used to drive the compressor, and away from other localized odors and contaminants. Activated charcoal may be used at the outlet of the compressor to remove odors and oil vapor. Desiccants or moisture-removal devices, however, are necessary for the air to pass through before it reaches the charcoal, since the charcoal is most effective if kept dry. The type of filtering device used must be capable of functioning efficiently at the maximum anticipated degree of contamination that might exist in the incoming air.

If compressed air is to be used at temperatures below freezing, excess water vapor should be removed to reach a dewpoint below the minimum temperature anticipated in order to prevent the condensation of moisture from the air. As the compressed air passes through valves and regulators from a higher to a lower pressure, the temperature of the delivered air will be *lower*.

HELIUM

Helium is seven times lighter than air. Of all the elements, only hydrogen is lighter. Helium is noncombustible, nonexplosive, poorly soluble in liquid, and a good conductor of electricity, sound, and heat. As a gas, helium is odorless and tasteless and is generally considered inert as it relates to the body.

One of the major sources of helium is the natural gas fields around Amarillo, Texas, which contain about 2% helium. Other sources are found in Saskatchewan, Canada, and areas near the Black Sea. The helium recovered from these natural fields is obtained by liquefaction and purification of the natural gas. Although helium can also be recovered from the atmosphere by fractional distillation, the amount recovered in this manner is so small that it is commercially impractical.

One of the most important commercial uses of helium is as a cooling agent in nuclear reactors. Helium is used in cold-weather fluorescent lamps and in arc-welding as a gas shield. Since it is lighter than air, it is also used in some types of aircraft as a lifting gas. It provides protection in the production of metals such as titanium and zirconium and is useful for tracing leaks in refrigeration and other closed systems.

Because helium is a rare and limited natural resource, the cost of administering it for medical purposes is very high. The most common uses of helium in the medical setting are in the pulmonary function laboratory (e.g., in the helium dilution test for functional residual capacity [*see* Chap. 10] and the VisoV̇ test [*see* Chap. 11]). Laboratory mixtures that contain helium have found limited therapeutic usefulness in medicine (e.g., in ventilating patients with extremely high airway resistance and in reducing massive subcutaneous and mediastinal emphysema). The most economical means of administration is with a rebreathing system, using a carbon dioxide absorption device, to prevent carbon dioxide accumulation. Since helium is physiologically inert, it must be administered with oxygen. Mixtures that contain helium and oxygen are supplied in several different compositions, of which the most common mixture is helium and 20% oxygen.

When administering the mixture, special flowmeters are required because the mixture is less dense than oxygen alone. If these special flowmeters are not available and regular oxygen flowmeters are used, one must calculate the error in the flowmeter. The 80%/20% mixture flows through restricted orifices 1.8 times more readily than does 100% oxygen. To get the proper total flow of an 80/20 mixture, one must multiply the flow that is shown on the flowmeter by 1.8. To calculate a desired flow rate, one needs to divide the desired rate by 1.8 and adjust the flowmeter accordingly.

CARBON DIOXIDE

Carbon dioxide is a colorless, odorless gas about 1.53 times as heavy as air. It is abundant and constant in the atmosphere and is generated by the combustion of fuels, by respiration, by fermentation, and by the decay of animal and vegetable matter. The unrefined gas may be recovered from the gases found in some natural wells and springs. It is also a byproduct of the commercial production of ammonia.

Large-scale carbon dioxide production takes place primarily in lime kilns. The limestone is heated to a red glow in closed containers. Superheated steam is forced in at the bottom of the chambers, and as it passes through the heated limestone the steam carries with it the liberated carbon dioxide. The gas then passes out of the top of the chambers into coolers and compressors.

Carbon dioxide can be refined and purified to 99.9% or higher and is used medically in combination with oxygen. The gas itself is not toxic; without sufficient oxygen, however, it causes asphyxiation. The mixture of oxygen and carbon dioxide is sometimes called "carbogen."

The critical temperature of carbon dioxide is 83°F and it is easily liquefied under pressure. When the pressure is released, part of the liquid vaporizes rapidly, but the rest solidifies into what is commonly called "dry ice." One of the most important commercial uses of carbon dioxide is as an expandable refrigerant. It is also used extensively to carbonate soft drinks and as a food preservative. Carbon dioxide is also used in metal welding and, in liquid form, is commonly used in fire extinguishers.

TRANSPORTATION OF GASES

The Federal Department of Transportation was established by Congress in 1967 to coordinate the executive functions of all transportation agencies into a single governmental department. The rules for the transportation of compressed gases and the requirements imposed on both the carriers and shippers fall under this department. The transportation agencies of greatest importance in the compressed gas industry are

1. the Federal Aviation Agency, which regulates shipment by air;
2. the Coast Guard, for transportaton by water;
3. the Federal Railroad Administration, for shipment by railroad; and
4. the Federal Highway Administration, for highway shipment.

Further discussion of these governmental agencies will be found later in this chapter.

Whenever compressed gases are transported in cylinders and where caps are provided for valve protection, the caps should not be removed until the cylinder has reached its destination and is ready to be used. During the transport of cylinders, protection against excessively high or low temperatures should be provided.

STORAGE OF GASES

CYLINDERS

Nonflammable medical gases include oxygen, nitrous oxide, medical compressed air, carbon dioxide, helium, nitrogen, and various mixtures of these gases. Strict regulations for locating and maintaining bulk oxygen systems have been established by the National Fire Prevention Association (NFPA), subject to further control by local community fire and building codes.[3]

Storage rooms for cylinders should be dry, cool, well-ventilated, and fire-resistant. Subsurface locations should be avoided, and cylinders should never be stored in or near a hospital operating room. The temperature within the room must not exceed 125°F, and any source of heat within the room should be located well away from the cylinders. Full and empty cylinders should be stored separately. The storage layout should be carefully planned so that older stock can be easily removed first, preventing unnecessary handling of the cylinders.

There must be separate storage areas for cylinders containing oxidizing gases that support combustion, such as oxygen and nitrous oxide, and for flammable gases. Such a precaution is critical. In the event of fire, the contents of the cylinders evacuate when the safety releases valves open. In such cases the oxidizing gases would then accelerate the combustion of any flammable gases in the area. As an added precaution, cylinders of carbon dioxide are in themselves good fire extinguishers.

Storage rooms for oxygen and nitrous oxide must be vented to the outside if the amount of gas to be stored is in excess of 200 cubic feet. The storage areas for these gases and flammable gases must have at least a 1-hour fire resistance rating and may not be used for any purpose other than the storage of cylinders. Under no circumstances should flammable materials be stored in these areas.

The storage area should contain racks on fasteners to prevent the cylinders from falling over, which could result in damage to cylinders or to persons who may be working in the area. Electric wall fixtures, receptacles, or switches must be installed not less than 5 feet above the floor as a precaution against damage to them from the cylinders.

Cylinders may be stored outside when necessary but should be protected from rusting caused by weather or contact with the ground. They should never be stored in areas where there is constant dampness, and they should be protected from continuous direct rays of the sun and excessive accumulations of ice or snow. Cylinders must never be stored where oil, grease, or other readily combustible materials may come into contact with them. They should also be protected against corrosive chemicals or fumes. It is good practice to store the cylinders in a locked area to prevent tampering by unauthorized persons.

BULK GAS SYSTEMS

The NFPA has also established regulations governing bulk oxygen systems for industrial or institutional use. A bulk oxygen system comprises an assembly of oxygen storage containers, pressure regulators, safety devices, vaporizers, manifolds, and interconnecting piping. By definition, the storage capacity of the system must be more than 20,000 cubic feet of oxygen, including reserves on hand that are not connected to the system.

Oxygen containers in the bulk system may be stationary or moveable, and the oxygen may be either gas or liquid. The bulk system ends at the point where the oxygen first enters the supply line. It consists of the main equipment that actually supplies the system (primary supply), a secondary system that takes over when the primary supply is used up, and a reserve system that will function in an emergency when the primary–secondary operating supply fails.

The system must be located outdoors or in a building of noncombustible construction with adequate ventilation to the outside. If the system is located in a building, the building must be used for no purpose other than to house the system. The bulk system must be located above ground and in a place that is easily accessible for the mobile equipment used to supply it. Of special importance is that the system be located well away from exposure to power lines, flammable or combustible liquid, or gas lines (Fig. 15-4).

Four basic types of bulk systems pipe oxygen to a central supply area within a facility. In the manifold system, large cylinders are banked together and replaced when empty. Another system uses fixed cylinders that are refilled on location from a truck that contains liquid oxygen and converts the liquid to gas for pumping into the cylinders. In the third system, large cylinders are permanently attached to a trailer, and the entire trailer unit is replaced when the oxygen supply is used up. In all three of these methods, oxygen is supplied in gaseous form.

When large volumes of oxygen are used, the most practical and economical method for storage is the liquid bulk supply system. Containers are constructed on the principle of a large thermos bottle, consisting of inner and outer steel shells separated by a vacuum that effectively blocks the transfer of heat into the liquid. The containers are kept under pressure not exceeding 250 psig and must be kept below −297°F, both in transportation and storage, to prevent the liquid from reverting to gas. Vaporizing units, consisting of finned tubing, are used to convert the liquid oxygen into gas. The size of the vaporizing unit depends on the rate of withdrawal from the vessel. Normally water vapor from the air will condense and freeze on these units over a period of steady use.

The location of the liquid storage system should be carefully planned. Again, the NFPA, along with local, state, and federal agencies, has created regulations, including safe limits for the distances between the system and various points of exposure. At least 3 feet of a noncombustible surface should be extended in all directions from the storage tank. The area under the liquid delivery connections should be at least as wide as the mobile supply equipment and should extend at least 8 feet in both directions to prevent hazards from any leakage while the system is being filled. This surface must not be of asphalt paving because this type of paving may be combustible.

Under normal operating conditions, the liquid oxygen remains in the liquid state and is automatically transformed into gas as it passes through the vaporizing portion of the unit upon demand by the user.

DISTRIBUTION OF GASES

OXYGEN PIPING

Since any bulk system ends at the point where the oxygen first enters the supply lines, a distribution system is necessary within the facility. This piped distribution system consists of a central supply area where manifold, bulk, or compressors are located, control equipment, and where piping extends to points in the facility where the gas is to be used (Fig. 15-5). Seamless type K or L copper or brass pipe is used in the medical oxygen piping system. These pipelines must not be supported by other piping, as a safety precaution, in the event that the supporting piping may be hot or may develop maintenance problems with damage to the oxygen piping occurring during the repairs. Pipe hooks or straps of the proper strength are necessary. Fittings used in copper tubing must be wrought copper, brass, or bronze made especially for solder or brazed connections. Piping is usually connected by welding. Fittings for oxygen systems should be free of corrosion or rust, and the pipes should be free of lacquer, paint, varnish, or any coating.

The system should be cleaned before it is used to remove any materials that may have collected in the

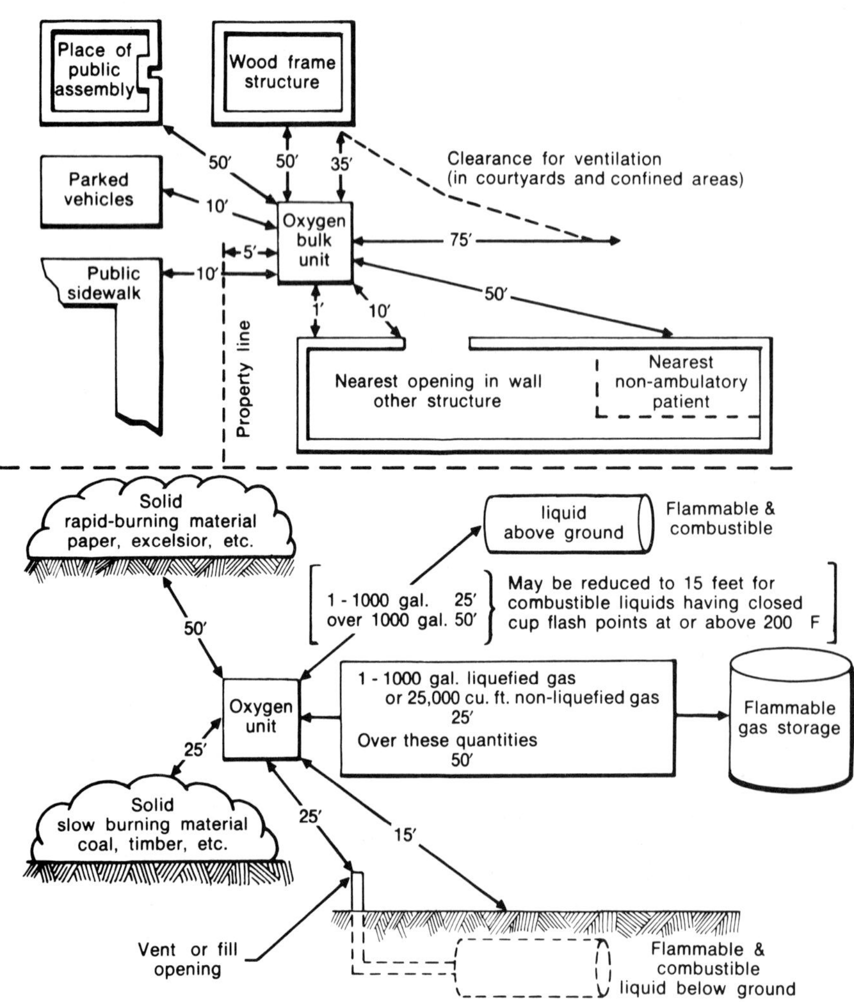

Fig. 15-4. Distance between bulk oxygen systems and various nearby structures (not to scale). (Reproduced with permission from *Bulk Oxygen Systems at Consumer Sites* [NFPA 50] © 1974, National Fire Protection Assn., Boston, MA 02210)

pipes. After cleaning, each section of the pipeline should be pressure-tested, using oil-free dry air or nitrogen at 1½ times the maximum working pressure (approximately 75 psi) of the pipeline system. This pressure is maintained for 24 hours. After the 24-hour test has been completed, the entire system should be pressurized with oxygen and all outlets opened, starting with the one nearest the source and progressing to the outlet farthest away from the source. The oxygen should flow from the outlets until the test gas has been completely purged from the system. Each outlet should be checked to see that 100% oxygen is present. Whenever any piping changes are made in the system, these pressure and priority checks must be repeated. Some states now require periodic oxygen outlet purity checks even though the system has not been modified in the interval.

CYLINDERS

Manufacture

The Department of Transportation (DOT) establishes regulations and specifications for the manufacture, marking, testing, and transportation of cylinders in the United States. This was formerly the responsibility of the Interstate Commerce Commission. DOT establishes what type of material is to be used in the construction of cylinders and the method of fabrication. High-pressure oxygen cylinders must be made of seamless steel, meeting certain chemical and physical requirements. Other cylinders may be formed of seamless, drawn, welded, or brazed tubing. In addition to these requirements, DOT also specifies the maximum wall stress permissible at test pressure and the service pressure at which the cylinder may be used.

Markings

All cylinders must carry certain easily recognized identifying marks that are stamped into the steel (Fig. 15-6). The marks must include the number of the specification by which the cylinder was manufactured, the authorized service pressure, a serial number, and the date of manufacture. There must also be symbols identifying the original owner of the cylinder, the manufacturer, and the independent agency that performed the tests required at the time of manufacture. Sometimes tare weights (*i.e.*, the weight of the cylinder full, making allowance for the weight of

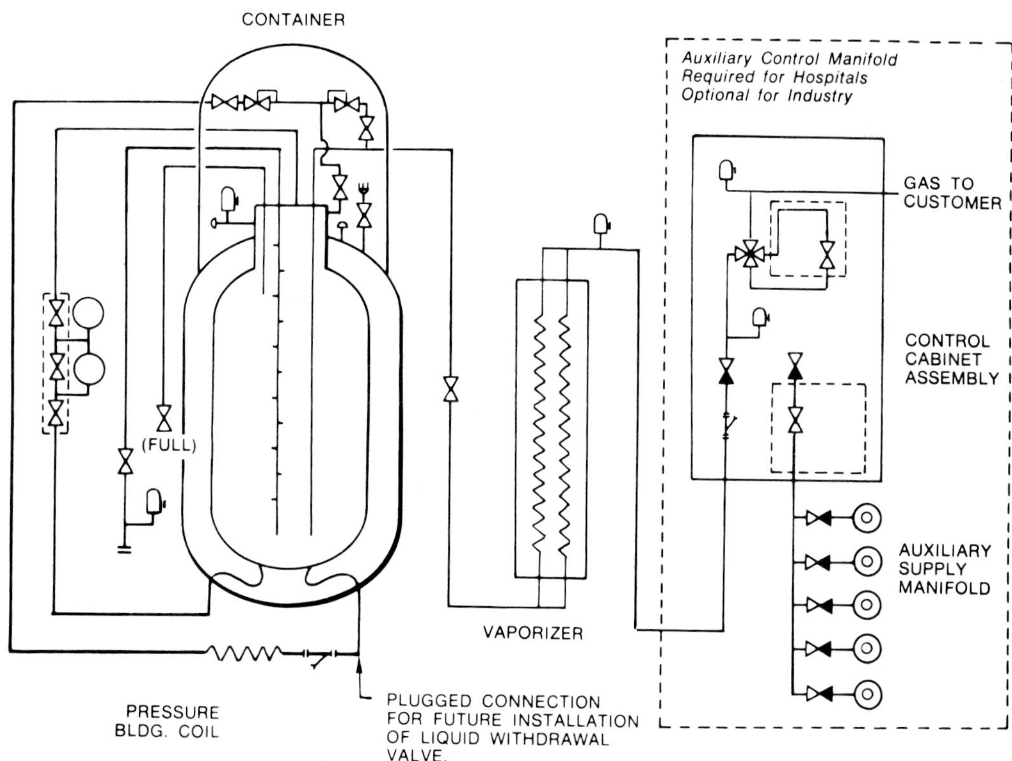

Fig. 15-5. Flow diagram of a customer station. (Compressed Gas Association)

the cylinder), water capacities, and the elastic expansion values of the cylinder are also included as if the cylinder is to be used to hold liquefied gas.

Most cylinders used in the United States are marked either DOT or ICC, to indicate that they conformed to the specifications in force at the time of the original test by the manufacturer. Some old cylinders, however, may be marked BE, indicating that they were made to specifications prepared by the Bureau of Explosives. In Canada, cylinders may be marked CRC (Canadian Rail Commission), BTC (Board of Transport Commission for Canada), or CTC (Canadian Transportation Commission) to indicate that they conform to Canadian specifications. Cylinders carrying any other markings are considered to be foreign and may be filled in the United States, but only for export, and the cylinder must have been hydrostatically tested within the past 5 years.

Following the letters ICC or DOT will be a combination of numbers and letters indicating the manufacture and testing specifications of that particular cylinder. These may be 3A, 3AA, 4B, 8AL, or any combination thereof. Each indicates a separate set of specifications for chemical composition, tensile strength, elongation of metals used, and method of fabrication. They also indicate the type of final acceptance test used, various inspections to be performed by an independent agency, and the cylinder service pressure limitation.

Cylinders marked 3A, 4B, and ICC8 are made of relatively low-strength steels and, as a result, have thicker sidewalls that make the cylinder heavier. Cylinders marked 3AA, 4BA, and DOT or ICC 8AL are made of lighter-strength steel and are lighter in weight, but cylinder cuts, gouges, or corrosion are more serious hazards. The thicker side-wall cylinder is made either of manganese or carbon, as compared to the alloy steel of the thinner-walled cylinder.

The serial number on a cylinder identifies it as part of a given lot produced for a specific owner and is the basis for a historical record of the life of the cylinder. It is part of the data recorded each time the

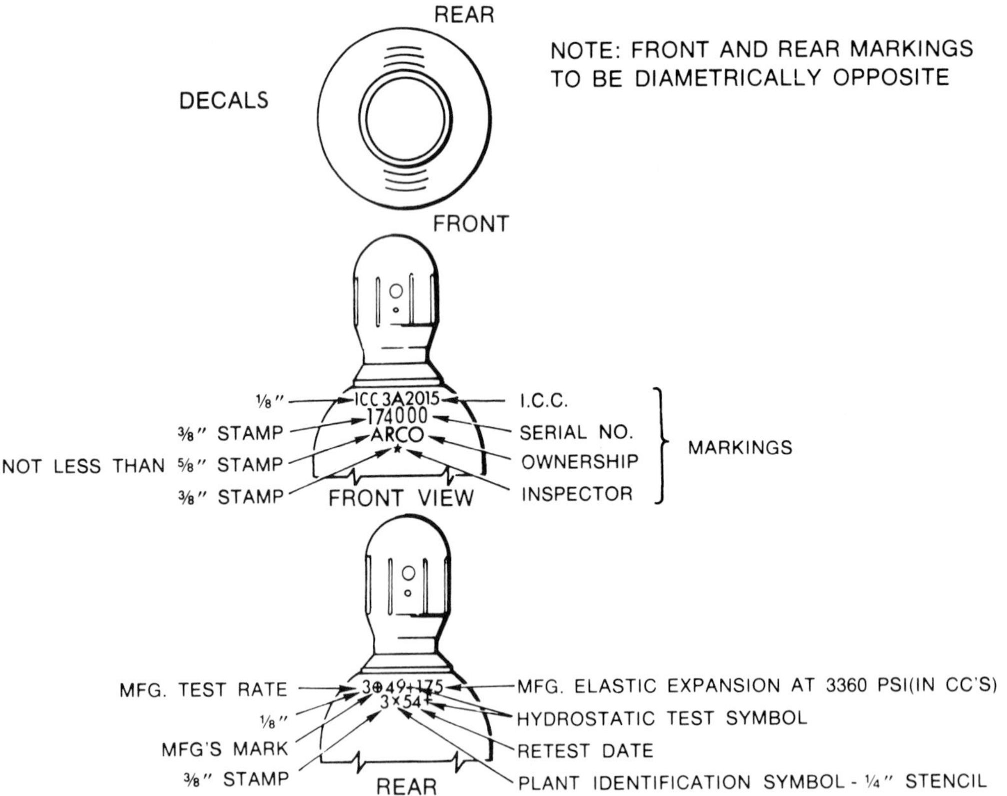

Fig. 15-6. Permanent markings required for Interstate Commerce Commission (ICC) or Board of Transportation Commission for Canada (BTC) specifications. (Compressed Gas Association)

cylinder is visually or hydrostatically retested, making possible a comparison of retest results and a subsequent evaluation of the rate of deterioration of the cylinder. The serial number is also important as a source of identification for any cylinder involved in an accident.

The ownership symbol or letters, used to identify the company or person for whom the cylinder was originally made, are registered with the BE. Regulations state that a container of compressed gas cannot be shipped unless it has been charged by, or with, the consent of the owner, and it is important that the filler or distributor know if he is legally permitted to fill and to ship the cylinder in filled condition. Since cylinders may change owners, the mark on the cylinder may not be positive proof of ownership, and any distributor should require proof of ownership before filling a cylinder.

Each cylinder is generally marked the same way. Markings on the front of the cylinder include the DOT or ICC mark, serial number, ownership, and inspector symbol. On the rear of the cylinder are found the manufacturer's mark, test date and elastic expansion values, the hydrostatic test symbol, the retest date, and the plant identification symbol. The original elastic expansion value of the cylinder, measured in cubic centimeters, is not required by DOT; however, it is valuable in providing a reference for subsequent retests.

Two other important marks are on every cylinder. Some cylinders are made from seamless tubing by forge-welding the bottom closure in a spinning process. The spinning process requires a high degree of manual skill to make sure the cylinders are tightly closed, and these cylinders must be tested for tightness using dry air. The letters SPIN are then marked into the shoulder of the cylinder.

Other manufacturers, as a final step in the process, drill and plug the bottom closure of the cylinders with pipe-threaded plugs. This type of closure may develop leaks from service impacts, and, since the plugs are not visible when the cylinder is in an upright position, the shoulder of these cylinders is marked PLUG so that the bottom closure will be checked at each filling.

Testing

Hydrostatic testing and retesting of cylinders are required by DOT. The most common method is the *water-jacket volumetric expansion test,* standard in the compressed gas industry for testing high-pressure gas cylinders (*i.e.*, those over 900 psig). This method is used to determine elastic expansion, which is directly related to the wall thickness of the cylinder. An increase in the elastic expansion will indicate a reduction in average wall thickness (Fig. 15-7).

In the water-jacket test the cylinder is suspended in a vessel of water. As pressure is applied to the interior of the cylinder, a volume of water is forced from the jacket. As the pressure is released from the interior of the cylinder, some of the originally displaced water returns to the jacket. The volume of water originally displaced represents the total expansion of the cylinder, and the final displaced volume represents the permanent expansion. Total expansion minus permanent expansion results in the elastic expansion value, giving a definite measure of the average wall thickness of the cylinder at a given pressure.

To determine whether the cylinder is still usable, the percentage of permanent expansion is then calculated by dividing 100 times the permanent expansion by the total expansion. If that percentage exceeds the allowable DOT specifications, the cylinder must be rejected. Some cylinders may originally have been tested for the specific purpose of being used for oxygen, and, at a later date, the retesting will no longer permit the cylinder to be filled to that capacity. Such a cylinder may be used for other gases for which the maximum pressure of a full cylinder is less.

There are several other acceptable but less commonly used cylinder tests. In *the direct expansion method,* expansion is determined by compressing a volume of water into the cylinder, but compensation for water compressibility and temperature are factors that must be taken into account. *The proof pressure method* may be used when DOT regulations do not require the determination of total and permanent volumetric expansion. *The pressure recession method* is practically obsolete.

The frequency and the type of periodic cylinder testing are regulated by DOT, depending on the specification to which the cylinder was manufactured and the gas for which it is to be used. Records showing the results of inspection must be maintained by the owner until the cylinder is due for retest or additional inspection. The cylinder is inspected externally for signs of damage or corrosion and internally for signs of corrosion (Fig. 15-8). When corrosion is severe, large quantities of loose scale will usually be in the bottom of the cylinder. The loose scale should be removed and the cylinder hydrostatically retested to be sure it is safe for continued service. Light rusting of the interior sidewalls where there is no localized cor-

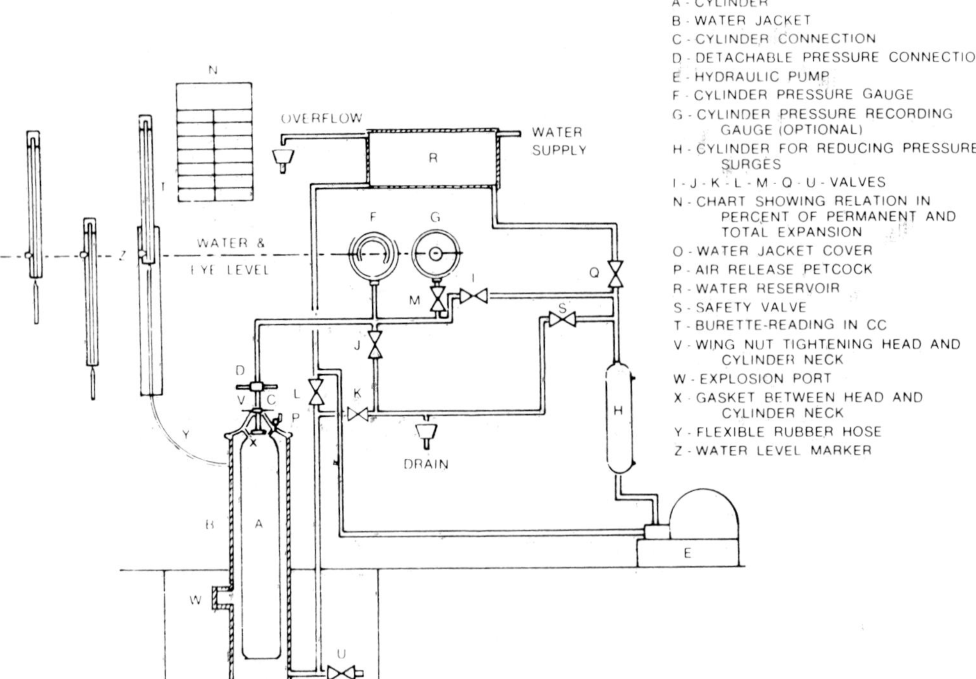

Fig. 15-7. Water jacket leveling burette method of testing cylinders consists essentially of enclosing the cylinder in a water jacket and measuring the volume of water forced from the jacket upon application of pressure to the interior of the cylinder, and the volume remaining displaced upon release of the pressure. These volumes represent the total and permanent expansions of the cylinder, respectively. To measure them accurately, a movable burette calibrated in cubic centimeters is positioned to maintain the water level at a uniform height when taking readings. (Modified from Compressed Gas Association: Handbook of Compressed Gases. New York, Reinhold, 1967)

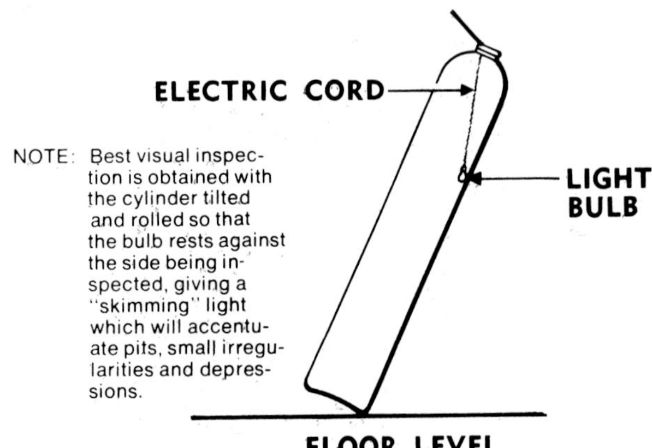

Fig. 15-8. Method for internal inspection of a cylinder with a drop light. (Compressed Gas Association)

rosion and very little scale in the bottom of the cylinder is not normally considered a cause for removal from service.

The hammer or *dead-ring test* should be performed on all cylinders every time they are refilled. Striking the cylinder lightly on the side should produce a clean, ringing tone that lasts 2 to 3 seconds. If the tone is flat or fades almost immediately, the cylinder may have suffered fire damage, may be severely corroded on the inside, or may contain a contaminant such as water or oil, in which case the cylinder should not be refilled until a complete inspection can be made.

Cylinders were originally made of low-yield tensile steel, and excessive corrosion could be detected with the hydrostatic test when the permanent expansion exceeded 10% of the total expansion. Later, around 1937, alloy steels were introduced in the manufacture of cylinders, and the specified 10% expansion limit was weakened. There could be a considerable amount of corrosion in the cylinder before the 10% permanent expansion test would show that the cylinder be rejected.

During World War II, a 10% increase in the filling pressure was authorized with no change in the test pressure of the safety device setting on the cylinders. Following this emergency measure, regulations were established authorizing the continued practice of 110% filling provided that the wall-stress limitations are based on the water-jacket hydrostatic test and that the unbacked frangible disc safety device is used. If the elastic expansion reading at minimum pressure does not exceed DOT specifications, the cylinder may then be examined internally and externally for objectionable defects and stamped with a plus sign following the test date to signify that the cylinder can be filled to 110% of the service pressure marking.

Cylinders made to the specifications of 3A and 3AA must be hydrostatically retested every 5 or 10 years at a pressure equal to five thirds of the service pressure. Originally, the test was used to prove that the stress at service pressure would not exceed five thirds of the yield strength of the steel. It was later found, however, that data used in this retest could also be used to determine loss of wall thickness due to wear and corrosion. The test, therefore, justified increasing the filling pressures of these cylinders to 110% of the service pressure, and DOT extended the 5-year retest period for 3A and 3AA cylinders to 10 years provided that the cylinders are used with only certain gases and are under specific inspection and

Table 15-1. Color Markings

INTENDED GAS	COLOR
Oxygen (O_2)	Green
Carbon dioxide (CO_2)	Gray
Nitrous oxide (N_2O)	Blue
Cyclopropane $(CH_2)_3$	Orange or chrome
Helium (He)	Brown
Ethylene (C_2H_4)	Red
Carbon dioxide and oxygen (CO_2/O_2)	Gray and green
Helium and oxygen (He/O_2)	Brown and green
Nitrogen (N_2)	Black
Air	Yellow
Mixtures of nitrogen and oxygen	Black and green

retest procedures. Such cylinders are stamped with a five-pointed star. Only cylinders under 35 years of age qualify for the retest permission, unless special permits have been obtained for older cylinders. The specifications of the various cylinders are listed in Figure 15-9; the color coding index is found in Table 15-1 (also see p. 354).

SAFETY

The terms "laws," "regulations," and "standards," used in dealing with medical gases, may, on the surface, appear synonymous. However, while the intent of the "law," "regulation," or "standard" may be aimed at accomplishing the same objective, their enforcement, initiation, and penalties may vary widely. It is therefore important to distinguish between these terms.

LAWS

A law requires the approval of some legislative body of the federal, state, or local government. This body of officials may be the Congress of the United States, a state assembly, or possibly a local city council. These laws may establish an agency within the government to enact the regulations or may state specifically what is to be governed and to what extent.

When an agency is appointed to promulgate the regulations, such action is usually referred to as "enabling" legislation. This means that the passage of a law establishes an agency that is enabled, or given the power, to write regulations.

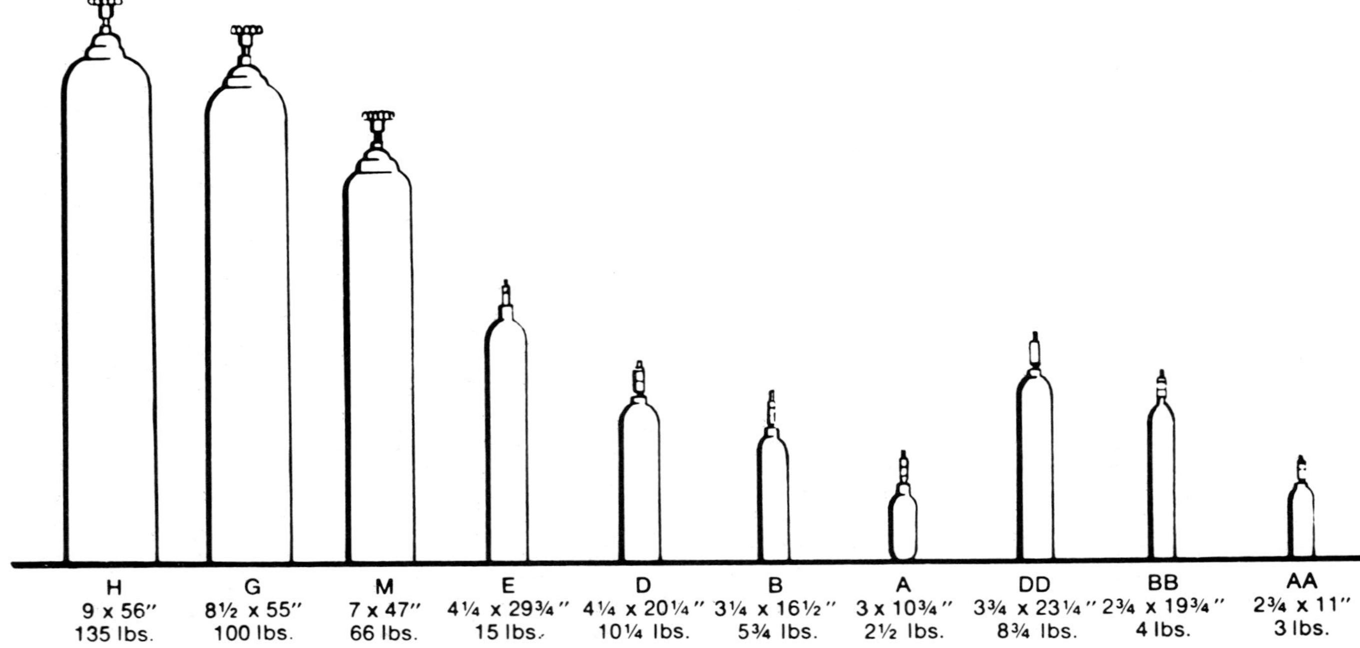
H
9 x 56″
135 lbs.
G
8½ x 55″
100 lbs.
M
7 x 47″
66 lbs.
E
4¼ x 29¾″
15 lbs.
D
4¼ x 20¼″
10¼ lbs.
B
3¼ x 16½″
5¾ lbs.
A
3 x 10¾″
2½ lbs.
DD
3¾ x 23¼″
8¾ lbs.
BB
2¾ x 19¾″
4 lbs.
AA
2¾ x 11″
3 lbs.

NET CONTENTS OF CYLINDERS FOR ALL GASES

	H	G	M	E	D	B	A	DD	BB	AA
CO_2		3200 gals. (12,112 liters) 48 lbs. 4 oz. 422 C.F.	2745 gals. (10,390 liters) 31 lbs. 4 oz. 367 C.F.	419 gals. (1,586 liters) 6 lbs. 9 oz. 56 C.F.	250 gals. (946 liters) 3 lbs. 14 oz. 33 C.F.	100 gals. (378 liters) 1 lb. 8½ oz. 13 C.F.	50 gals. (189 liters) 12½ oz. 7 C.F.			
CO_2/O_2		1400 gals. (5,299 liters) 18 lbs. 7 oz. 187 C.F.	800 gals. (3,028 liters) 11 lbs. 107 C.F.	165 gals. (625 liters) 2 lbs. 4 oz. 22 C.F.	95 gals. (359 liters) 1 lb. 5 oz. 13 C.F.	40 gals. (151 liters) 8 oz. 5 C.F.	20 gals. (75.7 liters) 4 oz. 2.5 C.F.			
$(CH_2)_3$								230 gals. (871 liters) 3 lbs. 5 oz. 31 C.F.	100 gals. (379 liters) 1 lb. 7 oz. 13 C.F.	40 gals. (151 liters) 9 oz. 5 C.F.
C_2H_4		2800 gals. (10,598 liters) 27 lbs. 5 oz. 374 C.F.	1600 gals. (6,056 liters) 15 lbs. 9 oz. 214 C.F.	330 gals. (1,249 liters) 3 lbs. 3 oz. 44 C.F.	200 gals. (757 liters) 2 lbs. 27 C.F.	100 gals. (378 liters) 15 oz. 13 C.F.	40 gals. (151 liters) 6 oz. 5 C.F.			
He		1100 gals. (4,164 liters) 1 lb. 8 oz. 147 C.F.	605 gals. (2,290 liters) 13 oz. 81 C.F.	131 gals. (496 liter) 3 oz. 17 C.F.	80 gals. (303 liters) 2 oz. 11 C.F.	28 gals. (106 liters) .6 oz. 3.7 C.F.	15 gals. (57 liters) .33 oz. 2 C.F.			
He/O_2		1126 gals. (4,262 liters) 15 lbs. 10 oz. 151 C.F.	620 gals. (2,347 liters) 8 lbs. 9 oz. 83 C.F.	134 gals. (507 liters) 1 lb. 14 oz. 18 C.F.	82 gals. (310 liters) 1 lb. 2 oz. 11 C.F.	29 gals. (110 liters) 7 oz. 4 C.F.	15 gals. (57 liters) 3 oz. 2 C.F.			
N_2O	4178 gals. (15,814 liters) 64 lbs. 557 C.F.	3655 gals. (13,834 liters) 56 lbs. 488 C.F.	2000 gals. (7,570 liters) 30 lbs. 10 oz. 267 C.F.	420 gals. (1,590 liters) 6 lbs. 7 oz. 56 C.F.	250 gals. (946 liters) 3 lbs. 13½ oz. 33 C.F.	100 gals. (378 liters) 1 lb. 8½ oz. 13 C.F.	50 gals. (189 liters) 12½ oz. 7 C.F.			
O_2	1825 gals. (6,907 liters) 20 lbs. 244 C.F.	1400 gals. (5,299 liters) 18 lbs. 7 oz. 187 C.F.	800 gals. (3,028 liters) 11 lbs. 107 C.F.	165 gals. (625 liters) 2 lbs. 4 oz. 22 C.F.	95 gals. (359 liters) 1 lb. 5 oz. 13 C.F.	40 gals. (151 liters) 8 oz. 5 C.F.	20 gals. (75.7 liters) 4 oz. 2.5 C.F.			

Fig. 15-9. Listing of dimensions and weights of empty cylinders, as well as the net contents of cylinders for all gases listed. The approximate dimensions and weights of empty cylinders include the valves. Note that tank sizes AA through E have flush-type valves and the larger tanks (M through H) have diameter-indexed valves. (Modified from Garrett DF, Donaldson WP: Physical Principles of Respiratory Therapy Equipment. Madison, Wisconsin, Ohio Medical Products, 1975)

REGULATIONS

Regulations do not require legislative approval for enforcement, but they have the same effect as law and are subject to penalties whenever there are violations. Federal, state, and local governments may delegate the writing and enforcement of laws to other persons or agencies, such as the state fire marshal or the local boards of standards and appeals.

STANDARDS

A standard is quite different from a law or regulation in that it may not have the effect of law. Standards may be prepared by technical agencies, by industry, or by any group of experienced persons that establishes a recognized acceptable procedure for a common purpose, such as safety.

Standards are intended to be followed voluntarily; however, they are frequently adopted by an enforcement agency, and then under their regulatory powers the standard may change from a strictly voluntary guideline to a law that is subject to the penalties under which the law was enacted. An example is Standard 50 of the NFPA, which provides for the instillation of bulk oxygen systems at consumer sites. This standard was developed by the Atmospheric Gases Committee of the CGA to promote uniform safety. It is important that the gas industry, as well as the users of such products, effectively control the standards by which they operate. If they do not accomplish this with effective and up-to-date standards, it becomes necessary for government agencies to enforce the standards. The important implication is that persons who are governed by these controls can and do have a large voice in the writing of standards, with a lesser voice in writing regulations, and often with little or no voice in the writing or changing of laws. It is therefore essential that we do an effective job in governing ourselves, or we may have unnecessary restrictions placed on our activities.

REGULATORY AGENCIES

The regulations of the federal agencies mentioned earlier not only establish the rules for the transportation of compressed gases, but also govern the packaging, marking, labeling, and shipping-paper preparation for the shipment of compressed gases and certain cryogenic liquids. There are severe penalties for failure to comply with these regulations, and they are enforced by field inspectors from the DOT and the BE.

One important distinction here is that the BE is not a government agency but rather an agency of the Association of American Railroads. Their inspectors do not have the police powers of the government inspectors and are not making inspections on behalf of the federal government.

Many states, such as Oregon, Washington, and California, have adopted the federal regulations to govern the shipment of compressed gases within the state. These states administer the regulations within the state through the state highway patrol, the Public Service Commission, the Public Utilities Commission, or the state fire marshal, depending on the state involved.

In addition to the above-mentioned agencies that govern the transportation of compressed gases are the regulations covered in the *Postal Manual* of the United States Postal Service. These regulations cover domestic and international mail shipment and generally place the responsibility for the shipment on the mailer.

The shipment of compressed gases must conform to the requirements of the Department of Transportation. These regulations cover such things as the qualification of drivers, the driving of motor vehicles, the parts and accessories needed for safe operation, the hours of service of the drivers, and the inspection, maintenance, and transportation of hazardous materials.

The Food and Drug Administration (FDA) of the Department of Health and Human Services (HHS) has for some time regulated the commodities used in the food, drug, and cosmetic industries. In 1962, however, certain changes were made, and for the first time a drug was defined as being anything listed in the *U.S. Pharmacopoeia* or the *National Formulary*. This list, at present, includes oxygen, nitrous oxide, cyclopropane, carbon dioxide, helium, ethylene, and mixtures of these gases, and it is anticipated that air for human respiration and nitrogen will eventually be added. These 1962 regulations also require that all producers or repackagers of drugs register with the FDA with heavy penalties for failure to comply. The significance of these regulations is that anyone who is filling, refilling, or "transfilling" cylinders (*i.e.*, filling one cylinder from another) must comply with these regulations. The FDA has field inspectors that evaluate establishments periodically for compliance with these regulations.

In 1966, the FDA also issued regulations for labeling certain hazardous substances that may cause substantial personal injury or illness to anyone handling them. These regulations appear under the Federal Hazardous Substances Labeling Act.

In addition to federal and state laws and regulations, many countries and municipalities have zoning laws, fire prevention codes, pressure-vessel regulations, hazardous-materials storage rules, and the like. In addition to these county and municipal safety laws and regulations, bridge, tunnel, and turnpike regulations govern the transportation of compressed gases over these facilities. These regulations are usually enforced by the state under the turnpike authority or the bridge authority.

The Occupational Safety and Health Act of 1970 (OSHA), sometimes referred to as the Williams–Steiger Act, was developed by the Occupational Safety and Health Administration of the Department of Labor in response to governmental recognition of the need for further reducing the incidence of occupational injury. The rate of occupationally related disabling injuries in the United States has been on an increase since about 1964. Under the provisions of this law it is the duty of every employer to furnish each of his employees with a place of employment free from recognized hazards causing, or likely to cause, serious physical harm or death to his employee. The basic concept in the Williams-Steiger Act is that the individual states will assume the responsibility for occupational safety and health standards. These standards, however, must be approved through the Department of Labor and are subject to modifications and monitoring by the federal OSHA.

Some of the OSHA standards were established before this act. Existing standards and regulations from the NFPA, National Electric Code, American National Standards Institute (ANSI), and others have been adopted by OSHA. These standards are enforced through a program of inspections. Compliance officers, trained by OSHA, have greater authority than those of almost any other enforcement officer. These compliance officers make inspections according to a priority schedule. Fatalities are given first priority, followed by serious injuries, employee complaints, high-risk target industries, and routine inspections. OSHA seeks to provide freedom from occupationally related injuries for all workers. Inspections and citations are a necessary part of the program; however, safety promotion through employee training and awareness, improvement, and management is stressed.

WARNING AND ALARM SYSTEMS

The NFPA recommends that audible and visual signals and pressure gauges be installed in the office or working area of the person responsible for maintaining any bulk oxygen system, and that a second alarm be located in an area where the system can be continuously monitored. This second system may be located at the telephone switchboard, security office, or other location where responsible people can monitor the system 24 hours a day. The system should be provided with an audible and visual alarm that will indicate that the oxygen supply has changed over to the reservoir system. A separate alarm system should be located in areas of vital life support, such as the recovery room and the coronary or intensive care units, that would indicate the amount of pressure located in the lines. These alarm systems again should be both visual and audible, and preferably located at the nurses' stations or other locations near these areas.

FIRE SAFETY

According to the NFPA, a fire requires the presence of a combustible or flammable material, an atmosphere that contains oxygen or other oxidizing agents, and a source of ignition in order for it to occur. Any of the mixtures of breathing gases used in respiratory therapy will support combustion. Materials that are combustible and flammable in air will ignite more easily and will burn more vigorously in an oxygen-enriched atmosphere, and materials that are not normally considered to be combustible in air may be considered combustible in an oxygen-enriched atmosphere.

Many combustible materials may be found near a patient receiving respiratory therapy, including oils, skin lotions, facial tissues, clothing, bed linen, oxygen tent canopies, rubber and plastic articles, suction and oxygen tubing, cyclopropane, ether, alcohols, and acetone. Another material that is highly flammable, even in air, is cellulose nitrate (nitrocellulose) base plastic. This may be found in such articles as eyeglass frames, mechanical pens and pencils, combs, and toothbrushes. Toys are occasionally made of this plastic.

Another hazard exists when high-pressure oxygen equipment becomes contaminated with oil, grease, or other combustible materials. These contaminants will ignite readily, burn much more rapidly in the presence of high oxygen concentrations, and make it easier to ignite less combustible materials with which they may come in contact.

In an oxygen-enriched atmosphere, sources that a person may not ordinarily consider hazardous may become significant. These include such things as open flames, smoking, electric heaters, the discharge of a cardiac defibrillator, arcing and excessive temperatures in electrical equipment, and defective electrical equipment. Under normal conditions the energy content of a static discharge will not be a source of ignition for a fire as long as the static discharge does not occur in the presence of items that are easily ignited, such as ether, cyclopropane, alcohols, acetone, oils, and grease.

Another potential fire safety hazard is from adiabatic compression. The rapid filling of an oxygen line from one pressure level to another will result in increased temperature of the oxygen gas within the line. To prevent this potential hazard, the lines should be pressurized slowly to minimize the temperature rise.

Compressed gas cylinders are heavy and bulky and are a potential hazard if not handled properly. Cylinders that are supplied with a cap should have it kept in place until the cylinder is ready to be used. Carriers specifically designed for use by cylinders are the only ones that should be used for moving the cylinder about, and the cylinder should be secured to a nonmovable object at all times when not being transported.

The improper maintenance, handling, or assembly of oxygen equipment may be another cause for personal injury, property damage, or fire. Electrical equipment must be in proper working order with adequate grounding.

Every effort should be made to eliminate any source of ignition during the administration of oxygen. Smoking materials should be removed from patients receiving therapy and their visitors, and the patient should be advised of potential fire hazards. Precautionary signs that are readable from a distance of 5 feet should be placed in conspicuous places at the site of administration, as well as in aisles or walkways leading to such an area. They are to be 8 inches by 11 inches and must also be attached to the doorway of the room where oxygen administration is taking place.

COLOR-MARKING AND PRECAUTIONARY LABELING

Compressed gases intended for medical use that are supplied in cylinders should be clearly identifiable for the type of gas that the cylinder contains. Since there is no existing U.S. standard for color marking of gas cylinders, the compressed gas industry has, for about 30 years, adhered to the *Simplified Practice Recommendation for Color Marking for Anesthetic Gas Cylinders* of the U.S. Department of Commerce.

Standard Z48.1 of the American National Standards Institute states that the only way to determine the content of any compressed gas cylinder is by means of the chemical name or other commonly accepted name that is marked legibly on the exterior of the cylinder. The Standard states further that the marking should be done by means of stenciling, stamping, or labeling and should not be readily removable. Certain precautionary information relative to the handling, storage, and use of the material should also be on the label. As stated previously, the FDA requires that specific warning statements be included in the labeling of any containers of gases intended for medical use. A secondary way of guarding against use of the wrong gas is by means of the standardized valve outlet connections that will be discussed in the next section. As a third means of guarding against inadvertently administering the wrong gas, the compressed gas industry uses color to designate certain cylinders for use with specific gases intended for medical use. Because of variations in color tones, chemical changes in paint pigments, various lighting effects, and differences in color perception by personnel, the color marking of the cylinders is not considered a reliable means for identifying the content of the cylinder (*see* Table 15-1 for usual color markings).

STANDARDIZED VALVE OUTLET CONNECTIONS

As mentioned in the preceding section, a secondary way of guarding against the inadvertent use of the wrong gas is by means of the standardized valve outlet connections. After World War I, the first efforts were made to standardize the valve threads on cylinders because of the difficulties that arose, both in industry and the military, owing to the multiplicity of connections then in use. Marginal progress was made in this area through the Gas Cylinder Valve Thread Committee of the Compressed Gas Manufacturers' Association, Inc. During the interwar years, several compressed gas manufacturers achieved virtual standardization; much of the progress in this area was due to the Federal Specifications Board. Although many manufacturers achieved standardization within their companies, these regulations were not fully coordinated with other related standards.

In October 1945, the standards association representing Great Britain, Canada, and the United States met in Ottawa to consider standardization of screw threads. In January 1946, an agreement was reached that resulted in final approval of a considerable num-

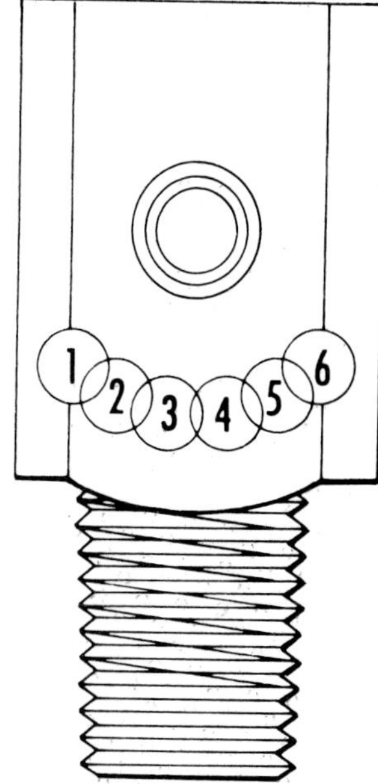

Fig. 15-10. The pin index safety system. The drawing shows details of the hole positions in a flush-type valve, in accordance with standards set by the Compressed Gas Association. The yoke with its matching pins is not shown. (Modified from Garrett DF, Donaldson WP: Physical Principles of Respiratory Therapy Equipment. Madison, Wisconsin, Ohio Medical Products, 1975)

Table 15-2. Pin Index System

INTENDED GAS	PIN COMBINATION
Oxygen	2 and 5
Carbon dioxide/oxygen (CO_2 7% or under)	2 and 6
Helium/oxygen (He 80% and under)	2 and 4
Ethylene	1 and 3
Nitrous oxide	3 and 5
Cyclopropane	3 and 6
Helium/oxygen (He over 80%)	4 and 6
Carbon dioxide/oxygen (CO_2 over 7%)	1 and 6
Air for human respiration	1 and 5

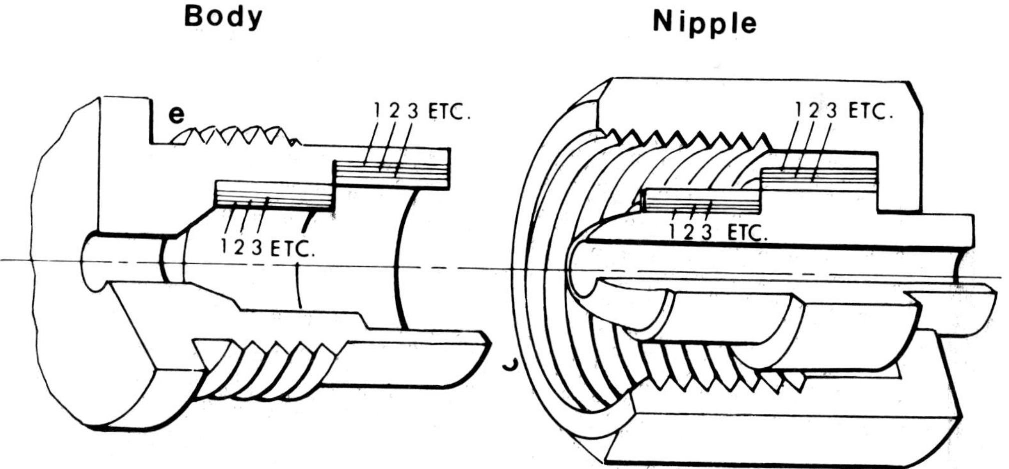

Fig. 15-11. The diameter index safety system standard low-pressure connection for medical gases, compressed air, and suction. The small bore in the body mates with the small diameter of the nipple, and the large bore in the body mates with the large diameter of the nipple. (Compressed Gas Association)

ber of additional gas cylinder valve threads; these data were included in the National Bureau of Standards' Handbook H-28. In January 1949, the Compressed Gas Manufacturers' Association, Inc., changed its name, and its Valve Thread Standardization Committee became known as the Valve Standards Committee of the Compressed Gas Association, Inc. Between 1946 and 1949 much progress was made in the area of standardization for valve threads, and in 1949 uniform standards were accepted by the American Standards Association and the Canadian Standards Association. The American Standard Compressed Gas Cylinder Valve Outlet and Inlet Connections (ANSI) are the OSHA standard for cylinder valves.

The standard is for large cylinders (sizes M through G), and the threaded outlets are separated into four basic divisions; internal, external, right-hand, and left-hand. Within each of the four divisions are further variations made by changing the diameter (*see* below) as well as the pitch of the threads. As far as possible, the different connections have been assigned to the different gases to prevent the interchange of connections that may result in a catastrophe. This standard is in the process of being revised, and it is hoped that with the new revisions the new version will be more inclusive.

Cylinder sizes E and smaller have what is known as *a pin index safety system*. As early as the spring of 1940, various medical societies, as well as the manufacturers of medical gases, determined that a system should be developed that would prevent the possibility of interchanging the medical gas cylinders that are equipped with flush-type valves. Various methods were studied, but the present pin index system has been adopted as an international standard. The system is designed to prevent the improper attachment of any regulator to a cylinder for which it was not intended. This is accomplished by the placement of two pins on the regulator yoke that are so arranged that only the correct gas cylinder valve will fit onto them. The specific gas is assigned a combination of pins that coincide with the yoke attachment on the regulator (*see* Fig. 15-10 and Table 15-2).

A system was developed by the CGA to provide a standard for noninterchangeable connections with individual gas lines of medical gas-administering equipment that operate at pressures of 200 psig or less. This system is known as the *diameter index safety system* (DISS) and is used on such low-pressure outlets as regulators and connectors for anesthesia, resuscitation, and respiratory therapy apparatus. This noninterchangeability of gas connections is achieved by a series of increasing and decreasing diameters in the connector, as well as by variations in thread size.

Each of the connections of the DISS comprises three parts: body, nipple, and nut. To achieve the noninterchangeability between the different connections, the two diameters on each part vary in opposite directions so that as one diameter increases, the other will decrease. Thus only the properly mated and intended parts will fit together (Fig. 15-11).

The safe use of medical gases requires an understanding of the nature of the gases on the part of those handling them. Accidents happen through carelessness and, perhaps, because those involved in the accident do not understand the potential dangers when regulations are not followed. Every effort should be made to ensure the safety of patients, employees, and visitors in medical institutions.

REFERENCES

1. Adriani J: The Chemistry and Physics of Anesthesia, 2nd ed. Springfield, Illinois, Charles C Thomas, 1962
2. Compressed Gas Association: Handbook of Compressed Gases. New York, Reinhold, 1966
3. National Fire Protection Association: Respiratory Therapy. NFPA no. 56B, Boston, 1973

BIBLIOGRAPHY

Adriani J: The Chemistry and Physics of Anesthesia, 2nd ed. Springfield, Illinois, Charles C Thomas, 1962

Brobner RH: Roi's Principles of Chemistry, 10th ed. St. Louis, CV Mosby, 1967

Brooks SM: Integrated Basic Science, 3rd ed. St. Louis, CV Mosby, 1970

Compressed Gas Association: Handbook of Compressed Gases. New York, Reinhold, 1966

Ent WL, Kitson FK: Filling procedures for compressed gases, including liquefied gases. Paper presented at the Distributor Safety Seminar. New York, Compressed Gas Association, 1973

Garrett DF, et al: Physical Principles of Respiratory Therapy Equipment. Madison, Wisconsin, Ohio Medical Products, 1975

Gilbert DL: Cosmic and geophysical aspects of the respiratory gases. In Fenn WO, Rahn H (eds): Handbook of Physiology, sec 3: Respiration, vol 1. Washington DC. American Physiological Society, 1964

Gilbert DL: Introduction: oxygen and life. Anesthesiology 37:100–111, 1972

Harris NC et al: Introductory Applied Physics, 2nd ed. New York. McGraw–Hill, 1963

Macintosh R et al: Physics for the Anesthetist, 3rd ed. Philadelphia, FA Davis, 1963

National Fire Protection Association: Manual for the Home Use of Respiratory Therapy NFPA no. 56HM, Boston, 1973

National Fire Protection Association: Bulk Oxygen Systems, NFPA no. 50, Boston, 1974

National Fire Protection Association: Fire Hazards in Oxygen-Enriched Atmospheres. NFPA no. 53M, Boston, 1974

National Fire Protection Association: Respiratory Therapy. NFPA no. 56B, Boston, 1973

National Fire Protection Association: Standards for the Use of Inhalation Anesthetics NFPA no. 56A, Boston, 1973

Pharmacopoeia of the United States of America, 18th ed. Easton, Pennsylvania, Mack Publishing Co, 1975

Pinney GG: OSHA, state and local employee safety standards. Paper presented at the Distributor Safety Seminar. New York, Compressed Gas Association, 1973

Senesky JS: Gas mixtures. Paper presented at the Distributor Safety Seminar. New York. Compressed Gas Association, 1973

Shaner RL: Production of Industrial Gases from the Air. Union Carbide Corporation, Linde Division, New York, 1969

Smith AL: Principles of Microbiology, 7th ed. St. Louis, CV Mosby, 1973

Spearman CB, Sheldon RL: Egan's Fundamentals of Respiratory Therapy. St. Louis, CV Mosby, 1982

Swope RL et al: Compressed gas containers. Paper presented at the Distributor Safety Seminar. New York, Compressed Gas Association, 1973

Tribolet R, Willoughby TE: Cryogenic-liquid containers. Paper presented at the Distributor Safety Seminar. New York, Compressed Gas Association, 1973

Van Volen L: The history and stability of atmospheric oxygen. Science 171:439–443, 1971

Willoughby TE: Safety laws, regulations, and standards. Paper presented at the Distributor Safety Seminar. New York, Compressed Gas Association, 1973

Young JA, Crocker D: Principles and Practice of Inhalation Therapy. Chicago, Year Book Medical Publishers, 1970

16

Physical and Physiological Principles of Aerosol Deposition and Mucociliary Clearance

David L. Swift • Mitchell Litt

The fluid–gas mixture that we take into our respiratory tract an average of 15 times a minute each day contains a great many substances. In addition to oxygen and other gases whose transport is the principal *raison d'être* of respiration, the inspired air contains other gaseous, liquid, and solid components that significantly affect the function of the respiratory system. Most important among these other substances is water, both in the gaseous vapor form and as liquid droplets that can contain dissolved or suspended contaminants. However, the air we breathe also contains other particulate matter, both liquid and solid, with whose behavior in the respiratory tract we shall be concerned here.

The behavior of water in the respiratory tract is complex because it can exist as a gas or liquid and because the respiratory mucosa itself is a source of water. The humidity, or *water vapor content*, of the air in the lower respiratory tract is such that the air is essentially fully (100%) saturated (*i.e.*, the air contains as much water vapor as is possible at the body temperature of 37°C). However, since the air we breathe is not at 37°C and is rarely saturated with water, clearly the respiratory system must, as one of its functions, serve to humidify as well as heat the inspired air to the desired physiological conditions. The increase in humidity and temperature occurs normally as the air flows through the upper part of the respiratory system. Although the respiratory system has considerable capacity for humidification, long-term breathing of dry air can have significant deleterious effects on the condition of the upper tract. Conversely, breathing of highly humidified gas may, under certain conditions, be beneficial in reversing water loss and can form the basis of rational humidification therapy. It is therefore important to understand and to quantify the behavior of water vapor in air and the interaction of this wet air with the respiratory system, both for an understanding of normal physiologic functioning and for possible applications to therapy.

The behavior of airborne particulate matter in the respiratory system is admittedly complex. The state of matter in which small particles (larger than molecular size but less than about 50 μm) are suspended in a fluid is called a *colloid*. A *sol* is a colloid in which the particles are free to move independently of each other but may interact with each other and the fluid through various forces. When the suspending fluid is a gas, the resulting substance is known as an *aerosol*. The important natural and man-made aerosols that interact in the human respiratory system contain particles ranging from about 0.05 μm to 50 μm in diameter. Typical natural aerosols include bacteria and other microorganisms, fog, plant spores and pollen, salt nuclei evaporated from the sea, and various natural smokes. Man-made aerosols include chemical mists and dusts generated from industrial operations, combustion smokes, and, of course, tobacco smoke. In addition, and of importance to the reader of *Respiratory Care*, are the man-made liquid aerosols intended for humidification and deposits of water and drugs in the respiratory tract.

Because natural aerosols are so widespread, the mammalian respiratory system has evolved a complex system for dealing with them, the *mucociliary clearance system*. This system constitutes a natural moving filter for the trapping and removal of aerosol particles and is generally quite efficient in dealing with natural aerosols. Respiratory disease, and often the increasing burden of man-made aerosols, can lead to overwhelming of this natural clearance mechanism.

Our aim herein is to discuss the interactions of humid air and aerosols with the respiratory system, in particular with regard to clearance, both in normal functioning and in disease. In this regard we must first present a description of aerosol properties, how they are generated and measured, and factors that will affect the stability of aerosols. The interaction of aerosols and of humidified air with the respiratory tract and mechanisms that determine where aerosols deposit in the respiratory system will then be discussed, followed by a description of the clearance mechanisms of the lung and of factors that may change normal functioning. Last, we shall present a brief introduction and critique of the use of aerosols in respiratory care, a subject discussed in greater detail in Chapter 17.

PROPERTIES OF AEROSOLS

The behavior of an aerosol depends on its physical properties. Some of the properties are associated with the particles themselves, whereas others are "system" or collective properties of the particle-gas dispersion.

PARTICLE PROPERTIES

Each particle in an aerosol has a chemical composition and an associated physical state related to the bulk properties of its component substances; the particle may be liquid, solid, or a mixture of states or compounds.

The primary physical properties of a particle are its "size" and shape. Liquid particles, which are under most conditions spherical because of surface tension, have only one important size parameter, *sphere radius* or diameter. Other particles may have a shape of such nature that it is difficult to describe the particle "size" with a single value. Although many solid particles are spherical or nearly so, others range in shape from plates to long fibers to dendritic (treelike) aggregates of smaller elements. Several methods have been used by investigators to describe the various shapes, but the characterization in terms of aerodynamic behavior, to be described below, is the most useful for this discussion.

Particle Density

Particle density (particle mass divided by particle volume) is another important property. For solid particles this must be determined experimentally; in many cases, even for particles of known composition, the particle density is *not* equal to the bulk "handbook" density of the substance because the handbook density is for a dense (often crystalline) solid, whereas the particle, depending on its mode of formation, may be quite porous or floclike. For liquids the handbook value is generally appropriate if the particles are of a single chemical substance or a known mixture.

Usually the particles in an aerosol carry electric charges; the number of unbalanced charges of either sign carried by a particle may significantly influence its behavior. Even if the net charge of an aerosol system is zero, which is not always the case, there can be a separation between individual particles, some having an excess of one or the other sign.

Vapor Pressure and Surface Tension

The vapor pressure and surface tension of liquid particles are important properties, particularly when these influence change of state. The *Kelvin equation* expresses the relation between particle vapor pressure and bulk vapor pressure as a function of particle diameter, surface tension, liquid density, and molecular weight of the particulate compounds:

$$ln \frac{P}{P_\infty} = \frac{2\gamma M}{RT\rho r} \quad (1)$$

P = vapor pressure of particle (atm)
P_∞ = vapor pressure of bulk substance at T (atm)
γ = surface tension (dynes/cm)
M = molecular weight (g/g mole)
R = gas constant (8.3×10^7 erg/g mole [°K])
T = absolute temperature (°K)
ρ = liquid density (g/cm^3)
r = particle radius (sm)

Table 16-1. Excess Vapor Pressure of Submicron-Sized Pure-Water Drops*

r μm	P/P_∞
1	1.001
10^{-1}	1.01
10^{-2}	1.11
10^{-3}	2.84

*Although the excess vapor pressure for micron-sized drops (of interest in aerosol therapy) is small, it is extremely important in determining stable aerosol particle size (*see* Aerosol Stability, p. 365).

In Table 16-1, we list P/P_∞ values for pure water at particle radii ranging from 1 to 10^{-3} μm.

COLLECTIVE PROPERTIES

The collective properties of an aerosol are of two kinds: those that describe a quantitative measure of particles per aerosol volume, and those that describe an average property taken over many particles having a distribution of values. The simplest collective property is the *number concentration* of particles, N, expressed as particles/cm³ of aerosol. Since the fractional volume of particles in most aerosols is much less than 1%, the number concentration can be expressed as particles/cm³ gas; it is customary to specify a standard condition for the gas, such as 1 atm, 70°F, or to specifically state the conditions.

If all the particles in an aerosol are of a single size (monodisperse), a particle property, such as mass, becomes a collective property in the sense that the aerosol particle mass/gas volume is simply the (mass/particle) × (number of particles/gas volume). The more common situation is that the particle sizes are distributed, and the collective properties are related to the distribution of sizes.

Let us assume that the aerosol being discussed is composed of liquid spheres of density ρ, so that the particle mass, volume, and surface area are simply related to the sphere radius, r. A size distribution function n(r) is defined such that for an infinitesimal size range $r \rightarrow r + dr$, the number of particles/cm³ gas is n(r)dr. In terms of the total particle concentration N,

$$N = \int_0^\infty n(r)dr. \tag{2}$$

From an experimental viewpoint, a more convenient function is the related function N(r) where

$$N(r) = \int_0^r n(r)dr. \tag{3}$$

N(r) gives the total number of particles/cm³ up to size r. One can conceive of a continuous function N(r) being generated from finite numbers of particles in finite size classes, then differentiated to obtain n(r):

$$n(r) = \frac{dN(r)}{dr}. \tag{4}$$

Once we have obtained n(r) we can determine the mean, or average, of several parameters in a straightforward manner. The *mean radius* $\bar{r}$ is defined as

$$\bar{r} = \frac{\int_0^\infty rn(r)dr}{N}. \tag{5}$$

The *mean surface area* for the distribution of spheres is

$$\overline{A} = \frac{\int_0^\infty 4\pi r^2 n(r)dr}{N}. \tag{6}$$

The *mean volume*, $\overline{V}$, and *mass*, $\overline{M}$, are

$$\overline{V} = \frac{\int_0^\infty \frac{4}{3}\pi r^3 n(r)dr}{N}; \tag{7}$$

$$\overline{M} = \frac{\int_0^\infty \frac{4}{3}\pi r^3 \rho n(r)dr}{N}. \tag{8}$$

For $\overline{A}$, $\overline{V}$, and $\overline{M}$, average particle radii can be obtained that are weighted toward area, volume, and mass:

$$\bar{r}_A = \frac{\overline{A}^{1/2}}{4\pi}; \tag{9}$$

$$\bar{r}_V = \frac{3\overline{V}^{1/3}}{4\pi}; \tag{10}$$

$$\bar{r}_M = \frac{3\overline{M}^{1/3}}{4\pi}. \tag{11}$$

Another useful parameter is the *median radius* of a distribution; this is often used in the literature to characterize an aerosol system. For the number distribution, the *number median radius*, r_{NMR}, divides the entire distribution into two equal populations:

$$\int_0^{r_{NMR}} n(r)dr = \int_{r_{NMR}}^{\infty} n(r)dr. \quad (12)$$

The other median particle size of interest is that for the mass distribution with respect to particle radius:

$$M(r) = \int_0^r \tfrac{4}{3}\pi r^3 \rho n(r)dr. \quad (13)$$

The *mass median radius*, r_{MMR}, is then the particle size for which

$$\int_0^{r_{MMR}} r^3\rho n(r)dr = \int_{r_{MMR}}^{\infty} r^3\rho n(r)dr, \quad (14)$$

which is to say that half of the mass is found in particle sizes larger than the MMR and half in sizes smaller. Twice the MMR is the mass median particle *diameter*, denoted "MMD."

Many aerosol systems have an experimentally determined distribution that can be well approximated by the log-normal distribution equation (*i.e.*, when the distribution function n(r) is plotted against log r, a gaussian or normal function is obtained). This is a convenience in that the log normal function is a simple function, and all of its properties are well described in elementary statistics textbooks.

The property of this function that describes the "spread" of the distribution is the geometric standard deviation, σ_g. It is obtained graphically from a normalized plot of N(r) (the cumulative size distribution) versus log r, in which N(r) is normalized by dividing by N, thus making the range of the new distribution function from 0 to 1. The σ_g is then defined as

$$\sigma_g = \frac{N\,(r_{84\%})}{N\,(r_{50\%})}. \quad (15)$$

For a perfectly monodisperse aerosol, $\sigma_g = 1.0$. Carefully prepared monodisperse aerosols (to be described below) have σ_g ranging from 1.05 to 1.2. Most other aerosol systems have significantly higher σ_g ranging from 1.5 to 2.5. *The practical implication of this large standard deviation is that the median size for the number distribution is very much smaller than the median size for the mass distribution, which is to say that most of the aerosol mass is contained in a relatively small number of large particles.*

GAS PHASE PROPERTIES: WATER VAPOR AND HUMIDITY

The behavior of an aerosol also depends on changes that take place in the gas phase, especially when the particulate phase is composed of liquid water droplets or can interact physicochemically with water vapor.

Of primary importance is the concept of water vapor saturation equilibrium for a given air temperature. For a given total pressure, which throughout we shall assume to be 1 atm (760 mm Hg), there exists at any temperature a single water vapor pressure in air attained by contact of air and liquid water at that temperature in a closed system. This is known as the *saturation vapor pressure*, and a plot of this saturation vapor pressure for different temperatures is shown in Figure 16-1 (the saturation vapor pressure for water at 100°C is 1 atm, its boiling point).

Air may contain less water vapor than saturation if it is not in contact with liquid water (subsaturation), but, if it contains more than saturation at any temperature, it is said to be supersaturated and cannot be in thermodynamic equilibrium. The usual consequence of this situation is condensation.

The content of water vapor in air, expressed as a mole ratio, g moles H_2O/g mole dry air, is known as the *absolute humidity*, H_A; this is directly related to the water vapor pressure through Dalton's law of partial pressures:

$$\frac{P_{H_2O}}{P_T} = \frac{n_{H_2O}}{n_T}. \quad (16)$$

P_{H_2O} = partial pressure of H_2O vapor (atm)
P_T = total pressure (atm)
n_{H_2O} = g moles of H_2O vapor
n_T = total g moles

If we assume the gas is just air and water vapor, then $n_{air} = n_T - n_{H_2O}$ and

$$H_A = \frac{P_{H_2O}}{P_T - P_{H_2O}}. \quad (17)$$

The *relative humidity*, H_R, is the ratio of the water vapor pressure to the saturation vapor pressure at the same temperature:

$$H_R = \frac{P_{H_2O,T}}{P_{H_2O,sat,T}}. \quad (18)$$

From this relationship, lines of constant relative humidity can be determined and are shown parallel to the saturation vapor pressure line on the psychrometric chart (Fig. 16-1).

When subsaturated air is in contact with bulk liquid water or water aerosol particles, evaporation of the liquid water takes place either until the air has been saturated or all the liquid has evaporated. Significant heat consumption effect is associated with evaporation *(evaporative cooling)*, 580 cal/g is evaporated, and, unless this is supplied by the environment, the temperature of the system will drop and a new equilibrium vapor pressure will be established. Similarly, when subsaturated air is cooled without addition of water vapor, it eventually reaches a temperature at which the vapor pressure equals the saturation pressure known as the *dew point*. Any further cooling will result in condensation, with the release of 580 cal/g, which will tend to warm the system to some extent, depending on the heat removal properties of the system. The significant cooling effect associated with the liquid-vapor transition for water is used in evaporative air conditioning, in which hot dry air is contacted with water to drop its temperature 10° to 20° and raise its relative humidity 10% to 20%.

HUMIDITY GENERATION AND MEASUREMENT

We have discussed the thermodynamics of air-water systems and have indicated the use of the psychrometric chart to determine equilibrium conditions toward which systems tend. Of equal importance with the equilibrium considerations is the rate of evaporation in humidification processes.

To transfer water from liquid to vapor state at a

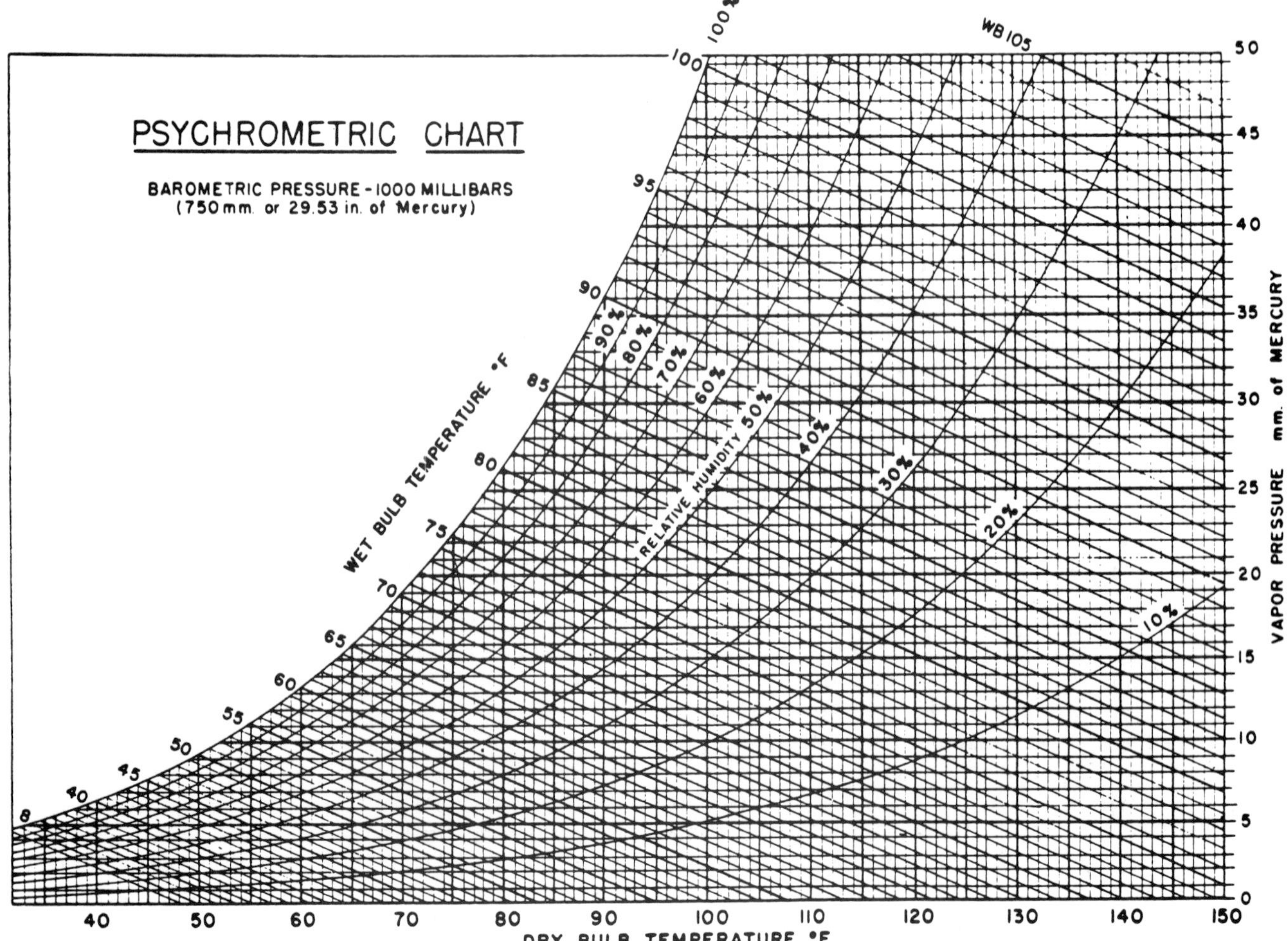

Fig. 16-1. Psychrometric chart. For details of application, *see* text.

reasonable rate, a large interfacial area must be provided, and the distance over which the vapor transfer rate is controlled by molecular diffusion must be made small. The first condition can be met by one of several methods: the water can be spread as a thin sheet over some sort of extended surface; the water can be dispersed as aerosol droplets providing large surface contact with air; or the air can be dispersed in the water as bubbles.

Reducing the molecular diffusion length is accomplished by providing high relative velocities between the gas and liquid and convective mixing in the bulk of the gas phase. In the vicinity of the interface, the vapor transport rate is described by Fick's law:

$$J = -D\frac{dc}{dz}. \tag{19}$$

J = vapor flux (g H_2O vapor/cm^2 sec)
D = molecular diffusion coefficient of H_2O in air (cm/sec)
dc/dz = vapor concentration gradient
c = vapor concentration (g H_2O vapor/cm^3 gas)
z = dimension along the direction of transport (cm)

For many situations the steady-state value of the gradient may be approximated as follows:

$$\frac{dc}{dz} = \frac{C_{\text{bulk}} - C_{\text{interface}}}{\Delta}, \tag{20}$$

where $C_{\text{interface}}$ is in equilibrium with the bulk liquid at its temperature and Δ represents the layer thickness of the region controlled by molecular diffusion.

Several commonly used methods measure the humidity of an air mass. The most direct way is to collect all the water vapor by passing a known volume of air through a desiccant and determining its mass gravimetrically; this method is unsuitable when aerosol particles of water are present because both gaseous and particulate water will be absorbed.

The more common method is the determination of the "wet-bulb" temperature of the air with a device such as a "sling psychrometer." In this method a water-soaked cloth wick is placed over the mercury bulb of a normal stem thermometer, and the thermometer is slung rapidly to provide rapid evaporative cooling of the water in the wick. The temperature indicated by this thermometer is lower than the "dry-bulb" temperature, reaching a maximum depression after a minute or so of slinging. The relative humidity is obtainable from the wet- and dry-bulb temperatures, either from a chart of depression or directly from the psychrometric chart. Diagonal lines on the chart are constant wet-bulb lines; the wet-bulb temperature is located on the saturation line, and the state location (vapor pressure and relative humidity) is the intersection of the diagonal wet-bulb line and the vertical dry-bulb line.

The psychrometric chart is useful in determining the consequences of temperature and vapor concentration changes of all kinds. If the temperature of an air mass is lowered, the state location moves horizontally leftward until it reaches the dew point at the saturation curve. Further temperature lowering moves the state of the air down the saturation curve with consequent reduction of vapor pressure, condensation of vapor, and release of heat.

AEROSOL GENERATION AND MEASUREMENT

Aerosol generation processes can be conveniently classified into two types: condensation processes, those proceeding from the molecular level upward to particles; and comminution processes, these proceeding from the macroscopic state downward to particles.

One type of condensation process begins with a subsaturated vapor in air. The air is cooled to produce a supersaturated vapor. Without walls or "nuclei" of another suitable substance, the vapor will undergo homogeneous nucleation at some degree of supersaturation known as the "critical supersaturation," determined by the thermodynamic properties of molecular clusters of the substance. More commonly, condensation aerosols are "grown" on preexisting nuclei by the process of heterogeneous condensation until saturation is reached at the new condition. The kinetics of particle growth is such that a very monodisperse aerosol can be generated from a polydisperse nuclei population as long as the final aerosol size is large with respect to the nuclei dimension. The other significant feature about such condensation aerosols is that the particles carry few or no electric charges.

Another type of condensation aerosol is that produced by chemical reaction of two gaseous substances to produce a solid reaction product. A typical reaction is that of ammonia gas (NH_3) with hydrogen chloride gas (HCl) to produce ammonium chloride aerosol, which is a solid of virtually no vapor pressure at room temperature. A related type of generation process is the oxidation of a metal at high temperature to produce a volatile oxide that condenses as it cools; this aerosol is the product of a gas–solid reaction.

Comminution or breakup of macrosized solids usually is accomplished in two steps: the mechanical disintegration of the macromatter to produce small particles; and the aerodispersion of these particles. Because the molecular forces are significant for solids, much energy is needed to accomplish mechanical breakup, and there is a practical limit to the minimum size attainable. Most aerosol generators used in clinical practice use this principle.

The mechanical comminution of liquids to produce aerosol droplets is accomplished similarly in that shear forces are applied to the liquid; in this case the viscous resistance to shear is much less than for solids, and the individual liquid particles are formed from an extended sheet of liquid through surface tension forces.

The simplest kind of liquid atomization occurs when liquid under pressure is forced at high velocity through a small orifice. The emerging stream of liquid becomes unstable and breaks up into droplets. This process is called *hydraulic atomization;* unless special steps are taken to apply a regular perturbing force for breakup (e.g., baffles), the resulting aerosol size distribution is polydisperse, with a minimum particle size of about 25 μm for low viscosity liquids such as water.

The most common type of comminution generator for therapeutic liquid aerosols is the pneumatic atomizer, also called an air blast, jet atomizer, or nebulizer. In the atomizer, a very high velocity air stream shears the liquid and produces a droplet distribution varying from a few micrometers to more than 50 μm. It is common in such atomizers to remove large droplets very near the generation point by an impaction body such as an appropriate size sphere; this makes the distribution somewhat more uniform at the expense of removing a significant fraction of the suspended liquid mass. Even so, the geometric standard deviation (σ_g) of such pneumatically generated aerosols is generally between 1.7 μm and 2.5 μm.

In most pneumatic atomizers the liquid is drawn up to the region of high gas velocity through a small diameter tube by the pumping action of the decreased static pressure (the Venturi effect). A significant improvement in the utilization of the high velocity gas jet was made in the design of Babbington,[5] in which the liquid passed over the exterior of a 1-cm glass ball as a thin film, and the gas flowed from the interior of the ball through a minute longitudinal slit. Near the slit, the thin liquid film was further thinned and atomized over the entire circumference of the slit. The result of this design is a liquid aerosol that has a size distribution similar to that of the conventional jet nebulizer but produces a significantly greater number of particles and mass concentration.

Another method for generating liquid aerosol particles is by applying ultrasonic energy. In this kind of device electrical energy is converted to ultrasonic pressure waves in a transducer shaped to bring the waves to a focus within the volume of liquid to be atomized. The transducer is usually operated at a frequency of 10 to 3000 kHz, the smaller mean particle size resulting from higher frequency. The practical lower limit is about 3 μm, number median diameter; if higher frequencies or power levels are used, the liquid becomes excessively overheated. The mass concentration of ultrasonic-generated aerosols is large compared to most pneumatic generators but is limited ultimately by particle coagulation.

Aerosols can also be produced by electrostatic repulsion at the tip of a dropping stream of liquid. If a large negative DC voltage is applied to a capillary from which a suitably nonconducting liquid flows by gravity, the charge repulsion at the surface of the emerging drop will cause microfilaments to form and break into aerosol particles. This aerosol has a high unipolar charge and will expand rapidly as a cloud or collect on surrounding surfaces unless the surface charge is quickly removed. Particles as small as 1 to 5 μm have been produced in laboratory experiments, but no clinically practical aerosol generators have been produced using this principle.

Other special methods employ other forces whereby liquids are broken down to produce practically monodisperse aerosols, which also are generally used only in research and have limited use for aerosol therapy. These include the spinning disc generator, in which a thin film of liquid breaks up as it is centrifugally propelled from a rapidly rotating disc; and the vibrating orifice generator, in which a liquid stream passing through a minute (10–20 μm) orifice is broken up by an impressed electromechanical vibration of the orifice.

Numerous methods to determine the size distribution of aerosols and the morphologic properties of individual particles have been developed. *Optical* and *electron microscopy* are widely used and must be considered as primary standards, but for volatile liquid drops neither method is suitable. Determination of the *terminal settling velocity* by microscopic observation in a cell is a method by which particles of unknown structure or density can be characterized according to their aerodynamic behavior. The terminal settling velocity of spherical particles of density

1 g/cm³ has been derived theoretically and checked experimentally for particle diameters greater than 0.1 μm. A particle of any other shape and density is said to have a given aerodynamic equivalent diameter if its terminal velocity is equal to that of a sphere of that diameter and has a density of 1 g/cm³. For an aerosol system comprising many particles, a number of settling velocity measurements will indicate the distribution of sizes.

Sizing methods and instruments can be divided into those that initially sort an aerosol into size intervals and those that do not. A widely used example of the first kind is the *cascade impactor*. In this instrument an aerosol is drawn through a series of slits, behind each of which is an impaction plate. The aerosol velocity increases from one slit to the next so that the largest particles are inertially removed on the first stage and successive size fractions are removed at successive stages. The impaction plates are removed after sampling a suitable quantity of aerosol, and various analyses may be performed, such as microscopy and gravimetric analysis. The cascade impactor is most suitable for solid aerosols or low volatility liquids; high vapor pressure liquids may undergo significant size change in passing through the impactor since there is a significant absolute pressure drop through the instrument.

An example of a sizing instrument in which no size selectively is used is one in which the light-scattering properties of particles are measured. Optical particle measuring instruments are of two types: those that look at a large number of particles at once, and those that look at a single particle.

If the aerosol being sized is of known distribution or is monodisperse, the scattering character of a number of particles can be used to determine the number concentration and the size. If this is not the case, a light-scattering instrument must be used in which a single particle is sensed at a time. This usually means that the number concentration must be less than 1000/cm³, and a significant dilution with clean air must be used if the initial number concentration is greater.

Optical particle measuring instruments can count and classify particles of known shape and refractive index from 0.3 μm to 20 μm. They are calibrated with aerosols of known properties and dimensions, and one must be careful when using other particles to know how changes in properties influence the calibration.

For particles smaller than 0.3 μm, in cases where electron microscopy is not feasible or convenient, the mean particle size may be determined by the diffusional loss of particles when passed through a tube or channel having a small diameter. Such a collection of equal size tubes is known as a *diffusion battery*; the number concentration before and after the diffusion loss can be determined in most cases by a condensation nuclei counter that causes small particles to grow up to a suitable size with condensed water and measures number concentration by the intensity of forward scattered light.

AEROSOL STABILITY

An aerosol system is inherently unstable, but the time scale over which significant changes take place depends on the particle and collective properties of the system as well as the motion of the diluent gas. If we define the state at time zero to be a distribution of particles in a certain configuration, the particles can "interact" with the boundaries of the system, resulting in cloud expansion or wall deposition; they can interact with each other; and they can interact with the gas phase components.

The first factor, boundary interaction, depends on the boundary configuration and the forces that act on the particles, such as gravity, electrostatic forces, inertial forces from gas flow, or gas molecule forces that produce a diffusional transport. These forces on particles depend on particle size and other particle properties such as density, charge, and shape. This means that in an aerosol of a broad distribution of sizes, some particles are much less stable than others, and there will be a selective removal.

The rate at which particles deposit on a boundary surface is generally expressed as

$$\frac{dN}{dt} = -kN, \tag{21}$$

where k = a "constant" related to particle, gas, and wall properties, and N = aerosol particle concentration/cm³ gas.

It is generally assumed that when a particle comes into physical contact with a solid surface, it "sticks," although there is undoubtedly, under certain conditions, particle bounce or resuspension. However, for liquid aerosols, the assumption is quite appropriate.

Particle–particle interaction where contact occurs and possible permanent aggregation exists is known as *coagulation*. The results of coagulation are a reduction of particle concentration and an increase in the mean size of the aerosol distribution. Coagulation rate is the time change of the particle concentration and is proportional to the square of the concentration:

$$\frac{dN}{dt} = k_c N^2, \tag{22}$$

where k_c = a coagulation constant, a function of particle properties, gas flow, and temperature.

Particles can interact in several ways: by random, Brownian motion; by fluid motion that produces relative particle velocities such as shear flow or turbulence; and by differential particle velocities resulting from size-dependent forces such as gravity, viscous drag, or electrical forces.

An overall particle concentration equation including coagulation and particle loss to walls is

$$\frac{dN}{dt} = -kN - k_c N^2. \tag{23}$$

It can be seen from this equation that, depending on the constants k and k_c, coagulation is the dominant term at high concentrations, and wall loss is dominant at low concentrations. If coagulation is dominant, the mean particle size increases, whereas if wall losses dominate, the effect on the particle distribution is more complex because of the above-mentioned size-selective removal. If Brownian motion coagulation is the prime particle–particle interaction, the value of $k_c \cong 10^{-10}$ cm³/sec and is important with respect to wall loss only if the concentration is greater than 10^5 particles/cm³.

The interaction of particles with the gaseous environment is perhaps most important for particles in humid air, particularly when the particles are partly water or are composed of a water-soluble substance. Condensation or evaporation can take place on the particles and significantly change their size, and thus their stability and behavior within the respiratory tract.

The tendency for particles to grow or evaporate in the presence of water vapor (humidity) depends on the difference between the vapor pressure of the water on the particle and the partial pressure of the water in vapor in the gas phase. If the water vapor partial pressure is greater than the vapor pressure of the drop, *condensation* will occur.

Three factors influence the vapor pressure of water at the surface of a drop: the temperature of the drop, which determines the vapor pressure of pure liquid over a plane surface; the drop diameter, which determines the pure vapor pressure over a curved surface according to the Kelvin equation; and the solute concentration, which lowers the vapor pressure for dilute solutions according to *Raoult's law.*

$$P_s = Px \tag{24}$$

P_s = vapor pressure of the solution
P = vapor pressure of the pure water
x = mole fraction of water in the solution

From this last equation it is evident that as a particle evaporates, the solute concentration increases and the water mole fraction decreases, lowering the effective vapor pressure. The presence of a solute (e.g., saline or propylene glycol) will therefore stabilize the particle size in a high-humidity gas (see below).

Having discussed the equilibrium considerations for the evaporation or condensation of solution particles in humid air, we must now look at rate expressions. For evaporation from a spherical liquid drop in still air, Maxwell gave the classic isothermal steady-state equation:

$$-\frac{dm}{dt} = \frac{4rDM(P_s - P_\infty)}{RT}. \tag{25}$$

m = droplet mass (g)
t = time (sec)
r = droplet radius (cm)
D = water vapor diffusion coefficient in air (cm²/sec)
P_s = droplet surface vapor pressure (atm)
P_∞ = bulk gaseous vapor pressure (atm)
R = gas constant (82.06 cm³/atm/g mole [°K]
T = absolute temperature (°K)
M = molecular weight of the water vapor (g/g mole)

This mathematical expression can be transformed to show that for constant droplet and bulk vapor pressures, the surface area of the droplet changes linearly with time.

To give a specific example, suppose a *pure* water droplet of radius 10 μm is brought into contact with *dry* air at 25°C. The time required for the drop to evaporate completely according to the above equation would be about 0.1 sec. For 50% H_R air surrounding the drop, the evaporation time would be 0.2 sec, whereas for 95% H_R, the time would be 2 sec.

If the assumptions made for this calculation hold, the indication is that particle diameter changes may occur very rapidly, *and that complete evaporation of drops can serve to bring dry air up toward saturation.* The almost universal presence of some dissolved substances in water is one important factor that limits the degree of evaporation by lowering the vapor pressure. Additionally, if a very large mass of water particles is present in a partially water-vapor-saturated atmosphere, the air may reach a condition of equilibrium with only a limited amount of evaporation.

To take a specific example of reaching equilibrium with limited evaporation, let us assume air is at 21°C and 50% H_R. From the psychrometric chart we can calculate the vapor mass content as 10.2 mg H_2O/liter air. To saturate completely the air at this temperature requires an additional 10.2 mg/liter. Suppose there are 10^6 particles/cm^3, all of 5-μm diameter. The mass concentration of particulates is 65.5 mg/liter air. The additional 10.2 mg/liter can be supplied by evaporation of about 15% of the mass of the aerosol, leaving a final particle diameter of 4.7 μm.

As an example of the effect of a dissolved substance, let us assume that a single 5-μm diameter particle of water containing 1% NaCl by weight is in the same atmosphere (21°C, 50% H_R). The droplet will evaporate as an NaCl solution until it becomes a saturated NaCl solution. Since the water vapor pressure at this point is still above the vapor pressure in air, the drop would evaporate to dryness, leaving a salt particle. Only if the H_R is quite high will the droplet stop evaporating at some point before becoming a saturated salt solution.

If the water vapor pressure in the bulk gas exceeds the equilibrium vapor pressure at the drop surface, vapor condensation will occur at a steady-state rate given by Maxwell's equation (25) in which (P_s − P_∞) is replaced by (P_∞ − P_s) and the mass differential becomes positive. If this occurs on a water-soluble substance, as water condenses and the solution becomes more dilute, the droplet surface vapor pressure rises according to Raoult's law, and the vapor pressure "driving force" decreases until equilibrium is reached.

The heat effects associated with evaporation or condensation of water vapor tend to retard the rates of change: in the case of evaporation the temperature of the droplet falls, lowering the equilibrium vapor pressure at the drop surface (and thus the vapor pressure driving force) until heat conduction or convection can return the system to its original temperature. Similarly, in condensation the heat released at the droplet increases the temperature (and the surface vapor pressure) and decreases the driving force for mass transfer.

In practice, when water or aqueous solution aerosols are produced by pneumatic or ultrasonic atomization, most of the vapor required to saturate the gas in the nebulizer comes from the bulk liquid solution, and in the case of dry air supply the temperature of the nebulizer at steady-state often runs 10°C to 15°C lower than the surrounding temperature because of the evaporative heat losses. If the gas is later warmed, it becomes subsaturated, and further particle evaporation may take place to resaturate the gas.

When an aerosol from a generator enters a therapy tent, the changes in particle size that occur during the time the particles are in the tent (before inhalation) depend on the state of humidification of the tent and the boundary temperature conditions. If room air backflow is prevented into the tent so that humidified air is continuously flowing through the tent and out, the tent temperature then depends on three factors: the aerosol mass content and temperature entering; the heat production of the patient; and the heat transfer away from the tent walls by convection and through the patient and bed by conduction.

If the core region of the tent (where aerosol enters and the patient breathes) is at a higher temperature than the nebulizer temperature, the equilibrium water vapor pressure will be higher; water will evaporate from the particles until the vapor pressure in the air is just equal to the vapor pressure at the particle surface. This system cannot reach full saturation at the tent temperature if the particles contain any reasonable quantity of a nonvolatile solute such as NaCl because, after some water evaporates from the particle, the solute concentration is increased, which further decreases the vapor pressure at the particle surface. When the particle–vapor-gas mixture leaves the tent, it will contact tent walls at room temperature (and colder), at which time condensation of vapor will take place on the walls.

AEROSOL BEHAVIOR IN THE RESPIRATORY TRACT

DEPOSITION COMPARTMENTS OF THE RESPIRATORY SYSTEM

In this section we will discuss the interaction of aerosols with the respiratory tract, and, for this purpose, a description of the structure of the respiratory tract is needed. Many different approaches describe the respiratory tract and divide its various components into manageable sections for description. For our purposes the most efficient division of the respiratory tract into its component parts can be made on a functional basis relevant to aerosol and water vapor transport and deposition. This leads to dividing the lung into three compartments in series: a *conditioning region* in which the incoming gases are air-conditioned and brought to the desired temperature and humidity and large particles are removed; a *conducting region* whose principal function is to conduct the gases to the periphery of the lung, although significant aerosol removal of smaller particles occurs here as well; and an *exchange region* consisting of the structures distal to the terminal bronchioles, which are actually involved in gas exchange.

Conditioning Region

The conditioning region, called by some authors the upper respiratory tract, comprises the nose, pharynx and trachea, and perhaps the larger bronchi. Both the gross anatomical configurations of this region and the histology of its epithelium are efficiently designed to carry out the principal functions of this region: to heat the incoming air to 37°C, to humidify the incoming gas to 100% relative humidity, and to remove as large a fraction as possible of airborne particulates. In this regard, in particular, the nose and pharynx are designed to optimize mass transport as well as deposition, the particulars of which will be discussed below.

Conducting Region

The principal function of the conducting region, comprising the bronchi and bronchioles down to the terminal bronchioles, is that of acting as a passage for air to the distal exchange region. In the normally functioning lung, air entering this region has been heated and humidified to optimal conditions but still contains a significant number of particulates of sufficiently small size to escape deposition in the conditioning region. The conducting region, like the conditioning region, is covered with a mucosal epithelium that functions to protect the airways and to remove the smaller particles deposited by the mechanisms to be discussed below. The gross structure of this region is of a dichotomous branching nature with short sections of length two to three times their diameter, with successively smaller diameters proceeding distally toward the periphery. The total cross-sectional area increases significantly as one proceeds toward the smaller airways, so that the velocities in each of the generations significantly decrease. The result of this flow behavior on deposition in the conducting region will be discussed below.

Exchange Region

The exchange region comprises the respiratory bronchioles and the associated passageways leading to the alveoli. This region is penetrated only by the smallest aerosol particles. Its mucosa is not lined with cilia, and clearance from this region is not well understood. Although the exchange region consists of very small structures, it constitutes the major portion of the respiratory system volume.

DEPOSITION MECHANISMS

For aerosol particles to deposit on the walls of the respiratory airways, there must be a movement of the particles across the air flow-stream lines in the airways. Investigations of the fate of particles in similar gas flow systems suggest that there are three major transport mechanisms: gravitational force; the inertial force of the particle; and the random forces of gas molecules on a particle producing Brownian motion.

The force of gravity on a particle is balanced by the viscous drag of the air, resulting in a steady downward particle velocity known as the *terminal settling velocity* (V_T). For a spherical particle of diameter d and density ρ, the value of this velocity for diameters between 1.0 and 70 μm is

$$V_T = \frac{d^2 \rho g}{18\eta}. \qquad (26)$$

g = gravitational constant (980 cm/sec²)
η = air viscosity (1.9×10^{-4} g/cm − sec at 25°C 1 atm)

For a 1-μm diameter sphere, this is 3.5×10^{-3} cm/sec, whereas for 70 μm it is 13.6 cm/sec. The rate at which aerosol particles deposit onto upward-facing surfaces depends on the particle size, the particle concentration, and the flow properties near the surface.

For nonspherical particles, no single theory of viscous drag covers all possibilities, and it is customary to express particle "size" of such a particle in terms of a sphere of density 1 g/cm³ that has an identical falling velocity; this is known as the *aerodynamic equivalent diameter* (AED) (*see* Equation 26 above).

The deposition of aerosol particles by inertial forces depends on changes in the fluid direction that particles cannot follow and thus move transverse to the fluid. The parameter that measures this tendency for a particle to move to a wall by its inertia is the "stopping distance" (X):

$$X = \frac{\rho d^2 v}{18\eta}, \qquad (27)$$

where v = fluid velocity (cm/sec).

The ratio of the stopping distance to a distance that must be traversed by the particle is a dimensionless ratio known as the *Stokes number*, which is an index of impaction probability. For a given geometric arrangement, the fractional loss of aerosol particles is a function of the Stokes number; in general, a high Stokes number means a high impaction probability and *vice versa*, but the specific range of the Stokes number is quite dependent on the flow geometry. For example, impaction probability of spherical particles on cylindrical fibers will depend on such variables as fiber diameter, orientation of fibers to each other, and distance between fibers.

The particle deposition tendency for both inertial impaction and gravitational settling increases with particle diameter, other things being equal, but the dependence of flow is different; gravitational deposition is favored by low flow rates and long residence times, whereas impaction is favored by high flow rates.

For particles smaller than 0.5 μm, these two mechanisms become vanishingly small, and the transport of particles by *Brownian motion diffusion* begins to be dominant as particle size decreases. The transport of particles by this mechanism is appropriately described by a Fick diffusion equation in which the particle diffusivity, D_p, is given by the Stokes–Einstein equation:

$$D_p = \frac{kT}{3\pi\eta d}. \qquad (28)$$

k = Boltzmann's constant (1.38×10^{-16})
T = absolute temperature (°K)

The role played by gas viscosity (η) in providing a retarding force is seen from this equation. As particle size decreases, the particle diffusivity increases and the transport by diffusion increases.

To estimate the deposition properties of particles in the human respiratory tract, one must combine the properties of the particles with the flow properties of air and the geometry of the airways. In the conditioning region, flow in the nasal airway is characterized by very high velocity (~10–15 m/sec at 30 lpm flow) in the anterior nares (where nasal hair is situated); lower flow and turbulent mixing in the main nasal passage; and changes in the flow direction at the posterior nares and the posterior nasal pharynx.

Flow in the oral pharynx is generally of lower velocity, depending on the configuration of the tongue with respect to the palate. Flow in the larynx is similar to that in an orifice: stable convergent flow up to the vocal cords, with a drop in static pressure owing to fluid acceleration followed by turbulent flow in the expansion at the top of the trachea.

The flow in the trachea and first three generations of bronchi of the conducting region continues to be influenced by turbulence generated at the larynx. The average velocity is moderately high (2–3 m/sec), and secondary flows across the main flow direction occur because of the direction changes that occur at the airway bifurcations. Beyond the third-generation bronchi there is a sudden increase in the total cross-sectional area of the airways with a concomitant decrease in average velocity. The flow becomes more dominated by the viscous nature of the gas, and at the terminal bronchiole level the average velocity is estimated from morphologic studies to be about 1 cm/sec.

In the respiratory bronchioles and alveolar ducts, the velocity drops further as the cross-section increases; the typical dimension for these airways is 0.02 to 0.05 cm, so that sedimentation could occur for large particles that reach this level.

Several notable models of aerosol deposition have been developed over the last 40 years, beginning with the work of Findeisen, who developed a simple nine-generation model of the respiratory tract starting at the trachea.[2] The approach was to calculate fractional loss in each generation by the three mechanisms (gravity, impaction, and diffusion) and use the exit concentration from one generation as the inlet concentration for the next. Simple expressions for deposition were developed based on highly simplified flow assumptions.

A somewhat more complete model including mouth and nasal passage was proposed by Landahl, who calculated deposition fractions in the 11 regions of his model for four conditions of breathing and five particle sizes: 20, 6, 2, 0.6, and 0.2 μm diameters.[4] At the larger sizes, deposition was calculated to occur primarily in the first five generations by impaction. As the size decreased, the particles penetrated deeper and deposited primarily by sedimentation, the fraction increasing with the time spent in the smaller airways. The minimum deposition fraction overall was calculated at 0.6 μm, with diffusional deposition increasing for the 0.2-μm aerosol.

Several different experimental techniques have been used to investigate the total and regional deposition fractions of aerosol particles in the human respiratory tract. The original methods involved aerosols having a wide size distribution in which the distributions of inhaled and exhaled aerosol were collected and measured. This did not prove to be as good as studies using a single-sized aerosol in which the fractional deposition could be determined by radioactive counting or by exhaled concentration measurement using light scattering.

Although the trends with particle size seem in relatively good agreement with the theory, the absolute and regional fractional depositions vary significantly from one investigation to another. Some of this lack of agreement may be a result of the difference in electrical charge on particles, but this factor remains to be investigated in human subjects.

Figure 16-2 shows the theoretical curves for nasal, tracheobronchial, and pulmonary deposition fraction for two conditions of breathing as a function of the particle diameter as calculated in the Task Group Report.[6] The predominance of impactive removal for large particles in the nasal passage can be clearly seen and is the reason that tracheobronchial deposition does not rise above 10% under these conditions of respiration.

All these calculations are made for nonvolatile, nonhygroscopic particles where no change in particle size is allowed for during their passage through the respiratory tract. There are many particles for which this is not the case (e.g., cigarette smoke particles, volatile liquid drops, and hygroscopic solids). It has been demonstrated for particles of hygroscopic solids and cigarette smoke that growth takes place under conditions simulating passage into the respiratory tract, and one would then calculate more deposition occurring higher up in the bronchial airways.

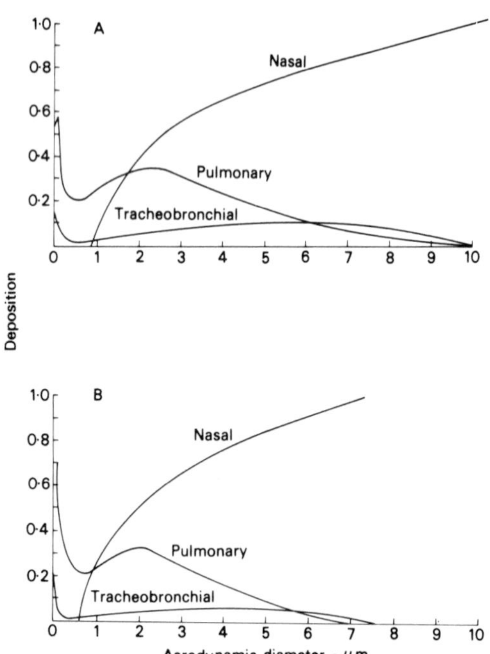

Fig. 16-2. Pulmonary deposition as a function of particle size: *(A)* 750 ml tidal volume; *(B)* 1450 ml tidal volume. (Adapted from Task Group on Lung Dynamics: Deposition and retention models for internal dosimetry of the human respiratory tract. Health Physics 12:173, 1966)

The fate of liquid drops in the human airways has been investigated in a few experiments in which the aerosols were produced by standard pneumatic generators. It is not clear from these experiments to what degree growth or evaporation took place, but it would seem from theory that the water vapor pressure of the droplet with respect to the vapor pressure of the airway fluid would be the critical factor.

Upper airway flow considerations and the availability of a large wet surface maintained near core temperature (37°C) suggest that the adjustment to body temperature and vapor saturation occurs in these airways, primarily in the nasal passage for nose breathing and in the mouth and trachea for oral breathing. Experiments carried out by Ingelstedt in which the temperature and relative humidity of inspired air were measured at the trachea indicated rapid equilibration to body core conditions of saturation at 37°C.[3] These experiments suggest that conditions are very good for rapid transport of heat and water vapor. The effect this would have on an inhaled aerosol is that very rapidly the particle environment would be at 37°C with a vapor pressure equilibrium with the fluid lining the airways at 37°C. This fluid is not pure water but contains 0.9% NaCl and a small amount of dissolved proteins, which would together depress the vapor pressure according to Raoult's law by about 1%.

Let us suppose that a pure water drop enters the respiratory tract in a gas at 25°C and 100% H_R. There will be immediate heat and moisture transfer from the walls occurring simultaneously to bring the air up to 37°C and to 99% H_R. Theoretically, the pure water will have a higher vapor pressure and will tend to evaporate, but the gradient of vapor pressure is so small (1% of the case for evaporation in dry air) that one would estimate a minimal change in particle size through the respiratory tract. It does not seem likely that the deficit in water vapor will be made up by particle evaporation but rather by wall vapor transfer, since the processes of heat and mass transfer for water vapor are equally rapid.

We have thus considered the factors that determine the deposition characteristics of inhaled particles in the human respiratory tract. We shall now consider the mechanisms involved in the removal of substances from the respiratory surfaces.

CLEARANCE

PROPERTIES OF MUCUS AND THE MUCOCILIARY ESCALATOR

The major clearance mechanism in the normal respiratory system is known as the mucociliary escalator, an apt description of a continuously moving layer of fluid that acts as the principal collector and clearer of deposited particulate material. The proper functioning of this clearance system depends on a complex interaction between the moving fluid, or mucus, and the underlying epithelium, which consists principally of cells equipped with the propulsive appendages called cilia. In this section we shall proceed with a description of each of these components in turn and with the mechanisms by which they are coupled.

Properties of Mucus

Chemically, mucus consists of an aqueous solution containing both low- and high-molecular-weight substances. Its low-molecular-weight components, including small proteins, are similar to those found in serum. However, the principal macromolecular components of mucous secretion are very high-molecular-weight, insoluble glycoproteins or mucins. These compounds are macromolecules having a protein core with a large number of oligosaccharide or short polysugar side-chains linked to the protein. A typical structure of a mucus glycoprotein is shown in Figure 16-3. These glycoproteins, or mucins, are unlike those found in the blood because they contain more than 50% carbohydrate. The carbohydrates include hexosamines, galactose, fucose, and sialic acid. Sialic acid, when present, is always terminal in the side-chain and is thought to play a significant role in the physical properties of mucus, although this is now being questioned.

Much of what is currently known about the detailed chemistry of mucins is based on studies of submaxillary and gastric mucins, which are relatively easy to obtain and are more soluble than bronchial mucins. Because the amount of mucus in the normal respiratory tract is quite small and spread out in a very thin layer, it has been quite difficult to obtain normal respiratory mucus for chemical and physical testing, so that to date very little is known about the detailed structure of normal human respiratory mucins. More is known about the composition of sputum, which can be defined as an expectorated mixture of mucus and saliva. However, since the mucus component of sputum is significant only in disease, information about sputum reflects significant changes owing to pathology and gives little information about normal respiratory secretions.

Physically, respiratory tract mucus behaves as a viscoelastic gel. Unlike a sol, a gel is a colloidal state of matter in which the molecules can interact strongly with each other either through direct chemical bonds or, in the case of the long-chain molecules that constitute mucins, by physical interactions and entanglements as well. The result is a material with very complex flow properties that cannot simply be classified as a fluid or a solid. Like a fluid, mucus, when stressed, will flow, with the component molecules moving relative to each other and to the solvent. However, because of the gel interactions, the mucus possesses solidlike properties, principally that of elasticity. When acted on by a force, mucus molecules can store energy and resist deformation. When the force is removed, such solutions can relax and recoil.

Those properties of matter that relate to their flow and deformation ability are known as *rheological properties*. Water is a rheologically simple material possessing only viscosity, or resistance to flow, under ordinary conditions. Mucus is a rheologically complex material possessing both viscous and elastic components. This behavior is intimately related to the chemical structure of the mucins and can be modified by factors such as pH, solids content, and other electrolytes that change the ionic interactions between the

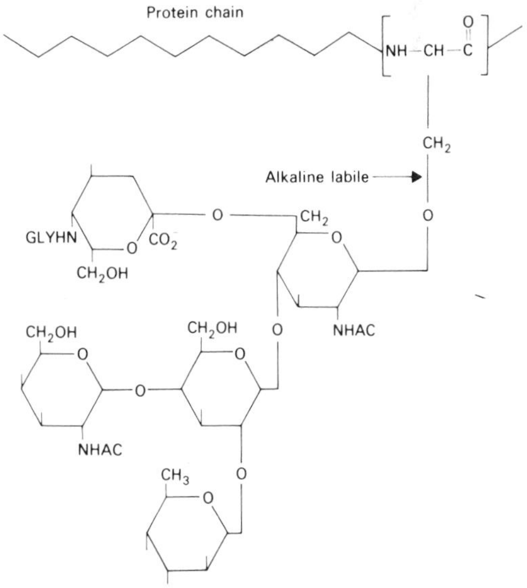

Fig. 16-3. Structure of a mucus glycoprotein. (Adapted from Lutz RJ, Litt M, Chakrin LW: Rheology of Biological Systems. Springfield, Illinois, Charles C Thomas, 1973. Courtesy of Charles C Thomas, Publisher)

mucus molecules. In addition the rheological properties of mucus *in vivo* are significantly changed by various pathologic processes that can cause the secretion of a more concentrated polymer solution, leading to significantly increased viscoelastic properties, or by contamination of the bronchial mucus with various cellular breakdown products such as bacterial DNA or cellular components from the lung itself.

Physiology of Mucus Production

Mucus is produced by the epithelial mucosa lining essentially all the surfaces of the conditioning and conducting compartments. A schematic representation of the surface of a typical ciliated epithelium is shown in Figure 16-4. This epithelium contains a number of different cell types, but we need to consider only the two principal types: the pseudostratified columnar ciliated cell and the goblet cell, which normally exist in a ratio of about 5:1, respectively. The ciliated cell has as its principal function the propulsion of the mucus layer, which will be discussed shortly. The goblet cell represents a surface mucous-secreting cell, as indicated by the secretory granules inside. These cells are very similar to goblet cells in the intestinal tract, which are the major producers of gastrointestinal mucus. Goblet cells synthesize mucus glycoprotein and periodically discharge their contents by expulsion directly to the surface of the epithelium.

In the human lung, however, the major source of mucus production is not in the mucosa but in glands situated in the submucosa (*see* Fig. 9-5). These simple tubular alveolar glands contain both mucus-producing and serous-producing cells. These glands, which discharge to the surface through ducts such as the one shown in Figure 9-5, are the principal source of respiratory mucus in the normal system. They are innervated by the autonomic nervous system, so that the secretion of mucus can be affected by nervous activity or by drugs affecting the autonomic system. In

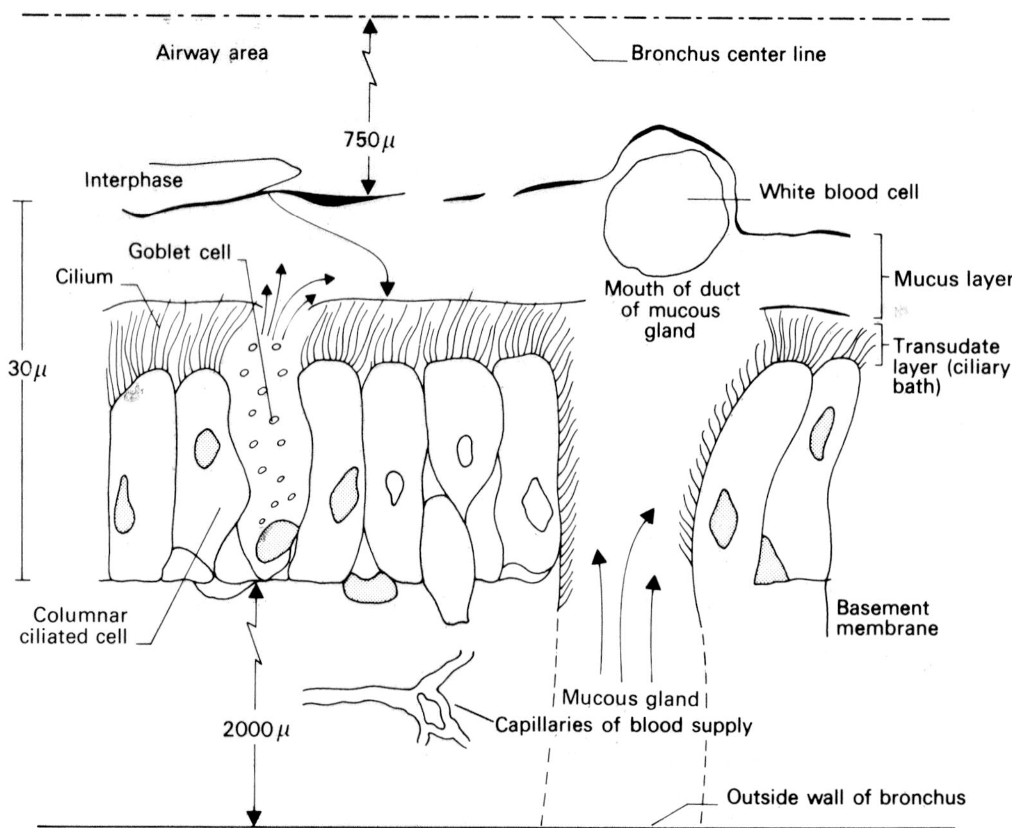

Fig. 16-4. Surface of a typical ciliated epithelium. (Adapated from Denton R, Hwang SH, Litt M: Chemical engineering aspects of obstructive lung disease. Chem Eng Progress 62(66):12, 1966)

addition, of course, the goblet cells may be affected by direct irritation. In pathologic conditions a metaplasia may take place in which ciliated cells are replaced by goblet cells that have the effect both of producing more mucus and reducing the ability of the epithelium to transport it. Also, a hyperplasia or increase in mass of the submucosal glands occurs that leads to greatly increased mucus secretion. This change in cell populations may be an important concomitant of obstructive pulmonary disease. In addition, because irritation results in stimulation of mucus production, local infection also may cause hypersecretion of mucus, resulting in airway obstruction.

In addition to mucus, the surface of the respiratory mucosa in the region surrounding the cilia is believed to consist of a serous or periciliary fluid whose composition is relatively unknown. The existence of this fluid as distinct from the mucus is based on histochemical preparations that indicate a non-mucus-staining region surrounding the cilia. Because of the presumed small volume of this material, it has not been subjected to collection and analysis. However, its existence is important to basic concepts of mucociliary flow, which we shall discuss in the next section.

Cilia

The luminal surface of the ciliated cell contains about 200 cilia per cell. Cilia are, on average, 0.2 to 0.3 μm in diameter and about 6 μm long. In cross-section the cilia show what is known as a "nine plus two" pattern, consisting of a ring of nine double filaments of contractile protein around the periphery surrounding a pair of single filaments. These filaments are thought to be connected to each other by small protuberances that may play a role in the bending motion of the cilia.

Each cilium possesses a characteristic beat consisting of an effective or power stroke, during which the cilium is almost straight, and a bending or recovery stroke, which constitutes the major part of the cycle. The position and shape of the cilium at each phase of this cycle are shown in Figure 16-5. However, the cilia of each cell and of adjacent cells are controlled in a coordinated manner so as to produce a "metachronal" wave that propagates along the ciliated epithelium and that provides the effective propulsive force for mucus transport. In the human respiratory system, the wave propagates in the opposite direction of the effective stroke of the cilia and is known as an antiplectic wave, with the effective force being directed centrally toward the trachea. The cilia are surrounded by the periciliary fluid mentioned earlier, which is believed to be of relatively low viscosity.

The mucociliary escalator comprises the metachronal wave of beating cilia surrounded by a low-viscosity sol layer of periciliary fluid and surmounted by the transported layer of gel mucus. Current concepts of mucociliary transport are based on this two-fluid layer model (Lucas–Douglas model of mucus transport). The details of this transport mechanism and of its structure are still somewhat in doubt and are based principally on histochemical evidence. It is not known, for example, whether the gel-like mucus exists in a continuous blanket covering the surface of the mucosa or whether islands of mucus float on the periciliary fluid. It is also not known how the secretions of the goblet cells and glands enter the overlying mucus layer, whether in a continuous stream or in discrete boli. It is known that the cells lining the exits of the gland ducts are also ciliated. It is also known that gel-like properties are required for mucus transport to take place (*i.e.*, the mucus must possess a certain degree of viscoelastic character to be efficiently coupled to the ciliary wave and to be transported). Most authors have assumed that the ciliary tips touch the overlying mucus and propel it; however, this is not essential, since flow of the periciliary fluid could induce shear, with resulting transport of the overlying mucus.

To summarize, mucus represents the principal filtering material of the respiratory system, serving to trap deposited particulates in the conducting and conditioning parts of the airways. The mucus viscoelastic properties are coupled to a metachronal wave of beating cilia in a complex two-fluid layer that produces a net flow of mucus from the lung and pharynx to the

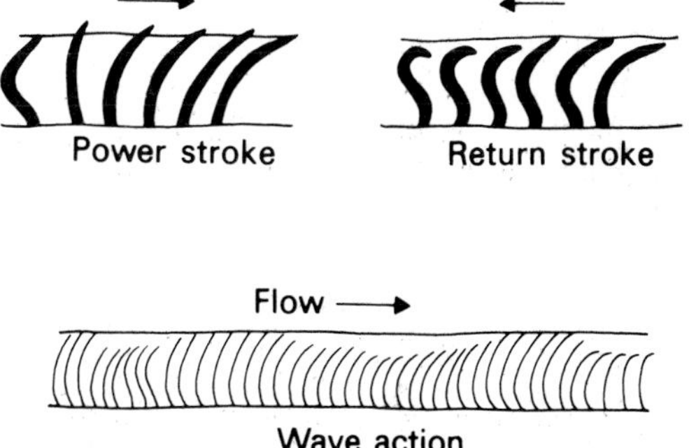

Fig. 16-5. Cilium at each phase of the beat cycle. (Adapted from Denton R, Hwang SH, Litt M: Chemical engineering aspects of obstructive lung disease. Chem Eng Progress 62(66):12, 1966)

glottis, where it is finally swallowed. In the normal lung, the volume of viscoelastic mucus is very small. Because the total surface area at each generation decreases as one moves from smaller airways toward the trachea, it has been thought that the mucus is concentrated by resorption of water to reduce the fluid volume during the ascent of the airway and that this perhaps would explain the strongly viscoelastic character of secretions obtained from the trachea. All of these factors may interact in pathologic conditions, resulting in reduced mucociliary transport. These factors will be considered in the last part of this chapter.

Alveolar Clearance

By definition the alveolar or exchange compartment of the lung contains none of the components of the mucociliary escalator and therefore cannot clear to the mucociliary system directly. The subject of alveolar clearance is still considerably open to question. Long-term clearance studies of solid particulates, which are known to have deposited in alveoli, indicate that the time scale of clearance is much longer than that associated with the mucociliary system.

Possible mechanisms for alveolar clearance include ingestion by alveolar macrophages recruited to the exchange area in response to deposited material. Presumably, these cells ultimately clear by way of lymphatics or possibly blood vessels. However, the findings of particle-laden macrophages in sputum indicate that macrophages can be cleared from the exchange compartment, although the mechanism for this is unknown. It has been suggested that the surface-tension gradient resulting from pulmonary surfactant may provide a means for clearing macrophages to the peripheral parts of the mucociliary escalator. However, the clearance of macrophages in mucus may represent only material from the more proximal ends of the exchange region.

COUGH

Although the mucociliary escalator is the principal mechanism for clearance of secretions and trapped aerosol particles, a second, completely separate mechanism exists in the form of *cough*. For clearance of secretions, cough is important probably only in cases of impaired flow or pathology; the only areas so cleared are the trachea and larger bronchi.

Clearance by means of the cough mechanism is due to high-velocity entrainment of the secretions during the cough and is thus an aerodynamic phenomenon. High velocities approaching the velocity of sound at tracheal conditions are produced by the apposition of the muscular posterior surface of the trachea to the anterior cartilaginous portion. The resulting reduction in tracheal cross-section produces a highly increased velocity during expiration, with resulting turbulent flow in the trachea and large bronchi. This turbulence results in very high wall shear forces that can entrain the secretions and carry them to the pharynx. However, because of the naturally large increase in airway cross-section as one proceeds distally, the increased velocity is effective only in the larger airways. In obstructive pulmonary disease the mucociliary system, although abnormal, is still the *only* mechanism for bringing secretions from the bronchioles and smaller bronchi to the region where cough may be effective.

Because cough is reflexive and may be induced by deposition of particles on the tracheal mucosa, the cough may represent a protective mechanism to clear larger particles deposited in the upper respiratory tract. Cough is also the principal means of sputum production in obstructive airways disease. Various methods of therapy designed to induce a productive cough, which could include aerosol therapy, postural drainage, and percussion, may be effective because of their ability to induce a cough and not by mobilizing secretions in any other way. However, while coughing provides an alternative mechanism of keeping open the larger airways, a functioning mucociliary system is still essential for clearance of the smaller conducting airways.

INTERACTIONS AND ALTERATIONS

Factors Producing Impaired Clearance

A cessation or reduction in mucus flow can be produced by a number of factors affecting the mucociliary escalator at various levels of operation. Indeed, because the proper functioning of the mucociliary system requires a well-balanced dynamic interacting system, there are several points at which function can be impaired. Some of these are discussed below.

Changes in Properties of the Mucus. Since viscoelastic properties of the mucus are essential to proper clearance, an alteration in mucus properties either due to altered synthesis or changes in mucus after secretion can act to impede mucus flow. For example, a complete loss of gel structure would eliminate the elasticity of the mucus and actually allow retrograde flow. Such behavior does occur, for example, with the thin watery secretions in the nose during a "cold." Such a change in mucus properties in the lung could produce a pooling of thin secretions, particularly in the lower lobes of the lung.

Conversely, a large increase in the elasticity of the mucus could also result in mucostasis. Such an eventuality could occur if the gelled mucus could not flow from the mouths of goblet cells or gland duct mouths, producing long elastic ropes that the metachronal action of the cilia would be insufficient to shear and flow. It is important to remember that while some solidlike properties are essential, a completely solid strand could not flow. In some pathologic conditions, inspissated solid mucus strands have been observed in gland mouths, which could account for the mucostasis that occurs.

Interestingly, changes in the rheological properties of mucus have long been associated with obstructive pulmonary diseases such as bronchitis and cystic fibrosis, but they have traditionally been associated with increases in mucus viscosity, owing to lack of awareness of the elastic nature of the material. It is indeed possible for increased viscosity *per se* to result in improved mucus clearance rather than impaired clearance. Therefore, when considering the effect of changes in rheological properties on mucus transport, the possible changes in both the elastic gel nature and viscous fluid nature must be considered.

These properties may be changed not only systemically but also by admixture of compounds found in the airway lumen. This is particularly true in the case of infection; bacterial cells, phagocytic cells that ingest the bacteria, and sloughed-off epithelial cells are all trapped on the mucosal surface. The local irritation caused by the infection results in stimulation of mucus production, presumably as a response by the system to provide clearance of the insult. However, with concurrent obstructive pulmonary disease, this simply exacerbates the situation, leading to increased airway obstruction. Treatment techniques intended to function by producing changes in the mucus must take these factors into account.

Changes in the Flow Mechanism. We have seen that normal mucociliary flow requires a two-fluid layer with the cilia bathed in a low-viscosity solution. Therefore any changes in either the properties or geometry of the system can result in impaired mucus flow. For example, water loss with a decrease in volume of the periciliary fluid or a large overburden of mucus could result in entangling of the cilia with the gel-like mucus and cessation of transport. There is evidence that cilia continue beating even with many times their normal burden of overlying mucus, so that interference with ciliary dynamics is not usually a problem. However, mucus flow would cease if mucus became completely entangled in the cilia.

On the other hand, hypersecretion of the periciliary fluid could also result in decreased transport. If contact of the cilia tips with the overlying mucus is essential, then an increased depth of ciliary fluid would eliminate this contact. However, even if contact were not essential, increased depth of the ciliary fluid would increase the layer of fluid that needs shearing to transport the mucus, and hence the efficiency of coupling between the cilia and the mucus would be significantly reduced, again leading to impaired clearance. Thus any change in the balance of the ciliary fluid could result in impaired mucociliary transport.

Transport would be affected directly, of course, if the ciliary beat itself were impaired. For example, various aerosols such as tobacco smoke may cause a cessation of transport by simply stopping the cilia during, and for some time after, the exposure. In this regard, the differential effects of short-term versus long-term exposure may be due to different mechanisms. In the short term, the cilia may stop beating; in the long term, hypersecretion of mucus may also be produced by various particulate pollutants. Local environmental conditions such as cold or drying of the mucosa can also impede ciliary beating. Finally, of course, injury to the mucosal epithelium itself with changes in the epithelium either due to chronic disease or acute insult will result in impaired clearance (see Fig. 9-6B).

The various manifestations of impaired mucociliary clearance are produced by factors that represent examples of chronic obstructive pulmonary disease. The classic example of this is chronic bronchitis, in which airway obstruction follows impaired mucus clearance. Chronic bronchitis has been produced in experimental animals by exposure to low concentrations of sulfur dioxide for long periods of time. This animal model is accompanied by all the concomitants discussed above: metaplasia of the mucosal surface, hyperplasia or increase in the volume of goblet cells, and the production of a very viscoelastic mucus. However, other types of obstructive respiratory disease are associated with impaired mucociliary clearance, including emphysema, bronchitis associated with pneumoconiosis, and bronchiectasis. Cystic fibrosis is perhaps the extreme example of obstructive respiratory disease in which a highly rubbery, gel-like mucus is produced. It is still uncertain whether secretion of this abnormal mucus is the primary cause of the airway obstruction or whether it is a secondary effect of infection or another biochemical effect of the primary genetic abnormality. However, the common feature of all these conditions is the hyperproduction of a more elastic and viscous material with gradually increasing obstruction of the smaller airways, leading eventually to atelectasis. While, as noted above, the larger airways can be cleared by the cough reflex, the blockage and impaired mucociliary clearance of the small airways ultimately become the focal point of the disease. With time, as obstructive disease progresses, even the cough reflex may be lost and the larger airways occluded with uncleared secretions.

Factors Relative to Improved Clearance

A rational attempt to restore impaired mucociliary clearance should be based on reversal of any of the many factors discussed above. These attempts could be either systemic, by attempting to intervene in the secretion process itself, or local, by topical administration of pharmacologic agents. This latter intervention is the basis for the use of therapeutic aerosols.

Systemic Modifications. Attempts to modify mucociliary flow systemically would be based on administration of drugs or an attempt to alter the body's water balance. Although some drugs given systemically have reportedly resulted in improved clearance, a rational experimental design to test such a system would require a far greater knowledge of the secretory process than we now have.

From a nonspecific point of view, the overall water balance must play a significant role in ability to clear mucus since the lung is a net loser of water. Aerosol therapy, which is based on local factors as discussed below, may actually benefit the patient by altering the water balance in the lung, but this also is still an unknown area.

Local Modifications. The local administration of various agents to improve airway clearance forms a large part of respiratory bronchial toilet and care. The types of agents used in these treatments are mucolytic or expectorant drugs designed to change mucus properties back to those more easily cleared; and continuous bland aerosol therapy, also designed to improve clearance.

Any treatment technique designed to affect mucociliary clearance locally must fulfill the following conditions: to be effective at all, it must be delivered to the desired site; it must remain pharmacologically active during the transport process and *in situ;* and it must produce a change in the mucus properties or functioning of the mucociliary clearance system that can result in improved mucus flow.

The major means of delivering various agents locally to the respiratory system has been the use of liquid aerosols. This includes not only drugs, but also the liquid itself (e.g., the use of water as a mucus-thinning agent). For completeness we should also include the delivery of saturated humidified gas such as those used in croup tents or vaporizers, but this use is principally for treatment of diseases that affect the upper respiratory tract.

Delivery to the Site of Action. In considering the use of aerosols to deliver a therapeutic agent to a specific section of the respiratory tract, one must consider the mass deposition rate of particulate matter as a function of particle size, and the region of the respiratory tract. Apparently in such a design the aerosol should have a mass median diameter such as to deposit a large fraction of the mass of particles in the desired airway region. To reach the smaller airways, which are the principal focus of chronic obstructive pulmonary disease, the aerosol should have a mass median diameter on the order of a few micrometers. Particles any larger than this will be principally deposited in the larger airways and not reach the desired site of action. However, such small particles have very little mass per particle, and the deposition of even large numbers of such particles does not add up to significant total mass. A number of studies of experimental deposition of liquid aerosols in the respiratory tract, even using mouth breathing with a mask, show that only a small percentage of the aerosol mass entering the respiratory tree is deposited in the peripheral airways. Where a tent is used, such as in continuous liquid aerosol therapy, the situation is much more complex because, as described above, particles may either evaporate or grow, both in the tent and in the respiratory tract; thus the particular particle size distribution found in the trachea and lower tract is unknown. It is therefore unlikely that very large mass deposition rates can be obtained in the smaller airways.

Pharmacologic Activity. The act of dispersing a drug onto large surface areas by aerosolization does not alter the pharmacologic activity of the drug itself. For example, a drug that is subject to oxidation such as N-acetylcysteine might be inactivated by aerosolizing it, since a much larger surface would be exposed to the gas by dispersion in an aerosol. Therefore tests of activity of drugs to be aerosolized must be conducted using the aerosolized material rather than carried out with the bulk form.[1] A material that is strongly mucolytic in the test tube may lose its activity after aerosolization.

Do Changes Result in Anything That Might Change Mucociliary Clearance? The final factor in attempting to alter mucociliary clearance by local deposition must involve changes in the rheological properties of the secretions or the properties of the airways that will cause increased mucus flow. In current therapeutic practice there are two types of such agents: mucolytic agents such as N-acetylcysteine, which are delivered to the local mucosa and which allegedly have the property of dispersing the mucus gel; and aerosol droplets, consisting principally of water designed to dilute the mucus gel and "improve" its flow properties.

Mucolytic agents such as N-acetylcysteine definitely do have mucolytic action *in vitro* and apparently *in vivo* as well. However, such agents, because they disperse proteins and carbohydrates generally, may prove quite irritating to the mucosa, and thus must be used with caution. In addition to mucolytic drugs, bronchodilators could be used to increase airway caliber and decrease resistance and might be used in conjunction with the mucolytic agent to improve delivery of the aerosol.

The use of water aerosols, generally on a continual basis, is based on the idea of "thinning" the secretions that are thought to be too "viscid." This is particularly a therapeutic method of choice in the United States in treating cystic fibrosis. However, even if sufficient water could be delivered to the mucus of the peripheral airways, which is doubtful, there is little evidence that the changes in the rheological properties of mucus would result in significant alteration of mucociliary transport. In particular, the highly insoluble mucus found in obstructive pulmonary disease is not dispersed by water or saline *in vitro* and is unlikely to be dispersed *in vivo*. It is also difficult to design an experiment *in vitro* that would adequately determine if added water would affect mucociliary flow, because of the two-fluid nature of the mucus flow. Addition of water directly to the mucus, if the mucus blanket is not continuous, would simply add to the periciliary fluid layer and would not significantly swell the mucus, since it is known from studies *in vitro* that this does not occur.

The use of aerosols for the local administration of therapeutic agents in chronic obstructive pulmonary disease can also be criticized on the basis of impaired air flow in such disease. It is important to recognize that the deposition patterns discussed earlier and the implicit assumption that particles will be uniformly deposited would be untrue in the case of obstructive disease. Indeed, the greatest deposition would occur in the area least obstructed, resulting in delivery of the therapeutic agent in inverse relation to the region where it is needed. Recent clinical studies of the efficacy of continuous water aerosol therapy in cystic fibrosis have not shown any significant effect on pulmonary function with use of the treatment.* However, it is unclear what significant pulmonary function tests one should use for assessing improvement in airway performance, and this field is currently the subject of considerable controversy.

SUMMARY

The interaction of aerosols with the respiratory tract is of considerable significance to the respiratory care practitioner, both with regard to the induction of insults by airborne aerosols and as a possible source of therapy using man-made therapeutic aerosols. Any rational design of therapy must take into account the basic physics of aerosols and what is currently known about their deposition in, and interaction with, the respiratory tract as outlined here.

The use of aerosols in therapy is still subject to considerable controversy. However, aerosol therapy is in widespread use, particularly in the United States for treatment of various manifestations of chronic obstructive pulmonary disease, and it therefore behooves the reader to be widely aware of these principles. Specific information on the generation of therapeutic aerosols and currently used methods of delivery are discussed in Chapter 17.

REFERENCES

1. Denton R, Kwart H, Litt M: N-Acetylcysteine in cystic fibrosis: Mechanical and chemical factors in treatment by aerosol. Am Rev Respir Dis 95:643, 1967

*See Bibliography under Aerosol Therapy.

2. Findeisen W: Ueber die kleiner Absetzung in der Luft suspendierten Teilchen in der menschlichen Lunge bei der Atmung. Arch Gesamte Physiol 236:367, 1935
3. Ingelstedt S: Studies on the conditioning of air in the respiratory tract. Acta Otolaryngol [Suppl] (Stockh) 131:1, 1956
4. Landahl HD: On the removal of airborne droplets by the human respiratory tract. Bull Math Biophysics 12:43, 1950
5. Litt M, Swift DL: The Babington nebulizer: A new principle for the generation of therapeutic aerosols. Am Rev Respir Dis 105:308, 1972
6. Task Group on Lung Dynamics: Deposition and retention models for internal dosimetry of the human respiratory tract. Health Physics 12:173, 1966

BIBLIOGRAPHY

Aerosol Physics

Dautrebande L: Microaerosols. New York, Academic Press, 1962

Davies CN: Aerosol Science. New York, Academic Press, 1966

Friedlander SK: Smoke, Dust and Haze—Fundamentals of Aerosol Behavior. New York, John Wiley & Sons, 1977

Fuchs MA: The Mechanics of Aerosols. Oxford, Pergamon Press, 1964

Green HL, Lane WR: Particulate Clouds, 2nd ed. London, E & FN Spon, 1964

Liu BYH (ed): Fine Particles—Aerosol Generation, Measurement, Sampling, and Analysis. New York, Academic Press, 1976

Mercer TT: Aerosol Technology in Hazard Evaluation. New York, Academic Press, 1973

Morrow PE: Aerosol characterization and deposition. Am Rev Respir Dis 110:88, 1974

Shaw DT (ed): Fundamentals of Aerosol Science. New York, John Wiley & Sons, 1978

Interaction of Aerosols with Respiratory System

Albert RE et al: Bronchial deposition and clearance of aerosols. Arch Intern Med 131:115, 1973

Altshuler B, Yarmus L, Palmes ED et al: Aerosol deposition in the human respiratory tract. AMA Arch Ind Health 15:293, 1957

Davies CN (ed): Inhaled Particles and Vapours, Vol 2. Oxford, Pergamon Press, 1966

Ferron GA: The size of soluble aerosol particles as a function of the humidity of the air application to the human respiratory tract. J Aerosol Science 8:251, 1977

Hatch T, Gross P: Pulmonary Deposition and Retention of Inhaled Aerosols. New York, Academic Press, 1964

Heyder J et al: Total deposition of aerosol particles in the human respiratory tract for nose and mouth breathing. J Aerosol Sci 6:311, 1975

Lippmann M, Albert RE: The effect of particle size on the regional deposition of inhaled aerosols in the human respiratory tract. Am Ind Hyg Assoc J 30:257, 1969

Morrow PE: Alveolar clearance of aerosols. Arch Intern Med 131:101, 1973

Stahlhofen W et al: Experimental determination of the regional deposition of aerosol particles in the human respiratory tract. Amer Ind Hyg Assoc J 41:385, 1980

Mucus and Mucociliary Clearance

Barton AD: Bronchial secretions and mucociliary therapy. Arch Intern Med 131:140, 1973

Camner P: Clearance of particles from the human tracheobronchial tree. Clin Sci 59:79, 1980

Jakowska S (ed): Interdisciplinary investigation of mucus production and transport. Ann NY Acad Sci 130(3):869, 1966

Keal EE: Physiological and pharmacological control of airway secretions. In Brain JD, Proctor DF, Reid L (eds): Respiratory Defense Mechanisms. New York, Marcel Dekker, 1977

Kilburn KH (ed): Symposium on pulmonary responses to inhaled materials. Arch Intern Med 126:415, 1970

Kilburn KH, Salzano JV (eds): Symposium on structure, function and measurement of respiratory cilia. Am Rev Respir Dis 93(2), Part 2, 1966

Proctor DF, Anderson I: Nasal mucociliary function in normal man. Rhinology 14:11, 1976

Rheology of Bronchial Secretions and Respiratory Function. Proceedings of Entretiens de Physio-Pathologie Respiratoire, 9th series. Bull Physiopathol Respir (Nancy) 9(1 & 2), 1973

Wanner A: Clinical aspects of mucociliary transport. Am Rev Respir Dis 116:73, 1977

Aerosol Therapy

Chang N et al: An evaluation of nightly mist tent therapy for patients with cystic fibrosis. Am Rev Respir Dis 107:672, 1973

Matthews LW, Doershuk DF, Spector S: Mist tent therapy of the obstructive pulmonary lesion of cystic fibrosis. Pediatrics 176:39, 1967

Miller WF: Aerosol therapy in acute and chronic respiratory disease. Arch Intern Med 131:148, 1973

Montoyama EK, Gibson LE, Zigas CJ: Evaluation of mist tent therapy in cystic fibrosis using maximum expiratory volume curves. Pediatrics 50:299, 1972

Proceedings of the Conference on the Scientific Basis of Respiratory Therapy. Am Rev Respir Dis 110(6), Part 2, 1974

Scherer PW, et al: Growth of hygroscopic aerosols in a model of bronchial airways. J Appl Physiol 47:544, 1979

Swift DL: Generation and respiratory deposition of therapeutic aerosols. Am Rev Respir Dis 122(5), Part 2: 71, 1980

Wolfsdorf J, Swift DL, Avery ME: Mist therapy reconsidered: An evaluation of the respiratory deposition of labeled water aerosols produced by jet and ultrasonic nebulizers. Pediatrics, 43:799, 1969

17

Applied Humidity and Aerosol Therapy*

H. Frederic Helmholz, Jr. • George G. Burton

The theory is complex, based in higher mathematics. Work on the manufacture, delivery, deposition, and clearance of aerosols, at least in animal models, seems to be proceeding apace (*see* Chap. 16). The reader will perceive, in reading this chapter, that the theory of *applied* humidity and aerosol therapy is not easily grasped at first reading, but at least the nomenclature is there, and the various interrelationships of temperature, water-vapor pressure, and so forth are fairly well worked out.

What is conspicuous by its absence, despite the urgings of three recent international, multidisciplinary conferences,[3,5,28,29] is a sound clinical basis for using bland aerosol and humidity therapy in medical practice. An attempted consensus view of the conferees at these sessions appears in Table 17-1. With the possible exception of ultrasonic nebulization, the use of humidity and aerosol therapy remains as clinically invalidated as ever, despite the use of millions of disposable and nondisposable humidity generators and despite thousands of mothers (and their pediatricians) who swear that the "steam" (or cool water vapor) from a hot (or cold) shower has saved many an infant's trip to the emergency room for conditions ranging from croup to bronchiolitis!

*The authors wish to thank Gary Lynch, RRT, Administrative Director, Respiratory Care Services, Hoag Memorial Hospital, Newport Beach, California, for his advice and contributions to this chapter.

Modern practice reflects the opinion of Spearman and Sheldon,[32] who have pointed out that the use of bland aerosols should probably be thought of as adjunctive therapy to other methods that improve removal of secretions (*i.e.*, bronchodilator therapy, systemic hydration, proper coughing techniques, postural drainage, and chest percussion and vibration).

For humidity therapy, particularly, one longs for scientific support or rejection of the modalities once and for all.

Like Darin,[9] we are surprised that no one has yet attempted to calculate the costs of aerosol- and humidity-generating devices in these fiscally conscious times. Perhaps the constraints of prospective reimbursement will determine the place of "fumes and smokes" and "vapors and mists," whose use dates from many years past.[7,8] Meanwhile, this chapter will concern itself with the current view of practical, safe methods of humidity and aerosol administration.

HUMIDITY THERAPY

TERMINOLOGY

In calculating humidity therapy, *temperature* is expressed in degrees Celsius (Centigrade; C) or in degrees Kelvin (K). Temperature in degrees Kelvin des-

Table 17-1. Clinical Effects* of Humidity and Bland Aerosol Therapy: Data as Summarized at Three Scientific Symposia

THERAPY	IMPROVEMENT OR POSITIVE EFFECT	QUESTIONABLE EFFECT	NO EFFECT	WORSENING
Humidity	**1.** Patients with bypassed upper airways (*e.g.,* endotracheal tubes)[4,6,30] **2.** Ventilator patients†[6,30] **3.** Patients on >2 liters/min or >30% oxygen therapy†	**1.** Croup **2.** Bronchiolitis		**1.** Asthma **2.** Anesthetized, intubated patients (USN with distilled water)[36]
Bland aerosol‡	**1.** Sputum induction for cytologic or bacteriologic studies **2.** Croup **3.** Patients with bypassed upper airways (*see* above) **4.** Postextubation or postbronchoscopy	**1.** Chronic bronchitis[27] **2.** Cystic fibrosis[2]	**1.** Emphysema[35] **2.** Pneumonia	**1.** Asthma§

*Criteria used included tests of respiratory function, mucociliary function, and improvement in subjective symptoms.
†Not reported specifically but alluded to in several presentations.
‡Bland aerosols: water; hypertonic, isotonic, and hypotonic saline.
§The bronchoconstrictor effect of bland aerosols can be prevented by prior or concomitant administration of β-adrenergic agents.[25] This is standard practice in many institutions (so-called sandwich therapy).

ignates the energy level of a substance. Zero on the Kelvin scale (absolute zero) is the level of no kinetic energy, at which all motion of molecules is said to cease, and everything is solid. Zero degrees Celsius (Centigrade) is equivalent to 273 degrees Kelvin (0°C = 273°K). Temperature conversions, including those from degrees Fahrenheit (F), are as follows:

Temperature in °F = (9/5 × °C) + 32

Temperature in °C = 5/9 (°F − 32)

Temperature in °K = °C + 273

The unit °K = unit °C = 1.8° in the Fahrenheit scale

The *critical temperature* of a substance, as explained by kinetic theory, is that energy level above which its molecules have the kinetic energy (energy of motion) necessary to overcome all the forces attracting molecules to each other. At or below the critical temperature, a substance can be liquefied by compression. At temperatures above the critical temperature, the substance is a gas, regardless of pressure.

The *critical pressure* is the vapor pressure of a substance at its critical temperature, that pressure required to liquefy a gas at its critical temperature, or that pressure required just to maintain a liquid at its critical temperature.

> *Example:* Carbon dioxide has a critical temperature of 31.1°C (304.1°K). Even though the pressure in a cylinder remains above the critical pressure of 73 atmospheres (55,480 mm Hg or 7396.7 kilopascals [kPa]*), the contents will be a gas at temperatures above 31.0°C. They will be part liquid and part gas below that temperature. *Note:* Below 31.7°C the CO_2 will boil, so that the CO_2 in the cylinder above the liquid can be defined as a gas because it is at, or above, the boiling temperature for that pressure.

The *boiling point* of a substance is that temperature at which the escaping tendency of the molecules (kinetic energy) equals the confining pressure of 1 atmosphere plus the adhesiveness of the intermolecular forces. At this temperature, as long as the pressure is 1 atmosphere or less, the substance will change completely to a gas (boil) as long as heat is added to maintain the temperature, while energy is used to change the liquid to a gas. The boiling point rises when total pressure rises and falls when total pressure falls.

The pressure at which a liquid will boil, at any given temperature, allowing all gas molecules to es-

*See Appendix F for an explanation of kPa.

cape as a gas, is called its *vapor pressure*. The boiling point is specifically defined as the temperature at which vapor pressure is 1 standard atmosphere and is characteristic of each substance.

A *vapor* is the molecular form of a substance below its boiling temperature, dispersed in a true gas (see above). Vapor will be present only if a true gas is also present. The vapor pressure of a liquid, however, at a specified temperature, is used to designate the escaping tendency of the molecules of that liquid that would at equilibrium produce an equal pressure of vapor in a gas phase, were it present. The vapor pressure of a liquid increases as temperature increases. Whenever ambient pressure is equal to or below its vapor pressure, a liquid boils (*i.e.*, becomes a gas).

Humidity is a term used to describe the water vapor *content* of environmental gases (Table 17-2). Various designations are used in speaking of humidity. *Absolute humidity* refers to the mass (weight) of water vapor in a given volume of gas. The absolute humidity of the air we breathe is usually maintained at a comfortable level by the balancing forces of nature (e.g., evaporation from bodies of water, rainfall, surface winds), although we are all familiar with the extremes of environmental humidity—the dry, parched air of the deserts and the "muggy," damp weather of the tropics. For purposes of respiratory therapy, absolute humidity is usually expressed as milligrams of water per liter of gas-vapor mixture.

Example: Usual air at room temperature (20°C or 293°K) has an absolute humidity of around 9 mg H_2O/liter) (0.5 mM/liter), whereas alveolar gas (at 37°C or 310°K) has an absolute humidity of 43.9 mg/liter (2.44 mM/liter).

Relative humidity, a percentage (Fig. 17-1), is 100 times the ratio of the amount of vapor actually present in the gas-vapor mixture (absolute humidity) to the potential amount of water (absolute humidity) that would be present were the same gas mixture in equilibrium with water at the designated temperature. The term "relative humidity" has no meaning unless the temperature of the gas-vapor mixture is also given.

Example: The room air described above (20°C or 293°K), having an absolute humidity of 9 mg/liter, has a relative humidity of 52%. This is derived by dividing the 9 mg/liter by 17.3 mg/liter—the absolute humidity of saturated gas at 20°C (203°K)—and multiplying by 100. One would therefore say that the room air had a relative humidity of 52% at 20°C.

Relative humidity can also be expressed as a percentage of saturation. In the above example, the room air would be described as 52% saturated at 20°C. If the room air containing 9 mg H_2O/liter were heated to a body temperature of 37°C (310°K), the relative humidity would now fall to 9 ÷ 43.9 × 100, or 21%. This gas would be described as 21% saturated at body temperature.

Table 17-2. Relation of Temperature to Water Content and Vapor Pressure in Saturated Gas

TEMPERATURE		WATER CONTENT (C_{H2O}) *mg/liter*	WATER VAPOR PRESSURE (P_{H2O}) *mm Hg*
Celsius	*Fahrenheit*		
0	32.0	4.85	4.58
5	41.0	6.80	6.54
10	50.0	9.40	9.20
15	59.0	12.83	12.79
16	60.8	13.64	13.62
17	62.6	14.47	14.51
18	64.4	15.36	15.46
19	66.2	16.31	16.45
20	68.0	17.30	17.51
21	69.8	18.35	18.62
22	71.6	19.42	19.79
23	73.4	20.58	21.02
24	75.2	21.78	22.32
25	77.0	23.04	23.69
26	78.8	24.36	25.13
27	80.6	25.75	26.65
28	82.4	27.22	28.25
29	84.2	28.75	29.94
30	86.0	30.35	31.71
31	87.8	32.01	33.58
32	89.6	33.76	35.53
33	91.4	35.61	37.59
34	93.2	37.57	39.75
35	95.0	39.60	42.02
36	96.8	41.70	44.40
37	98.6	43.90	46.90
38	100.4	46.19	49.51
39	102.2	48.59	52.26
40	104.0	51.10	55.13
41	105.8	53.70	58.14
42	107.6	56.50	61.30
43	109.4	59.50	64.59
44	111.2	62.50	68.05
45	113.0	65.60	71.66
50	122.0	83.20	92.30
55	131.0	104.60	117.85
60	140.0	130.50	149.19
100*	212.0*	598.00	760.00
121†	249.8†	1156.00	1530.00
374‡	705.2‡	400,000.00	165,452.00§

*Boiling point of water.
†Temperature, autoclave.
‡Critical temperature.
§Critical pressure (217.7 atm).

Water vapor capacity is often used to describe the absolute humidity of a gas sample when saturated at any given temperature. The contents of a liter of fully saturated gas (*i.e.*, its capacity) at various temperatures are given in Table 17-2.

Relative humidity at temperature T

$$= \frac{\text{water content of sample}}{\text{capacity of gas at temperature T}} \times 100$$

Relative humidity at temperature T

$$= \frac{\text{water vapor pressure of sample}}{\text{water vapor pressure of saturated gas at T}} \times 100$$

The *water vapor pressure* designates the partial pressure exerted by the water vapor present in vapor form in a gas sample. The fraction of water vapor in that gas sample may be obtained by dividing this vapor pressure by the total pressure.

Example: The vapor pressure in alveolar gas at 37°C (310°K) is 47 mm Hg (torr) (6.27 kPa). The fraction of water vapor in alveolar gas would then be 47 mm Hg (6.27 kPa) divided by 760 mm Hg (101.32 kPa) or 0.0619; thus the percentage of water vapor in alveolar gas is 6.19 at sea-level conditions.

Water vapor pressures in saturated gas are also given in Table 17-2.

If a gas-vapor mixture is cooled until "dew" condensates on the vessel or tubing containing it, the temperature at which this occurs is designated as the *dew point*. If one looks up the absolute humidity and vapor pressure of saturated gases at that temperature, one can find the water content and the vapor pressure of that sample.

Example: If the dew point is 37°C (310°K), the absolute humidity of the gas sample, whatever the temperature, will be 43.9 mg/liter. If the temperature of that gas sample had been 40°C, the relative humidity would have been 86% (43.9 ÷ 51.1 × 100) (see Table 17-1).

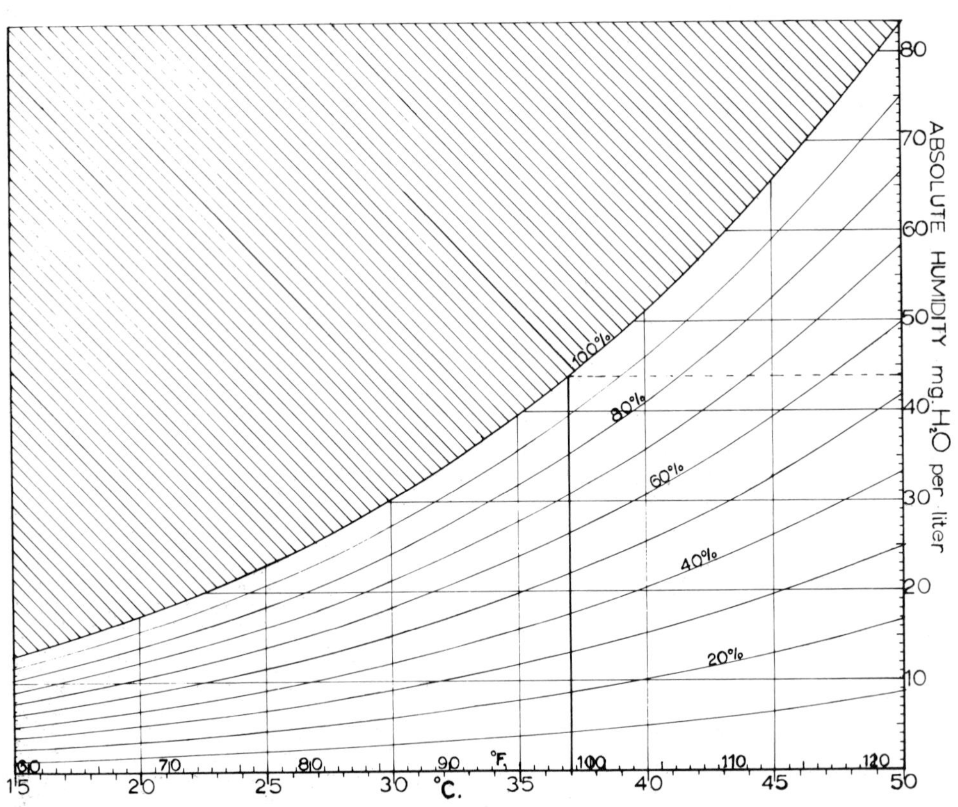

Fig. 17-1. The water content of air (absolute humidity) is depicted as a function of temperature. The shaded area indicates water content–temperature relationships not ordinarily found in nature. The various degrees of saturation are expressed as *relative* humidity (percentages) by the curved isopleths. The dotted line indicates absolute humidity at 100% body humidity, at normal body temperature.

By convention, 37°C (310°K or 98.6°F) is accepted as normal body temperature. Any gas having a water vapor content of 43.9 mg/liter (fully saturated gas at 37°C [310°K] and 100% relative humidity at 37°C [310°K] or having a dew point of 37°C) is said to have a *body humidity* of 100%. Any gas sample having a water vapor content of more than 43.9 mg/liter (e.g., saturated at a temperature higher than body temperature) will have a body humidity greater than 100%. Any gas sample containing less than 43.9 mg/liter will have a body humidity of less than 100%. The term *body humidity*, therefore, is useful in describing gas samples containing more than 43.9 mg H_2O/liter and is also helpful when one is talking about humidity deficits (see below).

By convention, whenever a gas sample contains insufficient water to provide for 100% body humidity (100% relative humidity at 37°C [310°K] or 43.9 mg/liter absolute humidity), it is said to have a *humidity deficit*. Theoretically, the body temperature of any patient in question should be measured, and humidity and saturated gas water content at the patient's temperature should be used, rather than the conventional 37°C. In practice, however, this refinement is unnecessary. One can speak of a humidity deficit of any gas sample that is not saturated, by giving the temperature of the sample in question. When no temperature is designated, body temperature is assumed, and the deficit is relative to body humidty.

Example: What is the humidity deficit in the gas described above under *relative humidity* (52% relative humidity at 20°C)? The absolute humidity is 9 mg/liter; 9 ÷ 43.9 × 100 = 21% body humidity; 100 − 21 = 79% humidity deficit. This can also be expressed as 43.9 − 9 = 34.9 mg/liter humidity deficit.

Heat capacity (or *specific heat*) is that amount of heat energy required to raise a unit weight of a substance 1°C or 1°K. The specific heat of water (cal/g/°C) can be considered to be 1.0.

The *heat of vaporization* is the heat energy required to change a unit mass of a liquid substance to a gas at the same temperature (usually defined for water as 539 cal to convert 1 g of water to 1 g of steam at 100°C [373°K]). The heat of vaporization is greater for water at temperatures below 100°C (e.g., when one perspires, the heat loss is greater than 539 cal/g of water loss). Heat loss from the respiratory tract mucosa owing to evaporation of water is likewise significant (579 cal/g H_2O loss).[33]

Under normal conditions in the respiratory tract, inspired air at 25°C and 50% relative humidity will be "air-conditioned," when a person is breathing through the nose, to produce an average relative humidity in the trachea of 70% at 34°C. Full saturation of the inspired gas is thought not to occur until the inspired gas has reached the third or fourth generation of airways (the so-called *isothermic saturation boundary*[11]). This boundary moves deeper into the lung with hyperventilation (e.g., during exercise).

THE THERMODYNAMICS OF HUMIDIFICATION

The three critical factors in humidification are temperature, the area of contact between the water and gas, and the time the gas and water are in contact. It is true that the higher the final temperature, the greater will be the water vapor concentration (or partial pressure) in equilibrium with water. It is also true that the greater the surface for evaporation, the more water will become a vapor in any given time, all other factors being equal. However, the *rate* at which equilibrium is approached and the *temperature at equilibrium* depends equally on the amount of heat available. Water requires more heat in changing from liquid to vapor than does any other substance familiar to man. If a dry gas and water are brought into contact, the temperature of both will fall unless heat is added to the system (evaporative cooling). No humidifier can produce 100% relative humidity at the temperature of the gas and water unless heat is also provided.

Example: Consider the humidification of 10 liters of dry oxygen at room temperature (20°C or 293°K) and 1 atmosphere pressure (760 mm Hg or 101.32 kPa). This 10 liters of oxygen weighs 13.31 g. Oxygen has a heat capacity of 0.2178 cal (0.911 joules*) per degree C. It will require 49.28 cal (206.24 joules) to raise the temperature of the gas to 37°C (13.31 × [37 − 20] × 0.2178). The increase in temperature will increase the volume to 10.58 liters (10 × 310 ÷ 293). When saturated with water vapor, the volume will increase further to 11.28 liters (10.58 × 760 ÷ 760 − 47). This volume of gas will contain 43.9 mg H_2O/liters or 495.08 mg. It will require 0.49508 × 17 × 1 or 8.42 cal (35.22 joules) to raise this water to 37°C. The amount of heat (heat of vaporization) required to change water at 37°C to a vapor at 37°C is 575.8 cal (2409.7 joules) per gram.

In this case, therefore, 285.07 cal (1193 joules) are used in evaporating the water. The above amounts of energy must be supplied from an external source or the temperature of the liquid and the gas involved will drop, thus preventing the required humidification. For example, were the gas to provide the energy required,

*See Appendix F under SI Units (Systeme International d'Unites) for an explanation of joules.

it would have to enter the system at 118.25°C above the 20°C, or at a temperature of 138.25°C. Were the water to supply the energy (*i.e.*, just that evaporated), it would have to be supplied at 692.4°C above the 20°C, or at 712.4°C. However, if a 100-ml reservoir of water were available, then a temperature of only 40.26°C would be required. Thus the easiest and most efficient way to provide the energy required for humidification is by heating the water in a reservoir. In this case, if the water in the reservoir is heated enough to supply 285.07 cal for every 10 liters of flow, without water temperature fall, the humidification will be continuous and at the same level. A large water reservoir is also a reservoir of heat.

To recapitulate, the humidification of 10 liters of dry gas in contact with water, all at room temperature (20°C or 293°K), will require (13.31 × [37 − 20] × 0.2178) + (0.49508 × 575.8) + (0.49508 × 17) cal to produce 11.28 liters of gas at 100% body humidity, or a total of 342.8 cal, or 1434.48 joules. Whenever evaporation takes place, the heat for evaporation must be provided, or a fall in temperature of the water and gas present will take place.

GAS AND FLUID DISPERSION: THE INCREASE OF SURFACE AREA

Since, by definition, a vapor cannot be present except in a true gas, evaporation of water can take place only at a gas interface. The vapor pressure is defined by its temperature. When there is no gas interface, however, no evaporation will take place. Vapor pressure expresses only the escaping tendency of the water molecules. The greater the area of the gas–water interface, the greater the number of escaping molecules. If heat energy is available, this rapid escape will continue. If no heat is available, a greater surface will simply increase the rate of temperature drop, which in turn decreases the rate of molecular escape (evaporation).

The airway system is a good example of an efficient means of increasing the water–gas interface. The trachea divides into the main bronchi, which in turn divide until, after 15 such divisions, there will be 16,384 branches. In the average lung, these thousands of bronchioles will have a diameter of approximately 0.6 mm each. The total cross-sectional area of the trachea is between 4.7 and 6.3 cm^2. The total cross-sectional area of the sum of the tubes after 15 divisions will have a cross-sectional area of 4.7 to 6.3 cm^2, whereas a similar length of the 15th generation tubes will have an area of 3088 cm^2.

By the time air reaches the alveolar level and division has taken place into millions of discrete chambers, the cross-sectional area is about 700,000 to 1,000,000 cm^2. Approximately 1.5 liters (at the end of a maximal exhalation) to 6.0 liters (at total lung capacity) of gas is thus exposed to a very large surface indeed.

Humidification is normally provided by the nose and upper airway, thus preventing mucosal drying and interference with normal clearance mechanisms of the lung (see Chaps. 16 and 21). The nose is also a heat and water conserver for the body. Inhaled gas must be heated and humidified except in exceptional circumstances. At nasal surfaces, water vapor and heat are added to the inhaled gas. These surfaces are cooled in the process. As exhalation begins, water condenses on the previously cooled surfaces and heat is returned. Exhaled gas is usually below body temperature as it leaves the nostrils, even though its relative humidity remains at 100%.

Efficient humidity and aerosol generation devices operate in much the same way as does the airway system. Whether one provides the increase in surface area by breaking up the air mass into tiny bubbles or breaking up the water mass into tiny particles, the surface area is increased exponentially. Thus devices that either break up gas into small bubbles in water or break up water into tiny particles in a gas provide tremendous surface for evaporation. If heat is added, the rate of humidification is proportionally increased. If heat is not added, the rate of cooling is proportionally increased.

Since the human airway is an ideal humidifier, one can ensure that secretions, if normal when produced, remain so if water loss is prevented. This can be done by providing at least 43.9 mg H_2O for every liter of inhaled gas, regardless of whether it is in the form of vapor (see section on Thermodynamics of Humidification) or liquid. For each liter of dry gas at room temperature, 49.5 mg H_2O are needed; thus the rounded-off figure of 0.05 g/liter or 0.5 cc of water per 10 liters of gas from a flowmeter is a useful rule of thumb. The airway itself will then evaporate the needed amount. The total amount of water needed is greater for the patient with a fever (see Table 17-2), if there is to be no humidity deficit.

EQUIPMENT FOR HUMIDIFICATION

When one attempts to classify humidification and aerosol therapy equipment in a fashion analogous to the classification of ventilators, immediate problems become apparent. The problem arises because devices that produce aerosols usually produce humidity (water vapor), whereas the reverse is less often true (i.e., many humidifiers produce only water vapor).

One simple classification contains two categories: "true" humidifiers, which add only water vapor to gases; and devices that add both water vapor and particulate water. This general classification, developed by Klein and coworkers,[19] is followed in our discussion.

TRUE HUMIDIFIERS

"Pass-over" Humidifiers

In "pass-over" humidifiers, gas is allowed to circulate over and around a water surface (Fig. 17-2A) or is made to flow through a water-containing vessel that also contains blotters, cloth, or other porous material. These materials may be stationary or moving through the water bath, as in the "rotating wick" humidifier (Fig. 17-2B). If heat is added to the water in any of these units, more efficient humidification for any given surface area will result.

"Bubblers"

In "bubbler" humidifiers, gas is broken into small particles as it passes through water. As emphasized above, the number of bubbles into which a given amount of gas is broken increases exponentially both the surface and the evaporation taking place. The efficiency of such "bubblers" is improved as the bubbles are made smaller. Humidifiers of this classification are most efficient at low flows (e.g., 2.5–5.0 liters/min) and characteristically have high airflow resistance (Fig. 17-3A). At these flow rates, they may be expected to humidify gas to between 38% and 48% relative humidity when warmed to 37°C. At higher flow rates, there is a dramatic and linear decrease in humidity output, since heat available becomes limiting and temperature falls until heat transfer equilibrium is established with the environment.[13,18,37] Devices in this classification include the Puritan Bubble/Jet, Ohio, Aqua-Pak 500, Hudson, McGaw, Ideal, and Inspiron units, some of which are disposable or prefilled with various solutions.

Unless heated, the water vapor output from bubble humidifiers is small (14.6–20.4 mg/liter) and is inversely proportional to flow, at least in four varieties of prefilled nebulizers recently tested.[10] Whether the molecular water contribution of unheated bubble humidifiers can correct a humidity deficit with eupneic breathing is debatable, but it is generally agreed that the humidity deficit is prevented from worsening during (otherwise dry) gas therapy.

Another type of "diffuser-bubbler" is that type of unit operating on the "cascade principle" (Fig. 17-3B). The efficiency of these units is considerably less flow-dependent, since the diffusers involved are of a lower resistance, allowing the production of more and smaller bubbles at higher gas flows. Such units are heated for more complete humidification and can be used in humidity tents, with high-flow oxygen enrichment systems, and in ventilator circuitry. Such units include the Bennett Cascade and Commonwealth Industrial Gases (CIG) humidifiers (permanent), and the McGaw and Aqua-Pak disposable devices.

MIST PRODUCERS AND "FOGGERS"

Mist producers and "foggers" constitute a category of devices that add both water vapor and particulate water to gas. High-density *fluid jets*, such as used by fire departments, are not used in clinical devices. In such units, extremely high fluid pressure forces fluid through small orifices into the gas, causing a fine "fog" that is ideal for smothering flames fed by highly combustible materials. The pressure and orifice size determine the particle size and volume of fog produced.

Atomizers

The term *atomizer* is conventionally used to apply to unbaffled devices producing a wide range of particle sizes, most of which are in the 30- to 100-μm range. Such units are ideal for depositing solutions on a surface in the path of the mist travel (Fig. 17-4). The usual

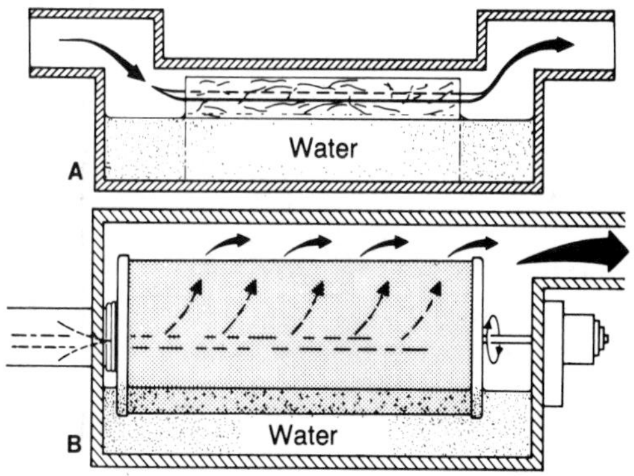

Figure 17-2. *A.* Section of "pass-over" humidifier. *B.* Section of rotating-wick humidifier. Gas passes through a porous cylinder that is kept wet by rotation through a water reservoir. High humidity cannot be produced by these types of devices unless heat is added. Type A can produce 10% to 20% relative humidity, and Type B can produce 30% to 40%, in desert or northern winter conditions, in relatively small (room-sized) areas.

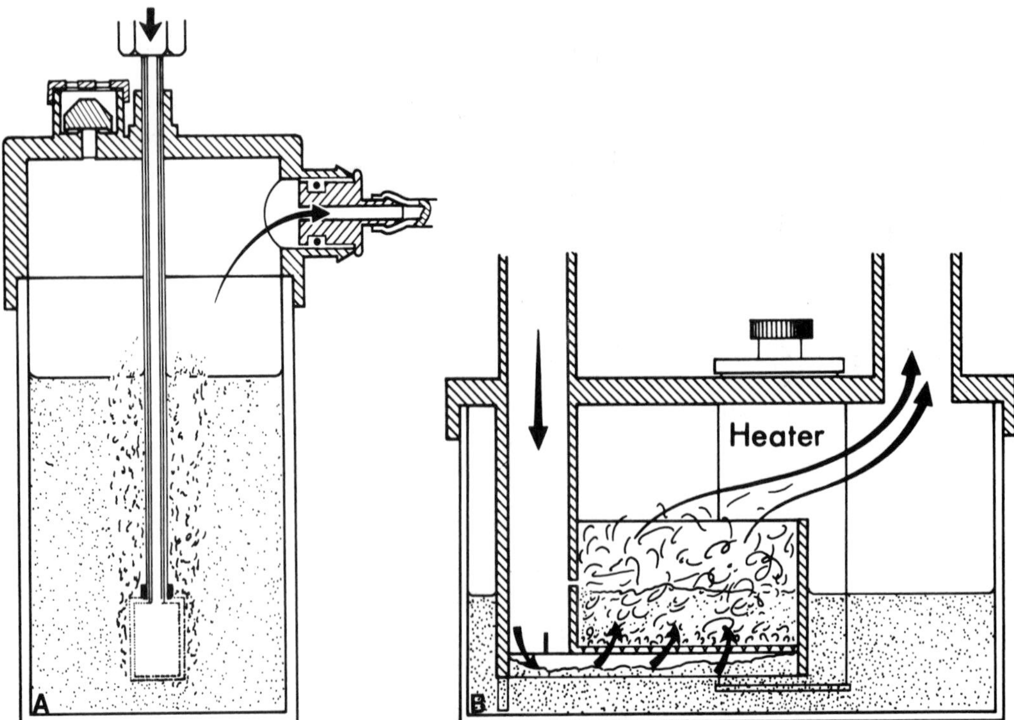

Figure 17-3. *A.* Section of a large-volume, "high-resistance" bubbler. These units are effective only when low gas flows are used, and even then produce only moderate humidification unless heated. These units are suitable for low-flow (masks, cannula, catheter) oxygen therapy. *B.* Section of a large-volume, "low-resistance" humidifier of the "cascade" type. These units may be heated. They allow higher flows than do "high-resistance" bubblers and may be used for high airflow oxygen enrichment therapy (with a Venturi mask) or in ventilator circuits. They must be heated to provide 100% body humidity.

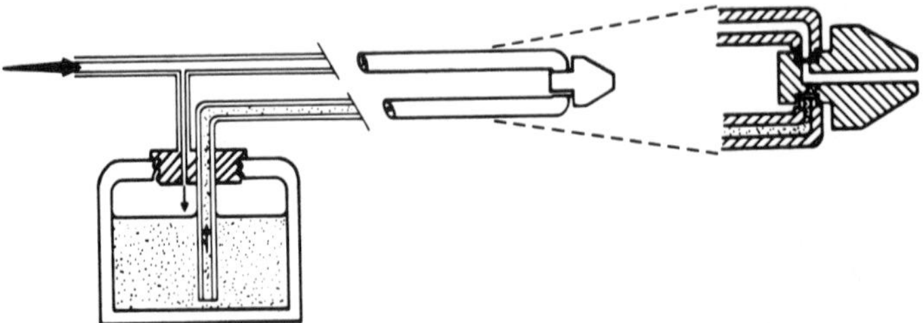

Fig. 17-4. Section of an atomizer, as commonly used in otolaryngology and endoscopy for application of local anesthetic. An enlargement of the air–fluid mixing nozzle is shown to the right. Most types of atomizers force fluid into a moving stream of gas and have a tip that can be rotated or angled to deposit fluid on desired surfaces. An atomizer is the basic unit of many nebulizers in which baffles are added.

hand-held atomizer forces fluid into the flowing gas stream at a mixing nozzle, where it exits as a mist. Other atomizers (not shown in Figure 17-4) function by drawing fluid into a jet as a result of the low boundary pressure produced (as explained by the Bernoulli theorem). Such units are conventionally called "Venturis," although the design is not quite that of Venturi's original device. Atomizers are effective devices that can provide adequate fluid for the body to use in humidification. The fact that particles of any size, once in the airway, will humidify is often ignored, and humidification too often is assumed to depend on the presence of small particles. Unless one wishes to guard against heat loss, introduction of larger particles of water into the airway provides the *most efficient* way of guarding against water loss.

Nebulizers

The term *nebulizer* is conventionally used to identify a baffled device that produces a relatively stable aerosol consisting of particles less than 30 μm in diameter.

Jet nebulizers entrain fluid from reservoirs of various sizes (as explained by the Bernoulli theorem) and are called "Venturis," particularly when also producing air entrainments to dilute carrier gas. The gas–fluid mixture impinges on a baffle (sometimes referred to as an impactor), which serves to fractionate or remove larger particles from the existing gas stream. Units such as those depicted in Figure 17-5 may produce heated or cold aerosols; some are disposable.

Another nebulizer is illustrated in Figure 17-6. This nebulizer uses the *Babbington* principle, which has been discussed in Chapter 16. A heated type of this unit is now available.

Ultrasonic nebulizers use fluid contained in a chamber that is shaken vigorously, producing a geyser of rapidly moving fluid that breaks into small particles (Fig. 17-7). Frequencies need not be ultrasonic, but particle size and nuisance value are reduced by increasing frequency to above the sonic range. Particles produced by physical vibration must be removed from the production chamber by a flowing gas. The physi-

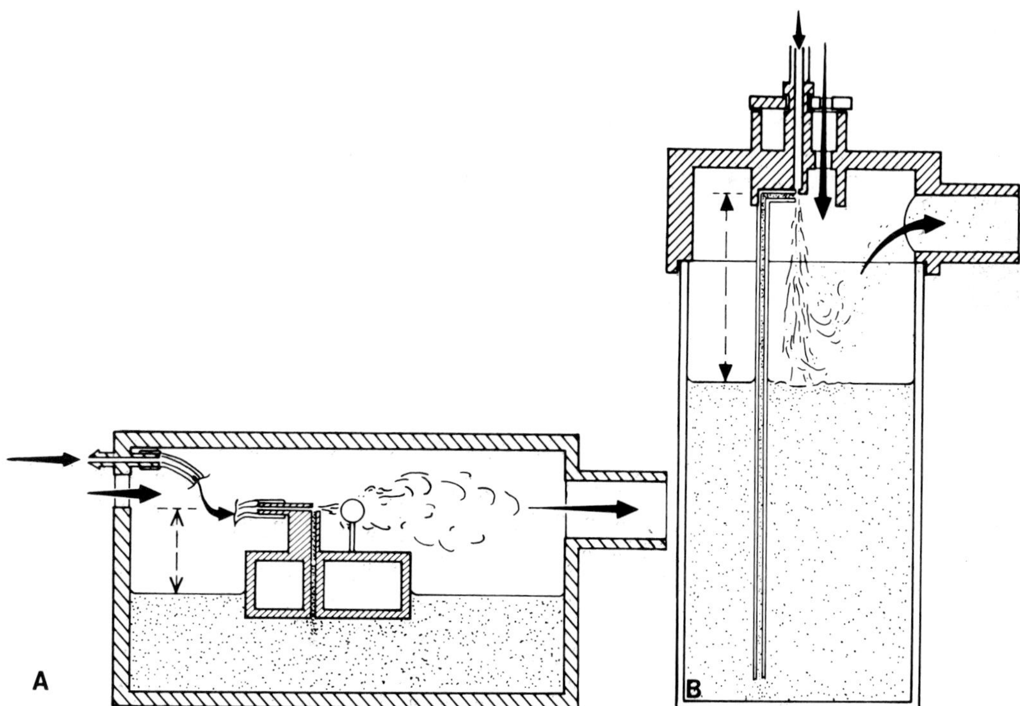

Fig. 17-5. Sections of jet nebulizers. *A.* A float type with a fixed fluid column length. *B.* A large-volume reservoir type, the fluid column of which becomes longer as the reservoir fluid level falls. In this type the output characteristics of the nebulizer change (for the worse) if the fluid volume in the reservoir falls below recommended levels. The vertical dashed line indicates the critical portion of the fluid column length.

cal motion imparted produces heat as well as dispersion. Unless evaporative heat removal is provided, the fluid will become very hot. The patient gas flow is generally sufficient to accomplish this purpose. This type of unit can produce a very dense fog and introduce entirely adequate amounts of water into the airway, even though the particle size is quite small.[1] Most jet humidifiers are not designed to do this. Thus, for preventing all evaporation, ultrasonic nebulizers are efficient without heaters, although the carrier gas itself may not be brought to full 100% relative humidity, even at ambient temperature.

Ultrasonic nebulizers have great usefulness in inducing sputum for cytologic or bacteriologic studies.[17,20] Sterile distilled water or hypertonic (10%) saline is used to promote coughing. Twenty percent propylene glycol was a favored aerosolized irritant for use in ultrasonic nebulizers, but its use has been abandoned since it inhibited the growth of *M. tuberculosis*.[39]

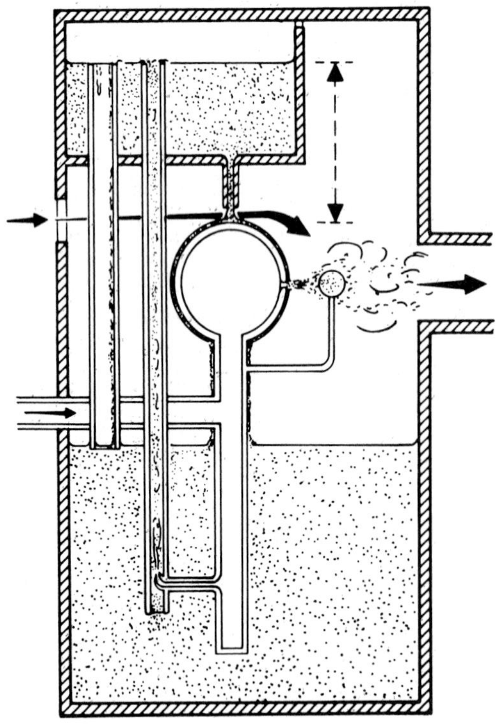

Fig. 17-6. Sectional diagram of a hydrosphere nebulizer that uses the Babbington principle. A thin film of fluid moves over the glass sphere toward a small orifice from which compressed gas escapes. At the gas–fluid interface, nebulization occurs by a highly efficient use of the Venturi principle: Fluid entrainment occurs around the entire circumference of the high-velocity gas jet. The aerosol is baffled in standard fashion. Such nebulizers may or may not be heated. The design allows increased fluid entrainment with increased gas flows (produced by increasing the pressure behind the orifice).

In a careful study by Malik and Jenkins,[22] patients with COPD complained of increased coughing and wheezing after inhalation of ultrasonically nebulized distilled water or 5% saline. Normal saline was generally better tolerated. There was a slight increase in airway resistance in those who tolerated the mist poorly, especially when 5% saline was used. These changes were short-lived and could be reversed by inhalation of isoproterenol. Lower levels of nebulizer output, preferably below 3.0 ml/min, were also better tolerated.

The amount of water introduced into the air stream is a function of the energy imparted to the fluid (other things remaining the same, this is proportional to the amount of current provided to the piezoelectric vibration generator) *and* the rate at which the existing carrier gas removes particles from the generator. Although the volume of water removed *per unit time* may increase as gas flow increases, the operating characteristics of most ultrasonic nebulizers are such that the actual volume of water removed *per volume of*

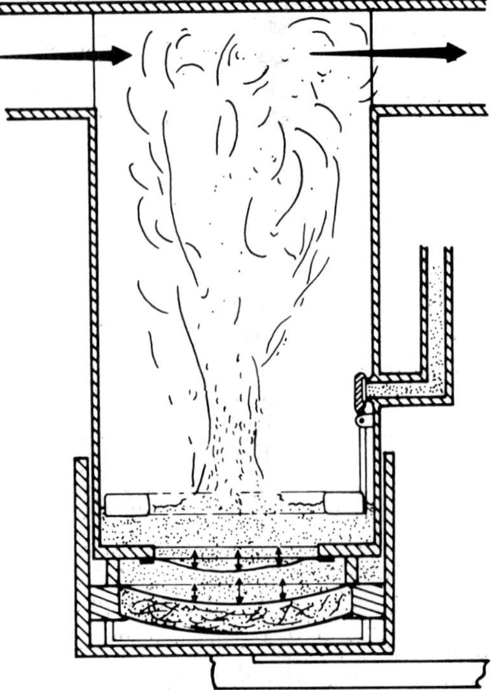

Fig. 17-7. Sectional diagram of an ultrasonic nebulizer. Small-sized (less than 5 μm in diameter) particles are produced by this type of nebulizer, which relies for its output on a ceramic or quartz diaphragm that responds to high-frequency alternating current (1.35 MHz) by the piezoelectric effect (*see* text).

carrier gas (aerosol density) may actually be reduced at higher gas flow rates.[19]

Centrifugal humidifiers operate on the principle of the centrifugal blower, which uses a rotating set of radially oriented blades that provide low pressure at the center and high pressure at the periphery. Water is raised by atmospheric pressure to the surface of a rotating disc (through a tube at the center with its lower end in water) on which the blades of the blower are mounted. The water is then flung, by centrifugal force, from the edges of the rotating disc against a screen set in the housing of the apparatus (Fig. 17-8). The generated gas stream picks up water broken up by the screen, and a mist-containing gas flows from the periphery of the rotating unit. The housing is channeled so that the mist may be blown into the room or into a tubing system. Such systems could be heated but usually are not, and are used allegedly to increase humidification in rooms. At best, some provide enough mist to prevent evaporation at body temperature in enclosures such as hoods or tents. "Centrifugal humidifiers" typify the problems with nomenclature when one attempts to classify such devices: here is a true nebulizer that functions most appropriately as a humidifier. The Defensor, DeVilbiss, Hankscraft, and Walton cool-spray humidifiers are examples of these units.

PRACTICAL CONSIDERATIONS

Although one can measure the humidity output of a device by rather complicated methods,[14,31] in the actual practice of respiratory therapy less complicated procedures are sufficient when used with understanding. The following two techniques are recommended.

1. When using a heated "true" humidifier, a thermometer should be put in the airway as close to the point at which the patient inhales as possible. If, at this point, the inflowing gas is at the same or a higher temperature than that of the patient and water is settling out in the tubing between the humidifier and the patient, the patient will get 100% body humidity. (*Note*: The temperature of the humidifier will necessarily be higher than that of the patient under these circumstances.) Thus measurement of temperature at the inhalation port in any apparatus is sufficient where a heated humidifier is raising the humidity of gas above 100% body humidity.

   Controversy still exists on the optimum temperature and water vapor content of humidified gases to be used in the patient with a bypassed upper airway. Sykes and coworkers[34] recommend between 80% and 100% relative humidity at between 32°–37°C for patients with artificial airways. If secretions are especially thick and tenacious, aerosolized solutions will need to be added to the treatment regimen (see below).
2. If particulate water is being provided, the entire set-up must be tested. The set-up (generator, water, and tubing system) to be used should be put on one pan of a large balance. This should be balanced against a large bottle of water by varying the water contained in the latter. The mist generator is then connected to an energy source or sources (electricity, compressed gas, or both) and run for a measured time, allowing gas and water to escape only at the point it will be provided to the patient.

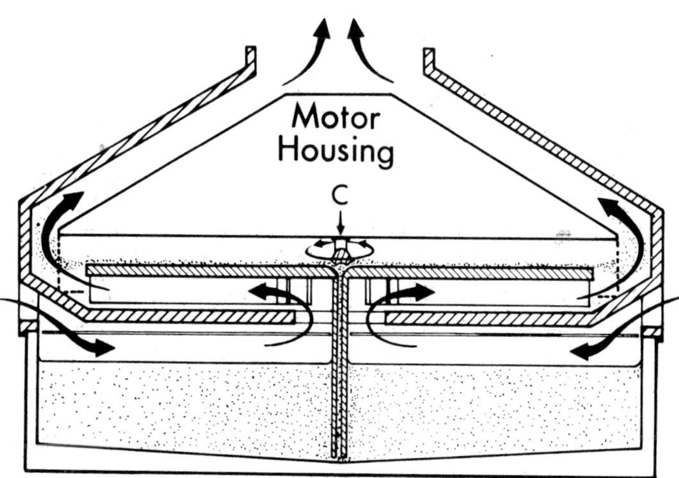

Fig. 17-8. Section of a spinning device, or centrifugal humidifier. Subatmospheric pressure is produced at the center of this device. Fluid rises from the reservoir to orifices around the central axle (*C*), where fluid is thrown peripherally against the baffling screen by centrifugal force. The aerosol generated is directed as desired by variations in design of the apparatus; the one shown is for room humidification.

Once again the set-up is balanced against the water-containing bottle. The water that must be removed from the bottle to achieve a balance will represent the water that will be provided to the patient during the time the apparatus was run during the test. Some care is needed in this procedure, if heated mists are used, to ensure that the test gives data at a stable temperature and not during warm-up or cooling-off periods.[3,19]

A word of warning: Measurement of humidity in the gas phase of a mist does not give an accurate measurement of the water available for humidification in the airway of the human being.[12,18] The relation of particle size to the amount of water vapor contained in a mist sample should be kept in mind (see Chap. 16).

Example: To provide 43.9 mg H_2O in 1 liter of gas (100% body humidity), the following numbers of spherical particles will have to be provided. (1 mg H_2O equals 1 mm^3, which equals 1×10^9 μm^3). If particles are 1 μm in diameter, 8.38×10^{10} particles per liter (8.38×10^7 particles per cm^3) are required (83,800,000 particles/cc). If particles are 10 μm in diameter, only 8.38×10^7 particles per liter ($8.38 \times 10^4/cm^3$) are required (83,000 particles/cc). If particles are 20 μm in diameter, only 1.05×10^7 particles per liter are required (10,500 particles/cc). If particles are 30 μm in diameter, 3.105×10^6 particles per liter are required (3000 particles/cc).

From the above one can readily appreciate why atomizers are quite satisfactory for providing water in particulate form for introduction directly into the airway of patients.

AEROSOL THERAPY

Man inhaled smoke (aerosols of a solid in a gas) before he discovered fire. Deposits of carbon, asbestos, and silica in the lungs bear witness to the fact that inhaled aerosols do indeed deposit material other than water in the airways and the alveoli. The purpose of this section is to review certain principles covered in Chapter 16, giving special attention to the inhalation of active materials for therapeutic purposes.

TERMINOLOGY

A *sol* is a mixture of colloidal particles suspended in a fluid. The particles may be another fluid or a solid. The term *aerosol* defines a suspension of colloidal particles in a gas or mixture of gases. *Smoke* is an aerosol in which the particles are solid. *Fogs and mists* are aerosols in which the particles are primarily water. In respiratory therapy, for some reason, the general term aerosol is used rather than the terms fog and mist.

The distinction between a true sol and a suspension from which the particles readily settle out has become blurred with use of the term aerosol. The spray generated by the usual atomizer is called by some an aerosol. Strictly speaking, a spray is distinguished from an aerosol by the former's content of large particles that are readily caused to settle out by gravity or to impinge on walls or baffles by their momentum as the gas stream is diverted.

FACTORS DETERMINING THE SETTLING-OUT OF PARTICLES IN SPRAYS AND AEROSOLS

Large particles are defined as those having a volume that is large relative to the surface area. Particles over 30 μm in diameter are considered large. These particles behave dynamically according to characteristics of systems with intermediate to large Reynolds' numbers.* The momentum of such particles (including their tendency to "settle out" owing to gravity) is a function of the mass of each particle. The forces acting on the surface that resist settling or movement in directions different from that of the gas stream are a function of gas density and viscosity, the particle surface area, and the velocity of the particle relative to that of the gas stream. If particles are the same size, those composed of denser materials will settle (sediment) more rapidly. Particles will also settle more rapidly in gases of lower density. Thus one can say that large particles influenced by gravity will settle out in a slow-moving gas in a horizontal channel and that they will tend to impinge on the walls when the tube is bent (i.e., when flow direction is changed) in fast-moving gas. This tendency to impinge (impaction) will be greatest when the velocity of the particle and the gas is greatest, and the terminal settling velocity attained by any particle relative to the gas will be a function of the density of the particle and the density of that gas.

When the dimensions of particles suspended in a gas are very small (less than 1 μm in diameter), the system is one characterized by a very small Reynolds' number. Under such circumstances, the important property of the gas is its viscosity, the density of both

*The Reynolds' number is a dimensionless number equal to

$$\frac{\text{velocity (cm/sec)} \times \text{diameter (cm} \times \text{density (g/cm}^3\text{)}}{\text{viscosity (Poise)}}$$

the gas and the material making up the particles having essentially no influence (the tendency of particles to move in this milieu is called *diffusion*). The primary determinants of the properties of such a system are surface effects. Very small particles suspended in a gas act in a characteristically viscous fashion. These particles develop practically no momentum, and any movement through the suspended gas causes enough drag to prevent rapid settling. When particles approach molecular size, the tendency to settle is entirely overcome by the intramolecular surface forces. Thus very small particles suspended in an inhaled gas will tend to be exhaled as well.

The characteristics of the airway that influence particle deposition have been discussed in Chapter 16. Certain conclusions can be drawn from those considerations. If large quantities of any material must be introduced into the smaller airways, either direct *spraying* of the materials is necessary or the materials should be *introduced as a liquid*. If the addition of a small amount of fluid would be beneficial, it can be introduced by an aerosol. If a chemical substance is remarkably active, it can be introduced as an aerosol. Bronchodilators, for example, are active in very low concentration. They can be given effectively by aerosol. Corticosteroids have been demonstrated to be effective when applied by this route.

Particles over 30 μm in diameter will almost uniformly settle out in the upper airway. Materials in solution deposited in these areas are absorbed through the mucous membranes. Particles less than 30 μm in diameter and greater than 5 μm in diameter tend to settle out in the airway at distances from the larynx that will be dependent on the velocity of inhalation and relation to gravity. Since the relative size of the airways and metabolic rates of individuals make the relative inhaled velocities quite uniform from person to person, the tendency for particles to settle in the airway can be generalized. Particles smaller than 30 μm will tend to enter the trachea; only particles of 5 μm or less enter the small airways, and particles smaller than 1 μm tend to be exhaled, avoiding deposition. This generalization applies to normal and moderately deep breathing patterns.[21,26]

As particle size decreases, the number of particles necessary to carry a certain amount of material rises by the power of two. Thus aerosols made up of very small particles will have to contain only very large numbers of particles per cubic centimeter to deliver a large quantity of material. This, together with the other factors mentioned above, makes it impossible to deposit large quantities of material in the small airways of the lung.[38]

Experience in the last 25 years has indicated that potent bronchodilators give best results with minimal side-effects if given by aerosol in dilute solution over 8 to 15 minutes. Concentrations used will depend on the potency of the material being given. Although concentrated solutions may give an immediate effect, the effect soon wears off. When a similar amount is given in a more dilute solution over a longer period, the effect may last several hours. Unfortunately, the exact details of the method of administration of bronchodilators by aerosol are rarely given in sufficient detail for one to judge with confidence the differences between administration of aerosols by the so-called T-tube technique (*see* below) and with intermittent positive pressure breathing devices.

EQUIPMENT FOR AEROSOL PRODUCTION

MEDICATION NEBULIZERS

At present many nebulizers on the market are designed to produce aerosols of medication (bronchodilators, mucolytics, and corticosteroids)[23,24] Examples of such units and descriptions of each are seen in Figure 17-9. Most can be hand-held, connected by a T-tube into a gas pressure source so that the delivery port held in the mouth will deliver aerosol when the other limb of the T is blocked. It has been amply demonstrated that bronchodilator administered by this technique is generally as effective as bronchodilator administered by any other method. To use this method, the person receiving the bronchodilator must use his thumb to block the T-tube just before inspiration begins; he must be capable of taking a slightly deeper than normal breath and be able to follow directions so as to avoid hyperventilation.

For any person incapable of the coordination necessary to block off the T-tube, the effort necessary to breathe a little deeper than normal, or the cooperation necessary to avoid serious hyperventilation, assistance to breathing is effective. Thus whenever assistance to breathing is necessary, intermittent positive pressure is the method of choice in giving a bronchodilator. Intermittent positive pressure has the advantage that the untrained person will receive some bronchodilator if the intermittent positive pressure machine is used properly. None of the other methods of giving bronchodilator medication can guarantee this.

With the advent of cromolyn sodium as an active agent in preventing asthmatic attacks, the use of

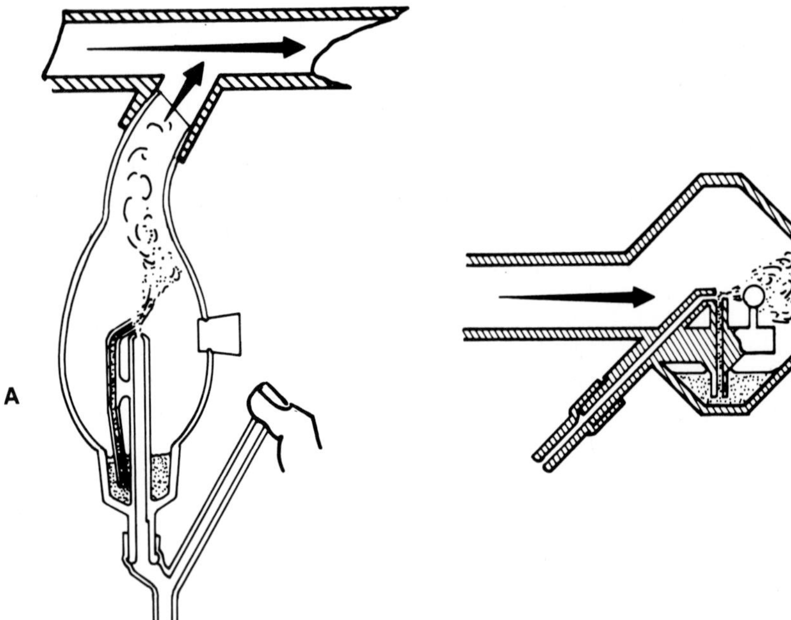

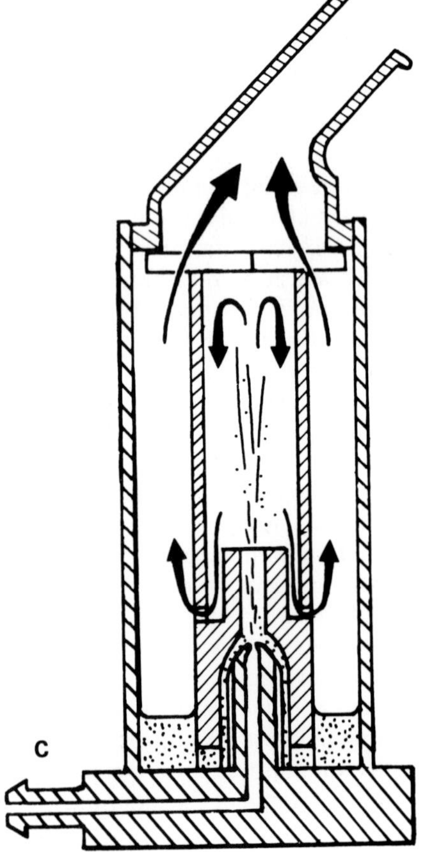

Fig. 17-9. Sections of medication nebulizers. *A.* Side-arm type, where mist is delivered into a moving gas stream. *B.* Mainstream unit; the total amount of mist delivered is influenced both by the flow of gas through the nebulizer and the flow in the mainstream. *C.* Nebulizer after a design by Dautreband. All of the above units can be used with a T-tube and air compressor, as is shown in *A.*

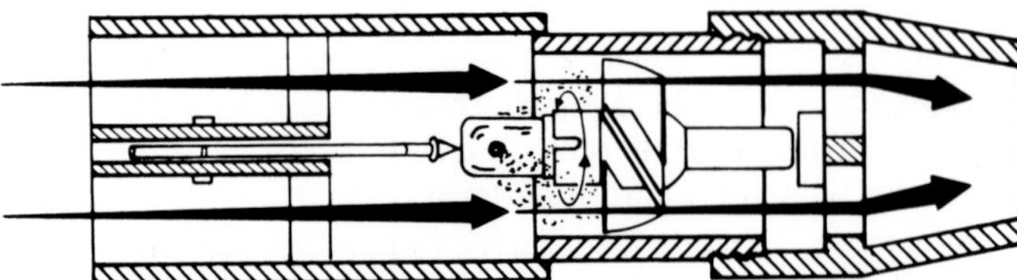

Fig. 17-10. Section of a spinning powder dispenser. Powder from a perforated capsule is spun into the inspiratory airflow, which causes the impeller vanes to rotate. Inspiratory flow produced by the patient both spins the vanes and the capsule and propels the powder into the airway.

equipment to disperse solids in the airstream has again come into vogue. Certain antibiotics were administered in this way at one time in the past. Suppliers should be consulted concerning this type of equipment. The rotating impeller and other devices used to disperse a powder during inhalation have proved effective (Fig. 17-10). Certain precautions are needed in using these devices that are adequately covered in the literature available with the apparatus.

Another popular method of administering aerosolized medication is by volatile propellants. A liquid with a boiling point well below room temperature (such as Freon), in which the material to be administered is soluble, is held in a pressure container and delivered through a small jet in bursts (Fig. 17-11). The propellant volatilizes, leaving behind tiny, dry particles that are then inhaled. It has been shown that bronchodilators are administered effectively this way. The units are designed to give a rather high dose of the bronchodilator in a single jet pulse. Multiple inhalations may lead to overdosage with adverse side-effects. Some of these side-effects, particularly cardiac arrhythmias, are thought to be due to the propellant itself.[5]

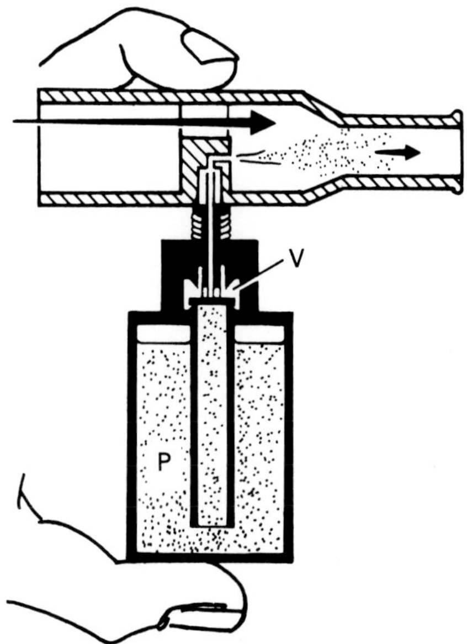

Fig. 17-11. Diagram of a gas-propelled hand nebulizer. The material to be delivered is dissolved in fluid with a boiling point below room temperature, confined in a pressurized container *(P)*. A valve is designed to release a measured volume of fluid *(V)*. Boiling liquid escapes and evaporates; particles of the active material continue in the airstream as dilute "smoke."

LARGE VOLUME FLUID NEBULIZERS

The patient's condition and tolerance for inhalation of larger quantities of aerosol vary greatly. For bland aerosol treatments, including sputum induction, inhalation periods of 30 to 60 minutes several times a day are usually recommended. In some conditions (e.g., croup, bronchiolitis, resolving pneumonias, particularly in childhood), nearly continuous therapy is recommended.

Equipment used for this type of aerosolization is depicted in Figures 17-5, 17-6, and 17-7. Large bore-tubing or tents are used so that "rainout" is minimal. Heated aerosols are generally used when lower airway secretions are a problem, as are cool aerosols for upper airway conditions. Repeated use tends to cause drying of the upper airway, owing to the desiccating effect of the propellant gas. Mucosal drying is associated with intensive use of the dry-powder inhalation devices as well.

DRUG RECONCENTRATION

A potential hazard of small-volume nebulizers is a phenomenon known as drug reconcentration. With operation of many nebulizers, droplets of medications (and diluent) return to the nebulizer because of baffling in the system. Glick[15] has demonstrated, in a study using acetylcysteine, that in a system using a dry carrier gas the diluent molecules are nebulized preferentially over those of the (heavier) drug. In 30 minutes' running time, the concentration of acetylcysteine rose from 20.5% to 40.1%, using ambient air. When humidified air was used, drug reconcentration did not occur. Evidently, this phenomenon is true with both jet and ultrasonic nebulizers and occurs in proportion to the molecular weight of the pharmacologic agent involved. If this is the case, the same might be expected to occur with saline solutions over time.

CONCLUSION

Operational characteristics of devices of all types are described by manufacturers. The foregoing material is designed to summarize principles that are applied by manufacturers in the design of their equipment. Before using any type of aerosol- or humidity-providing equipment, one must determine the principles involved so that rational use is ensured, proper precautions are observed, and malfunctions are avoided or identified and remedied.

REFERENCES

1. Abramson HA (ed): Proceedings of the Second Conference on Clinical Applications of the Ultrasonic Nebulizer. J Asthma Res 5:213, 1968
2. Barker R, Levison H: Effects of ultrasonically nebulized distilled water on airway dynamics in children with cystic fibrosis and asthma. J Pediatr 80:396, 1972
3. Brain J: Aerosol and humidity therapy. Am Rev Respir Dis 122(2):17, 1980
4. Chalon J, Ali M, Ramanathan S et al: Humidity and the anesthetized patient. Anesthesiology 50:195, 1979
5. Clark SW, Pavia D (eds): Lung mucociliary clearance and the deposition of therapeutic aerosols. Chest 805:789, 1981
6. Comer PB et al: Airway maintenance in patients with long-term endotracheal intubation. Crit Care Med 4:211, 1976
7. Communications relative to the datura stramonicum or thornapple: As a cure or relief of asthma. Edinburgh Med Surg J 8:364, 1812
8. DaCosta JM: Inhalations in the Treatment of Diseases of the Respiratory Passages, Particularly as Affected by the Use of Atomized Fluids. Philadelphia, JB Lippincott, 1867
9. Darin J: The need for rational criteria for the use of unheated bubble humidifiers. Respir Care 27:945, 1982
10. Darin J, Broadwell J, MacDonell R: An evaluation of water-vapor output from four brands of unheated, prefilled bubble humidifiers. Respir Care 27:41, 1982
11. Dery R: The evolution of heat and moisture in the respiratory tract during anesthesia with a non-rebreathing system. Can Anaesth Soc J 20:296, 1973
12. Dolan GK: Reply to letter to the editor. Respir Care 22:2, 134, 1977
13. Dolan GK, Zawadzki JJ: Performance characteristics of low-flow humidifiers. Respir Care 21:5, 393, 1976
14. Franks F (ed): Water—A Comprehensive Treatise, Vol 1, The Physics and Physical Chemistry of Water. New York, Plenum, 1972
15. Glick RV: Drug reconcentration in aerosol generators. Inhal Ther 15:179, 1970
16. Harris W: Aerosol propellants are toxic to the heart. JAMA 223:1508, 1973
17. Hensler NM, Spivey CG Jr, Dees TM: The use of hypertonic aerosol in production of sputum for diagnosis of tuberculosis. Chest 40:639, 1961
18. Hoover CM: Letter to the editor. Respir Care 22:2, 134, 1977
19. Klein EF et al: Performance characteristics of conventional and prototype humidifiers and nebulizers. Chest 64:690, 1973
20. Lillehei JP: Sputum induction with heated aerosol inhalations for the diagnosis of tuberculosis. Am Rev Respir Dis 84:276, 1961
21. Lourenco RV (ed): Inhaled aerosol symposium. Arch Intern Med 131:21, 1973
22. Malik SK, Jenkins DE: Alterations in airway dynamics following inhalation of ultrasonic mist. Chest 62:660, 1972
23. Mercer TT: Production of therapeutic aerosols—principles and techniques. Chest 80 [Suppl]:813, 1981
24. Mercer TT, Tillery MI, Chow HY: Operating characteristics of some compressed-air nebulizers. Am Ind Hyg Assoc J 29:66, 1968
25. Miller WF: Aerosol therapy in acute and chronic respiratory disease. Arch Intern Med 131:148, 1973
26. Morrow PE: Aerosol characterization and deposition. Am Rev Respir Dis 110:88, 1974
27. Pflug AE, Cheney FW Jr, Butler J: The effects of an ultrasonic aerosol on pulmonary mechanics and arterial blood gases in patients with chronic bronchitis. Am Rev Respir Dis 101:710, 1970
28. Pierce AK: Scientific basis of in-hospital respiratory therapy. Am Rev Respir Dis 122:1, 1980
29. Pierce AK, Saltzman HA (eds): Sugarloaf Conference on the Scientific Basis of Respiratory Therapy (section on aerosol therapy). Am Rev Respir Dis 110 [(6): Part 2]:1, 1974
30. Poulton TJ, Downs JB: Humidification of rapidly flowing gas. Crit Care Med 9:59, 1981
31. Ruskin RE (ed): Humidity and Moisture Measurement and Control in Science and Industry, Vol I. Principles and Methods of Measuring Humidity in Gases. New York, Reinhold, 1965
32. Spearman CB, Sheldon RL (eds): Egan's Fundamentals of Respiratory Therapy, 4th ed. St. Louis, CV Mosby, 1982
33. Strauss RH, McFadden ER, Ingram RH et al: Influence of heat and humidity on the airway obstruction induced by exercise in asthma. J Clin Invest 61:433, 1978
34. Sykes MK, McNicol MW, Campbell EJM: Respiratory Failure, 2nd ed. Oxford, Blackwell Scientific Publications, 1976
35. Taguchi JT: Effect of ultrasonic nebulization on blood gas tensions in chronic obstructive lung disease. Chest 60:356, 1971
36. Waltemath CL, Bergman NA: Increased respiratory resistance provoked by endotracheal administration of aerosols. Am Rev Respir Dis 108:520, 1973
37. Wells RE, Perera RD, Kinney JM: Humidification of oxygen during inhalation therapy. N Engl J Med 268:644, 1963
38. Woolsdorf J, Swift DL, Avery ME: Mist therapy reconsidered: An evaluation of the respiratory deposition of labelled water aerosols produced by jet and ultrasonic nebulizers. Pediatrics 43:799, 1969
39. Yue WY, Cohen SS: Sputum induction by newer inhalation methods in patients with pulmonary tuberculosis. Chest 51:611, 1967

18

Oxygen as a Drug: Chemical Properties, Benefits, and Hazards of Administration

Gene G. Ryerson • A. Jay Block

CHEMICAL PROPERTIES

Oxygen is a colorless, odorless, and tasteless gas that is essential for life of the human organism. The atmosphere contains 20.95% oxygen. This percentage of total pressure remains constant at higher altitudes as atmospheric pressure decreases. In both the free and combined forms, oxygen is one of the most plentiful chemical elements on earth. Oxygen makes up 89% of the weight of water; nearly half of the weight of rocks and minerals is oxygen.

An atom of oxygen has an atomic number of 8. Therefore its structure contains 8 nuclear protons and 8 orbital electrons. The extremely stable isotope O^{16} has 8 nuclear neutrons, resulting in an atomic weight of 16. Medical oxygen consists mainly of this isotope. In nature, however, the oxygen atom exists in 3 stable isotropic forms: O^{16}, O^{17}, and O^{18}, which occur in the approximate ratios of 1000:3.7:20, respectively.[16] The electron configuration of an oxygen atom allows electrons in the outer orbit to be shared with another atom (see Fig. 18-1). This outer orbit also allows room for 2 additional electrons, which accounts for the negative valence of 2. Two oxygen atoms combine to form molecular oxygen (O_2), with a molecular weight of 32. Molecules made of 3 oxygen atoms comprise the gas ozone (O_3). This allotropic form of oxygen results from the action of an electrical discharge or ultraviolet light on oxygen. Oxygen is extremely reactive and combines with many elements, resulting in a class of compounds called oxides.

The methods used to measure oxygen concentrations that are delivered to patients are based on physiochemical properties of the oxygen molecule.[25] Oxygen possesses unique *paramagnetic susceptibility*. When placed in a magnetic field, oxygen alters the configuration of the field. Nonparamagnetic gases such as ozone, carbon dioxide, and nitrogen are displaced out of the magnetic field. This special property of oxygen is due to its unpaired electron structure and forms the basis for paramagnetic analyzers. Bedside instruments can measure oxygen concentrations of 0.1% to 100%.

The *polarographic property* of oxygen is the basis for several electrochemical methods of measuring oxygen.[25] Electric cells are designed to analyze low concentrations of oxygen in either gas or liquid mixtures. The oxygen molecule will result in a flow of electrons, hence producing an electrical current. The electric cells are surrounded by an oxygen permeable membrane when dissolved oxygen is being measured in blood. Miniature electrochemical analyzers have even been designed to measure oxygen tension in blood vessels.

Mass spectrometry utilizes the ionization property of gases. In an ionization chamber, gas molecules,

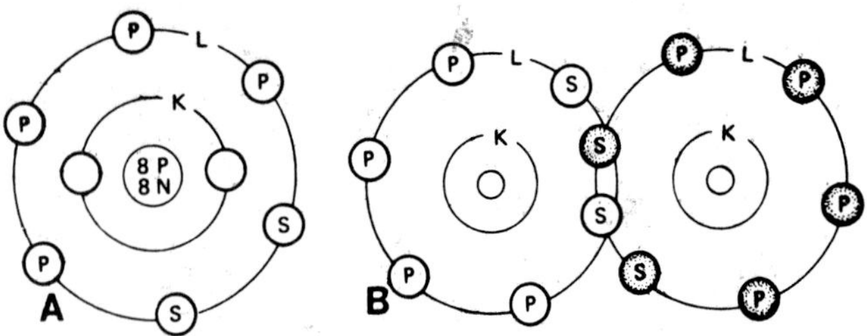

Fig. 18-1. Atomic structure of oxygen. *(A)* An atom of oxygen: The nucleus contains eight protons and eight neutrons; the electron configuration is composed of an inner *(K)* orbit of two electrons and an outer *(L)* orbit of six electrons. *(B)* A molecule of oxygen (two atoms). Note the sharing of the *s* electrons in the L orbit filling the capacity of that orbit.

including those of oxygen, are converted to positive ions by the loss of electrons. The gases are then separated according to the molecular mass of their ions.[45] The extremely rapid response time of spectrometers allows continuous, breath-by-breath oxygen analysis.

The primary commercial means of manufacturing oxygen is by liquefaction, followed by fractional distillation of air. This method utilizes differences in boiling points. A cooling process condenses air from the gaseous to the liquid state. As the temperature is slowly raised, nitrogen and inert gases evaporate before the boiling point of oxygen is reached. At atmospheric pressure, this boiling point of oxygen is −183°F. Liquid oxygen is then converted under high pressure to the gaseous state. Oxygen is stored in steel cylinders under a pressure of about 2000 pounds per square inch (psi). Characteristics of the most commonly used cylinders are listed in Table 18-1. The most frequently used are the D, E, G, and H cylinders. Emergency portable oxygen and anesthetic gases are most often stored in E cylinders. Since various gases are stored in cylinders, color coding is used for easy identification (Table 18-2). If oxygen is to remain in the liquid state, it must be stored at atmospheric pressure at a temperature below its boiling point.

ADVERSE EFFECTS OF OXYGEN THERAPY

HYPOVENTILATION

In certain clinical situations, the ventilatory drive that results from carbon dioxide stimulation of the respiratory centers is blunted. This phenomenon may be a consequence of a drug overdose, such as observed with barbiturates or heroin, or may result from chronic hypercarbia. Hypoventilation is of particular importance in patients with severe chronic obstructive pulmonary disease, where carbon dioxide retention and hypoxemia develop gradually over months. A major portion of these patients' ventilatory drive results from hypoxic stimulation of the carotid chemoreceptors. The arterial and cerebrospinal fluid pH usually shows at least a partially compensated respiratory acidosis. Thus the main stimulus for ventilation is hypoxemia. If this hypoxic drive is relieved, hypoventilation occurs and further carbon dioxide retention ensues. Although sometimes unavoidable, an important factor in carbon dioxide retention in patients with respiratory failure is the injudicious administration of excessive oxygen. Importantly, once carbon dioxide retention develops after oxygen administration, under no circumstances should oxygen be withdrawn or withheld. Without supplemental oxygen, dangerous hypoxemia will occur. If spontaneous ventilation becomes depressed, artificial ventilation should be instituted.

Table 18-1. Common Oxygen Cylinders

CYLINDER SIZE	EMPTY WEIGHT *lb*	OXYGEN VOLUME* *cu ft*	OXYGEN VOLUME* *liters*	AMOUNT OF OXYGEN AVAILABLE IN HOURS (APPROXIMATE), FLOW RATE 2 LITERS/MINUTE *hr*
D	10.25	12.6	356.0	3
E	15	22.0	622.0	5
G	100	186.0	5260.0	43
H–K	135	244.0	6900.0	56

*Measured at 70°F and 14.7 pounds per inch absolute.

Table 18-2. Color Codes of Compressed Gas Cylinders

GAS	UNITED STATES	ISO*
Oxygen (O_2)	Green	White
Air	Yellow	White and black
Carbon dioxide (CO_2)	Gray	Gray
Nitrous oxide (N_2O)	Blue	Blue
Cyclopropane (C_3H_6)	Orange	Orange
Helium (He)	Brown	Brown
Ethylene (C_2H_4)	Red	Violet
Carbon dioxide and oxygen (CO_2–O_2)	Gray and green	White and gray
Helium and oxygen (He–O_2)	Brown and green	White and brown

*International Standards Organizations recommendation for single color code for all cylinders.

ABSORPTION ATELECTASIS

Alveolar collapse may develop during inhalation of high oxygen concentrations. Nitrogen, an inert gas that is relatively insoluble in blood, maintains a residual volume in an alveolus. If oxygen replaces nitrogen, the gas volume within the alveolus is reduced because oxygen is rapidly absorbed into the blood. This is particularly likely in alveoli with low ventilation–perfusion ratios (perfusion in excess of ventilation). In pulmonary diseases that involve narrowing or obstruction of airways—for example, mucus retention—alveolar collapse may result within minutes after breathing pure oxygen.[44]

NORMOBARIC PULMONARY OXYGEN TOXICITY

Although the potential side-effects of oxygen were recognized for many years in animals, oxygen toxicity has only recently become a real clinical concern, primarily in intubated patients who require the delivery of continuous high concentrations of supplemental oxygen for long periods. Oxygen toxicity has been recorded to affect the lung, central nervous system, retina, hematopoietic system, and endocrine organs. Normobaric oxygen toxicity is most often manifested by pulmonary abnormalities and is therefore of greatest clinical importance.

Clinical and Pathologic Findings

The manifestations of lung toxicity can be separated into three clinical entities: tracheobronchitis; adult respiratory distress syndrome; and bronchopulmonary dysplasia, which is primarily a neonatal disorder.[11] It is not certain whether these syndromes are a progression of oxygen injury or are actually unique disorders. The earliest clinical findings in normal human volunteers after breathing 100% oxygen for 6 hours are cough and substernal chest pain.[37] This acute tracheobronchitis appears to result from an irritant effect of oxygen, which is transitory and tolerated by most patients. Bronchoscopic studies performed as early as 3 hours after breathing 90% to 95% oxygen have shown depressed tracheal–ciliary mobility and mucous clearance.[36] Pulmonary function, however, generally remains unchanged until 24 hours of oxygen breathing. At this point, the vital capacity progressively decreases. This dimunition appears to be the best objective index for the development of pulmonary oxygen toxicity.[6] Vital capacity, however, is a difficult maneuver to perform if the patient is unable to cooperate or has some type of mechanical limitation. The chest roentgenogram in these early stages usually remains normal, except for decreased lung volume. After 1 to 4 days of continued 100% oxygen exposure, patients develop progressive dyspnea, increasing hypoxemia, a productive cough, and a widened alveolar–arterial oxygen gradient. At this point, diffuse, patchy infiltrates first appear on the chest roentgenogram (see Fig. 18-2). Physical examination for the first time may show abnormalities of basilar rales.

In both humans and well-studied animal models, the pathologic pulmonary changes of hyperoxia are divided into an early exudative phase and a later proliferative phase.[46] Within 24 to 48 hours of oxygen exposure, exudative morphologic changes appear with the development of interstitial, perivascular and intraalveolar edema, hemorrhage, an influx of polymorphonuclear leukocytes, variable loss of type I alveolar pneumocytes, and necrosis of pulmonary capillary endothelium. After more than 72 hours of continued exposure and if the patient survives the acute phase, the proliferative phase begins, with reabsorption of early exudates and thickening of the alveolar septa. The relatively oxygen-resistant type II pneumocytes hypertrophy and increase in number. However, these surfactant-producing cells show signs of intracellular damage. Once this proliferative phase has been reached, total recovery is unlikely, and residual scarring is permanent with variable loss of lung function. The resulting clinical pattern is similar to that of pulmonary fibrosis. These chronic changes in the newborn are referred to as bronchopulmonary dysplasia.[1,33] Lung toxicity resulting from the administration of oxygen to infants with respiratory distress syndrome appears to be a major contributing factor for this disorder. The newborn lung possibly is more susceptible to the effects of oxygen toxicity.

Level of Exposure

The major determinants of hyperoxic lung injury are the partial pressure of oxygen in the inspired air ($P_{I_{O_2}}$) and the duration of exposure.[9,14] Although a high percentage of oxygen ($F_{I_{O_2}}$) is an important factor, this by itself is not toxic as long as the partial pressure is significantly low. Astronauts, for example, have tolerated many days of 100% oxygen, but at a barometric pressure of ⅓ of an atmosphere (about 250 mm Hg). The partial pressure of inspired oxygen ($P_{I_{O_2}}$) is the best guide of effective exposure. The $P_{I_{O_2}}$ is given by the equation $P_{I_{O_2}} = (P_B\text{-}47) \times F_{I_{O_2}}$, where P_B is barometric pressure in mm Hg, 47 is the partial pressure of water vapor at body temperature in mm Hg, and $F_{I_{O_2}}$ is the inspired oxygen concentration expressed as a decimal fraction. The $P_{I_{O_2}}$ is often stated in terms of atmospheres of oxygen as shown by the equation

$$\text{Atmospheres } O_2 = \frac{P_{I_{O_2}}}{760}$$

where 760 represents atmospheric pressure at sea level.

Pulmonary oxygen toxicity is a consequence of direct exposure of the lung parenchyma to excessive oxygen tension. Experimental studies in animals have demonstrated that the elevated alveolar oxygen concentration is the prime factor causing pulmonary oxygen toxicity, not the level of oxygen tension in systemic arterial blood (Pa_{O_2}).

The duration of exposure necessary to produce pulmonary oxygen toxicity is directly related to the $P_{I_{O_2}}$. In normal humans, there appears to be a threshold of 0.5 atmospheres of oxygen or an $F_{I_{O_2}}$ of 0.5% at sea level below which clinically apparent oxygen toxicity has not been reported. Despite variations in human susceptibility, there is little or no identifiable lung injury to humans exposed to 700 torr (approximately 100% oxygen at 1 atmosphere) for nearly 24 hours.

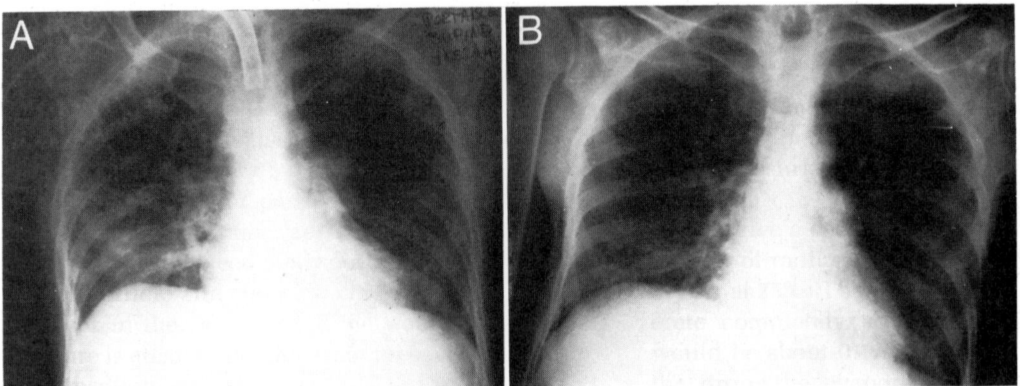

Fig. 18-2. *(A)* An AP roentgenogram of a patient exposed to 100% oxygen for 5 days. There is an alveolar-filling pattern in the lower half of the right lung and at the left base. These findings are consistent with oxygen toxicity. *(B)* In response to appropriate therapy the oxygen exposure was reduced to safe levels. The patient was eventually weaned from oxygen, and his roentgenogram at 6 weeks (shown here) had returned to normal.

Host Tolerance

Certain factors have been reported to potentiate the development of pulmonary oxygen toxicity, whereas others modify the syndrome.[6,43] Most experimental studies have been conducted in animal models, however, and therefore may not apply to humans. At present, prophylactic measures including various drugs have not been subjected to clinical evaluation and are therefore of no practical value. One notable exception is intermittent exposure to oxygen, which has been shown to delay the onset of pulmonary oxygen toxicity. If it is possible to reduce the FI_{O_2} for short periods every few hours during an exposure to a high oxygen tension, the duration of high tension exposure can be extended with a lessening of detrimental effects. In most clinical situations, this is not practical; however, intermittent therapy could be considered if high oxygen tensions are used to aid in the absorption of trapped body air such as is found in a pneumothorax. Another possible beneficial agent for preventing oxygen toxicity is the antioxidant vitamin E. Preliminary results in premature newborns who receive high fractional concentrations of inspired oxygen suggest that this vitamin may delay the onset of bronchopulmonary dysplasia.[10] This is a unique circumstance, however, in that newborns are vitamin E deficient. Since vitamin E deficiency is rarely encountered in adults, these results cannot be extended to older age groups.

Several factors appear to accelerate lung oxygen injury (*see* Table 18-3). Corticosteroids, sometimes used to treat critically ill patients, have had no beneficial effects in pulmonary oxygen toxicity. In fact, animal studies suggest that they may actually accelerate oxygen-induced lung damage.

Table 18-3. Factors Increasing Susceptibility to Oxygen Toxicity

Corticosteroids
Premature birth
Hyperthyroidism
Vitamin E deficiency
Hyperthermia
Adrenergic stimulation
Paraquat

Biochemical Mechanisms

The precise mechanisms of oxygen toxicity have not been well characterized in humans. The most widely accepted theory is that biologically active oxygen radicals induced by hyperoxia participate in this cytotoxic process.[14] Oxygen radicals are formed intracellularly by one of the many oxidase systems that donate an electron to oxygen. These oxygen metabolites, including superoxide, activated hydroxyl radical, hydrogen peroxide, and singlet oxygen, are all considered possible agents of hyperoxic tissue damage. These free radicals act to inhibit or inactivate sulfhydryl enzymes, disrupt DNA, or interact with membrane lipids, with resultant loss of membrane integrity. Superoxide is probably the radical most responsible for the biochemical alterations that result in the morphologic changes of oxygen toxicity (Fig. 18-3).[9]

Several natural cellular mechanisms are present in cells to protect themselves from oxidant damage. The three most important are superoxide dismutase; the sulfhydryl compounds; and antioxidant vitamins C and E. Superoxide dismutase is an enzyme whose sole function appears to be the inactivation of superoxide.[8] The most abundant sulfhydryl compound is glutathione, which acts to reduce compounds oxidized by oxygen or to be oxidized itself, hence acting as a scavenger of oxygen radicals. During prolonged hyperoxia, the production of activated oxygen mole-

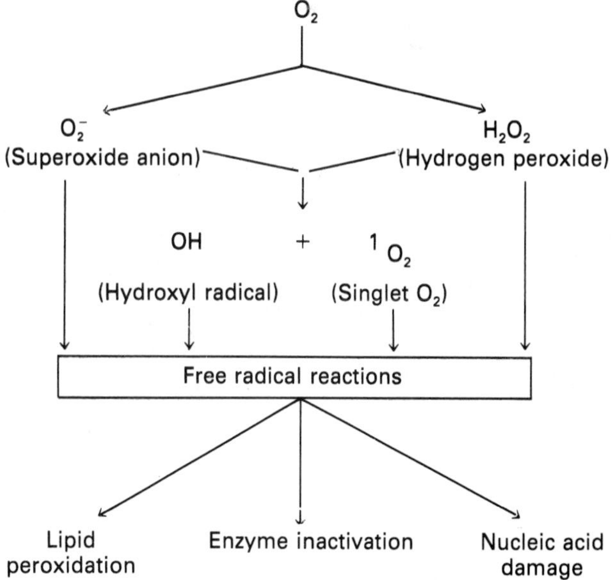

Fig. 18-3. Chemical mechanism of oxygen toxicity: free radical theory. (Drawn with suggestions by Dr. Edward R. Block).

cules may overwhelm natural antioxidant defenses, thereby allowing toxic morphologic changes in a lung to proceed unchecked.

Treatment

There is no specific therapy for pulmonary oxygen toxicity. The emphasis should be on prevention by adequate monitoring of the FI_{O_2}, employing the lowest level that allows adequate tissue oxygenation. One must be aware, however, of the relative dangers of hypoxia and hyperoxia. A patient should never be allowed to be exposed to hazardous levels of hypoxia because of the fear of producing oxygen toxicity. There is no evidence that a high FI_{O_2} causes any clinically significant damage when used for brief periods (i.e., during surgery or bronchoscopy). Clinical oxygen toxicity is a problem in the setting of prolonged severe respiratory failure. In these situations in which hyperoxic therapy is essential for managing an adult or neonatal patient, pulmonary oxygen toxicity can be avoided only by reducing the duration of exposure to high partial pressures of oxygen. This may be accomplished by using other techniques to improve gas exchange, such as positive end expiratory pressure (PEEP), mobilization of secretions, and decreasing bronchospasm.

HYPERBARIC OXYGEN TOXICITY

Under hyperbaric conditions, 100% oxygen accelerates the development of pulmonary oxygen toxicity. Exposure to pure oxygen at 2 atm of pressure results in the onset of dyspnea within about 8 hours. Vital capacity will begin to decrease after several hours (see Figs. 18-4, 18-5). However, the major toxicity of oxygen at a partial pressure of greater than 2 atm is a characteristic central nervous system syndrome. This

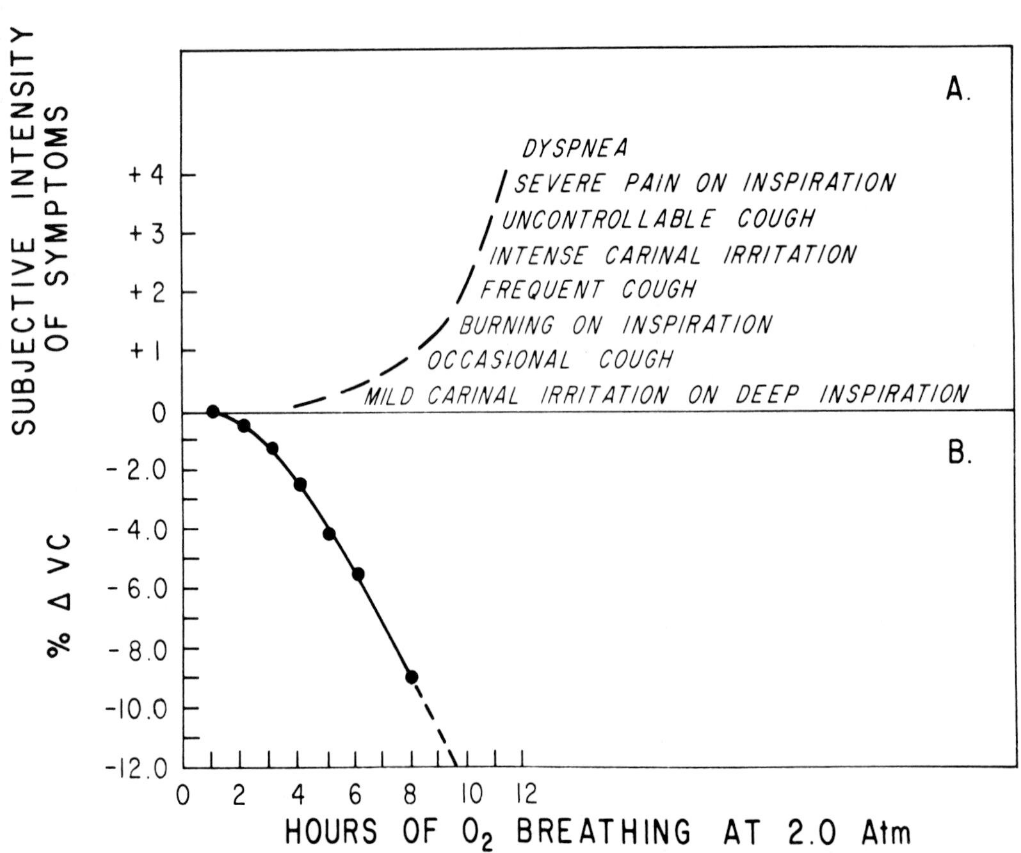

Fig. 18-4. The early clinical stage of oxygen toxicity. *(A)* Progression from mild (1+) to severe (4+) symptoms over the first 12 hours of exposure to 2.0 atm of oxygen. *(B)* Percentage of reduction of vital capacity (% ΔVC) with respect to time.

often appears as the first symptom in a hyperbaric environment.[7] Early manifestations are diverse and include muscular twitching, nausea, vertigo, paresthesias, and mood changes. Any of these minor symptoms may be rapidly followed by a grand mal seizure. If oxygen exposure is terminated at the onset of convulsions, there is usually no evidence of residual brain damage. Of course, physical trauma, especially in a debilitated patient, is a real danger during the seizure. The appearance of this syndrome is related to both the partial pressure of arterial oxygen and the duration of exposure. The symptoms may appear in less than 2 hours at 3 atm or in a few minutes at 6 atm of oxygen. The mechanism of this toxicity appears to be complex.

RETROLENTAL FIBROPLASIA

If excessive oxygen is administered to a premature newborn infant, immature retinal vessels constrict and endothelial cells are damaged.[18,32] Subsequent abnormalities, including disorganized vascular proliferation and retinal destruction, appear between the 3rd to the 6th week of life. These changes may progress to retinal detachment and blindness. The amount of retinal destruction depends on the degree of immaturity of the newborn, the length of exposure, and, importantly, the arterial P_{O_2}, not the inspired P_{O_2}.[18] It is not clear what the exact limits of oxygen tolerance are for the newborn retina; however, if the inspired oxygen concentration is adjusted to maintain the arterial P_{O_2} between 60 and 100 torr (the range of normal for the newborn), the risk of retrolental fibroplasia is minimized.[18,32]

Retinal injury can also occur in adults after exposure to 100% oxygen. This is especially true under hyperbaric conditions. Patients with previous retinal disease—that is, a history of retinal detachment causing compromised retinal circulation—are especially vulnerable.[28]

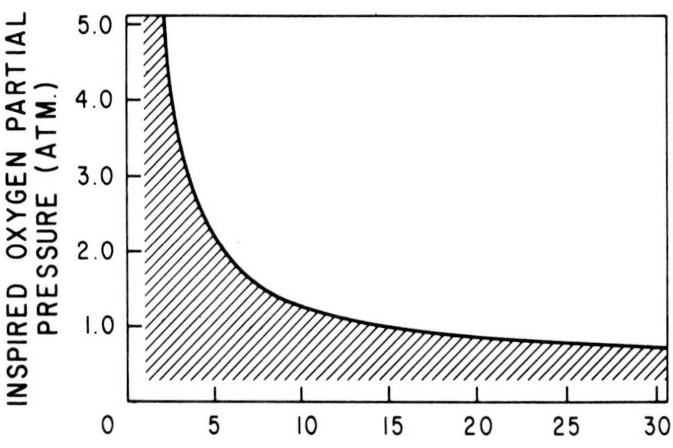

Fig. 18-5. Pulmonary oxygen tolerance curve in normal men based on a 4% decrease in vital capacity. Illustrated is a plot of the inspired oxygen partial pressure in atmospheres against duration of oxygen breathing in hours. Safe dose-duration combinations are indicated by the hatched area below the curvilinear line.

INDICATIONS FOR ACUTE OXYGEN THERAPY

Supplemental oxygen is widely used for various clinical disorders, both respiratory and nonrespiratory. Proper administration of oxygen should be based on sound physiologic principles. The primary therapeutic goal of oxygen is to prevent hypoxia, a deficiency of oxygen at the tissue level. Although hypoxemia, a deficiency of oxygen in arterial blood, is the most frequent index for estimating hypoxia, arterial P_{O_2} is only one of the variables of oxygen delivery. Adequate tissue oxygenation depends on several additional critical factors: hemoglobin level, the position of the oxyhemoglobin dissociation curve, cardiac output, and cellular oxygen uptake. The distinction between hypoxemia and hypoxia is important in managing patients. Although arterial hypoxemia is the most frequent cause of tissue hypoxia, tissue hypoxia may occur in the absence of hypoxemia.

ARTERIAL HYPOXEMIA

Arterial hypoxemia should be demonstrated and quantified before oxygen therapy is initiated, unless, of course, an emergency situation prevents measurement. The absolute level of hypoxemia at which supplemental oxygen is indicated for all patients is debatable. There is general agreement that an arterial P_{O_2} less than 45 mm Hg requires urgent treatment. However, on a physiologic basis, many patients receive supplemental oxygen at an arterial P_{O_2} of 60 mm Hg or less. Below this level, oxygen saturation rapidly drops for small decreases in arterial oxygen tension. In contrast, arterial P_{O_2} higher than 60 mm Hg may indicate a need for oxygen therapy in certain unstable patients with acute conditions such as pneumonia, pulmonary embolism, or a myocardial infarction. An arterial oxygen tension above 70 mm Hg will allow for abrupt changes owing to sudden deteriorations in gas exchange. Of course, the arterial oxygen tension that is miminally acceptable for each patient will be influenced by oxygen delivery, patient tolerance, and symptoms of hypoxia.

Arterial hypoxemia is the reason that most patients need supplemental oxygen. As reviewed in Chapter 12, there are four pathophysiologic mechanisms for hypoxemia: alveolar hypoventilation; a diffusion defect; ventilation–perfusion mismatching; and right-to-left intrapulmonary or cardiac shunt. Although more than one mechanism may be operative in a given patient with respiratory failure, one disorder often predominates. The most common physiological abnormality of hypoxemia in lung disease is mismatching of ventilation and perfusion. The next most frequent abnormality is intrapulmonary right-to-left shunts secondary to such diseases as pneumonia, atelectasis, or adult respiratory distress syndrome. These two common physiological mechanisms of hypoxemia can be distinguished acutely by increasing the inspired oxygen concentration. The arterial P_{O_2} increases readily in patients with ventilation–perfusion mismatching. In patients with right-to-left shunts, the arterial P_{O_2} does not improve significantly (see Fig. 18-6). Even increasing the inspired oxygen concentration to 100% will increase the arterial P_{O_2} by only a few mm Hg in severe shunting. Two contrasting examples of oxygen therapy for arterial hypoxemia will be discussed below.

Chronic Obstructive Pulmonary Disease

Ventilation–perfusion mismatching and alveolar hypoventilation are the primary mechanisms responsible for hypoxemia in acute respiratory failure secondary to chronic obstructive pulmonary disease. Controlled administration of oxygen is a cornerstone of therapy and an important therapeutic advance in managing this disease.[4] Since hypoxemia is mainly due to ventilation–perfusion mismatching, acceptable levels of arterial oxygen tension can be achieved at minimally elevated inspired oxygen concentrations. In addition, these patients are frequently less responsive to the respiratory stimulus of an elevated arterial carbon dioxide, and therefore depend on the hypoxemic effects of the peripheral chemoreceptors to preserve nonvoluntary respiration. Importantly, controlled oxygen does not depress the hypoxic drive to breathe. Figure 18-7 demonstrates how the shape of the oxyhemoglobin dissociation curve assists in correcting hypoxemia without promoting hypercapnia.

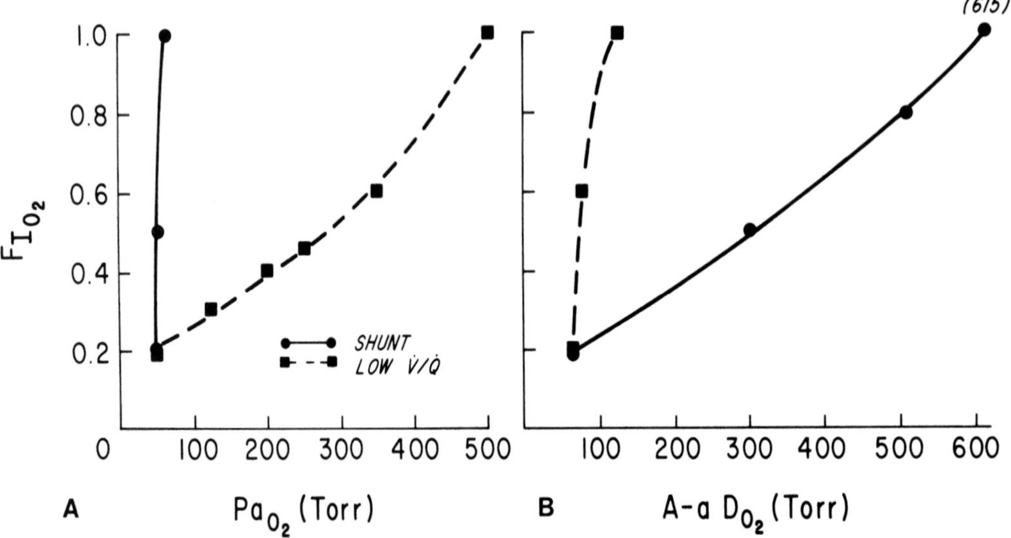

Fig. 18-6. *(A)* The effects of increasing fractional inspired oxygen ($F_{I_{O_2}}$) on arterial oxygen tension (Pa_{O_2}) in patients with shunt and low ventilation-perfusion relationships ($\dot{V}/\dot{Q}$). A patient with a 50% shunt has a change in arterial oxygen tension from 50 to 60 torr. By contrast, a patient with low $\dot{V}/\dot{Q}$ has a change in arterial oxygen tension from 50 to more than 500 torr. *(B)* The effects of increasing $F_{I_{O_2}}$ on alveolar–arterial oxygen difference (A-a D_{O_2}) in these two patients. In a patient with a shunt, raising the $F_{I_{O_2}}$ serves to markedly widen to A-a D_{O_2}. By contrast, in a patient with low $\dot{V}/\dot{Q}$ there is little widening of this gradient.

A small increase in arterial oxygen tension causes a large improvement in hemoglobin saturation when the initial oxygen measurements occur on the steep portion of this curve. This results in large increases in delivery of oxygen for a small change in arterial P_{O_2}. The hypoxic respiratory drive is functional when the arterial P_{O_2} is less than 60 mm Hg. In most cases, carbon dioxide narcosis occurs only if this level of arterial P_{O_2} has been exceeded. Furthermore, at an arterial P_{O_2} of 60 mm Hg, hemoglobin is about 90% saturated with oxygen. Since the upper portion of the dissociation curve plateaus beyond this point, additional increases in arterial P_{O_2} will only minimally increase hemoglobin saturation. Thus, in patients with acute respiratory failure associated with chronic obstructive pulmonary disease, the appropriate objective is to increase the arterial P_{O_2} to the 50 to 60 mm Hg range. This allows adequate tissue delivery of oxygen without depressing overall ventilation. Small increments of inspired oxygen can be delivered by nasal prongs at a low flow rate or by a Venturi mask. If a Venturi mask is used, arterial P_{O_2} can be predicted.[5] For example, on a 24% Venturi mask arterial P_{O_2} rises 8 to 10 mm Hg (Fig. 18-8). Although low concentrations of oxygen are used to produce an acceptable arterial oxygen level, other therapy for these patients is directed at reversing the factors that precipitated respiratory failure, such as bronchospasm or a superimposed infection. In most cases, patients do not require intubation or mechanical ventilation since they can be adequately treated with low-dose oxygen.

Adult Respiratory Distress Syndrome

Hypoxemia is part of a constellation of pathophysiological abnormalities that defines noncardiogenic pulmonary edema or adult respiratory distress syndrome. This diffuse lung injury results in increased capillary permeability and lung edema. Because of subsequent atelectasis and alveolar flooding, numerous alveoli are perfused but not ventilated. Therefore, the primary mechanism that decreases arterial oxygen tension is intrapulmonary shunting of blood. As is characteristic of a shunt, the hypoxemia of adult respiratory distress syndrome responds poorly to supplemental oxygen. On the other hand, elimination of carbon dioxide is generally not a problem early in the course of this disorder. Most patients exhibit hypoxemia with hypocarbia. Hence, oxygen therapy is not limited by respiratory depression, as is often the case in patients with chronic obstructive pulmonary disease. Instead, excessive inspired oxygen concentrations necessary

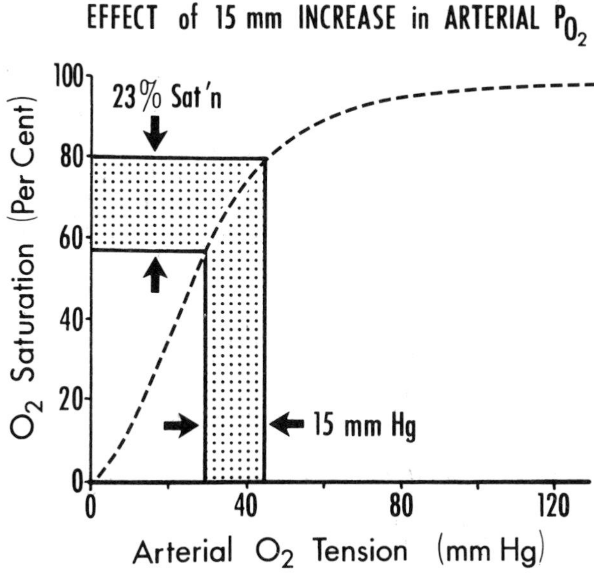

Fig. 18-7. Hemoglobin dissociation curve illustrating large increase in oxygen saturation for modest increase in arterial oxygen tension in the hypoxic patient who starts out on the steep portion of the curve. (From Block AJ: Management of pulmonary insufficiency. In The Acute Cardiac Emergency. Mt. Kisco, New York, Futura Publishing, 1972. Reproduced with permission.)

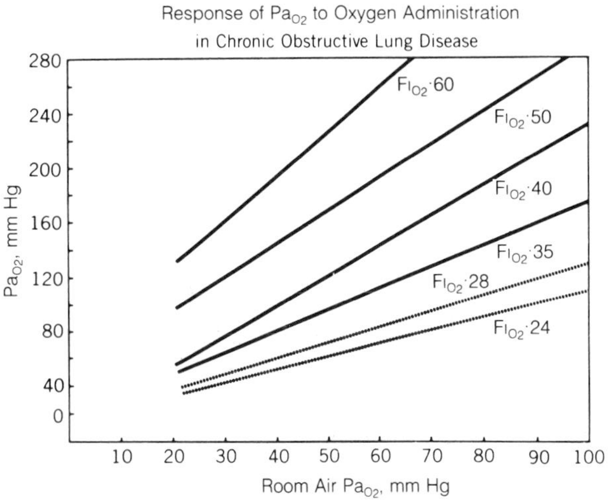

Fig. 18-8. Regression lines for different inspired percentage of oxygen (Fi_{O_2}). Each line gives the expected arterial oxygen tension and applied Fi_{O_2}. The relationship was obtained with patients in acute respiratory failure (*dashed lines*) and stable patients (*solid lines*). If a patient with chronic obstructive pulmonary disease presents with a certain arterial P_{O_2} on room air (*horizontal axis*), the resulting arterial P_{O_2}, after supplemental oxygen (*vertical axis*), can be predicted for an applied Fi_{O_2}. (From Bone RC: Arch Intern Med 140:1018, 1980. Reproduced with permission.)

to relieve hypoxemia increase the likelihood of pulmonary oxygen toxicity. If a patient does not have acceptable arterial oxygenation—for example, a Pa_{O_2} greater than 60 mm Hg with a nontoxic inspired oxygen concentration—other maneuvers such as PEEP with mechanical ventilation can be instituted.[21,42] Beneficial effects of this mode of therapy are attributable to an increase in lung volume, mainly the functional residual capacity, and the reestablishment of patency of airways and alveoli. This results in improved ventilation of gas exchange units; hence, shunting is decreased, arterial oxygen tension improves, and inspired oxygen concentration can be reduced.

TISSUE HYPOXIA WITHOUT HYPOXEMIA

Oxygen therapy is indicated in several clinical states in the absence of hypoxemia.[39] Since hemoglobin is near maximum saturation at a normal Pa_{O_2}, the only benefit of further increases in arterial P_{O_2} depends on dissolved oxygen. If an inspired oxygen tension of 100% is given, the arterial P_{O_2} is raised to nearly 650 mm Hg. At this level, about 2.1 ml of oxygen is dissolved in every 100 ml of blood. This dissolved oxygen can significantly enhance the amount of oxygen supplied to tissues. If a high concentration of oxygen is used, it must be supplied for brief periods to avoid oxygen toxicity. The indications for oxygen therapy in several hypoxic clinical situations will be reviewed below.

Anemic Hypoxia

Inadequate amounts of oxygen are delivered to tissue when the hemoglobin content of blood is markedly reduced, as in acute hemorrhage or anemia. The treatment should be aimed at increasing the hemoglobin level. However, immediate oxygen therapy is supportive until transfusions are available. Carbon monoxide poisoning is another example of anemic hypoxia in which the Pa_{O_2} may be normal. Oxygen is more than palliative, being the definitive treatment to reverse carboxyhemoglobinemia.

Circulatory Hypoxia

Oxygen therapy is generally recommended for patients with hypotension and congestive heart failure. In most cases, arterial oxygen tension is reduced. However, even in the face of a normal arterial P_{O_2}, inadequate tissue perfusion may result in tissue hypoxia. The mixed venous oxygen tension has been proposed as another index of measuring tissue oxygenation (see Chap. 12).[27] An increased inspired oxygen concentration is useful as palliative therapy until circulatory abnormalities can be corrected.

Cellular Hypoxia

Cyanide, a rapidly acting poison, is an example of agents that will cause cytotoxic hypoxia.[35] It reacts readily with the trivalent iron of cytochrome oxidase in mitochondria of cells. Cellular respiration is inhibited. Oxygen alone has only slightly beneficial effects in cyanide poisoning. However, oxygen may potentiate specific treatment, and therefore high concentrations should be used.[17]

CHRONIC OXYGEN THERAPY

Continuous low-flow oxygen at 1 to 4 liters per minute has emerged as an important aspect of outpatient respiratory therapy regimens, especially for managing patients with advanced chronic obstructive pulmonary disease (COPD). This oxygen therapy is supplied by both portable and stationary systems to selected patients with manifestations of sustained hypoxemia. Reports have shown that oxygen supplementation can improve exercise tolerance, decrease symptoms, return patients to ambulatory status, and prolong survival in patients with COPD.

EFFECTS OF CHRONIC OXYGEN THERAPY

In 1967, a study in Denver reported that six severely hypoxemic patients with COPD, who were bed-bound before therapy, markedly improved after 1 month of chronic oxygen administration via nasal cannula. The resting mean arterial P_{O_2} was raised from an initial level of 43 to 65 mm Hg with continuous oxygen. Five of the six patients were able to participate in rehabilitation programs.[24] In subsequent expanded studies, similar improvement in functional activity occurred; however, there was no measured improvement in these patients' pulmonary function. Further clinical studies, performed on groups of patients living at sea level, not only confirmed the initial Denver results, but also noted a decrease in the number of hospital admissions for oxygen-treated patients compared with control patients.[41]

Comprehensive neuropsychiatric studies on COPD patients treated with chronic oxygen therapy reveal significant changes after correction of hypoxemia. These improvements include intelligence, motor coordination, memory, and visual motor ability. Psychologic studies after correction of hypoxemia indicate that patients become more independent, less concerned with social problems, and better equipped to handle emotional stress. The relief of cerebral hypoxemia is postulated as the cause of this improved function.[23]

Polycythemia is an adaptive response due to chronic hypoxemia regularly found in altitude dwellers. However, the polycythemic response in hypoxemic COPD patients is unpredictable and appears to be inhibited by superimposed infections, iron deficiency, carbon dioxide retention, and congestive heart failure. If, however, secondary polycythemia develops in COPD patients, chronic oxygen therapy has reportedly been beneficial in reversing this compensatory mechanism.[24]

Pulmonary artery resistance and pressure increase in patients with COPD after induced hypoxemia and correlate inversely with the level of arterial saturation. The pulmonary hypertension in these patients is partly related to the vasoconstrictor response to the reduced arterial P_{O_2}. Studies have shown that the pulmonary artery pressure is reduced to normal in most patients with correction of arterial hypoxemia by domiciliary oxygen given over extended periods of 6 months or more. Several studies with small groups of patients have suggested that 15 to 18 hours of oxygen administration per day, but not 12 hours per day, can be effective in lowering pulmonary artery pressure.[40]

The National Heart, Lung, and Blood Institute recently conducted a controlled study of advanced COPD patients to determine whether 12 hours per day of oxygen (including the hours of sleep) might be just as effective as 24 hours per day of oxygen in terms of survival, neuropsychiatric function, and physiologic parameters, including reduction in pulmonary hypertension.[30] In this multicenter project, 203 patients were randomly allocated into either 12- or 24-hour per day oxygen groups. Patients entered this study only if they had clinically stable COPD with an FEV_1/FVC of less than 0.6 and a stable, resting arterial P_{O_2} of 55 mm Hg or less, or an arterial P_{O_2} of less than 60 mm Hg with associated evidence of tissue hypoxia such as polycythemia, cor pulmonale, or electrocardiographic evidence of right ventricular hypertrophy. Randomization resulted in close matching of the two groups, and the compliance to the oxygen treatment regimen was close to expected. The nocturnal group averaged 12 hours of oxygen per day, whereas the continuous group averaged 17.7 hours per day. The results revealed that continuous oxygen therapy is associated with a better survival than 12 hours per day or nocturnal therapy. In addition, the continuous group required fewer hospitalizations during the 2 years of observation. This study appears to indicate a beneficial effect on survival as well as improvement in physiologic and psychologic factors provided that chronic home oxygen is used for the major portion of the day (Fig. 18-9).

SELECTION OF PATIENTS AND DURATION OF TREATMENT

Chronic oxygen therapy has been most widely applied to patients with COPD, although the indications are certainly not confined to this disease. Whatever the underlying illness, arterial hypoxemia or tissue hypoxia must be documented. A committee of the American Thoracic Society has recommended criteria for home oxygen in COPD.[3] Candidates should have persistent resting hypoxemia with an arterial P_{O_2} of 55 mm Hg or less while breathing room air. The patient should be under optimal medical management, including treatment of bronchospasm, pneumonia, heart failure, and discontinuance of cigarette smoking. A single abnormal arterial blood gas measurement should not be the sole criterion for prescribing home oxygen. Some COPD patients with less severe arterial

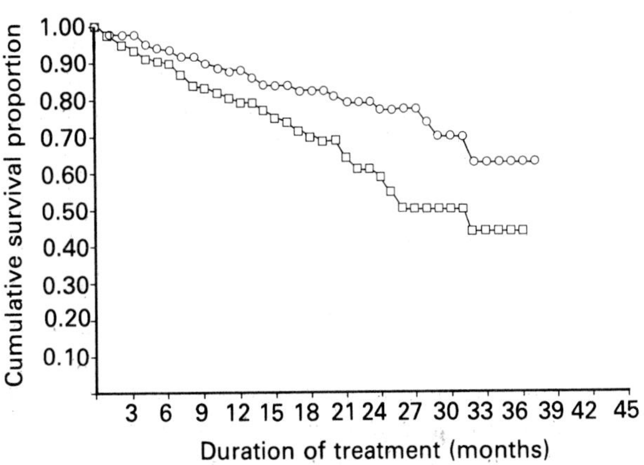

Fig. 18-9. Overall mortality of continuous oxygen therapy versus nocturnal oxygen therapy. Vertical axis is fraction of patients surviving; horizontal axis is time for randomization or duration of treatment. Open circles represent continuous oxygen, squares represent nocturnal oxygen. (From Nocturnal Oxygen Therapy Trial Group: Ann Intern Med 93:391, 1980. Reproduced with permission.)

hypoxemia are also candidates, but these patients must exhibit one or more manifestations of tissue hypoxia, including

1. pulmonary hypertension;
2. cor pulmonale;
3. increasing severity of arterial hypoxemia with exercise;
4. exercise limited by hypoxia but improved by oxygen administration; or
5. secondary polycythemia.

The arterial oxygen saturation decreases to very low values during sleep in some patients with COPD.[12] In some persons cor pulmonale apparently is potentiated by disordered breathing during sleep with frequent nocturnal apneic or hypopneic episodes. Some patients do not meet the criteria for continuous oxygen therapy on the basis of their arterial P_{O_2} while awake, yet might benefit from oxygen while asleep.[13] If cor pulmonale is present disproportionately to awake arterial blood gas findings, desaturation during sleep should be suspected. Confirmation can be obtained by monitoring arterial oxygen saturation during sleep.

The presence of carbon dioxide retention with chronic respiratory acidosis is not a contraindication to instituting chronic oxygen therapy; however, oxygen therapy should first be monitored in the hospital so that the oxygen flow can be adjusted and the effect on the patient's hypercapnia determined. Moreover, the patient must be informed and reliable regarding the dangers of high flow rates. At chronic low rates of flow that have been used in long-term oxygen therapy, a gradual rise in carbon dioxide tension does occur, but this hypercapnia has been well tolerated by patients.[41]

TECHNIQUES OF CHRONIC OXYGEN ADMINISTRATION

Oxygen is most often administered in the home using a nasal cannula at a predetermined low flow rate, usually 2 liters per minute. In patients with advanced COPD, this flow rate dose, however, may vary in the same patient depending on the ventilatory pattern. Mild increases in oxygen flows may be necessary during exercise or sleep. In the nocturnal oxygen trial, 1 liter per minute more oxygen was provided during exercise and sleep than during the rest of the day.[30] Goals of chronic oxygen therapy include improvement in the quality of life, allowance of an ambulatory existence, and, for some, prolonged survival. To accomplish this, both stationary and portable systems have been developed to provide practical, relatively inexpensive sources of oxygen. Portable systems allow the patient to be ambulatory and away from a large reservoir for up to 8 hours. Oxygen sources for home use are provided by conventional high-pressure oxygen cylinders, low-pressure liquid oxygen, or devices that concentrate oxygen from ambient air.[31,34]

Compressed Gas

Large oxygen tanks, usually of the H–K size, are preferable to smaller high-pressure oxygen cylinders because of the relative cost. Disadvantages of tanks include the heavy weight and the possible torpedo hazard. Either the tank or the valve apparatus is a potential projectile given sufficient damage to the valve end of the tank. Long extension tubing can be attached that will allow a patient some mobility within the home. Small portable tanks, containing nearly a 3-hour supply of oxygen at a flow of 2 liters per minute, are also widely available. These cylinders, some of aluminum construction, can be transfilled from a large reservoir tank at home. Transfilling must be done carefully because of a fire hazard that can result if any petroleum product lubricant is applied to the transfilling connectors.

Liquid Oxygen

The low-pressure liquid oxygen system comprises a reservoir cannister and a light-weight, readily transfillable portable device. Oxygen liquifies when its temperature is decreased to −183°F. The resulting volume of oxygen is less than 0.2% of an equivalent amount of oxygen at atmospheric pressure and temperature. Liquid oxygen is stored in a low-pressure, vacuum-insulated reservoir cannister that usually contains about 40 pounds of oxygen. This reservoir can provide a continuous flow of 2 liters per minute for 4½ days. Portable units that weigh about 11 pounds can supply enough oxygen to last about 8 hours at a flow rate of 2 liters per minute. The low pressure of the liquid oxygen systems allows lightweight construction of these portable units. This type of system allows the patient to be ambulatory and away from the reservoir for extended periods.

Concentrators

The most recent development for home oxygen is the oxygen enricher or oxygen concentrator. Ambient air is pumped either through banks of molecular sieves or a semipermeable membrane, which then preferentially separates oxygen from nitrogen. These devices can operate on household electricity and can deliver about 90% oxygen at a flow rate of 2 liters per minute. The oxygen concentrators are not portable, and small high-pressure tanks cannot be filled from these devices. However, this system is convenient for continuous oxygen therapy, and a 50-foot tube can allow ambulation in the home. A separate portable system may be necessary if the patient leaves his home. Disadvantages of the system are the added expense of electricity and the possibility of electrical outage. Patients should be advised to have a separate source of oxygen such as a compressed oxygen tank in the event of an electrical failure.

MODES OF OXYGEN DELIVERY

The many delivery devices available for supplemental oxygen can be divided into two major groups.[38] A *low-flow oxygen system* is an apparatus whose oxygen flow is not intended to provide the total inspiratory requirements of the patient. Each tidal volume contains a variable amount of room air. For this reason the inspired oxygen concentration is variable and is influenced by the patient's ventilatory pattern. This remains true even if the oxygen source for the apparatus is set at a high flow rate. A nasal cannula is an example of a low-flow oxygen system. On the other hand, a *high-flow system* has a reservoir and a total gas flow that supplies the entire inspired volume. The patient's ventilatory pattern has no effect on the inspired oxygen concentration. Under most circumstances, a Venturi mask falls into the high-flow category. In the intubated patient attached to a ventilator, a designated FI_{O_2} at levels ranging from that of room air to 100% can be prescribed. Because of the ventilator reservoir and flow rates, this is also a high-flow oxygen system. Several factors must be considered before selecting the technique of administering supplemental oxygen to patients. The desired range of the fractional oxygen concentration limits the type of the apparatus. If there is a danger of reducing the respiratory drive, especially in patients with hypercapnia, low concentration controlled oxygen therapy is warranted.

Commonly used methods of delivering oxygen in nonintubated patients will be described below (see Table 18-4).

Table 18-4. Oxygen Concentrations for Delivery Systems*

SYSTEM	O_2 FLOW RATE *(liters-min)*	FI_{O_2} RANGE
Nasal cannula	1	0.21–0.24
	2	0.23–0.28
	3	0.27–0.34
	4	0.31–0.38
	5–6	0.32–0.44
Venturi masks	4–6 (total flow = 105)†	0.24
	4–6 (total flow = 45)	0.28
	8–10 (total flow = 45)	0.35
	8–10 (total flow = 33)	0.40
	8–12 (total flow = 33)	0.50
Simple masks	5–6	0.30–0.45
	7–8	0.40–0.60
Masks with reservoirs	5	0.35–0.50
Partial rebreathing	7	0.35–0.75
	10	0.65–1.00
Nonrebreathing	4–10	0.40–1.00

*Values listed in this table are approximate.
†Values for total gas delivered are for the Accurox Venturi Mask.

NASAL CANNULA AND PRONGS

Low concentrations of inspired oxygen can be provided by nasal cannula or prongs, are generally inexpensive, well tolerated by patients, and are one of the most commonly used devices.[22] This simple system consists of delivering 100% oxygen through two prongs inserted 1 cm into each anterior nare (*see* Fig. 18-10A). The cannulas are made of unobtrusive, soft plastic and are generally comfortable for long-term use. The nasal passages should be patent. Mouth breathing does not, however, significantly affect the final oxygen concentration since inspired ambient air flow in the oral pharynx entrains oxygen from the nasopharynx. The prongs must also be positioned properly since malposition can reduce the FI_{O_2}.[29]

Because this is a low-flow oxygen system, the final concentration of oxygen received by the patient depends on a mixture of ambient air and oxygen and is therefore sensitive to changes in tidal volume and ventilatory pattern. If the tidal volume is large, the FI_{O_2} will be low; if the tidal volume is small, the FI_{O_2}

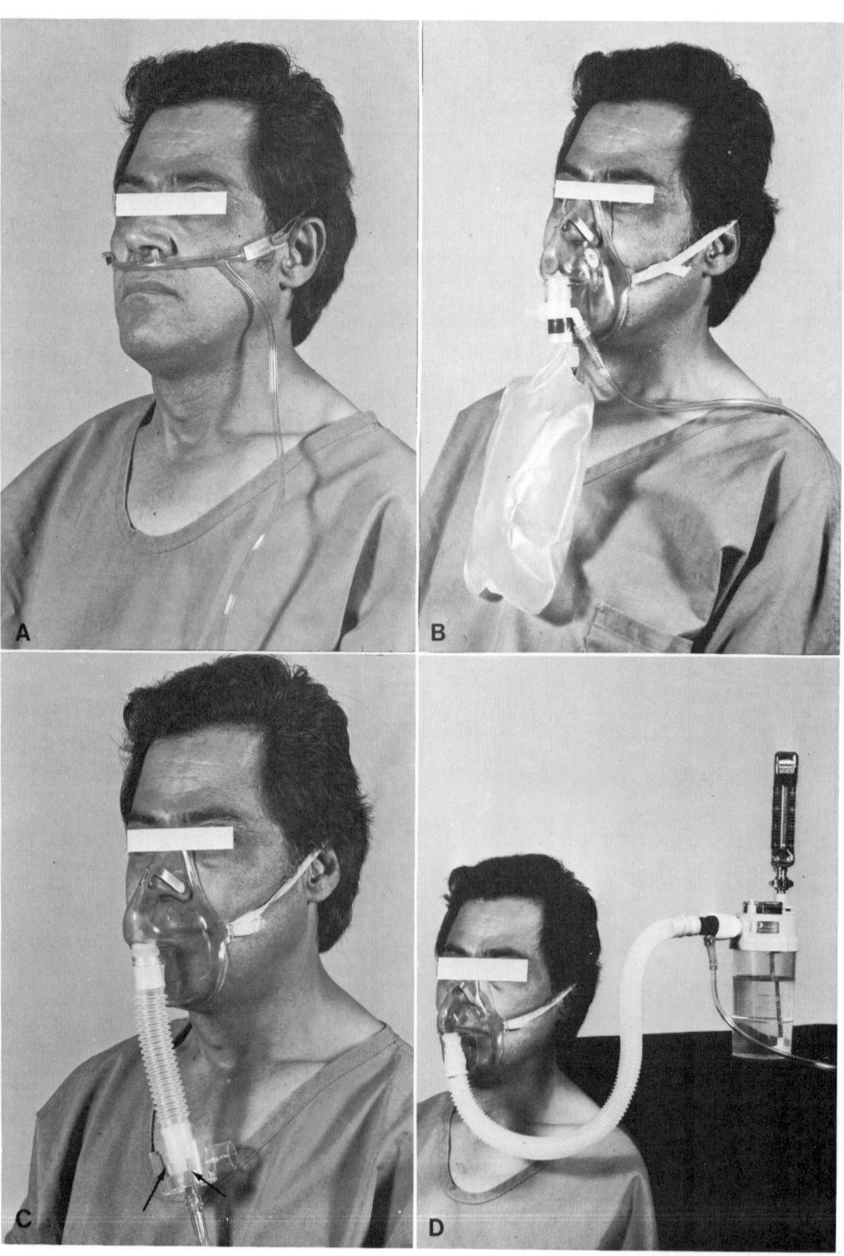

Fig. 18-10. *(A)* Nasal prongs. The patient is receiving 100% oxygen at a low flow rate (*i.e.,* 2 liters/min.). *(B)* Tight-fitting mask with reservoir bag. The patient is breathing 100% oxygen delivered by the thin tubing to both the mask and a reservoir bag. Note the mask contains two one-way expiratory valves to permit exhalation without FI_{O_2} dilution. The reservoir bag supports high flow rates. *(C)* Venturi mask. The source gas entering the thin tubing is 100% oxygen but is diluted down to a fixed FI_{O_2} (*i.e.,* 24, 28, 35, 40%) by the air as it enters the specially constructed openings (arrows) of the Venturi system. This unit is equipped with a humidification port as well. *(D)* High airflow oxygen enrichment with nebulization. Gas (air/O_2) at a high flow rate is provided from a Venturi-type nebulizer. Low flow-rate oxygen can be delivered through a side port, producing oxygen enrichment in the wide-bore tubing with resultant oxygen levels between 22% and 40% FI_{O_2}.

will be higher. A child will receive a higher FI_{O_2} with nasal prongs than will an adult given the same oxygen flow rate. This low-flow system does not provide a low concentration of oxygen if the patient is hypoventilating. On the other hand a hyperventilating, dyspneic patient may receive a reduced FI_{O_2} because of increased dilution with ambient air. Therefore if nasal prongs are selected for oxygen supplementation. the arterial P_{O_2} must be monitored frequently to measure the therapeutic effect.

Generally flow rates of 1 to 4 liters per minute are used with the desired FI_{O_2} ranging from about 24% to 40%. Higher flow rates by nasal cannula—that is, 7 to 8 liters per minute, should be avoided because they cause crusting of secretions and drying of the nasal mucosa. Despite these various practical limitations, nasal prongs have many valuable uses.

1. Chronic domiciliary oxygen
2. Patients without hypercapnia who require supplemental oxygen up to an FI_{O_2} of 40%
3. Patients who require low concentrations of controlled oxygen but who cannot tolerate mask devices

VENTURI MASKS

A technique based on the Bernoulli principle is one of the most accurate methods of delivering a prescribed dose of oxygen. These masks are engineered to provide controlled oxygen to the patient, which is achieved by flowing 100% oxygen through a narrowed orifice, resulting in a high velocity stream that creates a "subatmospheric" pressure after leaving the orifice. This in turn entrains room air through multiple open side ports at the base of the mask. Primarily by altering the orifice size, the FI_{O_2} can be varied (Figs. 18-10C, 18-11). Above a minimum oxygen flow, the flow rate can be altered without causing a significant change in the ratio of oxygen to entrained room air, and thus, in the resulting FI_{O_2}, Venturi masks can provide a range of specific oxygen concentrations from 24% to 50%. These masks are accurate to within 1% to 2% of the stated concentration on the base of the mask.[15] As a result of the entrainment of large quantities of air, a large volume of enriched gas is delivered to the patient. Therefore the pattern and volume of the patient's ventilation will not affect the specific inspired oxygen concentration delivered by these masks.

Venturi masks have wide clinical uses, and their value has been well proved. They are particularly efficacious in treating hypoxic–hypercapnic respiratory failure when there is a danger of respiratory depression from excessive inspired oxygen concentrations. Further, the 40% Venturi mask is particularly useful in patients without danger of respiratory depression but who require prolonged oxygen treatment at nontoxic oxygen concentrations. There are several disadvantages from this mask: a feeling of claustrophobia, especially in an anxious, dyspneic patient; the removal of the mask by patients so that they may ingest meals or expectorate; and discomfort. Also, because this system requires high-flow rates of oxygen, it is relatively expensive and not practical for chronic home use.

OPEN FACE MASK

Simple open face masks cover the nose and mouth and deliver oxygen concentrations up to 60%. Oxygen flow rates of 5 to 6 liters per minute are required so that the patient does not accumulate carbon dioxide within the mask. Open face masks do not allow precise inspired oxygen concentrations and are impractical in situations requiring controlled oxygen. If the mask is designed to fit the patient's face tightly, the amount of ambient air dilution with each inspiration will be lower; therefore, a higher inspired oxygen concentration will be achieved. One of the main uses for simple masks is humidification or aerosol therapy with oxygen. A disadvantage is that the FI_{O_2} is variable

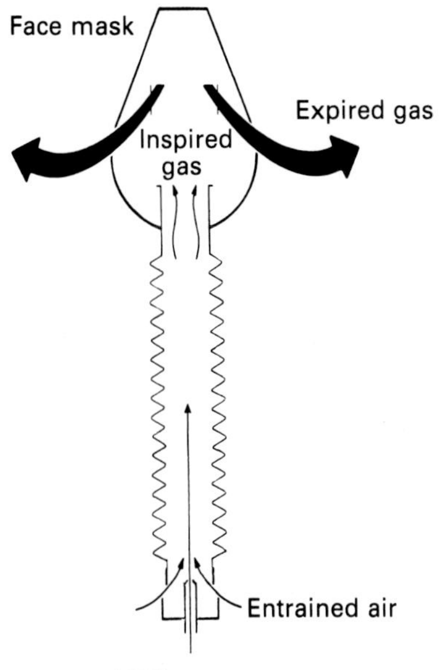

Fig. 18-11. Air flow diagram with Venturi mask. Arrows indicate direction of flow.

and depends on the ventilatory pattern. Other limitations are similar to those of all face masks, including discomfort and frequent removal.

PARTIAL REBREATHING MASK

To deliver greater than 60% oxygen to a nonintubated patient, a reservoir bag must be added to a tight-fitting mask. If there are no one-way valves between the mask and the bag, this is referred to as a partial rebreathing mask. However, this name is misleading because the bag serves as an oxygen reservoir, not as a carbon dioxide reservoir. An oxygen flow rate of approximately 5 to 6 liters per minute must be applied so that the bag does not completely collapse during inhalation. Then only a small portion of early exhaled gas will enter the bag as it is reinflated. This early exhaled gas, which primarily originates from dead space, contains very low amounts of carbon dioxide (Fig. 18-12). The rebreathing mask can provide adjustable inspired oxygen concentrations up to about 80%. Since minimal room air enters the system, the FI_{O_2} is fairly predictable, even if the patient's ventilatory pattern exceeds the flow rate of the oxygen source. This method is best suited for short-term support of a patient who requires a high FI_{O_2}.

NONREBREATHING MASK

The nonrebreathing mask differs from the partial rebreathing mask in that one-way valves allow the patient to inhale only from the reservoir bag and exhale through separate valves on the side of the mask (Figs. 18-10B, 18-13). If the mask has a tight seal over the face, it is designed to deliver 90% to 100% oxygen. Those masks that fit tightly are used less commonly because of discomfort.

HYPERBARIC OXYGEN THERAPY

The administration of hyperbaric oxygen requires a special facility with trained personnel familiar with specialized pressure chambers and the therapeutic applications of barometric pressure greater than sea level. Hyperbaric oxygen is provided in either a monoplace (single occupant) chamber or a larger multiplace chamber in which members of the medical team can work on and around the patient (see Fig. 18-14). Monoplace chambers are pressurized throughout with 100% oxygen. Multiplace chambers are pressurized with compressed air that the medical personnel breathes. The patient receives 100% oxygen

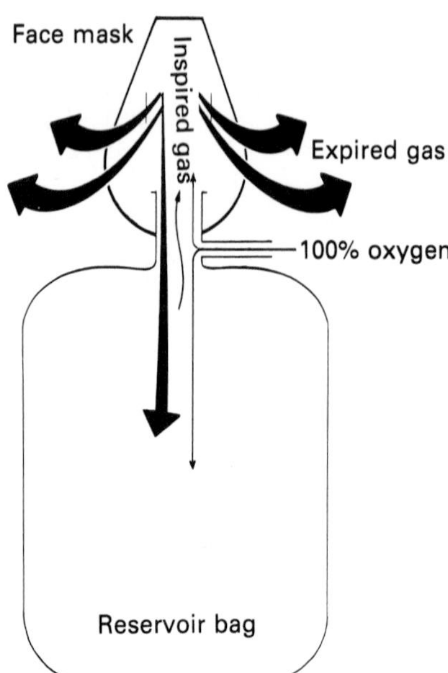

Fig. 18-12. Air flow diagram with partial rebreathing mask. Arrows indicate direction of flow.

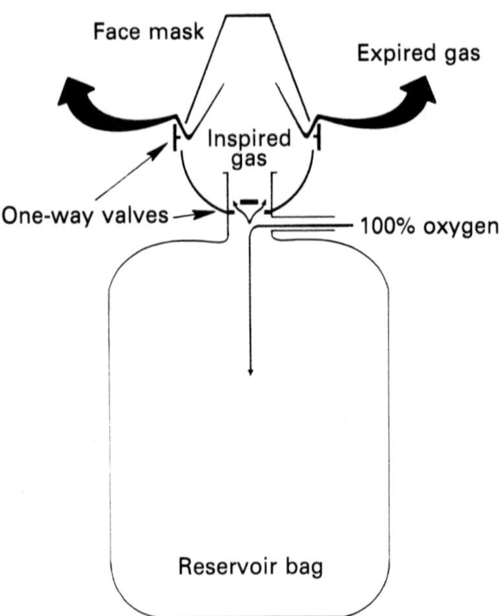

Fig. 18-13. Air flow diagram with nonrebreathing mask. Arrows indicate direction of flow.

usually by a tight-fitting face mask but occasionally by a head tent or endotracheal tube.

PHYSIOLOGIC EFFECTS

At normal barometric pressure when the arterial P_{O_2} is about 100 mg Hg, only a small portion of oxygen—that is, 0.3 ml O_2/100 ml blood—is dissolved in the plasma. Under conditions of increased barometric pressure, the amount of oxygen dissolved significantly increases. This follows Henry's law, which states that the degree to which a gas enters into physical solution is directly proportional to the partial pressure of the gas that is exposed to the liquid. At 3 atm of 100% oxygen, it is possible to carry in solution about 6 ml of oxygen in every hundred ml of blood. Normally, the difference between the oxygen content of arterial blood and the oxygen content of mixed venous blood (sampled from the pulmonary artery) is also close to 6 ml/100 ml of blood. This represents the mean tissue extraction of oxygen by all tissues of the body. Hyperbaric oxygen, therefore, can compensate for an inadequate hemoglobin oxygen content by delivering significant amounts of oxygen in physical solution to tissues (Table 18-5). Further, the high partial pressure of oxygen created by the hyperbaric state provides a gradient for delivery of oxygen to tissues. Not only does this improve the oxygenation of ischemic tissues, but also it promotes the reabsorption of trapped gases in tissues.

Hyperbaric oxygenation results in a number of cardiovascular changes. There is a slight reduction in the cardiac output primarily because of bradycardia. Increased arterial P_{O_2} causes generalized vasoconstriction that tends to decrease tissue perfusion. However, the enhanced oxygen available to tissues with a markedly increased Pa_{O_2} more than compensates, and tissue hypoxia is easily corrected. Despite vasoconstriction, the arterial blood pressure remains constant.

The elevated atmospheric pressure can have both beneficial and adverse consequences. According to Boyle's law, the volume of a gas is inversely proportional to its pressure, assuming a constant temperature. Loculated gas collections in the body will be

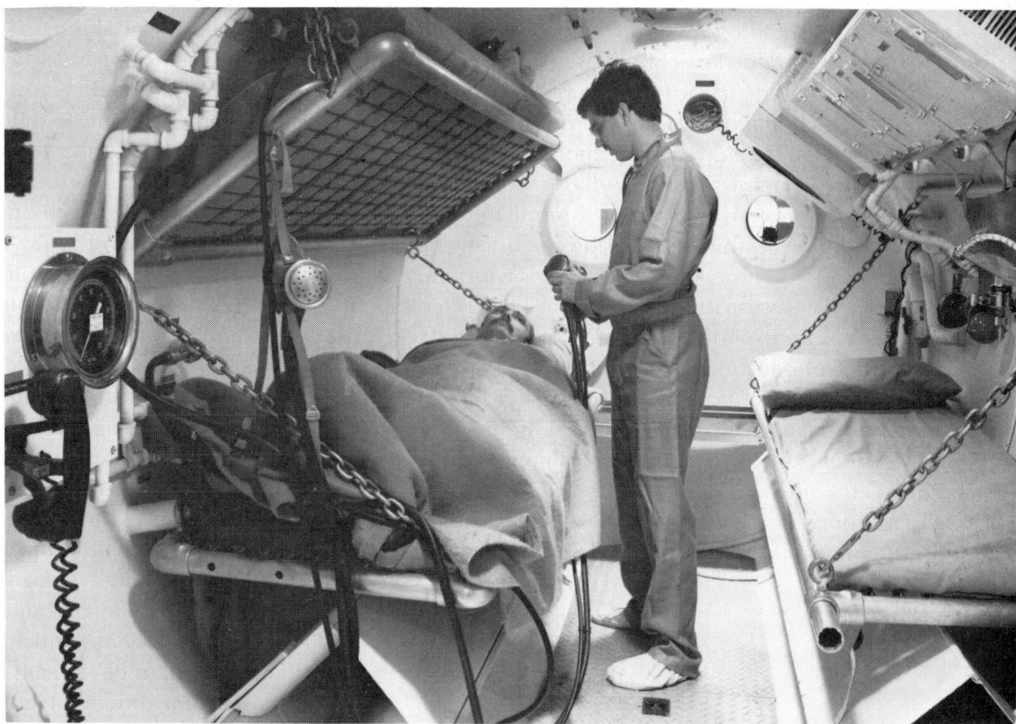

Fig. 18-14. Multiplace hyperbaric chamber at Shands Hospital of the University of Florida on loan from the National Aeronautics and Space Administration.

Table 18-5. Hyperbaric Effect on Oxygen Delivery*

	AMBIENT DRY AIR PI_{O_2} *torr*	ARTERIAL BLOOD Pa_{O_2} *torr*	HEMOGLOBIN SATURATION %	HbO_2† *ml O_2/100 ml blood*	DISSOLVED O_2‡ *ml/100 ml blood*
1 Atm					
(sea level)					
21% O_2	158	100	97	20.3	0.3
100% O_2	760	640	100	20.9	2.1
2 Atm					
(33 ft below sea level)					
100% O_2	1520	1313	100	20.9	4.6
3 Atm					
(66 ft below sea level)					
100% O_2	2280	2026	100	20.9	6.2

*Values are approximate.
†Assuming 15 g Hb/100 ml blood, and a maximum uptake of 1.39 ml O_2/g Hb.
‡Assuming about 0.3 ml dissolved O_2/100 ml blood for every increase in Pa_{O_2} of 100 torr.

reduced in volume during hyperbaric compression. This is beneficial in decompression sickness and gas embolism. In contrast, patients and staff who are unable to equilibrate pressure in their middle ear or sinuses can experience severe pain during compression. Nonemergent patients and staff with upper respiratory tract infections may have to avoid the chamber for this reason. Occasionally, in emergency situations, especially with an unconscious patient, bilateral myringotomies are necessary. Another consideration is managing an endotracheal tube under hyperbaric conditions. The pressure in the endotracheal cuff must be monitored. The cuff will decrease in size during compression, necessitating additional volume to maintain a tracheal seal; during decompression the expanding cuff will pose a danger to the trachea. Patients, as well as staff with obstructive airways disease such as emphysema or with a history of spontaneous pneumothorax, should avoid the chamber. During decompression, volume expansion of loculated gas spaces can result in alveolar rupture with subsequent pneumothorax or even possibly gas embolism.[2]

If air, rather than oxygen, is administered in the hyperbaric chamber, elevated partial pressures of nitrogen can result. Nitrogen can cause an anesthetic effect on both patients and attendants. Usually nitrogen narcosis is not evident until greater than 4 atm of pressure are reached, but there is individual variability in susceptibility to this effect. Therefore, when high pressures such as 6 atm are administered, the staff inside the chamber should not make management decisions without assistance.

Hemoglobin accounts for about 20% of the transport of venous carbon dioxide. If venous hemoglobin is 100% saturated with oxygen under hyperbaric conditions, it is unavailable for carbon dioxide transport. As a consequence, there is a slight rise in carbon dioxide levels. This, however, is a very minor problem because the bicarbonate buffer system and dissolved carbon dioxide assume the added load. The resulting elevated tissue carbon dioxide plays a beneficial role in reducing cerebral edema.

INDICATIONS

Many potential uses of hyperbaric oxygen therapy have been explored. However, the benefits in many situations still remain controversial and unproved. In an attempt to clarify which uses are justified, a committee of the Undersea Medical Society reviewed the clinical applications of hyperbaric therapy and has published a report that divides these disorders into four categories (Table 18-6).[20] Category 1 includes disorders for which hyperbaric oxygen is the primary mode of therapy. Clinical experience and research have demonstrated the efficacy of hyperbaric oxygen in these disorders. Category 2 includes disorders and situations for which animal or clinical experience is compelling, but controlled studies are needed to es-

Table 18-6. Examples of Hyperbaric Oxygen Therapy*

Category 1 lists situations in which there is no doubt about the efficacy of hyperbaric oxygen as primary or adjunctive therapy.

- Exceptional blood-loss anemia
- Acute carbon monoxide poisoning
- Acute cyanide poisoning
- Decompression sickness
- Acute gas embolism
- Gas gangrene
- Meleney ulcer
- Compromised skin grafts or flaps
- Smoke inhalation with chemical pneumonitis and presumption of carbon monoxide or cyanide poisoning

Category 2 includes disorders for which animal or clinical experience strongly suggests that there may be primary or adjunctive usefulness, but more definitive clinical data are needed.

- Acute peripheral arterial insufficiency
- Crush injury
- Bone and soft tissue radionecrosis
- Acute traumatic peripheral ischemia
- Acute thermal burns
- Suturing of several limbs
- Scleral buckling procedures in sickle cell retinopathy
- Acute cerebral edema
- Actinomyocisis

Category 3 includes conditions for which there is a theoretic indication, but definitive evidence is lacking

- Bone grafts
- Acute carbon tetrachloride poisoning
- Diabetic retinopathy
- Frostbite
- Sickle cell crisis
- Migraine headache
- Nonjoined or nonhealing fractures
- Lepromatous leprosy
- Cerebral arterial insufficiency or cerebrovascular accident

Category 4 includes those disorders for which there is no theoretic or scientific basis or for which there is only hearsay evidence of usefulness.

- Arthritis
- Emphysema
- Loss of normal hair color
- Multiple sclerosis
- Hypertension
- Loss of sexual vitality

*Recommendations from the Committee on Hyperbaric Oxygenation of the Undersea Medical Society.[20]

tablish that hyperbaric oxygen is the primary mode of therapy or an important adjunctive therapy. Category 3 is the most controversial in regard to indications for hyperbaric oxygen. Definitive evidence is still lacking for treatment of these disorders. There may be a theoretical indication, but further studies are needed. Category 4 includes conditions for which there is no theoretic or scientific basis for the use of hyperbaric oxygen.

Several established indications will be reviewed below.[26]

Decompression Sickness (Bends)

Decompression sickness is the most common indication for hyperbaric therapy and the primary reason for the existence of many hyperbaric chambers. Rapid decompression of divers or workers in tunnels causes nitrogen in the blood to come out of solution and form bubbles, with subsequent joint pain, central neurologic deficits, pulmonary gas embolism, and infarction of the spinal cord. Immediate recompression in a hyperbaric oxygen chamber decreases intravascular nitrogen bubble size. Then, during slow decompression, these bubbles that become filled with oxygen are gradually absorbed. Hyperbaric oxygen remains the primary method of treatment for this disorder.

Gas Embolism

Some deaths attributed to drowning, especially among scuba divers, likely involve cerebral gas embolism. If a diver holds his breath while ascending, air can inadvertently enter the vascular system from overdistention of gases in the lung. Other ways in which gas embolism can occur include pump oxygenation, cardiovascular surgery, and diagnostic catheterization. Emergency hyperbaric oxygenation gives satisfactory results in most cases and is the only definitive treatment for this disorder.

Clostridial Cellulitis and Myonecrosis (Gas Gangrene)

Along with antibiotics (penicillin) and surgical debridement, hyperbaric oxygen is a valuable adjunctive treatment of infections produced by *Clostridium perfringens*, the anaerobic bacillus that causes gas gangrene. Increasing oxygen pressure inhibits the production of toxin by these bacteria. Results in another anaerobic bacterial infection, tetanus, have been less spectacular. Tetanus toxin is apparently bound to neural tissue and is not affected by hyperbaric treatment, even though the bacterium itself is inhibited.

Carbon Monoxide Poisoning

Carbon monoxide combines with hemoglobin to form carboxyhemoglobin, which is then unavailable for transport of oxygen. Carbon monoxide attaches to the same binding site on hemoglobin, and with an affinity more than 200 times the affinity for oxygen. Elevated levels of carboxyhemoglobin also shift the oxyhemoglobin dissociation curve to the left, and hence decrease oxygen available to tissues. In addition to these two effects, recent evidence has shown that carbon monoxide also attaches to tissue mitochrondrial cytochrome oxidase. Hyperbaric oxygenation promotes removal of carbon monoxide bound to tissues, dissolves an increased amount of oxygen in solution in plasma, and results in a more rapid conversion of carboxyhemoglobin to oxyhemoglobin. The half-life elimination of carbon monoxide from hemoglobin is 5 hours and 20 minutes breathing room air, 90 minutes breathing 100% oxygen at 1 atm, and 23 minutes breathing 100% oxygen in a hyperbaric chamber under 3 atm of pressure. Indications for hyperbaric oxygenation in carbon monoxide poisoning are not universally agreed on. If a hyperbaric chamber is available, all cases with carboxyhemoglobin saturation of 25% or more should be treated, even though symptoms may be minimal. Patients with carboxyhemoglobin levels greater than 40%, or who are unconscious, should be transported immediately to a hyperbaric facility. Treatment must be based on clinical symptoms rather than carboxyhemoglobin level alone.[19]

REFERENCES

1. Banerjee CK, Girling DJ, Wigglesworth JS: Pulmonary fibroplasia in newborn babies treated with oxygen and artificial ventilation. Arch Dis Child 47:509, 1972
2. Bassett BE, Bennett PB: Introduction to the physical and physiological bases of hyperbaric therapy. In Davis JC, Hunt TK (eds): Hyperbaric oxygen therapy. Bethesda, MD, Undersea Medical Society, 1977
3. Block AJ, Burrows B, Kanner RE et al: Oxygen administration in the home. Am Rev Respir Dis 115:897, 1977
4. Bone RC: Acute respiratory failure and chronic obstructive lung disease: Recent advances. Med Clin N Am 65:563, 1981
5. Bone RC, Pierce AK, Johnson RL: Controlled oxygen administration in acute respiratory failure in chronic obstructive pulmonary disease: A reappraisal. Am J Med 65:896, 1978
6. Clark JM: The toxicity of oxygen. Am Rev Respir Dis (Suppl)110:40, 1974
7. Clark JM, Lambertsen CJ: Pulmonary oxygen toxicity: A review. Pharmacol Rev 23:37, 1971
8. Crapo JD, Tierney DF: Superoxide dismutase and pulmonary oxygen toxicity. Am J Physiol 226:1401, 1974
9. Deneke SM, Fanburg BL: Normobaric oxygen toxicity of the lung. N Engl J Med 303:76, 1980
10. Edwards DK, Dyer WM, Northway WH Jr: Twelve years' experience with bronchopulmonary dysplasia. Pediatrics 59:839, 1977
11. Fisher AB: Oxygen therapy: Side effects and toxicity. Am Rev Respir Dis 122(Part 2):61, 1980
12. Flick MR, Block AJ: Continuous in vivo monitoring of arterial oxygenation in chronic obstructive lung disease. Ann Intern Med 86:725, 1977
13. Flick MR, Block AJ: Nocturnal vs diurnal cardiac arrhythmias in patients with chronic obstructive pulmonary disease. Chest 75:8, 1979
14. Frank L, Massaro D: The lung and oxygen toxicity. Arch Intern Med 139:347, 1979
15. Gibson RL, Comer PB, Beckham RW et al: Actual tracheal oxygen concentrations with commonly used oxygen equipment. Anesthesiology 44:71, 1976
16. Grant WJ: Medical gases: Their properties and uses. Chicago, Year Book Medical Publishers, 1978
17. Isom GE, Way JL: Effect of O_2 on cyanide intoxication: Reactivation of cyanide-inhibited glucose metabolism. J Pharmacol Exp Ther 189:235, 1974
18. James LS, Lanman JT (eds): History of oxygen therapy and retrolental fibroplasia. Pediatrics (Suppl)57:591, 1976
19. Kindwall E: Carbon monoxide and cyanide poisoning. In Davis JC, Hunt TK (eds): Hyperbaric oxygen therapy. Bethesda, MD, Undersea Medical Society, 1977
20. Kindwall EP: Hyperbaric oxygen therapy—a committee report. Undersea Medical Society Pub. No. 30 CR (HBO). Bethesda, MD, Undersea Medical Society, 1979
21. Kirby RR, Downs JB, Civetta JM et al: High level end-expiratory pressure (PEEP) in acute respiratory insufficiency. Chest 67:156, 1975
22. Kory RC, Bergmann JC, Sweet RD et al: Comparative evaluation of oxygen therapy techniques. JAMA 179:767, 1962
23. Krop HD, Block AJ, Cohen E: Neuropsychologic effects of continuous oxygen therapy in chronic obstructive pulmonary disease. Chest 64:317, 1973
24. Levine BE, Bigelow DB, Hamstra RD: The role of long-term continuous oxygen administration in patients with chronic airway obstruction with hypoxemia. Ann Intern Med 66:639, 1967
25. McPherson SP: Respiratory Therapy Equipment. St Louis, CV Mosby, 1977
26. Hyperbaric oxygen therapy. Med Lett 20:51, 1979
27. Mithoefer JC, Holford FD, Keighley JFH: The effect of oxygen administration on mixed venous oxygenation in chronic obstructive pulmonary disease. Chest 66:122, 1974
28. Nichols CW, Lambertsen CJ: Effects of high oxygen pressures on the eye. N Engl J Med 281:25, 1969

29. Nicogossian A, Chusid EL, Miller A: Effect of positioning of nasal cannulae on efficacy of oxygen therapy. Respir Care 16:171, 1971
30. Nocturnal oxygen therapy trial group. Continuous or nocturnal oxygen therapy in hypoxemic chronic obstructive lung disease. Ann Intern Med 93:391, 1980
31. Petty TL: Home oxygen in advanced chronic obstructive pulmonary disease. Med Clin N Am 65:615, 1981
32. Phibbs RH: Oxygen therapy: A continuing hazard to the premature infant. Anesthesiology 47:486, 1977
33. Phillip AG: Oxygen plus pressure plus time: The etiology of bronchopulmonary dysplasia. Pediatrics 55:44, 1975
34. Roberts SD: Cost-effective oxygen therapy. Ann Intern Med 93:499, 1980
35. Robin ED: Dysoxia—abnormal tissue oxygen utilization. Arch Intern Med 137:905, 1977
36. Sackner MA, Hirsch JA, Epstein S et al: Effect of oxygen in graded concentrations upon tracheal mucous velocity. Chest 69:164, 1976
37. Sackner MA, Landa J, Hirsch J et al: Pulmonary effects of oxygen breathing: A 6-hour study in normal men. Ann Intern Med 82:40, 1975
38. Shapiro BA, Harrison RA, Walton JR: Clinical applications of respiratory care. Chicago, Year Book Medical Publishers, 1982
39. Snider GL, Rinaldo JE: Oxygen therapy: Oxygen therapy in medical patients hospitalized outside of the intensive care unit. Am Rev Respir Dis 122(Part 2):29, 1980
40. Stark RD, Finnegan P, Bishop JM: Long-term domiciliary oxygen in chronic bronchitis with pulmonary hypertension. Br Med J 3:467, 1973
41. Stewart BN, Hood CI, Block AJ: Long-term results of continuous oxygen therapy at sea level. Chest 68:486, 1975
42. Suter PM, Fairley HB, Isenberg MD: Optimum end-expiratory airway pressure in patients with acute pulmonary failure. N Engl J Med 292:284, 1975
43. Tierney DF, Ayers L, Kasuyama RS: Altered sensitivity to oxygen toxicity. Am Rev Respir Dis 115:(Part 2)59, 1977
44. Wagner PD, Laravuso RB, Uhl RB et al: Continuous distributions of ventilation–perfusion ratios in normal subjects breathing air and 100% O_2. J Clin Invest 54:54, 1974
45. Wilson RS, Laver MB: Oxygen analysis: Advances in methodology. Anesthesiology 37:112, 1972
46. Wolfe WG, DeVries WC: Oxygen toxicity. Ann Rev Med 26:203, 1975

BIBLIOGRAPHY

Chemical Properties

Grant WJ: Medical Gases: Their Properties and Uses. Chicago, Year Book Medical Publishers, 1978

McPherson SP: Respiratory Therapy Equipment. St Louis, CV Mosby, 1977

Adverse Effects of Oxygen Therapy

Fisher AB: Oxygen Therapy: Side Effects and Toxicity. Am Rev Respir Dis 122(Part 2):61, 1980

Indications for Acute Oxygen Therapy

Snider GL, Rinaldo JE: Oxygen Therapy in Medical Patients Hospitalized Outside of the Intensive Care Unit. Am Rev Respir Dis 122(Part 2):29, 1980

Chronic Oxygen Therapy

Block AJ: Low Flow Oxygen Therapy: Treatment of the Ambulant Outpatient. Am Rev Respir Dis 110:71, 1974

Petty TL: Home Oxygen in Advanced Chronic Obstructive Pulmonary Disease. Med Clin N Am 65:615, 1981

Modes of Oxygen Delivery

Shapiro BA, Harrison RA, Walton JR: Clinical Application of Blood Gases. Chicago, Year Book Medical Publishers, 1982

Hyperbaric Oxygen Therapy

Davis JC, Hung TK (eds): Hyperbaric Oxygen Therapy. Bethesda, MD, Undersea Medical Society, 1977

19

Infectious Disease Aspects of Respiratory Therapy

James J. Couperus • Harvey A. Elder

Microorganisms, not man, dominate the planet earth. This is a fact of biology. Human dominance is social, technical, intellectual, and spiritual. Usually *Homo sapiens* and microorganisms live in a close, mutually beneficial relationship called *mutualism*. To other microorganisms the human is a source of nutrition, and they exist upon his surfaces with neither invasion nor benefit to the host *(commensalism)*. The relationship between an organism and man that is harmful to man is called *parasitism*. Such relationships may result in overt disease and occasionally in death (Table 19-1).

This chapter will explore pulmonary infections, but at the outset one should appreciate several aspects of parasitism by microorganisms.

1. The diversity of microorganisms (in both kind and number) in the human environment is beyond human technologic ability to measure.
2. Microorganisms multiply only under special circumstances. If the temperature, concentrations of hydrogen, other ions, and oxygen are appropriate and carbon, nitrogen, and special nutritional requirements are met (necessary synthetic energy mechanisms may need to be supplied), the organism can multiply. Most microorganisms cannot multiply in the human environment; relatively few species can grow under conditions existing on or in humans. Those that can are potentially pathogenic (capable of causing disease), but in the past only a relative few of these species have been shown to cause human infection. Pulmonary infections can be caused only by some of the human pathogens. Thus, when focusing on pulmonary infections, we are considering only a minute fraction of all species of microorganisms—in fact, only a small fraction of the species that colonize humans.
3. The history of microbiology shows that the identity of many microorganisms has been discovered only recently, and they have undergone several name changes. The growth of microbiologic knowledge and understanding suggests that some important pathogens of the future may be organisms not now considered to be pathogens and may even be organisms not yet identified.
4. Continuous and intense colonization by microorganisms usually results in the absence of discernible human disease despite the fact that pathogenic organisms are present (*i.e.*, parasitism is an uncommon relationship; commensalism and mutualism are common).

Table 19-1. Effects of Man-Microbe Relationships in Nature

	RELATIONSHIP		
	Mutualism	*Commensalism*	*Parasitism*
Effect on microbe	Benefit	Benefit	Benefit
Effect on host	Benefit	None	Harm
Invasion	None	None	Invades the organism or alters its metabolism

5. The terms "pathogenic" and "nonpathogenic" are characterizations often attributed to different species of microorganisms. However, whether an organism is pathogenic (has a parasitic potential) may depend more on the host (the specific patient) than on the organism. Most people are not infected by nonpathogenic species. However, these species may cause disease in patients with impaired defenses against microbiologic invasion (e.g., patients with acute leukemia). If "healthy" young children contact pathogenic organisms (e.g., *Hemophilus influenzae)*, they may become acutely ill, whereas most "healthy" adults will not. Resistance to infection is acquired with maturation, partially because previous exposure to microorganisms has stimulated host resistance mechanisms (immunity).
6. Transmission of microorganisms can occur by many routes. Usually, but not necessarily, air-transmitted organisms are in respiratory secretions and cause diseases in the upper or lower respiratory tract, or both. Organisms transmitted by other routes may also cause respiratory diseases. *Salmonella typhi*, for example, is transmitted by ingesting material with fecal contamination. This organism causes typhoid fever, a systemic disease with an associated bronchopneumonia.

In *Homo sapiens*, initial high susceptibility to infection is associated with exposure to innumerable microorganisms. Parasitic relationships occur either with successful results (the human who recovers has in the process acquired increased resistance to the microorganisms) or unsuccessful ones (the human dies or is left seriously impaired, presumably even more susceptible to subsequent microbial invasion). The habitually successful, healthy human is unsuccessful either when new, highly pathogenic microorganisms are encountered and the human is without defense (a chance exposure to influenza) or because the human has lost his health and can no longer maintain a completely successful defense against microorganisms. This occurs because of some physiological impairment, such as recurrent chronic infection (e.g., recurrent pneumonia in the patient with emphysema and chronic bronchitis). Finally, rapid loss of host defense mechanisms may be manifested by the abrupt onset of overwhelming sepsis. An example of this is the child who presents with *Pseudomonas* (a low-virulence organism that is rarely a pathogen to healthy persons) pneumonia and septicemia because leukemia has just become manifest. In some diseases (e.g., tuberculosis), the extent of infection is affected to a great degree by the *number*, as well as the type, of infecting organisms.

MICROBIOLOGY

Before the discovery of the microscope, man found it relatively easy to assign all forms of life to one of two groups. Living forms were either animal or plant; hence biology, the study of life, was subdivided into zoology, the study of animals, and botany, the study of plants. All organisms large enough to be seen with the naked eye could be placed in one of these groups, based on visible characteristics.

Careful use of the microscope has revealed minute forms of life that have characteristics of both plants and animals. Some microorganisms, for example, are motile (characteristic of animals) but also use chlorophyll to perform photosynthesis (characteristic of plants). Microbiology encompasses life that is too small to be seen with the naked eye. It is subdivided (Fig. 19-1) to include the studies of algae (phycology), protozoa (protozoology), bacteria (bacteriology), fungi (mycology), viruses (virology), and host resistance (immunology). These subdivisions are based on specific differences in structure and function.

There are two different types of cellular organization. The kingdom Eucaryotae has complex, highly organized cells, including animal, protozoal, plant, and most algal and fungal cells. The kingdom Procaryotae has simpler cells that include the bacteria and blue–green algae (Fig. 19-2). Biologists assign all forms of life, with the possible exception of viruses, to one of these kingdoms. We will not elucidate the details of cellular classification in this chapter; however, a brief summary is provided because infectious disease therapy depends on the similarities and dissimilarities of various microbial and human cells.

BASIC CELL DIFFERENTIATION

All cells have a number of common structural characteristics, but the degree of their internal complexity varies. The eucaryotic cell, whether found in a multicellular organism such as man or in a unicellular organism such as the fungus, has a high degree of internal complexity, whereas the procaryotic cell is structurally less complex. While, for example, the genetic material of all cells is responsible for reproduction of genetically similar offspring, the genetic organization varies. The genetic information of both eucaryotes and procaryotes is contained in nucleic acids called deoxyribonucleic acids (DNA) of the cell nucleus. The cell nucleus of the eucaryote consists of multiple complete DNA molecules organized on functional subunits called chromosomes and is bound by a nuclear membrane, whereas the procaryotic nucleus is a single complete DNA molecule that is neither membrane-bound nor organized on chromosomes. Replication of the eucaryotic nucleus is more closely linked to cell division than is replication of the procaryotic nucleus.

Eucaryotic respiratory and digestive enzymes are found in membrane-bound, intracellular compartments (e.g., mitochondria), whereas procaryotic enzyme systems are not compartmentalized but are housed directly in the specialized cytoplasmic membrane surrounding the cytoplasm.

Another distinct structure, the cell wall, is found in some eucaryotic and most procaryotic cells, but the composition differs. Procaryotes contain a taxonomically significant group of molecules called peptidoglycans. This substance provides strength and shape for procaryotic cell walls but is not found in eucaryotes. Later in this chapter we shall indicate that human cells have no surrounding cell wall and are devoid of this unique peptidoglycan, and therefore specific therapy (e.g., penicillin) can be used because it interferes with the synthesis of the invading organism's procaryotic cell peptidoglycans, without affecting human cells.

Several other structural differences may explain the varying responses to antimicrobial therapy. Sterols are common to eucaryotic cells, such as those of fungi and man, but are rarely found in procaryotes. The dissimilarity of the eucaryotic ribosome to that of procaryotes may explain the differential binding of antimicrobial agents to ribosomes in some cells but not in others.

Finally, as if to confound an apparently logical classification scheme, the viruses differ from all known cellular organisms, not comfortably fitting into any scheme of cell classification. DNA is the source of genetic information. RNA translates the genetic information for synthesis and control of cellular functions. Because most bacteria have DNA and RNA as

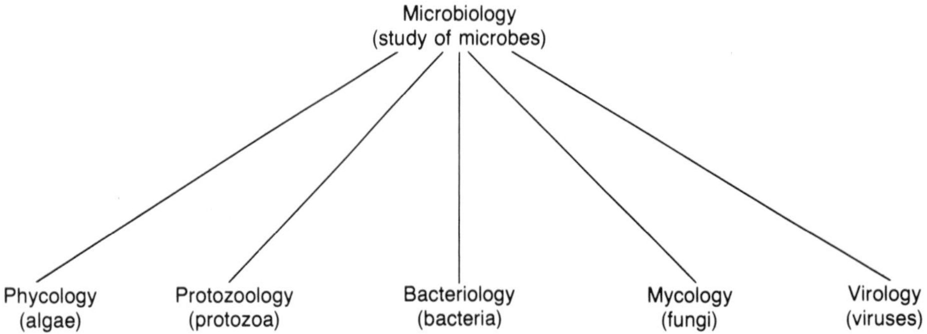

Fig. 19-1. Subdivisions of the field of microbiology. With the possible exception of algae, all these groups of organisms are important in human pulmonary disease.

well as other specialized structures, the cell can synthesize proteins, nucleic acids, lipids, and carbohydrates without depending on the host cell for assistance. In other words, they can grow in artificial media without other living cells present. *The virus has none of these specialized functions and contains only one type of nucleic acid, either DNA or RNA.* Thus the virus totally depends on the host cell for energetic and synthetic processes.

Although a virus consists of little more than a single type of nucleic acid with a protein coat, this submicroscopic subcellular agent can enter a host and begin directing the host cell to supply all the metabolic and synthetic needs of the virus. The infected cell may reproduce myriad numbers of new viruses.

These characteristics do not represent the only differences between procaryote, eucaryote, and viruses, but they are significant differences that may influence antimicrobial therapy or modify the ability of the cell to survive various environmental conditions. The student should realize that all cells have differences in needs and organization that allow them to survive and reproduce in various ecological niches (e.g., soil, mouth, or nares).

REQUIREMENTS FOR MULTIPLICATION

All cells are comprised of, and require, carbon, hydrogen, oxygen, nitrogen, and many other substances. As a group, microorganisms metabolize chemicals man cannot use. Humans, for example, use glucose for carbon and give off carbon dioxide as the end product of respiration, whereas certain bacteria use carbon dioxide as the sole carbon source for incorporation into various structural substances.

A limiting factor for the growth of most microorganisms is the gaseous environment. Humans are accustomed to breathing air containing about 21% oxygen. Those microorganisms that require or tolerate molecular oxygen are termed *aerobes*, whereas those that cannot use or even tolerate molecular oxygen are termed *anaerobes*. If molecular oxygen is an invariable requirement, the organism is an obligate or strict aerobe. If absolutely no molecular oxygen can be tolerated, the organism is an obligate or strict anaerobe. If the organism can multiply in the presence or absence of molecular oxygen, the organism is called facultative. Still other organisms prefer reduced amounts of oxygen. These organisms are described as microaerophilic.

The temperature range that supports growth also varies widely. There are three major groups based on temperature requirements. Organisms that grow optimally in the cold (15–18°C) are called psychrophiles. Psychrophiles may grow at temperatures near or below 0°C. At present there are no known psychrophilic pathogens. Organisms that grow best at 30°C to 45°C are called mesophiles. This group is able to multiply at human body temperatures, and hence are potential human pathogens. Other organisms prefer 55°C to 75°C and are called thermophiles. Certain thermophiles, while unable to multiply at human body temperature, are known to cause allergic reactions when man inhales the organisms grown outside the body.

Salt concentration is another factor affecting growth. Forms of microbial life can exist over a broad

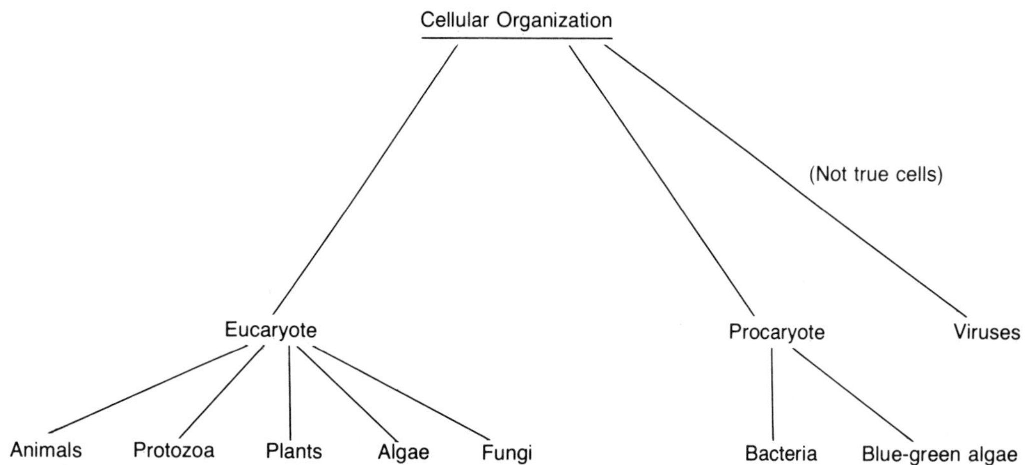

Fig. 19-2. Possible organizational relationships of microbes, animals, and plants.

range of salt concentrations. Certain microbes (e.g., *Halobacterium*) require at least 15% salt, others, such as *Pseudomonas*, require very little salt and can grow very well in distilled water.

Most organisms, including man, function and grow best within a narrow range of pH. Humans prefer a blood pH of 7.35 to 7.45, and changes of several tenths of a pH unit are poorly tolerated. Individual species of microorganisms are also limited by hydrogen ion concentrations, whereas certain varieties tolerate extremes in pH.

The examples cited illustrate a few factors that modify the ability of pathogens to invade man. Respiratory pathogens must be able to survive man's restrictive environment and combat various normal resistance factors. Since man's environment is in continual flux and the diversity of microorganisms is broad, man continues to be a suitable growth environment for a changing spectrum of microorganisms. Whether or not disease may follow is a consequence both of microbial growth and host defense.

The microbiologist may be called on to determine which microorganisms are residing in or invading the patient. The microbe might be transient and leave without medical treatment or may become a permanent resident, unable to be removed without intensive therapy. Medical personnel should know which organisms compose usual flora and which types usually lead to or cause disease. As will be explained later, organisms considered usual flora (mutuals and commensals) may invade (become parasites), thereby causing infection.

BASIC GROUPS OF MICROORGANISMS

Human infections are caused by microorganisms from four of the five major groups (*see* Fig. 19-1). Each group comprises a large number of diverse subgroups. Microbiologists usually can differentiate the four major groups (protozoa, fungi, bacteria, and viruses) rather quickly because, as a group, each of the four has a distinctly different appearance, as well as size (Table 19-2). Members of each group can be found in mixtures with any of the other groups, and infection resulting from one group can mimic the symptoms of the others. Fortunately, clinical evidence commonly suggests the type of culture to be requested. The microbiology laboratory does not routinely examine all specimens for each of the four groups. Therefore requests for laboratory examinations must accurately describe the required tests. A brief review is included to increase the student's awareness of the unique characteristics possessed by each group and to emphasize the wide diversity of organisms within a group.

Table 19-2. Size Approximations of Various Types of Cells

NAME OF CELL	SIZE (μm)*
Liver cell	20
Red blood cell	7.5
Protozoon	5–60
Yeast	2.5–6
Bacterium	0.5–0.75 × 1–6
Rickettsia	0.3–0.6
Chlamydia (infectious forms)	0.2–0.3
Virus	0.02–0.3

*1 micron (μm) = 1 millionth of a meter, or 10^{-6} m.

Protozoa

Protozoa are eucaryotic cells. They are unicellular microorganisms ranging in size from 5 to 60 μm and have no protective cell wall. Each species causes a specific type of disease. Amebic dysentery, caused by *Entamoeba histolytica*, can be complicated by amebic abscesses of the liver that occasionally rupture through the diaphragm, infecting the pleura and occasionally the lung. Few protozoa invade the lung primarily. Two species, *Pneumocystis carinii* and *Toxoplasma gondii*, can cause pulmonary infections in patients with serious underlying disease, such as leukemia. To diagnose respiratory infections secondary to protozoa, special stains or animal inoculation procedures may be required. The techniques are not performed routinely in the microbiology laboratory.

Fungi

Fungi are microorganisms belonging to the kingdom Eucaryotae. Most fungi possess either of two basic morphologies. The most noticeable morphologic form is mold, since mature mold is visible to the naked eye. Microscopically, molds consist of many branching multicellular filaments or hyphae that multiply and intertwine to form a mycelial mass of tiny hyphae. This mold or mycelial form produces tiny infective spores that are easily spread to new environments, including man.

The second basic morphologic form is that of yeasts. Yeasts are unicellular and reproduce by forming buds, which increase in size and at one or more locations separate from the parent yeast. They are microscopic cells ranging in size from about 2.5 to 6 μm.

Fungi generally exist in either the mold or yeast form, but certain fungi can convert from one form to the other. These are called dimorphic fungi because they possess two entirely different morphologies. Dimorphism is controlled by environmental conditions. Dimorphism allows systemic growth of some fungi in man. *Blastomyces dermatiditis* and *Blastomyces brasiliensis*, for example, exist as a mold if grown at 25°C but convert to a yeast if grown at 37°C (body temperature). Some species, such as *Histoplasma capsulatum* and *Sporothrix schenckii*, depend on both temperature and nutritional changes, whereas *Candida albicans* maintains the yeast phase only in the proper nutritional environment. Most systemic dimorphic fungi exist as a mold in nature and as yeast in man. *Coccidioides immitis* is an important exception because, following inhalation of spores from the mold form, conversion to large, thick-walled, nonbudding spherules (30–60 μm) containing numerous, tiny, infective endospores (2–5 μm) occurs. (These are not yeast forms.)

Most systemic fungal pathogens exist as either yeast or mold. These fungi invade deeper than the skin, often spreading to many organ sites. *Cryptococcus neoformans*, a systemic pathogen, remains in yeast form, generally characterized by a large slimy capsule surrounding each cell. Another potential systemic pathogen, particularly in compromised hosts, is *Aspergillus fumigatus*, which exists as a mold in man and nature. Fungi capable of causing systemic disease represent an extreme laboratory hazard and must be handled in properly equipped laboratories.

Fortunately, not all fungi are pathogenic. They are ubiquitous in nature, but only a few are known pathogens. Some fungi are of commercial value. *Penicillium* species are natural sources of penicillin antibiotics. *Saccharomyces* is important in the fermentation industry.

Unfortunately, any fungus that can grow at body temperature (37°C) must be considered a potential pathogen. The increased use of drugs, such as steroids to suppress inflammatory response and antibiotics to cure bacterial infections and the use of indwelling catheters and prosthetic devices result in fungal infections not previously encountered. *Candida albicans*, a yeast normally inhabiting many gastrointestinal tracts, has been isolated, on rare occasions, as a pathogen from infections in most body regions.

Fungal infections are a serious therapeutic problem. The fungal cell possesses functional similarities to the human cell, despite the presence of a cell wall composed of chitin and other polysaccharide polymers. This limits the therapeutic attack that can be mounted against fungi. The best antifungal drug (amphotericin B), for example, works by binding to sterols in the cell membrane. Human and fungal cells both contain sterols; hence treatment with amphotericin B is very hazardous.

Bacteria

Bacteria are procaryotic cells that come in all shapes and a broad range of sizes (from 0.5 μm in diameter to 6 μm in length). Most require a magnification of about 1000 times to be seen distinctly. The three basic shapes (morphologies) have several variations (Fig. 19-3). If a bacterium is spherical, it is called a coccus (plural: cocci); if it is shaped like a rod, it is called a bacillus (plural: bacilli); if it is hairlike and coiled in spirals, it is called a spirochete. Cocci have characteristic spatial arrangments. Cocci that occur in pairs are called "diplococci;" in chains, "streptococci;" and in grapelike clusters, "staphylococci." A Gram's stain can demonstrate morphology and show staining characteristics. Those that hold the blue dye (gentian violet or crystal violet) are gram-positive, and those that lose the blue dye (counter-stain red) are gram-negative.

This chapter cannot explore all the intricacies of bacterial classification. The details are constantly

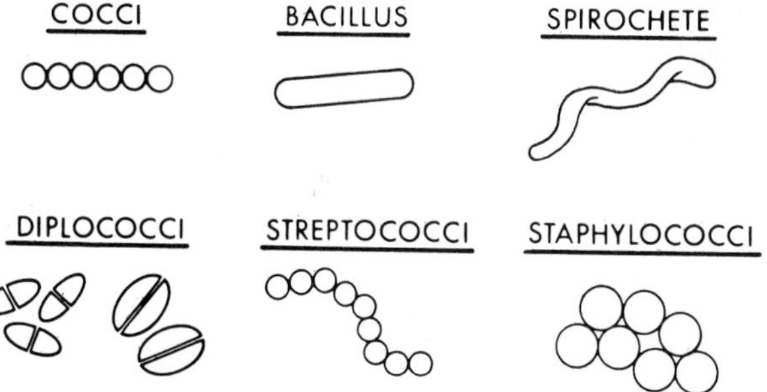

Fig. 19-3. Morphologic characteristics of bacteria. The individual bacterial shapes are round *(coccus)*, straight rod *(bacillus)*, or curved rod *(spirochete)*. The individual bacteria can group in pairs ("diplo," as with diplococci), in chains ("strep," as with streptococci), or in clusters ("staph," as in staphylococci).

evolving. Most groups of bacteria that can produce human disease have been classified on the basis of their oxygen requirements (aerobic, anaerobic, facultative), their morphology (coccus, bacillus, spirochete), the Gram's stain reaction (gram-positive or gram-negative), unusual growth requirements such as obligate parasitism, or other distinctive features.

Within each group further differentiation can be made by tests that identify the biochemical capability of the organism. All living cells, for example, have energy-yielding biochemical reactions called oxidation–reduction reactions. The most common test substrate for energy-yielding reactions is glucose, a sugar. The cells use glucose as an energy source by degrading it to other compounds through a series of oxidation–reduction reactions. In the process of glucose degradation, energy is released. Oxidation–reduction reactions that require molecular oxygen are utilized by bacteria called oxidizers (e.g., *Pseudomonas*). Oxidation–reduction reactions that occur in the absence of molecular oxygen are called fermentation, and bacteria using this method are called fermenters (e.g., *Klebsiella*).

The demonstrated biochemical capabilities of bacteria provide a "fingerprint" for identification. Test substrates range from simple sugars such as glucose to very complex environments containing gas mixtures or chemicals. Each biochemical test adds more evidence for the identity of the organism. The evidence eventually becomes definitive, and a name can be assigned to the organism. Gram-positive cocci, for example, growing in grapelike clusters aerobically and anaerobically on nutrient agar at 37°C, possessing the enzyme catalase to break down hydrogen peroxide and coagulase to coagulate plasma, and having the capacity to ferment glucose are *Staphylococcus aureus* (*S. aureus*). More tests could be performed, but *S. aureus* is adequately defined with these few tests. Occasionally it is necessary to differentiate various strains of the same bacteria. Sophisticated tests such as phage (a test of the bacteria's susceptibility to virus) and serologic typing (a test for antigenic identity) have been devised to distinguish individual strains of bacteria. Hence a specific *S. aureus* has a phage type and a serotype that distinguishes it from other strains of *S. aureus*.

Identification of a bacterial species is the result of a logical series of tests. Most bacterial groups are rather easy to isolate and identify, using a few simple techniques. At least three groups warrant further discussion because they differ significantly from typical bacteria: *Mycoplasma*, *Rickettsia*, and *Chlamydia*.

Mycoplasma. During the course of penicillin therapy, bacteria may lose their cell wall. Normally this causes the cell to lyse and die. If environmental conditions are optimal, some of the bacteria may be able to survive in the absence of the cell wall and are called L-forms. These are not to be confused with *Mycoplasma*, a genus of bacteria that *never* forms a cell wall. Bacterial L-forms will revert to normal bacteria when the environment becomes suitable. Mycoplasma never form cell walls, are a distinctly different group of bacteria, and present unique therapeutic problems. These organisms (formerly known as pleuropneumonia-like organisms—PPLO) are involved in a number of pathogenic processes. One species, *Mycoplasma pneumoniae* (Eaton agent), is a major cause of primary atypical pneumonia. Other species are found in respiratory secretions, but their etiologic role is uncertain. Isolation of mycoplasma from specimens is accomplished in a clinical laboratory if the unique growth requirements are met. They are not isolated on routine bacterial growth media, and most bacteriology laboratories are not prepared to culture for them. Hence the diagnosis is often based on clinical symptoms or serologic tests.

Rickettsia. *Rickettsia* is a genus of bacteria with properties that place them in a position intermediate to bacteria and viruses. They are smaller than most bacteria but larger than most viruses. They contain both DNA and RNA, have bacteria-like cell walls, and are susceptible to some antibacterial drugs. However, like viruses, they multiply only within living cells of certain animal species, implying that they are deficient in enzyme systems that allow growth on artificial media. Isolation of rickettsiae is difficult. Rickettsiae are dangerous to laboratory personnel; hence, isolation of rickettsiae should be attempted only in laboratories properly equipped for strict isolation. Diagnosis may be aided by serologic tests.

Chlamydia.* The chlamydiae, like the rickettsiae, were once thought to be viruses. They are intracellular parasites, requiring a living host cell to supply some of their needs. They possess both DNA and RNA, have cell walls like those of bacteria, and are susceptible to some antibacterial drugs. The unique characteristic of chlamydiae is their unusual method of reproduc-

*The taxonomy of *Chlamydia* is changing rapidly. Terms used previously to describe this genus include *Bedsonia*, psittacosis, lymphogranuloma venereum, *Miyagawanella*, and trachoma group.

tion. Most bacteria produce offspring that appear similar to the parent cell. The chlamydiae enter a host cell as small particles (0.2–0.3 μm) that reorganize within the cell to form large particles (0.5–1.0 μm). The host cell is arrested and used during the reorganization of the large particle to form small particles that are released as the host cell dies. The small particles (the infectious form) then reinitiate the cycle. The most common chlamydiae-induced respiratory disease is psittacosis (ornithosis), a pneumonitis caused by *Chlamydia psittaci*. Routine bacteriologic procedures are not useful in identifying these organisms. As with rickettsiae, these organisms pose a serious hazard to laboratory personnel and should be handled only by experienced workers.

Viruses

Viruses are not true organisms. Their structural organization is too simple to qualify as cells. They are infectious agents that can reproduce, but only within living cells. Viruses are distinguished from other microbes by their size (they require electron microscopy to visualize), lack of energy-generating or biosynthetic mechanisms, resistance to common antimicrobial drugs, and possession of only one type of nucleic acid, either DNA or RNA.

The techniques required for complete viral identification are more complex than the simple techniques used for most bacteria and fungi. Because viruses require living cells (tissue and organ culture) for growth and multiplication, biochemical characterization and antiviral drug testing are difficult. The two major groups of viruses recognized are DNA and RNA viruses. Current antimicrobial therapy is directed toward components of the microbial cell that are absent in the virus (e.g., ribosome, cell wall); hence, this therapy is not effective for viral infections. The incidence and severity of viral infections common during previous decades have been decreased by vaccines (influenza, polio, and measles), whereas elimination of insect carriers dramatically decreased other virus-mediated infections (e.g., encephalitis).

PROCESSING OF SPECIMENS

Proper identification of microorganisms begins at the bedside when the patient's symptoms are recognized, continues with collection and transportation of the specimen, and concludes in the laboratory when isolation and characterization of the infectious agent are accurately performed. To determine which infectious agent is present in a specimen, the microbiologist follows routine methods to detect common microbes and uses specialized procedures only if unusual organisms are suspected. Because of risk, time, and costs, specialized methods are not performed unless clinically or epidemiologically indicated, or if the clinical history and examination provide clues necessitating specialized procedures. Therefore, one must always include pertinent data when sending specimens to the laboratory for special studies. The more the consultation with the laboratory, the greater the likelihood that the right studies will be done and definitive answers given.

Collection and Transportation of Respiratory Specimens

Respiratory tract cultures must be collected, transported, cultured, and interpreted with care. A great number and diversity of microorganisms (aerobic and anaerobic) inhabit the nose, oral cavity, and pharynx of normal, healthy people, as well as compromised, sick, and infected people. This normal or usual flora may contain many or few pathogens, whether or not the patient is infected. Thus cultures of the upper and lower respiratory tract must contend with potential contamination from the residual flora. Only when correctly obtained directly *from the site of infection* does the culture reliably reflect the infecting agent. In other areas, the usual microbiota persist with greater or lesser numbers of the infecting pathogen. Sputum cultures containing pulmonary exudate but contaminated by mouth organisms can present difficulties in interpretation. Errors can result if the pulmonary exudate is not selectively examined to the exclusion of the oral contribution (e.g., the presence of pneumococci in the pharynx does not reveal the etiology of a pneumonia; *only if the pneumococci are in the pulmonary exudate is the etiology of the pneumonia likely to be pneumococcal*).

Pharyngeal Cultures. Throat cultures are usually obtained to diagnose the etiology of pharyngitis. (In children pharyngeal cultures may be useful when searching for the etiology of a lower respiratory infection.) The laboratory should be notified if diphtheria, pertussis (whooping cough), or gonorrhea are suspected. Throat cultures should be collected on a polyester, or calcium alginate swab. The tongue should be depressed with a tongue blade to visualize the pharynx clearly and to minimize contamination. The swab is then rubbed vigorously over the tonsils and posterior pharynx. If the swab is not inoculated directly on culture media, it is placed in a transport tube containing a medium that allows the organism to survive but not multiply, thus preserving the initial ratio of pathogen to usual flora. The specimen should be delivered to the laboratory *immediately* for culture.

Because viruses cannot grow on bacterial culture media, routine throat cultures do not diagnose viral infections. If viral detection is required, the adult gargles with sterile broth containing 0.5% gelatin and then collects the expectorate in a sterile cup. The specimen should be processed immediately or frozen until ready for processing. Since throat washings of children may be difficult to obtain, throat swabbings with throat or nasopharyngeal swab tips, previously moistened with the same broth, should be placed in a tube containing 5 ml of the broth. This sample is then processed as a throat washing.

Nasopharyngeal Cultures. Nasopharyngeal cultures provide information about the microbiologic flora of the upper respiratory tract. Nasopharyngeal specimens are collected with polyester or calcium alginate swabs on a flexible wire. The swab is gently passed through the nose into the nasopharynx and allowed to set for a few moments. It is then carefully removed and inoculated directly onto culture media or placed in a suitable transport medium. The specimen should be delivered to the laboratory promptly.

Sputum. Routine sputum cultures are the most common method used to diagnose the etiology of lower respiratory tract infection; however, recovery of organisms from expectorated secretions does not necessarily mean association with lower respiratory infection. Because of the large number and variety of anaerobic flora in the normal oropharynx and mouth, expectorated sputum is unsuitable for culture of anaerobes.

There is no suitable transport medium for sputum; it must therefore be transported to the laboratory immediately. Because trained microbiologists may be available only during the day, specimens received in the evening may not receive immediate and adequate attention. If significant, accurate microbiologic data are to be available, collection, delivery, and culture must be coordinated so that competent laboratory workers can process fresh, properly collected specimens. Obviously, communication with the laboratory is essential.

Laboratory Procedures

Preliminary Examination. After a properly collected specimen has been promptly delivered to the laboratory, it can be examined for gross and microscopic clues. A drop placed on a glass slide may be examined while wet for motility, shape, and size of larger forms, such as fungi, yeast, protozoa, ova of worms, or human cells. If any of these are seen, a drop of dye such as methylene blue or iodine may be added to increase the visibility of internal structures. Bacteria are too small to be seen clearly in wet preparations, and viruses can be visualized only with an electron microscope.

A thin, dry smear of the specimen should be prepared on a glass microscopic slide and stained. Stained smears allow better resolution of bacteria and internal structures of host cells than unstained preparations.

Staining Methods. The differential binding of various dyes is the basic principle of stain technology. The dye is applied for a time sufficient to stain all organisms uniformly. Solvent is added to remove all stain not permanently bound to the organisms. The solvent is rinsed off before the bound stain is removed Finally a stain of a different color (counter stain) is added to stain all organisms that did not bind the first stain. Gram's stain, developed by Hans Christian Joachim Gram in 1884, is the most commonly used stain in clinical microbiology. The dye is crystal violet, which stains blue and is further bound to the cell by iodine. Alcohol–acetone solvent quickly removes the dye from some, but not other, bacterial cell types. The solvent is removed by rinsing with water, and the slide is counter-stained with safranin, a red stain. After rinsing and drying, the slide is ready for microscopic examination. Depending on the structure of the cell wall, each organism will either retain the crystal violet stain and appear blue (Gram's stain positive or gram-positive) or be decolorized by the solvent and have the red color of safranin counter stain (Gram's stain negative or gram-negative). Gram's staining should be the very first microbiologic evaluation when making a bacteriologic diagnosis for most infectious diseases.

A second stain of major importance, especially in respiratory infections, is the acid-fast stain, also frequently referred to as the Ziehl–Neelsen's stain (named for Franz Ziehl and Friederich Karl Adolf Neelsen, who developed it in 1892). The first dye is carbol-fuchsin, a red dye used with a wetting agent or steamed so that the dye will penetrate the fatty substances in the cell walls of bacteria such as mycobacteria and *Nocardia*. Acid–alcohol is the solvent and methylene blue the counter stain. If the cell stains red, it is called acid-fast because the acid–alcohol solvent has been unable to remove the first stain quickly. If the cell stains blue, it is non-acid-fast. This stain provides a relatively fast screen for the presence of tubercle bacilli (mycobacteria), but culture should always be done to identify the species of organism, since not all acid-fast organisms are *Mycobacterium tuberculosis*.

Acridine orange is a fluorescent stain that binds to the lipid substances of mycobacteria and other acid-fast organisms. With fluorescent microscopy, the organism appears brilliant orange against a dark black background, making the organism easily seen in striking contrast to the field.

Culture. Microscopic observations provide a rapid statement of the presence, type, and relative numbers of organisms and are the basis for interpreting culture results. Stain results are *immediate* guides for therapy. Definitive and supporting results can be obtained only if specimens are cultivated in a manner that will grow the suspected microorganisms. No financially feasible system can identify all microbes present in all specimens; however, the stains may suggest organisms that require special culture methods.

To characterize the bacteriologic flora more fully, a specimen is cultured on artificial media, liquid or solid. A liquid medium is called broth; a solid medium is solid because agar, a solidifying agent, has been added to the broth. Many kinds of media with different nutrients have been developed. Enriched media contain extra nutrients to enable the nutritionally demanding (fastidious) organisms to grow. Commonly used enriched media include blood agar (a nutrient agar with blood added as enrichment). Differential or selective media have been developed to facilitate the isolation of one kind of organism despite the presence of many other kinds. Such media accentuate physiologic differences and inhibit the growth of unwanted forms. Commonly used differential media are MacConkey's agar and eosin-methylene-blue (EMB) agar. Both promote growth of gram-negative rods while inhibiting gram-positive organisms. Media that neutralize circulating antibiotics are now also in use.

If a specimen is appropriately spread over the surface of solid media (Fig. 19-4) and the environment (temperature, oxygen, and carbon dioxide) and nutritional requirements are met, a distinct colony of organisms will form wherever a single microbe has been

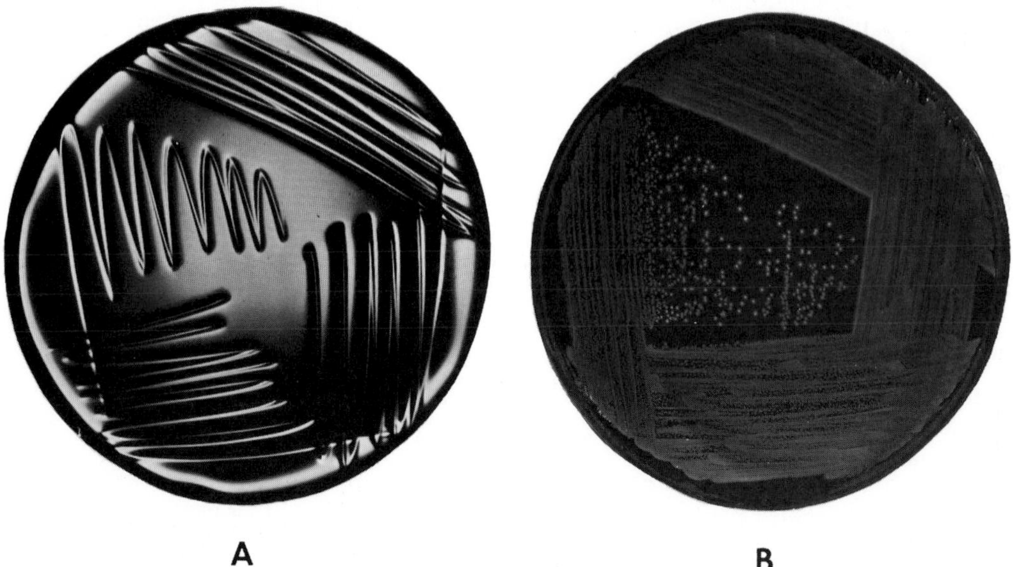

Fig. 19-4. Inoculation of a plate to isolate individual colonies. *(A)* The path of the inoculating loop that streaked the semisolid media. *(B)* The results are shown after 18 hours of incubation of a similarly streaked plate. Individual colonies are readily "picked off" the midzone of the plate for further study.

deposited. The colony morphology is often distinctive but rarely diagnostic for each type (genus). If the inoculum is quantitatively diluted, the microbiologist can estimate the relative frequency of each genera of organism and perform analyses, including microscopic, physiologic, and biochemical descriptions, that identify the exact species and antimicrobial susceptibility tests to guide therapy.

These procedures are only a sample of the methods used to characterize most microorganisms and are not applicable to viruses, protozoa, or some bacteria and fungi, which require more complex procedures.

DETERMINANTS OF MICROBIAL PATHOGENICITY

Infectious disease is the result of inoculating pathogenic microorganisms or their products into a susceptible host. Some organisms are very pathogenic and need only small numbers to initiate disease in healthy people, whereas others have a low order of pathogenicity, requiring large numbers to initiate disease and then only in highly susceptible patients who are already sick. The degree of pathogenicity is called virulence. Highly pathogenic organisms are virulent, whereas nonpathogenic organisms are avirulent (nonvirulent). Pathogenicity is usually applied to groups or species of microorganisms; virulence refers to the degree of pathogenicity of a specific strain within a group or species. *S. aureus*, for example, is considered a potential pathogen. A given strain of *S. aureus* may be virulent (a few organisms capable of initiating infection) or may be relatively avirulent (large numbers of organisms required to cause even a mild infection).

Virulence is usually the result of many factors. It depends on the ability of organisms to survive in the environment, penetrate host defense, and initiate a disease process. Many microbiologic mechanisms can serve as virulence factors. Microbes can injure host tissues directly by producing one or more toxic products; by the magnitude of the microbial load with its demand for space, respiration, nutrition, and removal of metabolic wastes; or indirectly by stimulation or other modification of the host immune system.

The toxic product may be one of many parts of the microbial cell itself or may be a product released from the microbial cell to the surrounding environment. The toxic component interacts with the host tissues and may interfere directly with host cell function, or it may initiate an immunologic response that inadvertently damages bystanding normal tissue.

Occasionally bacterial disease is the direct result of *toxin production*. Certain bacterial species produce readily identifiable toxic components. *Clostridium tetani*, for example, releases an exotoxin that can produce tetanus even in the absence of the organism. Certain other bacteria, such as *Salmonella typhi*, produce endotoxins, which are intimately associated with the bacterial cell. The release of endotoxins may be one pathogenic mechanism that occurs when structural components of the microbial cell interact with host tissues. In most microbial diseases, pathogenicity does not rely solely on toxin production. Viruses produce no recognized toxins, and pathogenesis is ultimately related to alteration or destruction of host cells resulting from intracellular growth and resultant cellular disruption in the host.

The relation between microorganisms and the host cell is vital to the pathogenicity of organisms that produce no demonstrable toxin. *Mycoplasma pneumoniae*, for example, has an ability to become and remain intimately attached to host cells. This relation causes the cilia of bronchial epithelial cells to stop their sweeping motion. Eventually there are changes in host cell metabolism and macromolecular synthesis with desquamation of the epithelial layer.

Pathogenicity may depend on the degree and type of host immune response elicited. Immunity can be both protective and destructive (as in the case of allergies). Fungi, for example, exist in nature as mutual symbiots or commensals and rarely invade human tissue. The severity of fungal disease varies largely with the degree of host resistance, although the species and route of inoculation are important variables. Hence debilitated patients have fungal infections with greater severity and frequency. Using a different pathogenic process, certain microbes, although unable to invade human tissue, can grow in the external environment (e.g., hay, paprika, tree bark) and, when inhaled, present an antigenic insult to the healthy lung with resultant hypersensitivity pneumonia. This is not an infection, but rather the immunologic response (allergy) is the pathogenic mechanism.

Although we will not discuss pathogenic mechanisms thoroughly in this chapter, we wish to emphasize the broad diversity of mechanisms (virulence factors) that can and do operate. Seldom do microorganisms rely for their effect on a single toxic product, such as the toxins responsible for tetanus and botulism. More commonly, virulence involves many factors. Thus, if the invasion is small or if host defense is brisk and adequate, the microbial invasion will be blocked or ended, and the host survives even the most virulent microbe. If the host defense is compromised, even mutual or commensal organisms may possess enough unopposed virulence factors to cause disease.

THE KILLING OF MICROORGANISMS

Seemingly miraculous powers are often attributed to chemicals called disinfectants and antibiotics. We shall list and discuss strict definitions that may clarify the functions and limitations of various agents. One should follow methods that maximize the effectiveness and minimize the hazards and cost of disinfectants.

DEFINITIONS

Sterilization

To the microbiologist, sterilization (from Latin *sterilis:* not fertile) is the complete destruction of all microorganisms. Either physical or chemical agents may be used to end permanently the metabolic activity and the capacity to reproduce for all forms of life, whether or not they are pathogenic. Although microbiologists claim sterilization is absolute, we shall point out later in this section that in practice this fact is difficult to demonstrate.

Disinfection

Disinfection (from Latin *infectus:* to taint, plus *dis:* apart) is freeing from infection; it is the destruction of potentially pathogenic microorganisms. Most disinfectants are chemicals. From the two foregoing definitions, note that disinfection is possible without *sterilization,* but not vice versa.

Antisepsis

Antisepsis (from Greek *septikos:* putrefying, plus *anti:* against) is the application to the body surface of chemicals that inhibit the growth and multiplication of pathogenic microorganisms. To be useful, antiseptics must not injure the skin or mucosa. Disinfectants that can safely be applied to the skin are also antiseptics.

Asepsis

Asepsis (from Greek *septikos,* plus *a:* not) is either the state of being free from pathogenic microorganisms or a description of techniques that prevent sepsis. Asepsis of inanimate surfaces is achieved by disinfection. Asepsis of body surfaces is achieved by antisepsis. Aseptic technique includes sterilization of supplies and equipment and antisepsis of the body surface and orifices.

Germicides

Germicides (from Latin *germin,* Old Latin *genmin,* stem of *gignere:* to beget, plus *cida,* from *caedere:* to kill) are agents that kill microorganisms. The term does not imply effectiveness or percentage killed, nor does it imply a particular spectrum of agent killed. (No effective disinfectant would be called by the nebulous term germicide.) Germicides can be divided into bacteriocides, virucides, fungicides, amebicides, and so forth. Because the term is nonspecific, it is not helpful in classifying commercially available agents.

Sanitization

Sanitization (from Latin *sanitas:* health) is the process of removing factors injurious to health. It is used to mean cleansing in order to lower microbiologic concentration, usually by removal of microorganisms. Because microorganisms are not necessarily killed, sanitizers may not be germicides. The most common method of sanitizing is to wash with soap. Thus a sanitizing agent is essentially a cleansing, not a killing, agent.

Antimicrobial Agents

Antimicrobial agents are chemicals that can suppress or destroy microbes (specifically chemicals that directly interfere with microbial metabolism and multiplication). To be useful, microbial interference must occur at concentrations readily and safely attained in host tissues.

Antibiotics

Antibiotics (from Greek *biotikos:* of life, plus *anti*) are antimicrobial agents of microbial origin (e.g., penicillin).

DETERMINATION OF STERILITY

The *classic definition* of sterility is absolute: the total killing of the microbiota. However, in practice, the only method for determining absolute sterility alters the product. After disassembly, for example, respirator parts can be homogenized with, or immersed in, broth that is then cultured. Microbes in corners and pits may be kept from the broth by surface tension so that cultures may not reveal the presence of these organisms. If the part is pulverized in broth, the organisms are more likely to be exposed and grow on culture media. (If a part is in poor repair with pits and cracks, it is difficult to determine its microbiologic sterility.)

A *pragmatic definition* of sterility is less stringent but allows the investigator to predict probability of sterility from the available facts. That probability is based on the following tests: First, the most resistant organism likely to colonize the product is determined. Second, the maximum number of the species that might be present is estimated. Third, the sterilization process is designed to kill one million times the maximum number of the most resistant organisms that might be present. When this sterilization process is used and it is demonstrated that this number of the resistant organisms *was* killed, then it can be said that the chance of contamination by a single bacterium is less than one on one million. This pragmatic statement on sterility causes virtual apoplexy in many classical microbiologists, who hold to the "baroque" idea that sterility (like pregnancy) is absolute, not partial.

Ordinary bacteria (aerobes and anaerobes) and fungi are the only potential contaminating microbes that can be cultured in artificial media. Viruses, rickettsiae, and chlamydiae require living cells for multiplication. Most protozoa do not multiply in artificial media (*i.e.*, broth, agar plates, or tracheostomy tubes). Bacteria and fungi, therefore, are the only contaminants that are recognized and commonly discussed. Hence sterility is an implied concept, but not necessarily a proven fact, since fact requires 100% proof of sterility.

Sterility Testing

In conducting a proper test for sterility, one must transfer all microbes from the product in question to the culture medium. Transfer is usually accomplished by disassembling the part and washing it in a solution (water or broth). If the part has many corners and crevices, then the part must be destroyed by grinding in a solution so that the microbes will be exposed and can be suspended in the solution. (The debris is discarded by any one of several methods.) It is usually convenient to concentrate the microbes on a filter disc (pore size of less than 0.45 μm), and the filter disc can be placed on an agar plate for culture. Universal neutralizer* is added to neutralize any substance that may have been used in the disinfectant process so that residual chemicals will not inhibit the growth of persisting bacteria or fungi.

An appropriate culture technique must sample every pertinent part of the product. In the case of respiratory therapy equipment, what is sampled must represent all parts of the device exposed to inhaled or exhaled air.

After sterilization is completed, a fraction of the devices (e.g., tracheostomy tubes) are disassembled in an appropriate sterile area and cultured. This is *end-product sterility testing* and follows the classical definition of sterility. If a sample of tracheostomy tubes (only a fraction of the entire lot) are cultured and found to be sterile, can one infer that 100% of the lot was sterile? With what confidence? This is a statistical problem. The higher the percentage of devices that one wants to say are sterile, the larger the number of devices (e.g., tracheostomy tubes) that must be sampled. In other words, if one wants to say that 100% are sterile, one must sample more devices than if one needs to say that only 50% are sterile. If one desires to be 100% certain that 100% of the tubes are sterile, one must culture all of the tubes. After this process, the tracheostomy tubes are no longer sterile and usable. They must be cleaned, repackaged, resterilized, and retested for sterility. By this time one would be out of business! Thus end-product testing for sterility, although useful as a quality control check, is not practical as the sole means of establishing sterilization procedures for respiratory therapy equipment and associated supplies.

End-product sterility testing is, however, a method commonly used commercially in the United States. Accordingly, one can assume that an occasional lot of products will contain a few (an uncertain number) contaminated units. The intravenous fluid industry has had several disasters when contaminated fluids have been released to the market, thus proving that end-product testing in the best of hands misses some batches with low-level contamination.

In practice, sterilization procedures that follow the pragmatic definition of sterility are more applicable. This method has already been briefly described. By way of example, if the most resistant organism anticipated is the enterococcus in concentrations as high as 10^5 organisms/ml, then the sterilization process

*Universal neutralizer is 0.5% Tween-80 and 0.07% soy lecithin.

should reliably kill all enterococci in concentrations of 10^{11} per milliliter. With every lot of material sterilized, a container with one million times ($10^5 \times 10^6 = 10^{11}$) the expected number of enterococci is included. If the container is sterilized, one can safely say that the chance for enterococcal contamination of the lot is one in one million. In this method the adequacy of the *process*, rather than end-product sterility, is tested.

Process plus periodic end-product sterility testing should be employed to assure maximum safety and that no changes in materials, techniques, procedures, or potential pathogenic flora have occurred.

Principles of Sterilization and Disinfection

Microbes (including viruses, chlamydiae, rickettsiae, and protozoa) are killed by denaturing their protein or destroying the cell membrane. Which molecules are denatured depends on the species of microbe and the physical or chemical process used in sterilization or disinfection. The time required to sterilize or disinfect depends not only on the temperature and process (which determines the rate of killing), but also on the original number of organisms. The logarithm of the number of surviving organisms (N_t) of a given species is directly proportional to the logarithm of the original number of organisms (N_o) and inversely proportional to the duration of exposure (T):

$$\ln N_t = \frac{\ln N_o}{KT}$$

With chemical sterilization and disinfection, the rate of killing (K) for a given number of bacteria also depends on the chemical, its concentration, and the temperature.

The technical differences between sterilization (all organisms including resistant spores killed) and disinfection (only the pathogens, most of which are relatively sensitive and usually present in lower number are killed) are twofold. First, the spores are more resistant forms and are killed more slowly, thus requiring a longer exposure to a higher concentration of sterilant. Second, the larger the number of organisms to be killed, the longer the necessary exposure to the sterilant. Inadequate concentrations of chemical or inadequate length of exposure negates disinfection. If a chemical sterilization process is used but the concentration of chemical is inadequate or the time of exposure is shorter than required, sterilization will not be achieved. Disinfection may not be achieved; in fact, even sanitization may not be accomplished.

Sterilization and disinfection occur only if the agent is in contact with the microbes. Physical methods must penetrate and produce the necessary changes in all parts of the product to achieve effective results. (Radiation must penetrate the wrapping; steam must penetrate the entire autoclave load, or the products will not be autoclaved and there will be no sterility.) Chemical agents can be prevented from reaching microorganisms by coverings of dirt or mechanical crevices because inadequate diffusion or surface tension prevents entry into the crevices and damaged or dirty parts of the apparatus.

Chemical agents can also be bound to dirt or other organic materials, decreasing the concentration of free chemical at the microbial surface. Low concentrations of the agent decrease its effectiveness and prolong the necessary duration of exposure. Quaternary ammonium compounds ("quats") may be inactivated by organic materials such as gauze, dirt, and blood.

If bacteria are allowed to multiply in a solution (e.g., fluid for nebulization) and the fluid is autoclaved before use, the bacteria will be killed. However, the lipopolysaccharide of the bacterial wall (endotoxin) may act as a pyrogen (fever-causing substance), and the patient may become febrile because of the toxin absorbed from the respiratory surfaces. Thus fluids for aerosolization must be not only sterile, but also pyrogen-free.

Methods of Sterilization

Physical Methods. Heat in sufficient quantity will denature the proteins of all organisms. Many pathogenic organisms are killed by as little as 62°C for 30 minutes (as with pasteurization, a form of disinfection), but spores are more resistant. They require higher temperatures for longer periods.

Incineration. If the contaminated product has no further use or the pathogens are of extreme virulence, incineration is a preferred method of sterilization. The proper fuel and air mixture must be used so that temperature is adequate, combustion complete, and air contamination prevented.

Autoclave. High temperatures (121°C) are achieved by using steam at the two atmospheres of pressure necessary to achieve this temperature. Moisture increases conduction of heat and rate of killing. To use the autoclave properly, the air must be exhausted so that steam can replace air. The temperature achieved is related to the pressure. If the vessel contains two atmospheres of pressure, the boiling point of water is 121°C. The autoclave must be properly packed. Any covered containers must be loosely capped (never completely filled with liquid), and the autoclave time must be adequate to allow complete penetration of all packs by steam. Instruction in the technique of packing an autoclave can be obtained in most central service departments or from the manufacturer's literature or training films. Autoclaving causes deterioration of rubber, many plastics, and many solutions (especially if they contain dextrose) and dulls the sharp edge of many instruments.

Dry Heat. Because organisms are more resistant to dry temperature, the temperature needed to obtain sterility must be hotter (160°C) and longer (1–2 hours). In addition, dry heat is conducted less well than moist heat, so that the process must be prolonged if sterilization is to be achieved. Dry heat does not dull edges and is usually reserved for metal and glass objects.

Ionizing Radiation. Many hospital products are sterilized by the manufacturer with ionizing radiation. The radiation penetrates well; however, the dose required produces minor changes in some products (see Chap. 21). The basic radiation equipment and shielding are expensive; hence, this process is usually reserved for special installations and commercial establishments and is rarely used by individual hospitals.

Filtration. Some solutions are changed or destroyed by heat. Filtration through minute pores (e.g., nitrocellulose, porcelain, or sintered glass filters) can be used to remove some microbes. The simpler nitrocellulose filters (e.g., Millipore) can be used to concentrate microorganisms and have been mentioned previously.

Chemical Methods. *Gas Sterilization.* Ethylene oxide (ETO) is a gas widely used to sterilize many heat-sensitive products, including plastics. Many hospital devices are gas-sterilized. The gas penetrates well and is effective at lower temperatures (58°C) than is water vapor. Activation increases at higher temperatures, taking less time to sterilize. However, if the temperature is above 60°C, polymerization of the ETO occurs and no sterilization takes place. ETO is more effective in the presence of water; therefore, a humidity of 50% should be maintained. In the presence of 90% carbon dioxide, ETO is not explosive. ETO leaves a residual substance that is toxic to human tissues unless removed. The residual substance is removed by aerating the equipment with sterile air. The aeration time necessary to remove the residua is decreased if the temperature of aeration is increased and vacuum utilized (see Chap. 21). The basic equipment for ETO sterilization is more expensive than are similar steam autoclaves.

Aldehydes. Alkaline or (acid) aqueous solutions of gluteraldehyde (2% solution) and formaldehyde (8%) in 70% alcohol are two widely used chemical agents. They are broadly bactericidal, killing vegetative bacteria (gram-positive and gram-negative organisms), spores, and *M. tuberculosis.* They kill viruses readily. Gluteraldehyde is useful as a sterilant for medical and surgical instruments damaged by ETO or autoclaving. These chemicals must be used in adequate concentration and for long periods—about 10 to 24 hours, depending on the equipment to be sterilized. Adequate rinsing in a sterile environment, using sterile pyrogen-free water, is needed. There must be appropriate drying and packaging to prevent recontamination. Aldehydes are very irritating to the skin and mucosa. Exposure of patients to the chemicals can be controlled by careful rinsing to remove all residua. Exposure of employees can be controlled by using sterile gloves and good exhaust ventilation. Aldehydes penetrate dirt poorly and thus do not sterilize organisms embedded in dirt. They are too expensive and toxic to be used as a valid alternative to autoclaving. It is difficult to monitor the sterilization process and demonstrate that sterility has been accomplished. Moreover, aldehydes are corrosive. Nonetheless they are popular at many hospitals, possibly because they promise sterilization. Unfortunately, they are seldom used correctly so that, in fact, sterilization is rarely accomplished.

METHODS OF DISINFECTION

Physical Methods

Pasteurization. Pasteurization involves the application of heat to the equipment being disinfected (62°C for 30 minutes or 72°C for 15 seconds). These temperatures will kill vegetative bacteria and tuberculosis organisms but do not kill spores. The effects on viruses are not uniform.

Pasteurization is a practical means of physical disinfection. Many liquids (e.g., milk, wine) do not deteriorate when exposed to these conditions. The heat-sensitive parts of many medical instruments (including respiratory therapy and anesthesia equipment) tolerate these temperatures with little evidence of deterioration. Pasteurization equipment and the necessary monitoring devices are relatively simple.

Chemical Methods

Aldehydes. Formaldehyde in alcohol and gluteraldehyde (as discussed above under sterilization) are disinfectants if used in more dilute concentrations for shorter periods (see instructions for the use of the particular chemical) on clean objects free of organic material. These chemicals are corrosive. After disinfection the objects need to be rinsed in sterile, pyrogen-free water to remove all residual matter and dried appropriately before being packaged, so that the products do not become recontaminated.

Alcohols. With increasing chain length, aliphatic alcohols are associated with increasing bactericidal activity until the carbon chain is about eight. Compared with ethyl alcohol (ethanol), isopropyl alcohol is more rapidly bactericidal and less dependent on water for action. Ethyl alcohol is more corrosive. The optimal concentration is 70% for ethyl and 90% for isopropyl alcohol. Both are rapidly bactericidal for vegetative forms, especially tuberculosis organisms. They are viricidal but do not necessarily kill hepatitis viruses. Alcohol is not sporicidal. Thus, regardless of the duration of exposure, these alcohols are not sterilants but are effective disinfectants of clean objects that have been exposed for more than several minutes.

The alcohols are effective antiseptic agents of clean skin if the alcohol is applied with vigorous friction so that it can remove the surface scale and dirt. The common practice of touching the skin surface with small pledgets of alcohol-wetted cotton material before intravenous or arterial puncture is to be avoided. The skin must be vigorously scrubbed with the alcohol for at least 1 minute before the intravascular puncture.

Iodines. Iodine is a rapid germicide and is effective against vegetative organisms, tuberculosis (especially in the presence of alcohol), some viruses, and fungi. At concentrations usually available, the action is effective in 5 minutes. It is necessary to check the instructions with the particular preparation used to be certain that exposure is adequate. As commonly used, iodines are "waved" at the microbes and not brought into contact with them for adequate periods of time. Contrary to traditional belief, iodines are not magic; they work by oxidizing selective enzymes, which takes a certain time (see below).

Available iodine preparations include 70% alcohol with 0.2% iodine, and iodophores, which are organic iodine complexes that slowly release free iodine, the active disinfecting agent. A solution of alcohol and iodine is a rapid disinfectant for use on some clean surfaces; it can stain or corrode some materials. It is also a safe and cheap antiseptic; however, it further injures damaged tissue surfaces. Iodophores are effective disinfectants and antiseptics that cause less skin irritation and thus are better tolerated; iodophores are less likely to result in iodine sensitivity. For iodophores to be effective, they must be in contact with the surface for several minutes before removal so that enough free iodine is released. (Check the directions for the specific preparation used.) All iodine preparations are partially deactivated by the presence of dirt or other organic materials; therefore, the surface must be clean before attempts at disinfection or antisepsis.

Chlorhexidine. Chlorhexidine is an antiseptic recently released in the United States. The gram-positive spectrum includes *Mycobacteria* and *Nocardia;* the gram-negative spectrum includes the important nosocomial causes of sepsis *(Pseudomonas, E. coli, Klebsiella,* and *Serratia).* The fungal spectrum includes *Candida* but excludes *Aspergillus* and other important species. According to available data, chlorhexidine cannot be considered an effective virucide. The preparation available in the United States is a 4% detergent solution that should not be diluted further. Chlorhexidine is inactivated by soap and slightly inactivated by pus, blood, and other organic materials. When used several times a shift (at least three), there is accumulative and residual action (as with hexachlorophene). The currently available preparation has a low order of dermal sensitization, and with frequent use the skin rarely chafes. Although recently introduced into the United States, long experience elsewhere suggests that chlorhexidine will be an important agent for hand scrub and wash.

Phenols. Phenolic preparations are good bactericides and are effective against vegetative forms of bacteria and tuberculosis organisms. They are viricidal against some agents and are also fungicidal. Phenols, however, are not sporicidal; they do not kill hepatitis virus reliably and are inactivated by dirt and organic compounds. Alcohols and soap decrease their effectiveness, but neutral detergents and acid *p*H increase their effectiveness.

Many modern agents are substituted phenols that give more rapid bactericidal action, broader spectrum, less aroma, and more residual activity. Such substituted phenols are widely used disinfectants. Many are irritating to the skin and, of course, are not useful as antiseptics.

Hexachlorophene. Hexachlorophene is a halogenated bisphenol of great popularity. It is a good antistaphylococcal agent but is relatively ineffective against several gram-negative pathogens. (*Klebsiella* and *Serratia* have been grown from bottles containing hexachlorophene.) It works slowly, is only bacteriostatic, and is neither a true disinfectant nor an antiseptic, although it is frequently misused for these functions. If used regularly for 2 to 4 days, it will build up a residuum on the skin that decreases staphylococcal colonization. In addition to its low order of effectiveness, hexachlorophene is absorbed through the skin and is neurotoxic. Hexachlorophene has no distinct value for respiratory therapy services.

Quaternary Ammonium Compounds ("Quats"). "Quats" are cationic detergents that kill by disrupting the cell membrane. They are rapidly bactericidal and virucidal but have a limited spectrum. *Pseudomonas* can multiply in the concentrated solutions of many "quats."

Quaternary ammonium compounds are rapidly neutralized by dirt and other organic materials, including soap. Many important hospital organisms are resistant. Several serious epidemics have been traced to the improper use of "quats" as disinfectants or antiseptics. "Quats," however, are fairly effective sanitizers.

ANTIMICROBIAL DRUGS

PRINCIPLES OF ACTION

Antimicrobials are chemicals that kill microbial cells by attacking a point in metabolism or multiplication where the microbe differs from the mammalian host. Procaryotes (bacteria) have cell walls; mammalian eucaryotes do not. Penicillins, semisynthetic penicillins (e.g., ampicillin, methicillin), and cephalosporins interfere with the synthesis of the bacterial cell wall.

Some metabolic pathways may represent crucial, rate-limiting biosynthetic steps for the microorganism. Many pathogens, for example, synthesize folinic acid but cannot transport it across the cell membrane. The combined drug trimethoprim–sulfamethoxazole, which interferes with folinic acid synthesis, is a case in point. Mammalian cells transport folinic acid and do not need to synthesize it. On the other hand, certain organisms (e.g., *Pneumocystis carinii*) do need to synthesize folinic acid and are "metabolically paralyzed" without it—hence, the efficacy of combined drug therapy with trimethoprim and sulfamethoxazole.

Bacteriostatic antimicrobial agents (such as tetracycline or erythromycin) block bacterial multiplication. When the antimicrobial agent is withdrawn, the bacteria can continue to multiply, unless the antibacterial defenses of the host contain and kill the microbe. Bactericidal antimicrobials in high, but achievable, concentrations kill bacteria. Penicillin, semisynthetic penicillins, cephalosporins, and aminoglycosides such as kanamycin, gentamicin, tobramycin, and amikacin are examples of commonly used bactericidal antimicrobial agents.

For most antimicrobials to be effective, the bacteria should be rapidly multiplying. If the bacteria are in high concentration but not multiplying (as in an abscess or behind an obstructed bronchus), antimicrobial agents may not kill the bacteria, even though the bacteria may be susceptible *in vitro*. If the abscess is drained or the bronchial obstruction removed, the nonmultiplying bacteria are eliminated, new tissue fluids move into the area, residual bacteria multiply, and their susceptibility to the antimicrobials will again be apparent.

USE OF ANTIMICROBIALS

The antimicrobial agent of choice is the one least likely to cause toxicity and, on the basis of susceptibility data (from the literature or clinical laboratory testing), most likely to be effective against the suspected invading organism. The dose of antimicrobial should provide drug levels in the host cells low enough to avoid toxicity but levels in the infectious site high enough to cause microbial death, or at least high enough to inhibit microbial multiplication. Because data from tissue sites are not readily available, most studies use blood levels as crude estimates. The ratio between effective drug concentrations and drug toxicity is called the *therapeutic index*.

Antimicrobial agents are distributed in various fluid compartments. Blood levels are achieved by drug absorption (from the gut or parenteral injection site) or by direct intravenous infusion. Blood levels are decreased as the drug is distributed throughout the body. Drugs diffuse or are transported and carried through extracellular and intracellular fluid compartments. Drug levels at various sites depend on drug diffusion, drug binding to protein or other cell structures, active transport (as by the kidney), and permeability barriers such as the blood–brain barrier or blood–sputa barrier.

Most antimicrobial agents are given in an active form. A few formulations (usually less desirable) must be metabolized to become active. Many drugs are metabolized to less active forms (usually by the liver) and are excreted by the kidney (free or metabolized), the liver (into the bile), or the colon (into the stool).

The frequency of dose depends on the rate of loss of active drug from the body. Those drugs lost quickly, such as penicillin, must be given at frequent intervals. Drugs lost slowly, such as amphotericin B, can be given less frequently.

If organs that metabolize or excrete the drug are impaired, the frequency of dose must be decreased. Gentamicin, for example, is excreted by the kidney. If kidney impairment occurs, the drug will be excreted more slowly; therefore, the drug should be given less frequently. (Instead of every 8 hours, it is given every 12 to 24 hours, or even less frequently.)

When drugs are given by routes other than oral, they should never be mixed. *Drug incompatibility* means that the presence of drugs A and B in the same syringe or intravenous infusion alters the physical or chemical properties of one or both drugs. This results in altered distribution, excretion, and therapeutic activity. In the past, incompatibility meant gross physical changes in the solution, such as precipitate. Today incompatibility means any alteration in therapeutic effectiveness or pharmacokinetics.

The listing of incompatibilities is long. It is easier to accept the truism "Don't mix," unless testing shows that the two drugs in a specific solution have no effect on the kinetics or efficacy of each other.

Types of Drug Reactions

Drug Toxicity. Drug toxicity is a predictable pharmacologic action (e.g., nervousness with epinephrine; altered renal function with kanamycin). Low doses may prevent toxicity, but it may be necessary to accept some toxicity to achieve a necessary benefit in critically ill patients (e.g., increased serum creatinine in patients receiving amphotericin B).

Idiosyncratic Reactions. Idiosyncratic reactions are reactions that are not predictable. Often they are allergic in nature (e.g., anaphylactic reactions to penicillin; pulmonary fibrosis secondary to nitrofurantoin). To a certain extent, idiosyncratic reactions may be predicted by identifying the patient's previous drug reactions and allergy history and making careful assumptions. Idiosyncratic reactions can be prevented only by avoiding the use of the inciting drug. Low doses may not prevent idiosyncratic actions. When a drug is indicated and the patient's history predicts an idiosyncratic reaction, then a clinical decision must be made. Rarely should the drug be used. Other agents should be substituted when possible.

Superinfection. Superinfection can occur when antimicrobial agents change the bacterial flora of the mouth, respiratory tract, gut, or vagina. Susceptible bacteria are killed and resistant bacteria multiply in the ecologic vacuum. The susceptible bacteria may have been mutuals and the resistant bacteria may be pathogenic; thus, by replacing mutual organisms with pathogenic organisms, antimicrobial agents can *cause* infections. These are called superinfections.

RESPIRATORY INFECTIONS

COLONIZATION VERSUS INFECTION

In discussing microorganism–host interactions, three words need to be defined: colonization, infection, and disease. *Colonization* describes the behavior of organisms when they grow on the surface or lining of the host without invasion, alteration of tissue, or any host response to toxin; this includes mutual and commensal relationships. *Infection* occurs when microorganisms or their toxins invade the host. Tissue changes may or may not occur. The responsible microorganism is called etiologic. This is a parasitic relationship. *Disease* is decreased health produced by changes in the host's physiology, biochemistry, and histology. In the absence of symptoms, the disease is subclinical. (Microbes, of course, are only one group of causes for disease.) A few examples are in order. Pneumococci can colonize the upper airways but not the lower airways in the absence of abnormality (e.g., chronic bronchitis). A patient with chronic bronchitis may have pneumococci in the pharynx and in the sputum. However, the pneumococci are not playing a role in the etiology of the chronic bronchitis; the organisms are almost certainly only colonizing the airway. If the sputum becomes more purulent and viscid and the patient more symptomatic while the pneumococci persists and the chest roentgenogram shows an infiltrate in the right lower lobe, then pneumococcal pneumonia may be diagnosed. In this case the colonizing organism has invaded the tissues and caused an infectious disease.

M. tuberculosis rarely colonizes but does infect, as shown by a positive skin test (evidence of cell-mediated immunity). If the patient has a normal chest roentgenogram, negative sputa cultures, and no other abnormality, this would be called infection without disease. If the patient has a positive chest roentgenogram and positive skin test but no symptoms, this is asymptomatic disease. Active tuberculosis (positive chest x-ray and sputum culture) may be asymptomatic even though it is contagious.

Factors Affecting Colonization

Microbiologic ability to grow on a particular surface depends on many factors already discussed. Environmental factors such as pH, nutrients, and partial pressure of oxygen may be controlled by the host or other microbes. These factors encourage some organisms and stop the growth of others. The normal flora make antimicrobial products that prevent growth by other organisms. Antimicrobials kill normal flora, allowing new microbes to colonize—microbes that are resistant to the antimicrobial agent. The new microbes may be pathogens and cause disease. Alpha-hemolytic streptococci in the mouth, for example, normally block *Pseudomonas* multiplication and are part of the candidicidal (*Candida*-killing) system of the mouth. Occasionally the administration of tetracycline kills many resident alpha-hemolytic streptococci. Oral candidiasis (thrush) and *Pseudomonas* colonization frequently result.

Exudates: Hallmarks of Infection

Pus from an infection consists of serum proteins, living and necrotic polymorphonuclear cells, and the infective agent. Because polymorphonuclear cells exude from the tissue, pus is also called an exudate. An *uncontaminated exudate* occurs if the infection is in an otherwise sterile area (subcutaneous tissues) and stays protected from colonizing flora (e.g., a closed abscess). Then the organisms in the pus are the organisms that caused the infection. On the other hand, if the pus is open to colonizing organisms (an open wound), the organisms in the pus are those that have growth potential in necrotic tissue or pus. The organisms initiating the infection continue to invade tissue but may be killed in the exudate by colonizers. Thus, in a *contaminated exudate*, both Gram's stain and culture will give information about the colonizers, but not necessarily the invading organisms. Accordingly, technically accurate microbiologic data colonizers can be erroneously interpreted as referring to invaders.

While still at the infective site, *sputum*, which is the pus of lungs and bronchi, contains the infecting organism usually uncontaminated by colonizers. As the sputum travels up the tracheobronchial tree to the larynx, it has a slight (but definite) chance to become contaminated. Above the larynx oropharyngeal flora are added in concentrations 10 to 100 times that of the invading organisms in the lung pus. Quantitative enumeration of organisms in the expectorated sputum will result in information that can be erroneously interpreted.

Principles of Interpretation of Exudate (Pus and Sputum). Subsequently we shall discuss the interpretation of sputum samples, but here we shall review some of the general principles for recognizing etiologic agents for infections usually caused by a single etiology (e.g., pneumonia).

1. If a common etiologic agent (e.g., pneumococci) for an infection (pneumonia) is identified in the pus (sputa), and if the infection is consistent with the etiology clinically, radiologically, and pathologically (the disease looks like pneumococcal pneumonia), then the demonstrated organism is accepted as the etiologic agent and antimicrobial therapy is directed against the organism. (Penicillin is given to treat the pneumococcal pneumonia.)
2. If several common organisms are obtained, contamination should be assumed and the approach described below initiated.
3. If pus is contaminated, whether at the source or in traveling to an orifice (expectorated sputum), vigorous attempts should be made to collect an uncontaminated specimen. If it is impossible to obtain pus without contamination from the source, it may be necessary to obtain a tissue biopsy. To obtain pus or sputum without transient contamination (oropharyngeal), one should take the specimen between the site of infection (lungs) and the site of contamination (mouth) by, for example, obtaining a

transtracheal aspirate or bronchoscopic specimen.

4. If the identified organism is not a common etiologic agent for the infection under investigation, one must prove that it is the infecting agent. The role of contamination should be ruled out by meticulously collecting the specimen as described above.

If the organism is infecting tissue (e.g., pneumonia), an appropriate stain (e.g., Gram's stain) should show the microbe in the tissue with an appropriate inflammatory reaction (polymorphonuclear cells and bacteria in the alveoli). If the agent has not been previously described as a known etiologic agent for that infection, then one must prove that the organism can cause the observed disease.

PATHOGENESIS OF RESPIRATORY INFECTION

Disease is a rare result of the human–microorganism interface. Whether invasion occurs depends on the relation between host defense mechanisms and the number and virulence of the organisms. In this section we shall define respiratory infections and examine the human changes that accompany invasion of the respiratory tract by pathogenic bacteria. We shall describe the various mechanisms operative during infectious pulmonary disease in humans.

Pneumonia is defined as an infection of pulmonary tissues involving the interstitial space and alveoli, often with bronchiolar and bronchial involvement. Pneumonia results in edema of the alveolar septa and intra-alveolar exudate (Fig. 19-5). Early hy-

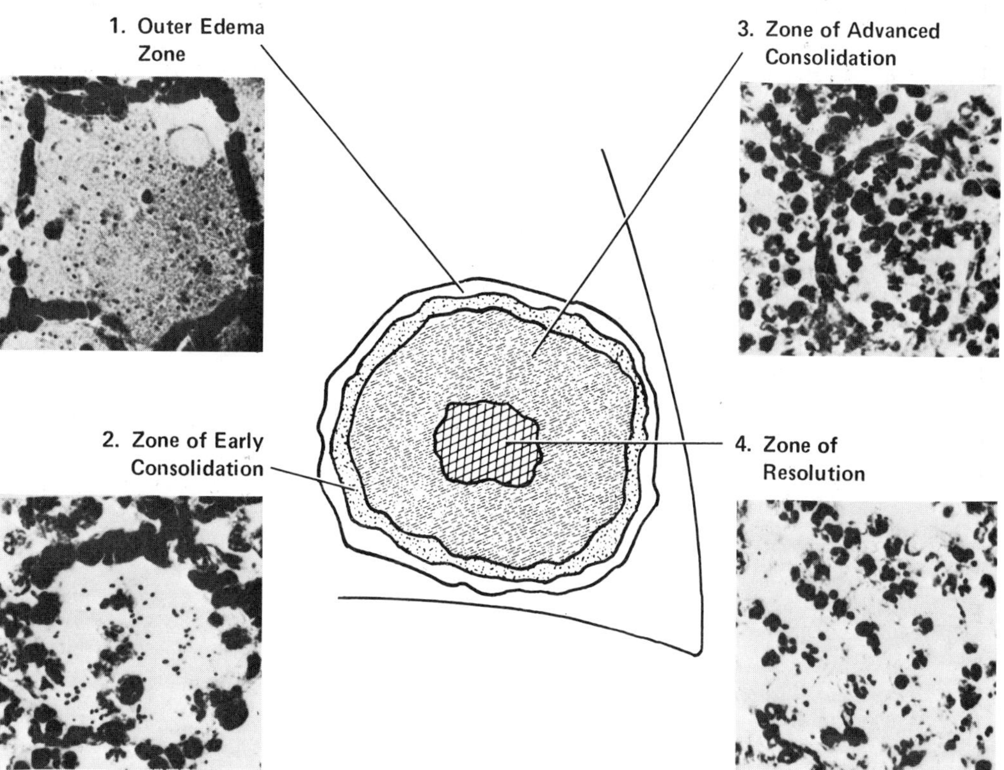

Fig. 19-5. Four stages of pneumonia. Edema (zone 1) is the first change caused by pneumococcal pneumonia. With early exudation (zone 2), there is associated engorgement of the capillaries. With increased consolidation (zone 3), mononuclear cells infiltrate and polymorphonuclear cells are less prominent. The capillary bed is relatively bloodless. During resolution (zone 4), cellular exudate is removed. Fibrin is either removed or becomes dense scar and part of the repair mechanism.

peremia (increased blood flow) is followed by vascular sludging and diminished capillary blood flow. The products of inflammation are drained by the lymphatics and may overflow into the venous circulation. The invading organism may obtain access to the bloodstream by overwhelming the lymphatics, thus causing septicemia.

Bronchitis is an infection of the bronchi with proliferation of the goblet cells, epithelial metaplasia, submucosal edema, polymorphonuclear infiltrate, and increased purulent secretions. The process often results in narrowing of the bronchial lumen and bronchospasm.

To be a successful pathogen, the organism must survive the geometric defenses of the branching airways, the mucociliary escalator, and secretory antibody. Then either by attachment, lytic enzymes, or other toxins the organism must penetrate the mucosa or reach the alveolus, evading alveolar macrophages long enough to multiply with subsequent "irritation," formation of edema fluid, and other evidences of inflammation. In the alveoli the inflammation thickens the alveolar wall and edema fills the air sac, protecting the organisms from further phagocytosis and carrying the organisms to other alveoli. Thus the pathogen has an established area for multiplication, free from the ravages of phagocytosis, at least for a short time.

With microbial multiplication, the pool of organisms extends to uninvolved respiratory tissues, increasing the magnitude of infection. The initial host response is usually vasodilation with edema formation: polymorphonuclear cells marginate along the arterioles and capillaries; then, with diapedesis, they leave the vessels, reach the tissue, and migrate to the site of the organisms. Several substances are known to be important in the sequence of vascular dilation, diapedesis, and chemotaxis of polymorphonuclear cells. Several of the substances in the complement cascade (whether activated by antibody or properdin) are chemotactic. Several of the substances in the clotting cascade initiate and maintain altered vascular reactivity. Bradykinin seems to play an important yet largely undefined role.

The extent of pulmonary involvement after microbial invasion depends on the specific defense and on general defenses. (Because general defense mechanisms against pneumococci are often inadequate, before the age of antimicrobial therapy, pneumococcal pneumonia was a common cause of death.) In an impaired host, bacteria can multiply, protected from host defenses. For example, multiplying anaerobic organisms necrose tissue (necrotizing pneumonia) to form an abscess and continue erosion until the bronchial wall is perforated and the abscess empties, leaving a pulmonary cavity.

Local Pulmonary Physiologic Effects

Structural Changes. Microbial invasion results in a transient polymorphonuclear exudate followed by a mononuclear infiltrate and a contraction of the protein matrix, with the formation of fibrin. This gives an x-ray shadow with loss of air space. These subacute changes may resolve slowly or may persist as a permanent scar.

Sputum reflects the inflammatory exudate of pulmonary disease. There is an acute outpouring of polymorphonuclear cells into the bacteria-filled fluid. The bacteria among the pus in the sputum are the infectious agents (if the specimen is collected and interpreted properly). In nonbacterial pulmonary infections, the sputum is often relatively free of bacteria. As the acute stage passes, the sputum has fewer polymorphonuclear cells, and a higher percentage of cells are macrophages and other round cells. During the reparative phase, desquamative bronchial epithelial cells are present in the sputum, and the concentration of cells decreases further.

Functional Changes. The edema of inflammation stiffens the lung, decreasing compliance and vital capacity. The exudate filling airways or alveoli cause a shunt type of ventilation/perfusion defect with resultant hypoxemia. Infection *per se* increases the metabolic demands with a secondary tachypnea. Decreased surfactant production results in atelectasis. The protein matrix that becomes fibrinous during resolution decreases compliance, with reduced lung volume. In such situations, spirometry will demonstrate a restrictive defect.

Systemic Effects

Inflammatory Changes. Infections often cause *fever*. The phagocytes (both polymorphonuclear and mononuclear) release a chemical called endogenous pyrogen (EP) when ingesting particles. EP carried by the blood to the hypothalamus turns up the body thermostat. With the temperature-regulating center set to a higher level, the body raises its temperature by preventing heat loss through decreased circulation in the superficial skin vessels, and increasing heat production through increased muscle work (shaking chills) and increased metabolism.

Cardiovascular Effects. Because of increased metabolic demand, *tachycardia* occurs. The blood pressure may be decreased because of increased peripheral vasodilatation and decreased circulating blood volume secondary to dehydration. In addition, the systemic effects of complement, clotting cascades, and bradykinin also decrease blood pressure. Cardiac function may be impaired by products of infection, hypoxemia, or increased metabolism, and the patient may develop *congestive heart failure* or *shock*. Cardiac irritability may be increased because of inadequate tissue oxygenation or changing carbon dioxide or hydrogen ion concentration. All of these factors increase the possibility of serious *arrhythmias*.

Hematologic Effects. Infections may cause increased breakdown of red cells and often block erythrocyte maturation. Antimicrobial drugs may cause red blood cell hemolysis by any one of several mechanisms. Patients may thus become *anemic*. In response to the infection, marginated polymorphonuclear cells immediately mobilize, and the splenic reserve is rapidly poured into circulation, all resulting in an *increased white blood cell count*. If the bone marrow cannot make new polymorphonuclear cells at this rate (either because of the infection or for other reasons), immature polymorphonuclear cells will be released (a shift to the left), and occasionally the white blood cell count may fall.

Hepatic Effects. Fever, red blood cell hemolysis, and other products of infection increase the metabolic demands on the liver. The infection itself, or antimicrobial agents, may have a direct hepatotoxic action.

Renal Effects. Dehydration and peripheral vasodilation decrease total blood flow through the kidney. The kidney becomes susceptible to toxins and to free hemoglobin released from hemolyzed red blood cells. The blood urea nitrogen concentration often increases as tissue is broken down to become a source of energy and amino acids for repair. Antimicrobial agents are often nephrotoxic, causing further damage to the susceptible kidneys.

Effects on Water and Electrolyte Metabolism. Many febrile infections increase water loss through the kidneys. Fever and hyperpnea cause the patient to lose additional water through the skin and respiratory tract, with subsequent *dehydration*. Conversely, pulmonary infection may cause the body to retain water by the mechanism of inappropriate antidiuretic hormone release, and the patient can become *water-overloaded*. Thus the water balance may need to be protected. It cannot be assumed that a patient on intravenous feedings, catheterized, and unable to take fluids *ad libitum* will maintain a normal water or electrolyte balance without close monitoring.

The patient may lose excess potassium in the urine or, because of associated vomiting and diarrhea, lose electrolytes from the gut, with resultant *electrolyte disturbances*.

Metastatic Infection

Since infection frequently causes bacteremia, hematogenous (blood) spread of infection to distant sites may occur. By uncontrolled local multiplication, the infection may enlarge until the organisms invade contiguous structures. *Pulmonary infections* may involve the pleura with *pleuritis, pleural effusion* (fluid in the pleural space), or *empyema* (pus in the pleural space). Multiple pulmonary lobes may become involved.

Pleural infections may extend to include the pericardium, producing *pericarditis*. Hematogenously spread bacteria may infect the heart valves, causing *endocarditis* with catastrophic results. A few viral species cause pulmonary infections and affect the myocardium *(myocarditis)*, with associated myocardial irritability and decreased cardiac output.

Pulmonary Infection in the Compromised Host

Patients with preexisting pulmonary disease and other defense disorders are prone to develop significant pulmonary infections. Compared to unimpaired patients, those with emphysema, chronic bronchitis, bronchial asthma, and bronchiectasis may develop pneumococcal pneumonia, pneumonia caused by *H. influenzae, Staphylococcus, Klebsiella*, or *Enterobacter*. If the patient is on nebulizer therapy, infection (commonly *Pseudomonas* or *Serratia*) may occur secondary to the use of contaminated equipment. These patients are much more at risk to complications of influenza virus disease and its secondary bacterial infections. Because these patients already have pulmonary impairment, the etiologic diagnosis for the bronchopulmonary infection should be made quickly. Invasive techniques to obtain sputum are often necessary. Diagnostic precision is needed, since delay in etiologic diagnosis with use of incorrect antimicrobial agents for a period of time will allow additional lung destruction, chronic physiologic worsening, and additional spread of metastatic infection.

In endobronchial disease, recurrent pneumonias at the same location are frequently caused by pneumococci. The episodes must be recognized as recurrences so that additional studies can be performed to identify the lesion. The endobronchial disease must be properly treated to control and to obviate the problem of recurrent pneumonia.

Children with cystic fibrosis have thick, abnormal sputa with frequent pulmonary infections secondary to *Pseudomonas* or other very resistant organisms, including *Staphylococcus.*

Congenital or acquired *antibody impairment* may result from protein-losing gastrointestinal disease or from loss of ability to make antibody, as in chronic lymphocytic leukemia or multiple myeloma. These patients have recurrent pneumonia secondary to *Pneumococcus* (often of the same serotype), *H. influenzae*, and *Streptococcus pyogenes.*

Patients with impaired cell-mediated immunity have many infections not limited to the lungs. Impairment of cell-mediated immunity is rarely a congenital abnormality. More often it is acquired and is associated with Hodgkin's disease, lymphosarcoma, high-dose steroid therapy, or cancer chemotherapy. This impairment may be associated with tuberculosis, other mycobacterioses, disseminated deep fungal diseases, herpes zoster, cytomegalovirus, and *Pneumocystis carinii* infections.

Because of drug toxicity, malignancy, or other causes, the mature polymorphonuclear cell count may drop below 500/mm^3. These patients with severe *neutropenia* are more susceptible to disease caused by *Klebsiella, Pseudomonas,* and other gram-negative rods, *Staphylococcus, Candida, Cryptococcus, Aspergillus,* mucormycosis, and *Toxoplasma gondii.*

DIAGNOSIS OF RESPIRATORY INFECTION

Respiratory infection is diagnosed by answering a series of questions. First it is necessary to determine whether there is an infection. If an infection is present, we must attempt to answer these questions: (1) What is the etiology (based on criteria from sputum examination and clinical characteristics)?; (2) What structures are infected (based on clinical evaluation and radiologic data)?; and (3) What are the physiologic impairments (based on clinical evaluation, clinical laboratory and pulmonary function laboratory testing)? In specific cases other questions may be pertinent.

SPUTUM

Sputum examination is important in diagnosing respiratory infections. In a healthy state, sputum is a mixed gel and sol that contains alveolar macrophages and bronchial epithelial cells. About 100 ml of this sol-gel mixture is manufactured by the respiratory mucous glands daily. The normal nonsmoker has no productive cough and swallows the sputum.

In bronchopulmonary illnesses the sputum contains cellular debris from the disease process. In bronchogenic carcinoma, tumor cells may be in the sputum. In acute infection, polymorphonuclear cells are present in large numbers. As the respiratory infection begins to resolve, the cells decrease in number, polymorphonuclear cells (which die quickly) are not replaced, and round cells (which live many days to years) predominate. (Round cells include lymphocytes, monocytes, alveolar macrophages, and plasma cells.)

Problems in Evaluating Sputum

Because sputum originates in the lungs, bronchi, and trachea, it may contain material from the entire length of the respiratory tree. In patients without pulmonary disease and with no history of smoking, the lungs below the carina are sterile. If the patient develops an acute bacterial infection of the lungs, this area will shed bacteria in concentrations of 10^6 to 10^7/ml (10–100 organisms per oil immersion field [OIF]), mixed with the polymorphonuclear cells and round cells of the sputum.

As mentioned earlier, contamination of bronchial specimens may occur before the sputum is expectorated. Bacteria from the normal flora of the pharynx and mouth will be mixed with the sputum. Any bacteria from infected gums, pharynx, or sinuses may be added to the sputum. If the patient has a tracheostomy, the purulence induced by the tracheostomy tube and associated bacterial flora can easily mix with sputum from the lower airways. Thus the original exudate may well be contaminated by cells and bacteria added to the sputum that emerges from the bronchi, but these do not represent true pulmonary infection.

If sputum is not evaluated while fresh, three simultaneous processes occur. With stasis, [1] the polymorphonuclear cells become deformed and rupture;

[2] some bacteria (primarily gram-negative rods) multiply, so that they appear to be the predominant flora in the specimen; and [3] the pH of the sputum becomes more acidic, and pH sensitive gram-positive cocci such as pneumococci and streptococci are killed, lose their staining properties, and appear to be gram-negative cocci. Stasis with these changes can occur in pulmonary cavities, in the specimen jar at the bedside, during transportaton to the laboratory, or in the laboratory. *Unless the sputum is to be examined while fresh (and still warm), interpretation may be unreliable.*

Sources of Material. Normal, healthy bronchi and lungs do not produce sputa for expectoration. Most adults with chronic bronchitis have excess sputum production containing mixed bacterial flora of uncertain significance. Generally, when such patients are uninfected, a Gram's stain of their sputa shows either bacteria mixed with a few pus cells or pus with rare bacteria. A few of these patients, while "stable," will have both bacteria and pus. It is not clear whether these patients should be diagnosed as "infected" or "not infected."

The mouth has a great plethora of bacterial types. Pulmonary infections (except anaerobic infections) are usually of one or two bacterial types: If the specimens show many morphologic types of bacteria, probably the bacteria are from the mouth, not the lungs. This statement is especially true if the chest roentgenogram shows no evidence of an anaerobic infection (e.g., abscess).

The saliva has great numbers of squamous epithelial cells. If the sputum has large numbers of squamous epithelial cells, it is probably a specimen of saliva. Even if the specimen has low numbers of squamous epithelial cells, the cells and bacteria immediately surrounding a squamous epithelial cell (within 5 OIF diameters) are ignored since it is assumed that this area reflects mouth flora.

Finally, if the unimpaired patient able to mobilize polymorphonuclear cells has a pulmonary infection, the sputum will contain a dense purulent exudate. If the concentration of pus in sputum is not significant and the patient has a peripheral white blood cell count with more than 1000 polymorphonuclear cells per cubic millimeter, it should be assumed that the specimen is not sputum, and a better specimen should be obtained.

In summary, a valid specimen of sputum with Gram's staining should have no evidence of stasis, minimal or no evidence of mouth bacteria or cells, and many polymorphonuclear cells with bacteria (10–100/OIF) scattered among the pus.

Techniques for Collecting Specimens

The several techniques for collecting specimens from the lung vary in specificity, invasiveness, and ease of performance. Ideally, the teeth should be brushed and the mouth rinsed to remove debris and other contaminating materials. A deep, vigorous cough produces material that should not be allowed to remain in the patient's mouth while he is "catching" his breath. (As soon as the material gets to the mouth, it should be expectorated.)

Expectorated Sputum. Sputum may be tenacious and difficult to expectorate or, because of stasis, be inappropriate for examination. The sputum that can be expectorated should always be collected and a Gram's stain performed. If it is unsatisfactory (as often is the case), an induced specimen can be obtained.

Induced Specimens. The patient inhales sterile, nebulized pyrogen-free water or 5% saline for up to 30 minutes. Both of these substances induce bronchorrhea and cause the patient to cough. The bronchorrhea results in a thinner, less tenacious specimen, tending to provide a vehicle in which the pulmonary exudate can travel. (The same precautions stated above as to collection, transportation, and evaluation must be followed.) If sputum is induced in a patient with a very contagious pneumonia (e.g., tuberculosis, chicken pox), then the patient should be in a properly isolated environment and the therapist protected by mask and gown. Induction is a fast, simple, and usually reliable method of getting satisfactory sputum specimens.

Orotracheal or Nasotracheal Specimens. If the patient is not alert enough to cough, a suction catheter may be passed into the trachea through the nose or the mouth. If the patient has an endotracheal tube for control of ventilation or secretions, this route can be used for aspirating a sputum specimen. Since the tube travels through the pharynx, some pharyngeal flora will be carried into the trachea and aspirated into the collection. Orotracheal and nasotracheal specimens are not satisfactory for anaerobic culture.

Transtracheal Specimens. A number 14 catheter placed through the cricothyroid membrane following local anesthesia of the area is threaded down the trachea and a specimen aspirated (Fig. 19-6). Because the catheter is below the larynx, bacterial flora unrelated to the pulmonary lesion are usually negligible. This technique can be used to obtain specimens for anaerobic culture. Although the technique is simple, rapid, and usually successful, it is invasive, and about 1% have serious complications, including significant subcutaneous emphysema, bleeding, or infection. A specimen obtained through a tracheostomy tube will sample the flora associated with the tracheostomy tube plus the organisms of the pulmonic lesion.

Bronchoscopic Specimens. Flexible bronchoscopy can remove a specimen directly from a specific distal bronchus. Thus the specimen can be correlated with the appearance of the bronchial mucosa and the roentgenogram of the lung. The technique requires a skilled operator and temporarily increases the patient's work of breathing. Unless care is taken (occasionally supplemental oxygen is needed), hypoxemia may occur during the procedure.

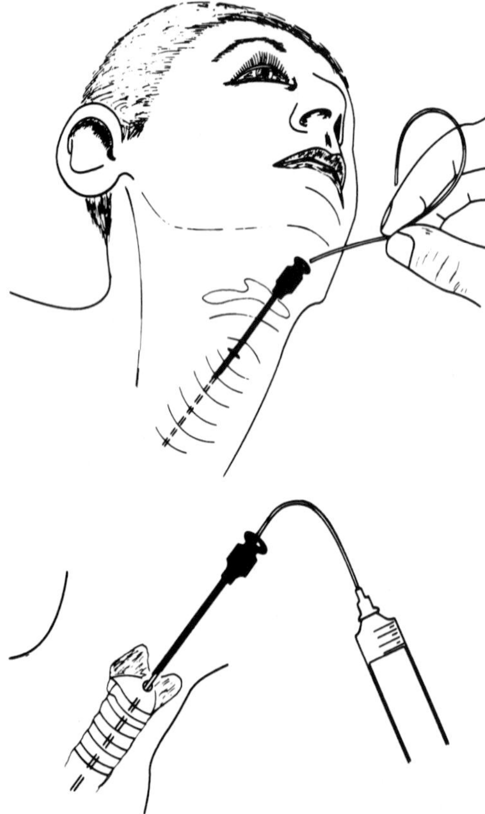

Fig. 19-6. Transtracheal aspirate. Entry is through the cricothyroid membrane with a needle catheter, which allows the catheter to be advanced toward the carina. If aspiration produces no secretions, a bolus (2–5 ml) of sterile pyrogen-free saline (no preservative added!) may be injected and then aspirated.

Transthoracic Specimens. A transthoracic specimen is obtained by aspirating through an aspiration or cutting needle directed into the lesion, usually under fluoroscopic control. This technique, which is regaining popularity, can be used to obtain a specimen for anaerobic cultures. The technique is not universally available and cannot be performed if the patient either is unable to cooperate or has a bleeding diathesis.

Additional Sites for Culture. If the patient is septic or physiologically impaired, a blood culture should be drawn immediately and repeated every 30 to 60 minutes until three cultures have been obtained. This will not significantly delay antibiotic therapy, and crucial data may be obtained, should an organism causing bacteremia be found.

If the patient with pulmonary infection also has a pleural effusion, this should be tapped and the fluid examined by Gram's stain; anaerobic, aerobic, fungal, and tuberculosis cultures; cell count; and protein and sugar determinations.

In summary, because of the range of techniques available, it is usually possible to obtain satisfactory material for Gram's stain and culture.

Preparation of Specimens for Evaluation

The need to transport the properly collected specimen to the laboratory for *immediate* processing cannot be overemphasized.

Washing of Specimens. If saliva contaminates the specimen, often the saliva can be diluted out. In the presence of water, saliva thins, but sputum maintains itself as a viscid gel/sol. By shaking sputum in isotonic saline, using a special container, the surface saliva is diluted and thinned, whereas the cells and bacteria in the sputum gel are not disturbed.

Microscopic Evaluation of Sputum

The recommended procedure for examining sputa treated with Gram's stain is outlined in the following sequence.

1. Estimate the number of squamous epithelial cells. If there are more than 25 squamous epithelial cells per slide, the slide is probably too

contaminated with saliva to evaluate, and a washed specimen or new sample is prepared.

2. Look at the polymorphonuclear cells; they should be present in significant numbers (more than 5/OIF) and should appear well-formed. If the cells look deformed, the specimen may be old. If the number of polymorphonuclear cells is small (no more than 3–5/OIF), the specimen is not from an area of inflammation and there is no evidence of infection. If the concentration of polymorphonuclear cells is inadequate, there is no need to study the Gram's stain further or to perform sputum cultures. (If the patient has severe neutropenia, this rule should not be followed.)
3. Look at the bacteria: if they are present in large clumps of morphologically similar organisms, this is probably due to stasis. If multiple microbiologic forms are present in large numbers, this is probably saliva, especially if the chest roentgenogram does not show evidence of anaerobic pneumonia or cavity formation. Try to obtain a better specimen.
4. Look at the organisms among the polymorphonuclear cells that are *not* near squamous epithelial cells. The bacteria should be present in concentrations between 10 and 100 organisms per oil immersion field. (The number of bacteria present should be approximately equal to the number of pus cells.) These bacteria are probably etiologically related to the infectious process; they are significant and should be described.
5. When appropriate areas are found for evaluation (*i.e.*, areas 5 or more OIF diameters away from squamous epithelial cells), note the dimensions of the purulent area. It should be a minimum of 5 OIF diameters. If the only areas showing appropriate material for evaluation are less than 5 × 5 OIF diameters in minimum dimensions, the slide is inadequate. Prepare another slide or obtain another specimen. If no more than two satisfactory areas are available, a preliminary report can be given, but a fresh specimen should be repeated and evaluated. *Never try to use an inadequate specimen. The only reliable data are from a reliable specimen. An unreliable specimen should be discarded and a new, proper specimen obtained.*
6. Certain terms or guides to classification are used to semiquantitate the slide: "Rare" means that the object is seen less frequently than once in every 5 OIF diameters. It is rarely significant; "occasional" means that one of the objects is seen less frequently than once per OIF diameter but more frequently than once in every 5 OIF diameters. This is usually not significant; "1+" means that there are 1 to 5 items per average OIF when looking in an appropriate area; "2+" means that there are 6 to 15 items per average OIF for most of the slide, or that there are several satisfactory areas (at least 5 × 5 OIF diameters in minimum dimension) with 15 to 50 items per average OIF; "3+" means that there are 16 to 50 items per average OIF for most of the slide, or that there are several satisfactory areas that are loaded with the items (greater than 50/OIF); "4+" means that most of the slide is satisfactory and contains a large number of items (greater than 50/OIF).*
7. The morphology of bacteria, which has been discussed in an earlier section, may be used to evaluate Gram-stained sputum, as the following examples demonstrate. If gram-positive cocci are in pairs or short chains, they are presumed to be *Streptococcus pneumoniae* (*see* Plate 19-1C). If the gram-positive cocci are in a grapelike cluster, the organisms are presumed to be staphylococci. Gram-positive bacilli in sputum, which are branched, suggest *Nocardia*. Gram-negative bacilli include the small pleomorphic (multiform) bacilli *Hemophilus influenzae*, or the larger bacilli that can be *Klebsiella*, *Pseudomonas*, *Providencia*, *Serratia*, or *E. coli*, among others. Gram-negative cocci in pairs are probably *Neisseria;* some are significant but usually are oral commensals of no pathogenic interest. Occasionally there will be a halo surrounding the bacteria. This is usually an artifact of the staining method but can indicate the presence of capsule. If there are gram-positive diplococci with a capsule, it is likely to be *Streptococcus pneumoniae*. If the bacteria are gram-negative bacilli with capsules, they are likely to be *Klebsiella*.

*In our laboratory, bacteria are quantitated in the same manner as are pus cells.

1. High concentrations of bacteria indicate that they may be of salivary origin.

2. Although 4+ pus is more significant than 1+ pus (in that more inflammation is present), 4+ bacteria are less significant than 2+ bacteria.

3. Bacteria close to squamous epithelial cells (closer than 5 OIF diameters) should not be evaluated.

Quellung Reaction. The quellung (German "swelling") reaction, also known as Neufeld's reaction, is probably the most sensitive and specific test for the presence of pneumococci. Interpretation of the test results can be difficult if the specimen examined is not sputum from the lungs or bronchi, but rather oral secretions where the presence or absence of pneumococci may be irrelevant to the diagnosis of pulmonary infection. If stasis of sputum occurs, autolysis of pneumococci will occur, and the pneumococcal polysaccharide capsule leaves the bacteria and diffuses into the gel, where it can still bind the antibody but not show a quellung reaction in the presence of pneumococci. In other words, the antibody binds to the free polysaccharide. In the sputa and surrounding the pneumococcus, there is no halo.

Culture Results. If the organisms that grow agree with results seen on the Gram's stain, then culture and stain results confirm each other. The cause of the infection is probably thus ascertained. If the organism that grew was *not* seen on the Gram's stain, two explanations can be put forward (assuming the Gram's stain and culture were done competently): [1] only a few colonies grew, so that the concentration of bacteria was too low to be seen on the Gram's stain (recall that untreated pulmonary infections have 10–100 bacteria per OIF); or [2] the bacteria originated from parts of the sputum not examined. When reading the Gram's stain, selected areas were studied and other areas reflecting mouth flora ignored. The cultured bacteria may have come from the saliva attached to the sputa and may have been ignored when reading the Gram's stain.

If the cultured organisms are small gram-negative rods (*Hemophilus* or other unusual organisms), the Gram's stain should be carefully reviewed to be certain that these organisms were not missed. In most circumstances when culture results do not confirm the Gram's stain, the culture results are less reliable, probably representing saliva. The Gram's stain is a more reliable test if performed properly. If culture and stain do not agree, new specimens should be obtained wherever possible. By following the principles given above, reliable results can be obtained most of the time.

Susceptibility Testing. Antibiotic susceptibility testing should not be performed unless the specimen is reliable. Susceptibility testing on all organisms yields useless and confusing data. Susceptibility testing becomes vital when a patient is not improving on antibiotic therapy to which his infecting organisms "should" be susceptible. Susceptibility testing may be to the *kind* and *serum concentration* of the antibiotic.

Additional Cultures. *Blood Cultures.* Organisms present in all samples represent a reliable indication of the infecting organism. If an organism is present in only one specimen (of all cultures taken), contamination is possible, and the results should be examined in view of the sputum Gram's stain and clinical criteria.

Pleural effusion cultures are usually negative. If positive, they usually demonstrate the etiology of the pulmonary process and are reliable.

EPIDEMIOLOGIC CONSIDERATIONS IN RESPIRATORY DISEASE

Evaluation of the infectious problems that may be associated with respiratory therapy is part of the broad field of epidemiology. In this section we shall first define some of the important terms and discuss approaches. Then we shall look at specific epidemiologic problems. The following terms are noteworthy.

1. *Epidemiology* (from Greek *epi:* on, plus *demos:* populace): The dynamic study of the occurrence and determinants of health and disease.
2. *Epidemic* (from Greek *epidemos:* prevalent): An increased number of cases in defined areas and defined time.
3. *Endemic* (from Greek *endemos:* native): An approximately constant rate of occurrence in a defined area during a defined time.
4. *Sporadic:* Single or isolated (scattered) cases of a disease.
5. *Pandemic* (from Greek *pandemos:* of or belonging to all the people): A disease spread widely and in high frequency (either of high frequency in defined areas or epidemic in almost all areas).
6. *Nosocomial infection* (from Greek *nosokomos:* one who tends the sick, hence Latin *nosocomium:* hospital): Hospital-associated infection with onset after hospitalization and not incubating at the time of admission.

THE BASIC EPIDEMIOLOGIC INVESTIGATION

Epidemiologic investigations seek to identify the reservoir and mode of transmission of organisms and to determine the populations at risk so that effective methods of eradication or interruption may be devised. By characterizing the infection and the organism, the reservoir and mode of transmission can often be hypothesized and tested. The occurrence time and the time course of the epidemic are important: If the exposure is a single event lasting a short time, it is usually from a "common source" with transmission of contaminated material from a single reservoir by a single route of transmission to the portal of entry of many hosts. The time course is short because the duration of exposure is short. Usually the epidemic begins abruptly and ends spontaneously, except for a few secondary cases. The "common source" is usually contaminated food or water or some other source used by a group of people that included the infected patients. It could be a contaminated batch of respiratory equipment or a contaminated multidose medication vial. Each of these could result in the rather sudden occurrence of a cluster (group) of respiratory infections. New primary cases would stop when the contaminated equipment or supplies were identified and cleaned (or used up). Apparently what is considered the endemic respiratory infection rate (about 1–4% of hospitalized patients) may include recurrent, common-source epidemics owing to poor decontamination procedures for equipment or an inadequate medication additive program. The problem can be solved if the exposed group is defined accurately so that the infected material can be identified.

If spread is "person-to-person," onset is prolonged and more gradual as the microbes are transmitted from one to the next potential patient, usually by indirect contact or by air. After an "incubation period," the patient may spread the organism to additional people. Thus the onset is less dramatic, and discovery of the contaminated persons and route of transmission may be difficult. Potentially, person-to-person spread may result in a prolonged epidemic, often involving many people. The time course for an epidemic is an important clue to this type of transmission.

There are other important questions: [1] Who is infected? [2] What are the patient's age, sex, commonalities, and other obvious characteristics? Certain hospital factors are important, such as ward or medical service location, procedures performed, including respiratory therapy, tracheostomy, arterial puncture, or surgery. Additional information may be needed, including the type of respiratory equipment involved, which employees cared for the patient, and where the patient went for additional studies (e.g., x-ray, radioisotopes, pulmonary function testing, or physical therapy).

From these data a hypothesis is formed and a control population chosen similar to the infected group but differing by the hypothesized factor. A study similar to that described above is performed on the control group. The control group is compared with the infected patients for an excess presence or an excess absence of each of the items studied.

An example may help to clarify this idea. Suppose that preliminary data indicate that seven staphylococcal pneumonias occurred in patients receiving IPPB. An additional search for staphylococcal cases indicates one staphylococcal septicemia. All patients are on the general surgical service, all have been in the surgical intensive care unit, and all have had respiratory therapy. Hypothesis might suggest that the critical factor in transmission is a person (e.g., a surgical intensive care employee, a surgeon, or a respiratory therapist); a piece of equipment, such as one of the respirators or nebulizers; or a particular surgical technique.

A control population would separate between these two groups in the following manner. When studies comparing control subjects and infected patients are completed, the investigator will have infection rates for each surgeon, anesthesiologist, surgical intensive care unit employee, and respiratory therapist, as well as for equipment, medication, and surgery. If patients exposed to a particular person have the highest infection rate and those not exposed to the person have the lowest infection rate, this would suggest that the person in question could be involved in the bacterial transmission. The hypothesis can then be confirmed by appropriate bacterial cultures.

NOSOCOMIAL PULMONARY INFECTIONS

Hospital-associated (nosocomial) infections occur in 5% to 10% of all hospitalized patients. The most common infections are of the urinary tract and lungs (pneumonia and bronchitis), each explaining nearly one third of the infections. Nosocomial infections prolong hospitalization by an average of 3 days. The dollar cost of these hospitalizations is upwards of $500 million per year, with total economic loss estimated at $5 to $10 billion per year. Since nosocomial *pulmonary* infections occur in 1% to 4% of all hospitalized patients, respiratory care workers are potentially involved in a massive infectious disease problem. In this section we shall develop some general principles on nosocomial infections (using lower respiratory infections as examples). Later we shall address ourselves directly to the question, What can be done to prevent nosocomial pulmonary infections? Only after the questions are understood can the answers be appreciated and comprehended.

Nosocomial infections occur because hospitals have host defense impaired patients; procedures that bridge host defenses are performed during diagnosis and therapy, further impairing the patient; and hospital bacteria are characterized by virulence (they *come* to the hospital as the etiology of an infection) and resistance (they *persist* in the hospital because they are resistant to antibiotics).

The impaired host has already been discussed. Recall that bacteria entering the body at any point because of any defect in host defense can spread by means to the blood to the lungs. Pneumonia is a frequent metastatic complication of other sepsis.

Procedures that bypass host defenses increase the risk of sepsis. Examples include intravenous or intraarterial cannulas, chest tubes, endotracheal tubes, urethral catheters, and Swan–Ganz or hyperalimentation catheters. Procedures that carry particles into the body may overwhelm the normal defense mechanisms of the body if the particles are contaminated. Water particles, for example, containing *Pseudomonas* (nebulized by IPPB) can overload the mucociliary escalator and alveolar macrophage defenses. Again, the *number* of infecting organisms is critical. The nebulized water *may*, of course, accelerate mucociliary clearance. If the equipment is clean and the water essentially sterile, the risk of the procedure is minimal. If these standards are *not* met, the risk may be very high.

Hospital bacteria have been "preselected." The air and patients of hospitals are frequently exposed to antimicrobial agents. This is a proven method for inducing resistance. The common nosocomial bacteria are in a continuous state of flux. In many hospitals, coagulase-positive *Staphylococcus* are of decreased importance, but *Escherichia coli*, *Pseudomonas*, *Klebsiella*, *Enterobacter*, *Serratia*, *Proteus*, and *Providencia* are of great importance. *Candida* is the most common fungus to cause pulmonary nosocomial infections.

Soon after patients are hospitalized, the flora changes depending on the intensity of medical care. This may follow intensive care and multiple procedures (including respiratory therapy) that increase the size of inoculation, or flora change may follow antimicrobial use that creates an ecological vacuum, quickly filled by hospital bacteria.

Problems Caused By Respiratory Care Procedures

A look at specific procedures done by respiratory care personnel may clarify some of the potential infectious disease problems.

Pulmonary Function Testing. Tests that collect expired gases utilize a reservoir that is, or can become, moist and inoculated by organisms in the patient's exhalate. The significance of this is potential and becomes real only when the air from these devices is inhaled and the air contains nebulized water or respiratory secretions. To our knowledge, despite the thousands of pulmonary function tests done yearly in tuberculosis sanitoria and in patients with diseases such as cystic fibrosis (and associated *Pseudomonas* colonization), documented cases of infection spread from pulmonary function equipment to patients are rare. The problem of infection spread by contaminated nebulized water, however, is separate and will be discussed later.

Respiratory Therapy Treatment Without Humidity or Nebulization. Air transmits organisms carried on extraneous material such as fomites, water, medication droplets, or oil. Particle deposition depends on particle size. Large particles deposit in the upper airways and small particles in the smaller airways (*see* Chap. 16). The occurrence of infection depends on host defense, the number and virulence of the microbes on the particles, and the irritation produced by the particles.

Nebulizers and Humidifiers. Fluids and medications *are* lifted and suspended in the liquid phase as aerosols that can be carried to the lungs. The particle size of the nebulizer output is small, so that deposition will occur in the distal airways. *All nebulizer systems have the potential to carry large amounts of "bacterial soup" into the airways.* Bacteria from humidifying reservoirs are *rarely* lifted into the airstream, but recent work has indicated that this too can occur, the risk being proportional to the reservoir inoculum.[1] Even prefilled reservoirs should be periodically cultured against this hazard.

Intubation. Endotracheal tubes (including tracheostomy tubes) provide direct access to the usually sterile areas of the tracheobronchial tree (*see* Chap. 21).

These devices impair pulmonary clearance. Tubes also create the potential for inhaling dry air, with secondary inspissation of secretions and further impairment of the mucociliary stream.

Intravascular Punctures. Arterial and venous punctures provide a pathway from the skin surface directly to the bloodstream. Such punctures represent an opportunity to put dirt or a skin plug directly into the circulation! Hematomas resulting from the puncture represent defenseless bits of nutritional fluid. Small hematomas may resolve before infection; however, large hematomas resolve slowly with a greater infection risk.

Cannulas. Intravascular cannulas and catheters are foreign bodies and, as such, are a potentially serious problem. Fibrin deposits on the intravascular edges begin within 30 minutes of placement and continue to enlarge throughout the cannulation period, even in the presence of anticoagulants.[2,4] Circulating microorganisms or those entering between the cannula and skin can enter the clot and receive protection from the humoral and phagocytic defenses of the host. Indwelling arterial lines are recognized as important causes of infection.

THE HUMAN FACTOR IN THE SPREAD OF BACTERIA

The concentration of airborne microbes depends on the number aerosolized into the air by such items as mechanical or human nebulizers and the number removed from the air by the ventilation system. Exhaled air contains microbes bound to particles of various sizes. Quiet breathing adds the least number of particles, whereas talking, whistling, and singing add larger numbers of small particles. The person with no obvious secretions aerosolizes less than the person with excess secretions. The coughing individual gives the greatest velocity to the aerosol created.

Aerosolized particles are either droplets or droplet nuclei (Table 19–3). *Droplets* are particles so large that they fall before they dry. After drying they are probably bound to dust or dirt. The microbe on the droplet can be resuspended by resuspending the dust or dirt *(fomites)*. Small droplets that dry before they fall form *droplet nuclei*. Because these dried particles have a high ratio of surface area to weight, they no longer fall but remain suspended in the air until removed by the ventilation system. Only droplet nuclei (and the microbes attached to them) can reach the alveoli. Alveoli are the only part of the respiratory system highly susceptible to tuberculosis, and only droplet nuclei can carry mycobacteria to the alveoli. Thus tuberculosis is spread not by droplets or fomites but by droplet nuclei. On the other hand. most viral illnesses (including influenza) are carried by droplets, fomites, and droplet nuclei, which can settle anywhere in the upper respiratory tract, tracheobronchial tree, or alveoli. Compared to tuberculosis, the transmission of viruses such as influenza occurs at least 1000 times more readily.

The outer layers of skin are called epithelium. Cells continuously formed at the deepest epithelial layers move outward, becoming dry and ready to *shed*. Peeling after sunburn is an exaggeration of the normal epithelial shed. In a healthy state, hundreds of thousands of cells are shed per day; during episodes of certain skin diseases, shedding increases

Table 19-3. Comparison of Particles

	DROPLETS	DROPLET NUCLEI	FOMITES
Content	Primarily water	Dry	Dry
Source	Oral-respiratory secretions	Dried oral-respiratory secretions	Dried secretions, squames, and other dusts
How formed	Nebulized particles from voice, cough, etc.	Dried suspended droplets	Dust particles
Rate of fall	30–60 cm/min	1–2 mm/min	50 cm/min
Size	50–100 μm	0.5–12 μm	>50 μm
Removal of particles	Ventilation (becomes either a fomite or droplet nuclei)	Ventilation + filtration	Cleaning, ventilation
Deposition if inhaled	Nasopharynx	Nasopharynx, tracheobronchial tree, and alveoli	Nasopharynx

manyfold. Attached to the shed skin cells (called *squames*) are the organisms of the skin: coagulase-negative staphylococci, diphtheroids, and probably some potential pathogens that were in a commensal relationship. Squames drop with gravity but are part of the resuspendable fomite population. Some normal people have coagulase-positive staphylococci as part of their skin flora. These people shed squames that contain coagulase-positive staphylococci. People with skin abscesses (boils) have many more coagulase-positive staphylococci on their skin and shed these pathogens in high densities. Bandaging and clothing are only cosmetic and have little effect on shedding. People with eczema or other skin diseases may have severe problems because they shed large numbers of squames, often populated with coagulase-positive staphylococci, that contaminate an extended space.

Personnel with skin abscesses should not work in critical care areas that have susceptible patients (ICU, postrecovery, surgery, nursery, and so forth). Some argue that they should not work around patients at all.

PRINCIPLES FOR CONTROLLING THE SPREAD OF INFECTION

Infection control begins with *cleanliness* (*i.e.*, in the presence of filth, no infection control is possible). Specific techniques of disinfection and sanitization have been discussed, but basic cleaning requires "elbow grease." There is not now, and never has been, a substitute for soap, water, and a scrubbing brush. The hands should be washed at the beginning of each shift and periodically thereafter. In addition they should be washed before and after each patient. Cleaning the equipment should be the first step in all decontamination procedures.

The problems of microbial shed by squames and aerosols are increased by the high density of people in intensive care units. Procedures that control contamination and that decrease the microbial and fomite load in the air include [1] proper design of the facility; [2] control of the traffic pattern used by visitors and employees; [3] air exchange (to dilute the microbes); [4] appropriate filtration and exhaust ventilation of isolation rooms; [5] masks (for patients and all personnel) to block aerosolized microbes from persons who are shedding pathogenic organisms from the mouth or nares; and [6] gowns to cover exposed skin and clothing to decrease the attachment of organisms to the body surface or personal clothing.

The specific details for isolation will be covered separately. From these suggestions can be taken those procedures necessary to accomplish a specific task. In some cases where the infection rate is low, a simple approach is adequate. In special situations where the infection rate is high, stringent approaches may be indicated.

Cultures taken during epidemics may show that healthy employees are colonized by the organism in question. This raises two possibilities: Did the employee acquire the organism from a patient? Or did the employee shed the organism to the patient? Extensive surveys have indicated that two thirds of hospital employees are carriers of coagulase-positive staphylococci at any given time. Carriage is temporary in half the carriers and persistent in the other half. No simple, effective treatment is certain to stop persistent carriage.

If the carrier gets "sick," with increased nasal secretions (if a nasal carrier) or with return of dermatitis (if a skin carrier) or if an abscess develops, then the shed of organisms (coagulase-positive staphylococci) increases manyfold. The shedding person is a potential risk. Staphylococcal nasal or skin carriers with minimal bacterial shed are minimal risks without some abnormality (as discussed above) that changes them so that they shed large numbers of the pathogens.

ISOLATION TECHNIQUES

Indirect and direct contact and the airborne route are the major mechanisms for transmission of many infectious diseases. Isolation is designed to break the chain of transmission to and from susceptible patients. Indirect transmission of microbes by the clothing or hands of employees to and from patients must be prevented. The air must be clean, which is accomplished by five basic isolation procedures.

1. *Separate rooms:* If air-spread plays a role in transmission, the shedding or aerosolizing patient must have a separate (isolation) room with exhaust ventilation that is not recirculated to other parts of the hospital. (Direct contact transmission may not require a separate room.) If the patient needs a separate room, the door must be shut!
2. *Masks:* Masks block the exit or entrance of pathogens through the nose and mouth. The properly applied, effective mask will remove most of the microorganisms that pass out or enter through, the mouth and nose. A moist

mask is useless because organisms pass through it with ease. Modern masks are effective for about 45 minutes and then need to be changed.

3. *Handwashing:* Hands are contaminated by touching contaminated articles (e.g., bedding, used linen, sputa cups) or patients themselves. The contamination may be spread from patient to patient (indirect contact) and across the ward. The sequence of indirect contact can be interrupted by handwashing before and after each patient contact (whether or not the patient is in isolation). The hands of respiratory care workers should be washed well at the beginning of each shift, before going home, and regularly between visits to patients. The particular type of soap or antiseptic probably is less significant.
4. *Gloves:* Most people have small, insignificant wounds on their hands. Often they have small infections that harbor large numbers of bacteria. These wounds make them susceptible to infections such as hepatitis. Although the role of the hands in indirect spread of infection can be controlled by handwashing, this is not always reliably performed. Gloves are worn to protect the employee from direct inoculation of small hand wounds by the patient's exudate and blood and to protect the patient from bacterial colonization by the employee's wounds. Gloves are always required if the hand can be a direct or indirect agent of transmission, such as in oral-fecal spread or direct inoculation.
5. *Gowns:* The gown prevents contamination of the employee's clothing to decrease indirect transmission to other patients or to the employee's colleagues and home. All employee clothing should be able to withstand the hospital laundry (temperatures greater than 63°C with high concentrations of disinfectants). The home laundry rarely exceeds 41°C and does not kill microbes, but spreads them to all other laundered articles. Clothing that becomes contaminated directly or through an isolation gown should be changed immediately and never laundered at home.

Removal of Equipment from Isolation Rooms

Generally there is little problem in removing respiratory equipment from an isolation room. It is adequate to enclose the equipment in impervious plastic so that it can be transported safely to the decontamination areas. The external surface of the equipment should be cleansed by scrubbing with soapy water and brush, then rinsed and disinfected. The respirator circuits and small parts should be decontaminated as described above.

Who Should Be Isolated?

The decision to isolate is a balance between the risk of transmission and the *potentially* decreased quality of care received with psychologic and sociologic isolation. Patients who have been colonized should rarely, if ever, be isolated. Patients with diseases caused by an epidemic strain of organisms representing a significant risk to other patients or employees should be isolated. Decisions about patients who represent minimal risks are difficult. There is no simple guide that can be followed vigorously and adhered to blindly. Most hospitals have guides and procedures taken from the public health code of their state or the Centers for Disease Control in Atlanta, Georgia. *These should be intelligently followed.*

PROTECTIVE AND PROPHYLACTIC MEASURES

Vaccination is a means of stimulating immune defenses so that the worker or patient will be relatively or absolutely resistant to the given disease, without suffering the effects or consequences of illness. Vaccination may cause a person to resist colonization and thus not be part of the spread of disease.

Influenza is a devastating illness when it produces respiratory impairment. Respiratory care workers should have influenza vaccinations regularly, so that they are less likely to infect uninfected patients. Moreover, they are less likely to be ill during an influenza epidemic and can respond to the increased work load that they must carry during such an emergency.

Respiratory care workers not known to be tuberculin-positive should be *skin-tested* every 12 months. If the skin test converts, the therapist should receive 1 year of prophylactic isoniazid hydrazide (INH).

Whenever possible, respiratory therapists' *assignments should limit the number of wards* worked during one shift. Employees should not go from infected cases to highly susceptible patients in areas such as the recovery room, the ICU, or the nursery. Thus, if the therapist is an agent of transmission, he rarely should be moving throughout the hospital, disseminating infection.

SURVEILLANCE

Surveillance consists of collecting precise data, arranging them appropriately so that they are readily understood, and disseminating the data to those who will use them for decision making. Respiratory infections and microbial colonization of respiratory equipment are the two surveillance concerns pertinent to the respiratory care worker. For surveillance purposes, these respiratory infections are defined as infections of the trachea, bronchi, and lung parenchyma. They are identified by the presence of purulent sputum, and, if pneumonia has occurred, there will be an appropriate infiltrate on x-ray. By identifying each patient who presents with, or develops, purulent sputum or who presents with an infiltrate on chest roentgenogram and other certain basic details, it is possible to determine the infected patients, the infecting organism, and the respiratory care associated with the infections.

If the line listing shown in Figure 19-7 is used, it will be possible to determine on a periodic basis [1] the number of infections on each hospital ward; [2] the number of infections that occur with and without respiratory therapy modalities; and [3] the infecting agent. By reviewing mortality data, patient out-

Name	Hospital Number	Ward and Room	Physician[1] Service	Age[2]/Sex	Admission		Respiratory[4] Impairment
					Date	Diagnosis[3]	

Respiratory[5]					Other[6]			Onset Date	Diagnosis[7]/Organism (Culture No.)
Nebulizer	IPPB	Intubate	Trach	Other[6]	Bladder	IV	Other[6]		

Fig. 19-7. Example of a line listing (to be viewed as a continuous chart). The usual parts of a line listing include identification (name, number, culture number); demography (ward, service, age, sex, date admitted); host factors (admitting diagnosis, host susceptibility); hospital procedures; and infection (date, diagnosis, organism). The sequence shown is typical but not critical. The fields shown are not always needed. These are suggestions that would apply to patients receiving respiratory therapy or to patients developing nosocomial respiratory infections. Certain headings on the chart (with superscripts) require further explanation.

1. Usually a physician admits to only one service, and service would not be entered. If the physician admits to several services, the service entry is added.
2. Age or birthdate can be entered, but birthdate is more accurate.
3. The diagnosis heading refers to that of the major reason for admission; thus all the diagnoses are not listed.
4. Only significant respiratory impairments, if any, are listed. If no such impairment is known, a dash is used to show that the field has been completed.
5. For each listed procedure, only the date started is given. Only procedures started before the onset of the nosocomial infection should be indicated. Procedures not given during the 7 days before the nosocomial infection are not listed. Line listings for patients receiving respiratory therapy should include more detail about the therapy and should indicate all patients receiving the therapy, whether or not they had infections.
6. Procedures of a nonrespiratory nature and onset dates are listed under the "Other" heading.
7. Nosocomial infection diagnosis is made by strict definitions. Included are the day of onset for the infection, the name of the infection, and the infecting organism. The culture number is also included so that additional data can easily be obtained if needed.

come can be determined. If the number of patients for each ward and the number of patients receiving respiratory therapy are known, then the infection rate can be determined.* The hospital's rate of respiratory infection should be reviewed at least monthly, the relationship to specific modalities of respiratory care noted, and the etiologic agents reviewed.

When interpreting such data, one cannot assume that normality is a zero infection rate. Based on factors already discussed, the baseline is above zero and will depend on the characteristics of the hospitalized patients. If the rate increases from month to month or if most infections are caused by a single agent, then there is a problem that needs investigation. The techniques of epidemiologic investigation have been outlined earlier in this chapter. If *Pseudomonas*, *Klebsiella*, or other gram-negative rods are the cause of infection, the problem may be related to contaminated water, medication, or equipment. If the infecting agents are usually staphylococci or pneumococci, the problem may be related to personnel who are transmitting the pathogen.

Microbiologic surveillance of respiratory therapy equipment should be performed to determine the effectiveness of policies governing disinfection, sterilization, and utilization routines. Samples of equipment *already sterilized* and ready to be distributed to the wards should be cultured periodically by mechanisms discussed in the previous section. Such data will document the quality of the disinfection/sterilization process. Appropriate results should show the equipment to be free of gram-negative rods with only a few (if any) gram-positive organisms present.

*Infection rate is the quantitative measure of the occurrence of infection corrected to a population size of 100:

$$\text{Infection rate} = \frac{\text{number of occurrences}}{\text{total population}} \times 100.$$

Occurrence rate for patients receiving respiratory therapy =

$$\frac{\text{Number of occurrences in patients receiving respiratory therapy}}{\text{patients receiving respiratory therapy}} \times 100.$$

Occurrence rate in patients *not* receiving respiratory therapy =

$$\frac{\text{Number of occurrences in patients not receiving respiratory therapy}}{\text{(total number of patients) minus (patients receiving respiratory therapy)}} \times 100.$$

Equipment in use should be monitored to demonstrate the adequacy of policies regarding the duration of use between equipment and tubing changes. In use, the number of gram-negative rods and gram-positive cocci should be small. If the numbers increase, the equipment is not being changed frequently enough. During use, equipment can be cultured by bubbling effluent air from the device through broth containing universal neutralizing agent (*see* p. 428) or by removing the terminal length of tubing that connects to the nebulizer and rinsing it with broth. In either case, the broth can be filtered through a disc and the disc cultured on a simple medium (blood agar plate). This will give a semiquantitative statement of the number and types of bacteria recovered. Usually the total number of organisms rinsed from a 4-foot length of tubing is less than 5. (This will be discussed in more detail later.)

The disinfection/sterilization *reports* should be reviewed regularly for precise documentation of compliance with established procedures. If there has been compliance, then the culture results should show essentially sterile equipment; otherwise, the disinfection/sterilization procedures need to be updated.

CONTROLLING BACTERIAL INOCULATION OF RESPIRATORY THERAPY EQUIPMENT

Respiratory therapy equipment is used in a microbiologic arena which has, in the foregoing sections, been described as crowded. Already infected patients may be further colonized or superinfected with other virulent organisms during their hospitalization, as a result of direct inoculation, nosocomial infection, or antimicrobial manipulation of their own respiratory flora. The basic principles of cleaning, drying, sterilization, and storage have already been discussed. This section deals with application of these principles to respiratory therapy departments *per se*.

GENERAL METHODOLOGY

Layout of Decontamination Area

The basic layout of a central supply unit, with a dirty entrance and a clean exit, should be used. There should be no traffic of equipment, carts, personnel, or other supplies between the dirty and clean areas. Dirty equipment should go directly to, and only to, the dirty area. Various embellishments of the room (e.g., dividers and doors) may be needed to separate dirty from clean and to enforce the need to decontaminate before leaving the dirty area.

The decontamination area should have its own air exhaust. This air should not be recirculated to any other parts of the hospital. The airflow should be such as to change the air in the unit at least six times per hour.

Disassembly. All equipment exposed to patient exhalate, fluid, and aerosols should be broken down into its smallest parts and checked for surface pitting or other defects that can protect microbes. If defective, the piece should be repaired or discarded. Every item in the dirty area should be decontaminated before it leaves the area. Respiratory therapy equipment and supplies should be disinfected or sterilized, as should all carts and containers. Personnel should wash with antiseptic solutions and dress again before they leave the dirty area.

Washing. From the basic principles discussed earlier, it is apparent that washing is the most important step in decontamination. Clean material may well be safe, even though not sterile. Dirty material cannot be sterilized or adequately disinfected and is never safe. The design of tubing and parts should allow easy scrubbing with brush and soap. Tubing should be in short lengths so that it can be scrubbed with a brush and rinsed before the sterilization/disinfection step.

Sterilization and Disinfection. Directions for use of autoclaves, gas sterilizers, glutaraldehyde, and chemical disinfectants are provided with the equipment or chemical concentrates. They should be followed exactly. The preparation of packs for the autoclave and arrangement of packs within the autoclave are additional critical areas. If great care is not exercised with packing the autoclave, air will become trapped, the steam autoclave will not reach a temperature of 121°C, or the ethylene oxide sterilizer will not achieve the minimum concentration of ethylene oxide, and sterilization may not occur.

Rinsing and Drying. The sterilizing agent of the steam autoclave is steam, and thus it needs no rinse. After a proper steam autoclave cycle the equipment is dry, and it can be directly packaged and sealed. After gas (ETO) sterilization, the equipment is dry but must be adequately aerated to remove all traces of ethylene oxide, which is irritating to the skin, the mucosa of the trachea, the bronchi and lungs of the patient, and the hands of employees. Sterility can be maintained during ETO aeration because the equipment is already in its final package.

Pasteurization leaves no residua, but chemical sterilization/disinfection does, and this must be removed, or serious irritation can occur to therapists using the equipment and patients receiving treatments. Proper methods of removing the residua have been discussed. The equipment must be taken to the drying area without contamination; employees must wear caps, masks, gloves, and gowns. For the drying cycle, tubing should hang full length and not be coiled. Filtered, warm, dry air should be forced through and around all parts and tubing until they are known to be dried. The drying time depends on the equipment load and dryer efficiency.

Packaging. Autoclaved equipment can be sealed in plastic immediately after autoclaving. Gas-sterilized equipment is sealed before sterilization with a plastic porous to the ETO. (Such packages can be sterilized and aerated.)

Items from the dryer should be handled by properly trained, masked, capped, gloved, and gowned personnel. The equipment should be assembled and packaged in a dry, clean area. Arguments favoring a horizontal laminar airflow area for these activities can easily be made.

Labeling. A labeling system that ensures rapid turnover of equipment with "first-in, first-out" should be used. Items should not remain on the shelf longer than the safety of the package and seal protects against contamination.

WATER FOR NEBULIZATION

If a container of sterile water is opened in the hospital setting, it will become contaminated, probably by *Pseudomonas*, within 24 hours. To maintain a safe, pyrogen-free supply of water is not simple. Sterile, pyrogen-free water should be obtained in containers holding no more than a 24-hour supply. Commercial bottled water not certified as "sterile, pyrogen-free" is not necessarily sterile. Many commercial concerns do not include cultures for the water organisms (e.g., *Pseudomonas*) in their quality-control program (Most tests are only for stool organisms such as *E. coli*.) If water certified free of fecal organisms is available, it may be used. If water is to be autoclaved in small jars, it should be filtered before autoclaving; otherwise, the sterile water may contain dead organisms with their endotoxin released into the water. Endotoxin can stimulate leukocyte endogenous pyrogen, and the patient may have a febrile response.

Distilled and deionized water, used in many hospital plumbing systems, often contains high counts of water pathogens. Water faucets and aerators become contaminated rapidly and may contain high concentrations of water pathogens. Theoretically, in-hospital systems for continuous, sterile, pyrogen-free water can probably be constructed. At present, however, probably no hospital has a system that is entirely reliable.

Water reservoirs for humidifiers and nebulizers should be changed at least every 24 hours and, optimally, every shift. Water reservoirs are never to be refilled; rather they are to be replaced with reservoirs that have been disinfected and dried and that are free of water-borne pathogens before reuse.

NEBULIZER MEDICATIONS

Multiple-dose medication vials are contaminated after puncture and usually allow multiplication of water pathogens. Withdrawal of medication from such vials should be made by a person trained in an appropriate setting. The sterility of the vials should be monitored both as "process" and "end-product" determinations.

HANDLING OF LARGE EQUIPMENT

Large equipment, such as isolettes and oxygen tents, should be appropriately covered and bagged before being taken to the decontamination area. There these pieces of equipment are scrubbed with soap and water, then disinfected with an appropriate disinfectant, such as alcohol, alcohol iodine, or a phenol, following the instructions of the disinfectant manufacturer about concentration, duration of application, and method of drying. When dry, these large pieces of equipment can be properly enclosed with impervious plastic to await reuse.

REASONABLE REQUIREMENTS AND CRITERIA FOR EQUIPMENT STERILIZATION/ DISINFECTION PROCEDURES

Monitoring Washing. Some method of checking for mucus and other exudate should be devised. If debris is present in any piece after washing, the entire lot should be rewashed.

Monitoring the Sterilization/Disinfection Process. For each lot that is sterilized or disinfected there should be documentation details of the process, signed by the supervisor in charge of decontamination and regularly reviewed by the technical director of the department.

Autoclaving. For each cycle there is a time–temperature record and a chemical detector within the packs, indicating that the load was hot enough. These records must be maintained by lot number. Spore tests (or suspensions of *B. subtilis* and *B. stearothemophilus*) should be added to the load at regular intervals so that it can be shown that the autoclave conditions were so severe that even these resistant spores were killed. The records must be maintained and reviewed regularly.

Gas Sterilizing. For each cycle there should be a time–temperature and "gas present" record. These documents must be maintained for each lot sterilized. In addition, spore tests, as in autoclaving, should be performed at regular intervals and the records maintained with the lot control number.

Glutaraldehyde. The lot number of glutaraldehyde, the volume of concentrate and volume of diluent added, the time the lot was added to the solution, and the time the lot was removed from the solution should all be recorded and maintained as part of the permanent record for each lot sterilized.

Pasteurization. The water temperature and duration of exposure should be recorded and the records maintained for the lot.

Chemical Disinfection. The specific chemical, the manufacturer and lot number, the volume of concentrate, the volume of diluent, and the time in and out should be recorded and all these data maintained with the batch number.

Removal of Chemical Sterilants or Disinfectants. The method for removing chemical sterilants or disinfectants should be described in writing. The time and duration of rinse for each batch should be recorded.

Monitoring Dryness. The appearance of equipment at the end of the dry cycle (if a separate drying step is required) is not an adequate guide to the presence of dryness. There should be some means of determining that the flow of air was more than adequate to dry a maximum load completely. The data demonstrating dryness should be recorded, signed by the supervisor, and made part of a permanent record for that batch.

Monitoring the Air Filter in Drying Equipment. The pressure across the air filter in the drying equipment will rise as the filter becomes clogged. This does not increase the risk of contamination; rather it decreases the efficiency of the filter and increases drying time.

Random Culturing. Sterilized or disinfected parts should be cultured near the end of their shelf-life. Cultures should be randomly taken so that on any day, any piece (tubing, nebulizer, small parts) has an equal chance of being cultured. Sampling should check results from each cleaning shift. Cultures should be taken at least every week, examining various parts, various shifts, and various days. This will not dispense with "process sterilization," previously described; rather it will show the adequacy or inadequacy of the policy on packaging, storage, and shelf-life.

Culturing Equipment in Use. Equipment in use should be cultured to determine the adequacy of policies regulating the duration of use for the equipment. If the total number of gram-negative rods in the tubing or nebulizer is greater than 10, either the equipment was dirty before use or was in use too long before replacement.

If contamination has been no problem, the assembled equipment can be cultured as a unit. If there has been contamination, the separate pieces must be cultured to identify the batch and parts contaminated and the lot in which they were decontaminated. Unfortunately, most of the batch will be used before culture results are known, thus emphasizing the need for process sterilization.

Table 19-4. Microbial Surveillance of Respiratory Equipment

	TOTAL COUNT FOR ALL ORGANISMS	
ORGANISMS	*Maximum Allowable*	*Usual*
Staphylococcus epidermidis	10	0–2
Other gram-positive organisms (*Bacillus* sp.)	10	0–5
Gram-negative rods (not water pathogens)	10	0–1
Water pathogens	5	0–1

Methods for Culturing in the Respiratory Therapy Department. Among culturing methods having specific application to the needs of a respiratory therapy department, the following are noteworthy:

1. A specific volume of effluent gas from the equipment can be bubbled through liquid media containing universal neutralizer (see p. 428). For good contact and reliable culture results, the bubble size should be small; however, this causes a foaming problem.
2. A specific volume of effluent gas can be impacted on agar plates. This requires a special impaction device and is relatively slow.
3. Tubing or other equipment can be rinsed with broth (containing universal neutralizer) using a constant shaking technique, then filtered, and the filter disc cultured. This is cheap, rapid method.
4. Nebulized fluid can be collected, filtered, and the filter disc cultured, but this is a slow process.
5. If broth is used to entrap the organisms, it can be filtered through a membrane and the membrane directly cultured. This will give semiquantitative results, indicating the approximate numbers and species of organisms present.

With each lot, records of the sterilization/disinfection process should document that the process was adequate and fulfilled policy. Culture results should show that water pathogens are not multiplying and that only small numbers of organisms (if any) are present in the equipment (Table 19-4).*

CARE OF HOME RESPIRATORY THERAPY EQUIPMENT

Owners and those responsible for the daily cleaning and maintenance of respiratory therapy devices at home must understand the principles of cleanliness,

*In our laboratory we culture by rinsing the effluent tube with broth, pulling the broth through a membrane filter, and culturing the filter.

dry equipment, and safe water. The organisms colonizing a home therapy machine will be the patient's flora, in addition to *Pseudomonas*, *Serratia*, or *Flavobacterium* from water. *The decontamination needs of home care are for clean, not sterile, equipment.* Thus avoidance of water pathogens, removal of bacteria by cleaning, and inhibition of bacterial multiplication by drying equipment will usually suffice.

The home-care visitation team should periodically evaluate the equipment in use. If simple equipment is grossly dirty, patients should not be trusted with more complicated types of home-care equipment. If the equipment is clean and dry, they may be using it properly. Guidelines for cleaning home equipment appear below.

It is wasteful and superfluous to culture dirty equipment. We doubt that microbiologic results will motivate patients to clean their equipment better. If the patient does not have recurrent infection and the equipment looks clean and properly maintained, we do not believe that the home equipment should be microbiologically monitored. The emphasis should be on cleaning and drying, not on the "magic" of microbiology.

Dilute medication to be nebulized should be made up at a properly administered "additive center,"[3] or the patient should dilute the medication himself just before use. If sterile medication is contaminated, organisms will grow in the dilute solutions. Without adequate refrigeration, bacterial multiplication will be even faster. All solutions should be refrigerated. Patients who must learn to mix their solution must do so with aseptic technique.

HOME CLEANING AND STERILIZATION OF RESPIRATORY THERAPY EQUIPMENT*

1. Each night wash manifold, tubing, mouthpiece, nebulizer, and other parts in mild detergent; scrub equipment thoroughly.
2. Rinse equipment well, making sure all remaining soap is removed.
3. Soak equipment in vinegar solution containing 2 parts white distilled vinegar and 3 parts distilled water; soak for 20 minutes.
4. Rinse after soaking in vinegar solution.
5. Drain dry on clean towel; do not wipe or dry with towel.
6. Remember to remove all water from tubing.
7. Reassemble when equipment is dry; store, ready for use, in plastic bag or dust-free area.

*Statement by the Committee on Therapy, American Thoracic Society.

INFECTIOUS HAZARDS OF THE INTENSIVE CARE UNIT

The intensive care unit (ICU) patient is at enormous risk of acquiring a nosocomial infection. Each person with a function in the intensive care unit environment can increase or decrease the risk. The ICU cares for seriously impaired patients, each with an individual microbial flora; often this contains virulent pathogens that can invade other patients in the ICU. These pathogenic organisms are spread throughout the ICU in the air (disseminated by coughing, suctioning, e.g.) and by employees' hands. Shortly after arrival in the ICU, new patients acquire organisms with an ecologic advantage. Most ICUs are crowded, with an air turnover no greater than other parts of the hospital. In addition to patient crowding, there is employee crowding, since it is necessary for many hospital workers to be present in the ICU (e.g., nurses, medical staff, laboratory technicians, x-ray technicians, respiratory therapists and technicians, physical therapists, pharmacy personnel, maintenance personnel, and housekeepers). Not only do these workers crowd the ICU, adding their own microbial load, but many have just come from other parts of the hospital, bringing "hospital-based" microbes with them.

When "codes" are called and cardiopulmonary resuscitation is undertaken, the number of people in a small space increases further. Family members, students from each school associated with the hospital, observers, visiting dignitaries, and the curious are all likely to wander by. The ICU can become a very densely populated area—a valid case of "people pollution" of the environment. To limit this, a good operating rule is that *people should not enter the ICU without legitimate and compelling reasons.*

Proper design of ICUs could lessen some of the overcrowding common to these units. Ventilation could be increased. Air return should not draw air past patients. General traffic flow for necessary personnel should exclude patient areas. It should be possible to get to each patient without entering the "airspace" of another, and it should be possible to observe patients without entering the traffic areas. There should be multiple sinks for handwashing. Clean and dirty areas should be so located that dirty and contaminated material can be removed without risk of contaminating clean areas.

The role of human fluids and hands in the spread of microbial disease is not adequately appreciated. Blood may be a source of microbes. Every year hospital personnel acquire syphilis and hepatitis because of carelessness in handling blood. The bedding must be seen as potentially contaminated with feces. When bedding is touched by hands or clothing, the patient's fecal organisms spread. Patients with oral secretions or sputum are shedding droplets and droplet nuclei, further contaminating air and bedding with their organisms.

If the patient has skin lesions, the skin flora are shed at an exaggerated rate into the environment. If the patient has an infection affecting the skin, eyes, mouth, gingiva, respiratory tract, perineum, or gut, the number of virulent organisms shed to the environment (*i.e.*, organisms already causing a disease) is 100 to 10,000 times the usual number of bacteria shed. Therefore, the bedding, gown, skin, and air around the patient are heavily contaminated. Unless care is taken, ICU personnel will quickly contaminate their clothing, hands, and face and will carry the bacteria to the next patient, thus unwittingly spreading virulent organisms as an unrecognized part of their "tender loving care."

Urine provides a rich medium for bacterial growth. Any urine exposed to air will have a high concentration of bacteria within a few hours. If a urine device (catheter, output bags, measuring cups) is handled, the bacteria can transfer to hands and be carried to the next patient.

INFECTION CONTROL PROBLEMS

The major aspect of infection is indirect transmission by the *hands*. Air and contaminated equipment, previously discussed, are also important. The same pair of hands may do endotracheal suctioning, straighten bedclothes (with their layer of fecal organisms), place and remove the urinal, empty catheter bags, measure urine output, massage the back, adjust the i.v. rate, stabilize the i.v. needle, measure the CVP, care for tracheostomy sites, give i.m. injections, and give eye and mouth care. Because of the many demands, ICU personnel go from contaminated to susceptible sites in a continuous whirl of activity. If the hands are not microbiologically clean, they are disseminating bacteria to every site not yet colonized by those bacteria.

Intravascular devices bridge the host defenses, puncturing skin and traveling to the bloodstream, there providing bacteria with niches within thrombi on the catheter, protected from phagocytes and antibodies. Cannulas, even if placed skillfully, are associated with a rapidly increasing incidence of bacteremia over a period of 48 hours. Thus peripheral cannulas should be changed before there is associated inflammation and tenderness secondary to thrombophlebitis. The puncture site should be protected from bacterial contamination.

Central cannulas are placed only when the patient's life depends on the system. As a "lifeline," it should be placed under aseptic circumstances with meticulous technique, and it should not be used for obtaining blood samples or for transfusions. (Blood greatly increases the risk of infection.) Central catheters should have the puncture site meticulously maintained. Careful change of solutions, filter, and the i.v. line for central catheters should be performed only by specially trained persons.

Intra-arterial lines, Swan–Ganz catheters, and heparin locks require the same care as do other central catheters. Blood-drawing and infusion should not be performed through the same lines as pressure measurements, if at all possible. The puncture sites should be maintained with meticulous, aseptic technique and the tubing fixed so that there is no movement. The heparin lock and other interfaces should be meticulously maintained to prevent contamination. Only devices (including syringes) with sterile interfaces should be connected.

Intravascular infusion material should never be assumed to be sterile, even if the bottle has not been opened. The bottle should be inspected for cloudiness, precipitates or other suspended material in the solution, and cracks. Solutions with additives should be refrigerated until used and infused as rapidly as is consistent with good treatment. If any adverse effects suggest possible contaminated solutions, the bottle, tubing, filter, lot control numbers, and all relevant hospital samples should be completely identified and properly stored so that microbiologic and other epidemiologic studies can be performed by the county or state epidemiologist or the FDA.

In emergencies, infection control is less important than preservation of life. In such cases, sterility should not interfere with survival. However, much of life is not an emergency. We should not let the standards set for CPR set codes for infection control. Skill allows preservation of asepsis even during CPR. Technical ability decreases tissue injury, hematoma formation, and contamination. When the resuscitative effort is over and the patient is stable, it is often desirable to replace potentially contaminated devices with sterile equipment.

GOALS FOR RESPIRATORY THERAPY IN THE TREATMENT AND PREVENTION OF RESPIRATORY INFECTIONS

This section will not deal with the indications for IPPB and other forms of respiratory therapy. Rather, we shall identify certain therapeutic goals claimed by advocates of the various respiratory therapy modalities and assume that the goals can be accomplished. If present methods fall short, we call for more effective techniques. If goals are reached, we applaud their appropriate uses in patients with pulmonary infections.

Pulmonary infection impairs ventilation/perfusion ($\dot{V}/\dot{Q}$) ratios, increases bronchospasm, and fills bronchi with mucus plugs. These factors affect host defense against infection in various ways, through a series of complex, intertwined pathways.

The primary lung defense against bacteria is the alveolar macrophage. Hypoxia and acidosis impair macrophage phagocytosis. Pneumonia first causes hyperemia in the infected area, followed by decreased perfusion. Local factors affect the involved vessels and bronchi. The abnormal $\dot{V}/\dot{Q}$ with reduced oxygen and carbon dioxide transport impairs local primary host defense mechanisms, increasing the possibility of bacterial spread to other lung segments and thus causing more extensive $\dot{V}/\dot{Q}$ abnormality, with increased local susceptibility and progressive disease.

Bronchospasm modifies airflow with altered deposition of inhaled microbes. Again $\dot{V}/\dot{Q}$ is altered, with areas of alveolar dead space secondary to decreased perfusion, and local hypoxia with acidosis results. Thick secretions decrease the effectiveness of the mucociliary escalator, thus favoring bacterial persistence with possible infection.

Bronchial obstruction exaggerates and extends the effects of bronchospasm. Ventilation is decreased, and a tendency to atelectasis and secondarily decreased perfusion develops. This decreases the host's ability to clear the emerging infection and to oxygenate the phagocytes optimally. With decreased perfusion and obstructed bronchi promoting abscess formation, the contained bacteria persist in an area impermeable to antibiotics. If the organisms are not multiplying, they are in the stationary phase, and as such are not susceptible to antibiotics, even if antibiotics could diffuse into the area.

Two primary goals of respiratory therapy are to mobilize secretions, thus decreasing bronchospasm and atelectasis and increasing the removal of organisms; and to wet and remove bronchial plugs, further decreasing bronchospasm and emptying intrabronchial collections of bacterial soup, thus allowing antimicrobials to reach infecting organisms that have again begun to multiply and become susceptible to antibiotics. The mucociliary escalator can return to normal function, although perhaps slowly. Relief of bronchospasm and removal of bronchial plugs will help to improve $\dot{V}/\dot{Q}$, increase compliance, and improve ventilation, resulting in better oxygenation and acid–base status. These factors work to improve pulmonary host defense and aid in limiting pulmonary infectious diseases.

The objectives of respiratory therapy are

1. *to mobilize secretions:* Nebulized fluids, postural drainage, coughing, and forced expiration are all done for the purpose of mobilizing secretions and clearing endobronchial plugs.
2. *to control bronchospasm:* Systemic and nebulized agents are given to reverse bronchospasm and allow better mobilization of secretions and normalization of $\dot{V}/\dot{Q}$.
3. *to improve ventilation:* Ideally, respiratory therapy will increase compliance, improve the $\dot{V}/\dot{Q}$, and decrease dead-space ventilation and shunt perfusion so that ventilation will be more efficient, requiring less patient effort and support.

SUMMARY

Human colonization is usually by mutuals and commensals. A defect in host defense mechanisms can allow one or more of these strains to establish a parasitic relationship that can often be corrected by removing the defect and reestablishing the host's health. Use of unclean respiratory therapy equipment can, on occasion, overwhelm even the most competent of host defense mechanisms. By not correcting host defects and only altering colonizing species, antimicrobials often determine which agent will cause infection but do not determine whether an infection will occur. That depends on correcting host defects such as postoperative hypoventilation, ineffective cough, thick secretions, intrabronchial mucus plugs, bronchospasm, suboptimal ventilation, and abnormal blood gases. The respiratory care worker must be sure that his contribution to the care of the patient is microbiologically helpful, not deleterious.

REFERENCES

1. Ahlgren, EW, Chapel JF, Dorn GL: *Pseudomonas aeruginosa* infection potential of oxygen humidifier devices. Respir Care 22:383, 1977
2. Hoshal VL et al: Fibrin sleeve formation on indwelling subclavian central venous catheters. Arch Surg 102:353, 1971
3. National Coordinating Committee on Large Volume Parenterals: Recommended methods for compounding intravenous admixtures in hospitals. Am J Hosp Pharm 32:261, 1975
4. Nejad MS et al: Clotting on the outer surfaces of vascular catheters. Radiology 91:248, 1968

BIBLIOGRAPHY

Johanson WG Jr: Infectious complications of respiratory therapy. Respir Care, 27:445, 1982

20

Drugs Used in Respiratory Therapy

Irwin Ziment

Many of the drugs used to treat disorders of the lung can be administered by nebulization or by instillation into the respiratory tract. Drugs given directly are not always prescribed by physicians in precise dosages and concentrations. The actual administration of the medication is performed by a nurse or a respiratory therapist or by the patient himself. A ridiculous legalistic quibble occasionally is voiced, expressing doubts as to the legal propriety of respiratory therapists mixing and delivering prescribed drugs. Since obviously the patient can be instructed in safe self-therapy, there can be no serious questioning of the trained therapist's capability as a provider of pharmacologic therapy in the hospital setting. Indeed, the educated therapist generally knows more about respiratory aerosol pharmacology than does the average physician or nurse; in fact, it would be reasonable to expect the nonspecialist physician to consult with a therapist about the details of aerosol drug administration.

Relatively few drugs are used in aerosol therapy, and it is essential for therapists to be completely familiar with the pharmacology of these agents and to know the indications and contraindications for their use, as well as the complications that may arise during their administration. The main emphasis herein will be placed on drugs commonly given by aerosolization, and comparatively less detail will be provided for the other drugs used to treat respiratory disease. Many drugs given by inhalation can also be given orally, and in the future probably more developments will occur in the latter field, since oral therapy is cheaper and easier to administer. The well-educated respiratory therapist should therefore maintain a strong interest in all respiratory pharmacologic preparations, not simply those given by nebulization.

Relatively few new respiratory drugs have been introduced in the United States since the first edition of *Respiratory Care* was published.

AEROSOL THERAPY

The use of inhalational drug therapy developed empirically, and numerous controversies about the value of such therapy still exist. Prescribers and providers of aerosols should recognize the advantages and limitations of the technique.

ADVANTAGES OF AEROSOL THERAPY

The main advantage of delivering a drug by aerosol is that relatively small quantities of the drug can be given, with maximal pulmonary effect and minimal extrapulmonary side-effects. The onset of action is rapid, and repeated therapy with small doses can be given at relatively frequent intervals, according to the patient's needs, with little risk of toxicity. The use of aerosols may be preferable in situations where oral or intravenous medications are difficult to give because of the unavailability of these routes. Certain drugs are specifically designed for aerosolization and cannot be given by other means.

ADVANTAGES OF AEROSOL THERAPY

1. Topical administration results in rapid therapeutic effect.
2. Only a small total dose of potent drug need be nebulized.
3. Minimal extrapulmonary side-effects are produced.
4. Individual dosage titration is possible.
5. The respiratory route is always available for drug delivery.
6. Certain drugs (e.g., cromolyn) cannot be given by other routes.
7. Humidification and bland droplet therapy are essential for tracheostomized and intubated patients and are soothing and probably beneficial for most patients with respiratory disease.
8. Administration of aerosol therapy in the hospital involves the respiratory therapist, with the attendant benefits of skilled attention to the respiratory tract.
9. Patients develop faith in nebulizers and derive psychological benefits from their use.
10. Aerosol therapy may provide patients with an oral-inhalational substitute for smoking.

DISADVANTAGES OF AEROSOL THERAPY

1. Special, expensive equipment is often required.
2. Patients must be able to cooperate in taking synchronized deep breaths (unless intubated).
3. Precise drug dosage is often not achieved; underdosage and overdosage are readily produced.
4. Only a small proportion of a nebulized drug is retained in the lung.
5. Oropharyngeal deposition of an aerosol results in appreciable systemic absorption.
6. Oropharyngeal irritation by the aerosol can result in gagging, nausea, vomiting, or aerophagia.
7. Tracheobronchial irritation by the aerosol can result in bronchospasm, coughing (thus limiting the inhaled dose), and possibly tracheobronchitis.
8. The inhalational adjuvants may cause detrimental side-effects (e.g., oxygen, Freon).
9. Nebulizers readily become dirty, thus losing effectiveness, and possibly become sources of infection.
10. Aerosol therapy results in unreasonable complexity (involving patient, equipment, and personnel factors) that is greatly reduced if oral administration is used instead.

DISADVANTAGES OF AEROSOL THERAPY

The major problem in inhalation treatment is that, unless the trachea is intubated, patients must be able to cooperate by breathing deeply in coordination with the administration of the aerosol by mouthpiece or mask. Oral therapy with a pill or liquid is much simpler in most cases because no expensive or cumbersome equipment is required. In contrast, aerosol therapy necessitates nebulizers of various degrees of complexity, which makes the modality expensive; moreover, in most hospitals skilled personnel are required to operate and to maintain the more complex pieces of machinery, such as positive pressure respirators. Domiciliary equipment suffers from dual disadvantages: Difficulty in operation and maintenance may discourage patients from using the more expensive machines, yet accessibility of ready relief from simple nebulizers may result in overuse of potent drugs. Much money can be spent on domiciliary nebulization devices that are not indicated and are probably not used correctly by patients, who would do just as well with oral medications or simple, inexpensive humidifiers. An additional concern about aerosol therapy is based on the experience of Great Britain in the 1960s: The death rate from asthma in children greatly increased because of overuse of metered aerosol bronchodilators.[48]

Thus aerosol therapy suffers from disadvantages that include overuse, underuse, and misuse of the prescribed medications. Further, even when drugs are administered appropriately, there is a lack of knowledge as to what the appropriate dosage of most inhalational agents should be. More precise dosing would be attained if clinicians prescribed drugs in milligrams, rather than in milliliters or in percentage strengths of solutions. Not only are drugs prescribed imprecisely, but many physicians and therapists fail to appreciate that the dose delivered can be extremely variable. The cooperative patient given an aerosol through a mouthpiece by IPPB probably retains only 5% to 10% of the prescribed amount of the drug in the respiratory tract, whereas more efficient aerosolizing devices can result in much larger doses being delivered, for example, metered units with spacers.

The problem of droplet size is still a controversial topic, and it is difficult to know if any one of the conventional nebulizing units offers significant advantages over its competitors.[56] The less effective equipment delivers droplets of larger diameter, which are deposited mainly in the mouth and upper airways. Many patients treated with bronchodilator aerosols provided by such equipment may actually obtain the bronchospasmolytic effect as a result of systemic absorption of the drug through the oropharyngeal or gastric mucosa. Similarly, the very dyspneic asthmatic who is unable to take a deep breath and hold it may resort to excessive use of the nebulizer, since pharmacologic relief is derived only from systemic absorption of large amounts of drug deposited in the mouth. Further, the hypoxemic asthmatic may become even more hypoxemic after aerosolizing drugs such as isoproterenol, since systemic absorption causes vasodilation of pulmonary vessels disproportionate to the bronchodilation achieved, resulting in an increased shunt effect through poorly ventilated areas of the lung.

There are other disadvantages to administering drugs as aerosols. Many patients find that the taste and the oropharyngeal irritation of the droplets cause gagging and nausea, whereas the irritant effect of the aerosol on reactive airways can cause deterioration in respiratory variables (e.g., oxygen transport, dynamic compliance) and may result in bronchospasm. The latter problem is likely to arise with any pharmacologic aerosol, and, for this reason, incorporation of a bronchodilator drug with other classes of drugs is usually necessary when giving treatment. Unfortunately, bronchodilators are not entirely compatible with all other inhalational drugs; many inhalational drugs are alkaline, whereas bronchodilators are acidic and undergo fairly rapid breakdown in an alkaline medium.

A further disadvantage of aerosol therapy is that the nebulizer readily becomes contaminated with microorganisms. Thus inhalational apparatus is a potential source of serious nosocomial infections. This fact is so well known that elaborate precautions are taken, including the use of disposable equipment and the employment of complex cleaning and sterilizing protocols in hospitals. The expense of such methods constitutes a major factor in the relatively poor cost-effectiveness benefits of aerosol therapy. Further, the more complex and "effective" an aerosol generator may be, the more expensive it is to keep clean and in good working order. In such circumstances, one wonders whether a drug such as acetylcysteine, delivered by a highly trained respiratory therapist using a pressure respirator equipped with an oxygen blender and an ultrasonic nebulizer, is more effective than a simple home humidifier steaming out an aromatic vapor and costing perhaps 1% as much as the more complicated apparatus!

PHARMACOLOGY OF RESPIRATORY DRUGS

The most important and frequently administered drugs in aerosol therapy are agents used to improve mucociliary clearance (mucokinetic agents) and agents used to relieve bronchospasm. Relatively few other categories of drugs are given by nebulization; they include antiasthmatic agents, mucosal vasoconstrictors, local anesthetics, and antibiotics. The major drugs in these categories will be considered in this chapter.

MUCOKINETIC AGENTS

Drugs in this category include mucolytics, expectorants, and other agents found in "cough medicines." The most important mucokinetic agent is actually water.

The end result of successful mucokinetic therapy is usually seen in a sputum receptacle by the bedside or in the suction bottle in an intensive care unit. Sputum is a complex fluid consisting of mucoprotein (including mucopolysaccharides), electrolytes, water, cellular debris, and, in the case of expectorated specimens, oropharyngeal secretions (i.e., saliva, food particles, and bacteria). The respiratory tract secretions originate from two major sources (Fig. 20-1): The goblet cells that produce a gelatinous secretion, mainly in response to irritation, and the bronchial glands that secrete a more watery solution and are under vagal control. Infected sputum contains, in addition, deoxyribonucleic acid (DNA), which is liberated from polymorphonuclear (white) blood cells and bacteria. This material gives a yellow or green color to the secretions, which it renders highly viscous.

The normal mucus blanket has two layers: the more watery sol layer in which the cilia beat, and the superficial viscous gel layer. The ciliary activity serves to waft the gel layer proximally up the respiratory tract against gravity. Problems with sputum expectoration occur when there is increased production of viscous secretions in airways having damaged cilia and impaired architecture which interferes with effective coughing.

Although pharmacologic agents can alter the consistency of mucus, subsequent mucokinesis requires the presence of an effective cough; otherwise, loosened, hypoviscous secretions can gravitate down the airways, causing the patient to "drown in his secretions." If a patient is unable or unwilling to cough, then postural drainage or, alternatively, tracheobronchial suctioning will be required. Thus, effective mucokinesis requires more than active drug therapy, and pharmacologic agents contribute only the first half of the process: Physical therapy is equally or, at times, more important.[30]

Mucokinetic Drugs Suitable for Aerosolization

Water. The addition of water to mucus results in decreased viscosity of sputum. If relatively large quantities of water are added, the sputum is simply diluted; however, smaller amounts of water can become incorporated into mucus to reduce the adhesiveness of gelatinous secretions. In the case of retained secretions within the respiratory tract, mucokinesis may be improved by the addition of water to a depleted sol layer, since this allows the cilia to beat more effectively, thereby contributing to the proximal propulsion of the viscous gel layer.

There is considerable question as to whether water provided in the form of an aerosol or as humidity (e.g., in "croup tents") has a significant effect on mucociliary clearance;[18] certainly, the nebulization of 2 ml of water (resulting in the actual deposition of

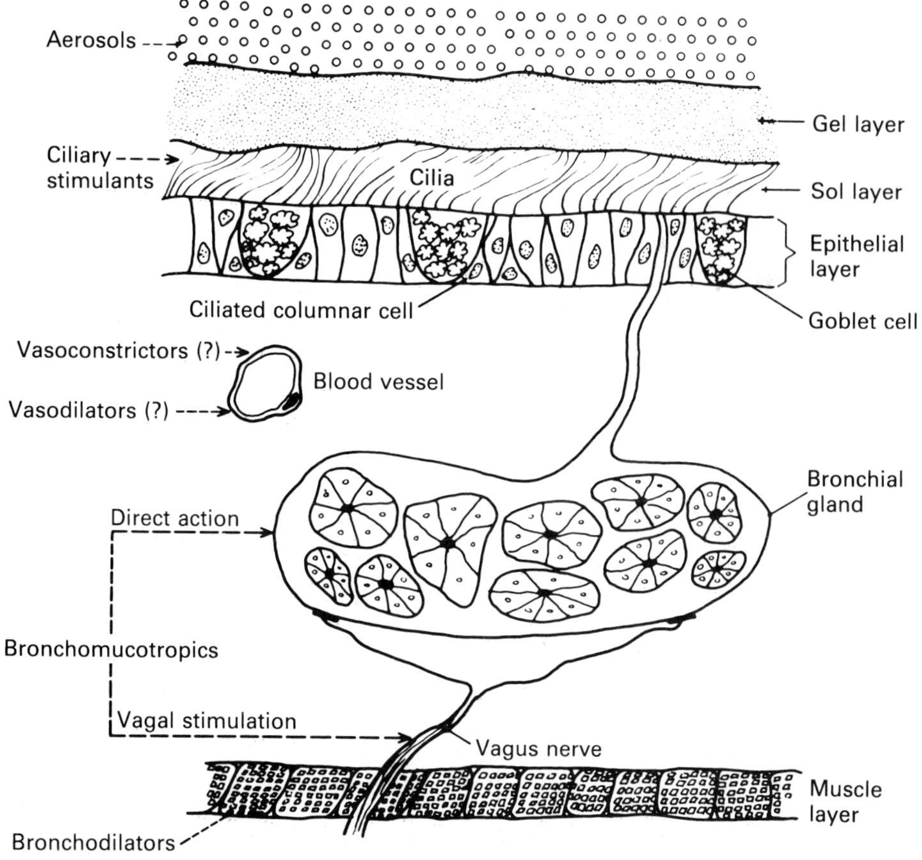

Fig. 20-1. Schematic diagram illustrating the sites of action of various classes of pharmacologic agents within the wall and lumina of the respiratory tract.

FACTORS INVOLVED IN MUCOKINESIS

Natural
- Respiratory tract secretions of adequate amount and consistency
- Maintenance of appropriate sol–gel relationship
- Ciliary activity and coordination
- Patent airways and adequate airflow
- Muscular coordination with laryngeal activity and effective cough

Pharmacologic
- Hypoviscosity agents and diluents
- Bronchomucotropic agents
- Mucolytics
- Detergents and surfactants
- Bronchodilators
- Mucosal constrictors

Mechanical
- Cough stimulation (*e.g.,* IPPB, pharyngeal catheter)
- Postural drainage
- Physical therapy (*e.g.,* percussion–vibration, rocking bed)
- Suctioning
- Psychic stimulation, encouragement, and teaching of patient

less than 0.2 ml in the respiratory tract) may do no more than add an imperceptible amount of fluid to the gel-layer coating of the tracheobronchial tree.[35] In contrast, secretion of a watery fluid by the bronchial glands may serve to replenish the sol layer from below, and thereby to loosen adherent inspissated secretions from attachment to the ciliated epithelium. Correction of cellular dehydration by oral or systemic administration of water could be expected to improve bronchial gland activity; this method of treatment may be much more effective than the nebulization of minute amounts of this valuable mucokinetic agent (see Table 20-1).

A further criticism of plain water as a topical inhalational agent is that the low osmolality of the fluid may cause it to be absorbed by the respiratory mucosa with an adverse effect on airway flow mechanics. However, it is not certain that aerosols of plain water have this effect in practice, since droplets that are aerosolized into the lungs may rapidly evaporate to smaller sizes, and may not deposit at all.[31] For these reasons, plain water is not favored as a mucokinetic for nebulization therapy, although it does have a valuable prophylactic effect in preventing dehydration of the secretions in the upper airway during normal respiration. Thus, plain water in inhalational therapy subserves a "demulcent," soothing effect, rather than acting as a mucokinetic, and should be given as humidification therapy or as hot or cold mists.

Saline. Various concentrations of sodium chloride (NaCl) in water are used in aerosol therapy, either as primary drugs or as diluents or carriers for other drugs.

Normal saline (0.9% NaCl, which is isotonic with tissue fluids) is generally favored as a "bland" aerosol solution.

Half-normal saline (0.45% NaCl, hypotonic saline) is sometimes preferred, particularly for use in ultrasonic nebulization. The aerosol droplets of half-normal saline are thought to undergo some evaporative concentration when they reach the warmth of the respiratory tract; thus the droplets that impact are almost isotonic.[32] Although proof is as yet lacking, this supposed behavior of half-normal saline may result in a bland nonirritating aerosol.

Hypertonic saline (e.g., 1.8–15% NaCl) offers a theoretically more effective form of mucokinetic therapy. Deposition of hypertonic droplets on the respiratory mucosa results in the osmotic attraction of fluid from the mucosal blood vessels and tissues into the airway. Thus a "bronchorrhea" is induced, and the watery solution helps to dilute the respiratory tract secretions and to increase their bulk, thereby augmenting expectoration. Further, there is evidence that hypertonic saline has a direct effect on mucoprotein-DNA complexes, and by reducing the cohesive intramolecular forces the salt helps to decrease the viscous properties of the mucoid fluid.

Hypertonic saline is most useful as a sputum-inducing agent. A heated aerosol of 10% to 15% sodium chloride with 10% to 20% propylene glycol is an effective stimulus to expectoration in patients who have little spontaneous sputum production, and such mixtures are recommended for use when induced sputum specimens are needed for cytologic and microbiologic studies.

Although various concentrations of sodium chloride can be used without significant untoward effects in inhalation therapy, certain precautions should be taken. For purposes of irrigation or instillation into the tracheobronchial tree, normal saline and perhaps half-normal saline are favored because they are relatively nonirritating to the airways. If hypertonic saline

Table 20-1. Important Aerosol Mucokinetic Drugs

TRADE NAME (MANUFACTURER)	MAIN CONSTITUENTS	USUAL AEROSOL DOSAGE	COMMENTS
Mucomyst (Mead Johnson)	N-acetyl-L-cysteine (10–20%)	2–5 ml q 6 hr	Breaks disulfide bonds, causes mucolysis. Malodorous and may cause bronchospasm. 20% solution should be diluted with an equal volume of isotonic saline or sodium bicarbonate.
Dornavac* (Merck, Sharp and Dohme)	Pancreatic dornase (desoxyribonuclease)	100,000 units t.i.d. Range: 50,000–100,000 units 1–4 times a day	Enzyme: depolymerizes DNA and is indicated for purulent secretions only. May be irritating; can cause hypersensitivity reactions. Suitable for short-term use only. Dissolve in 1–2 ml normal saline.
Tryptar* (Armour)	Trypsin	100,000 units t.i.d. Range: 25,000–100,000 units 1–3 times a day	Enzyme: digests mucoprotein. May be irritating; can cause hypersensitivity reactions. Suitable for short-term use only. Dissolve in 3 ml normal saline.
Alevaire* (Breon)	Tyloxapol (0.125%), sodium bicarbonate (2%), glycerin (5%)	2–5 ml q 6 hr Range: 0.5–10 ml q 3–8 hr	Wetting agent. Usually given with other medications (*e.g.*, bronchodilators, antibiotics) to help improve their distal deposition.
	Sodium bicarbonate (1.4–7.5%)	2–5 ml q 6 hr Range: 1–10 ml q 2–8 hr	Wetting agent in low concentrations, bronchomucotropic in higher concentrations. May be combined with other drugs for immediate use.
	Sodium chloride	2–5 ml q 6 hr Range: 1–10 ml q 2–8 hr	Hypotonic solution penetrates well, especially when given by ultrasonic nebulization. Hypertonic solutions stimulate cough and may have mucolytic effect. Normal saline is a standard diluting agent.
	Propylene glycol (2–25%)	2–5 ml q 4 hr Range: 1–10 ml q 1–8 hr	Soothing demulcent for tracheobronchitis (2% solution). Stabilizes droplets; used with medicational aerosols to improve distal deposition. Effective for cough induction (15% or stronger solution).

*These products are no longer available in the United States.

is used, not more than 10 ml a day should be given for not more than a few days; excessive use is not only irritating to the respiratory tract, but absorption may occur, and patients who cannot handle the sodium load may develop edema, heart failure, or hypertension.

Sodium Bicarbonate. For many years, solutions of sodium bicarbonate ($NaHCO_3$) have been used as surgical irrigating fluids and for cleaning tracheostomy tubes. The salt was introduced into inhalation therapy in Alevaire: This product contained 2% sodium bicarbonate in combination with 0.125% tyloxapol (a "wetting" agent or "detergent") and 5% glycerin (used as a hygroscopic agent for stabilizing droplets and for "soothing" the respiratory mucosa). There is no satisfactory evidence that Alevaire is more successful than hypertonic sodium bicarbonate alone,[4] and for this reason it is no longer promoted. Bicarbonate solutions can be given by aerosolization or by direct instillation; the higher concentrations may be somewhat irritating.

The success of sodium bicarbonates seems to be related partly to its alkaline pH (whereas sodium chloride is provided as an acidic solution), and sputum may be less adherent in an alkaline medium.[25] The hypertonic solutions also have a bronchorrheic effect, and possibly a direct salt effect, that helps disrupt some of the complex molecular bonds in mucus.

A minor disadvantage of sodium bicarbonate is that added bronchodilators (which have an acid pH) undergo more rapid breakdown in the alkaline solution. However, if a bronchodilator is added to a solution of sodium bicarbonate immediately before nebulization, effective therapy without adverse effects can be achieved, although the material that is subsequently expectorated or suctioned from the respiratory tract may be colored pink because of the presence of breakdown products (adrenochromes) of the catecholamine. Sodium bicarbonate makes a particularly suitable diluent for acetylcysteine, since this mucolytic agent is more effective in an alkaline medium.

Acetylcysteine. Acetylcysteine (N-acetyl-L-cysteine sodium salt, Mucomyst) is currently the most powerful mucolytic agent in use in inhalation therapy. Like its parent compound, the amino acid cysteine, acetylcysteine contains a thiol group, and the free sulfhydryl radical of this group is a strong reducing agent that ruptures the disulfide bridges that serve to give stability to the mucoprotein network of molecules in mucus. Agents that break down these disulfide bonds produce the most effective mucolysis in laboratory studies.[21] The most powerful thiol compound is dithiothreitol, which is too toxic to be used therapeutically but is valuable as a laboratory mucolytic. Interestingly, the main constituent of garlic, which is a traditional expectorant, is the compound S-allyl-L-cysteine sulfoxide (also known as alliin); however, this agent does not have the mucolytic properties of acetylcysteine.

It has not been clearly demonstrated that nebulization of thiol compounds in small amounts can produce the same degree of mucolysis as that seen in test tube experiments. Indeed, the well-documented effect of acetylcysteine as a mucokinetic agent may depend more on the irritative qualities of the compound, which may thus simply induce bronchorrhea and stimulate coughing, thereby increasing expectoration. A further consideration is that acetylcysteine should be used as the 20% solution with the addition of an equal volume of sodium chloride or, preferably, sodium bicarbonate, since the resulting 10% solution is as effective as the higher concentration. Before instituting a course of acetylcysteine therapy, one should make certain that this expensive and irritating agent is more effective than the use of the diluent on its own. Once a bottle of the agent has been opened, it must be stored in a refrigerator; it should be used within a few days, since its potency rapidly declines.

Acetylcysteine is an irritant to the respiratory tract: It can cause mucosal changes and may induce bronchospasm. In addition, it can inhibit ciliary activity. These side-effects may be obviated by pretreating with an aerosol bronchodilator or by using the combined product, Mucomyst with Isoproterenol, which is 10% acetylcysteine with 0.05% isoproterenol.

Acetylcysteine has a sulfurous odor and an unpleasant taste, and on nebulization can irritate the oropharynx and may induce gagging and nausea or vomiting. However, the drug has no serious toxicity and, indeed, can be given with a fair degree of safety orally or even intravenously. In Europe and South America, oral acetylcysteine is a very popular mucolytic, since the product is tasteless and odorless and does not cause irritation of the airways. In the United States, interestingly, oral acetylcysteine is recommended in treating acetaminophen poisoning.

Enzymes. Currently, enzymes are out of favor in respiratory therapy. Generally, the various enzymes that have been used do not seem to be any more effective than acetylcysteine. Enzymes are relatively expensive and are much more toxic than other mucokinetic agents. They tend to cause irritation of the mouth and throat, and for this reason a mouth rinse is advised following nebulization of one of these agents. They are also irritating to the respiratory tract and can induce bronchospasm; more prolonged use may result in tracheobronchitis. Many patients develop febrile and hypersensitivity responses to enzymes; these may include rashes, asthma, pulmonary infiltrates, and fever.

Deoxyribonuclease (pancreatic dornase, Dornavac) is obtained from beef pancreas. It can break down DNA, and was therefore advised for treatment of patients with thick, purulent secretions. There was some worry that the enzyme might be damaging to lung tissue, but this has not been shown to be the case, even in patients with $alpha_1$ antitrypsin deficiency. Dornavac is no longer available in the United States.

Trypsin has an antifibrin digestive effect. It was formerly used to treat fibropurulent exudates in the lung and in alveolar proteinosis, but proof as to its value is scanty. The drug is no longer marketed.

Streptokinase and streptodornase were sometimes used in a combined preparation for inhalation. However, the use of these enzymes is no longer promoted.

Hygroscopic Agents. Several agents are incorporated into proprietary aerosols as soothing demulcents or as droplet-stabilizing adjuvants. Propylene glycol is probably the best of these agents and can be used with sodium chloride as a sputum-inducing aerosol. Glycerol (glycerin) is more irritating and cannot be recommended.

Alcohol. Many respiratory therapists believe alcohol is a useful mucokinetic agent. However, alcohol is an irritant, and any increase in respiratory tract secretions that follow nebulization with this agent probably results from bronchorrhea. Prolonged use of this drug causes tracheobronchitis, and, since alcohol also inhibits ciliary activity, the adverse effects of injudicious use might actually be seen in the form of mucus retention. One must not assume that the mucokinetic effect of an irritant agent is necessarily beneficial; after all, cigarette smoking is a prime means for stimulating mucus production, but obviously smoking should not be encouraged. Likewise, alcohol should not be used as a means of improving expectoration.

The main use for ethyl alcohol in respiratory therapy is in managing foaming pulmonary edema. Alcohol, as a vapor or droplets, acts to reduce the stability of the edema bubbles, and thereby results in rapid dispersion of the foam.[34] The alcohol can be used in the form of vodka diluted with one or two parts water. Since this form of therapy is rarely needed today, one should be suspicious of a respiratory therapy department that uses more than a fifth of vodka a year for "medical" purposes!

Other Mucokinetic Agents. Various other drugs are advised for use in loosening respiratory tract secretions (Table 20-2).

Table 20-2. Classification of Mucokinetic Drugs

CLASS	ACTION	EXAMPLES
Drugs that increase the depth of the sol layer	1. Topical diluents 2. Stimulators of bronchial glands or respiratory mucosa a. Direct b. Blood-borne c. Via vagal reflex 3. Osmotic effect on mucosa	1. Water,* electrolyte solutions* 2. Bronchomucotropics (bronchorrheics) a. Irritants* (*e.g.,* smoke, alcohol, aromatic vapors, ultrasonic aerosols) b. Iodides (other oral expectorants?) c. Emetics (*e.g.,* guaifenesin, ipecac) 3. Hypertonic salt solutions*
Drugs that alter the consistency of the gel layer	1. Topical diluents 2. Drugs that break down mucoprotein or DNA a. Thiols (split disulfide bonds) b. Enzymes (digest DNA, etc.) c. Decomplexing agents (break mucoprotein-DNA complexes) d. Mucoregulators (alter mucoprotein secretion) e. Activators of natural proteases f. Reducing agents g. Amide effect h. Calcium binders	1. Water,* electrolyte solutions* 2. True mucolytics a. Acetylcysteine* b. Dornase,*† trypsin,*† streptokinase*† c. Sodium chloride,* sodium bicarbonate* (*i.e.,* salt effect/alkalinity) d. S-Carboxymethylcysteine,† bromhexine† e. Iodides, electrolytes* f. Ascorbic acid* + copper*† g. Urea (topical effect)† h. L-Arginine,*† chelating agents,† hypertonic saline*
Drugs that decrease the adhesiveness of the gel layer	1. Wetting agents 2. Surfactant effect	1. Sodium ethasulfate,*† water* 2. Tyloxapol,*† sodium bicarbonate,* propylene glycol,* glycerin*†

*Usually given by inhalational route.
†Not marketed in the United States.

Tergemist was formerly promoted in the United States: It contained 0.125% sodium ethasulfate (a "wetting" agent) and 0.1% potassium iodide. The manufacturer withdrew the preparation because it was difficult to prove its efficacy. However, potassium iodide may be of value when given by nebulization.

Traditional Remedies. Interestingly, traditional household inhalational remedies have never become popular in modern hospital practice. Thus agents such as menthol, eucalyptus, camphor, and benzoin are still popular as home remedies, and years of apparently satisfactory experience suggest that steam, rendered aromatic by the addition of one of these essential volatile oils, may be an effective, inexpensive, and pleasant mucokinetic. Many such agents are available as proprietary products—for example, Vick's Vaporub and Friar's Balsam.[7]

Urea is an effective topical mucolytic under laboratory conditions, but the amount required is so great as to preclude its being of value in clinical practice. Therefore this compound has never been used in respiratory therapy.

L-Arginine can reportedly reduce the viscosity of sputum in patients with mucoviscidosis (fibrocystic disease). It is thought that this amino acid combines with calcium, thereby reducing covalent bonding in mucoprotein. Aside from an increased amount of calcium in the respiratory tract secretions in mucoviscidosis, no basic abnormalities have been clearly identified to be the cause of the highly viscous mucus that characterizes this disease.[43]

Noninhalational Mucokinetic Drugs

Most of the noninhalational drugs, besides water, are given orally and are generally classified as expectorants. Although the mechanism of the effect of such drugs has not been clearly established, Boyd and others give evidence to suggest that these agents stimulate afferent receptors in the stomach.[6] These postulated receptors result in a vagal reflex, which may relay through a "mucokinetic" medullary center, which possibly lies between the respiratory center and the vomiting center. The efferent arc of the reflex is thought to be provided by vagal fibers to the lungs; similar vagal fibers supply the stomach. Strong stimulation of this reflex results in vomiting; the act of vomiting includes salivation and sometimes expectoration. A lesser stimulus by a subemetic dose of a vagal stimulant does not cause vomiting but does result in increased expectoration, presumably by activating the bronchial glands (*i.e.*, the gastropulmonary mucokinetic vagal reflex). The submucous glands are under vagal control, and a suitable stimulus results in the output of a watery secretion. Accordingly, small doses of emetic drugs have a bronchomucotropic action (*i.e.*, they result in augmentation of the secretory output of respiratory tract fluid).[57]

Certain drugs are preferentially concentrated by the bronchial glands, which are then stimulated to secrete. These drugs attain their effect after being absorbed by the stomach into the bloodstream, after which they reach the bronchial glands from the supplying blood vessels. Some agents, when secreted into the respiratory fluid, have a direct or indirect mucolytic effect on the mucoproteins. The complete mechanism has not yet been defined, but evidence can be assembled to enable one to postulate a means by which oral drugs affect the respiratory secretions.

In the following section, the more important oral mucokinetic drugs will be discussed briefly (Table 20-3).

Potassium Iodide. For many years, a saturated solution of potassium iodide (SSKI) has been favored as a mucokinetic agent. There are several ways in which iodides may have an effect.

1. The drug stimulates the gastropulmonary mucokinetic vagal reflex, thereby activating the submucosal bronchial glands. Excessive dosage with potassium iodide causes nausea and vomiting.
2. The bronchial glands selectively concentrate circulating iodide, which then stimulates the glands to secrete. The salivary, nasal, and lacrimal glands act similarly, and iodotherapy may cause salivation, rhinorrhea, and lacrimation. The stimulus to the salivary glands can be so great that they actually enlarge to produce a mumps-like appearance. Moreover, iodide concentrated in and then secreted by the salivary glands results in a characteristic metallic taste of the secretions, which patients often notice.
3. There is evidence that iodides stimulate natural proteolytic enzymes in the respiratory secretions, thereby enhancing the digestive breakdown of mucoprotein.[26] Thus iodide can have a direct mucolytic effect.
4. There is some evidence that potassium iodide can stimulate ciliary activity, thereby improving mucociliary clearance.[10]

Table 20-3. Some Oral Mucokinetic Agents

AGENT	USUAL DOSAGE	NOTES
Water	Variable	Essential
Potassium iodide (SSKI)	5–20 drops (300–1200 mg) 3 or 4 times a day	Probably most effective mucokinetic. Toxicity: rashes, metallic taste, parotid swelling, lacrimation, rhinorrhea, nausea, thyroid suppression
Sodium iodide	1–3 g/day intravenous	
Syrup of ipecac	½–2 ml 3 times a day	One of more effective agents. May cause nausea and vomiting
Ammonium chloride	0.3–1 g 3 times a day	Probably effective. Nauseating
Guaifenesin (glyceryl guaiacolate)	400 mg 4–6 times a day	Probably ineffective if less than 2400 mg per day is used. Toxicity: nausea, vomiting, drowsiness
Terpin hydrate	300 mg 4 times a day	Probably ineffective
Bromhexine	8–16 mg 3 times a day	Not available in the United States
S-Carboxymethylcysteine	375–750 mg 4 times a day	Not available in the United States. Note similarity to alliin found in garlic
Acetylcysteine	200 mg 3 times a day	Oral form not available in the United States

5. Iodide may have an anti-inflammatory effect, thus aiding in the resolution of conditions such as bronchitis, pneumonitis, and asthma.[42]

Iodide is usually administered as a saturated solution of the potassium salt (SSKI), 5 to 10 drops in a glass of water; as many as 20 to 30 drops may be given in this way three or four times a day. Unfortunately, iodide may cause an acneiform eruption, and many patients develop rashes while taking the drug; it should be used with particular care in adolescents prone to acne. Long-term administration of the drug may affect thyroid function, and for this reason the TSH and T_4 tests for thyroid function should be checked after the first 2 or 3 months of therapy. Hypothyroidism coexisting in patients with chronic obstructive disease is not always clinically apparent, and thyroid function tests should always be performed at the first suspicion of hypothyroidism in patients taking protracted courses of iodide medication.

If oral therapy is contraindicated, *sodium iodide* can be given intravenously. The dose is 1 to 3 g/24 hr by continuous drip. This form of therapy seems to be particularly valuable in patients with status asthmaticus.

Syrup of Ipecac. Syrup of ipecac is best known as an emetic agent. However, it has long been used, in small doses, as a mucokinetic agent. The appropriate dose for adults is 0.5 to 2 ml three to four times daily; at this low dosage nausea should not be a problem.

Salts. Various salt solutions are suitable for oral use as vagal stimulants. Thus concentrated solutions of sodium chloride, ammonium chloride, sodium citrate, and similar salts are used on their own or incorporated into proprietary expectorant mixtures. Any osmotic cathartic, used for its effect on the bowel, may also have a beneficial effect on respiratory tract fluid by means of the postulated gastropulmonary mucokinetic vagal reflex. Any of these agents may be contraindicated in patients with electrolyte problems, particularly subjects who retain sodium.

Guaifenesin. Guaifenesin was formerly called glyceryl guaiacolate. It is still one of the most popular expectorants, being present in proprietary "cough medicines" such as Robitussin. The drug is derived from creosote, which was formerly used as an expectorant.

There is evidence that guaifenesin acts both as a vagal stimulant and by direct stimulation of the bronchial glands. The drug is absorbed from the stomach and is concentrated by the bronchial glands, which rapidly secrete it into the respiratory tract. The recommended dose for adults is 100 to 200 mg four times daily, but it is doubtful whether this dosage has any beneficial effect.[20] The drug is also present in bronchodilator mixtures such as Bronkotabs and Quibron, but the amount is less than 100 mg per dose, which is unlikely to have any mucokinetic effect. A more appropriate dosage would be 500 to 1000 mg, but such amounts may produce vomiting and can cause cerebral depression.

Terpin Hydrate. Terpin hydrate is a volatile oil related to turpentine, and it supposedly has similar actions to those of guaifenesin. However, the conventional dosage of 5 ml (85 mg) is probably without effect, and the drug should be regarded simply as a flavoring agent for use with other "cough medications."

Bromhexine. Bromhexine (Bisolvon) is used in Europe, where it has gained a reputation of being one of the most successful oral mucokinetic agents.[8] Evidence suggests that bromhexine acts on the bronchial glands to increase their secretions, thereby causing an augmented volume of sputum of decreased viscosity in bronchitic patients. The drug may also have a mucolytic action, since it can produce depolymerization of mucopolysaccharides *in vitro*.

S-Carboxymethylcysteine. S-Carboxymethylcysteine (Mucodyne) is the most recent oral mucokinetic to have been introduced in Great Britain. Although it is related to acetylcysteine, the molecular structure is such that its thiol group is not free (*i.e.*, it is "blocked"), and thus the molecule cannot directly rupture disulfide bonds. It is thought that this agent acts directly on the bronchial glands to induce secretion of an increased amount of sialomucins, thereby producing fluid of relatively low viscosity; this action has been called a mucoregulator effect. Interestingly, this drug is closely related to alliin, the parent compound of garlic, which is also believed to be an effective oral mucokinetic agent, probably because it has mucoregulator properties (Fig. 20-2).

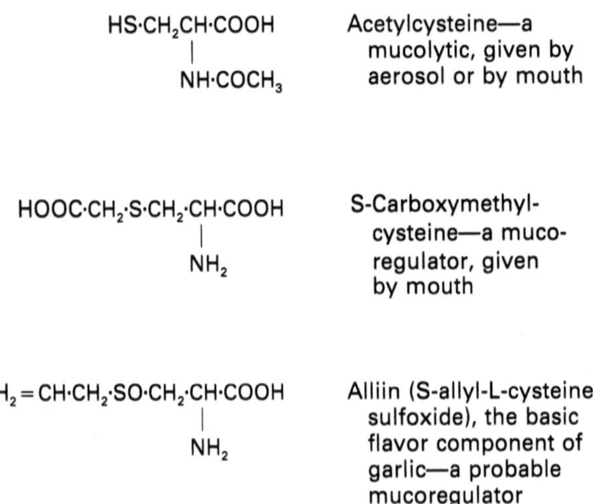

Fig. 20-2. Chemistry of some related cysteine derivatives with mucokinetic properties.

Miscellaneous Oral Mucokinetic Drugs. Other orally administered drugs are credited with mucokinetic properties, although substantiation is needed. Among the more popular of such agents are *anise, camphor, chloroform, licorice, paregoric* (camphorated tincture of opium), *senega, squill,* and *tolu balsam*. Many of these agents are still incorporated into proprietary "cough medicines."

Garlic has already been discussed, and this spice is still credited with expectorant effects in several national pharmacopoeias. Some evidence suggests that various foods and spices favored in folk medicine do have a mucokinetic effect, as does chicken soup.[59] Since agents such as pepper, mustard, and horseradish can cause lacrimation and rhinorrhea, not surprisingly they can cause an appreciable augmentation of tracheobronchial secretions; perhaps vagal stimulation is involved.

Parasympathomimetic drugs are powerful stimulants of the bronchial glands. However, although they can produce mucokinesis, they may also cause bronchospasm and other harmful parasympathetic effects. Apparently, no cholinergic drug has been found suitable as a therapeutic mucokinetic agent. In contrast, antiparasympathomimetic drugs such as atropine have an antimucokinetic action and can cause drying of the respiratory tract mucosa when given systemically in large doses.

BRONCHODILATORS AND ANTIASTHMA DRUGS

Most drugs used to manage bronchospasm act on the biochemical mechanisms that control bronchial muscle tone. In recent years it has been clearly shown that the "second messenger," cyclic 3′,5′-adenosine monophosphate (cAMP), is required to reverse bronchospasm (*see* Fig. 20-3 and Table 20-4). Intracellular levels of cAMP are increased by either of two mechanisms: stimulation of the enzyme *adenyl cyclase* catalyzes the conversion of the precursor adenosine triphosphate (ATP) to form cAMP; and inhibition of the enzyme *phosphodiesterase* prevents the rapid breakdown of cAMP to inactive metabolites. The major bronchodilators have their effect on one or the other of these two mechanisms.[36] *Catecholamines* and similar sympathomimetics stimulate adenylate cyclase, whereas *methylxanthines* are phosphodiesterase inhibitors. At present, only the catecholamines and related compounds are routinely given by both oral and inhalational routes.

Cyclic AMP is also important in allergic asthma, since increased intracellular concentrations of this messenger inhibit antigen-induced release of mediators, such as histamine and slow-reacting substance of anaphylaxis, that induce the pathophysiologic response. The release of these mediators is enhanced by cholinergic (*i.e.*, vagal) stimuli that produce increased concentrations of intracellular cyclic 3′,5′-guanosine monophosphate (3′,5′-GMP); this is a further messenger, which, in effect, has the opposite action to that of cAMP and results in bronchospasm.[39]

SYMPATHOMIMETIC DRUGS

The natural hormonal transmitters of the sympathetic nervous system are norepinephrine and epinephrine. These hormones are chemically related to catechol and are known as catecholamines; they are also classified as sympathomimetic agents, adrenergic agents, or adrenoreceptor stimulators. These chemicals have various categories of effects on autonomic function, and at present most of these effects are artificially subdivided into alpha, beta-1, and beta-2 properties, depending on the anatomical sites of the various receptors that are stimulated. The bronchial muscle receptors are termed beta-2 adrenergic receptors, and stimulation of these activates the adenyl cyclase mechanism, leading to cAMP production and resulting bronchodilation.

Stimulation of beta-1 receptors of the heart and blood vessels results in undesired side-effects, including tachycardia, possible arrhythmias, and blood pres-

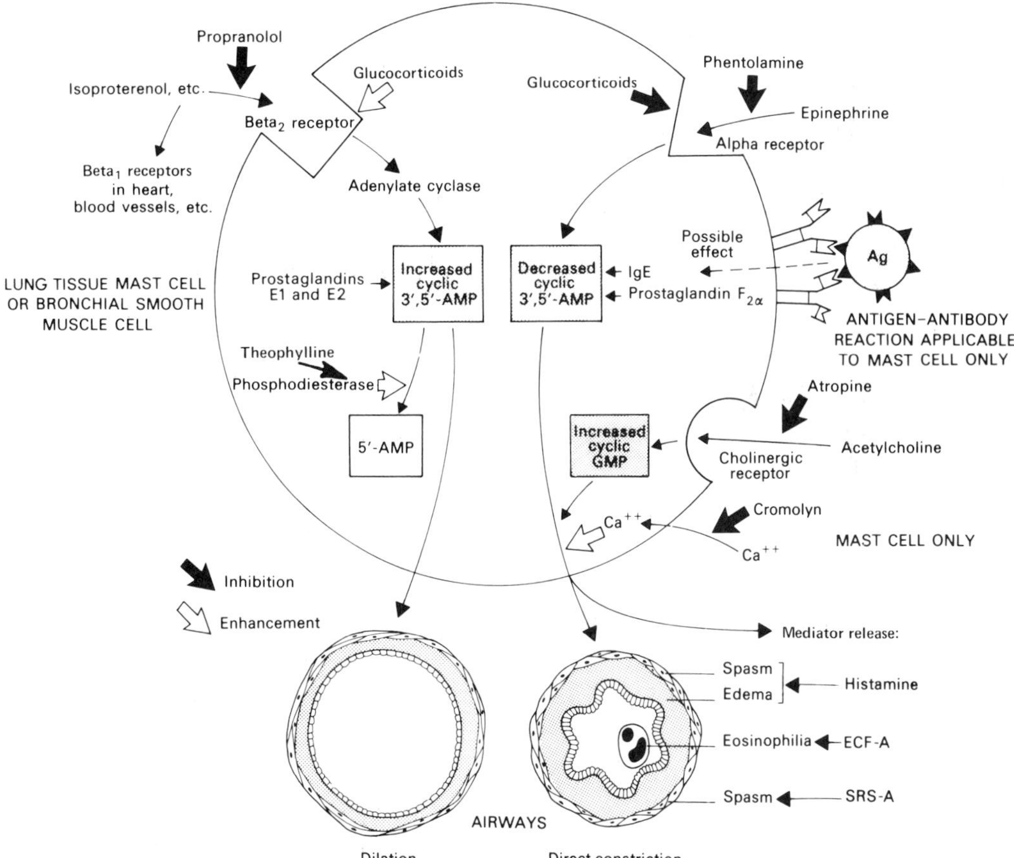

Fig. 20-3. Schematic representation of the pharmacologic control of bronchial tone and allergen-induced release of chemical mediators. Cholinergic or alpha-adrenergic stimulation in the presence of beta-adrenergic blockade results in bronchial constriction directly, as well as enhanced release of mediators from lung tissue. This may result in an amplification phenomenon since both enhanced release of mediators as a result of allergens reacting with IgE and an enhanced bronchoconstricting effect of such mediators on the bronchi occur. (Adapted from Townley RG: Pharmacologic blocks to mediator release: Clinical applications. Adv Asthma Allergy *2*(3):7, 1975)

Table 20-4. Pharmacology of Autonomic Modulation*

EXAMPLE OF REACTANT	SITE OF ACTION	CYCLIC NUCLEOTIDE EFFECT	MAST-CELL MEDIATOR RELEASE	BRONCHIAL END-ORGAN RESPONSE	EXAMPLE OF BLOCKER
Isoproterenol	Beta adrenergic receptor–adenyl cyclase stimulation	↑ cAMP	Inhibited	Bronchodilation	Propranolol
Epinephrine†	Beta adrenergic receptor–adenyl cyclase stimulation	↑ cAMP	Inhibited	Bronchodilation	Propranolol
Norepinephrine	Alpha adrenergic receptor-ATPase (?) stimulation	↓ cAMP	Enhanced	Bronchoconstriction (?)	Phentolamine
Theophylline	Phosphodiesterase inhibition	↑ cAMP	Inhibited	Bronchodilation	
Acetylcholine and analogues	Cholinergic receptor–guanyl cyclase stimulation	↑ cGMP	Enhanced	Bronchoconstriction	Atropine

*Adapted from Wilson AF, Galant SP: Recent advances in the pathophysiology of asthma. Calif Med 120:463, 1974
†Also has alpha-adrenergic activity, but in the lung beta activity is dominant.

sure changes. Blood vessels are supplied with beta-2 receptors; stimulation results in vasodilation. The blood vessels of the respiratory mucosa are also supplied with alpha receptors, the stimulation of which causes vasoconstriction, which may be valuable in treating bronchospasm, especially that associated with edema and cellular infiltrates as a result of inflammation. A further sympathomimetic effect, which is unwanted, is stimulation of the nervous system, causing nervousness, sleeplessness, and tremor; this effect is inevitable with drugs that are potent beta-2 stimulators.

Epinephrine is the prototype of the catecholamines. It has alpha, beta-1, and beta-2 effects and thus, in addition to being a very effective bronchodilator, has unwanted cardiovascular and nervous system side-effects. Epinephrine also has the powerful beta effect of releasing glucose from the liver (glycogenolysis). The molecule of epinephrine contains hydroxyl groupings in the 3 and 4 positions of the benzene nucleus, and thus is susceptible to degradation by at least two different enzyme systems.

1. In the bowel wall, and to some extent in the liver, are enzymes that degrade epinephrine and related catecholamines by mechanisms such as sulfatization. For this reason, epinephrine and isoproterenol are relatively ineffective as bronchodilators when given orally.
2. In various tissues, including the lungs, the enzyme catechol-O-methyl transferase (COMT) causes inactivation of the 3,4-hydroxysympathomimetics by O-methylation.

The amino group of the ethylamine side-chain is responsible for the alpha and beta stimulatory properties of the catecholamines. The addition of alkyl substitution radicals in the amino group leads to a progressive increase in beta-2 activity, with a corresponding decrease in beta-1 and alpha potency. The amino group is deaminated by monoamine oxidase (MAO) during metabolic breakdown. As a result of these metabolic processes, the catecholamines are finally excreted in the urine as ethereal sulfates, glucuronides, and vanillylmandelic acid (VMA).

Although the activities of the various catecholamines and derivatives used in therapeutics have been carefully evaluated, their effects are complex since they not only have multiple sites of action, but also their primary actions are complicated, in the intact animal, by reflex responses. It is therefore difficult to compare the bronchodilator potency of the various sympathomimetics and to determine the comparative beta-2 receptor selectivity of these agents. The therapeutic response to an agent is also affected somewhat by the route of administration, but generally the best bronchodilator side-effect ratio is obtained by aerosolization rather than by oral administration.

In the following section, the various sympathomimetic agents best suited for respiratory therapy are described. Most, but not all, of these drugs can be given by inhalational administration. Norepineph-

Table 20-5. Classification of Adrenergic Receptors

	ALPHA	$BETA_1$	$BETA_2$
Distribution of receptors			
Airways			
Muscle	Yes	No	Yes
Blood vessels	Yes	Yes	No
Heart	Yes	Yes	No
Systemic blood vessels	No (?)	No (?)	Yes
Central nervous system	?	?	Yes (?)
Result of receptor stimulation			
Bronchial muscle	Weak contraction	No effect	Relaxation
Bronchial glands	Inhibition (?)	?	Stimulation (?)
Cilia	?	?	Stimulation
Blood vessels (general)	Constriction	?	Dilation
Cardiac muscle	Excitation	Stimulation	No effect
Skeletal muscles	?	?	Excitation
Central nervous system	?	?	Excitation
Liver and muscle	?	?	Glycogenolysis
Adipose tissue	?	No effect	Lipolysis
Physiologic effects*			
Bronchospasm	Slight increase	No effect	Decrease
Respiratory tract secretions	Slight decrease (?)	No effect	Slight increase (?)
Cough	?	No effect	Decrease
Airway resistance	Decrease (?)	No effect	Decrease
Heart rate	Reflex slowing (may cause ectopy)	Increase	No effect
Blood pressure			
Weak stimulus	May increase	Varies	Varies
Strong stimulus	Increase	May decrease	Uncertain
Skeletal muscle	No effect (?)	No effect (?)	Tremor
Central nervous system	?	?	Stimulation

*The effect on human adrenergic receptors depends on factors such as route of administration, total dose given, time measurement is made, and reflex responses, among other variables.

rine, which has an unsubstituted amino group, is a powerful alpha-receptor stimulator and also has strong beta-1 effects; however, clinically it has no beta-2 activity and is not a bronchodilator, although it is a powerful pressor agent. A tentative classification of adrenergic receptors is given in Table 20-5.

Sympathomimetic Drugs Suitable for Aerosolization

Epinephrine. Epinephrine (adrenaline) is a natural sympathomimetic hormone that has been recognized as a bronchodilator for more than 70 years. It is rarely used in modern respiratory therapy because of its marked beta-1 effects, although it remains popular for self-therapy because it is available without prescription in several proprietary metered inhalers. For inhalational therapy, a 1:100 solution is used; this solution is too concentrated for subcutaneous administration (*see* Tables 20-6, 20-7, and 20-8).

Racemic Epinephrine. Racemic epinephrine (Micronefrin, Vaponefrin) is obtained synthetically; it is a racemic mixture of dextro- and levo-epinephrine, whereas the natural hormone exists only in the levo form. The racemic mixture is claimed to have adequate beta-2 potency, with less beta-1 and alpha activity than epinephrine. Although the manufacturers suggest that racemic epinephrine is a more suitable drug for use in respiratory therapy, no adequate controlled comparison of the two drugs has been reported.

Table 20-6. Structure and Actions of Common Bronchodilator Catecholamines and Derivatives*

								Relative Effects on Adrenergic Receptors			
								Vasoconstriction	*Cardiac Stimulation*	*Bronchodilation, Nervous System Stimulation, Vasodilation*	*Persistence of Effect of Aerosol*
	2	3	4	5	β	α	NH	α	β_1	β_2	*hr*
Epinephrine	H	OH	OH	H	OH	H	CH_3	+ + +	+ + + +	+ + +	1–2
R-Epinephrine	H	OH	OH	H	OH	H	CH_3	+ + (+)	+ + + (+)	+ + (+)	1–2
Isoproterenol	H	OH	OH	H	OH	H	$CH(CH_3)_2$		+ + + +	+ + + + (+)	1–2
Isoetharine	H	OH	OH	H	OH	C_2H_5	$CH(CH_3)_2$		+ (+)	+ + + (+)	2–4
Ethylnorepinephrine	H	OH	OH	H	OH	C_2H_5	H	+ +	+ +	+ + (+)	2–4
Metaproterenol	H	OH	H	OH	OH	H	$CH(CH_3)_2$		+ (+)	+ + + (+)	3–5
Terbutaline	H	OH	H	OH	OH	H	$C(CH_3)_3$		+ (+)	+ + + (+)	4–7
Albuterol	H	CH_2OH	OH	H	OH	H	$C(CH_3)_3$		+ (+)	+ + + + (+)	4–5
Ephedrine	H	H	H	H	OH	CH_3	CH_3	+ + (+)	+ + +	+ + +	4–6

*The relative effects are not established accurately, and therefore the above information is only approximate. The actual result obtained depends on the total dose given, the route and rate of administration, the presence of disease and other drugs, and factors such as tachyphylaxis. The measured response will also vary with time, since initial pharmacologic effects result in reflex adjustments. For these reasons, the actual findings at any time in a given patient may show major departures from this schema.

The presence of alpha-receptor activity makes racemic epinephrine a useful drug when mucosal congestion requires treatment. The drug has been recommended for aerosolization in managing croup and epiglottitis, but the validity of favorable reports is questionable. Clinical experience has shown that the drug is a useful bronchodilator, whether given by simple aerosolization or by IPPB. In recent years, the drug has become relatively obsolescent and is rarely used in routine respiratory therapy.

Isoproterenol. Isoproterenol (isoprenaline, Isuprel) was once the most popular inhalational bronchodilator. The drug is a synthetic derivative and appears to be one of the most potent beta-2 stimulators. Oral preparations are available, but absorption is unreliable; intravenous administration in asthmatic patients may be effective, but there is a risk of dangerous inotropic and chronotropic cardiac stimulation.

The marked beta-1 activity of isoproterenol makes it a less than ideal bronchodilator, and its inhalational use may be complicated by unwanted effects on the heart and blood pressure. Moreover, since the drug has no alpha effect (see Table 20–6), its unopposed beta-2 effect causes vasodilation in the pulmonary vasculature. This may result in mucosal congestion, and the increased blood flow leads to rapid systemic absorption of the drug with resulting shortening in the length of the bronchodilator response and increased risk of extrapulmonary side-effects. A further problem is that systemic absorption can cause pulmonary vasodilation in poorly ventilated lung areas which increases the shunt effect in the lungs, and this may be manifested as a fall in the Pa_{O_2}.

Isoproterenol, when given by nebulization, is one of the shortest-acting bronchodilators. Patients with severe asthma frequently have to take inhalations of the drug every 1 to 2 hours, and by so doing they run the risk of inducing *tachyphylaxis*: This is a phenomenon whereby responsiveness to the bronchodilating effects of a drug becomes progressively smaller, although beta-1 effectiveness may be maintained. As a result, the patients who overuse the aerosol may develop cardiac side-effects, including tachycardia, tachyarrhythmias, and even myocardial necrosis.

Table 20-7. Metered Aerosol Bronchodilators

DRUG	CONTENT PER CARTRIDGE	DOSES PER CARTRIDGE (APPROXIMATE) *no.*	AMOUNT OF DRUG DELIVERY PER INHALATION *mg*
EPINEPHRINE			
Asthma Haler (Norcliffe–Thayer)	15 ml	300	0.16
Asthma Meter (Rexall)	15 ml	300	0.20
Bronitin Mist (Whitehall)	15, 20 ml	300, 400	0.16
Bronkaid Mist (Winthrop)	15, 22.5 ml	300, 450	0.16, 0.27
Medihaler-Epi (Riker)	15 ml	300	0.16
Primatene Mist (Whitehall)	15, 22.5 ml	300, 450	0.20
Primatene Mist Suspension (Whitehall)	10 ml	200	0.16
ISOPROTERENOL			
Isoproterenol (generic)	15 ml	300	0.125
Isuprel Mistometer (Breon)	15, 22.5 ml	300, 450	0.131
Medihaler-Iso (Riker)	15, 22.5 ml	300, 450	0.080
Norisodrine Aerohalor (Abbott)	10 mg	220	0.045
Norisodrine Aerohalor (Abbott)	25 mg	230	0.110
Norisodrine Aerotrol (Abbott)	15 mg	350	0.120
ISOPROTERENOL-PHENYLEPHRINE			
Duo-Medihaler (Riker)	15, 22.5 ml	300, 450	
Isoproterenol			0.137
Phenylephrine			0.126
ISOETHARINE			
Bronkometer (Breon)	10, 20 ml	200, 400	0.340
METAPROTERENOL			
Alupent (Boehringer)	15 ml	300	0.65
Metaprel (Dorsey)	15 ml	300	0.65
ALBUTEROL (SALBUTAMOL)			
Proventil (Schering)	17 g	200	0.090
Ventolin (Glaxo)	17 g	200	0.090

These adverse effects are particularly dangerous in patients who have underlying heart disease or blood-pressure problems, and the concomitant presence of hypoxemia may increase the danger of a fatal arrhythmia or a cardiovascular catastrophe.[48]

When the drug is given by IPPB, the therapist should watch for evidence of toxicity. The patient may complain of palpitations, anxiety, flushing, or tinnitus or may experience faintness or a throbbing headache. The pulse should be checked during and after therapy, and, in patients at particular risk, monitoring of the electrocardiogram and blood pressure is advisable. Rinsing the mouth and throat may decrease systemic absorption through the oropharyngeal and gastric mucosa and may reduce the incidence of unwanted beta-1 complications. In all cases overuse and overdosage with isoproterenol must be avoided.

The main value of isoproterenol aerosol is in the pulmonary function laboratory, where it can be used to evaluate the reversibility of obstructive airway disease. However, it can also be useful for occasional aerosol therapy for younger asthmatics with no car-

Table 20-8. Bronchodilator Preparations Available for Aerosolization Using Simple Nebulizer, IPPB, or Compressor

		INITIAL DOSAGES*	
DRUG	CONCENTRATION	*Hand Nebulizer No. of Inhalations*	*Compressor Amount in ml*†
EPINEPHRINE			
Adrenalin (Parke–Davis)	1%	2–3	0.25–0.7
RACEMIC EPINEPHRINE			
MicroNEFRIN (Bird)	2.25%	2–3	0.2–0.4
Vaponefrin (Fisons)	2.25%	2–6	0.25–0.7
ISOPROTERENOL‡			
Aerolone (Lilly)	0.25%	6–12	0.3–1
Dispos-a-Med (Parke–Davis)	0.25%, 0.5%	6–12	0.25–1
Isuprel (Breon)	0.5%	5–15	0.5
Isuprel (Breon)	1%	3–7	0.25
ISOETHARINE‡			
Bronkosol (Breon)	1%	3–7	0.25–1
Bronkosol Unit Dose (Breon)	0.25%	3–7	2
Dispos-a-Med (Parke–Davis)	0.5%, 1%	—	0.25–1
METAPROTERENOL			
Alupent (Boehringer)	5%	5–15	0.3
Alupent Metered Dose (Boehringer)	6.6%	—	2.5

*These dosages are based on manufacturers' recommendations and illustrate the imprecision in prescribing that exists.

†The recommended amount can be diluted with 1–3 ml saline. Prepackaged unit dose preparations are available with various diluents.

‡Generic preparations are marketed in various concentrations. Each manufacturer's information should be used in determining dosages.

diovascular abnormalities. If low-dose aerosolization is followed by mouth rinsing with water, few, if any, side-effects will be experienced.

An attempt has been made to enhance the usefulness of isoproterenol by including phenylephrine in the product (e.g., as Duo-Medihaler). The strong alpha effect of phenylephrine may counteract the vasodilator effect of isoproterenol on the respiratory mucosa, thereby reducing the systemic absorption of the drug, thus serving to prevent some of the cardiac effect while prolonging the local bronchodilator effect in the lungs. The pharmacologic principles on which this combination therapy is based appear to be reasonable. A further possible advantage of the combination is that the aerosol is less likely to cause a fall in Pa_{O_2}, thus suggesting that the combination of drugs in the Duo-Medihaler offers a more suitable bronchodilator preparation than does isoproterenol alone for patients with hypoxemia.

The appropriate dosages of isoproterenol preparations are given in Tables 20-7 and 20-8.

Isoetharine. The catecholamine isoetharine (also known as Dilabron) is available as a proprietary aerosol, which formerly also contained phenylephrine. Isoetharine differs from isoproterenol in having an ethyl group on the alpha-carbon atom, and as a result it has somewhat less of a beta-2 effect than does isoproterenol, and much less beta-1 activity (Table 20-6). The addition of phenylephrine, which is a powerful alpha-receptor stimulator, may have served to reduce mucosal vasodilation and to prolong the bronchodilator effect of the isoetharine. However, proof of these possible benefits was lacking, and Breon laboratories chose to remove the phenylephrine.

Isoetharine has become very popular as a metered preparation (Bronkometer), as well as for use with IPPB (Bronkosol). The product is particularly useful for bronchospastic patients who are hypoxemic and who have tachycardia and underlying coronary artery disease. In such patients Bronkosol is much less likely to cause serious cardiac side-effects than is isoproterenol.

Although isoetharine is effective when given orally, no oral preparation is marketed in the United States; however, a tablet form (Numotac) is available in the United Kingdom. Curiously this drug has never become popular as an inhalational bronchodilator in Europe, whereas it deservedly remains a favored bronchodilator in the United States.

Recommended dosages of isoetharine are provided in Tables 20-7 and 20-8.

Metaproterenol. Metaproterenol (orciprenaline, Alupent, Metaprel) is available as a metered aerosol and as a tablet; it recently became available as a unit dose for nebulization. It is chemically related to isoproterenol, but the hydroxy groups, which occupy the 3 and 4 positions in the benzene nucleus of isoproterenol, are in the 3 and 5 (meta) positions (Table 20-6). This configuration renders metaproterenol immune to sulfatization in the bowel, and it is therefore effective when given orally. The molecule is not inactivated by COMT, and consequently the drug has a more sustained bronchodilator effect.

When used by aerosol, metaproterenol causes few side-effects; it is less likely to cause tachycardia than is isoproterenol. The effect of the aerosol usually lasts 3 to 4 hours or more, and it is usually required four times daily.[3] Dosages of the aerosol are listed in Tables 20-7 and 20-8.

Protokylol. Several years ago protokylol was marketed in the United States as an aerosol (Caytine). It was withdrawn from the market but reintroduced as a 2-mg tablet (Ventaire). The product is similar to ephedrine, but the 2-mg tablet is equivalent as a bronchodilator to 25 mg of ephedrine and appears to have fewer nervous system side-effects. However, the drug again has fallen into disuse.

Terbutaline. Terbutaline (Brethine, Bricanyl) was introduced into the United States several years ago. Since that time, surprisingly, the aerosol form has not achieved FDA approval, and only the subcutaneous form and oral preparations are currently available. Aerosol dosages are listed in Tables 20-7 and 20-8, but there is no justification for giving the subcutaneous form by aerosol, since other authorized aerosol bronchodilators are preferable.

Albuterol. Albuterol (salbutamol) is the latest selective bronchodilator to enter the U.S. market, with the names Proventil and Ventolin. It is very similar to terbutaline but appears to be more potent; it is somewhat shorter acting and may have a greater tendency to cause hypoxemia. Albuterol resembles terbutaline in having a tertiary butyl substitution in the amino group, and therefore it has similar beta-2 selective properties. The drug is protected from sulfatization and from COMT, since the hydroxyl group in position 3 of the catechol nucleus has been replaced by a CH_2OH group that interferes with the activity of these enzymes.

Albuterol is currently the most popular bronchodilator in many countries, both as an aerosol and as an oral drug[19] and for intravenous use in status asthmaticus. Although it is doubtful that albuterol will become as popular in the United States, it certainly merits a constituency because it is safe and effective.[28,44]

Noninhalational Sympathomimetic Drugs

Several inhalational drugs for treating bronchospasm are also commonly given by alternative routes of administration. A few sympathomimetics are not suitable at all for inhalation, and these will also be considered in this section.

Epinephrine. Epinephrine is available as the hydrochloride and as the bitartrate; there are no significant differences between these preparations. In status asthmaticus 0.1 to 0.5 ml of the 1:1000 aqueous solution can be given subcutaneously and repeated after half an hour if necessary. An aqueous solution for intramuscular administration (Sus-Phrine) has a longer-persisting effect that lasts up to 8 hours. If the response is not satisfactory, further reliance on this drug is probably not warranted, and other forms of treatment should be initiated. A 1:5000 solution in oil is available for intramuscular injection: 0.2 to 1.0 ml can be given and may have an appreciable effect for 8 to 16 hours.

Isoproterenol. Isoproterenol is rarely given by the noninhalational route for the treatment of asthma. An oral preparation is available, but absorption is erratic. Sublingual tablets are effective, and, although it is difficult to regulate the dose when using this route of absorption, sublingual isoproterenol may be a useful emergency drug for selected asthmatic patients. The drug has been given intravenously to adequately oxygenated patients with status asthmatics; however, cardiotoxicity precludes this treatment by those inexperienced in its use.

Metaproterenol. Currently, metaproterenol is the oral sympathomimetic bronchodilator of choice. The drug is only about 40% absorbed in the bowel, but effective bronchodilation usually lasts at least 3 to 4 hours, and as long as 6 hours or more. It is advisable to start with a dosage of 10 mg every 6 to 8 hours in adults, and then to gradually increase the dosage every few days to reach an optimal schedule; this is likely to be 20 mg every 4 to 6 hours for more severe asthma, whereas 10 mg three times daily suffices in milder cases. If lower dosages are initiated and increased over the next 1 to 2 weeks, side-effects are likely to be fewer, and the need for the higher doses can be evaluated. Generally, side-effects are not severe, but nervousness, tremor, and palpitations may occur. Maintenance therapy with oral metaproterenol can be effective for many months or years without significant intolerance, and tachyphylaxis leading to loss of bronchodilator responsiveness is uncommon.

Metaproterenol is marketed as Alupent and Metaprel. It is available for oral intake as 10-mg and 20-mg tablets and as a syrup containing 10 mg of the drug per 5 ml. No subcutaneous or intravenous forms are available in the United States, and it is unlikely that such preparations will be introduced. The drug is approved for use in children, but particular caution is needed when giving it to those under 6 years of age.

Terbutaline. This drug is the longest acting bronchodilator currently available, with an effect that may persist for more than 7 or 8 hours.[40] However, this relative potency is accompanied by a relatively high incidence of side-effects; tremor is the most troublesome complaint and is particularly likely to be a problem in older patients. The drug is not yet recommended for use in children under 12, for whom its safety needs to be proved.

Terbutaline is available as Brethine and Bricanyl, which are marketed as injectable solutions for subcutaneous use and as 2.5-mg and 5-mg tablets. Initially one 2.5-mg tablet should be taken every 8 hours; if the effect is inadequate but the drug is well tolerated, then the 5-mg tablet can be taken as often as every 6 hours. The subcutaneous injection preparations contain 1 mg/ml of solution; the usual adult dose is 0.25 mg, which can be repeated if necessary in 15 to 30 minutes. It had been hoped that this product would be better tolerated than subcutaneous epinephrine; unfortunately, it seems that terbutaline causes equivalent side-effects, although its bronchodilator action does persist longer.

Ephedrine. Ephedrine is the longest-established oral agent for treating bronchospasm; curiously, it has not proved to be suitable for inhalational use. The drug is a strong stimulator of beta-2 receptors but also has a marked effect on beta-1 and alpha receptors.

The oral dose of 15 to 50 mg (given three or four times daily according to individual needs of the bronchospastic patient) usually causes disturbing stimulation of the central nervous system, and therefore it has been thought that concurrent tranquilizer administration is needed. In a further effort to reduce unwanted effects, manufacturers have produced proprietary preparations in which 12 to 25 mg of ephedrine is combined with 50 to 130 mg of theophylline and a tranquilizer, either a barbiturate (e.g., Amesec, Bronkotabs, Quadrinal, Tedral) or hydroxyzine (e.g., Marax). The dose of theophylline alone probably has as much bronchodilator effect as does that of some of the combination preparations.[53]

Ephedrine has other disadvantages: it can cause urinary retention in men with prostatic hypertrophy and is ineffective in severe asthma. Moreover, the long-term effectiveness of this drug cannot be relied on, since tachyphylaxis readily develops, apparently because ephedrine works, in part, by releasing catecholamines from neuronal storage vesicles, which eventually become depleted.

Methoxyphenamine. Methoxyphenamine (Orthoxine) is a rarely used oral bronchodilator. It is related to methamphetamine chemically but has only slight central stimulatory actions. It is thought to be a more potent bronchodilator than ephedrine and to have fewer cardiovascular side-effects.

Ethylnorepinephrine. Ethylnorepinephrine (butanephrine, Bronkephrine) is a further example of a marketed bronchodilator whose probable value greatly exceeds its present popularity. It is a less potent beta-2 stimulator than epinephrine but has much less beta-1 activity; it does have appreciable alpha activity. The drug is suitable for inhalational as well as systemic use but is only marketed as a 0.2% solution for intramuscular or subcutaneous use, the dose in adults being 0.3 to 1.0 ml.

Other Sympathomimetic Bronchodilator Drugs. The pharmaceutical industry keeps searching for the ideal bronchodilator: a potent, moderately long-acting drug with few side-effects when given in the therapeutic dosage range. It must be suitable for aerosol, oral, or parenteral administration, and predictable dose-response effects must be achieved. Thus far, no contender for the title has appeared, although the new agents fenoterol (Berotec)[23,59] and pirbuterol[16] may possess some of the desired advantages. Other less impressive bronchodilators have been reported, including rimiterol, carbuterol, salmefamol, hexoprenaline, reproterol, and clenbuterol.

NONSYMPATHOMIMETIC BRONCHODILATORS AND ANTIASTHMA DRUGS

A number of nonsympathomimetic drugs have been used to manage bronchospasm. These agents can be classified as phosphodiesterase inhibitors (methylxanthines); mucosal constrictors; antiallergy agents; immunosuppressives; prostaglandins; and a miscellaneous group.

The important drugs in these categories will be discussed in the following section. Some of the agents are suitable for inhalational administration, although most are not given by this means.

Methylxanthines

Methylxanthines are important to respiratory therapists, since theophylline and aminophylline are of major value in treating bronchospasm, although they are not inhalational agents.[36] The methylxanthines are phosphodiesterase inhibitors; they increase the availability of cAMP by inhibiting its breakdown by the intracellular enzyme phosphodiesterase. Although tea, coffee, chocolate, and cola beverages all owe their characteristic taste and properties to their content of methylxanthine, they do not have any significant inhibitory effect on phosphodiesterase, and thus are not of pharmacologic value for bronchospasm.

Theophylline. *Properties of Theophylline.* The major pharmacologic use of theophylline and a few related compounds is in treating bronchospasm. Theophylline is a potent bronchodilator and has numerous less impressive, but generally beneficial, effects.[59] Therapeutic doses can produce cardiac stimulation, resulting in a slightly increased heart rate, but arrhythmias may occur with slightly larger doses. Cardiac performance and left ventricular output may be improved in patients with heart failure, but in normal people cardiac output is not significantly affected. Generally, theophylline appears to be a vasodilator, and it may cause a useful decrease in vascular resistance in pulmonary and coronary arterial vessels. However, the drug is believed to be a vasoconstrictor of the cerebrovascular supply, and indeed theophylline was formerly used to treat hypertensive and migraine headaches. This is difficult to reconcile with the experience, particularly of pediatricians, that theophylline can cause headaches. A final possible benefit of theophylline (well known to beverage drinkers) is its diuretic effect.

Theophylline has no beneficial effect on the gastrointestinal tract; on the contrary, therapeutic levels may cause adverse reactions, including increased gastric acid secretion, which results in indigestion, vomiting, gastric irritation and reflux; abdominal pain, diarrhea, and even gastric bleeding may result. Certain oral products are better tolerated than others, but the symptoms are related to the concentration of the drug in the blood rather than to the direct irritative effect of the preparation in the bowel.

Stimulation of the nervous system is produced by the methylxanthines, which accounts for their popularity in beverages. Normal serum levels of theophylline may produce anxiety and tremulousness in susceptible patients, whereas excessive levels may result in potentially lethal seizures.

Dosages of Theophylline. A partial bronchodilator response may be produced by a serum level of theophylline of about 5 μg/ml (0.5 mg/dl), whereas a full response is usual with a serum level of 10 to 20 μg/ml. However, some patients require higher levels (20–25 μg/ml), and, although such concentrations are potentially dangerous, there are patients who tolerate these levels without signs of toxicity. Thus, in practice, the therapeutic range for theophylline is 5 to 25 μg/ml (see Table 20-9).

The clearance of theophylline from the body occurs mainly as a result of enzymatic degradation in the liver. Any condition that impairs hepatic function

Table 20-9. Correlations of Serum Levels of Theophylline with Responses

SERUM LEVEL $\mu g/ml$	CORRESPONDING BRONCHODILATOR EFFECT	CORRESPONDING POSSIBLE SIDE-EFFECTS
5	Partial	Side-effects unusual
10	Moderate	Vague discomfort
15	Usually optimal	Gastrointestinal problems
20	Usually maximal	Anxiety, tremor
25	These levels are required for	Tachycardia
30	occasional patients	Arrhythmias
40+	This level is never therapeutic	Convulsions

will decrease the clearance rate; hepatocellular failure, hypoxia, and venous congestion have all been shown to prolong the presence of the drug in the body. Stimulation of liver enzymes can increase the clearance rate, and this can result from the effects of constituents in cigarette smoke, smog, and barbecued protein; certain drugs, such as phenytoin, barbiturates, and marijuana, also increase theophylline clearance. Generally, children clear theophylline more rapidly than do adults, and in very old patients clearance rates may be decreased. Dosages for theophylline depend on many factors,[53] and guidelines for reaching a serum level of 10 to 20 μg/ml are suggested in Table 20-10.

Now that serum levels of theophylline are becoming more available, there has been a tendency to order studies in a nondiscriminatory fashion. When theophylline therapy is initiated, the serum level gradually builds until a relatively stable level has been reached after about 36 hours: serum levels before this will not necessarily be in the therapeutic range. If a short-acting preparation is being given every 6 hours, a peak level can be obtained about 1 hour after the drug has been taken. If a slow-release preparation is given every 12 hours, a relatively constant plateau is assured, and a serum level can be taken at any time. In a few cases, where rapid metabolism is suspected, one should determine whether the trough level has dipped too low just before the routine next dose is to be given. The time the specimen is taken and the time the previous theophylline dosage was taken should always be recorded, so that meaningful information will be available to the physician responsible for adjusting the dosage.

Numerous brand and generic preparations of theophylline have been marketed. In recent years, long-acting products have become extremely popular, since they result in smoother bronchodilation and encourage better compliance. The main preparations are listed in Table 20-11. Combination products with ephedrine cannot be recommended, although very mild bronchospasm may respond adequately to such preparations.

Aminophylline. The main disadvantage of theophylline is that it is relatively insoluble in water. This is the reason why this hazardous drug is not suitable for inhalation, since the solution would be too dilute to be effective. Long ago, it was discovered that theophylline is 20 times more soluble in the ammoniacal solvent ethylenediamine; the resulting solution is aminophylline. Ethylenediamine is not inert; one benefit is that it can stimulate the respiratory center and thereby correct some cases of Cheyne–Stokes breathing.

The average dosage of aminophylline is 5 to 7 mg/kg as a loading dose, to be given over 15 to 30 minutes intravenously; this is followed by 0.5 mg/kg/hr given as a continuous intravenous drip. A smaller loading dose is needed if the patient has recently taken a theophylline preparation. In contrast, some patients with status asthmaticus (particularly young smokers) need and tolerate a larger loading dose.[53] If in doubt as to the appropriate maintenance dosage, one should obtain a serum level, but generally the first day or two of hospital therapy can be provided without such information, and after the second day most asthmatic patients can be managed with oral theophylline.

Aminophylline has the same side-effects as theophylline as well as some individualistic ones. Although aminophylline is available for oral use as tablets, theophylline preparations seem to be better tolerated and are generally preferred. Rectal preparations of aminophylline are available but are rarely used because they irritate the mucosa and are unreliably absorbed. Inhalational aerosols of aminophylline may provoke bronchospasm, and, in practice, nebulization is not of therapeutic value. The ethylenediamine component of aminophylline presents one additional, poorly recognized hazard: it is a potent sensitizing agent, and occasionally sensitive people develop skin reactions after administration of the drug. Of greater concern is that, rarely, bronchospasm may be induced by ethylenediamine when the drug is given intravenously.

Table 20-10. Theophylline and Aminophylline Dosages*

	THEOPHYLLINE	AMINOPHYLLINE
LOADING	*mg/kg*	*mg/kg*
Initial		
Average	5	6
Range	2.5–7.5	3–9
MAINTENANCE	*mg/kg/6 hr*†	*mg/kg/hr*‡
Average adult		
Nonsmoker	2.4	0.5
Smoker	4.2	0.9
Neonate	0.6	0.12
Young child	2.4–4.8	0.5–1.0
Geriatric	2.1–3.6	0.26–0.50

ADJUSTMENTS

Increase Dosage		*Decrease Dosage*	
Cigarette smoking	80%	Liver failure	50%
Marijuana smoking	50–80%	Cimetidine therapy	30–50%
Phenytoin	50%	Heart failure	30%
High protein diet	?	Cor pulmonale	30%
Barbecued food	?	Hypoxemia	10–30%
Smog exposure	?	High carbohydrate diet	?
Oral contraceptive use	?	Viral upper respiratory infection	?
Barbiturate use	?	Macrolide antibiotic therapy	?
Benzodiazepine use	?	Allopurinol	?
Ethanol use	?	Propranolol	?

(*Note:* When in doubt, serum levels should be obtained as a guide to dosage requirements for individual patients.)

*Dosages should be based on ideal weight in obese, but in some patients larger dosages will be needed.

†Two times this dosage should be given when slow-release products are being administered every 12 hours.

‡Given as a continuous infusion.

Intravenous aminophylline has resulted in a number of deaths, usually caused by rapid infusion of the drug; hazards can be avoided by injecting the drug slowly or by giving it as a continuous infusion. The explanation for the fatal reaction is unknown, but both hypotensive and hypertensive cardiac failure and arrhythmias have been invoked. Similarly, fatalities have occurred after the administration of excessive dosages of aminophylline per rectum (as suppositories or solutions) to young children.

Dyphylline. Dyphylline (hyphylline, Dilor, Lufyllin) is the only substituted derivative of theophylline; it has only 70% of the effect of theophylline. It can be given intramuscularly, since, unlike other theophylline preparations, it is very soluble and does not cause tissue irritation. Dyphylline is also available as tablets and liquid for oral administration, the recommended adult dosage being 400 to 800 mg four to six times daily. Recently, it has been suggested that the drug is suitable for intravenous use in acute asthma.[27] If given after food, gastric irritation appears to be minimized, although this problem may arise when doses in the upper range are administered.

Perhaps surprisingly this very soluble, nonirritating methlyxanthine has not been established as an

Table 20-11. Examples of Theophylline and Derivatives

ROUTE OF ADMINISTRATION OF THEOPHYLLINE AND DERIVATIVES	AVAILABLE FORMULATIONS	RANGE OF CONTENTS IN MARKETED PREPARATIONS
THEOPHYLLINE 100%*		
Oral	(a) Liquids, syrups, elixirs, suspension	100–250 mg/15 ml
	(b) Quick release tablets, capsules	80–300 mg
	(c) Slow-release tablets, capsules	60–500 mg
Rectal	No longer available	
Aerosol	Microphyllin, 1.25% solution	12.5 mg/ml
AMINOPHYLLINE (theophylline ethylenediamine) 79–84%*		
Injection	(a) Intravenous	250 mg/10 ml
	(b) Intramuscular	500 mg/2 ml
Oral	(a) Tablets	100, 200 mg
	(b) Slow-release tablets	225–300 mg
	(c) Elixirs, liquids	100–315 mg/15 ml
Rectal	Solutions, suppositories	250–500 mg/unit
DYPHYLLINE (hyphylline, dihydroxypropyl theophylline) 70%*		
Oral	(a) Liquids, elixirs	100–300 mg/15 ml
	(b) Tablets	200, 400 mg
	(c) Slow-release tablets	400 mg
Injection	Intramuscular	250 mg/ml
Aerosol	Not approved	
CHOLINE THEOPHYLLINATE (oxtriphylline) 64%*		
Oral	(a) Tablets	100, 200 mg
	(b) Elixir, syrup	50, 100 mg/5 ml
	(c) Sustained action tablet	400, 600 mg

*Content of theophylline.

inhalational drug, although recent studies have demonstrated its effectiveness and safety in animals.[22] This product or a similar one may eventually become part of the respiratory therapy armamentarium.

Oxtriphylline. Oxtriphylline (Choledyl) is the choline salt of theophylline, but claims that it is better absorbed in the gastrointestinal tract with less irritation are not convincing enough to support its use. The appropriate dose for adults is 400 mg four times daily; 400 mg provides the equivalent of 250 mg of theophylline, since oxtriphylline has only 64% anhydrous theophylline content.

Mucosal Vasoconstrictors

Mucosal vasoconstrictors have alpha-receptor stimulating properties. Drugs in this category are mainly used to treat the swollen nasal mucosa, but several of them are used in inhalation therapy. Their main value in the respiratory tract is in decreasing vascular engorgement and the accompanying edema of the mucosa, and also in delaying absorption and dispersion of topical bronchodilator drugs. There is a slight fear that the alpha stimulator can contribute to bronchospasm, but this does not appear to be of practical significance.

Phenylephrine. Phenylephrine (Neo-Synephrine) is the most popular nasal decongestant. It may be reasonable to administer 0.5 to 2 ml of 0.25% phenylephrine by nebulization into the tracheobronchial tree in managing inflammatory conditions such as bronchitis, tracheobronchitis, or postextubation tracheitis. There is no evidence that rebound congestion occurs in the lung following use of phenylephrine, although this problem may arise in the nasal mucosa after treatment with nose drops or spray. In suitable cases, the drug may be added to a bronchodilator for pulmonary aerosol therapy.

Cyclopentamine. Cyclopentamine (Clopane) was incorporated into the proprietary bronchodilator Aerolone at the recommendation of Dautrebande[15]; this product originally contained isoproterenol, procaine hydrochloride, atropine, and propylene glycol as well as cyclopentamine, but the present product contains only propylene glycol and isoproterenol. The original mixture was an interesting example of a combination preparation based on sound pharmacologic principles, and this bronchodilator product deserved further consideration as a therapeutic agent. Cyclopentamine is a moderately strong alpha stimulator, and it also has some beta-1 activity.

Antiallergy Agents

Since asthma is not infrequently allergic in its etiology, one would expect that *antihistamines* and other popular agents for treating allergic rhinitis would be valuable in managing asthma. However, practical experience has shown that the antihistamines are rarely beneficial in adult asthmatics, although they may be useful adjuvants in children. Perhaps some of these drugs would be of greater value if given by inhalation, but investigations have failed to establish the value of topical antihistamines in respiratory therapy.[12]

The main antiallergy drugs for asthma are the corticosteroids, but in the last few years the new drug cromolyn has been available. These drugs, and some less important ones, will be discussed below.

Corticosteroids. The adrenal cortex secretes various natural hormones, including cortisol (hydrocortisone) and cortisone; the pharmaceutical industry has produced an additional bewildering array of synthetic corticosteroids (Table 20-12). These drugs have an extraordinary variety of effects and are used to treat innumerable diseases, even though the mechanism by which they help is not always understood. In respiratory medicine the corticosteroids are mainly used to manage allergic diseases and are of particular value in severe asthma.

The beneficial actions of corticosteroids in asthma have not been fully worked out, but the following important actions are involved: inhibition of antibody formation, thereby preventing antigen-antibody reactions; inhibition of formation or storage of messenger agents such as histamine, which are involved in the asthmatic response; and inhibition of various cellular mechanisms involved in bronchoconstriction by a nonspecific anti-inflammatory action. Additionally, there is evidence that corticosteroids potentiate sympathomimetic agents, probably by acting directly on the beta-2 receptors, and can cause muscle relaxation, probably by directly increasing the intracellular concentration of cAMP. Thus, the anti-inflammatory steroids (glucocorticoids) can be of value not only in preventing allergic asthma, but also in managing status asthmaticus of any cause.

Unfortunately, the glucocorticoids can cause numerous long-term side-effects that are dramatically serious. They may result in a constellation of bodily changes, known as cushingism; these unpleasant features include excessive weight gain, truncal obesity, hirsutism, acne, ecchymoses, striae, plethora, and edema. The more dangerous side-effects include psychosis, hypertension, impairment of ability to fight infection, diabetes, cataracts, glaucoma, sodium retention, potassium loss, osteoporosis, and stunted growth; in some patients, peptic ulcer disease may be induced. Moreover, once a patient becomes dependent on steroid therapy, withdrawal of the drug may be difficult; the patient feels ill, and the disease exacerbates if dosage is lowered too quickly. Evidence of inadequate adrenal and pituitary function may also appear.

Corticosteroid preparations are given intravenously in the treatment of severe asthma (status asthmaticus), and oral preparations are used for long-term therapy. Over many years attempts have been made to treat asthma with inhalational steroid preparations, but not until relatively recently has a product, beclomethasone, gained considerable acceptance in the United States (Table 20-13).

Corticosteroids that have been used in respiratory therapy will be emphasized below. However, these powerful drugs are not suitable for IPPB administration because very precise dosage is needed, which can be provided by metered devices but not by free nebulization.

Beclomethasone (Vanceril, Beclovent) is marketed as a metered inhaler that delivers 50 μg per puff. Investigations suggest that up to 2 mg per day may be given without significant systemic steroid absorption, and thus without serious side-effects. Responsive patients seem to do well on much smaller doses, and steroid-dependent patients have been successfully transferred from oral preparations, which cause cushingism, to the relative safety of beclomethasone aero-

Table 20-12. "Older" Corticosteroid Preparations

GENERIC NAME	TRADE NAMES	TOPICAL ANTIALLERGY POTENCY	APPROXIMATE EQUIVALENT DOSE (ORAL) *mg*	USUAL DOSAGE (ORAL OR I.V.) *mg/day*	NOTES
SHORT-ACTING (Plasma half-life less than 2 hours)					Short-acting agents have more sodium retaining potency
Hydrocortisone (cortisol)	Cortef, Solu-Cortef	1	20	80–120	Hydrocortisone has been given by inhalation in doses up to 30 mg/day; this is not recommended
Cortisone	Cortone	0.8	25	100–150	Used for replacement therapy in adrenal insufficiency
INTERMEDIATE-ACTING (Plasma half-life 1–4 hours)					
Prednisone	Meticorten, Deltasone	3.5	5	5–80	Standard oral drug
Prednisolone	Meticortelone, Delta-Cortef	4	5	5–80	Oral drug; may be indicated if patient has liver insufficiency
Methylprednisolone	Medrol, Solu-Medrol	5	4	4–80	Parenteral alternative to hydrocortisone; may cause less electrolyte disturbance
Triamcinolone	Aristocort, Kenalog	5	4	4–80	Triamcinolone diacetate (Aristocorte Forte) has been given to prevent asthma, *e.g.,* 3–48 mg i.m. once a week

Table 20-13. Corticosteroid Preparation Suitable for Aerosol Administration

GENERIC NAME	TRADE NAMES	TOPICAL ANTIALLERGY POTENCY*	DOSE PER PUFF OF METERED CARTRIDGE *mg*	AEROSOL DOSAGE *mg/day*
Beclomethasone dipropionate	Beclovent, Vanceril	20–500	0.042	0.12–0.84
Betamethasone valerate	Bextasol	25–360	Not available	0.6–0.8
Dexamethasone sodium phosphate	Decadron Respihaler (for lungs), Decadron Turbinaire (for nose)	30	0.084	0.33–1
Flunisolide	–	–	Not available	1–2
Triamcinolone acetonide	Kenalog	5–100	Not available	0.8–2

*Compared to hydrocortisone having a potency of 1.

sol therapy. A potential problem with this drug, and with other aerosolized steroids, is seen in some patients who develop oropharyngeal *Candida* infections, which are generally not severe and are easily treated.

Beclomethasone may be effective enough if it is administered only once or twice a day. It is very effective topically and is poorly absorbed, and thus does not produce systemic effects. For individual patients, it is uncertain as to how many administrations a day will be needed, but initially the aerosol is used four times daily, two to four puffs at a time.

Betamethasone is another long-acting steroid that is suitable for topical therapy. In England the drug is available as a metered aerosol inhaler, Bextasol, and it appears to be similar to beclomethasone. This inhaler delivers 100 μg per puff; the dose required by asthmatic patients is almost the same as that for beclomethasone, and this dosage is delivered by half as many puffs of the Bextasol inhaler.

Dexamethasone (Decadron) was the first metered preparation of a corticosteroid available for inhalation in the United States; it has also been given by IPPB. The drug has lost popularity because effective dosages for asthmatic patients seem to lead to appreciable systemic absorption with resultant side-effects. A metered preparation is also available for aerosol therapy of the nasal mucosa, and this may be valuable in treating allergic or vasomotor rhinitis; however, irritation and dryness of the mucosa often occur, and nasal septal perforation has been reported.

Triamcinolone (Aristocort, Kenalog) was reported on favorably by Williams and coworkers, who used it as a micronized preparation of the acetonide packaged in an investigational metered dispenser to manage asthmatics.[55] Further experience is required before this preparation can be expected on the market. The long-acting depot preparation (Aristocort Forte) is sometimes given as a weekly injection in the prophylaxis of asthma. The appropriate dosage has not been defined, and the overall benefit of this treatment requires evaluation.

Hydrocortisone (cortisol) is a valuable corticosteroid for general use in many diseases. It can be given orally and systemically and also as a cream and by injection into joints. The usual oral dose is 10 to 80 mg per day, and the intravenous dose for conditions such as status asthmaticus is 250 to 500 mg initially, followed by 100 to 250 mg every 3 hours.

Hydrocortisone has been given as an inhalational aerosol to asthmatic patients in the form of Solu-Cortef, and although it may be effective this drug appears to have no advantage in this type of therapy, since systemic absorption occurs.

Cortisone is occasionally used to treat asthma, but the drug is primarily of value in replacement therapy for patients with adrenocortical insufficiency. There is no reason for using this drug in respiratory therapy.

Prednisone and prednisolone are similar synthetic drugs that are suitable for oral maintenance therapy in asthma and in many other diseases. These two drugs are similar to hydrocortisone but are about four times as potent. The maintenance dose is 5 to 20 mg a day, and cushingism can develop with prolonged use. Many asthmatic patients do well on alternate-day dosage; this form of therapy markedly decreases the incidence of unwanted side-effects.

Phenobarbital increases the rate of metabolism of steroids such as prednisone and dexamethasone.[9] If an asthmatic patient being maintained on one of these drugs is started on a preparation that contains a barbiturate (e.g., Amesec or Tedral), the steroid dose may need to be increased. Extra caution is therefore required if barbiturates are given to asthmatic patients on steroid therapy. In contrast, the macrolide antibiotics, such as erythromycin, appear to potentiate steroids.

Numerous other steroid preparations are available for oral and parenteral use, but it is doubtful whether these agents offer important advantages in managing respiratory disease. One corticosteroid, *methylprednisolone* (Solu-Medrol), is allegedly of special value in treating adult respiratory distress syndromes such as shock lung; however, further work is needed to determine whether this is true.

Cromolyn Sodium. A few years ago, a new drug was discovered that was related to the chromone khellin, which had been known as a weak bronchodilator for many years. The new chromone was called disodium cromoglycate in England and had the remarkable property of being able to prevent allergic asthma when given prophylactically by inhalation. The powder was subsequently introduced into the United States as cromolyn sodium (Aarane, Intal—but only Intal is currently marketed). It is packaged in capsules, and a special Spinhaler is needed to release the powder when an inhalation is taken from the device. The content of cromolyn in each capsule is 20 mg.

Cromolyn is not a bronchodilator, and, in fact, since it is a powder, inhalation may cause reactive airways to develop bronchospasm. Cromolyn is only of prophylactic value and can be used instead of corticosteroids in some asthmatic patients who are steroid-dependent. Cromolyn is also effective in preventing exercise-induced bronchospasm. Patients must recognize that the drug will not relieve acute attacks of bronchospasm.

Unlike the steroids, cromolyn is remarkably free from side-effects, although occasionally patients develop transient allergic rashes when they use the drug. Some patients find the powder is irritating to the throat; the cause of this may be the large particles of lactose present in the capsules that are marketed. The particles of cromolyn are less than 10 μg in size, and the larger lactose particles are included to improve the flow properties of the powder. The lactose tends to deposit in the oropharynx and trachea, whereas the cromolyn impacts further down the airways.

The drug is believed to act by interfering with the antigen–antibody effect on tissue mast cells (so-called "stabilization" of mast cells). In the allergic patient, this results in a decreased release of messengers such as histamine. The mechanism by which cromolyn prevents exercise-induced asthma has not been fully elucidated.

Cromolyn is usually given four times daily for the first 2 to 3 weeks, and if a beneficial effect is obtained the dosage may be reduced. Some asthmatics do well with only one or two capsules a day, and steroid therapy may be discontinued. Several days or even weeks of therapy may be needed before the benefits of cromolyn become manifest. Prophylactic bronchodilator therapy (e.g., inhalation of isoproterenol) may be needed before each inhalation of cromolyn to prevent reactive bronchospasm.

The drug seems to be most successful in younger patients. It may be unsuitable for very young children, since several vital-capacity breaths followed by breath-holding are required to empty out a capsule, and small children who are dyspneic may not perform the maneuver correctly. An oral equivalent to cromolyn will probably eventually be developed.[46] A soluble preparation suitable for IPPB or simple aerosol administration has been introduced recently.

As shown in Figure 20-3, cromolyn may have a basic action on calcium flux: By interfering with the entry of calcium into the cell, subsequent reactions resulting in release of mediators are prevented. Other new drugs that interfere with calcium flux may prove to be of value in asthma, especially that induced by exercise—for example, *verapamil, nifedipine*.[11,37] Another related antiasthma agent of interest is the mast-cell stabilizing drug ketotifen.[14,47]

Diethylcarbamazine. Diethylcarbamazine (Hetrazan) is a piperazine derivative used to treat parasite infestation with microfilariae. Inhalation of diethylcarbamazine pamoate may act like cromolyn in preventing exercise-induced asthma. The drug appears to act by preventing the release of bronchospasmogenic messengers, such as slow-reacting substance of anaphylaxis (SRS-A).

Immunosuppressive Drugs. Many drugs, including corticosteroids, are used to suppress immunologic reactions, and such therapy is mandatory for patients with transplanted organs to prevent rejection reactions. Several of these drugs are also of value in immunologic diseases such as periarteritis or rheumatoid arthritis, and a number of these agents have been tried on asthmatics (e.g., chloroquine, chlorambucil. 6-mercaptopurine, thioguanosine, and azathioprine). However, these immunosuppressive drugs do not seem to have been of significant benefit in the treatment of asthma.

Prostaglandins. The body produces a series of potent natural hormones called prostaglandins, since the prostate gland is a particularly rich source. The agent identified as prostaglandin F (PGF) is a potent bronchoconstrictor (especially $PGF_2\alpha$), whereas prostaglandins E (PGE_1 and PGE_2) are potent bronchodilators. Aerosolization of PGE_1 has reportedly resulted in 10 to 100 times as much bronchodilation as the same weight of isoproterenol. These agents appear to cause increased cAMP activity, but the mechanism involved is uncertain. Prostaglandins of the E series may eventually find a role in respiratory therapy, although no progress has been made during the past few years.

Anticholinergic Agents. One of the earliest forms of treatment for bronchospasm was provided by derivatives of plants such as *Datura;* a good example is the jimson weed or thornapple, *Datura stramonium.* These solanaceous plants contain a number of anticholinergic agents, including atropine, scopolamine, and l-hyoscyamine. Extracts from various parts of the plant have been used, including stramonium cigarettes or powders, which release the active drug in the smoke created by slowly burning them.[13] Asthmatic patients around the world still use these herbal preparations—for example, Asthmador cigarettes.

Atropine is dl-hyoscyamine, and it is the best known anticholinergic drug. It is a potent inhibitor of the neurotransmitter acetylcholine at the cholinergic receptor sites of the parasympathetic postganglionic system. This type of cholinergic stimulation is classically caused by muscarine, the agent in poisonous mushrooms, and therefore atropine is classified as an antimuscarinic drug. The muscarinic parasympathetic sites of relevance in the lung are the vagal nerve efferents to the bronchial muscles and the bronchial glands; stimulation results in bronchospasm and mucus secretion, respectively.

Atropine is administered parenterally for the preanesthetic preparation of a patient to decrease the production of respiratory secretions that would otherwise occur with general anesthesia. For many years, in many countries, atropine has been used in the aerosol management of bronchospasm, but this well-established form of therapy has only stimulated interest in the United States during the past few years, and the drug is still unapproved for this purpose. Nevertheless, knowledgable physicians do prescribe atropine for patients whose bronchospasm does not respond adequately to more conventional therapy. The effectiveness of atropine is attributed to the concept that asthmatic bronchospasm is a result of increased cholinergic tone in the airways, probably caused by an irritant-receptor reflex stimulation of bronchial muscle (*see* Chap. 30).

The appropriate dose of atropine sulfate for aerosolization is not firmly established but lies in the range of 0.005 to 0.075 mg/kg three or four times daily.[29] The drug is available in many different concentrations and as powders and tablets that can be dissolved in normal saline. The optimal concentration is probably a 1% solution, providing 10 mg/ml; for the average adult, a dosage of 0.025 mg/kg is reasonable, and this is achieved by nebulizing about 0.1 to 0.2 ml of the 1% solution. Major side-effects are dry mouth and tachycardia; these problems can be severely exacerbated if sympathomimetic drugs are given concurrently. Drying of respiratory secretions is not usual after atropine aerosolization in asthmatic patients, and the drug is particularly well tolerated in bronchitis.

Ipratropium (SCH 1000) is an investigational derivative of atropine that will shortly be released under the name Atrovent. It appears to be a very effective, relatively long-lasting aerosol bronchodilator with less potential for cardiac side-effects than atropine.[52] Ipratropium may also provide effective treatment for the blocked nose and rhinorrhea of the common cold and related conditions.[5] The formal introduction of this agent will provide a welcome extension of the inhalational armamentarium.

Miscellaneous Agents. Other agents have reportedly been effective in some cases of asthma, but further studies are needed to establish the validity of these reports.

Phentolamine is a blocker of alpha receptors and thus has a similar action to beta-2 stimulators. This drug has been given orally and by inhalation and has reportedly prevented exercise-induced asthma. Other alpha blockers may have a similar effect in some patients with bronchospasm.

Ascorbic acid (vitamin C), the controversial agent advocated by some for the prevention of colds, does have definite effects on the respiratory tract. In addition to being a component of the mucolytic preparation Gumox (which contained copper sulfate, sodium percarbonate, and ascorbic acid), ascorbic acid has been shown to inhibit histamine-induced bronchospasm. However, no convincing evidence justifies its use for the prevention or treatment of colds or asthma.

Pituitary extract (both anterior and posterior lobe hormones) is used in England in various combination inhalants that also include drugs such as atropine, papaverine, and epinephrine; all these constituents allegedly act synergistically as bronchodilators.

Marijuana has a long history of use in therapeutics and has been studied to determine what effect it has on the pulmonary function of asthmatic patients. Without doubt, smoked marijuana and oral ingestion of its principal psychoactive ingredient tetrahydrocannabinol (THC) both produce bronchodilation. Although the effect is not as great as that of isoproterenol, the decrease in airway resistance lasts longer.[51] Unfortunately, this proven value of marijuana cannot be taken as an endorsement of its use by asthmatic patients, since the smoke may lead to the development of bronchitis.

Erythromycin is an antibiotic often used to treat pulmonary infections. Erythromycin estolate can lead to improved asthmatic symptoms, particularly in patients on corticosteroid therapy. The related macrolide antibiotic *triacetyloleandomycin* (TAO), which is more toxic, may be more effective as a potentiator of the action of corticosteroids in asthma.

ANTIBIOTICS

At various times the support for the inhalational use of antibiotics and other antimicrobic agents waxes, but generally there seems to be waning enthusiasm. Relatively little evidence suggests that the topical administration of antibiotics into the respiratory tract is of value in established infections, whereas there is, of course, an abundance of proof in favor of systemic therapy. There is a valid argument for giving small doses of antibiotics topically if the agents are very expensive or very toxic, since the relatively small amount required by aerosolization can reduce both the dose and the danger. However, there is no reason to give inexpensive or relatively safe antibiotics by this route; thus, agents such as penicillin, tetracyclines, erythromycin, sulfonamides, and similar antimicrobics should not be given by inhalation. Further, inhalational administration of antibiotics carries risks of inducing hypersensitization and of causing bronchospasm and mucosal irritation. Whether more consideration should be given to nebulizing either dangerous drugs such as amphotericin and kanamycin or expensive drugs such as clindamycin and carbenicillin awaits further studies.

Probably the best established use for aerosol antibiotic therapy is in managing persistent airway colonization by a potentially dangerous organism, such as *Pseudomonas*. Many patients, particularly those who are intubated or those with bronchiectasis, grow a pathogenic organism on repeated sputum cultures, yet show no clinical, laboratory, or radiologic evidence of established respiratory infection. Under such circumstances the organism is simply growing in the airway secretions without invading the mucosa. A course of inhalation therapy with a suitable topical antibiotic may help eliminate the danger that the organism could become invasive.

Antibiotic drugs may be given by nebulization, although this is a relatively clumsy form of therapy; direct instillation may be preferable.[24] In all cases, reactive bronchospasm must be guarded against by giving a bronchodilator. Some practitioners advocate nebulization or instillation of topical antibiotics to treat sinus or nasal infections, and topical antimicrobic treatment is used to manage tracheostomy wounds that are colonized or infected.

Table 20-14 summarizes the available data on topical antimicrobial therapy for respiratory tract colonization or infection. The dosage ranges provided for most agents show a huge spread, reflecting the uncertainty as to whether most of these drugs are truly effective. This element of uncertainty accounts for the lack of general support for topical antimicrobial therapy of the lungs.

Miscellaneous Antimicrobial Agents. Other antibiotic and sterilizing agents have been given in respiratory therapy. However, proof as to their efficacy is generally inadequate, and, since most agents can be given by other routes in clearly established dosage regimens, the uncertainties of dosage and the unreliability of effect mean that inhalational administration constitutes an experimental approach.

Iodides are known to have an antifungal effect, and sodium iodide as a 1% to 2% solution has been used to treat pulmonary aspergilloma by means of an endobronchial drip. Whether nebulization therapy with sodium or potassium iodide would be valuable in treating other fungal problems in the lungs remains to be determined. However, the aerosol probably would have a mucokinetic effect similar to that attributed to Tergemist.

Table 20-14. Topical Antimicrobial Agents in Respiratory Therapy

AGENT	ANTIMICROBIAL SPECTRUM	USUAL DOSAGE RANGE*
Amikacin	Gram-negative bacteria	Uncertain
Amphotericin B	Fungal infections	1–20 mg
Bacitracin	Staphylococci	5,000–200,000 units
Carbenicillin	*Pseudomonas*	125–1000 mg
Cephalosporins	Not recommended for use	
Colistin	Gram-negative bacteria	2–300 mg
Gentamicin	Gram-negative bacteria	5–120 mg
Kanamycin	Gram-negative bacteria†	25–300 mg
Neomycin	Gram-negative bacteria	25–400 mg
Nystatin	*Candida, Aspergillus*	25,000–50,000 units
Penicillins	Not recommended for use	
Polymyxin	Gram-negative bacteria	5–50 mg
Tobramycin	Gram-negative bacteria	50 mg

*Dosages are poorly established. The drug should be dissolved in 2 ml of saline and each dose administered two to four times daily after initial bronchodilator therapy.
†Not suitable for *Pseudomonas*.

Acetic acid has been claimed to be a useful sterilizing agent for use in respiratory therapy. A solution of 0.25% acetic acid can be used as a decontaminating fluid for nebulizers; nebulization of 10 ml through the equipment effectively eliminates gram-negative bacterial contaminants. Some workers have nebulized 0.25% acetic acid into the lung; apparently the agent is well tolerated and can kill colonizing bacteria. Whether topical acetic acid should be used prophylactically in tracheostomized or intubated patients remains to be determined.

Copper and other metals can suppress the growth of many bacteria in water by an "oligodynamic" bactericidal effect. Copper mesh has been used by some workers as a prophylactic measure; the material is left in nebulizers and humidifiers which are at risk of being contaminated. The subsequent nebulization of the solution (which probably contains ionic copper) does not appear harmful to the lungs; however, there is insufficient evidence to endorse this form of nebulization therapy for its prophylactic or antibacterial value.

LOCAL ANESTHETICS

The popularity of fiberoptic bronchoscopy has resulted in increased use of topical local anesthesia in the respiratory tract. Various methods of administration are used, including direct application of the agent to the upper respiratory tract and ultrasonic nebulization or direct instillation into the larynx, trachea, and lower airways. Anesthesia can also be produced by injection, carefully placed to cause blockade of the glossopharyngeal nerve and its recurrent branch.

Local anesthetics may cause initial bronchospasm, but generally no significant adverse effect seems to be produced on pulmonary function. These drugs may also inhibit mucociliary activity, although low concentrations of some agents have allegedly improved ciliary action. Certain agents may have a bacteriostatic effect, and specimens of secretions taken for culture after exposure to local anesthetics may not yield their full microbial content.[38] However, this does not seem to be a major concern in practice.

Cocaine. Cocaine is favored by some endoscopists because it is potent as an anesthetic, it suppresses cough, and its vasoconstrictive action limits absorption. The dosage used varies, but 5 ml of a 10% solution should be diluted to give a 2% to 4% concentration, which can be safely used. The dose given should not exceed 3.3 mg/kg (i.e., 225 mg for a 150-lb adult).

Lidocaine. Lidocaine (Xylocaine) is used most frequently in bronchoscopy. The drug is one of the safest of the local anesthetics and can be given in concentrations varying from 1% to 20%. It is available as a Freon-powered metered aerosol of a 10% solution in Canada, but in the United States it is usually given as a 4% solution by machine nebulization, as an ultrasonically generated aerosol, or by direct instillation, with a total dose of 10 to 20 ml. Epinephrine in concentrations of 1:250,000 to 1:50,000 may be added; this helps to prevent instrument-induced bronchospasm and constricts the mucosal vessels, thereby decreasing the systemic absorption of the lidocaine. Further, the presence of epinephrine prevents or stops bleeding during instrumentation of friable mucosa.

In recent years, lidocaine has been shown to act as a bronchodilator in some asthmatic patients when given by aerosol or intravenously.[54] The drug may also be valuable in some cases of intractable cough caused by persisting damage to the tracheobronchial tree.

Dyclonine. Dyclonine (Dyclone) has been recommended for topical airway anesthesia. Up to 30 ml of a 1% solution can be given by ultrasonic nebulization or direct instillation. However, this drug may be less safe and less effective than lidocaine.

Miscellaneous Local Anesthetics. Other local anesthetics are used mainly as topical preparations for endoscopic procedures and in bronchography. Some of these agents, besides lidocaine, have also been given intravenously to suppress cough.

Local anesthetics are also used in various oral "cough medications," such as tablets that dissolve in the oropharynx; the mucosal anesthesia may interrupt irritative cough reflexes. Some agents are taken systemically for their cough-suppressing effects. *Benzonatate* (Tessalon), chemically related to the local anesthetic tetracaine, may owe part of its antitussive activity to its action on cough receptors in the lung. In contrast, most cough suppressants (other than dextromethorphan) are narcotics, related to morphine; they act centrally, and thus many of them cause some respiratory center depression.

AEROSOL PROPELLANTS

The metered aerosol bronchodilator preparations have become very popular, although there is some controversy about the safety of the devices generally and the propellants particularly.

Most propellants used in the United States are encompassed by the trade name Freon (the corresponding product in England is Arcton). Freon consists of a number of haloalkanes (fluoroalkanes), which are fluorocarbon derivatives of methane and ethane. The important agents in use are FC 11 (trichloromonofluoromethane), FC 12 (dichlorodifluoromethane), and, to a lesser extent, FC 113 (trichlorotrifluoroethane). These gaseous agents are liquefied by pressure, and metered cartridges contain the active bronchodilator as a suspended powder or solution in the liquid Freon. When the product is released from the cartridge, the Freon becomes gaseous, and a cloud of droplets of the bronchodilator is created.

Aviado has performed extensive work on the toxicity of propellants, and he classifies them as follows.[2]

Class 1: low-pressure propellants of high toxicity that cause tachycardia and hypotension. Included in this class are FC 11 and FC 113.
Class 2: low-pressure propellants of intermediate toxicity that influence either circulation or respiration, or both.
Class 3: high-pressure propellants of low toxicity that cause bronchoconstriction. FC 12 is in this class.
Class 4: high-pressure propellants of low toxicity.

The propellants in Freon do have definite toxic potential. FC 11 (CCl_3F) is the most potent agent in Class 1 and also has respiratory-depressant action. FC 12 (CCl_2F_2) is also the most potent drug in its class, and in addition to causing bronchoconstriction can also cause respiratory depression, tachycardia, and hypotension.

The most toxic propellant is FC 11, which is believed by some workers to cause fatal cardiac side-effects in patients who use metered bronchodilator aerosols excessively. Patients who do overuse inhalers in this way may suffer equally or more from the concomitant overdosage of the bronchodilator.

THE ADMINISTRATION OF RESPIRATORY DRUGS

Physicians generally have greater familiarity and security with the administration of oral and intravenous drugs than they do with inhalational drugs. Accordingly, oral and intravenous drugs are prescribed with relative accuracy and appropriateness, whereas inhalational drugs do not receive the same consideration from most physicians. Respiratory therapists and nurses who administer inhalation therapy carry a considerable responsibility when they receive a physician's order, since the prescription must be interpreted and monitored with active awareness of the desired effects and the possible side-effects.

Dosages of Drugs. The appropriate dosages for inhalational drugs are, in fact, quite variable because many factors influence the effectiveness of the different agents. The reliability and efficiency of the equipment and the cooperation of the patient profoundly influence the amount of drug deposited in the lungs.[58] The response to an individual dosage varies in each patient, particularly when catecholamines are given, since tachyphylaxis or converse effects may obviate the expected result. Side-effects are very variable and may be related to the positive pressure, the gaseous vehicle, the diluent, or the droplets rather than to the drug itself.

For all these reasons therapists should not be overly surprised or concerned when a physician prescribes an "inappropriate," excessive amount of drug. If the physician, for some reason, is unwilling to change the prescription when the error is brought to his attention, the therapist or nurse can administer the drug, but they should carefully monitor the patient for any adverse response; if evidence of toxicity appears, then the treatment can be stopped short before all the prescribed amount of the drug is given, and the fact should be recorded in the patient's chart. Similarly, when an "appropriate" recommended dosage is prescribed, the patient should nevertheless be monitored for an idiosyncratic or individualistic adverse response.

Evaluation of Therapy. Unfortunately, the recognition of "adverse effects" is not cut and dried. Thus, when a bronchodilator is used, an increased pulse rate from 70 to 110 may be tolerable, whereas an increase from 110 to 125 may not. Similarly, it is difficult to recognize a meaningful change in blood pressure, since observations are not easy to make and changes in systolic and diastolic values may vary independently. Thus, epinephrine in small doses may cause a small increase in systolic pressure with a fall or no change in diastolic pressure, whereas larger doses (such as probably cannot be attained with inhalation therapy) result in more marked changes in both values. The individual physician should request the therapist to check blood pressure before, during, and after bronchodilator administration in those selected patients in whom these changes may be detrimental. However, it is unreasonable to expect a therapist to worry about the effect on the blood pressure in every patient given an aerosolized sympathomimetic.

Rational aerosol therapy requires a recognition of the therapeutic objectives, skillful administration of appropriate dosages, and accurate recording of the effects of treatment. In most patients, bedside pulmonary function evaluations of vital capacity, peak flow rate, or forced expiratory volumes can be used to assess bronchodilator responsiveness. The patient's subjective feelings, volume of sputum production, and monitoring of the pulse and auscultatory findings in the lungs should be routinely evaluated to determine whether desired effects or undesired side-effects have been obtained. The patient's subjective response is often the best indicator of adverse effects, and more objective measurements may be less helpful.

When a mucokinetic drug is given, it is the therapist's responsibility to ensure that a therapeutic response occurs. Thus, relying uncritically on the drug alone is inadequate; the patient must be encouraged to cough and to expectorate, and some chest percussion and postural drainage may be needed to facilitate the process. The therapist should record the amount of sputum produced and note the color and consistency. In many cases a variety of mucokinetic agents should be added to samples of the mucus to determine which one has the greatest mucus-loosening effect.

Administration of Aerosolized Drugs. When bronchodilator therapy is initiated for the hospitalized patient, it is conventional to prescribe treatment by means of a respirator if the patient requires ventilatory support, or IPPB if the patient is very dyspneic, and then to follow with simple air-driven nebulizer therapy once the patient improves. Using any of these techniques, much of the drug in the nebulizer may be lost in the apparatus or in the air, unless a special delivery device is used. Most studies suggest that aerosolization by means of a gas-driven nebulizer results in deposition of 5% to 10% of the drug in the lungs, whereas an equal amount might be deposited in the mouth and swallowed, thereby resulting in systemic effects. However, different techniques of drug delivery may produce greater or lesser aerosol deposition in the lungs and oropharynx, and therefore the effect of any prescribed dose can vary. Similarly, if the drug is nebulized through an endotracheal tube, more drug is deposited in the lungs, whereas none enters the gastrointestinal tract.

When a metered aerosol is used, the amount deposited in the respiratory tract is extremely variable and is related to the competency of the patient's technique. Indeed, it is all too common to see patients who exhale while nebulizing the aerosol, thereby assuring that none of the drug gets into the body. With the best technique, it is unlikely that more than 60% to 70% of the "puff" of aerosol is deposited in the lungs, and the average patient is more likely to deposit 30% to 40% of the metered dose. As shown in Table 20-15, manufacturers take this into account in their instructions, which advise that about five to seven times as much drug should be measured into a nebulizer as is released by a standard treatment using the metered product.[58]

Therapists should become very familiar with the appropriate technique to be used with each aerosol device (see list below), and the last day or two of a respiratory patient's stay in hospital should be used to teach and to supervise the patient in the correct technique to be used following discharge home. Different metered dispensers should be used in different ways depending on their individual design. In all cases, the patient must inhale the sprayed drug deeply and then hold his breath to encourage maximal deposition. If side-effects are troublesome, then rinsing out the mouth and throat with water may help remove the excess drug whose systemic absorption accounts for the side-effects. Further important concerns are that the patient should be instructed to keep the nebulizing unit clean and that overuse of the aerosol should be avoided.

Multiple drugs are often prescribed in respiratory therapy, and fortunately most agents are compatible when mixed in the nebulizer. However, bronchodilators are relatively unstable, which is why they are stored in dark bottles and maintained at an acid pH. When the drugs are placed in a nebulizer and exposed to light and oxygen, they slowly break down to reddish-brown adrenochromes. Although these products are probably not harmful, their presence suggests that the mixture has diminished bronchodilator activity, and thus should be discarded.

Patients should be warned that their secretions may be stained pink by a bronchodilator and that this should not cause alarm.

Administration of Nonaerosolized Drugs. When drugs are given intravenously, the major respiratory agents can be mixed without any apparent adverse effects. Thus saline, dextrose, aminophylline, corticosteroids, and sodium iodide are all compatible.

Table 20-15. Comparative Dosages Achieved Using Metered and Inhalant Solution Preparations of Bronchodilators

	METERED DEVICE			INHALATIONAL SOLUTION			
	Dose per Puff mg	*Dose Delivered with Three Puffs mg*	*Probable Amount Deposited in Lungs (i.e., 33%) mg*	*Potency of Solution %*	*Usual Dose ml*	*Usual Dose mg*	*Probable Amount Deposited in Lungs (i.e., 5%) mg*
EPINEPHRINE							
Medihaler-Epi	0.16	0.48	*0.16*				
Vaponephrin				2.25	0.25	6	*0.30*
ISOETHARINE							
Bronkometer	0.34	1	*0.34*				
Bronkosol Solution				1	0.5	5	*0.25*
Bronkosol Unit Dose				0.25	2	5	*0.25*
ISOPROTERENOL							
Isuprel Mistometer	0.13	0.39	*0.13*				
Isuprel Solution				1	0.5	5	*0.25*
METAPROTERENOL							
Alupent Inhaler	0.65	2	*0.65*				
Alupent Solution				5	0.3	17	*0.85*
TERBUTALINE							
Bricanyl Inhaler*	0.25	0.75	*0.25*				
Bricanyl Solution				0.1	2	2	*0.10*

(*Note:* The probable amounts of each drug deposited varies considerably depending on whether IPPB (or other aerosolizer) or metered cartridge is used. The figures provided are based on typical recommended dosages. A metered device treatment delivers more isoetharine or terbutaline than does IPPB or other aerosolizer treatment, whereas the reverse occurs with epinephrine, isoproterenol, and metaproterenol.

*Not available in the United States.

However, some antibiotics may be incompatible with various drugs, and they should be given through an independent setup.

TECHNIQUE FOR USING METERED AEROSOL DEVICES

1. Shake the canister, unless manufacturer's brochure suggests that this is not necessary.
2. Hold upside down, with mouthpiece held either between closed lips or about ½ to 1 inch away from wide open mouth. (The latter technique may be better, but most patients feel less comfortable using this method.)
3. Exhale normally but not forcefully.
4. Inhale deeply and at the same time release a puff of bronchodilator.
5. Hold breath for several seconds before exhaling. (Note: If beclomethasone is used, exhale through the nose to deposit steroid on the nasal mucosa, thereby treating any nasal allergy that may be present.)
6. Breathe normally, and wait for up to 5 minutes to evaluate response.
7. Repeat with one, two, or even three inhalations over the next 20 minutes if needed and if tolerated.
8. Rinse out mouth after each inhalation of drug to prevent side-effects from oral absorption.

9. Do not overuse any preparation; if more than 16 inhalations a day are needed, then a different treatment regimen or a change in drug is advisable.
10. Keep the dispensing unit clean by frequently rinsing it in warm water.

Most oral drugs used in respiratory therapy are compatible with one another and are often administered in combination preparations. Alcoholic elixirs are potentially hazardous when given to alcoholics and are contraindicated if the patient is on disulfiram (Antabuse) or a similar type of drug. Epinephrine, when given subcutaneously (and perhaps when given by inhalation), may interact with various drugs (e.g., with monoamine oxidase inhibitors) to cause hypertension and excitability; with digitalis glycosides to cause cardiac arrhythmias; or with hypotensive drugs to cause the reverse effect of hypertension. Epinephrine may also interfere with the action of insulin and oral antidiabetic agents since catecholamines tend to cause a rise in blood sugar level.

APPENDIX: DOSAGES OF INHALATIONAL DRUGS

VOLUMES

The amount of solution delivered from an uncalibrated dropper is very variable and depends on the characteristics of the dropper, the method of use, and the nature of the solution. One drop approximates 1 minim of an aqueous solution, or 0.5 minim of an alcoholic solution, or 2 minims of a viscous solution. There are about 15 minims (or 15 drops of an aqueous solution) in 1 ml of water.

For practical purposes the following approximate conversion table can be used for dilute aqueous solutions.

1 minim = 1 drop
15 minims = 1 ml (1 cc) = 1 g
60 minims = 1 teaspoonful = 4 ml (approx)
240 minims = 1 tablespoonful = 15 ml (approx)
480 minims = 30 ml = 30 g = 1 oz

Abbreviations

ml = milliliter (1000 ml = 1 liter [l])
cc = cubic centimeter
mg = milligram (1000 mg = 1 gram)
g = gram (1000 g = 1 kilogram [kg])
1000 micrograms (μg or mcg) = 1 mg
1,000,000 micrograms = 1 g

Apothecary versus Avoirdupois. Since these two systems of weights and measures differ, *pints* and *pounds* (lb) should not be used as pharmacologic units. The apothecary pint contains 16 oz, but there are only 12 ounces to the pound in the apothecary scale, whereas there are 16 ounces to the pound in the avoirdupois scale.

PERCENTAGES

Inhalational solutions are commonly labeled according to a percentage or ratio scale. The following scales may be used.

Weight-in-weight (w/w): e.g., g/100 g
Weight-in-volume (w/v): e.g., g/100 ml
Volume-in-volume (v/v): e.g., ml/100 ml

Most frequently, a w/v percentage is used.

1% = 1:100 = 1 g/100 ml = 1 g/dl
(*i.e.*, 1000 mg/100 ml or 10 mg/ml)
5% = 5:100 = 5 g/100 ml
(*i.e.*, 5000 mg/100 ml or 50 mg/ml)
Thus, 0.1% = 1:1000 = 0.1 g/100 ml
(*i.e.*, 100 mg/100 ml or 1 mg/ml)

Various expressions can be used, for example,

0.5% = 5:1000 or 1:200
= 1 g/200 ml, or 0.5 g/100 ml, or 500 mg/100 ml, or 500 mg/dl, or 5 mg/ml, or 5 g/liter.

EXAMPLE

A mixture of 0.25 ml of 1:200 isoproterenol in 2.5 ml of water contains

0.25 ml of 0.5% isoproterenol
= 0.25 ml of a solution containing 1 g isoproterenol in 200 ml (or 5 mg/ml)

$$= \frac{0.25}{200} \times 1000 \text{ mg} = 1.25 \text{ mg.}$$

Thus the mixture contains 1.25 mg (1250 μg) of isoproterenol in 2.75-ml solution. If this solution is nebulized by IPPB, about 10% will be retained in the lungs, providing about 0.125 mg (125 μg) of isoproterenol. This is similar to the amount delivered by one activation of a metered aerosol of isoproterenol.

REFERENCES

1. Amory DW, Burnham SC, Cheney FW: Comparison of the cardiopulmonary effects of subcutaneously administered epinephrine and terbutaline in patients with reversible airway obstruction. Chest 67:279, 1975
2. Aviado DM: Toxicity of propellants. Drug Res 18:365, 1974
3. Beck GJ: Controlled clinical trial of a new dosage form of metaproterenol. Ann Allergy 44:19, 1980
4. Barton AD: Aerosolized detergents and mucolytic agents in the treatment of stable chronic obstructive pulmonary disease. Am Rev Respir Dis 110(6, Part 2):104, 1974
5. Borum P et al: Ipratropium nasal spray: A new treatment for rhinorrhea in the common cold. Am Rev Respir Dis 123:418, 1981
6. Boyd EM: A review of studies on the pharmacology of the expectorants and inhalants. Int J Clin Pharmacol Ther Toxicol 3:55, 1970
7. Boyd EM, Sheppard EP: Friar's balsam and respiratory tract fluid. Am J Dis Child 111:630, 1966
8. Editorial: Bromhexine. Lancet 1:1058, 1971
9. Brooks SM et al: Adverse effects of phenobarbital on corticosteroid metabolism in patients with bronchial asthma. N Engl J Med 286:1125, 1972
10. Carson S, Goldhamer R, Carpenter R: Mucus transport in the respiratory tract. Am Rev Respir Dis 98(2):86, 1966
11. Cerrina J et al: Inhibition of exercise-induced asthma by a calcium-antagonist, nifedipine. Am Rev Respir Dis 123:156, 1981
12. Chai H: Antihistamines and asthma. Do they have a role in therapy? Chest 78:420, 1980
13. Charpin D, Orehek J, Velardocchio JM: Bronchodilator effects of antiasthmatic cigarette smoke (*Datura stramonium*). Thorax 34:259, 1979
14. Craps L, Greenwood C, Radielovic P: Clinical investigation of agents with prophylactic anti-allergic effects in bronchial asthma. Clin Allergy 8:373, 1978
15. Dautrebande L: Microaerosols, p 98. New York, Academic Press, 1962
16. Ence TJ, Tashkin DP, Ho D et al: Acute bronchial and cardiovascular effects of oral pirbuterol and metaproterenol. Ann Allergy 43:29, 1979
17. Feeley TW et al: Aerosol polymyxin and pneumonia in seriously ill patients. N Engl J Med 293:471, 1975
18. Gibson LE: Use of water vapor in the treatment of lower respiratory disease. Am Rev Respir Dis 110(6, Part 2):100, 1974
19. Grimwood K, Johnson–Barrett JJ, Taylor B: Salbutamol: Tablets, inhalational powder, or nebulizer? Br Med J 282:105, 1981
20. Hirsch SR, Viernes PF, Kory RC: The expectorant effect of glyceryl guaiacolate in patients with chronic bronchitis. Chest 63:9, 1973
21. Hirsch SR, Zastrow JE, Kory RC: Sputum liquefying agents: A comparative in vitro study. J Lab Clin Med 74:346, 1969
22. Hirshman CA et al: Dyphylline aerosol attenuates antigen-induced bronchoconstriction in experimental canine asthma. Chest 79:454, 1981
23. Huhti E, Poukkula A: Clinical comparison of fenoterol and albuterol administered by inhalation. Chest 73:348, 1978
24. Klastersky J et al: Endotracheally administered antibiotics for gram-negative bronchopneumonia. Chest 75:586, 1979
25. Lieberman J: Measurement of sputum viscosity in a cone-plate viscometer. II. An evaluation of mucolytic agents in vitro. Am Rev Respir Dis 97:662, 1968
26. Lieberman J, Kurnick NB: The induction of proteolysis in purulent sputum by iodides. J Clin Invest 43:1892, 1964
27. Lawyer CH et al: Utilization of intravenous dihydroxypropyl theophylline (dyphylline) in an aminophylline-sensitive patient, and its pharmacokinetic comparison with theophylline. J Allergy Clin Immunol 65:353, 1980
28. Light RW, Taylor RW, George RB: Albuterol and isoproterenol in bronchial asthma. Arch Intern Med 139:636, 1979
29. Marini JJ, Lakshminarayan S: The effect of atropine inhalation in "irreversible" chronic bronchitis. Chest 77:591, 1980
30. Miller WF: Aerosol therapy in acute and chronic respiratory disease. Arch Intern Med 131:148, 1973
31. Morrow PE: Aerosol characterization and deposition. Am Rev Respir Dis 110(6, Part 2):88, 1974
32. Muir DCF: Clinical Aspects of Inhaled Particles, chaps. 1 and 9. Philadelphia, FA Davis, 1972
33. Murad F: Mechanism of action of some bronchodilators: Cyclic nucleotide metabolism in tracheal preparations. Am Rev Respir Dis 110(6, Part 2):111, 1974
34. Obenour RA et al: Effects of surface-active aerosols and pulmonary congestion on lung compliance and resistance. Circulation 27:888, 1963
35. Parks CR et al: Effect of water nebulization on normal canine pulmonary mucociliary clearance. Am Rev Respir Dis 104:99, 1971
36. Paterson JW, Woolcock AJ, Shenfield GM: Bronchodilator drugs. Am Rev Respir Dis 120:1149, 1979
37. Patel KR: Calcium antagonists in exercise-induced asthma. Br Med J 282:932, 1981
38. Ravin CE, Latimer JM, Matsen JM: In vitro effects of lidocaine on anaerobic respiratory pathogens and strains of *Hemophilus influenzae*. Chest 72:439, 1977
39. Reed CE: Mechanisms of hyperreactivity of airways in asthma. Eur J Respir Dis (Suppl)117:87, 1982
40. Roth MJ, Wilson ALF, Novey HS: A comparative study of the aerosolized bronchodilators, isoproterenol, metaproterenol and terbutaline in asthma. Ann Allergy 38:16, 1977
41. Sackner MA, Greeneltch N, Silva G et al: Bronchodilator effects of terbutaline and epinephrine in obstructive lung disease. Clin Pharmacol Ther 16:499, 1974
42. Siegal S: The asthma-suppressive action of potassium iodide. J Allergy 35:252, 1964
43. Solomons CC, Cotton EK, Dubois R: The use of buffered L-arginine in the treatment of cystic fibrosis. Pediatrics 47:384, 1971
45. Stewart BN, Block AJ: The trial of aerosolized theophylline in relieving bronchospasm. Chest 69:718, 1976
46. Stokes TC, Morley J: Prospects for an oral Intal. Br J Dis Chest 75:1, 1981
47. Tanser AR, Elmes J: A controlled trial of ketotifen in exercise-induced asthma. Br J Dis Chest 74:398, 1980
48. Stolley PD: Asthma mortality: Why the United States was spared an epidemic of deaths due to asthma. Am Rev Respir Dis 105:883, 1972
49. Sturgess JM: Mucous secretion in the respiratory tract. Pediatr Clin N Am 26:481, 1979
50. Taplin GV, Gropper AL, Scott G: Micropowdered aminophylline or theophylline inhalation therapy in chronic bronchial asthma. Ann Allergy 7:513, 1949.
51. Tashkin DP et al: Bronchial effects of aerosolized Δ 9-tetrahydrocannabinol in healthy and asthmatic subjects. Am Rev Respir Dis 115:57, 1977
52. Ward MJ et al: Ipratropium bromide in acute asthma. Br Med J 282:598, 1981

53. Van Dellen RG: Theophylline: Practical applications of new knowledge. Mayo Clin Proc 54:733, 1979
54. Weiss EB, Patwardhan AV: The response to lidocaine in bronchial asthma. Chest 72:429, 1977
55. Williams MH: Corticosteroid aerosols for the treatment of asthma. JAMA 231:406, 1975
56. Wood M: Production of therapeutic aerosols. Respir Ther 5:19, Jan/Feb 1975
57. Ziment I: What to expect from expectorants. JAMA 236:193, 1976
58. Ziment I: Bronchodilator aerosol therapy. Respir Ther 12:59, July/August 1982
59. Ziment I (ed): Practical Pulmonary Disease, Chs 3, 5, 6, and 9. New York, John Wiley & Sons, 1983

BIBLIOGRAPHY

General Reviews of Drugs Used in Inhalation Therapy

A.M.A. Drug Evaluations, 5th ed. Chicago, American Medical Association, 1983

Aviado DM: Krantz and Carr's Pharmacologic Principles of Medical Practice, 8th ed. Baltimore, Williams & Wilkins, 1972. (Aviado is the outstanding pharmacologist in the respiratory field, and this general textbook is excellent.)

Dautrebande L: Physiological and pharmacologic characteristics of liquid aerosols. Physiol Rev 32:214, 1952. (A classic account of aerosol therapy, with an extraordinary range of information.)

Gilman AG, Goodman LS, Gilman A: The Pharmacologic Basis of Therapeutics, 6th ed. New York, Macmillan, 1980. (The chapters on the autonomic nervous system and bronchodilators are extremely good.)

Martindale: The Extra Pharmacopoeia, 28th ed. London, The Pharmaceutical Press, 1982. (This compendium provides an extraordinary amount of information, including traditional and international drugs.)

Miller WF: Aerosol therapy in acute and chronic respiratory disease. Arch Intern Med 131:148, 1973. (An excellent, short practical account.)

Muir DCF (ed): Clinical Aspects of Inhaled Particles. Philadelphia, FA Davis, 1972. (This is a very good comprehensive review, with a good chapter on therapeutics.)

Osol A, Pratt R (eds): The United States Dispensatory, 27th ed. Philadelphia, JB Lippincott, 1973. (Excellent monographs on most drugs.)

Ziment I: Respiratory Pharmacology and Therapeutics. Philadelphia, WB Saunders, 1978. (A comprehensive practical guide to drugs used in inhalation therapy and pulmonary medicine.)

Mucokinesis

Respiratory Tract Secretions and Mucociliary Clearance

Boyd EM: Respiratory Tract Fluid. Springfield, Il, Charles C Thomas, 1975. (This book gives a comprehensive review of Boyd's considerable reasearch on sputum and the agents which affect the material.)

Dulfano MJ (ed): Sputum: Fundamentals and Clinical Pathology. Springfield, IL, Charles C Thomas, 1973. (This book provides an encyclopedic account of sputum and its structure, examination, properties, and management.)

Okeson GC, Divertie MB: Cilia and bronchial clearance: The effects of pharmacologic agents and disease. Mayo Clin Proc 45:361, 1970

Wanner A: Pulmonary defense mechanism: Mucociliary clearance. In Simmons, DH (ed.): Current Pulmonology, Vol 2, Chap. 12. Boston, Houghton Mifflin Professional Publishers, 1980.

Mucokinetic Agents

Barton AD: Aerosolized detergents and mucolytic agents in the treatment of stable chronic obstructive pulmonary disease. Am Rev Respir Dis 110(6, Part 2):104, 1974

Boyd EM: Expectorants and respiratory tract fluid. Pharmacol Rev 6:521, 1954.

Boyd EM: A review of studies on the pharmacology of the expectorants and inhalants. Int J Clin Pharmacol Ther Toxicol 3:55, 1970

Gunn JA: The action of expectorants. Br Med J 4:972, 1927

Hirsch SR: What role expectorants? Drug Ther 4:179, 1975.

Lieberman J: The appropriate use of mucolytic agents. Am J Med 49:1, 1970.

Lish PM, Salem H: Expectorants. *In* Salem, H. and Aviado, DM (eds): International Encyclopedia of Pharmacology and Therapeutics, Vol. 3, Sec 27. New York, Pergamon Press, 1970.

Marin R, Litt M, Marriott C: The effect of mucolytic agents on the rheologic and transport properties of canine tracheal mucus. Am Rev Respir Dis 121(3):495, 1980.

Ziment I: Mucokinesis—the methodology of moving mucus. Respir Ther 4:15, March/April 1974.

Bronchodilator Therapy

General

Aviado DM: Regulation of bronchomotor tone during anesthesia. Anesthesiology 42:68, 1975

Lichtenstein LM, Austin FK (eds): Asthma: Physiology, Immunopharmacology, and Treatment. New York, Academic Press, 1977

Middleton E: A rational approach to asthma therapy. Postgrad Med 67:107, 1980

Weinberger M, Hendeles L, Ahrens R: Pharmacologic management of reversible obstructive airways disease. Med Clin North Am 65:579, 1981

Weiss EB (ed): Status Asthmaticus. Baltimore, University Park Press, 1978

Weiss EB, Segal MS (eds): Bronchial Asthma: Mechanisms and Therapeutics. Boston, Little, Brown & Co, 1976

Wilson AF, Galant SP: Recent advances in the pathophysiology of asthma. Calif Med 120:463, 1974

Sympathomimetic Agents

Avner SE: β-Adrenergic bronchodilators. Pediatr Clin North Am 22:129, 1975

Brittain RT, Dean CM, Jack D: Sympathomimetic bronchodilator drugs. Pharmacol Ther B 2:423, 1976

Carlstrom S et al: Studies on terbutaline, a new selective bronchodilating agent. Acta Med Scand [Suppl] 512:1, 1970
Leifer KN, Wittig HJ: The beta-2 sympathomimetic aerosols in the treatment of asthma. Ann Allergy 35:69, 1975
Lyons HA et al: Symposium on isoproterenol therapy in asthma. Ann Allergy 31:1, 1973
Mallen MS et al: Salbutamol. Postgrad Med J [Suppl] 47:1, 1971
McFadden RR: Aerosolized bronchodilators and steroids in the treatment of airway obstruction in adults. Am Rev Respir Dis 122(5, Part 2):89, 1980
Paterson JW, Woolcock AJ, Shenfield GM: Bronchodilator drugs. Am Rev Respir Dis 120(5):1149, 1979
Webb–Johnson DC, Andrews JL: Bronchodilator therapy. N Engl J Med 297:476, 758, 1977
Ziment I: How to select an appropriate respiratory drug. Geriatrics 36:89, 1981

Methylxanthines

Grover FW: Oxtriphylline glyceryl guaiacolate elixir in pediatric asthma: With a theophylline review. Ann Allergy 23:127, 1965
Hendeles L, Weinberger M: Theophylline: A "State of the Art" review. Pharmacotherapy 3:2, 1983
Libby DM, Smith JP: Clinical considerations in determining theophylline dosage in the adult. Pract Cardiol 6:84, 1980
Tong TG: Aminophylline, review of clinical use. Drug Intell Clin Pharm 7:156, 1973
Weinberger M, Riegelman S: Rational use of theophylline for bronchodilation. N Engl J Med 291:151, 1974

Prostaglandins

Fanburg B: Prostaglandins and the lung. Am Rev Respir Dis 108:482, 1973
Hyman AL, Spannhake EW, Kadowitz PJ: Prostaglandins and the lung. Am Rev Respir Dis 117:111, 1978

Antiallergy Agents

Altounyan REC: Review of clinical activity and mode of action of sodium cromoglycate. Clin Allergy 10:481, 1980
Aviado DM, Carrillo LR: Anti-asthmatic action of corticosteroids: A review of the literature on their mechanism of action. J Clin Pharmacol 10:3, 1970
Sahn SA: Corticosteroids in chronic bronchitis and pulmonary emphysema. Chest 73:389, 1978

Antibiotics

Miller WF: Antibiotic aerosols. In Kagan BM (ed): Antimicrobial Therapy, 2nd ed. Philadelphia, WB Saunders, 1974
Wanner A, Rao A: Clinical indications for and effects of bland, mucolytic, and antimicrobial aerosols. Am Rev Respir Dis 122(5, Part 2): 79, 1980
Williams MH: Steroid and antibiotic aerosols. Am Rev Respir Dis 110(6, Part 2):122, 1974

Additives

Tiersten S: RT pharmacology: Where has it been and where is it going? Respir Ther 4:23, 1974
Wood M, Ziment I: Additives and combinations. Respir Ther 4:19, 1974

21

Artificial Airways

Sandra L. Caldwell • Kent N. Sullivan

Airway management is critical to the success of respiratory care; indeed, all members of the respiratory care team must be skilled in the procedures necessary for quality airway management. This chapter will review the various kinds of artificial airways, stressing the techniques for their insertion and maintenance, indications, contraindications, and complications.

Airway access and control may be achieved by simple means such as the use of oral nasal or esophageal airways, or by direct nasotracheal or orotracheal intubation. In emergency situations, a cricothyroidotomy may be performed. In this procedure, a surgical opening is made in the cricothyroid membrane. Cricothyroidotomy is alleged to be safe, quicker, and more simple than emergency tracheotomy.[41] Its role as an elective procedure is controversial.[5,6]

If intubation appears to be required for a prolonged period of time, a tube may be inserted through an incision in the neck, directly into the trachea (tracheotomy).

ORAL AIRWAY

In certain clinical situations (such as the immediate postanesthetic period or in coma with redundancy of the tongue), simple insertion of an oral airway (Fig. 21-1) often suffices, allowing easy respiration (assisted or spontaneous) and suctioning of the oropharynx as necessary. The use of oral airways has become so commonplace in medical practice that they are considered innocuous devices, and usually are. Stauffer and Petty have published a case report in which a patient developed cleft tongue and ulceration of the hard palate from an oral airway used in conjunction with an oral endotracheal tube.[48] Although this is an unusual complication, the case points to the need for constant awareness of the hazards and limitations of oral airways and the need for early recognition of problems. The oral cavity should be inspected at least daily. An airway size should be chosen that holds the tongue in its normal anatomical position. Care must be taken to avoid trapping the oral airway between teeth. The airway should be long enough to alleviate soft tissue obstruction by the posterior position of the tongue.

NASAL AIRWAY

Nasal airways, such as the straight red-rubber Reusch tube, are useful for short-term airway management when the oral route is inaccessible (Fig. 21-2). Such may be the case in the immediate management of lower facial and oral trauma or in the patient with an extremely sensitive gag reflex. These tubes extend through the nose into the hypopharynx. They are uncuffed; accordingly, ventilation through them will be achieved only if the mouth and the opposite nares are closed. If prolonged use for suctioning is necessary, as in some cases of mandibular fracture, the tubes should be rotated between the nares every 48 hours. Use of a water-soluble lubricant facilitates passage of these tubes. Effective nebulization therapy is not practical through nasal airways.

Some nasal airways do not have a well-enough structured phalange at the external nares to prevent aspiration of the airway. With these tubes, a large safety pin inserted off-center through the phlange end so that it does not obstruct the lumen solves the problem.

In our experience, nasal airways are most easily tolerated by patients when the airways are allowed to lie freely instead of being taped in place. Allowing the airway to move freely with swallowing seems to cause less patient discomfort and stimulation of the gag reflex.

ESOPHAGEAL AIRWAYS

Esophageal obturator airways (*see* Fig. 38-11) are modified endotracheal tubes designed to be inserted into the esophagus instead of the trachea. There is an inflatable cuff just proximal to the occluded distal end. When the cuff is inflated, the esophagus is obstructed under most normal conditions. Located in the upper third of the tube are 16 openings. The sum of the diameter of these openings exceeds the diameter of the tube itself. When in place, the openings are located in the posterior portion of the mouth and the upper portion of the pharynx. A self-sealing mask is used with the obturator to prevent air leakage from the mouth and nose. The mask can be removed when the patient resumes spontaneous respiration, but the obturator should be left in place until the patient reacts and is conscious enough to allow extubation with the appropriate safeguards. These airways should never be used in a conscious patient.

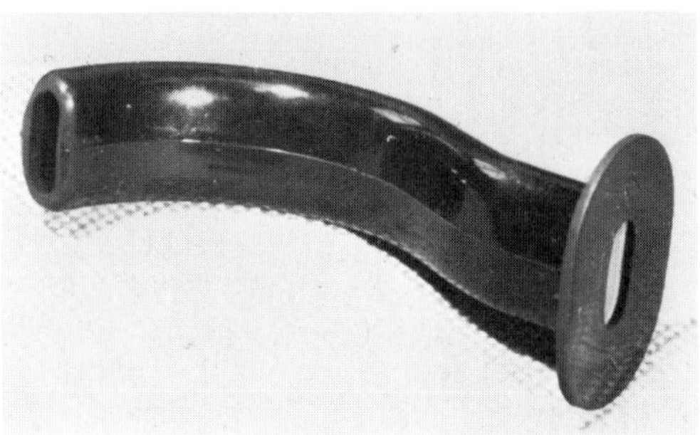

Fig. 21-1. S-shaped or Guedel oral airway.

The patient frequently vomits when the obturator is removed. The cuff should not be deflated until adequate suction is available to clear the airway. A modification of the original esophageal (obturator) airway (the esophageal gastric tube airway) allows for decompression of the stomach before removal of the airway.

Esophageal obturators are available in only one size for adults. The inflatable cuff (maximum volume 30 cc of air) always lies proximal to the carina and will not extend into the stomach even in short people.

Complications encountered with the use of esophageal obturators include inadvertent tracheal placement resulting in total airway obstruction and gastric distention, vomiting and aspiration on removal, rupture of the esophagus from overdistention of the cuff, and esophageal laceration from withdrawing the cuff without deflating it.

The attractions of esophageal obturator airways are their simplicity and the ease with which they can be inserted following only minimal training. An endotracheal tube can be inserted with an esophageal obturator in place. Since the level of skill required for endotracheal intubation is much greater than that for an esophageal intubation, these devices offer another option for obtaining a patent airway in a less controlled environment or whenever the level of skill necessary for endotracheal intubation is not readily available.[43,50]

Further indications for use of esophageal obturator airways, guidelines for their insertion and maintenance, and complications associated with their use are discussed in Chapter 38.

ORAL ENDOTRACHEAL TUBES

Most experts agree that oral endotracheal intubation is indicated during cardiopulmonary resuscitation. In most hands, oral intubation can be accomplished more rapidly than nasotracheal intubation because of better visualization of the vocal cords. Clearly there is less tissue destruction with oral or nasotracheal intubation than with performance of an emergency tra-

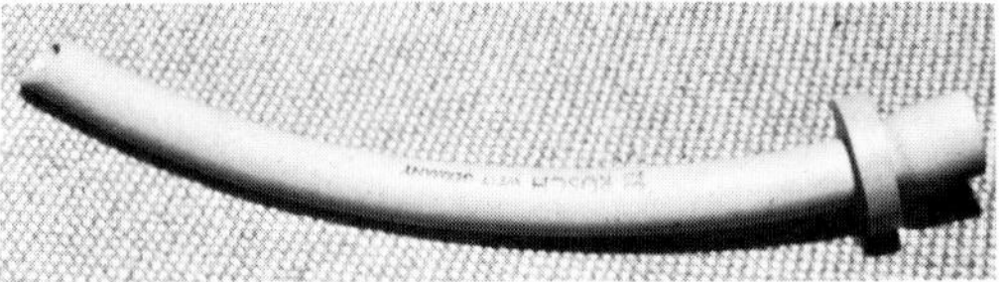

Fig. 21-2. A straight Reusch nasal airway.

cheotomy. If the first attempt at orotracheal intubation is unsuccessful, repeated attempts can be performed after appropriate intermittent periods of oxygenation.[53]

One of the primary objections to oral endotracheal intubation relates to activation of the gag reflex once the patient has regained consciousness. A further problem is the tendency of patients to bite down on the oral endotracheal tube, necessitating a bite block to keep the tube from being occluded. Equipment manufacturers are now aware of this problem, and endotracheal tube holders are available that incorporate bite blocks. Oral endotracheal tubes are less likely to kink than are longer nasotracheal tubes because of their lesser angle of curvature. They also have less resistance to airflow and to the passage of a suction catheter or fiberoptic bronchoscope. An oral tube is usually one size larger than a nasal tube used in the same patient.

The techniques of endotracheal intubation are discussed in Chapter 38. Nasotracheal intubation has an advantage over oral endotracheal intubation in that it can more easily be performed "blind," without directed visualization of the larynx, although some trauma to the nasal passages may occur, particularly if the procedure is done quickly.

Many practitioners believe that oral intubation requires high doses of sedatives in order for the patient to tolerate the endotracheal tube. In practice, this is not necessarily the case, especially if the patient has been given accurate, simple descriptions of his care. In actual practice, patients requiring prolonged ventilation with oral endotracheal tubes in place can often be managed without sedation, unless they have pain from another source.

Good oral hygiene is important in patients with any type of artificial airway. Oral hygiene procedures should be performed at least every 4 hours, with thorough inspection of the mouth and pharynx. Any signs of mucous membrane lesions should be reported to the physician immediately. Such lesions may reflect mechanical pressure (necrosis) or infection with *Candida* or herpes simplex. Utmost care must be given to either endotracheal or tracheostomy tubes so that as little torsion or traction as possible is transmitted to the tracheal mucosa.

The length of time oral intubation may be used remains debatable. Some practitioners believe that it must be terminated at 48 hours and a tracheotomy performed. Others continue oral intubation up to 5 or 6 *weeks*. These would seem to be the extremes. In clinical practice, the decision as to whether endotracheal intubation will be continued or tracheotomy performed is usually made around the fifth or sixth day of intubation. If the patient is recovering at a fairly rapid rate, he should probably be continued on an endotracheal tube to reduce the trauma, scarring, and possible complications of tracheotomy. If it is obvious on or before the sixth day that the patient will probably not recover for some time, then a tracheotomy should probably be performed.

No large prospective studies have assessed the relationship of complications to duration of intubation exceeding 3 weeks, and only three studies have been carried out over periods longer than 10 days.[13,14,47] There are little data to suggest that injury at the site of the cuff differs between endotracheal and tracheostomy tubes as a function of duration of use.

Stauffer and Silvestri suggest that "tracheotomy should not be performed routinely simply because an arbitrary number of days of intubation has elapsed." They suggest instead that the following four questions be answered based on factors relevant to each patient:

1. What is the estimated duration of need for the artificial airway?
2. How well is the patient tolerating endotracheal intubation?
3. Is it likely that care of the airway and the total patient will be improved by tracheotomy?
4. What is the likely morbidity, mortality, and expense of tracheotomy for this patient?[49]

NASOTRACHEAL TUBES

At times nasal intubation is preferable, such as when oral surgery is being performed or when fractures of the face are being set. The indications for nasal intubation are basically the same as those for orotracheal intubation, the prime one being to secure and to maintain a controllable airway.

Care of a nasal tube mandates compulsive care of the nares, since one of the major complications of this type of tube is necrosis of the nasal mucosa.[56] Since the tube is introduced blindly through the nares, kinking of the tube may occur but can easily be discovered by failure to pass a suction catheter through the tube into the tracheobronchial tree. Nasal endotracheal tubes are longer than oral tubes and do not allow the standard catheter to pass as deeply into the tracheobronchial tree for suctioning. These tubes are purportedly more comfortable and are preferred by many for long-term ventilation. On the other hand, in the case of the patient who has experienced facial trauma or with nasal pathology, it may be necessary to pass a small-diameter, high-resistance tube, which makes ventilation more difficult.

Laryngeal ulceration is half as common with nasal intubation as with oral intubation.[18] Also, self-extubation and endobronchial dislocation are less likely.[39]

TRACHEOSTOMY TUBES

The student is referred to standard surgical textbooks for techniques of tracheotomy. Preformed tracheostomy dressings should be used until most of the serosanguineous drainage has subsided. During this period, the dressings should be changed at least every 2 hours, and more frequently if they are saturated, since a moist dressing acts as a breeding ground for bacteria. The type of drainage from a recent tracheotomy should be noted. The incision should be carefully inspected each time the dressing is changed, and cleaning should be accomplished with hydrogen peroxide and sterile water. If signs of local infection are present, nitrofurazone (Furacin) ointment or gauze may be applied.

Many of the tracheostomy tubes used will have an inner and outer cannula as well as an obturator (Fig. 21-3). The inner cannula should optimally be removed every 2 to 4 hours for the first 24 hours, cleaned with a tracheostomy brush and hydrogen peroxide, and rinsed with sterile water. Another sterile tracheostomy tube of the same size should always be available at the patient's bedside.

Following tracheotomy, suctioning should be carried out frequently based on the volume and character of the patient's secretions. Physicians should be encouraged to write suctioning orders as p.r.n. orders. In this manner, the patient is not routinely suctioned every hour if it is not necessary, but he is suctioned as frequently as is necessary. Some patients, for example, may need almost constant suctioning initially (e.g., in fulminant pulmonary edema). On the other hand, unnecessary suctioning may lead to undue irritation of the tracheobronchial mucosa and actually cause extensive production of mucus. Suctioning techniques are discussed later in this chapter and in Appendix H.

Tracheostomy tubes should be changed regularly approximately every 7 days. This allows for total inspection of the tracheal stoma and the tube itself and allows the opportunity for judging adequacy of tube care and inspection for early signs of infection. Therapists and nurses should, if possible, be present when the tracheotomy is performed so that the anatomy of

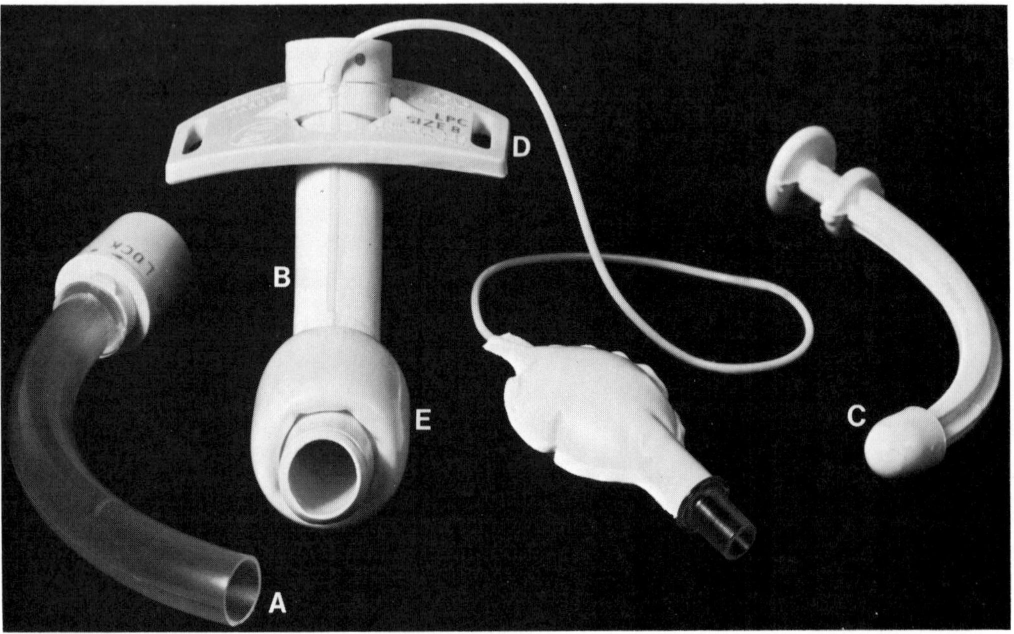

Fig. 21-3. A standard tracheostomy tube showing *(A)* inner cannula, *(B)* outer cannula. *(C)* obturator. *(D)* flange, and *(E)* cuff. (Reproduced with permission of Shiley Laboratories, Inc.)

the area is well known to them. Routine changing of tracheostomy tubes should be considered one of the duties of nurses or therapists once they have been properly taught how to perform the procedure. The first tube change should be performed by a physician, however, unless more than 7 days have elapsed since the tracheotomy.

With an artificial airway in place, the functions of the upper airway have been bypassed. Therefore, the body no longer has an entirely intact means of humidifying, filtering, or warming inspired air or of evacuating bronchial secretions. These functions must then be augmented by artificial means. Adequate humidification is of the utmost importance and is most often accomplished by the continuous use of a nebulizer of some type, propelled by oxygen or compressed air as the needs of the patient indicate.

Tracheostomy provides the best route for long-term airway maintenance and avoids the oral, nasal, pharyngeal, and laryngeal complications of endotracheal intubation. The tracheostomy tube is shorter, wider, and less curved than an endotracheal tube. There is minimal resistance to airflow and passage of suction catheters or endoscopes. Malnutrition presents less of a problem, and the patient may be able to communicate more easily.

However, tracheotomy has greater morbidity and mortality than does endotracheal intubation. The operation carries a high complication rate, particularly when performed on an emergency basis in suboptimal conditions. Complications tend to be more severe and numerous than do complications of intubation.[47] Severe complications may be life-threatening. Permanent scarring is unavoidable. Finally, a tracheostomy tube often lulls the staff into complacency about decannulation. Some tracheostomy tubes are left in place too long, perhaps as a security to the medical staff.[49]

SPECIAL-PURPOSE TRACHEOSTOMY TUBES

A tracheostomy *button* is an appliance used to maintain a tracheostomy stoma when there is some doubt as to the patient's ability to permanently maintain his airway without a tracheostomy tube (Figs. 21-4, 21-5, and 21-6) or during weaning from ventilatory support. The appliances are available in cannulated and uncannulated versions. The inner cannula is provided with a standard 15 mm universal adapter for IPPB treatments or hyperinflation with a manual resuscitator.

The tracheostomy button is short and occupies only the distance from the skin to the inside of the tracheal wall. Placing the inner cannula into the outer cannula causes the flanges on the outer cannula to open, holding the tube in place. The purpose of this appliance is to keep the tracheal stoma open for suctioning or, in emergencies, for ventilating the patient.

If ventilation is performed through this opening, the upper airway must be sealed, since the button is not cuffed and air will leak out through the mouth. As a replacement for the tracheostomy tube of a pa-

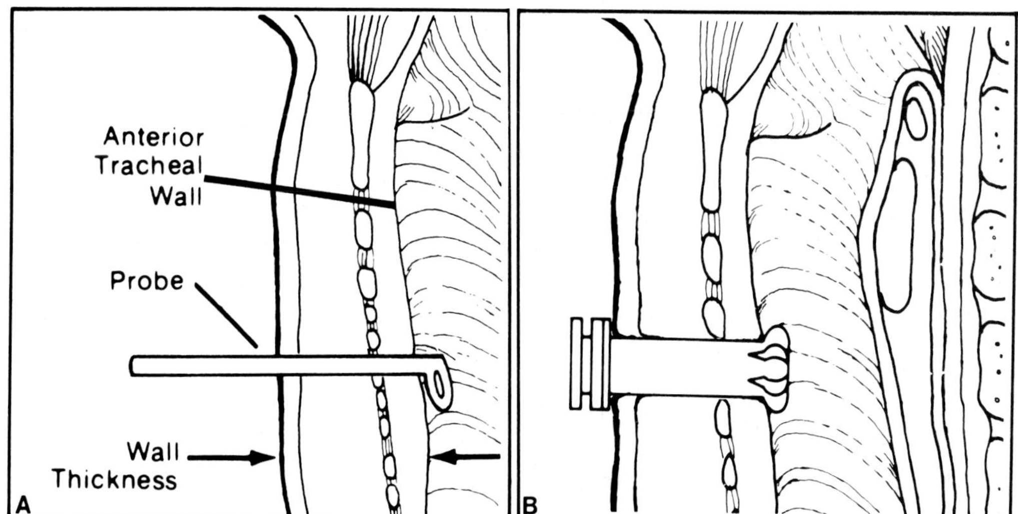

Fig. 21-4. A tracheostomy button. A probe is used to measure the length from the anterior tracheal surface to the skin of the neck. Spacers are used for length adjustment.

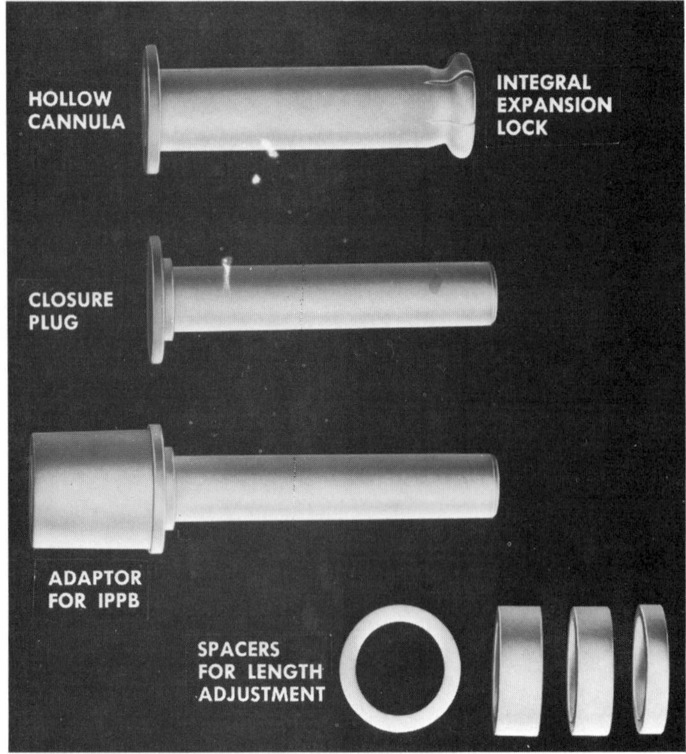

Fig. 21-5. Parts of the tracheostomy button.

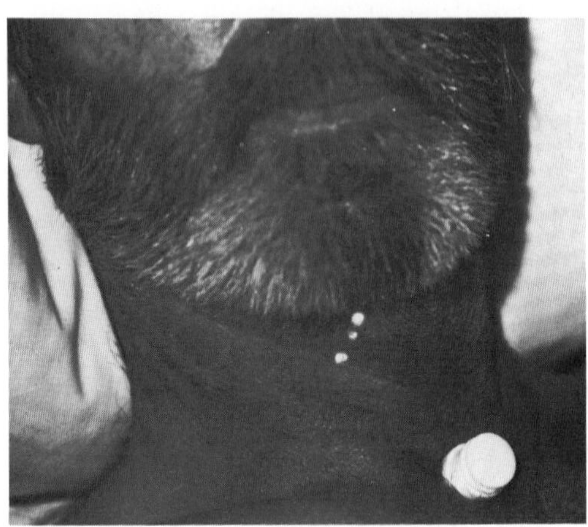

Fig. 21-6. The tracheostomy button in place.

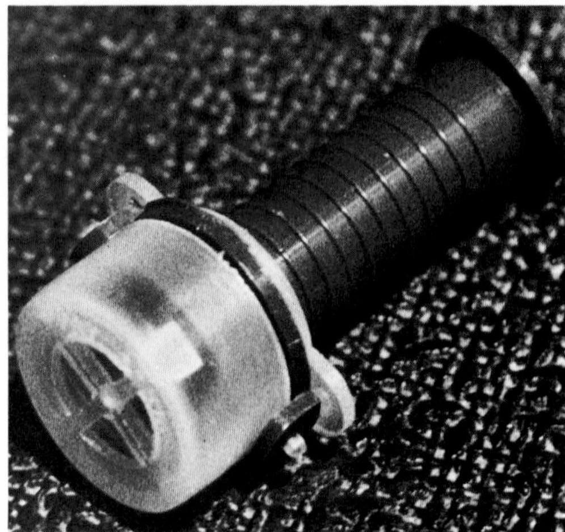

Fig. 21-7. Kistner plastic tracheostomy tube.

tient who has been extremely ventilator-dependent or in whom repeated suctioning is necessary, the tracheostomy button has found favor.

If standard tracheostomy tubes are left in place and plugged, even though the tube cuff is deflated or absent, airway resistance is still increased compared to normal, making it more difficult for the patient to expectorate secretions and also making phonation difficult. By removing the tracheostomy tube and preserving the stoma with a tracheostomy button, the patient can cough more readily, talk normally, and does not experience the increased resistance to breathing that a regular plugged tracheostomy tube provides.

Other devices have been designed to achieve the same ends. The Kistner plastic tracheostomy tube and the Olympic Trach-Talk are designed to reduce tracheobronchial inflammation and retention of secretions that collect in the lower respiratory tract. These one-way valves allow air to be taken in through the tube on inhalation (Figs. 21-7 and 21-8) but close on expiration, forcing the air out through the upper trachea. This allows the patient to build sufficient intrathoracic pressure to produce an effective cough. Kistner caps do not fit most standard tracheostomy tubes without adaptation; and the Trach-Talk has both 15-mm and 9-mm ends that insert into any tracheostomy tube or standard adapter.

Another such adaptation of the standard tracheostomy tube, which allows breathing through the upper respiratory tract and thus phonation and some humidification, is the fenestrated tracheostomy tube (*see* Chap. 25). One interesting innovation is the Gabriel Tucker sterling silver tracheostomy tube, which has a valve built into the inner tube that opens on inhalation, during which time the patient inhales through the tube. On exhalation, the valve leaflet closes, forcing air up through the trachea, nose, or mouth. All of these devices have their application in weaning patients from ventilator support. Trach-Talk devices and tracheostomy buttons have also been used in patients with recurrent aspiration and dysphagia.[31]

LARYNGECTOMY TUBES

A laryngectomy is a surgical procedure in which the larynx is removed and a permanent fistula between the skin and the trachea formed. A laryngectomy is usually performed for malignancy in or near the larynx. Such patients usually return from surgery with both jaw and neck bandaged and with a cuffed tracheostomy or a special, shorter laryngectomy tube in place. These tubes will ensure airway patency in the face of unusual postoperative swelling.

Despite preoperative instruction, it is not possible to prepare such patients totally for what they will experience postoperatively. Vocal silencing can be a tremendously emotional and traumatic procedure. Some patients, no matter how well informed, cannot accept the inability to speak or the appearance of the laryngectomy. Supportive care is clearly needed in such a situation. After the patient gains the equanimity to accept the laryngectomy, he usually learns how to care for himself very rapidly.

Patients are taught to cough using stimulation of cough receptors and dynamic chest compression. If

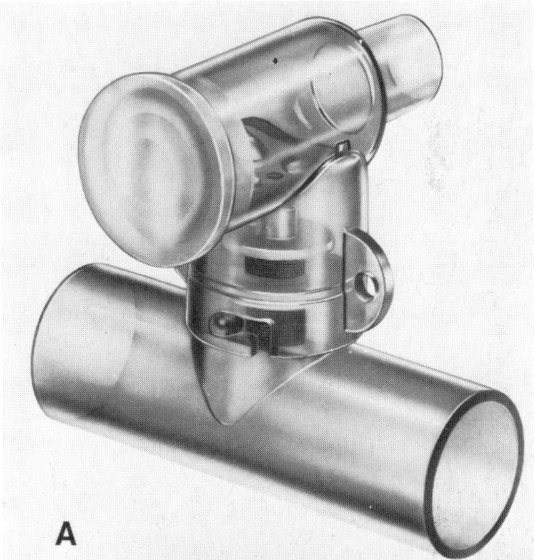

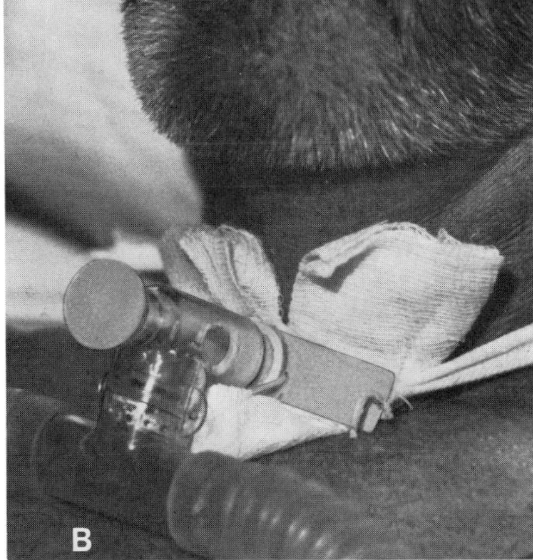

Fig. 21-8. An Olympic Trach-Talk.

suctioning is necessary, these patients can be provided with an Adams aspirator, a portable, inexpensive, and easy-to-clean device.

Proper postlaryngectomy humidification is critical. Since such patients have had their normal upper airway humidification mechanism bypassed, they will have to develop a *humidification membrane* in the area of the tracheal stoma. This humidification membrane is a poorly understood physiologic occurrence about which the following clinical observations have been made:

1. The tracheal epithelium goes through a minor metamorphosis, forming the humidification membrane, approximately 2 weeks to 2 months after laryngectomy.
2. Adequate humidification seems to be provided by the membrane except during hyperventilation.
3. Humidification membranes appear only to provide humidity and do not perform a particulate filtration function.

Laryngectomy patients are taught to watch for signs of infection, such as changes in secretion volume, color, or consistency. If the sputum becomes viscid, they are taught to intensify accessory humidification processes by humidification of inspired air or by increased oral fluid intake.

A number of ways of teaching laryngectomy patients vocal communication have been developed. A new device, the Blom–Singer Voice Prosthesis, is currently gaining attention. Since it does not have to be inserted at the time of surgery, it offers another option to patients who have been unsuccessful at learning other forms of speech.[26,45] A small tracheoesophageal fistula is created and a catheter inserted to act as a stent until the tract epithelializes (about 1–2 weeks). The catheter is removed and the prosthesis inserted into the fistula. The prosthesis is only about ½ cm across and has a small plastic tube with a slit on the distal end. The patient inhales, occludes the laryngectomy stoma, and forces air by intrathoracic pressure through the device, causing the leaves of the plastic tube to vibrate.[46,52,54] The sound produced does not sound like normal speech.

Despite the size range available, a tight fit of the appliance is sometimes a problem to maintain, and some cases of aspiration have been reported. Allergy to the adhesive that secures the device to the neck has also been reported. The prothesis is easily removed, but, because of its small size, some patients have difficulty reinserting it. Whether such devices should be used in tissue that has been irradiated is debatable.[38]

On the horizon for laryngectomy patients is a microelectronic device that attaches to the roof of the mouth and is activated by the tongue. The power comes from body heat, and, when available, the voice chip will produce a normal-sounding voice tone.[35,38]

INDICATIONS FOR USE OF ARTIFICIAL AIRWAYS

TRACHEAL INTUBATION

The indications for tracheal intubation include [1] failure of less complicated devices to maintain a patent airway or to achieve effective suctioning; [2] the need for long-term ventilation of the patient by means of a controlled airway; [3] repeated aspiration of gastric or oropharyngeal contents despite optimum management; and [4] trauma to the upper airway (e.g., tracheoesophageal fistula or following laryngeal surgery). Basically the indications for, and complications of, oral and nasal endotracheal tubes are common to both. Nasal intubation carries with it the additional hazard of fracture of the nasal turbinates or floor of the sinuses and blockage and infection of the nasal airway passages. With the exception of the specific circumstances cited, the choice of oral or nasal endotracheal tubes is largely a matter of personal preference and experience.

TRACHEOTOMY

Tracheotomy is indicated in situations where long-term respiratory support is necessary. If possible, tracheotomy should be considered an elective procedure done in an operating room under controlled conditions. Intubation should be accomplished before tracheotomy. According to Safar, fewer than 1% of those in need of tracheotomy cannot be intubated before the procedure.[41] Once tracheal intubation has been performed, the tracheotomy may be done more slowly and safely. Tracheotomy carries with it very definite surgical risks. Mortality from the procedure itself is estimated at about 3%. In one series, serious complications were estimated to occur in nearly 50% of cases.[30]

Tracheotomy is indicated in cases [1] where prolonged artificial ventilation is necessary; [2] when nasotracheal intubation or orotracheal intubation does not allow effective suctioning of secretions; [3] to bypass obstruction of the upper airway when it cannot be managed from above; and [4] as a prophylactic measure during radiation therapy of the larynx. An incidental benefit of tracheotomy is a significant reduction in anatomical dead space; thus the work of breathing is modestly diminished, at least temporarily.

COMPLICATIONS OF ARTIFICIAL AIRWAYS

Complications that occur with either *oral* or *nasal endotracheal intubation* (Table 21-1) include [1] inadvertent placement of the tube into the right mainstem bronchus or esophagus; [2] fracture of teeth during intubation; [3] positioning of the distal tube orifice against the carina or tracheal wall, causing partial or total airway obstruction; and [4] tissue damage to the oropharynx and upper airway, including the vocal cords.

Long-term complications that may occur are those secondary to the tube and its mouthpiece. These involve [1] damage to one or both of the vocal cords; [2] laryngeal or tracheal edema; [3] mucosal damage resulting in tracheal stenosis; and [4] occlusion of the tube with inspissated secretions, since thorough cleaning of endotracheal tubes is impossible without removing and replacing them. Frequently, the mucosal damage and necrosis are due to poor cuff handling techniques (*see* below). If tracheal stenosis significantly affects the patient's ability to breathe, tracheal dilatation or reconstructive surgery may ultimately be necessary.

Patients requiring endotracheal intubation should have a portable AP chest roentgenogram taken immediately after intubation and at serial intervals thereafter to check for tube placement. Care should be taken to ensure that the patient's head is in the same position during each X-ray so that no false impression of tube placement is imparted.

Tracheotomy carries with it many of the complications common to both oral and nasal intubation (Table 21-2). A dry, hoarse, hacking cough and blood-streaked mucus when the tracheostomy tube is manipulated and suctioned may indicate *tracheitis* and perhaps impending tracheal erosion. *Bleeding* is not an uncommon complication, with an incidence of 0.5% to 1%. The tracheostomy site, often near the thyroid gland, is very vascular. Hyperemia in the area of the stoma is frequently present because of mechanical and perhaps infectious factors. Major systemic vessels lie nearby. All bleeding sites should be carefully attended to at the time they are recognized. Bleeding may occur at any time during the course of tracheotomized patients and represents a life-threatening emergency. A pulsating tracheostomy tube may be a sign of impending exsanguination.[27]

Subcutaneous emphysema occurs when air escapes from the tracheal incision into the tissues, dissects up and under the skin, and accumulates around the face, neck, and thorax. Subcutaneous emphysema may occur immediately after tracheotomy, or later, particularly if the tracheostomy tube used is too short. The patients's face, neck, or supraclavicular area may appear puffy, and slight finger pressure will allow one to feel a crackling sensation (crepitation) under the skin when air is present.

Subcutaneous and mediastinal emphysema may be associated with pneumothorax. The etiology of these conditions is not entirely clear since they may occur with any form of mechanical ventilation, even if a tracheotomy has not been performed. In this instance, dissection of air probably occurs around peribronchial and perivascular planes into the mediastinum and then into the soft tissues of the neck and thorax. These complications usually are not life-threatening.

Pneumothorax is also a complication of tracheotomy, directly or indirectly related to the surgical procedure itself. This complication occurs in struggling, dyspneic patients or in ones who have serverely overexpanded lungs. The presence of a pneumothorax can be recognized by an abrupt decrease in the intensity of, or lack of, breath sounds. An even greater threat to the patient is the development of increased intrapleural pressure (tension pneumothorax), with a shift of the mediastinum and reduced cardiac output.

Two types of cardiovascular collapse have been described with tracheotomy:

1. Immediate-onset cardiac arrest is usually encountered during the process of an emergency tracheotomy under less than optimal conditions. It was originally believed that this was a vagal response, and the true cause—severe and profound hypoxia—was overlooked. Because tracheotomies are becoming more and more elective procedures, this complication tends to occur less frequently.
2. Delayed-onset cardiac arrest, occurring after a good airway has been established, has been attributed to a sudden reduction in Pa_{CO_2} *below* the patient's usual value, with resultant respiratory alkalemia, arrhythmias, and hypotension. However, this entity is poorly described, and the mechanism of occurrence is still only presumed.[22] Both of these types of cardiovascular collapse tend to speak in favor of endotracheal intubation and controlled ventilation before tracheotomy.

Table 21-1. Selected Complications of Endotracheal Intubation

COMPLICATIONS DURING TUBE PLACEMENT

Patient discomfort
Dental accidents
Facial trauma
Nasal/oral soft-tissue injuries (hemorrhage, laceration, edema)
Pharyngeal soft-tissue injuries (hematoma, perforation, laceration)
Retropharyngeal/hypopharyngeal perforation
Esophageal intubation
Laryngeal trauma
Laryngospasm
Intubation of the right main-stem bronchus
Bronchospasm
Pulmonary aspiration
Barotrauma
Cardiac/respiratory arrest
Cardiac arrhythmias
Hypoxemia
Cervical spine and cord injuries

COMPLICATIONS WHILE TUBE IS IN PLACE

Patient discomfort (pain, retching, salivation, difficulty in communicating)
Malnutrition
Nasal/oral soft-tissue injury (mucosal ulceration, infection, edema, hemorrhage)
Lip ulceration
Sinusitis
Otitis media
Laryngeal injury (ulceration, edema, inflammation, submucosal hemorrhage)
Laryngeal muscle dysfunction
Subglottic edema
Pneumonia
Pulmonary aspiration
Mechanical problems with the tube (kinking, obstruction, disconnection from ventilator, biting the tube, difficulty in suctioning secretions, and so forth)
Mechanical problems with the cuff (cuff laceration, cuff leak, herniation over tube tip, compression of the shaft of the tube, excessive pressure)
Tracheal injury (ulceration, inflammation, submucosal hemorrhage, tracheomalacia, cartilage and mucosal necrosis)
Laryngeal/tracheal web formation
Laryngeal/tracheal granuloma
Tracheal dilatation
Irritation of the carina
Tracheoesophageal fistula
Spontaneous dislocation of the tube (into right mainstem bronchus, too high in trachea, self-extubation)
Atelectasis
Reduction in mucociliary transport
Squamous metaplasia of respiratory epithelium
Ineffective cough

COMPLICATIONS DURING EXTUBATION

Patient discomfort (hoarseness, sore throat, dysphagia)
Upper-airway obstruction (laryngospasm, laryngeal edema, and so forth)
Bronchospasm
Aspiration
Glottic injury
Cardiac arrest

COMPLICATIONS AFTER EXTUBATION

Nasal stricture
Dysphagia
Laryngeal/tracheal granuloma
Laryngeal stenosis (glottic, subglottic)
Laryngeal motor dysfunction (vocal cord paralysis)
Crico-arytenoid ankylosis
Laryngeal/tracheal web
Laryngeal chondritis, perichondritis
Tracheal stenosis
Tracheomalacia
Tracheal dilatation

(Reprinted with permission from Stauffer JL, Silvestri RC: Complications of endotracheal intubation, tracheostomy, and artificial airways. Respir Care 27:417, 1982)

Table 21-2. Selected Complications of Tracheostomy

COMPLICATIONS DURING THE OPERATION	
Hemorrhage	Pneumothorax
Thyroid injury	Placement of the tube in pretracheal space
Tracheostomy too low or too high	Tracheoesophageal fistula
Injury to recurrent laryngeal nerve	Cuff laceration during tube placement
Subcutaneous emphysema	Cardiac arrest
Mediastinal emphysema	
COMPLICATIONS WHILE TRACHEOSTOMY TUBE IS IN PLACE	
Patient discomfort	Pseudomembrane formation
Infection of wound	Irritation of the carina
Infection of trachea	Tracheoesophageal fistula
Hemorrhage (mild: skin vessel; major: tracheoarterial fistula)	Mediastinitis
	Sepsis
Tracheal injury (inflammation, submucosal hemorrhage, ulceration, cartilage and mucosal necrosis)	Atelectasis
	Pneumonia
	Pulmonary aspiration
Tracheal dilatation	Subcutaneous emphysema
Tracheal granuloma	Mediastinal emphysema
Tracheal web formation	Pneumothorax
Tracheal perforation	Self-decannulation
Mechanical problems with the tube (obstruction, disconnection from ventilator, difficulty in suctioning secretions, and so forth)	Reduction in mucociliary transport
	Squamous metaplasia of respiratory epithelium
	Ineffective cough
Mechanical problems with the cuff (same as for endotracheal intubation)	
COMPLICATIONS DURING DECANNULATION	
Difficult decannulation (tight stoma)	Patient discomfort
COMPLICATIONS AFTER DECANNULATION	
Scar	Tracheomalacia
Keloid	Tracheal granuloma
Persistent open stoma	Tracheal web formation
Dysphagia	Tracheal dilatation
Tracheal stenosis	

(Reprinted with permission from Stauffer JL, Silvestri RC: Complications of endotracheal intubation, tracheostomy, and artificial airways. Respir Care 27:417, 1982)

The most common early complication of *laryngectomy* during the postoperative period is tracheoesophageal fistula, which occurs in about 10% of cases. Such fistulas usually will heal spontaneously. If a fistula develops, the patients are always fed in the extreme upright position. A nasogastric tube is left in place, instead of being removed and reinserted again at the time of each feeding. Patients are taught either to cough vigorously or to suction themselves after feeding to be sure that they have not aspirated. Tracheoesophageal fistula usually is a self-limiting complication that need not cause the patient any additional embarrassment or discomfort. Patients generally do well when they are fully prepared before they are sent home and are seen regularly thereafter by their physician.

Malignancy may recur after laryngectomy. In this situation, patients usually are given a second course of radiation therapy to the site of involvement. The decision as to whether further surgery is indicated is made by the physician, the patient, and his family. Should malignancy occur on the contralateral side, the outlook for the patient is bleak.

COMPOSITION OF ARTIFICIAL AIRWAYS

HISTORY

In the 16th century, Paracelsus attached a fireplace bellows to a tube placed in a patient's mouth to assist ventilation. Vesalius, in 1542, and Robert Hook, in 1667, were both experimenting with endotracheal intubation in animals. Reports of such activities continued through the 17th and 18th centuries, and, in 1880, Macewen described for the first time the successful use of endotracheal intubation in two patients for periods up to 36 hours.

By 1946, special tubes for special purposes were being described, particularly for persons suffering from facial injuries. There was, however, considerable hesitancy regarding the use of these tubes for prolonged intubation because of earlier reports of pressure necrosis, which was attributed to uncuffed endotracheal tubes. In 1950, the first case of prolonged respiratory support via endotracheal tube was reported by Briggs.[7] The patient died on the 42nd day, and autopsy showed ulcerations over each arytenoid and in two small areas of the trachea. It was thought that the ulcerations were of minor consequence and would have healed promptly had the patient lived.

Endotracheal and tracheostomy tubes were in the process of rapid evolution. The first tracheostomy tube was made of silver, as is the Jackson tracheostomy tube today. Early endotracheal tubes were made of natural rubber. After processing, rubber is generally impermeable to a number of vapors (mostly gases) and to water. However, rubber is affected by solvents such as oil, aromatic hydrocarbons, chloroform, ether, and carbon tetrachloride. Many of these substances are used as anesthetic agents and cause the rubber endotracheal tube to soften or dissolve partially in use.[24]

"Natural" rubber is not a pure chemical entity; the way it is collected, handled, and dried makes it an impure product. Even as synthetic rubberlike materials were discovered and cuffed tubes came into use, it was found that many of the additives of synthetic rubber leached into the trachea and produced damage.

Even more profound effects resulted from the cuff that was applied to early tubes. The cuff was made of natural latex and was often more toxic than the tube itself. The early cuffs were of low compliance, requiring high inflation pressures. Little was known at that time about the effects of cuff pressure on the tracheal submucosal circulation.

Investigators studying tubes made of various materials concluded that some form of standardization and testing needed to be developed. Since there was no agency available to monitor such matters, most manufacturers voluntarily agreed to have their products meet the requirements of what was then called the U.S.A. Standards Institute, Committee Z-79. The Z-79 Committee is still in operation today; however, it now operates under the American National Standards Institute (see below).

METAL TUBES

Although metal tracheostomy tubes (often silver or silver-plated), were used initially and continue to be manufactured today, there were many objections to hard, rigid tubes. Some of the objections involved [1] pressure necrosis; [2] stimulation of mucus production attributed to the metal; [3] patient discomfort; and [4] local tissue irritation, probably caused by the oxidation that takes place when sterling silver is exposed to air or the questionable irritant effects of silver polishes.

There are clinical situations where a metal tube may still be the tube of choice for an individual patient. Many laryngectomy tubes are made of metal and usually are comprised of three pieces: an outer cannula, an inner cannula, and an obturator. Laryngectomy tubes are much shorter than normal tracheostomy tubes because the distance from the skin to the trachea is small. Use of such a tube allows the patient to remove the inner cannula, clean it, and replace it without difficulty.

Metal tracheostomy tubes of several designs are still manufactured. Mostly three-piece tubes, the main differences between them are the angle at the flange and the presence or absence of a factory-applied 15-mm adapter as a permanent part of the inner cannula. In general, all metal tubes are being used less and less frequently because of the disadvantages mentioned above.

POLYVINYL CHLORIDE (PVC) TUBES

PVC is the material most commonly used for endotracheal tubes. Standards for the composition of plastics used in medical practice have been established by the

Z-79 Committee. PVC is not necessarily the same compound from manufacturer to manufacturer: PVC is an accepted generic term that has never been well defined. Pure PVC resin is hard, brittle, inflexible, and translucent. PVC in commercial use is a combination of a PVC resin and chemical agents that are added to increase the flexibility (plasticizers) and stability (stabilizers) of the plastic. Both heat and pressure are used to form the final device. PVC itself tends to degrade thermally, resulting in yellowing or darkening of the material. Chemical stabilizers have been added to retard these processes, some of which are toxic in themselves. Ethylene oxide, commonly used in sterilization of such tubes if they are to be reused (see below), degasses from PVC very slowly, particularly if the tubes are wrapped in materials such as polyethylene (Fig. 21-9).

SILASTIC (SILICONE RUBBER) TUBES

Silastic tubes seem to be gaining popularity. They have been used in pediatrics for several years but are now being used increasingly in adults because of their relatively low tissue toxicity. Silastic tubes are opaque and very flexible, which sometimes interferes with easy insertion unless the design is modified or an obturator is used. At present, there are few manufacturers of silastic tubes, and those tubes that are manufactured have a limited size range. Only a few silastic tubes are available with cuffs.

NYLON TUBES

Nylon is a generic term for a material developed by the DuPont Company. According to their own admission, the composition of tubes made of nylon can vary widely. Nylon tubes are rigid and usually of three-piece design. The tubes are light-weight and easy to clean and change; the inner cannula is removable. Patients find them more comfortable than metal tubes; they are nontoxic to tissues and can be steam autoclaved.

TEFLON TUBES

Teflon is the trade name of another class of plastic materials also developed by the DuPont Company. This plastic can be boiled, steam autoclaved, or

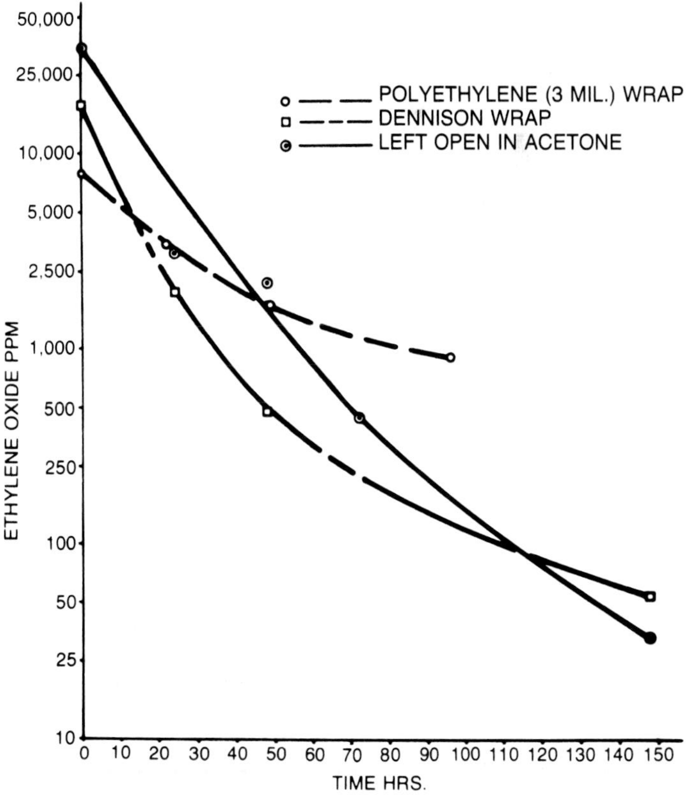

Fig. 21-9. Ethylene oxide degassing of PVC endotracheal tubes.

cleaned with an antiseptic solution without significant change in its properties. It does evoke a very minimal tissue reaction that has been attributed to the rigidity of the plastic. Because it is hard and rigid, Teflon has found little use as a tracheostomy tube material, but it is used in the form of tracheostomy buttons (e.g., the Olympic tracheostomy button).

CRITERIA FOR SELECTION OF TUBES (TUBE VARIABLES)

Clearly, tube selection must meet the needs of the patient. Just as the type of therapy performed on a patient should be specifically indicated, so the type of artificial airway chosen should reflect the patient's anatomic and physiologic requirements. For example, one would be unrealistic to think that the same tube could satisfy the needs of a patient with a laryngectomy, a patient with an elective tracheostomy receiving radiation therapy, and a patient needing long-term controlled mechanical ventilation with a cuffed tube. One type of tracheostomy tube could not meet the needs of all three patients. This section will discuss the variables necessary for intelligent tube selection in the individual patient.

THE CUFF

Cuff specifications and performance characteristics are critical. Despite many studies showing that high-pressure, low-compliance cuffs are deleterious to the patient, little has been written to help the therapist recognize the difference between a high-volume, low-pressure cuff and a low-volume, high-pressure cuff.

High-pressure (low-compliance) cuffs exert considerable lateral wall pressure on the tracheal mucosa with resultant necrosis, stricture, or formation of tracheoesophageal fistulas. Cuffs were being made from many materials that all had the same fault in common: when inflated they were narrow, spherical structures that had a very limited contact area with the trachea. Because the contact area was so small, very high pressures were transmitted against the tracheal wall by the cuff, not only interfering with the natural contour of the trachea, but also interrupting its blood supply. Not until 1969 did Geffin and Pontoppidan describe the now commonly used "prestretched" cuffs.[21] They described warming tubes with polyvinyl chloride cuffs, overinflating the warmed cuff, leaving the cuff inflated, removing it from the warm water, and allowing it to cool before it was deflated. This seemed to alter permanently the structure of the cuff, allowing it to inflate, and remain inflated, at relatively low pressures. This finally led to the design of the currently used low-pressure, high-compliance cuffs, which produce considerably less tracheal wall damage.

Essentially what had occurred was a change of cuff *shape* from spherical to sausagelike. This allowed the pressure to be transferred to the trachea over a wider area, resulting in lower tracheal lateral wall pressure at any one point. Inside the trachea, prestretched cuffs attempt to conform to the normal anatomical shape of the trachea, instead of trying to reform the trachea to match the outside diameter of the cuff.

Fig. 21-10 shows the current theory of how high intracuff pressure results in tracheal injury.[49] The high compliance of soft cuffs allows transmission of a relatively high fraction of total intracuff pressure across the cuff to the lateral tracheal wall. But because of their high volume, soft cuffs seal the airway with intracuff pressures of only 15% to 30% of those required by hard cuffs. Despite the greater transmission of pressure, the soft cuff's much lower intracuff pressure results in less lateral tracheal wall pressure than does that produced by hard cuffs.[10,16,32] This benefit of soft cuffs is lost if the cuff is overinflated. Only a few milliliters of air above minimal occluding volume may cause intracuff pressures to rise into the range seen with hard cuffs.[9,10] Some prediction of serious tracheal damage may be made by a cuff-diameter/tracheal-diameter ratio above 1.5/1.0 on serial radiographs during the period of intubation.[29]

Both the composition and design of the cuff need to be discussed. Many modern tubes and their cuffs claim to have low-pressure characteristics, when in fact they do not. Such misrepresentation makes it even more critical for the purchaser and the user to know how to tell the difference. For instance, should the cuff expand asymmetrically, no matter how pliable (compliant) the material from which it is made, there would be an area exerting high presure against the tracheal mucosa, resulting in possible tracheal wall damage. Inspection of the cuff material will give some indication of its compliance characteristics, but close inspection of the manufacturer's literature is usually the best way to obtain the needed information.

Although other factors such as esophageal contractions and turbulence of air flow in the tracheal tube itself may affect tracheal lateral wall pressures to a minor extent, clearly the cuff inflation pressures and the characteristics of the cuff itself are the most critical. Even with low-compliance cuffs, some pressure must be applied to the trachea before the cuff on the tube reaches "seal." If, in addition, the cuff stretches asymmetrically, this seal pressure is distributed to the tracheal wall unevenly, causing even greater damage. These factors would seem to explain the damage to the mucosa that occurs even when the cuff does not totally seal the space between the tube and the trachea.

All available evidence indicates that intracuff pressure at seal in highly compliant cuffs is a reasonable guide to the pressure applied to the tracheal wall and that if it approximates zero, the risk of arterial compression and ischemic necrosis is essentially eliminated (Figs. 21-11 and 21-12).[19] Although occlusion pressures that preclude adequate submucosal circulation have been said to be in the range of 25 to 35 mm Hg, the exact critical pressure in any given patient may vary widely. It is safe to say that the less sidewall pressure the better and that if a seal can be obtained with pressure outside the cuff as low as is absolutely necessary, the better it will be for the patient. Clearly, in patients with poorly compliant or highly resistant lungs, higher seal pressures will be necessary to prevent back-flow of air around the tracheal tube.

Several newer tubes use cuffs that are either major modifications of existing principles or entirely new operational principles designed to minimize the pressure exerted on the tracheal mucosa. As with all pieces of equipment, it is particularly important that the therapist understand the operational principles of these cuffs and any hazards that they may hold for the patient. This information is readily available on the packaging material or in informational material available from the manufacturer. Two examples of the evolution in low-pressure cuff design are the Shiley PRV and Kamen–Wilkenson Fome-Cuff tubes.

The Shiley PRV tube has a pressure relief valve incorporated with a thin-wall compliant cuff design. This valve is designed to prevent intracuff pressures in excess of 25 mm Hg. During cuff inflation, any volume of air injected into the cuff that creates a pressure above 25 mm Hg is vented to atmosphere. Once the syringe has been removed from the valve, the relief valve is closed (*i.e.*, if a change in tube position or tracheal diameter occurs that causes cuff pressure to rise, the valve will not vent this excess pressure to atmosphere).

The Fome-Cuff is a self-inflating unit that generates zero intracuff pressure. The cuff is designed with a foam material inside the cuff so that it is always expanded. To insert the tube, one must evacuate all the air from the cuff. Once the tube has been inserted, the pilot tube is opened to atmosphere to allow the foam to reexpand. When the cuff has expanded itself, the pilot tube is left open to atmosphere and will cor-

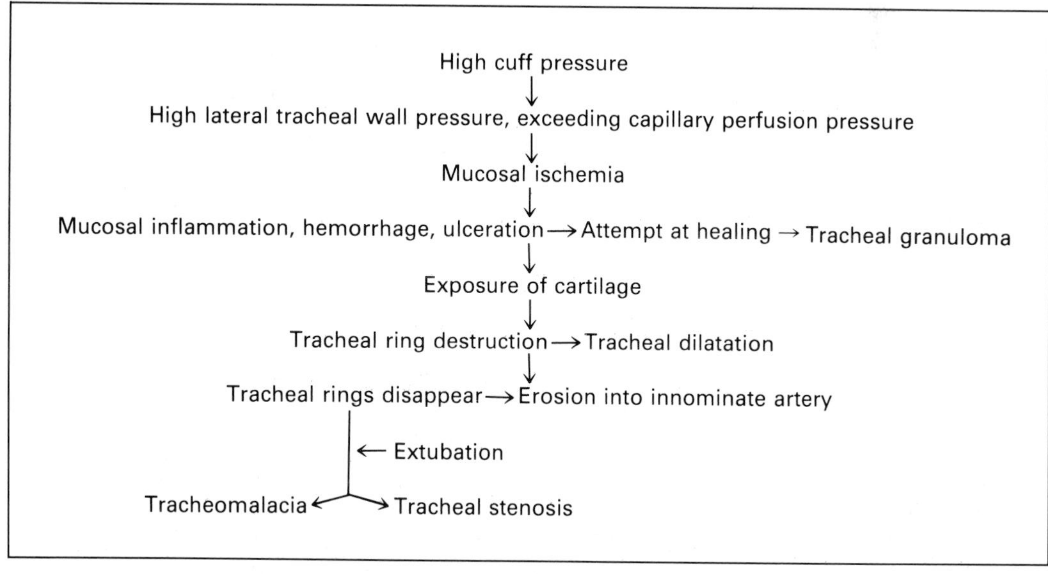

Fig. 21-10. Current theory of cuff-pressure-induced tracheal injury. (Reprinted with permission from Stauffer JL, Silvestri RC: Complications of endotracheal intubation, tracheostomy, and artificial airways. Respir Care 27:417, 1982)

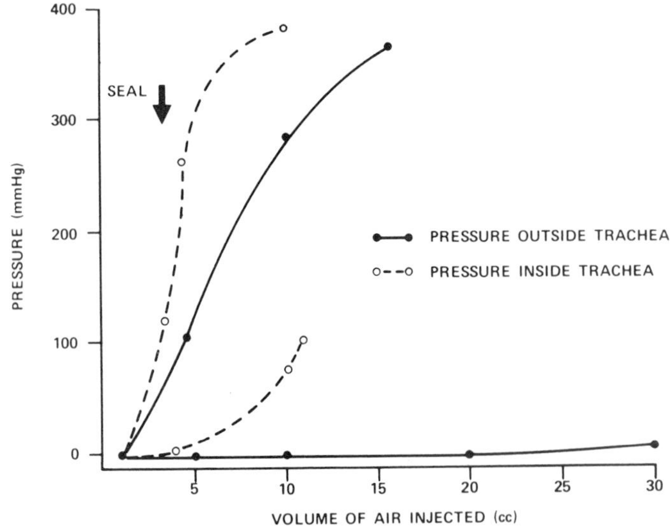

Fig. 21-11. Pressure-volume curves of low-compliance cuff (two curves to left) and high-compliance cuff (two curves to right) before and after placement in trachea. Seal = volume at which there was no leak when 40 cm H_2O pressure was applied to tracheostomy tube. (Dunn CR, Dunn DL, Moser KM: Determinants of tracheal injury by cuffed tracheostomy tubes. Chest *65*:128, 1974)

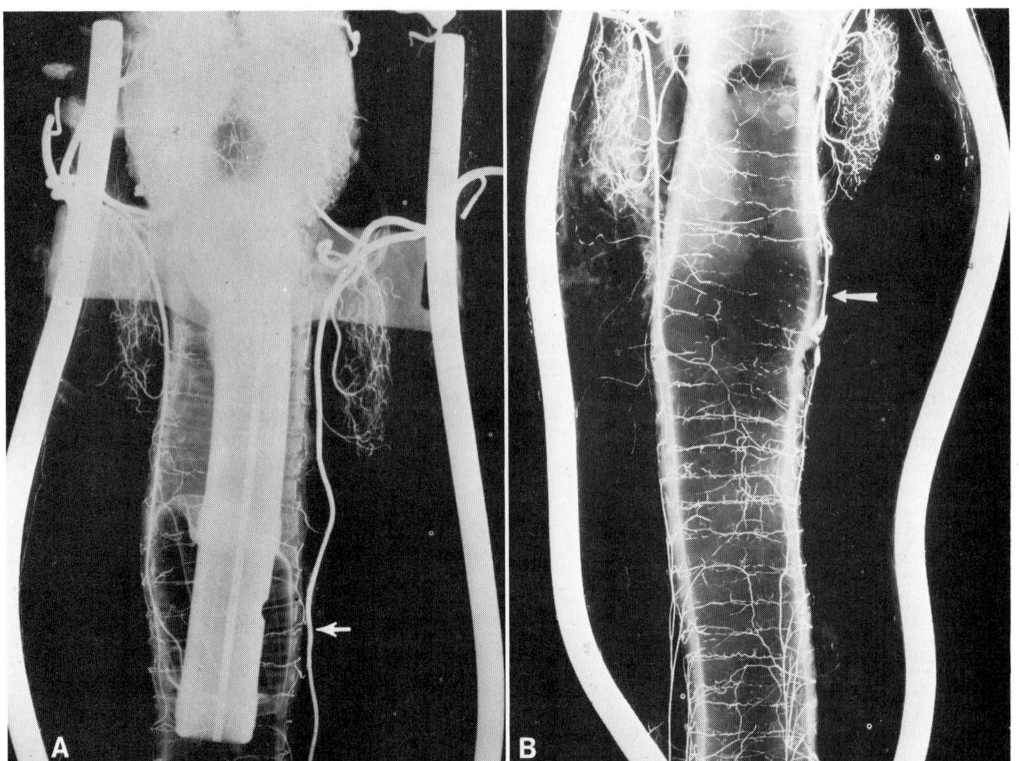

Fig. 21-12. *A*. Tracheal arteries in a dog with a prestretched cuff (pressure outside cuff essentially zero). Arterial vessels appear intact *(arrow)*. *B*. Roentgenogram of tracheal arteries injected with silicone rubber-tantalum after removal of a nonprestretched cuff *(arrow)* that had been inflated for 18 hours (pressure > 100 mm Hg). (Dunn CR, Dunn DL, Moser KM: Determinants of tracheal injury by cuffed tracheostomy tubes. Chest *65*:128, 1974)

rect its internal volume if the tube position or tracheal diameter changes. This tube, like any other, requires proper sizing to function properly. If air is inserted into this cuff, it takes on the same characteristics and problems of other air-filled cuffs.

Another evolution in low-pressure cuff design is incorporated in the "Lanz" tube. Its contribution is in the form of a pressure-regulating valve and external pilot balloon reservoir. This system allows air to be injected into the external balloon; the distal cuff then self-fills simultaneously, owing to equalization of the pressure (Fig. 21-13). (Once the syringe has been removed and the valve closed, pressure in the distal cuff can rise because the flow of air becomes one way from the external balloon. It is not possible to measure cuff pressure accurately with this tube unless the valve is kept unseated continuously. This can be done by inserting a stopcock, turned to the off position, into the pressure regulating valve.)

TUBE CONFIGURATION AND STANDARDIZATION

In the early 1970s, it became apparent to many workers in the field that standardization of health devices and appliances was a real necessity. Accordingly, in 1972, a committee of the American National Standards Institute, Inc. (ANSI) was convened under the auspices of the American Society of Anesthesiologists. The purpose of this committee was to draw up standards for endotracheal tubes and cuffs. These standards are discussed below in some detail.

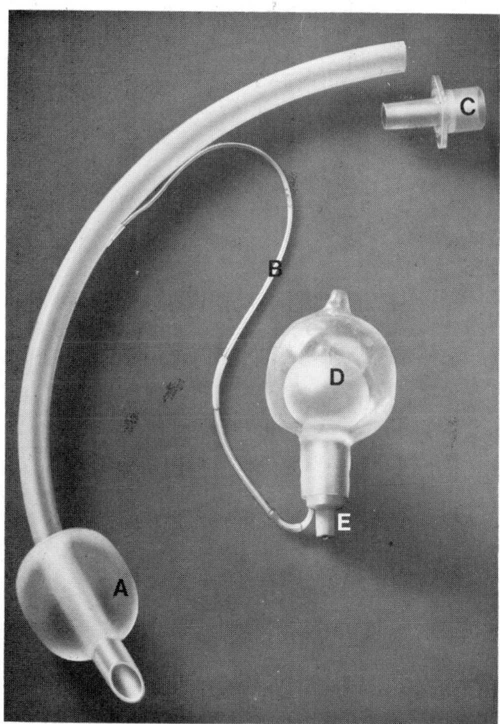

Fig. 21-13. Lanz endotracheal tube: *(A)* tracheal cuff, *(B)* pilot line, *(C)* 15 mm adaptor, *(D)* pilot balloon reservoir. *(E)* pressure-regulating valve.

The existence of these standards does not prohibit the manufacture, marketing, or use of products not conforming to ANSI standards. The standards are subject to periodic review and updating. The Z-79 Committee was specifically entrusted with the development of these standards for tracheal tubes and cuffs. The reader is referred to the entire standard report for details of standardization procedures for tracheal tubes and cuffs. Only the more important regulations will be mentioned here.

The definitions of various portions of endotracheal tubes (Fig. 21-14) are as follows:

1. *Bevel:* the slanted end of the tracheal tube.
2. *Inflating tube:* the tube provided for inflating the tracheal tube cuff.
3. *Machine or proximal end:* the end of the tracheal tube, which is intended to project from the patient.
4. *Patient or distal end:* the end of the tracheal tube, usually beveled, which is intended to be inserted into the patient's trachea.
5. *Pilot balloon:* a small balloon that may be fitted to the inflating tube to indicate inflation of the tracheal cuff.
6. *Tracheal tube cuff:* the inflatable sleeve that may be applied to the patient end of a tracheal tube to provide an effective, leak-resistant fit between the tube and the trachea.

The dimensions and tolerances of tracheal tubes are important and should be understood by all therapists. The metric system is the system of measurement used. The internal diameter (ID) of the tube is marked on the outside of each tube. The length of each tube bears a definite relationship to its internal diameter (Table 21-3).

Both oral and nasal tracheal tubes have a radius of curvature of 14 cm ± 10% according to the Z-79 standard. Oral tubes have a bevel at the distal end of 45° in relation to their long axis, and nasal tubes have a bevel angle of about 30°, except for tubes less than 6 mm in diameter, which have a bevel angle of about 45°. Oral-endotracheal tubes have the bevel opening facing the left when the tube is viewed from the concave aspect, but nasal tubes may have the bevel facing in either direction. Package labeling usually describes which type of tube is in hand.

The Z-79 Committee also has standards for cuff dimensions and performance characteristics. The maximum length of the cemented end of cuffs should not be more than 10 mm. The cuff length itself ranges from 20 mm ± 10% in a 5.0-mm ID tube to 40 mm ± 10% in an 11.0-mm tube. Recommended sizes for endotracheal tubes and suction catheters for various age groups are found in Table 21-4. Another standard of importance is the length of the tube distal to the cemented end of the cuff, which should be less than 13 mm, except in tubes smaller than 5 mm in diameter, where it should be between 5 and 6 mm.

The Z-79 Committee requires that the packaging of endotracheal tubes include the ID size printed in large type near the lower right front corner of the package. Packaging should also describe the suggested method of sterilization (unless resterilization is prohibited by the manufacturer), and the tube itself should be marked with the word "oral" or "nasal." For tubes smaller than 6.0 mm ID, the actual outside diameter (OD) in millimeters should also be shown.

Both the tubes and cuffs should be made of nontoxic materials that meet the rigid specifications of the Z-79 Committee. They should maintain their required curved shape when not in use and be relatively resistant to agents used in chemical cleansing and sterilizing. They should resist deterioration when autoclaved, if the tubes are intended for reuse.

Implant testing (IT) is a method of laboratory evaluation to ensure that tissue toxicity does not occur with the given product. Two methods of materials testing have been found to be sensitive, simple, and inexpensive. The first method, and that accepted by the Z-79 Committee, is rabbit muscle implantation. Small slivers of the material to be tested are placed into the beveled end of a 15-gauge needle and implanted percutaneously into the paravertebral muscle of anesthetized rabbits. After several pieces of material to be tested have been implanted, a known toxic plastic is implanted in two additional sites, and a known nontoxic control in two other sites. Seven days later, the animal is sacrificed, and the sites of implantation are examined both grossly and microscopically by a pathologist certified by a national certifying body. If the substance implanted is highly toxic, a zone of tissue necrosis appears around the shaft of the implant; nontoxic materials cause no damage to the tissues.

The second method of implant testing is that of *cell cultures*. A combination of mouse fibroblasts and cells from 10-day chick embryos is grown as a monolayer in a nonreplicating cell line. Once the cellular monolayer is healthy and well established, it is placed in a container with 1% agar. The agar provides a rigid substrate for the weight of the material being tested. The cultured cells are stained with 0.01% neutral red solution, which is released by dead, but held by living, cells. Using aseptic technique, samples of the

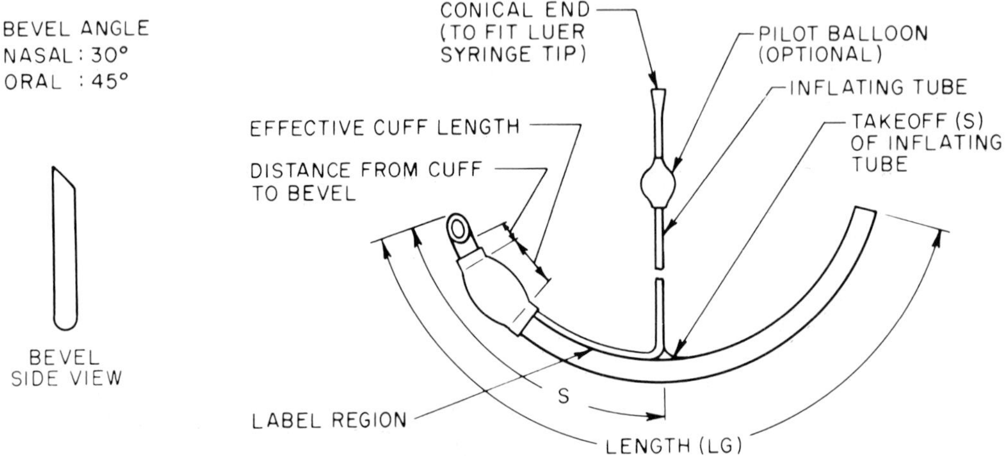

Fig. 21-14. A typical endotracheal tube with bonded cuff. Components of the tube are named using the nomenclature of the American National Standards Institute. (This material is reproduced, with permission, from American National Standard Tracheal Tubes and Cuffs, Z79.1, copyright 1974 by the American National Standards Institute, copies of which may be purchased from the American National Standards Institute, 1430 Broadway, New York, New York 10018.)

Table 21-3. Tracheal Tube Internal Diameters and Lengths*

INTERNAL DIAMETER OF TUBE			
Normal Size mm	*Tolerance mm*	MINIMUM TUBE LENGTH *mm*	PRECUT LENGTH† *mm*
2.5	±0.15	140	100
3.0	±0.15	160	110
3.5	±0.15	180	120
4.0	±0.15	200	130
4.5	±0.15	220	140
5.0	±0.15	240	150
5.5	±0.15	270	160
6.0	±0.15	280	180
6.5	±0.20	290	200
7.0	±0.20	300	210
7.5	±0.20	310	220
8.0	±0.20	320	235
8.5	±0.20	330	240
9.0	±0.20	340	250
9.5	±0.20	350	260
10.0	±0.20	360	260

*This material is reproduced, with permission, from American National Standard Tracheal Tubes and Cuffs, Z79.1, copyright 1974 by the American National Standards Institute, copies of which may be purchased from the American National Standards Institute, 1430 Broadway, New York, New York 10018.

†Manufacturers desiring to market prepackaged, sterilized orotracheal tubes with connectors may be guided by the lengths shown. The user, however, is cautioned that anatomical variations, conditions of use, length of tube inserted, or other factors may well result in use of a tracheal tube either too long or too short for a given patient. Use of a tracheal tube precut to a standard length should not, under any circumstances, be substituted for expert clinical judgment in selecting tube size and length.

material to be tested are placed on the surface of the agar. A known toxic material and a known nontoxic control are used. The cultures are incubated at 37° C in a 5% CO_2-air atmosphere for 24 to 48 hours. Since the agar layer is only about 1 mm thick, toxic materials diffuse rapidly and come in contact with the cell test system. A clear zone around the material under testing indicates the presence of toxic material. This test is extremely valuable because of the rapidity with which information can be obtained. With highly toxic materials, the clear zone appears within 24 hours; with mildly toxic materials, it appears within 48 hours.

Even though agreement between the cell culture technique and rabbit muscle implantation is generally excellent, only materials shown to be nontoxic on implant testing can bear the IT designation on Z-79 approved materials.

Additional Z-79 standards exist for other equipment used in respiratory therapy. In all, nearly 6000 standards exist.

Table 21-4. Recommended Sizes for Endotracheal Tubes and Suction Catheters*

AGE	ENDOTRACHEAL TUBE INTERNAL DIAMETER *mm*	SUCTION CATHETERS *Fr*
Newborn	3.0	6
6 months	3.5	8
18 months	4.0	8
3 years	4.5	8
5 years	5.0	10
6 years	5.5	10
8 years	6.0	10
12 years	6.5	10
16 years	7.0	10
Adult (female)	8.0–8.5†	12
Adult (male)	8.5–9.0†	14

*National Conference Steering Committee: Standards for cardiopulmonary resuscitation and emergency cardiac care. JAMA 227:852, 1974. Reproduced with permission of the American Heart Association.

†One size larger and one size smaller should be allowed for individual variations.

ANGLE AT THE FLANGE

The flange is that proximal part of a tracheostomy tube to which ties are secured to fasten it to the neck of the patient. The angle of flange surface to the centerline of the trachea that is most optimal is controversial and mainly comes down to physician preference and specific patient anatomy. Angles available range from 65° to 90°. The use of tracheostomy tubes with incorrect flange angles makes it possible to damage the posterior wall of the trachea with the posterior tube edge ("snowplowing").

One example of a situation where the flange angle might be crucial would be in the patient who has recently undergone laryngectomy. Since the trachea has been brought out to form a right angle with the skin, a tube with a 90° angle (also forming a right angle) could be the tube of choice for that patient.

With the wide variety of tubes manufactured today, the angle at the flange is not a major problem but is one of the considerations that should go into the selection of tracheostomy tubes. Tubes with adjustable flange angles, such as Shiley tubes, are available.

DISPOSABLES VERSUS REUSABLES

Except for a metal tracheostomy tube, most artificial airways are now so inexpensive as to be manufactured as "single patient use" items (*i.e.*, they are disposable). Good practice follows these economic concerns on scientific grounds as well, since effective cleaning of such devices is often more costly and less efficient than their replacement cost warrants.

EASE OF INSERTION

As mentioned above, endotracheal tubes are packaged in a slight curve, and, if they meet Z-79 standards, are maintained in this curve indefinitely. This process allows the tube to be introduced directly into the airway, often without a stylet or obturator.

With tracheostomy tubes, it is more difficult to evaluate the ease of insertion of a given tube because of the various materials from which they are made, their individual design, and the anatomic variations of given patients. If the tube is made from a rigid material, then it may need an obturator to be passed safely in order to avoid tissue damage. Should the tube be made of a softer material, an obturator may not be necessary and may actually be a hindrance. Obturators are not provided with many tubes made of silastic material.

TUBE SIZE

Correct endotracheal or tracheostomy tube sizing is necessary. Should the tube be too small in relation to the inner diameter of the trachea, then the volume of air needed in the cuff to ensure airway seal will, of necessity, be greater than if a tube of appropriate size had been selected. If too large a tube is selected, pressure necrosis of the tracheal wall may result with even minimum inflation of the cuff itself. A common rule of thumb is that the OD of the tube should be approximately two thirds of the ID of the trachea. Further, since resistance to air flow through a tube is a reciprocal function of its radius (Poiseuille's law), the larger the tube, the less air flow resistance will be encountered. Larger tubes also facilitate easier suctioning and are less easily occluded by mucus and foreign bodies such as suction catheters.

As is shown in Table 21-3, however, the internal diameter and length of endotracheal tubes, and, for that matter, tracheostomy tubes, bear a definite relationship to one another. Fairshter and coworkers have recently demonstrated that long tracheostomy tubes impinge upon the carina or, less commonly, inadvertently intubate the right mainstem bronchus, with resultant atelectasis of the left lung.[20] Guidelines for selection of endotracheal tubes of correct size for neonates have recently been reported.[34]

In a well-equipped department, a wide variety of tube sizes, styles, configurations, and composition should be available. For adults, endotracheal tubes should range from approximately 5 mm ID to 10 mm

Table 21-5. Dimensions of Low-Pressure Cuffed Tracheostomy Tubes (in Millimeters)*

KAMEN–WILKINSON (BIVONA)			LANZ			SHILEY		
ID	*OD*	*L*†	*ID*	*OD*	*L*	*ID*	*OD*	*L*
						5.0	8.5	74 (60)
6.0	8.7	75 (70)	6.0	8.0	96 (73)			
7.0	10.0	95 (84)	7.0	9.0	102 (78)	7.0	10.0	83 (68)
8.0	11.0	100 (90)	8.0	11.0	111 (84)			
						8.5	12.0	90 (71)
9.0	12.3	117 (105)	9.0	12.0	116 (88)	9.0	13.0	90 (71)
9.5	13.3	117 (105)						
			10.0	13.0	121 (92)			

*Fairshter RD, Litt MO, Wilson AF: Complications of long tracheostomy tubes. Crit Care Med 4:271, 1976

†To standardize measurements, lengths of tracheostomy tubes were measured along the outer circumference from flange to tip of tube. Data obtained from manufacturers are shown in parentheses. Since these lengths were apparently measured differently they are not directly comparable.

ID in 0.5-mm increments. They should be identified as to size and whether they meet the Z-79 specifications. For pediatric services, the size ranges are between 2.5 and 5.0 mm ID. The dimensions of some of the newer, low-pressure, high-compliance cuffed tracheostomy tubes are shown in Table 21-5.

Some tracheostomy tubes are produced in French sizes with the millimeter size stamped somewhere on the flange. The range for adults is from 24 French to 42 French, with incremental rises of three French units. Conversion from millimeter size to French and Jackson size is illustrated in Table 21-6. In adult tracheostomy tubes, French size = 3 × OD in millimeters.

STERILITY

Sterility and sterilization of respiratory therapy devices have been discussed in detail in Chapter 19. It is important not only that endotracheal and tracheostomy tubes be sterile before use, but also that the user know how that sterilization was performed.

If a PVC tube was sterilized originally by gamma ray irradiation, it could be resterilized safely by ethylene oxide (ETO), but this adds another variable and requires altered aeration time. The reason for this is that PVC contains free chloride ions that combine with ETO to form the product 2-chloroethanol (sometimes called chlorohydrin). Once chlorohydrin has formed, it is time-consuming and expensive to remove by standard aeration techniques. This toxic byproduct can leach into tissues and has a deleterious effect on mucous membrane, muscle, subcutaneous tissue, and skin.

Ethylene oxide readily combines with water to form ethylene glycol, a substance that is toxic to tissues. Most sterilizers require a humidity level of about 50% for efficient operation. If the materials being ETO-sterilized are porous enough to retain water after drying, then the potential for ethylene glycol formation exists. Small traces of ethylene glycol may be formed in or on devices undergoing ETO sterilization, given the proper conditions, and ethylene glycol may then diffuse from plastic to the tissues. Ethylene glycol is the principal component of antifreeze.

PVC products exposed to ETO sterilization have an unpredictable aeration period (see Fig. 21-9) varying up to 210 hours, depending on the type of wrapping used, the air flow through the aerator, and the temperature. If ETO is to be used as the method of sterilization for endotracheal and tracheostomy tubes, then an extremely large inventory of tubes is going to be needed to allow for adequate aeration. Therefore, it is recommended that the methods of sterilization of different chemical compounds being used today, for both endotracheal and tracheostomy tubes, be thoroughly understood by those using and purchasing them. Disposal of presterilized tubes may be the only realistic solution in many clinical settings.

Table 21-6. Tracheostomy Tube and Cuff-Size Conversion Chart

JACKSON SIZE	OUTSIDE DIAMETER* *mm*	FRENCH*	INTERNAL DIAMETER* *mm*
00	4.3	13	2.5
0	5.0	15	3.0
1	5.5	16.5	3.5
2	6.0	18	4.0
3	7	21	4.5–5.0
4	8	24	5.5
5	9	27	6.0–6.5
6	10	30	7.0
7	11	33	7.5–8.0
8	12	36	8.5
9	13	39	9.0–9.5
10	14	42	10.0
11	15	45	10.5–11.0
12	16	48	11.5

*Sizes given are approximate.

ARTIFICIAL AIRWAY CARE TECHNIQUES

TOTAL OCCLUSION OF THE TRACHEA ("NO-LEAK" TECHNIQUE) (MINIMAL OCCLUDING VOLUME)

Some clinical situations require total occlusion of the space between the tracheal wall and the tracheostomy tube or endotracheal tube cuff to the point where no air can escape past the cuff even at peak inspiratory pressure. This method may be desirable in patients who have poorly compliant lungs, those who aspirate repeatedly,[1,37] or when high levels of PEEP are necessary. Methods of ventilator parameter manipulation mentioned elsewhere in *Respiratory Care*, however, are more and more obviating the need for the "no-leak" technique. When this technique is used, meticulous monitoring of cuff pressure and volume variables must be done frequently.

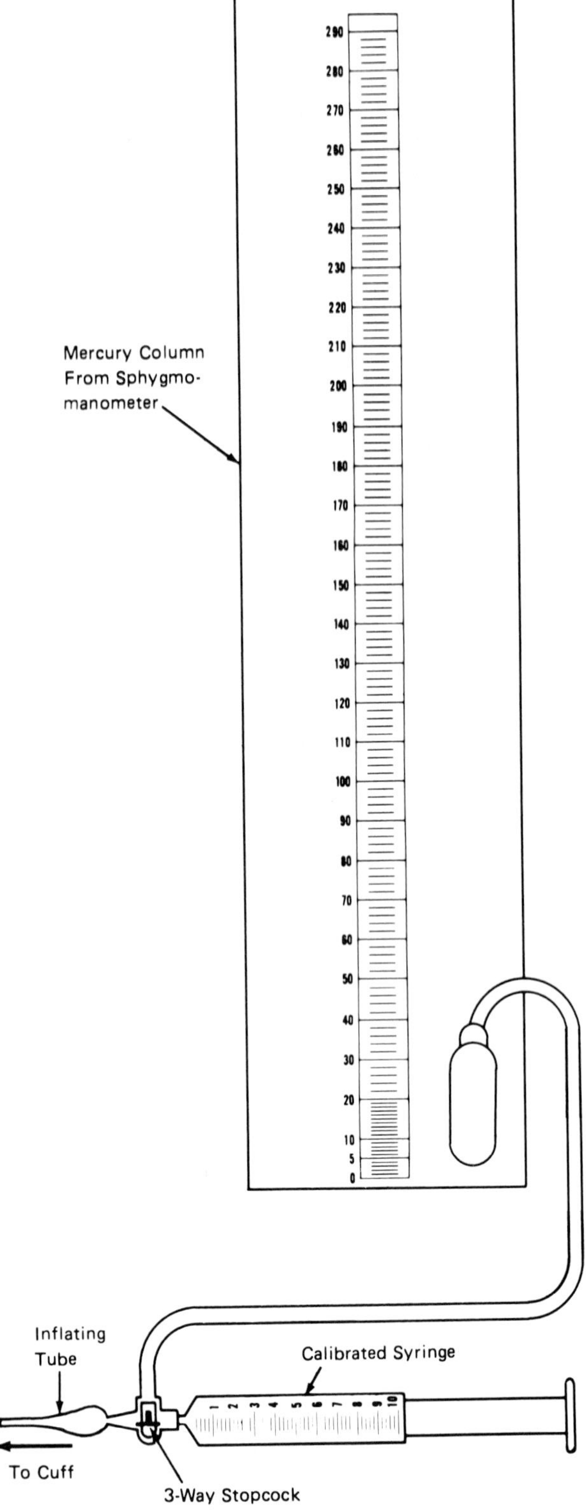

Fig. 21-15. Schema of equipment used to measure endotracheal and tracheostomy tube cuff pressures.

Development of cuff pressure-volume (compliance) curves can be accomplished with equipment as simple as a blood presure cuff and a calibrated syringe (see below). This should be done particularly when the total occlusion method is used to assure that high pressures are not maintained any longer than necessary, or that a high-pressure, low-compliance cuff is not mistakenly used. The cuff should be cared for by persons trained to do so. Absolutely minimum pressures and volumes should be used, and the cuff inflation and deflation routine should be dictated by the ventilatory needs of the patient. The volume and intracuff pressure should be checked and charted at regular intervals by trained personnel to assure that no one has inadvertently hyperinflated the cuff and to assure that the cuff has not ruptured or that tracheomalacia is developing. If one handles the cuffs carefully, such complications will rarely occur.

MINIMAL LEAK TECHNIQUE

By no means do all patients require total occlusion of the space between the tracheal wall and the tube cuff. The minimal-leak occlusion technique is finding increasing favor in such situations. Long before much was known about lateral tracheal wall pressures, the use of high-volume, low-pressure cuffs in conjunction with the minimal leak technique helped to reduce the incidence of tracheal damage.

With positive pressure applied to the airway, the cuff is inflated until total occlusion of the space between the cuff and the tracheal wall occurs. Air is then slowly removed from the cuff, until a small air leak is heard at maximum inspiratory ventilator pressure. Since the air leaking from the nose and mouth is part of the ventilator tidal volume, it then becomes necessary to adjust the tidal volume setting to compensate for the leak in this system. The only way to assess effective alveolar ventilation using this, as any other respiratory care technique, is to measure the arterial blood gases serially.

INTRACUFF PRESSURE AND VOLUME PRESSURE

Serial intracuff measurements require no special equipment and provide a useful method of following cuff and tracheal wall status. The equipment necessary for the measurement of intracuff pressure is a mercury manometer, a three-way stopcock, and a calibrated syringe (Fig. 21-15). The stopcock is inserted into the inflating tube (pilot line) in the closed position so that no air can escape from the cuff. The tubing from the mercury manometer is attached to the second stopcock opening and a syringe attached to the third opening. The pharynx is then well suctioned to remove any secretions that may have accumulated above the cuff. The stopcock is next rotated to allow passage of air from the cuff into the syringe. The entire volume of air is aspirated and the volume measured. The air is then reinserted into the cuff.

The stopcock is next rotated to allow the pressure in the cuff to be read on the manometer. That pressure reading is noted. If the initial pressure reading is taken as the true pressure reading for the intracuff pressure, it will be falsely low. The stopcock is once again rotated into a position that allows aspiration of the air from the cuff into the syringe. The volume obtained this time will be lower than before because of the trapped volume of air filling the pressure-measuring system, which has now been filled by some of the air that was in the cuff.

Additional air is then added to the cuff to compensate for the volume lost in the system, and the stopcock is once again turned to the position where pressure can be read on the manometer. The pressure this time will read higher than before; this reading is actually the intracuff pressure, compensated for the volume of air in the pressure-measuring system.

SUCTIONING

When an artificial airway is inserted, many of the normal mechanisms for warming and humidification of inspired air and clearance of secretions are bypassed (e.g., the cough mechanism no longer functions). Under these circumstances, it becomes necessary to institute other means by which these ends can be accomplished (e.g., airway hydration, chest percussion, postural drainage, and suctioning).

Suctioning is an example of Hagen–Poiseuille's law governing flow of fluids through tubes, although not often thought of in these terms. With respect to suctioning, negative pressure in the suction jar or trap generates flow and thus removal of secretions. The pressure difference between the proximal and distal ends of the tube is directionally proportional to flow when flow is laminar.

If the negative pressure in the suction jar is doubled, the flow of air through the tube will also be doubled. If flow is turbulent, suction flow more nearly equals the square root of the difference in pressure. At high (turbulent) flow rates, the negative pressure in the suction jar must be increased nearly four times in order to double the flow through the catheter (Fig. 21-16). The diameter and other design parameters of the suction catheters determine whether laminar or turbulent flow exists at a given negative pressure. Suction flow depends on the diameter of the catheter itself (Fig. 21-17) and on its length (Fig. 21-18).

Various suction catheter tip modifications have been introduced to provide more efficient suctioning at lower negative pressures. Such tip modifications include the open-ended catheter, whistle-tip catheter, modified whistle-tip catheter, Coudé modification, and the Argyle Airflow catheter tips (Fig. 21-19). Each of these catheter designs has its advocates and it is beyond the scope of this chapter to detail the merits of each catheter.

WHEN DOES THE PATIENT NEED TO BE SUCTIONED?

Suctioning has become such a routine part of respiratory care that there is a tendency to forget the complications and even the disasters that it can initiate. Even when done properly, it *is* a complicated, hazardous, and perhaps life-threatening procedure that should be undertaken only by those who know the complications, the patient, and the technique.

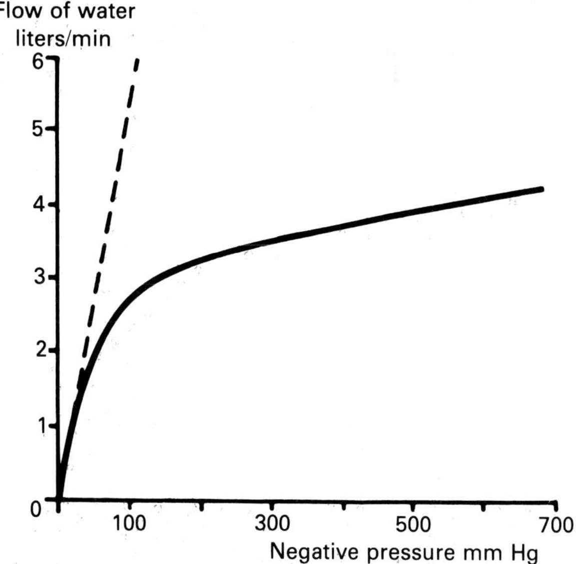

Fig. 21-16. Experimental data showing flow of water through tube at 5.8 mm ID, 2.0 m long, as negative pressure is increased. The dotted line indicates theoretical flow, had flow remained laminar.

Since the stethoscope has become part of the armamentarium of every nurse and respiratory therapist, time-specific suctioning orders are no longer indicated; p.r.n. or standing orders should suffice. Even with orders written properly in this fashion, the patient's breath sounds should be checked at least as frequently as his vital signs to determine whether suctioning is necessary. This then puts the onus of responsibility on the person caring for the patient to be sure that he understands chest auscultation clearly enough to know when suctioning is indicated (see Chap. 13). Indications for suctioning include the visible presence of secretions in the oropharynx or at the tube orifice, gurgling respiratory sounds, the sudden onset of dyspnea, and coarse tubular breath sounds or rales on auscultation.

THE SUCTIONING PROCEDURE

For many years, suctioning has been treated as an entirely sterile procedure. However, whenever a sterile object is introduced through a contaminated orifice such as the mouth, "sterility" seems to be an inappropriate description of the existing conditions. Suctioning is actually a "clean" procedure but not a sterile one. The use of sterile, disposable items is encouraged, however, to keep the procedure as clean as possible. Before suctioning, all equipment should be assembled:

1. Suction catheter of appropriate size
2. Sterile disposable gloves for one hand
3. Oxygen source, flowmeter, and connecting tubing
4. A non-self-inflating anesthesia bag
5. Vacuum source and connecting tubing
6. Sterile water
7. Disposable cup
8. A 5- to 10-ml syringe with saline for injection

TECHNIQUES FOR SUCTIONING THROUGH ENDOTRACHEAL AND TRACHEOSTOMY TUBES

Step-by-step instructions and an illustrative protocol for suctioning are found in Appendix H. The technique will clearly vary from patient to patient and from institution to institution. Each hospital needs to have its own established protocols and procedures that have been reviewed by appropriate physicians and all involved respiratory care personnel.

Before starting any suctioning procedure, one must use good hand washing technique with an antimicrobial preparation, except in emergencies. The

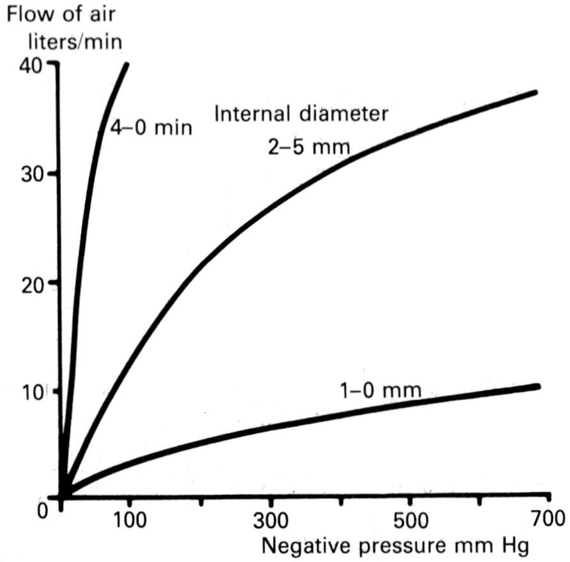

Fig. 21-17. Effects of suction tube internal diameter on airflow rate.

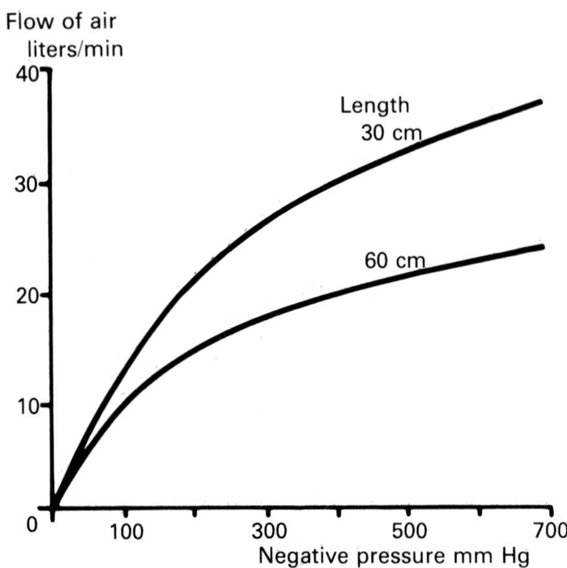

Fig. 21-18. Effect of suction tube length on airflow rate.

National Centers for Disease Control (NCDC) favor the use of iodophor preparations over those containing hexachlorophene, since some hexachlorophene preparations have been shown to support the growth of *Pseudomonas* species.

Aside from the step-by-step protocol outlined in Appendix H, one must consider the fact that effective oxygenation must *not* be interrupted during the course of the suctioning procedure. High-volume suctioning may actually withdraw enough oxygen from the patient, particularly if a large-bore suctioning catheter is used in a small-bore endotracheal tube, to cause him to become hypoxemic. A rule of thumb is that the suction catheter should not occupy more than half the internal diameter of the tube in place. Arrhythmia monitoring during the suctioning procedure is indicated, especially during nasotracheal suctioning.

Periodic hyperinflation of the lungs during suctioning is strongly urged, as is limited chest physical therapy to the areas being suctioned, as a preliminary measure.

If the patient has tenacious secretions, 5 to 10 ml of normal saline may be instilled into the endotracheal tube at the beginning of the suctioning procedure. After this, hyperinflation of the lungs should be achieved by having the patient take deep breaths or with a manual resuscitator. After the patient has been hyperoxygenated, suctioning may be resumed.

Suctioning, when performed correctly, should be an essentially atraumatic experience. Even minimal bleeding in the average patient is an indication of overly vigorous suctioning technique and the application of unacceptably high suctioning pressures. Rotation and gradual withdrawal of the suctioning catheter, catheter repositioning, and modification of the secretions themselves by instilled saline as mentioned above are all more effective ways of removing secretions from an obstructed patient than simply turning up the suctioning pressure.

One commercially available suction device provides an alternative to the traditional suctioning procedure. The TRACH-CARE Suction System is a self-contained device that can be inserted into a ventilator circuit and used for 24 hours. It contains a 14 French catheter enclosed in a sealed plastic envelope and has external suction controls (Fig. 21-20). Since the catheter is advanced into the tube using the external plas-

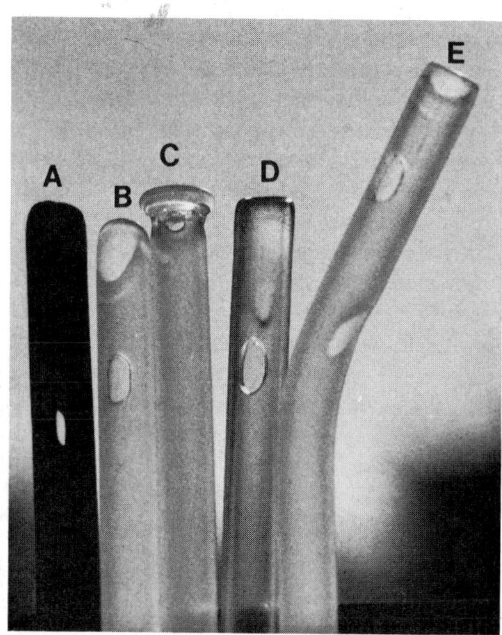

Fig. 21-19. Photograph of various catheter tips: *(A)* open-ended. *(B)* whistle-tip, *(C)* Argyle Airflow, *(D)* modified whistle-tip, *(E)* Coudé.

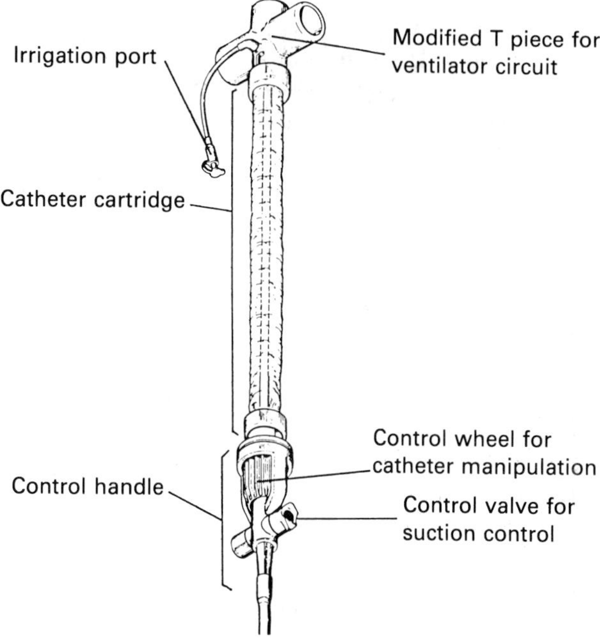

Fig. 21-20. Schema of the TRACH-CARE Continuous Use Suction System.

tic envelope, use of gloves is not necessary (Fig. 21-21).

During 2 years of clinical use in a major university regional referral burn/trauma/critical care facility, the TRACH-CARE Suction System has been found most useful in those patients whose cardiovascular system is unstable, those requiring high inspired O_2 concentrations (50–80%), and high levels of PEEP (10 cm or greater). In about 75% of those patients, use of this suction system has successfully eliminated bradycardia and hypotension associated with suctioning. This device is now routinely used on all patients who require PEEP at this facility.

NASOTRACHEAL SUCTIONING

Compared to other forms of suctioning, nasotracheal suctioning is technically more difficult to perform and is fraught with potentially greater hazards. In addition, the distance from the nares to the larynx is often too great to allow deep suctioning from the tracheobronchial tree, in which case nasotracheal suctioning may be worse than no suctioning at all.

The hypopharynx contains vagal afferents that, when stimulated, may induce abnormalities of cardiac rate (bradycardia), rhythm disturbances, and hypotension. These may be prevented by the use of atropine.

The trauma of nasal introduction of a catheter into the airway may result in catecholamine release, which, with attendant hypoxia, increased work of breathing, and vagal stimulation, may result in arrhythmias. Oxygen should be administered during nasotracheal suctioning even more frequently and more rigorously than during other types of suctioning.

The patient should usually be positioned in Fowler's position (intermediate or high) for nasotracheal suctioning to be easily performed. The equipment needed is essentially the same as that used in tracheal suctioning, as is the procedure (described in Appendix H), with the addition of water-soluble lubricant to facilitate passage of the nasal catheter, and cardiac monitoring capability at hand. For patients who experience considerable discomfort from nasotracheal suction, lubrication of the catheter with 1% xylocaine jelly may be helpful.

The catheter is slowly advanced through the nares to a point just above the larynx. Air flow sounds can be heard at the proximal end of the catheter. When air flow is felt to be strongest and respiratory sounds are loudest, the tip of the catheter is immediately above the epiglottis. If the catheter is advanced too far, it will usually have entered the esophagus. This will be recognized because sound and air flow will both stop. Slowly withdrawing the catheter to the level where the flow of air is felt will promptly reposition the tip of the catheter above the larynx, and reintroduction into the trachea may again be attempted.

If a successful tracheal intubation has been achieved, the cough will become hoarse and the patient will be unable to talk in a normal tone, usually not louder than a whisper. After the vocal cords have

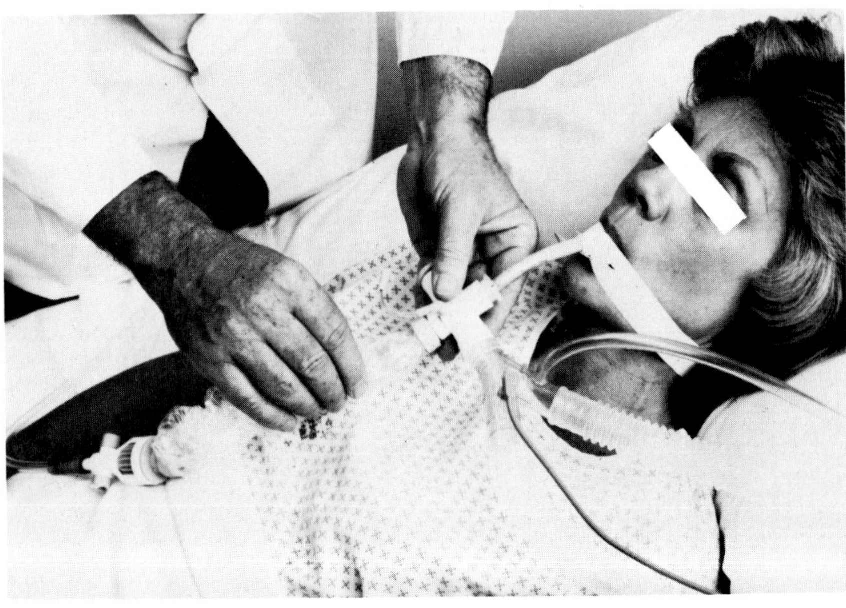

Fig. 21-21. The TRACH-CARE Continuous Use Suction System in use. Note that the suctioning procedure can be done without the usual necessity for gloving, while relative asepsis is still maintained (*see* text).

been passed, a few deep respirations are allowed while the patient is reoxygenated. Suctioning is then begun as in the standard suctioning protocol. In most patients, violent continuous coughing will be elicited once the catheter has passed into the trachea. It is extremely important that the person performing the procedure be aware of this and that he explain it to the patient before starting the procedure.

Although once believed to be the case, it is now becoming increasingly clear that head position has little to do with *predictable* positioning of the endotracheal catheter. Rotation of the catheter and rotation of the head should be attempted nonetheless during the suctioning procedure.

Probably the most significant benefit the patient derives from nasotracheal suctioning is mobilization of secretions by cough into the central airway, where they can then be effectively removed by suctioning itself. Nasotracheal suctioning should not be performed without reoxygenation for more than 15 seconds at a time. If patients are encouraged to breathe through the mouth during the nasotracheal suctioning period, the sensation of suffocation and feeling of gagging will be controlled fairly easily. If nasotracheal suctioning is to be performed frequently, a nasopharyngeal airway should be used, if possible.

COMPLICATIONS OF SUCTIONING

Hypoxia

Suctioning removes not only secretions but also the gases in the tracheobronchial tree and alveoli. Accordingly, during the process of suctioning, the alveolar oxygen available to be taken up by the arterial blood may be greatly diminished. *The maximum allowable time for continuous suctioning is 15 seconds.* Should suctioning continue for a prolonged time, hypoxemia may result and constitute a real threat to the patient's life.

Vagal Stimulation

Receptors for the vagus nerve are found throughout the tracheobronchial tree, down to the level of the carina. Stimulation of this nerve produces slowing of the heart rate. When suctioning a patient on a cardiac monitor, one frequently sees arrhythmias of many types, including marked bradycardia. Should slowing of the pulse occur during suctioning, continuation of the suctioning may lead to cardiac arrest.

Tracheitis

Tracheitis can be recognized by a dry, hoarse, hacking cough whenever the trachea is stimulated.

It is not unusual to have some small amount of bleeding from irritation of the tracheal mucosa. The most common cause of tracheitis is frequent or overly vigorous suctioning in the absence of secretions. Prolonged use of acetylcysteine by direct instillation or via IPPB may be another cause of tracheitis.

When tracheitis occurs, the patient should be encouraged to cough as vigorously as possible to bring secretions up into the tube. If he cannot cough, the instillation of 5 to 10 ml of sterile normal saline usually stimulates sufficient coughing to raise secretions into the tube. Attempts should not be made to suction past the end of the tube unless absolutely necessary.

If the patient continues to have paroxysms of coughing after suctioning has ended, instillation of 1 ml of 1% lidocaine every 2 to 4 hours p.r.n. helps to control the cough until the tracheitis subsides. Topical steroids have also been used with good effect in this situation.

Damage to the Mucous Membrane

Even though attempts have been made to design suction catheters that produce less trauma to the trachea, almost all patients will suffer some degree of damage to their mucous membranes during repeated suctioning. This occurs even in the presence of secretions but tends to occur more frequently when patients are suctioned in the absence of secretions. When suction is applied to a catheter, the negative pressure generated may cause the tracheal mucosa to be drawn into the catheter holes. As the catheter is moved, the mucosa that has been caught up by the catheter may literally be torn loose from the tracheal wall. One may sometimes see such pieces of tissue floating in the suction trap.

Occlusion of the Tube with the Catheter

Airway occlusion with oversized catheters has been mentioned as a cause of both hypoxemia and atelectasis. Sudden application of excessive negative pressure results in a large increase in venous return and subsequent increases in left atrial pressure upon release of the suctioning pressure. The heart may not be able to cope with this sudden increase in cardiac return, and again cardiac arrhythmias or arrest may ensue. *Suction catheters should not have an OD greater than two thirds of the ID of the tube being suctioned.*

Sudden Death

Although the exact mechanism of sudden death during suctioning has not been defined, one or more of the complications discussed above could be responsible for this occurrence. Whatever the mechanism, sudden death has occurred during suctioning and is indeed a potential complication of the procedure.

REFERENCES

1. Bernhard WN, Cattrell JE, Sivakumaran C, Patel K, Yost L, Turndorf H: Adjustment of intracuff pressure to prevent aspiration. Anesthesiology 50:363, 1979
2. Bernhard WN, Yost L, Turndorf H, Danzinger F: Cuffed tracheal tubes—physical and behavioral characteristics. Anesth Analg (Cleve) 61(1):36, 1982
3. Bishop MJ: Endotracheal tube lumen compromise from cuff overinflation. Chest 80:100, 1981
4. Black AM, Seegobin RD: Pressures on endotracheal tube cuffs. Anaesthesia 36(5):498, 1981
5. Brantigan CO, Grow JB Sr: Cricothyroidotomy: Elective use in respiratory problems requiring tracheotomy. J Thorac Cardoivasc Surg 71:72, 1976
6. Brantigan CO, Grow JB Sr: Cricothyroidotomy revisited again. Ear Nose Throat J 59:26, 1980
7. Briggs BD: Prolonged endotracheal intubation. Anesthesiology 11:29, 1950
8. Burns HP, Dayal VS, Scott S, vanNostrand AWP, Bryce DP: Laryngotracheal trauma: Observations on its pathogenesis and its prevention following prolonged orotracheal intubation in the adult. Laryngoscope 89:1316, 1979
9. Ching NP, Ayers SM, Paegle RP, Linden JM; Nealon TF Jr: The contribution of cuff volume and pressure in tracheostomy tube damage. J Thorac Cardiovasc Surg 62:402, 1971
10. Ching NPH, Nealon TB Jr: Clinical experience with new low-pressure high-volume tracheostomy cuffs: Importance of limiting intracuff pressure. NY State J Med 74:2379, 1974
11. Cooper JD, Grillo HC: Experimental production and prevention of injury due to cuffed tracheal tubes. Surg Gynecol Obstet 129:1235, 1969
12. Cooper JD, Grillo HC: Analysis of problems related to cuffs on intratracheal tubes. Chest 62:215, 1972
13. Deane RS, Mills EL: Prolonged nasotracheal intubation in adults: A successor and adjunct to tracheostomy. Anesth Analg (Cleve) 49:89, 1970
14. Deane RS, Shinozaki T, Morgan JG: An evaluation of the cuff characteristics and incidence of laryngeal complications using a new nasotracheal tube in prolonged intubations. J Trauma 11:311, 1977
15. Demers RB, Saklad M: Intratracheal inflatable cuffs: A review. Respir Care 22:29, 1977
16. Dobrin P, Canfield T: Cuffed endotracheal tubes: Mucosal pressure and tracheal wall blood flow. Am J Surg 133:562, 1977
17. Donnelly WH: Histopathology of endotracheal intubation: An autopsy study of 99 cases. Arch Pathol 88:511, 1969
18. Dubick MN, Wright BD: Comparison of laryngeal pathology following long-term oral and nasal endotracheal intubations. Anesth Analg (Cleve) 57:663, 1978
19. Dunn CR, Dunn DL, Moser KM: Determinants of tracheal injury by cuffed tracheostomy tubes. Chest 65:128, 1974
20. Fairshter RD, Liff MO, Wil AF: Complications of long tracheostomy tubes. Crit Care Med 4:271, 1976
21. Geffin B, Pontoppidan H: Reduction of tracheal damage by the prestretching of inflatable cuffs. Anesthesiology 31:462, 1969
22. Greene NM: Fatal cardiovascular and respiratory failure associated with tracheostomy. N Engl J Med 261:846, 1959
23. Grillo HC, Cooper JD, Geffin B, Pontopidden H: A low-pressure cuff for tracheostomy tubes to minimize tracheal injury: A comparative clinical trial. J Thorac Cardiovasc Surg 62:898, 1971
24. Guess WL: Rubber for tracheal tubes. Int Anesthesiol Clin 8:815, 1970
25. Guess WL: Safety evaluation of medical plastics. Clin Toxicol 12(1):77, 1978
26. Johns ME, Cantrell RE: Voice restoration of the total laryngectomy patient: the Singer–Blom technique. Otolaryngol Head Neck Surg 89(1):82, 1981
27. Jones JW, Reynolds M, Hewitt RI, Drapanas T: Tracheo-innominate artery erosion: Successful management of a devastating complication. Ann Surg 184:194, 1976
28. Kambic V, Radsel Z: Intubation lesions of the larynx. Br J Anaesth 50:587, 1978
29. Khan F, Reddy NC: Enlarging intratracheal tube cuff diameter: A quantitative roentgenographic study of its value in the early prediction of serious tracheal damage. Ann Thorac Surg 24:49, 1977
30. Kuner J, Goldman A: Prolonged nasotracheal intubation in adults versus tracheostomy. Dis Chest 51:270, 1967
31. Larsen GL: Conservative management for incomplete dysphagia paralytica. Arch Phys Med Rehabil 54:180, 1973
32. Leigh JM, Maynard JP: Pressure on the tracheal mucosa from cuffed tubes. Br Med J 1:1173, 1979
33. Lewis FR Jr, Schlobohm RM, Thomas AN: Prevention of complications from prolonged tracheal intubation. Am J Surg 135:452, 1978
34. Loew A, Thebeault DW: A new and safe method to control the depth of endotracheal intubation in neonates. Pediatrics 34:506, 1974
35. Lowry LD: Artificial larynges: A review and development of a prototype self-contained intra-oral artificial larynx. Laryngoscope 91(8):1332, 1981
36. MacKenzie RA, Gould AB Jr, Bardsley WT: Cardiac arrhythmias with endotracheal intubation. Anesthesiology 53:S102, 1980
37. Pavline EG, Van Ninwegan D, Hornbein TF: Failure of high-compliance low-pressure cuff to prevent aspiration. Anesthesiology 42:216, 1975
38. Larsen G: Personal communication, 28 June 1982
39. Ripoll I, Lindholm C–E, Carroll R, Grenvik A: Spontaneous dislocation of endotracheal tubes. Anesthesiology 49:50, 1978
40. Roberts RB: Gamma-rays + PVC + EO = OK. Med Instrum 13(2):107, 1979
41. Safar P: Respiratory Therapy. Philadelphia, F A Davis, 1965
42. Safar P, Penninckx J: Cricothyroid membrane puncture with special cannula. Anesthesiology 28:943, 1967
43. Schofferman J, Dill P, Lewis AJ: The esophageal obturator airway: A clinical evaluation. Chest 69:67, 1976
44. Sellery GR, Worth A, Greenway RE: Late complications of prolonged tracheal intubation. Can Anaesth Soc J 25:140, 1978
45. Singer MI, Blom ED: An endoscopic technique for restoration of voice after laryngectomy. Ann Otol Rhinol Laryngol 89 (6 Pt 1):529, 1980

46. Stallings JO: Surgical voice restoration—a 20th century reality. Ear Nose Throat J 60(6):250, 1981
47. Stauffer JL, Olson DE, Petty TL: Complications and consequences of endotracheal intubation and tracheotomy: A prospective study of 150 critically ill adult patients. Am J Med 70: 65, 1981
48. Stauffer JL, Petty TL: Cleft tongue and ulceration of hard palate: Complications of oral intubation. Chest 74:317, 1981
49. Stauffer JL, Silvestri RC: Complications of endotracheal intubation, tracheostomy and artificial airways. Respir Care 27:417, 1982
50. Stephenson HE Jr: Cardiopulmonary resuscitation. In Burton GG, Gee GN, Hodgkin JE (eds): Respiratory Care: A Guide to Clinical Practice, 1st ed, p 924. Philadelphia, J B Lippincott, 1977
51. Taryle DA, Chandler JE, Good JT Jr, Potts DE, Sahn SA: Emergency room intubations—complications and survival. Chest 75:541, 1979
52. Taub S: Air-bypass voice prosthesis for vocal rehabilitation of laryngectomees. Ear Nose Throat J 60(6):273, 1981
53. Weg JG: Prolonged endotracheal intubation in respiratory failure. Arch Intern Med 120:679, 1967
54. Wetmore SJ, Johns ME, Baker SR: The Singer–Blom voice restoration procedure. Arch Otolaryngol 107(11):674, 1981
55. Whited RE: Laryngeal dysfunction following prolonged intubation. Ann Otol Rhinol Laryngol 88:474, 1979
56. Zwillich C, Pierson DJ: Nasal necrosis: A complication of nasotracheal intubation. Chest 64:376, 1973
57. Zwillich CW, Pierson DJ, Creagh CE, Sutton FD, Schatz E, Petty TL: Complications of assisted ventilation: A prospective study of 354 consecutive episodes. Am J Med 57:161, 1974

22

Physiological Basis for Mechanical Devices That Aid Lung Inflation

Gennaro M. Tisi

A ventilator is a mechanical device that performs the function of ventilation (*i.e.*, the movement of air). Such devices of themselves do not assure the adequacy of respiration. In actuality a ventilator may be used to ventilate a cadaver, in which there is obviously no true respiration, a term implying gas exchange. A ventilator may initiate the movement of a normal tidal volume, which given normal distribution, perfusion, and diffusion within the lungs, will result in normal arterial blood gases. To assess the adequacy of ventilation, one must evaluate variables such as the rate of breathing (frequency), the depth of breathing (tidal volume), the rate of inspiratory and expiratory airflow, the duration of inspiration to expiration, and the length of the apneic period. To assess whether a particular grouping of ventilator settings is accomplishing normal respiration, however, one needs to measure arterial oxygen and carbon dioxide tensions.

This chapter is intended to be a general introduction to the three chapters on respirator and ventilator use that follow.

A SPONTANEOUS BREATH

The physiologic variables of a normal, spontaneous breath provide the basis that should underlie the rational clinical application of ventilators (Fig. 22-1). During this breathing cycle four simultaneous variables are plotted with reference to time, including pleural pressure (Ppl) in cm H_2O; alveolar pressure (PA) in cm H_2O; flow ($\dot{V}$) in liters per second; and volume (V) in liters. Review of this cycle raises a basic question: Why does air flow into and out of the lungs? Before inspiration begins, under conditions of zero flow, Ppl is about -5 cm H_2O, owing to the resting opposed recoil of the lung and chest wall. Under this condition of zero flow, PA is zero. As inspiration begins, the inspiratory muscles contract and the diaphragm descends. As a consequence, the volume of the thoracic cage increases and Ppl becomes more negative (more subatmospheric). With an expanding thoracic cage, alveolar volume increases and PA becomes negative. The change in Ppl *leads* that in PA (*i.e.*, at any point in time, the rate of change in Ppl is greater than that for PA). The answer to the question asked above should now be apparent: Air flows within the human lung because of differences in pressure. During inspiration, since PA is negative with respect to atmospheric pressure at the mouth, air flows into the lung. The integral ($\dot{V}$/time) of this airflow into the lung is the resultant inspiratory tidal volume. During expiration this sequence is reversed. The inspiratory muscles relax, the lung recoils, and the diaphragm ascends. Ppl returns toward the pressure at the lung's resting position (approximately −5 cm H_2O); PA becomes positive with respect to atmospheric pressure; expiratory flow occurs; and the tidal volume is exhaled.

Four additional features about Figure 22-1 should be stressed:

1. At the resting position of the lung, a unique volume is contained within the lung—the functional residual capacity (FRC). Accordingly, all depicted volume changes in Figure 22-1 occurred above FRC.
2. PA is zero or atmospheric at three points in the cycle (points of zero flow): preinspiration, end inspiration, and end expiration.
3. The PA and $\dot{V}$ variables are essentially sine wave functions in phase (cyclic variations occurring in the same direction).
4. To move a larger tidal volume, a more negative Ppl would have to be generated. Changes in Ppl are the primary events. As a more negative Ppl is generated, a greater pressure is exerted across the lung, resulting in a larger tidal volume. This point cannot be overstressed: *Volume is a function of pressure.*

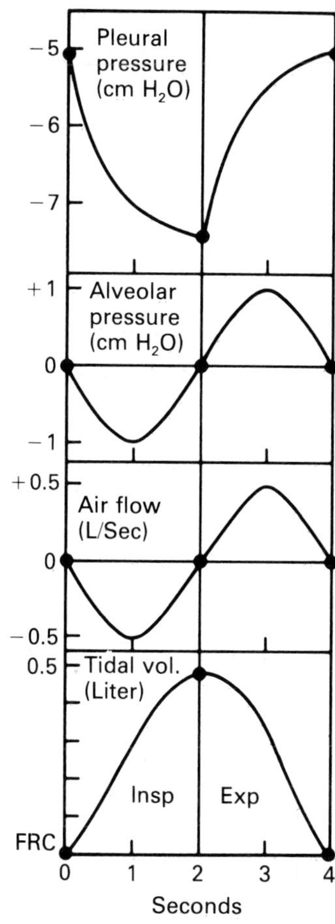

Fig. 22-1. A spontaneous breath. The variables of pleural pressure in cm H_2O, alveolar pressure in cm H_2O, flow in liters per second (L/Sec), and volume in liters are plotted as a function of time in seconds during a single, spontaneous breathing cycle. All volume changes are plotted above resting lung volume, the functional residual capacity *(FRC)*. Each pressure is graphed with reference to atmospheric pressure, expressed as zero pressure. Accordingly, pressures greater than atmospheric are positive (+) and those less than atmospheric are negative (−). INSP = inspired; EXP = expired.

This description of a normal, spontaneous breathing cycle provides the physiologic basis for the clinical application of ventilators, since during the cycle produced by a ventilator there will be an interplay between these same variables.

CLASSIFICATION OF VENTILATORS

For classification purposes, ventilators can be separated into three types: pressure-cycled, volume-cycled, and time-cycled. For each type the variables remain the same: flow ($\dot{V}$), volume (V), pressure (P), respiratory frequency (f), and ratio of inspiratory and expiratory time (I/E). Since the pressure-cycled and volume-cycled ventilators are the ones most commonly used in clinical practice, we will selectively deal with an overview of the general characteristics of these two types of ventilators. The differences between the two relate to which of the variables the operator can manipulate—in other words, expressed as a question, which variables can the operator control or set, and which become *determined variables* as a result of the settings (Table 22-1)? Let us review pressure- and time-cycled ventilators in terms of this concept.

Table 22-1. Characteristics of Pressure and Volume Ventilators

VARIABLES	PRESSURE VENTILATOR	VOLUME VENTILATOR
Flow	Control setting	Control setting
Volume	Determined variable	Control setting
Pressure	Control setting	Determined variable
Frequency	Control setting	Control setting
I/E ratio	Determined variable	Determined variable

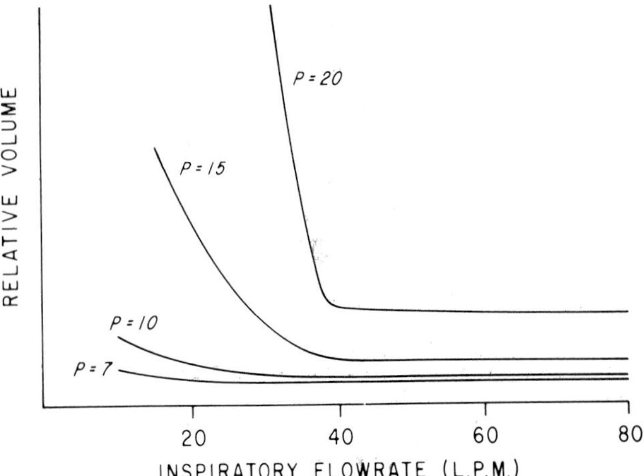

Fig. 22-2. Relationship between relative volume, inspiratory flow, and driving pressure. These data were obtained with a standard pressure-cycled ventilator and a test lung system. Flow and pressure settings were varied, and the volume delivered to the test system was determined. Volume was plotted proportional to the highest volume achieved at any pressure-flow setting. Inspiratory flow is in liters per minute *(L.P.M.)* and pressure *(P)* in cm H_2O.

PRESSURE-CYCLED VENTILATORS

For a pressure-cycled ventilator there are control settings for flow, pressure, and frequency. As a result of particular settings of these three, the variables of $\dot{V}$ and the I/E ratio become determined variables (see Table 22-1). The interplay between these variables becomes apparent in Figures 22-2 and 22-3. A standard pressure-cycled ventilator was used to obtain these data when a set of model lungs of normal compliance (elasticity) with normal resistance (normal airway caliber) was ventilated.

In Figure 22-2, relative-volume is plotted on the vertical axis and inspiratory flow rate ($\dot{V}$I) in liters per minute (liters/min) on the horizontal axis. There are four isoplots for pressures of 7, 10, 15, and 20 cm H_2O. Three features of the interdependence between $\dot{V}$I, P, and V should be apparent from Figure 22-2.

1. At any given pressure setting, as inspiratory flow rate was increased, relative inspiratory volume decreased. At any given pressure setting, the higher volumes were achieved at the lower flow rates.
2. As pressure was increased, relative volume was accurately determined by a narrow range of inspiratory flow rates. At 7 cm H_2O wide fluctuations in $\dot{V}$I produced a minimal change in relative volume, whereas at 20 cm H_2O narrow fluctuations in $\dot{V}$I (*i.e.*, between approximately 35 and 40 liters/min) produced large changes in relative volume.
3. As pressure was incrementally increased from 7 to 20 cm H_2O, relative volume increased.

In summary, the higher relative volumes were achieved at higher pressure and lower inspiratory flow-rate settings. The clinical message is that to increase the volume delivered by a pressure-cycled ventilator, there are two options: increase pressure or determine the optimal $\dot{V}$/P settings. This can be done by measuring expired tidal volume with a spirometer in series with the expiration limb of the ventilator circuit. As pressure is increased and as $\dot{V}$/P settings are varied in an individual patient at the bedside, the effects on volume can be reflected and measured breath-by-breath by means of suitable spirometers.

In Figure 22-3, inspiratory time in seconds (sec) is plotted on the vertical axis and inspiratory flow rate ($\dot{V}$I) in liters per minute on the horizontal axis. Once again there are isoplots for pressures of 7, 10, 15, and 20 cm H_2O. Three features of the interplay between $\dot{V}$I, P, and inspiratory time should be apparent from Figure 22-3.

1. At any given P as $\dot{V}$I was increased, the inspiratory time shortened. At any given P setting, longer inspiratory times were achieved at the lower flow rates.
2. As P was increased, inspiratory time was accurately determined by a narrower range of $\dot{V}$I.

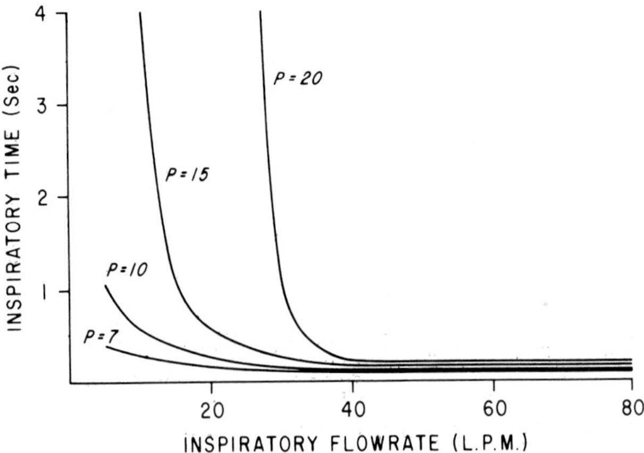

Fig. 22-3. Relationship between inspiratory time in seconds, inspiratory flow in liters per minute *(L.P.M.)*, and driving pressure *(P)* in cm H_2O in a pressure-cycled ventilator.

At 7 cm H_2O, wide fluctuations in $\dot{V}I$ produced minimal changes in inspiratory time, whereas at 20 cm H_2O narrow fluctuations in $\dot{V}I$ (*i.e.*, between approximately 30 and 40 liters/min) produced large changes in inspiratory time.
3. As pressure was increased from 7 to 20 cm H_2O, inspiratory time was increased.

In summary, the shorter inspiratory times were achieved at the lower pressures and the faster flow-rate settings. The clinical message is that to shorten the inspiratory phase of a pressure-cycled ventilator there are two options: lower pressure or increase flow rate.

In most pressure-cycled ventilators, the actual number settings on the dials controlling $\dot{V}$, P, and f are relative and not absolute numbers (*i.e.*, a setting of 20 on a $\dot{V}$ knob does not necessarily correlate with a flow of 20 liters/min, but a change from 20 to 80 would indicate a significant increase in relative flow).

This description provides an overview of the physiologic basis for the clinical application of pressure-cycled ventilators, and these principles apply to each of the commercially available products. A point-by-point analysis of the specific features of one of the prototypic pressure-cycled ventilators (Bird Mark 6) is included in Chapter 24 (Tables 24-2; Figs. 24-18 to 24-20).

VOLUME-CYCLED VENTILATORS

A volume-cycled ventilator has control settings for flow, volume, and frequency. Pressure and I/E become determined variables (see Table 22-1). These ventilators are so classified because the operator can "dial in" desired volume. This basic difference between the two ventilators is that in the pressure-cycled ventilator the operator sets pressure, and *volume* becomes the determined variable, whereas in the volume-cycled ventilator the operator sets volume, and *pressure* becomes the determined variable.

A point-by-point analysis of the specific features of several of the more commonly used volume-cycle ventilators appears in Chapter 24.

VARIABLES AFFECTING VENTILATOR ADEQUACY

The foregoing discussion developed the critical interplay between the V, $\dot{V}$, P, f, and I/E ventilator settings. However, at any given group of ventilator settings, the distribution of the delivered inspired volume depends on the regional elastance and resistance characteristics of the patient's lungs. Elastance (E) is the transpulmonary pressure (ΔP) required to produce a unit change in lung volume (ΔV). The elastance of the lung is about 5 cm H_2O/liter (BTPS). The terms elastance and compliance (C) are reciprocal terms. Increased elastance correlates with decreased compliance (*i.e.*, stiff lung); decreased elastance correlates with an increased compliance (*i.e.*, emphysema). Resistance (R) may be defined as opposition to motion. The resistance of the human airways depends on their geometric structure, including the variables of length, diameter, and area. In disease states, regional changes in R and C affect the regional distribution of ventilation (Fig. 22-4).

Although the ventilator settings may be the same in each of these clinical states, the distribution of ventilation in these simplistic, two-way compartmental lung models would be greatly disparate. In each of these examples, the dichotomous system of airways is diagrammatically represented by a Y tube and the two lungs by two air sacs. In Figure 22-4A, there is a narrowing of the airway to the right lung (the reader's

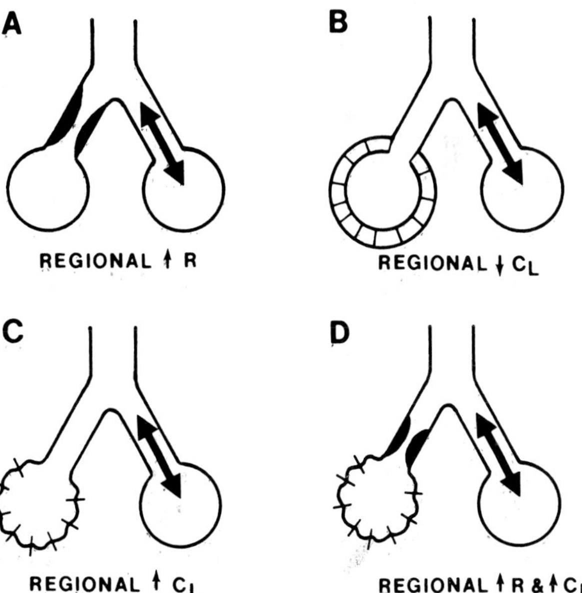

Fig. 22-4. Effect on distribution of ventilation in two-compartment lung models. *(A)* Increased resistance *(R)* of the lung on the left. *(B)* Decreased compliance of the lung on the left. *(C)* Increased compliance of the lung on the left. *(D)* Increased resistance and increased compliance of the lung on the left. Although some air flow would still go to the abnormal lung, most ventilation *(arrows)* in each case is to the opposite (normal) lung.

left), as might occur in asthma, in bronchitis, or with an intraluminal obstruction. This would produce a regional increase in R of this airway, with the result that the lion's share of the ventilation would go to the left lung. In Figure 22-4B, there is a decreased compliance of the right lung (as might occur with a fibrothorax, unilateral atelectasis, interstitial edema, and so forth), with the result that most of the ventilation would go to the left lung. In Figure 22-4C, there is an increased compliance of the right lung (as might occur in unilateral emphysema, the Swyer–James–MacLeod syndrome). This lung will quickly achieve a near maximal lung volume at FRC (i.e., it will become overinflated). As a consequence, most of the exchange of ventilation will occur in the left lung. In Figure 22-4D, there is increased R and increased C of the right lung (as might occur with combined bronchitis and emphysema), with the result that most of the ventilation will go to the left lung. In each of these simplistic examples, a two-compartmental lung model (right versus left lung) has been used, but regional differences in R and C between smaller lung subunits (i.e., lobes, segments, subsegments, and so forth) will similarly affect the distribution of ventilation.

The ventilator, then, affects the volume delivered; the regional R and C characteristics of the patient's lungs affect the distribution of ventilation, and the match of ventilation to perfusion ($\dot{V}/\dot{Q}$) in his lungs will determine the arterial oxygen (Pa_{O_2}) and carbon dioxide (Pa_{CO_2}) tension. More explicitly, the function of the ventilator can be described in terms of the $\dot{V}$, V, P, f, I/E ratio, but the efficacy of the ventilator operating in concert with the patient's lungs (the adequacy of the resultant respiration) requires close monitoring of arterial blood gases.

HEMODYNAMIC EFFECTS OF POSITIVE PRESSURE VENTILATION

There is a normal phasic variation in stroke volume of the two ventricles of the heart during normal breathing. During inspiration venous return is increased with increased filling of the right ventricle, resulting in an increased stroke volume of the right ventricle. During expiration pulmonary venous return is increased to the left atrium with increased filling of the left ventricle and a resultant increased stroke volume of the left ventricle. During positive pressure-cycled ventilation, normal phasic variation is altered. Inspiration is no longer a negative pressure event; both inspiration and expiration are now positive pressure events. Since inspiration is now a positive pressure event, venous return to the right ventricle may be retarded, which could be reflected in terms of a reduced cardiac output and hypotension. The overall effect of positive pressure-cycled ventilation on these hemodynamic variables will depend on the patient's baseline cardiovascular status and the mean airway pressure being produced by the ventilator. Mean airway pressure is defined as the average pressure over a series of breathing cycles (Fig. 22-5). Mean airway pressure can be increased by

1. increasing driving pressure, airway pressure (Paw) (Fig. 22-5A);
2. increasing frequency, resulting in a shortening of apneic time (Fig. 22-5B);
3. production of an inspiratory hold (Fig. 22-5C);

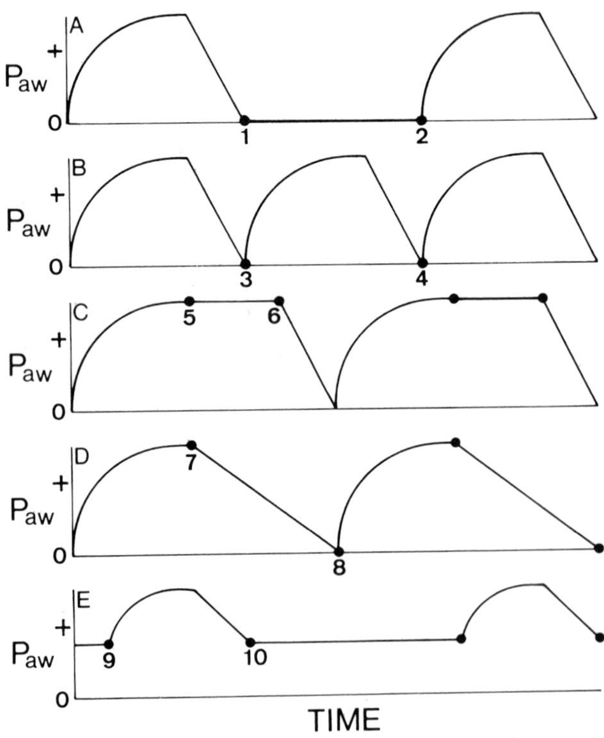

Fig. 22-5. Effects of cycle variations on mean airway pressure. Airway pressure *(Paw)* in cm H_2O is plotted as a function of time over several ventilatory cycles. Each cycle variation increases mean airway pressure: *(A)* increased Paw; apneic period occurs between points 1 and 2; *(B)* increased frequency; an additional respiratory cycle occurs between points 3 and 4, obliterating the apneic period; *(C)* inspiratory hold; that is, between points 5 and 6; *(D)* expiratory retard; that is, between points 7 and 8; *(E)* continuous positive pressure ventilation; that is, between points 9 and 10.

4. production of expiratory retard (Fig. 22-5D); and
5. continuous positive pressure ventilation (ventilation in which at end expiration a positive pressure is maintained) (Fig. 22-5E)

In patients with borderline hemodynamic status, increasing mean airway pressure may decrease the patient's cardiac output further so that he becomes a candidate for vascular volume expansion, vasopressors, or other hemodynamic support. An increase in cardiac output and systemic blood pressure can often be accomplished by *decreasing* any of the variables presented in Figure 22-5.

OTHER MECHANICAL DEVICES THAT AID LUNG INFLATION

Changes in the rhythmicity of breathing reportedly have major physiologic consequences. Mead and Collier originally reported that in dogs breathing spontaneously or ventilated with a pump, when periodic hyperinflation or sighing maneuvers were stopped, the lungs became progressively stiffer (*i.e.*, pulmonary compliance decreased with time by an average of 33%).[5] The gross appearance of the dogs' lungs postmortem provided direct evidence that this decrease in compliance was due to small airway closure.

These observations in dogs were substantiated by the observations of Ferris and Pollard in normal adults and convalescent patients with muscle paralysis due to poliomyelitis.[4] These workers showed that, after a series of deep breaths, shallow breathing in the tidal volume range resulted in decreased compliance of 26% to 40%. Two or more deep breaths to the limit of inspiration after the period of shallow breathing produced increased compliance that could be eliminated by a forced expiration.

INCENTIVE SPIROMETRY

A sigh has been defined as a maneuver that produces an inspiratory volume at least three times that of a normal tidal volume—that is, the volume of a sigh should exceed 1500 cc. As a subject sighs, the transpulmonary pressure becomes more negative (see Fig. 22-1). The pulmonary airways are exposed to this more negative pressure—that is, there is an increased pressure difference between the inner and outer walls of the airway (an increased transmural pressure). The above described investigations and those of others have established that periodic sighs and the attendant increase in transmural airway pressure are necessary to maintain airway patency. Postoperatively, pain and analgesic medication decrease the frequency of sighing. Such patients become susceptible to airways closure, clinically defined as atelectasis, and to a progressive decrease in pulmonary compliance.

In the early 1960s, the concept of intermittent positive-pressure breathing (IPPB) was introduced to postoperative care, despite the above described physiologic evidence on the interrelationships between changes in compliance, hyperinflation, and sighing. The central question was whether IPPB was the optimal approach to the problem of airway closure.

In the latter part of the 1960s and the early 1970s, the role of a deep, sustained inspiration (sigh or yawn) in the management of atelectasis was rediscovered.[1,3,6] Bartlett and coworkers recently compared expiratory maneuvers, CO_2-induced hyperinflation, IPPB, and voluntary maximal inhalation to the ideal respiratory maneuver that would reverse the pathophysiologic features of airway closure.[2] This work provides the basis for the development of the incentive spirometer, a device that encourages a patient to perform a voluntary hyperinflation maneuver that is sustained at peak inspiration for 5 to 10 seconds (Fig. 22-6). The number of times the maneuver is per-

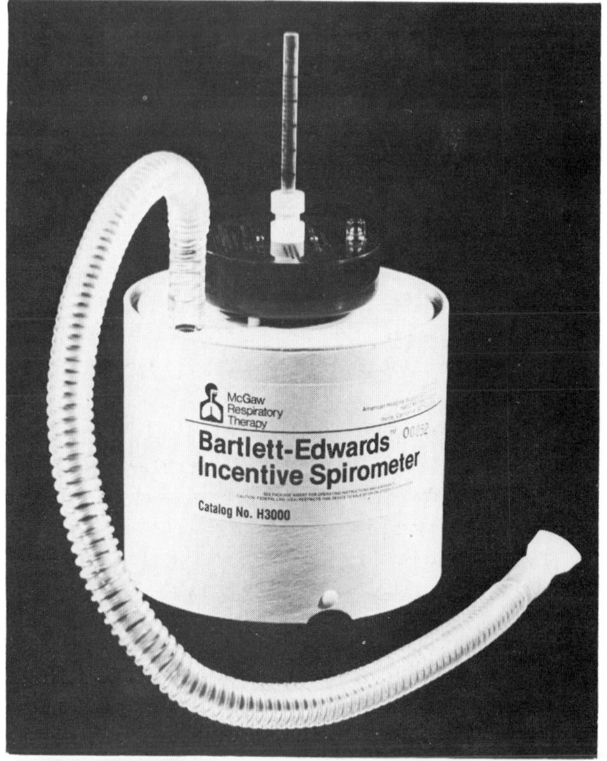

Fig. 22-6. A representative incentive spirometer.

formed is recorded, providing a feedback "carrot or the stick" system for the patient.

SUMMARY

The physiologic variables that occur during a normal, spontaneous breathing cycle provide the physiologic basis for the clinical application of ventilators. This chapter stresses the point that the difference between the two types of most commonly used ventilators (pressure-cycle and volume-cycled) relates to which of the variables of $\dot{V}$, V, P, f, and I/E the operator can manipulate. Appropriate clinical application of ventilators requires a basic knowledge of the mechanical properties of the lung, ventilation/perfusion relationships, and arterial blood gases. The hemodynamic consequences of ventilator therapy are related to mean airway pressure and the underlying hemodynamic status of the patient.

Intermittent sighing is necessary to maintain airway patency and to prevent atelectasis. Incentive spirometry is one technique for reproducing a sigh and is therefore a means of potentially treating, or preventing, atelectasis.

REFERENCES

1. Bartlett RH, Gazzaniga AB, Geraghty T: The yawn maneuver: Prevention and treatment of postoperative pulmonary complications. Surg Forum 22:196, 1971
2. Bartlett RH, Gazzaniga AB, Geraghty T: Respiratory maneuvers to prevent postoperative pulmonary complications: A critical review. JAMA 224:1017, 1973
3. Bartlett RH, Krop P, Hanson EL et al: Physiology of yawning and its application to postoperative care. Surg Forum 21:222, 1970
4. Ferris BG Jr, Pollard DS: Effect of deep and quiet breathing on pulmonary compliance in man. J Clin Invest 39:143, 1960
5. Mead J, Collier C: Relation of volume history of lungs to respiratory mechanics in dogs. J Appl Physiol 14:669, 1959
6. Ward RJ, Danziger F, Bonica JJ et al: An evaluation of postoperative respiratory maneuvers. Surg Gynecol Obstet 123:51, 1966

23

Intermittent Positive Pressure Breathing

Irwin Ziment

Since the first edition of *Respiratory Care* was published, intermittent positive pressure breathing (IPPB) has continued to occupy center stage as the villain that we love to hate in the ongoing saga, "What Is Wrong with Respiratory Therapy?" Despite all the hisses and boos that have been directed at IPPB, surprisingly few studies during the last 6 years have added to our understanding of this controversial modality. The opening statement that introduced this chapter in the first edition of *Respiratory Care* is no longer true: "Much of the daily activity of respiratory therapists is devoted to the administration of . . . IPPB. . . ." Indeed, there are now numerous therapists in hospitals across the country who never give IPPB, and recent school graduates may regard positive pressure respirators as being living fossils of an ignoble past era of nonscientific and unscrupulous exploitation of respiratory patients by means of these mechanical bandits.

Although IPPB had been criticized for many years, the respiratory community suddenly voiced its collective *mea culpa* in 1974 when the lack of rationale underlying the use of IPPB was given forceful publicity by the Sugarloaf Conference on the Scientific Basis of Respiratory Therapy.[32] It was hoped that the next few years would produce a clearer understanding as to how IPPB should be used, but unfortunately little in the way of additional useful information has become available. Indeed, at the follow-up conference sponsored by the National Heart, Lung, and Blood Institute (NHLBI) in 1979, which was directed at the Scientific Basis of In-Hospital Respiratory Therapy, IPPB received comparatively little attention, and no new therapeutic guidelines emerged.[29]

Recently, a collaborative study was published by the IPPB Trial Group, which conducted a multicenter clinical evaluation under the sponsorship of the NHLBI. Nearly 1000 outpatients with chronic obstructive pulmonary disease were treated for an average of 33 months with three times a day self-therapy using IPPB or a compressor nebulizer. It was concluded that if any advantage exists for IPPB in this setting, it must be marginal.[12a]

In this chapter, it is not possible to provide definitive answers as to the role of IPPB in the 1980s, and there is some doubt as to whether full scientific evaluation of this modality can be expected in the next few years. Thus, this review will be based on older concepts about positive pressure breathing, with the addition of some newer information on advocated approaches to the use of IPPB. Clearly, however, a major fault with intermittent positive pressure breathing is the emphasis on "positive pressure," since the principle involved in intermittent breathing treatments with a respirator should be based on the delivery of augmented volumes, with considerably less emphasis on the pressure being used.

Anyone who analyzes the literature on IPPB will recognize that most studies have assumed that there is a standard protocol for the use of positive pressure therapy; this is certainly not so. In most reports, there has been no description of the volume delivered, of the breathing rate and pattern, whether pauses were allowed for coughing and expectoration, and exactly what dosages of drugs were nebulized; on the other hand, most investigators have emphasized the pressure that was used, thereby demonstrating a preoccupation with the least relevant variable. Of even greater concern in any study should be the competence, enthusiasm, and reliability of the therapist who delivers the IPPB, but generally this vital factor has been ignored.[44] Considerations such as these illustrate that detailed documentation and rigorous controls must be reported in any study on IPPB if meaningful conclusions are to be drawn from the results obtained. Unfortunately, most of the literature lacks such requisites, and thus the clinical value as well as the therapeutic effects of IPPB remains controversial.

WHAT IS IPPB?

The concept of positive pressure respiration was first carefully investigated and developed by Barach, who introduced the modality into the management of various pulmonary disorders.[2] His studies on intermittent positive pressure breathing found an important application in the methods of delivery of oxygen to pilots flying at high altitudes during World War II. Around that time, Bennett developed a suitable valve that permitted the intermittent delivery of oxygen under pressure during inspiration, and subsequently the Bennett family of respirators was introduced into respiratory medicine as a result of the studies of Motley and his colleagues.[26,27] By 1950, IPPB had started its meteoric career as a major type of therapy for various disorders of the lungs, and the popularity of the modality in the United States rapidly outgrew the rather meager efforts to discern its scientific validity. The entry of the Bird pressure-cycled respirators into the medical field led to a form of competition in which the operational characteristics of the rival machines became the major considerations, whereas the actual therapeutic value of IPPB ceased to attract critical attention.

The present concept of IPPB therapy is one of repeated administration of a series of augmented inhalations of variable volume delivered by a pressure-cycled respirator, each followed by the subject exhaling to atmospheric pressure. The machines in use are readily triggered by the patient's inspiratory effort, and the sensitivity can be adjusted to ensure that minimal effort is required. The respirator can deliver air, oxygen, or a combination of these, or any other therapeutic gas that is selected (e.g., a mixture of oxygen and helium). Usually, concomitant nebulization of either a "bland" or a "therapeutic" aerosol is provided. Most frequently the patient is treated for 10 to 20 minutes during an IPPB session, and these sessions are generally given three or four times daily, although administrations may be given as often as every hour. If more frequent treatment is given, the patient will usually be intubated or tracheostomized; of course, if continued respirator inhalations are delivered, this no longer constitutes IPPB therapy but must be regarded as ventilatory support. IPPB is usually administered by means of a mouthpiece, although a well-fitting face mask is occasionally used. In an intubated or tracheotomized patient, the machine can be connected to the endotracheal tube for each IPPB session.

Portable respirators are available for home use, and various devices are incorporated into the different models that may confer additional benefits. There is little evidence to suggest that one particular model is outstandingly advantageous among the popular devices currently marketed for routine treatments.

The major requirements of any IPPB respirator have been identified by Motley and coworkers.[27] The device should be simple, and there should be a sensitive cycling mechanism, high instantaneous flow potential, and an adjustable flow rate. In all cases, adequate humidification of the inspired gas must be provided for; if the possible drying of secretions is a major concern, a suitable humidifier or nebulizer must be incorporated.

SCALE OF USE OF IPPB

At the Sugarloaf Conference in 1974, Baker reported that 5% to 10% of patients admitted to general hospitals receive IPPB treatments, with a relative preponderance of IPPB given to surgical patients.[1] The use of IPPB at different institutions varied considerably. The charge per treatment in the hospitals responding to Baker's inquiry varied from $3.75 to $7.50 or more, but it has recently been reported that charges in one area varied from $8.33 to $18.00.[12] Although this is an example of inflationary trends, the more important lesson is that hospitals often use IPPB in very individualistic ways to generate revenue, and thus have exposed the modality to severe criticism. In recent years, there has been a marked, but not universal, trend to decrease the amount of IPPB given, but this has not resulted in overall declines in income of respiratory therapy departments.[4] Indeed, the question of cost-effectiveness of IPPB has still not been resolved.

The frequency of administration of routine IPPB therapy is also variable, and convention, rather than science, has resulted in the customary 15 to 20 minutes of therapy given three or four times daily. Most physicians are relatively lax in their orders, and the length of each session is generally left to the judgment of the therapist or nurse giving the IPPB or to the patient who accepts or self-administers the treatment.

PHYSIOLOGICAL EFFECTS OF IPPB

The effects of substituting the inspiratory *negative* pressure in the airway that occurs during normal breathing (*see* Chap. 22) with *positive* pressure during IPPB have been carefully evaluated by numerous workers. Although findings have varied somewhat depending on the exact method of delivery of the positive pressure, some clearly defined effects can be summarized.

Since IPPB results in a positive intrathoracic pressure during inspiration, the most important difference in physiological consequences is seen in the pulmonary circulation (Fig. 23-1). The enhanced venous return that accompanies the inspiratory cycle in normal breathing is reversed during IPPB. Venous return is diminished and the total thoracic blood volume decreased. Blood in the pulmonary vasculature is "squeezed" into the left ventricle and cardiac output temporarily augmented. If the positive pressure is maintained, however, the pulmonary blood flow soon decreases because venous return remains impeded, and the initial enhancement of cardiac output is succeeded by a gradual decrease to less than normal, whereas pulmonary vascular pressure increases.[37]

In effect, positive pressure breathing acts as an intrathoracic tourniquet and results in peripheral venous pooling. If the inspiratory phase is prolonged sufficiently, marked circulatory changes may be induced, and a significant fall in blood pressure may occur, particularly if the patient has concomitant cardiovascular inadequacy or hypovolemia. The circulatory

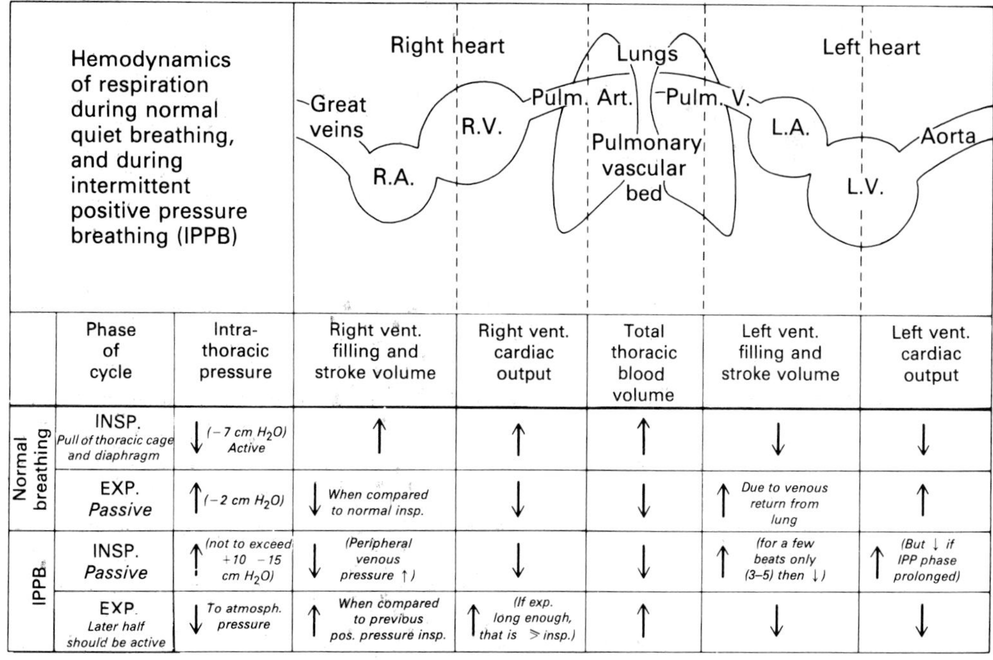

	Phase of cycle	Intra-thoracic pressure	Right vent. filling and stroke volume	Right vent. cardiac output	Total thoracic blood volume	Left vent. filling and stroke volume	Left vent. cardiac output
Normal breathing	INSP. *Pull of thoracic cage and diaphragm*	↓ *(−7 cm H_2O) Active*	↑	↑	↑	↓	↓
	EXP. *Passive*	↑ *(−2 cm H_2O)*	↓ *When compared to normal insp.*	↓	↓	↑ *Due to venous return from lung*	↑
IPPB	INSP. *Passive*	↑ *(not to exceed +10 − 15 cm H_2O)*	↓ *(Peripheral venous pressure ↑)*	↓	↓	↑ *(for a few beats only (3–5) then ↓)*	↑ *(But ↓ if IPP phase prolonged)*
	EXP. *Later half should be active*	↓ *To atmosph. pressure*	↑ *When compared to previous pos. pressure insp.*	↑ *(If exp. long enough, that is > insp.)*	↑	↓	↓

Fig. 23-1. Comparison of the effect of spontaneous and artificial ventilation on cardiovascular hemodynamics. Whether the artificial ventilation is produced as IPPB or IPPV, the qualitative changes in hemodynamics are the same. (Adapted from Sheldon GP: Pressure breathing in chronic obstructive lung disease. Medicine *42*:197, 1963)

changes are further increased during IPPB if the subject breathes out against a resistance, such as an expiratory retard valve.

As has been discussed in Chapter 22, to ensure that the effects on the circulation are minimized, one must use relatively low pressures with an adequate flow rate during the administration of IPPB. An additional requirement is that the respirator can provide a rapid, instantaneous initial flow during inspiration. The dry gas source should be able to provide a similarly high instantaneous flow of at least 100 liters/min. In practice, any of the more popular pressure respirators delivers adequate IPPB, and no published comparison has suggested that either the flow patterns or any of the other attributes of any machine results in significantly superior therapy. Although many therapists give considerable attention to the flow patterns generated by individual machines, these patterns are in fact extremely variable, and most physicians give little heed to them.

BENEFICIAL EFFECTS OF IPPB ON THE RESPIRATORY TRACT

IPPB is used primarily to produce "beneficial" changes within the lungs, but additional benefits may be produced in the cardiovascular system and in the patient's psyche.

The principal effects of IPPB resulting from administration of gas under pressure must be differentiated from those attributed to nebulization therapy. For the pressure effects of IPPB to be of value, each inspiration must deliver a tidal volume equal to or greater than that of the patient breathing spontaneously. Unfortunately, rarely is there any certainty that an augmented volume has been achieved, *unless the therapist or nurse takes the trouble to monitor the volume delivered.* Ideally, IPPB respirators should possess gauges that register the volume delivered to enable adjustments to be made in achieving the appropriate tidal volume. A major fault with most IPPB treatments is that the therapist does not measure objectively whether this requirement is being achieved. The valuable studies by Yanda illustrate that, generally, such quality control with regard to IPPB administration is woefully inadequate.[45,46]

Assuming an adequate volume is delivered at an appropriate frequency (8–10 breaths per minute in an adult with a modest increase in airway resistance), using the lowest possible flow rates, certain physiological changes can be expected.[35,37] These are discussed below.

EFFECT ON $\dot{V}/\dot{Q}$

Increased tidal volume will result in better delivery of gas to areas of the lung that are relatively hypoventilated during normal breathing. In a patient with airways disease, the augmented inspiratory volume will result in improved ventilation to the most compliant areas, such as nonatelectatic areas (see Fig. 23-2). However, expansion of these alveoli causes impaired blood supply, and thus IPPB may result in an actual worsening of local $\dot{V}/\dot{Q}$ relationships. Changes in the $\dot{V}/\dot{Q}$ matchings in different zones of the lungs are difficult to measure but appear to be insignificant in practice.[28]

EFFECTS ON VENTILATION

Improved ventilation will enable an overall increase in equilibration of oxygen to occur in the alveoli and across the alveolar–capillary membrane. Thus, it has been shown that for any concentration of inspired oxygen, hypoxic respiratory patients will usually attain a higher Pa_{O_2} with IPPB than when breathing the same oxygen concentration spontaneously at ambient pressure. Generally, the improvement is short-lived. The increase in tidal volume and in minute ventilation generally achieved with appropriately given IPPB causes a decrease in Pa_{CO_2} that may be transient or may persist for several hours, depending on the state of the diseased lung and the respiratory pattern of the patient.

EFFECT ON AIRWAY RESISTANCE

The entry of gas under positive pressure causes dilation of the airways, thereby resulting in decreased airway resistance during inspiration if low flow rates are used. If bronchospasm is simultaneously decreased (by bronchodilator aerosol) and mucus loosened, a progressive fall in airway resistance may be attained with each of a number of breaths. There is also evidence that decreased compliance caused by abnormal breathing patterns may be reversed by IPPB.[29]

EFFECT ON WORK OF BREATHING

If the patient is taught to relax while taking IPPB treatments, thereby allowing the machine to deliver the gas volume without continued inspiratory effort by the patient, the work of breathing can be decreased. The sensitivity of the respirator should be adjusted so that the patient need make only a slight inspiratory effort to trigger the machine into cycling, after which only minimal voluntary effort is required. If the respirator delivers low flow rates at low pressures, the severely obstructed patient may be able to effect gaseous exchange with less work of breathing during the IPPB treatment. Significant sustained decreases in the work of breathing may be produced by several IPPB treatments daily in patients with chronic disorders that decrease chest wall or pulmonary compliance, such as with kyphoscoliosis, obesity, or interstitial lung disease.[29] A decrease in the work of breathing is achieved, however, only if the patient can relax and allow the machine to inflate the lungs. This will not occur unless he is taught how to take the IPPB treatment; skilled supervision is needed to ensure that the machine settings (and thus the gas inflow rate) and the patient's breathing technique are appropriately matched. If these optimal circumstances are not achieved, and particularly if the patient "fights" the machine, then the work of breathing may be considerably increased.[40]

EFFECT ON RESPIRATORY TRACT SECRETIONS

As a consequence of the increased tidal volume and the decreased airway resistance produced by IPPB, trapped mucus that is inspissated may be removed. The mechanical expansion of the air passages stretches and breaks rings of mucoid material, thereby allowing gas to enter occluded bronchi. Further, some gas may enter atelectatic acini in the bronchial tree by circumventing the occluded airway, perhaps by crossing through the canals of Lambert and the pores of Kohn.[19]

When inspired gas is delivered in this manner to poorly ventilated distal segments of the lung, it may undergo compression during expiration and exert positive force on proximally sited plugs of secretions. The inspissated material can then be affected by cephalad-moving forces such as coughing or suctioning. Accordingly, one can readily visualize a mechanism by which IPPB may result in the movement of secretions from occluded bronchi up the tracheobronchial tree (Fig. 23-2).

EFFECTS ON PULMONARY FUNCTION

Yanda demonstrated that the only pulmonary function variable that could be accurately determined by clinical observation during IPPB was the respiratory rate![45] Moreover, optimal ventilation cannot be distinguished from nonoptimal by simple clinical observation. Although it is generally considered that *tidal volume* is increased by IPPB, this is not necessarily so, and unless the therapist monitors the treatment and measures the expired volume, in many cases the tidal volume will be inadequate.[34] This is more likely

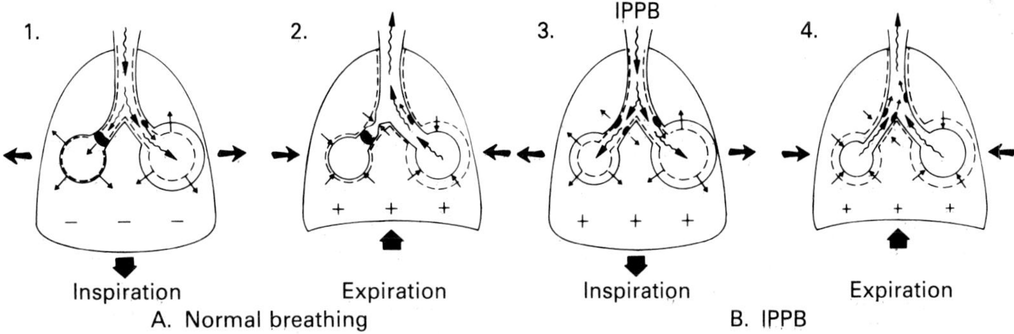

Fig. 23-2. Theoretical effect of IPPB on secretions. *(A)* Normal breathing. 1. The plug of inspissated secretions associated with a partially atelectatic lung module is drawn distally during inspiration as a result of the negative intrapleural pressure. The nonatelectatic area expands during inspiration, and a mucus plug in the supplying bronchus tends to be moved distally to a slight extent by the incoming breath. 2. During expiration the positive intrapleural pressure tends to cause compression of the bronchus supplying the atelectatic module, and the plug is not moved proximally. The nonatelectatic module compresses the air, and exhalation occurs forcefully, moving the mucus plug proximally. *(B)* IPPB. 3. During inspiration the positive pressure wave tends to expand the airway supplying an atelectatic area, as well as a nonatelectatic area. The dilatation of the airway breaks up the mucus plug and allows air to enter the atelectatic module. Mucus plugs tend to move distally. 4. During expiration the positive intrapleural pressure compresses the air in the ventilated lung units. The air is expelled forcefully, and mucus is moved proximally up the tracheobronchial tree from the atelectatic area as well as from the normally ventilated area.

to occur if the patient is in pain or is very dyspneic, has low pulmonary compliance or high airway resistance, or if either the patient or the therapist has inadequate training or ability.

Only about one half of patients obtain a transient but significant increase in vital capacity after IPPB. Obviously, *minute ventilation* may be affected by many variables, and an increase cannot be guaranteed by using IPPB without rigorous controls. Although IPPB has been shown to cause variable alterations in *ventilation/perfusion* matching, it is rarely clear, particularly with the diseased lung, whether IPPB causes a more significant increase in alveolar ventilation or in decrease in perfusion of lung units.

Other changes in pulmonary function caused by IPPB have been reported. Several workers have shown that the uniformity of *alveolar ventilation*, as measured by the nitrogen washout, may not be improved by IPPB; further, any improvement was similar to that obtained during voluntary hyperventilation. The *dead space/tidal volume* (V_D/V_T) ratio remains unaffected if the alveolar ventilation does not change much with IPPB; however, hyperventilation may increase the ratio.[20] Although normally V_D/V_T decreases as V_T rises in patients with lung disease, IPPB is more likely to produce an increased V_D/V_T.

Most studies on the *spirometric effects* of IPPB show that there is marked improvement in *bronchospastic* subjects with obstructive pulmonary disease only if bronchodilators are aerosolized (Fig. 23-3). If plain saline is nebulized, then spirometric measurements may worsen, and if IPPB without any aerosol is given, the same adverse result may be obtained.

Several workers now have shown that IPPB with bronchodilator drugs does not produce any significant long-term improvement in spirometry, even when administered for many weeks, in patients with chronic obstructive pulmonary disease.[6,17]

The overall conclusion is that IPPB, *without concomitant aerosol therapy*, may result in adverse changes in pulmonary function, particularly in patients who have underlying lung disease. In situations where IPPB produces subjective improvements in a patient's airway function, there is rarely any objective evidence of persistent beneficial changes in pulmonary function testing. Further, most benefits attribut-

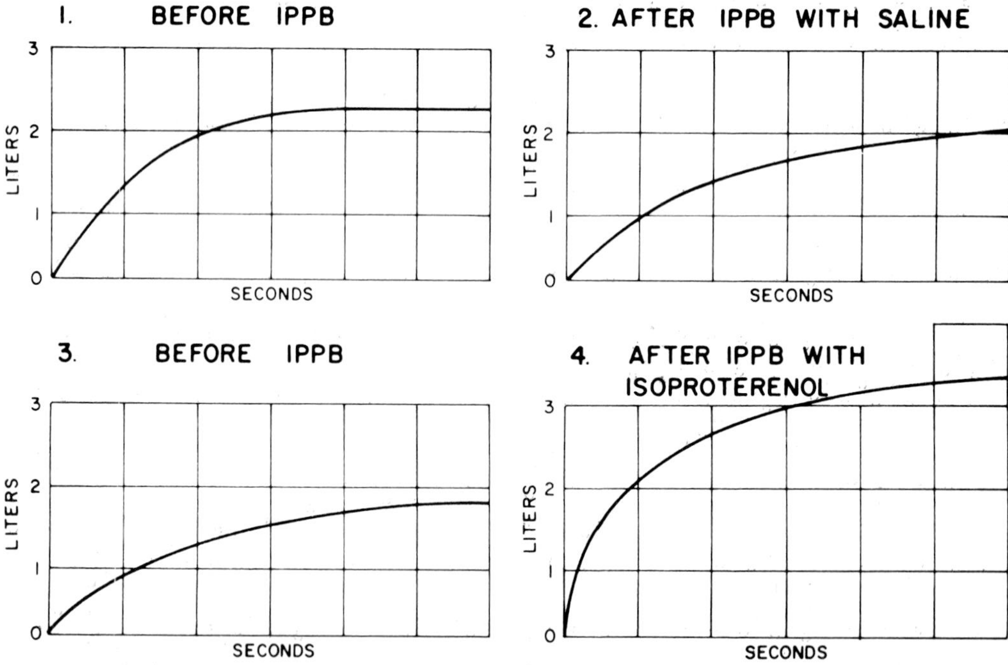

Fig. 23-3. Effect of IPPB therapy on spirometry. This figure is based on the actual spirometry of a cooperative asthmatic patient who received aerosol by a Bird Mark 8 respirator. *(1)* Spirogram before nebulization. *(2)* Spirogram obtained after nebulization of 2 ml of normal saline by IPPB: The flow and vital capacity have decreased. *(3)* A few minutes later increased spirometric deterioration had occurred. The subject was then given nebulization of 0.5 ml of isoproterenol in 1.5-ml normal saline, using the same IPPB machine. *(4)* Following the isoproterenol, improvement in flow and vital capacity was found.

able to IPPB are caused by concomitant bronchodilator administration, and other, simpler methods of nebulizing these drugs produce equally acute changes in spirometry. Finally, long-term use of IPPB in patients with chronic, stable obstructive disease does *not* produce measurable benefits in pulmonary function, and may in fact be accompanied by progressive spirometric deterioration, although this does not necessarily imply that IPPB is the cause.[7,16]

OTHER PHYSIOLOGICAL EFFECTS OF IPPB

FLUID BALANCE

When humidified gas is delivered into the respiratory tract, insensible water loss is decreased and water may, in fact, be absorbed, resulting in a positive fluid balance. If saline is given by nebulization, appreciable quantities of sodium chloride may be absorbed and may even result in hypernatremia. In some patients, peripheral edema may develop, particularly if the person has cardiac, renal, or hepatic disease or is taking corticosteroid drugs. Of course, this adverse effect is partly due to the swallowing and gastric absorption of saline deposited in the oropharynx.

A further interesting effect of IPPB, which might be a secondary consequence of the increased venous pressure, is the development of an antidiuresis, resulting in further fluid retention.[8] This may be mediated by stimulation of osmoreceptors in the hypothalamus, resulting in increased secretion of antidiuretic hormone (ADH) by the posterior lobe of the pituitary gland.[15] An appreciable antidiuretic effect does not occur commonly, and in fact the opposite effect, diuresis resulting from IPPB, has been reported.

CEREBRAL FUNCTION

Patients may experience various changes in nervous system function when they receive IPPB therapy. The mystique of mechanized medical practice can have a profound psychic effect, and psychologic consequences, both good and bad, may occur. Undoubtedly, one of the arts of respiratory medicine is to convince the patient that therapy is of value, and such conviction results in a grateful, appreciative recipient. Without doubt, psychologic responses are at least as relevant as physiological effects in many patients.

There can, however, be pure neurophysiologic responses during respiratory therapy. Changes in the blood gases occurring rapidly or slowly as a result of IPPB may result in improved cerebral function. Thus, an appropriate increase in Pa_{O_2} and a decrease in Pa_{CO_2} with restoration of the pH toward 7.40 will have marked benefits in subjects with acute, uncompensated respiratory failure. However, rapid blowing-off of CO_2 will result in an acute respiratory alkalemia and may cause the patient to experience lightheadedness, fatigue, dizziness, anxiety, and paresthesias; in extreme cases, epileptiform seizures and cardiac arrhythmias may occur.

If a patient receives a prolonged session of positive pressure therapy, or frequent IPPB, decreased venous return to the heart may result, to a minor degree, in the superior vena caval syndrome. The patient experiences a full-headed sensation and may develop a headache, and there will sometimes be evidence of impaired cerebral function. A patient on continuous respirator support may actually develop evidence of cerebral edema, and the "intensive care unit syndrome" that often develops in respiratory patients may, in part, be related to this effect. The possible hazard of IPPB in neurosurgical patients is discussed in Chapter 34.

INDICATIONS FOR IPPB

IPPB is currently used for a heterogeneous collection of specific and nonspecific pulmonary conditions, ranging from "atelectasis" to "wheezing." Ideally, the physician should specify the particular, quantifiable physiological or pathologic abnormality to be corrected and then decide whether positive pressure alone or gas therapy, a drug, or bland aerosolization can be expected to reverse or alter the specific problem. On this basis a rational prescription should be developed and appropriate therapy given under competent supervision. Further, it should be expected that therapists or nurses will make contributions and observations that will enable the physician to determine whether the objectives of therapy have been achieved. The well-trained therapist must play an active role in evaluating whether the prescribed treatment has been appropriate, and further suggestions for modifying the therapeutic regimen should be made by those giving the treatment.

Beneficial effects can be obtained with IPPB *only* if it is used correctly.[48] When a sick, hospitalized patient is first introduced to a respirator, the immediate relationship is unlikely to be a happy one. Indeed, the patient may be upset by the machine, and careless "treatment" is likely to cause deterioration in the pa-

INDICATIONS FOR IPPB

General Requirements

1. Simpler, less expensive modalities not suitable or not effective enough for patient.
2. Ability of patient to use modality appropriately and with subjective benefit.
3. Adequate supervision, instruction, and technical assistance to ensure correct use of the total modality.
4. Assurance of maintenance and reliability of equipment.
5. Periodic objective evaluation of effects of IPPB therapy.

Entities to Be Treated

1. Hypoventilation owing to inadequate tidal volume.
2. Mucostasis owing to hypoventilation, inadequate cough, hyperviscous secretions, airway obstruction.
3. Atelectasis owing to hypoventilation and mucostasis.
4. Bronchospasm inadequately relieved by aerosol therapy administered without positive pressure.
5. Respiratory distress resulting from weakness, impaired chest bellows, anxiety, or panic superimposed on lung disease.
6. Pulmonary edema with foam in airways.

tient's condition. Thus the therapist has to work with the patient and persuade the unwilling subject to relax and cooperate with the machine's cycling. Indeed, relaxation is so important a requirement that a guru specializing in yoga may be more successful than a respiratory therapist!

The benefit that a dyspneic patient obtains from initial IPPB treatment is more often attributable to the calming influence of the therapist or nurse than to the qualities of the respirator. A good therapist is more valuable than a good machine, and many doctors would rather have more of the former and less of the latter. It has been well said that the respiratory therapist should concentrate more on "inspiration" when treating a patient.

In 1980 the Respiratory Care Committee of the American Thoracic Society attempted to provide rational guidelines for the use of IPPB.[36] Most of the concepts embodied in the ATS Guidelines are given consideration throughout the remainder of this chapter.

IMPROVEMENT OF OXYGENATION

It is well known that IPPB will generally increase the Pa_{O_2} in a subject with respiratory disease, even if no supplemental oxygen is delivered. If IPPB delivers a volume of air greater than that which the patient obtains during spontaneous breathing, then the relative hyperventilation will usually improve oxygenation. This effect is particularly likely to occur if a patient has areas of atelectatic change caused by shallow breathing, retention of secretions, airways disease, or restrictive disorders.

In the hospital setting, most IPPB treatments are given with oxygen-driven pressure respirators, since piped-in oxygen is generally available in hospital rooms. The use of wall oxygen to drive an IPPB unit usually results in delivered oxygen concentrations well in excess of 40%.

Without the use of an "oxygen blender," the actual concentration of oxygen delivered by a Bird respirator varies directly with pressure and inversely with flow, and, as pointed out by Fairley and Britt, the F_IO_2 can exceed 90%.[9] Consequently, most patients not only obtain improved oxygenation as a result of the increased tidal volume provided by the IPPB but actually may become temporarily *hyperoxygenated* as a result of the high F_IO_2. Since most respiratory patients require less than 40% oxygen and many such patients rely on a hypoxic drive to maintain breathing, the hyperoxygenation resulting from IPPB may be detrimental rather than beneficial. Indeed, if the only consideration in treating a patient is to improve oxygenation, then the correct way to achieve this is to deliver a precisely measured amount of oxygen by cannula or mask rather than to deliver an imprecise and excessive amount with a respirator. Further, 15 to 20 minutes of improved oxygenation every 4 to 6 hours, which is achieved with IPPB, hardly contributes meaningfully to the management of the hypoxic patient.

IMPROVEMENT IN VENTILATION

Undoubtedly IPPB can result in an increased minute ventilation achieved by administering augmented tidal volumes. This can result in a lowering of Pa_{CO_2} as a consequence of improved intrapulmonary gas mixing, and this change is usually similar to the simultaneous change (increase) in Pa_{O_2} that positive pressure produces.[36,40] A small contribution to the fall in Pa_{CO_2} may be attributed to the decrease in metabolic production of CO_2 that occurs if the patient happens to decrease the work of breathing significantly during the IPPB session.

Although decreasing the Pa_{CO_2} is a definite benefit in a patient with acute respiratory failure, where the unstable Pa_{CO_2} is undergoing a rapid decrease, there is less rationale for trying to lower the Pa_{CO_2} in a chronic, stable, fully compensated, hypercarbic patient. If the patient has a Pa_{CO_2} of, for example, 60 torr with a pH of 7.36, there is little reason for attempting to lower the Pa_{CO_2} to a more "normal" level, since the 15 or 20 minutes of hyperventilation with IPPB will simply be followed by a period of post-IPPB hypoventilation that will restore the Pa_{CO_2} back toward 60 torr. The patient will continue to maintain this level of CO_2 until the next IPPB session a few hours later, when the cycle of events will be repeated. Most evidence demonstrates that there is no sustained decrease in Pa_{CO_2} in patients with chronic stable hypercapnia.[16]

IPPB can be of value in the *initial* treatment of acute respiratory decompensation. Many patients with rapidly increasing CO_2 retention can be spared intubation and total ventilatory support by the use of frequent IPPB. Some patients will tolerate hourly treatments with IPPB sessions, each of 10 to 15 minutes, and may cooperate for periods of 24 to 48 hours during acutely unstable episodes; by so doing, these patients avoid the necessity for, and the disadvantages of, intubation.

Whether IPPB is the only way to effect a reduction in Pa_{CO_2} depends on the particular situation. Since the major means whereby IPPB lowers the Pa_{CO_2} is by achieving a state of hyperventilation for a few minutes, evidently other means of inducing an increased tidal volume could be just as effective. There are many ways in which such augmented breathing maneuvers can be achieved. Chapter 36 discusses some of these maneuvers.

Although *voluntary deep breathing* can reduce the Pa_{CO_2} in persons with normal lungs, the attempt will be less effective in patients with obstructive airway disease. Hyperventilation can be physiologically induced by having a normal person *breathe CO_2* or by the rebreathing of expired air. Devices that enforce this type of activity include the Dale–Schwartz tube and the Adler rebreather (Fig. 23-4). Although this method can result in deeper breathing, the net effect may be an increased Pa_{CO_2}, particularly if the subject has hypercarbia to begin with, since such a person has to expend considerable work to achieve hyperventilation.

Expiratory maneuvers using blow bottles or blow gloves (Fig. 23-4) have been used to improve ventilation, but the Pa_{CO_2} will not be affected unless the subject inhales deeper before exhaling. Such methods are unlikely to be effective unless enforced by an interested therapist, and it is still doubtful whether a patient with significant airways obstruction could appreciably lower his Pa_{CO_2} by these maneuvers. A similar concept employs *sustained maximal inspiration* with devices such as an incentive spirometer (Fig. 23-4); again, it is unlikely that a hypercarbic patient would succeed in decreasing the Pa_{CO_2} as effectively or for as long by such means as would be achieved by the use of correctly administered IPPB.

Although a plethora of simple devices designed to encourage patients to take deep breaths has filled the therapeutic gap resulting from the decline in popularity of IPPB, these devices are being used for those very indications that could *not* be justified when man-

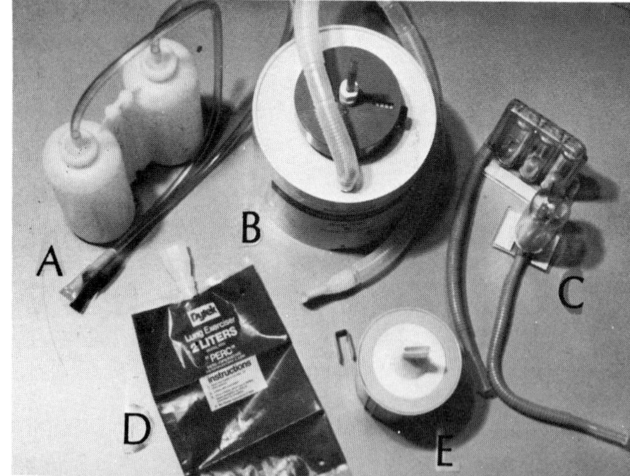

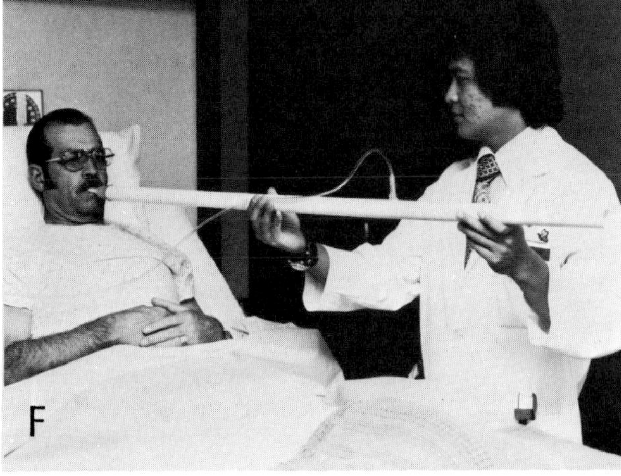

Fig. 23-4. Deep breathing devices. *(A)* Spiroflo blow bottle set (Chesebrough Pond's, Inc.). *(B)* Incentive spirometer (Bartlett–Edwards–McGaw Laboratories, Model 3000). *(C)* Uniflo and Triflo respiratory exerciser (Chesebrough Pond's, Inc.). *(D)* Dytek lung exercise. *(E)* Adler rebreather (Model AR 1). *(F)* Rebreathing tube of the Dale–Schwartz type with supplemental oxygen added.

aged by IPPB. Although the concept of device-assisted preoperative and postoperative hyperinflation of the lungs has never been shown to be of value[33]—and this led to the condemnation of much of the IPPB given in former years—this has not discouraged physicians and therapists from using incentive spirometers, respiratory exercisers, and motivators (as these simplistic devices are euphemistically labeled) with even greater lack of restraint than that which characterized the IPPB era. Not only are there little data to suggest that these "sons of IPPB" are of any value, but also general observation suggests that they are rarely used appropriately by patients or therapists.

When one examines the changing scenario in terms of cost-effectiveness, there is no evidence that the decline of IPPB led to the introduction of more economic respiratory therapy.[4] Few therapists have lost jobs, and most respiratory therapy departments have continued to show respectable gains in profits. Since most hospitals owned enough respirators to provide all the IPPB that was appropriately prescribed, the abandonment of these machines and the subsequent purchase of the newer, less expensive devices nevertheless resulted in overall increases in expenditure. Further, IPPB could be used to provide both augmented breathing and nebulization therapy; the post-IPPB era has used both hyperinflation devices and aerosol devices, thus further increasing costs. Finally, since the major economic factor has always been the time of the technician, the provision of appropriate hyperinflation treatment and of separate aerosol therapy may well result in increased expense to the patient who could have received more careful, combined treatment delivered by IPPB. Thus even if IPPB were overused, its recent eclipse with overused and poorly used alternatives may be equally scandalous, suggesting that the overreaction in favor of alternatives to IPPB now needs to be reversed so as to enable IPPB to find its rightful level of use in reducing Pa_{CO_2} and in serving as part of the "stir-up" regimen for patients at risk of pulmonary complications following major surgery, as discussed later.

PROVISION OF VENTILATORY SUPPORT

A patient may develop hypercapnia or hypoxemia for various reasons. The most rapid and the most lethal changes occur in apnea or in severe hypoventilation. Obviously, respiratory support is required in such emergencies, and sometimes IPPB with a face mask may provide sufficient ventilation to carry the patient through an apneic episode, such as might occur with a cardiac arrest. In less acute cases, frequent use of IPPB may help the patient maintain reasonable blood gas levels; thus IPPB is of value in certain conditions of hypoventilation short of a total respiratory arrest. Such conditions include primary hypoventilation, respiratory center depression caused by brain trauma or drugs, and neuromuscular insufficiency (e.g., severe kyphoscoliosis, chest injury, or massive obesity).

In all these conditions the patient may maintain a fairly satisfactory respiratory status with spontaneous breathing, but IPPB treatments every few hours may help prevent progressive deterioration in the blood gas levels. However, patients in this group more commonly need prolonged respiratory support, which can be given by a pressure-cycled or volume-cycled respirator through an endotracheal tube or by means of an external respirator. Good clinical judgment is needed to determine whether respiratory support is periodically required and to establish whether IPPB offers sufficient support.

IMPROVEMENT OF EXPECTORATION

Perhaps the greatest use for IPPB in current practice is to help loosen sticky secretions in patients with chronic sputum retention. Most patients who need help in expectoration have chronic bronchitis, but retention of tenacious secretions may be a major concern in diseases such as asthma, bronchiectasis, cystic fibrosis, pneumonia, and emphysema as well as in atelectasis. There is conflicting evidence attesting to the value of IPPB in these situations, and scientifically controlled trials comparing IPPB with other modalities are conspicuously lacking.

Unfortunately, exact studies on expectoration are difficult to carry out, since sputum production is not readily quantifiable. The patient who "expectorates" after inhalation therapy may do so because of increased salivation or bronchorrhea or because of increased coughing, and there need be no loosening of inspissated secretions to account for this "effect."

Although there may be some dispute about the apparent expectorant efficiency of IPPB, several independent factors might contribute to a therapeutic effect, but the independent role of each is difficult to determine. Thus, in most situations where IPPB is used, it is not clear whether the delivery of gas under positive pressure physically loosens the secretions or whether the distal deposition of aerosols causes pharmacologic mobilization of mucus. In actuality, the psychologic impression that the respirator makes on the patient and the active encouragement and physical participation of the therapist may contribute most to the coughing and expectoration that accompany an IPPB treatment. Most probably, it is the interaction of all these variables that results in an effective outcome.[23]

Certainly if IPPB results in an augmentation of the patient's tidal volume, poorly ventilated areas of the lung will tend to be exposed to gas exchange during positive pressure inhalation. Secretions retained in poorly ventilated or atelectatic areas will be disturbed by the movement of air and by the dilating effect on the airways. Plugs of secretions tend to become inspissated if the distal lung unit beyond the plug is poorly ventilated because absorption of air in the occluded area gradually occurs, thus creating a negative pressure that will draw the mucoid material distally. Moreover, if there is little air exchange in a lung zone, there is no forward propulsion of air generated during expiration that might drive the secretions proximally.

During the course of a 15- to 20-minute treatment with IPPB, conceivably the obstructed airways will be opened and the negative pressure in the semiatelectatic lung segment distal to the plug released, thereby reducing the suction force drawing the secretions distally. If the lung areas distal to the secretions become expanded during inspiration, the gas will be compressed during subsequent expiration, and as the airways narrow, the secretions will be exposed to a pressure gradient, with greater than atmospheric pressure on the distal side of the plug (see Fig. 23-2). Thus by opening up and aerating blocked segments of the lung, IPPB may help move secretions up the tracheobronchial tree. This process is enormously enhanced if the patient coughs effectively; once air enters alveolar zones distal to a plug, coughing maneuvers will generate a positive pressure behind the secretions that will help move the material toward the trachea.

As indicated above, there are adequate theoretical reasons for believing that positive pressure breathing *does* help mobilize secretions. Usually, however, nebulized water, electrolytes, or more sophisticated drugs are supplied as part of the therapeutic IPPB session. It is difficult to determine what proportion of the overall contribution is made by the mucus-loosening medications; indeed, some of these agents stimulate bronchorrhea and thus cause increased expectoration without necessarily loosening any of the inspissated secretions. Further, if the drugs do help liquefy secretions, this may have an adverse effect on expectoration; if the secretions lose their stickiness, they may simply run down the gravitational path into the basal parts of the lungs. Overly effective liquefaction of secretions in a patient with a poor cough can result in the virtual drowning of the victim in the resulting fluid. There is considerable doubt as to the value of IPPB administration of mucus-loosening agents in patients who do not cough during or after treatment, since such patients do not expectorate and may suffer increased blockage of airways by the more fluid secretions.

Thus IPPB may have special value as a loosener of sputum and as an augmenter of expectoration only in persons who appear to cough appropriately but who find that coughing is not effective enough to raise the viscid secretions. In contrast, persons who retain secretions only because they do not cough enough simply need to be persuaded to cough by any means available. Physical therapy, aerosol masks, coughing devices, pharyngolaryngeal stimulation with a catheter, persuasion, and coercion may be just as effective as IPPB.

PREVENTION AND TREATMENT OF ATELECTASIS

The loosening and the clearance of respiratory secretions are important in treating atelectasis. Inspissated secretions are often the main cause of atelectasis, and this problem is most likely to occur in a patient who never takes breaths of more than tidal volume size. Shallow breathing is a characteristic finding in many patients with metabolic, pharmacologic, or other forms of organic brain impairment and is a particularly common occurrence in postoperative patients with painful abdominal or thoracic wounds. Atelectasis can be forestalled in many such patients if one is aware of the liability of the person to this problem.

In the *preoperative preparation* of patients with chronic lung disease, many physicians who order IPPB treatments cannot logically justify their orders. Generally, two reasons are offered for the preoperative ritual: The bronchopulmonary cleaning effect of IPPB allegedly improves pulmonary function and lessens the liability to postsurgical atelectasis; and the patient may require IPPB after the operation, and it is therefore a sensible precaution to introduce the cooperative individual to the respirator before surgery, rather than trying to teach its use to a drowsy, sedated, uncooperative patient after the operation.

Although it is reasonable to try to improve pulmonary function in a respiratory patient before anesthesia, there is surprisingly little agreement that IPPB before surgery serves to decrease the incidence of subsequent atelectasis and other pulmonary complications. Although some studies suggest that preoperative IPPB is of value in respiratory patients, a greater number of studies suggest that no significant improvement is obtained. In summary, the value of IPPB in preventing postoperative atelectasis remains controversial.

Since the objective in preventing atelectasis is to remove secretions and to improve ventilation, it is not surprising that routinely administered IPPB may not be effective. Unfortunately, the uncontrolled way in which IPPB is administered in most hospitals fails to guarantee an increase in tidal volume or the removal of secretions. Since the patient awaiting elective surgery is not acutely ill, the respiratory therapy is usually delivered in a more casual and less effective manner when given prophylactically than when given for an established complication. Various methods of augmented breathing (e.g., Dale–Schwartz tubes, incentive spirometers, blow bottles [*see* Fig. 23-4]) and chest physical therapy may be more successful than IPPB in preventing postoperative atelectasis, although satisfactory evaluation of these alternative modalities has not been carried out in comparison with IPPB. Again, one must agree with Loehning and his colleagues who point out that "the routine preoperative use of IPPB is time-consuming, expensive, potentially harmful when improperly administered, and therefore impractical."[19] Further, evidence from McConnell and coworkers, among others, suggests that routine IPPB after surgery is of no more prophylactic value than simple deep breathing with or without a mechanical device.[22]

In contrast to the controversy about prophylactic IPPB, there is more general agreement that IPPB can be of real value in treating atelectasis once the condition has developed.[30] However, there is some doubt as to the value of the positive pressure itself, in contrast to the various bronchodilator and mucolytic drugs administered by IPPB. Certainly, the drugs may play a major role in loosening the inspissated secretions; in intubated or tracheotomized patients, these drugs may be given by direct instillation rather than by nebulization under positive pressure. Indeed, acetylcysteine may be more effective when given by instillation than when it is nebulized.[18]

Atelectasis can be managed without IPPB, either by drug administration using simple aerosolization or instillation, or by bronchoscopy. Intratracheal drug administration may be very successful, particularly if followed by postural drainage and vigorous percussion. In addition, augmented inspirations can be used in a cooperative patient. If the patient is intubated, a resuscitation bag can be used to produce large tidal volumes in the form of frequent "sighs." Another technique that may be of use is to encourage the patient to cough effectively while the surgical wound is supported. However, experienced therapists may argue that IPPB offers a more reliable way of producing large tidal volumes accompanied by aerosolization.

Thus IPPB, although very efficacious as a means of treating established atelectasis, is only one of several modalities that may be used. Once again the success of IPPB totally depends on the skill of the therapist and the cooperation of the patient, and in circumstances where one or the other is lacking, various alternatives such as chest physical therapy, drug instillation or simple nebulization, or bronchoscopy may be more suitable and at least as effective.

ADMINISTRATION OF AEROSOL THERAPY

Although most physicians regard IPPB as principally a highly effective means of delivering topical aerosol therapy, there is still considerable controversy as to how effective the modality is compared to simpler methods of nebulization.[5,24] Further, it is disturbing to find how little the average prescriber really appreciates the intricacies of aerosol pharmacology (see discussion in Chapter 20.) Consequently, the prescriptions used are sometimes very gross and often inappropriate.

Various topical drugs are considered in Chapter 20, but a few further comments will be offered here. Mucokinetic drugs are given less often by aerosol than they were a few years ago, and several of these agents have been withdrawn from the market. Of those still in use, the most popular are water alone and various concentrations of saline solutions. Other drugs, including acetylcysteine, are more controversial, and many authorities rarely use them. The question as to the effectiveness of topical mucokinetic therapy has not been completely resolved, and the quandary as to whether their administration by IPPB is of more value than mucokinetic therapy administered by other means (e.g., oral SSKI) still persists. Adequate hydration, oral drugs (such as acetylcysteine or S-carboxymethylcysteine, or SSKI), and chest physical therapy with postural drainage and percussion may serve the patient just as well as does the administration of mucokinetic agents by IPPB.

Bronchodilator aerosol therapy, in contrast, is accepted universally as an extremely effective form of topical treatment for the respiratory tract. Many studies, however, show that correct use of metered cartridges, squeeze-bulb nebulizers, or air-compressor-driven nebulizers can be just as efficient as IPPB for delivering bronchodilator drugs and that the therapeutic results show little difference between the different modalities.[39] Of interest, however, is the fact that IPPB administration of the newer, more selective drugs has become popular in England for treating severe bronchospasm.[3]

If one chooses to use IPPB, several observations must be taken into account.

1. Aerosol therapy by IPPB is very inefficient, and only about 10% to 20% of the amount of medication measured into the nebulizer will be retained in the body.[47] Of this, about half will be deposited in the airways, and the rest is likely to be swallowed and can result in systemic absorption (Fig. 23-5).
2. The conventional method of measuring out bronchodilator dosage in drops leads to further imprecision in topical therapy. IPPB aerosolization results in variable dosage; generally, the dose delivered is totally unpredictable and, moreover, essentially undeterminable.
3. Most patients with bronchospasm can successfully use metered aerosol bronchodilator preparations if the airways are not too obstructed. These patients should probably use the metered product or a hand-bulb nebulizer, since more precise dosage can be administered by a few puffs with much less trouble and expense.[14] With a somewhat more dyspneic, uncooperative, or uncoordinated patient, an air-compressor-driven nebulizer provides a simple and cheap alternative to IPPB; this form of nebulization is essential if large amounts (several milliliters) of a mucokinetic agent are to be given, since the simpler devices cannot be used to deliver more than a few puffs. Further, some medications are not available in metered-dose cartridges.
4. The main advantages of IPPB aerosolization are seen in patients who are unable to use simpler devices effectively.[5] IPPB may also offer an advantage in patients who cannot take a deep breath and hold it unless the pressure respirator is used to control the pattern of breathing (e.g., patients with status asthmaticus).
5. Aerosolization of mucokinetic agents with IPPB may be tried when simpler measures (such as aerosol mask therapy and physical therapy) fail to produce optimal expectoration. However, IPPB aerosolization usually constitutes only half the treatment, and this might be worse than no treatment at all. To complete the full treatment, aerosolization should be accompanied by supervised coughing efforts and should be followed by postural drainage if ex-

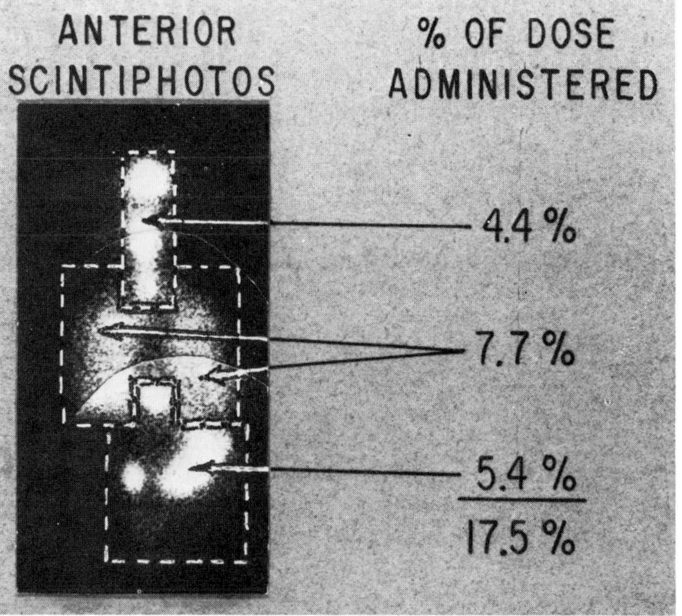

Fig. 23-5. Distribution of aerosol delivered by IPPB in an experienced patient who received a routine IPPB treatment, using 2 ml of a solution of normal sodium chloride containing a radioactive tracer. Immediately after the completion of the nebulization, the patient underwent scanning. The anterior scintiphotos were made into a composite photograph, which showed that only 17.5% of the original radioactive tracer was retained in the body. Less than 10% of the original amount was deposited in the lungs, and a greater amount was deposited in the mouth and pharynx and was then swallowed.

pectoration cannot be induced with the patient in the upright position. It is a great error to rely on IPPB aerosolization alone to produce expectoration in a weak, badly obstructed, or poorly motivated patient. Chest physical therapy, with or without IPPB, is needed by such patients.

6. A mainstream nebulizer may deliver more drug into the lung than a sidestream nebulizer, and Sheldon suggests that greater dilution of a bronchodilator is needed if a mainstream nebulizer is used.[38] Surprisingly, however, the validity of this recommendation has not been established.
7. Although it is conventional to dilute bronchodilator drugs for nebulization over the course of 10- to 20-minute intermittent positive pressure breathing treatment, equal results may be obtained in many patients by using undiluted drug and giving just 1 to 2 minutes of IPPB nebulization. This more economical form of therapy should be preferred for the average patient with bronchospasm.

TREATMENT OF PULMONARY EDEMA

In the 1960s, IPPB was recommended for treating pulmonary edema, and some of the explanations for its apparent success are listed in Table 23-1. The introduction of potent, rapidly acting diuretics and the improved prophylactic management of patients at risk has reduced the need for IPPB to be used as a major modality in treating congestive heart failure. However, IPPB may still be of adjunctive value in managing patients who present in acute pulmonary edema with severe airway obstruction and hypoxemia. The value of nebulized alcohol to break up the foam in the airways should be kept in mind.

USES OF IPPB

Table 23-1 summarizes the important uses of IPPB. The major explanations for the effectiveness of IPPB in each condition are summarized and the possible disadvantages listed. Although there are few valid indications for IPPB, its apparent successes are not always susceptible to mechanistic explanation, and a placebo effect may often be involved.[10]

The concept of the placebo effect deserves further consideration. The term "placebo" implies that a therapy is given solely to please the patient. Quite obviously, much of medical care is based on this ideal, and a therapy can be orthodox and acceptable even if no physiological benefit other than a placebo effect is detected. If the placebo succeeds in making the patient feel better and thereby reduces the patient's dependency on emergency medical services and on hospitalization, it may be fully justified. Obviously, one would not prescribe IPPB for backache or for dyspepsia, and yet massage may help backache without there being a physiological explanation, whereas aspirin seems to appeal to many patients with dyspepsia despite pharmacologic evidence that it should not. The physician who is forced to prescribe therapy that he may not fully believe in will nevertheless strive to provide the appropriate placebo for the specific disease. On this basis, IPPB is the ideal placebo for chronic respiratory disease in patients who obtain better results from the modality than from the use of simpler alternatives. In such cases we should perhaps be looking at nonphysiological parameters; perhaps IPPB releases endorphins in respiratory patients, thereby resulting in subjective improvement! If judicious use of IPPB in suitable patients reduces hospitalization or panic calls for emergency help, then its placebo value might be economically justified, since the alternatives are usually much more expensive. Thus the placebo effect of IPPB should not be scorned but should be used thoughtfully and deliberately in selected cases.

HAZARDS OF IPPB THERAPY

When IPPB is used appropriately under expert supervision, the potential dangers are minor. Unfortunately, however, much, if not most, IPPB therapy is given less than optimally. In this section the reasons why IPPB is often not given optimally will be examined and the hazards associated with such therapy enumerated.

WHY IPPB IS NOT GIVEN OPTIMALLY

Suboptimal therapy occurs at several levels: those of the physician, the patient, the therapist or nurse, and the machine.

The Physician's Role

Although IPPB is ordered by all categories of physicians in clinical practice, very few have expert knowledge on the scientific use of IPPB. Most standard textbooks in medicine and surgery fail to give *any* useful directions on the use of IPPB, and even the specialty textbooks in respiratory medicine provide little in the way of practical information and guidance.[47] Accordingly, physicians prescribe IPPB routinely and often thoughtlessly, hoping that the interaction of the machine and therapist with the patient will be beneficial. Most of the prescriptions are incomplete and inadequate; all too often the physician simply orders "IPPB q.i.d. with saline" without defining any other parameters to be used. This problem is discussed in further detail in Chapters 4 and 20.

The Patient's Role

Many patients are also impressed by complex forms of treatment, and in a society where machines such as automobiles, telephones, and television have an important effect on everyone's life, not surprisingly the delivery of medication by a compact machine authoritatively decorated with knobs, dials, and hoses offers more therapeutic promise than a simple hand-bulb nebulizer. It is not unreasonable to assume that respiratory patients in the United States react to medications delivered by IPPB machines in similar augmented fashion as would a less sophisticated patient in a foreign culture to the same medication tendered by a witch doctor flaunting feathers, rattles, and face masks! The psychologic benefits offered by a 20-minute IPPB treatment with bronchodilator obviously outweigh the therapeutic benefits that would be achieved by giving an equivalent dose of the drug in the form of a tablet or capsule. Moreover, the machine becomes a replacement symbol for the physician, particularly in the patient's home where the physician is rarely seen, and it can also serve as a sort of perverse status symbol when it becomes part of the domiciliary decor.

Although a patient may be able to use a machine correctly, most elderly, weak, and perhaps confused respiratory patients who have need for therapy cannot take a treatment correctly without constant supervision. It is an all too frequent experience to see such a patient sucking on the mouthpiece while breathing simultaneously through the nose, resulting in nothing more than a normal tidal volume and aerosolization therapy of the throat. Many chronic respiratory patients are given IPPB respirators for home use. It can easily be determined that, in many cases, the machine is used inappropriately, suboptimally or, perhaps, not at all.

The Role of the Therapist or Nurse

Although much time is spent on the education of respiratory care workers, no doubt the average technician has confused and inaccurate concepts about IPPB. Most textbooks of respiratory medicine (including those written for respiratory therapists) give surprisingly little practical information on how to deliver optimal IPPB treatments. Nurses, who are less informed in this area, generally will have the same problems to a greater degree. Moreover, since routine IPPB therapy is often regarded as a boring technical process, there is a great tendency for the nurse or therapist to provide less than adequate supervision of the treatment. A further problem is that no one on the health team is quite certain as to what results can be expected from treatment of the typical elderly patient with end-stage emphysema, for example, who has little motivation or interest in the treatment; consequently, the treatment is often given perfunctorily.

The Role of the Machine

Some still argue the merits of one respirator as compared to another. Probably any of the more popular pressure respirators can deliver an adequate treatment if used correctly. The Bennett respirators are easier for unskilled personnel to operate, whereas well-trained therapists often prefer Bird respirators. However, it is doubtful whether any respirator has qualities that make it the respirator of choice in all situations. There is little evidence that any of the wave-form characteristics of the more popular machines offer substantial therapeutic advantages over their competitors.

The major disadvantages of most respirators are as follows.

1. There is no way of determining what volume is delivered by the respirator into the patient's lungs unless this is measured. Since routine measurements of tidal volume and minute ventilation are relatively onerous to determine and are rarely made, most therapists have no precise knowledge as to what volume of gas the patient is receiving. Indeed, one wonders why volume respirators were not developed for the delivery of IPPB therapy!
2. Pressure-cycled respirators deliver variable concentrations of oxygen when this gas is used as the driving source. When air is entrained, the machines deliver a minimum of 40% oxygen; if there is a high resistance in the delivery line (e.g., if the patient has marked bronchospasm or low compliance), less air is entrained, and the concentration of oxygen delivered may rise to as high as 90%.

Table 23-1. Uses of IPPB

EFFECT	HOW IPPB WORKS	DISADVANTAGES OF IPPB
Increased Pa_{O_2}	1. Increased tidal volume 2. Improved ventilation of low-compliance lung units 3. Use of oxygen to drive respirator (*i.e.,* increased F_IO_2)	1. Simple O_2 supplementation with cannula or mask may result in the same degree of oxygenation 2. Hyperoxygenation may occur with depression of hypoxic drive 3. F_IO_2 may not be controlled readily 4. Increasing the Pa_{O_2} for a few minutes several times a day is of little value 5. Bronchodilators when given by IPPB may actually cause a fall in Pa_{O_2}
Decreased Pa_{CO_2}	1. Hyperventilation 2. Improved ventilation of low-compliance lung units 3. Decreased work of breathing	1. Overventilation may occur, resulting in respiratory alkalemia 2. Of real value only in patients with acute unstable CO_2 retention (*i.e.,* not of value in chronic stable respiratory failure) 3. Simple methods involving deep breathing may be equally effective 4. Lowering of Pa_{CO_2} may not occur unless tidal volume is increased
Improved clearance of secretions	1. Ventilation of partially obstructed lung units 2. Loosening of adherent secretions 3. Stimulation of cough 4. Delivery of aerosols and humidity	1. Simple aerosol and physical therapy are required and may work quite adequately without IPPB 2. Loosened secretions may move distally and cause worsening of $\dot{V}/\dot{Q}$, with a fall in Pa_{O_2} 3. IPPB and aerosol drugs may cause bronchorrhea rather than causing lysis of retained secretions 4. IPPB with dry gas or without bronchodilators may cause bronchospasm and inspissation of secretions
Prevention or treatment of atelectasis	1. Ventilation of atelectatic units directly and by collateral air flow 2. Loosening of secretions and stimulation of coughing 3. Stimulation of surfactant production by hyperventilation 4. Allowance of increased tidal volume with less pain in postoperative patient	1. Other simpler methods of augmented ventilation are as good or better in preventing atelectasis 2. Physical therapy (with percussion and postural drainage) may be more successful and makes better use of therapists' skills 3. Bronchoscopy may be more reliable treatment for atelectasis if due to foreign body or mucous plug 4. IPPB with large volumes may result in postoperative gastric distension or meteorism
Delivery of aerosol drugs	1. Increased tidal volume distributes aerosol distally 2. IPPB devices produce optimal aerosol particles for distal deposition 3. Treatment for 10–20 minutes gives time for airway improvement, allowing increasingly more effective drug delivery	1. Simple devices may be just as effective in practice and more tolerable if patient is dyspneic 2. IPPB is wasteful of drugs and results in extremely imprecise dosages 3. About 50% of the nebulized drug that is retained in the body is deposited in the mouth and may be swallowed; systemic absorption may occur 4. Hypoxemia may be worsened after aerosolization of bronchodilators

Table 23-1. Uses of IPPB *(continued)*

EFFECT	HOW IPPB WORKS	DISADVANTAGES OF IPPB
Treatment of pulmonary edema	1. Decreased venous return 2. Increased $F_{I}O_2$ improves oxygenation 3. Augmented tidal volumes improve oxygenation, resulting in better cardiac activity 4. A slowed breathing pattern is more efficient, leading to decreased work and better gas exchange 5. Delivery of aerosolized alcohol, which helps disperse pulmonary edema foam	1. Diuretics, oxygen, morphine, and cardiac drugs are more effective than IPPB 2. Very dyspneic patients may not be able to tolerate IPPB 3. IPPB may induce hypotension or arrhythmias in patients with cardiac failure 4. High pressures may theoretically worsen pulmonary edema 5. Effects of alcohol on pulmonary edema fluid controversial
Decreased work of breathing	1. Lungs are inflated passively 2. Opening of obstructed airways improves gas flow 3. Improved gaseous admixture allows more effective ventilatory exchange	1. If patient does not relax, work of breathing is not decreased 2. If patient resists therapy, work of breathing is increased 3. IPPB can induce coughing, which will increase work of breathing 4. Reducing the work of breathing for a few minutes several times a day is of no benefit to most patients
Improved pulmonary function tests	1. Improved blood gases owing to improved gaseous admixture 2. Decreased airway resistance owing to improved drug delivery and opening of airways	1. No measurable improvement may be produced above that attainable with simple aerosol therapy 2. No long-term improvements are produced in chronic stable obstructive pulmonary disease. IPPB without bronchodilator may cause increased airway resistance 3. Air-trapping may be produced, with measurable worsening of pulmonary function 4. Loosened secretions may impact distally, causing a fall in Pa_{O_2}

3. If inspired concentrations of oxygen of 21% are desired (and, in fact, this is generally the case), then an air source or electricity should be used to drive the machine. Accurate delivery of an FI_{O_2} in excess of 21% can be achieved, at a price, by the use of blenders that permit the choice of any concentration of oxygen greater than that of room air. However, both oxygen and air have to be supplied to the blender. For the domiciliary patient, it is both difficult and expensive to provide IPPB with controlled oxygen therapy. Regrettably, all too many domiciliary patients have been given gas-driven machines, thus increasing the expense inordinately while possibly decreasing the quality of the treatment.
4. Machines and software must be kept clean, sterile, and in good working order. This entails a lot of work for a respiratory therapy department in a hospital and constitutes a near impossibility for many domiciliary patients. The potential hazards of malfunctioning or dirty equipment often outweigh the advantages of the IPPB treatment.

All of the above-mentioned drawbacks *are* preventable or remediable within limits.

HAZARDS ASSOCIATED WITH THE USE OF IPPB

Numerous potential specific hazards can occur when IPPB is given in hospitals, and even more hazards may accompany domiciliary IPPB. The dangers are associated with the physiological effects of positive pressure breathing, the alterations in the patient's blood gas status, the effects of the medications, and the overall consequences of IPPB use. Further hazards are caused by accidents such as a malfunctioning machine, the administration of dry, nonhumidified gas, or, even worse, the delivery of dry, heated gas. The hazards are summarized in the outline on page 547, and the major ones are described in the following section; others have already been discussed in the preceding sections.

Pulmonary Effects

The main hazard attributable to IPPB is *barotrauma* (*i.e.*, overdistension of the lung). Obstruction in an airway may be bypassed during the inspiratory cycle, but during expiration the obstruction may serve as a check valve; in this way, *hyperinflation* of the distal lung unit may occasionally be produced. This phenomenon may result in growth of a bullous lesion or a cyst, with worsening of the patient's pulmonary status.

Pneumothorax is a rare complication of IPPB, but this serious event is particularly likely to occur when large volumes are delivered at high pressure to a lung that develops regional air-trapping.[13] There may be a particular danger of pneumothorax when IPPB is given to a patient with damaged lung parenchyma, such as may accompany a recent pulmonary infarction. Similarly, high-pressure IPPB may "blow" open a repaired lung following surgery if the tissue is poor or healing is compromised. Unfortunately, it is difficult to predict whether a patient is at particular risk of developing a pneumothorax, and therefore, as a general rule, caution dictates that pressures greater than 20 cm H_2O should not be given during a treatment, even though some patients may need and can tolerate pressures twice as great as this, and normal expulsive coughing pressures are many times greater than 20 cm H_2O.

A further interesting complication of high-pressure inflation has been demonstrated in laboratory animals, which may develop *pulmonary edema*.[43] This phenomenon can be prevented by the use of end-expiratory pressure, and the exact explanation as to the cause of the edema remains to be determined. This particular complication has not been shown to be a practical problem in humans, but it is reasonable to assume that high-pressure inflation may cause damage to the alveolar–capillary membrane and to the surfactant mechanism.

The inappropriate use of high flow rates is believed to be a major explanation for many of the reports of adverse consequences of IPPB. Aerosol distribution and distal lung unit ventilation are impaired when high flow rates are used. Many patients cannot tolerate high flows and are unable to obtain adequate ventilation; this leads to the patient "*fighting*" the machine, and the work of breathing will be increased. Under such circumstances, not only is little or no benefit obtained from the treatment, but also every measurable parameter might actually show deterioration, and the patient may experience dyspnea.

When IPPB is given to an inexperienced patient without adequate supervision or monitoring, hyperventilation may occur to a detrimental degree. The objective of therapy is to produce a certain amount of hyperventilation, but excessive hyperventilation as a result of incorrect use of the respirator is potentially hazardous and may result in respiratory alkalosis and seizures. There is a much smaller risk that a patient may hypoventilate while receiving improperly administered IPPB; the patient may then experience dyspnea and will often refuse further treatment.

If a patient with chronic lung disease does hyperventilate during an IPPB session, hypoxia and hypercapnia can be reversed. As a result, the patient will be left in a hyperoxic, relatively hypocapneic state, and therefore the chemical drive to respiration may be blunted.[41] Subsequently, the patient will hypoventilate just long enough to return the blood gases close to their pre-IPPB level. Following the IPPB, the patient may be tired, will have lost his ventilatory drive, and may eventually become more hypoxic if the secretions that were loosened during the IPPB are not expectorated. The busy therapist who tries to get such a patient to struggle through a treatment before rushing on to the next patient may not observe the phenomenon of *post-IPPB hypoventilation* into which the exhausted patient lapses.

Numerous reports attest to the importance of using slow inspiratory flow rates to avoid turbulent flow and rapid rise in intratracheal pressure, which may result in premature cessation of inspiration. It has been shown that too rapid an increase to a high pressure does not allow sufficient time for passive filling of lungs that have obstructed airways.[42] Such treat-

HAZARDS OF INTERMITTENT POSITIVE PRESSURE BREATHING THERAPY

- **I.** Adverse Effects of Positive Pressure
  - **A.** Pulmonary effects
    - **1.** Hyperinflation with air trapping may result in
      - **a.** dyspnea and discomfort in chest
      - **b.** growth of bullae
      - **c.** pneumothorax
    - **2.** Pulmonary edema, if very high pressures are used
  - **B.** Circulatory effects
    - **1.** Decreased venous return may result in
      - **a.** hypotension
      - **b.** increased intracranial pressure
    - **2.** Physical (and pharmacologic) disturbance of heart may cause
      - **a.** arrhythmias
      - **b.** coronary insufficiency
    - **3.** Changes in fluid balance
      - **a.** diuresis
      - **b.** fluid retention, as from increased antidiuretic hormone secretion
      - **c.** secondary electrolyte imbalance
  - **C.** Gastrointestinal effects
    - **1.** Gastric insufflation
    - **2.** Abdominal distension, with possibility of adverse effects on abdominal incisions
    - **3.** Nausea, vomiting, pulmonary aspiration
  - **D.** Effects on blood gases
    - **1.** Hypoventilation with deterioration in blood gases
    - **2.** Hyperventilation may result in
      - **a.** hyperoxia with depression of hypoxic respiratory drive
      - **b.** hypocapnia with depression of respiratory drive
      - **c.** respiratory alkalemia, causing paresthesiae, lightheadedness, liability to seizures, and so forth
- **II.** Adverse Effects of Aerosols
  - **A.** Bronchodilators
    - **1.** Systemic side-effects, such as tachycardia, arrhythmias, nervousness
    - **2.** Tachyphylaxis (with overly frequent use)
  - **B.** Mucokinetics
    - **1.** Toxic effects, such as nausea, bronchial irritation
    - **2.** Loosening of secretions with distal retention, causing hypoxemia
    - **3.** Sodium chloride retention may result in hypernatremia
  - **C.** Danger of delivering unhumidified gas that dries mucosa
  - **D.** Danger of delivering hot, dry gas if heated humidifier becomes empty, causing dehydration, irritation, and crusting of mucosa
  - **E.** Danger of delivering infected aerosol, resulting in nosocomial pneumonia
- **III.** General Adverse Effects
  - **A.** Patient may become claustrophobic or distressed by IPPB
  - **B.** Patient may not relax and may fight machine, resulting in dyspnea, increased work of breathing, and deterioration in pulmonary function
  - **C.** Patient may become "addicted" to machine, resulting in overuse and dependency

ment may be detrimental to the patient, whose work of breathing may be increased in these circumstances.

Cardiovascular Effects

Positive pressure during inspiration will reduce the venous return and can thereby result in decreased cardiac output.[21] These changes are particularly likely to occur with the use of high pressure and when the inspiratory time equals, or exceeds, the time allowed for expiration. If the patient's cardiovascular system is precariously balanced, reflex compensation for the fall in cardiac output may not occur, and *hypotension* may ensue. Other cardiac changes may include *tachycardia* and *arrhythmias*, which may result from reflex responses to the fall in blood pressure or as an autonomic response to hyperinflation of the lung. If a sympathomimetic bronchodilator is nebulized, there is a further risk of inducing tachyarrhythmias pharmacologically.

Danger of Infection

The contaminated IPPB setup provides an ideal vehicle for inducing a pulmonary infection. Needless to say, even if the IPPB treatment does not help the patient, it should not be harmful.

The various requirements to assure the sterility of the apparatus are discussed in other chapters. Probably the greatest risk to most patients is that the machine may serve as a culture site for the person's own organisms, which can then be returned in vastly increased numbers (since proliferation occurs in the tubing or nebulizer) during subsequent treatments. Although many domiciliary patients fail to keep their equipment sterile, surprisingly few seem to develop serious infections as a consequence. The probable explanation is that a stable patient in his home environment has considerable ability to resist infection from his "own" organisms, whereas the sick patient in the more vicious bacteriologic environment of the hospital has less chance of resisting a superinfection. Nevertheless, prudence demands that cleanliness and sterility of equipment be maintained both in domiciliary practice and in the institutional setting.

Miscellaneous Complications

Other complications may be induced by IPPB. Irritant aerosols may cause *bronchitis* and may result in excessive *bronchorrhea*, with the risk of distal migration of loosened secretions. Overdosage with drugs may result in problems such as *tachyphylaxis* and extrapulmonary *side-effects*. Some patients swallow air when they use IPPB, which can produce *gastric distension* or *meteorism* (insufflation of small bowel); there is then an additional risk of *vomiting*, which can be complicated by *aspiration*. Finally, the patient may develop adverse psychologic responses, such as *claustrophobia*.

CONTRAINDICATIONS FOR IPPB

Although guides to IPPB therapy generally list a number of contraindications, most of these seem to be based on unsubstantiated impressions rather than on clearly evaluated observations. Apart from untreated pneumothorax, there are hardly any *absolute* contraindications; more important in everyday practice are the few *relative* contraindications (*see* list following). Several dubious contraindications should also be mentioned.

RELATIVE CONTRAINDICATIONS

The few everyday contraindications for the use of IPPB are related to factors involved in the provision of this form of therapy more than to the dangers of optimally delivered treatment.

Lack of Expertise

In situations where there are no experienced respiratory therapy technicians, nurses, or physicians, the practical disadvantages of delivering IPPB to a patient outweigh the potential advantages of the treatment. The patient who most clearly requires IPPB is most susceptible to the harmful effects of poorly delivered treatments, and in such circumstances alternative forms of respiratory therapy are safer and more beneficial. In the United States, the requisite expertise is readily available in most hospitals, except perhaps in the smallest ones.

Lack of Service

IPPB can be hazardous if the respirator and associated equipment cannot be maintained in safe working condition. In many areas of the United States, the patient who is in an extended care facility or is at home may be unable to obtain help in keeping the machine and its various parts in optimal working condition. Under such circumstances, the patient cannot be expected to obtain the benefits of IPPB that may have been provided in the acute hospital setting. In practice, domiciliary IPPB should be regarded as contraindicated unless the patient or other responsible house members understand how to give therapy and how to maintain the equipment in reasonable condition. The physician who prescribes the therapy should order the simplest effective equipment, and, generally the respirator should be powered by electricity, thereby obviating the various difficulties associated with the use of tanks of gas in the home. Periodic home visits by a respiratory therapist are desirable.

CONTRAINDICATIONS FOR IPPB

1. *Acute pneumothorax* that is being managed without an intercostal tube.
2. *Intubated pneumothorax* with persistent leak (*e.g.,* bronchopleural fistula).
3. *History of pneumothorax*: spontaneous or secondary to IPPB.
4. *Subcutaneous or mediastinal emphysema* may worsen with IPPB.
5. *Tracheoesophageal fistula*: IPPB may cause gastric insufflation and vomiting.
6. *Inadequate facilities*: IPPB should not be used if lack of equipment, personnel, or adequate finances prevent optimal therapy.
7. *Bullous disease*: IPPB should not be given if it results in evidence of air-trapping (*e.g.,* dyspnea, feelings of hyperinflation, x-ray changes, worsening of pulmonary function).
8. *Cardiovascular insufficiency* (*e.g.,* hypotension, hypovolemia, arrhythmias, coronary artery insufficiency): if IPPB causes evidence of exacerbation of condition.
9. *Subjective deterioration*: if patient cannot use IPPB correctly or if the treatment causes the patient distress.
10. *Availability of simpler therapy* (*e.g.,* physical therapy, simple aerosols, and so forth), if these can be shown to be effective.

Availability of Simpler Therapy

IPPB tends to be overused simply because of the availability of machines and personnel in the hospital. Thus many patients, such as young asthmatics, are given IPPB in the hospital where it simply functions as an expensive technique for aerosolizing medication. Such patients generally obtain adequate relief from the proper use of simple hand nebulizers, and respiratory therapists would be providing a less expensive and more useful service if they supervised the periodic and correct use of these nebulizers in such cases rather than spending much more time in giving the patient IPPB treatments.

Many acutely ill patients who seem to benefit from the use of IPPB when admitted to the hospital no longer need this therapy when the acute immediate problem is resolved. Frequently, however, IPPB is prolonged for many more days than can be justified by the therapeutic results. Further, there is a tendency to prescribe IPPB for indefinite use at home, whereas a simple nebulizer or humidifier may be quite adequate, safer, and less expensive.

Bullous Disease

Many patients with obstructive pulmonary disease feel worse after an IPPB treatment, although evidence of any adverse effect is rarely more than transient. In some patients with large bullae, however, repeated IPPB treatments may result in radiologic evidence of growth of a bulla. Although this serious complication of IPPB is uncommon, it is important that high inspiratory pressures in subjects with bullous disease be avoided and care taken to detect increasing air trapping within a bulla. The use of an expiratory retard device when giving IPPB to patients with bullous disease may help forestall this complication, but it must be used with great care.

Cardiovascular Insufficiency

Patients with low blood pressure from any cause may suffer a further decrease in blood pressure during IPPB therapy. For this reason, IPPB is often said to be contraindicated in states of shock and in patients with myocardial disease (including infarction and coronary insufficiency, particularly when associated with arrhythmias). Certainly, prolonged inspiration using large volumes and high pressures can result in a sufficient decrease in venous return to jeopardize the cardiac output and blood pressure in such patients.

DUBIOUS CONTRAINDICATIONS

The various lists of contraindications found in guides to IPPB suffer from inadequate documentation and explanation of the reasoning behind the interdictions. In the following section, arguments for and against the usual proscriptions will be examined.

Pneumothorax

There is very little published evidence that routine IPPB can cause a pneumothorax,[31] yet the fear of causing or worsening a pneumothorax is frequently implied. If a patient has a history of a spontaneous pneumothorax, there is certainly a good chance that such an event may occur again. There is little reason to believe, however, that appropriately administered IPPB therapy increases that risk.

If a patient suffers a tension pneumothorax, the condition may be acutely and severely worsened by positive pressure therapy. The appropriate management of such a hazard is the prompt emplacement of a chest tube; once this is in place, low-pressure IPPB can be given with reasonable safety. However, it should then be determined whether the IPPB is really necessary. Whether cautious IPPB treatments in pneumothorax patients who have functioning chest tubes result in delay in the healing of the lung remains to be determined.

Patients with cystic or bullous disease are prone to develop a pneumothorax. These patients often have IPPB prescribed for management of associated airway obstruction. Practical experience clearly suggests that the potential hazard of a pneumothorax is very small. Thus the theoretical *liability* of a pneumothorax is, in practice, not regarded as a contraindication for IPPB. The same considerations apply to the patient who is a potential pneumothorax victim as apply to any person receiving IPPB: The treatment must be given correctly, using low flow rates and low pressures. The therapist must carefully observe the patient to make sure that the treatment is well accepted and no evidence of complications develops.

Mediastinal and Subcutaneous Emphysema

The patient who develops mediastinal emphysema spontaneously is similar to the patient who suffers a spontaneous pneumothorax. Although IPPB should probably be avoided in such cases, if respirator treatment is deemed necessary, it should be given carefully, watching the patient for evidence of further complications. In practice, most patients with mediastinal emphysema probably can manage without IPPB, and this opportunity for conservativism should not be resisted. The same remarks, of course, apply to every situation in respiratory medicine: If the patient can do equally well without IPPB, there is no need to give it!

With regard to subcutaneous emphysema, similar considerations apply. In practice, subcutaneous emphysema does not dissuade one from using a respirator if it is needed.

Tuberculosis

It has been frequently stated that a person with active tuberculosis should not be given IPPB. Unfortunately, there is no ready explanation for this injunction. Presumably it was feared that IPPB might help disseminate tuberculosis throughout the lungs, although there is no evidence to suggest that such a phenomenon occurs in practice. In any case, if the patient is on appropriate chemotherapy, there is no risk whatsoever of "spreading the tuberculous infection" with IPPB. It is also most unlikely that the exposure of the infected lung to positive pressure will result in any undesired structural change, although conceivably cavities might, in rare instances, be adversely affected. As yet, no documentation exists as to whether IPPB can spread other infections, such as fungal pneumonia, throughout the lung, although this remains a possibility.

A more relevant concern is that the use of an IPPB machine on an infected patient could result in cross-infection of other patients subsequently exposed to the equipment. This particular risk applies to various bacterial infections of the respiratory tract but is not a practical concern when an adequate cleansing and sterilizing program exists for respiratory therapy equipment (*see* Chap. 19).

Hemoptysis

Although it has been widely stated that IPPB is contraindicated in the presence of hemoptysis, neither explanation nor evidence supports such advice. Presumably, the injunction is based on the same considerations as for the proscription of IPPB in tuberculosis, but it is equally unlikely that positive pressure will adversely affect the patient who is coughing up blood. In fact, personal experience suggests that IPPB with oxygen may be beneficial in such circumstances. Indeed, if a patient suffers a severe, potentially lethal hemoptysis, intubation and respiratory support may be necessary while preparations are made for emergency surgery.

Tracheoesophageal Fistula

The presence of tracheoesophageal fistula, a rare condition, may be a contraindication for IPPB, since positive pressure breathing could result in gastric insufflation. This would increase the tendency of the patient to regurgitate and to aspirate gastric contents into the lung. In practice, this entity either requires surgical correction or is a preterminal condition, and in these circumstances IPPB is unlikely to be an important measure in managing the patient unless the trachea is first intubated, thereby bypassing the fistula.

Miscellaneous Contraindications

Other dubious contraindications for IPPB may be noted. *Psychologic dependency* may be a contraindication,[28] but certain patients should preferably vent their dependent need for support on an uncomplaining machine rather than on an all-too-human physician.

When IPPB is used to deliver bronchodilators with vasodilator properties, there is a danger of increased *hypoxemia*[11]; this is readily compensated for by using oxygen to drive the machine. *Inappropriate drug dosage* is certainly a risk of IPPB, since individual patients vary in their responsiveness to the "standard" dose. However, this concern does not contraindicate the use of IPPB but does emphasize the need for careful, individualized prescribing and for knowledgeable, watchful supervision of the patient's response to therapy.

In summary, there are few definite contraindications for IPPB when the treatment is indicated, but there are certain circumstances where the potential risks are a particular worry. However, all patients started on a course of IPPB are likely to have unsuspected adverse effects. The health care team must be aware of these possibilities, and those who supervise the treatment must be alert to the development of complications. Fortunately, most patients who develop adverse effects will give some obvious indication of distress, and usually the unpleasant experience will result in a refusal to continue the treatment. *All personnel responsible for giving IPPB should be aware that a patient who claims that the treatment is not helpful may be absolutely correct.* It is inappropriate, in such circumstances, to reassure the complaining patient and to insist on continuing the treatment.

RECOMMENDATIONS FOR ADMINISTRATION OF IPPB

IPPB can be given only if ordered by a physician. Before prescribing the treatment, the physician should give thought to the following questions.

1. *What is the objective of the therapy?*
   a. To increase the Pa_{O_2}?
   b. To decrease the Pa_{CO_2}?
   c. To improve mucociliary clearance?
   d. To relieve bronchospasm?
   e. To decrease mucosal congestion?
   f. To relieve atelectasis?
   g. To prevent atelectasis?
   h. To treat pulmonary edema?

If the physician is unable to specify which of these objectives is to be achieved, then possibly the treatment is not justified, except perhaps as a relatively expensive form of placebo psychotherapy.

2. *Can the objectives be realistically achieved by IPPB?*
   a. Will the patient be able to take an adequate treatment?
   b. Will anyone be available to give a skillful treatment and monitor the effects?
   c. Does the available equipment offer effective, safe treatment?

If the answer to any of these is negative, then an alternative to IPPB should be provided.

3. *Can the therapeutic objectives be attained by simpler and cheaper methods?*
   Metered bronchodilator dispensers, simple aerosol therapy, physical therapy, and enhanced tidal volume breathing (such as can be encouraged by an incentive spirometer) should be considered.

The physician who wishes to use respiratory therapy is usually able to make reasonable decisions regarding the prescription, but if there are difficulties, a respiratory therapist or respiratory physician should be invited to consult on the case and direct the treatment. In all situations where respiratory therapy is needed by the patient, the respiratory therapist should be expected to use clinical and technical judgment and to offer consultative advice on how to maximize the benefits of the treatment.[48]

The prescribing physician should, ideally, write a prescription that embodies the following details.

1. Objectives of the therapy (e.g., to improve expectoration)
2. Suggested physical method (e.g., deep breathing, using any suitable technique, and coughing)

3. Drug therapy (*i.e.*, precise drug dosages)
4. Suggested equipment (e.g., aerosol mask)
5. Frequency and times of delivery (e.g., q.i.d., after pain medications have been given)
6. Precautions (e.g., monitor pulse rate, watch for arrhythmias)
7. Posttreatment observations to be made (e.g., record FEV_1, describe sputum)
8. Other treatments (e.g., percussion/postural drainage)

In practice, it is advisable for medical directors of respiratory therapy to establish standard protocols listing standard IPPB settings. If IPPB is to be given as part of the treatment (unless the prescribing physician specifies other machine settings), the standard protocol should serve as a guide for the therapist. The following details should be covered in the protocol for standard IPPB treatments.

1. *The machine*. Generally, any of several devices can be used, without any manufacturer's brand being specified.
2. *Volume*. In most treatments with IPPB, an augmented tidal volume must be delivered to ensure improved gas mixing, peripheral deposition of drugs, and enhanced mucokinesis. Ideally, the spontaneous tidal volume of the patient should be measured with a respirometer or a collection bag, after which the patient should be coached to allow a large volume to be delivered by the machine, which should also be measured. The objective of therapy is to obtain an increase in tidal volume of at least 25%; some patients can obtain much larger volumes with IPPB by slowing their breathing rates and relaxing, although it may be beneficial if the patient makes a supplementary minimal inspiratory effort to help ensure maximal expansion.[34,44] Some recently introduced respirators provide a plateau hold at the end of inspiration, which offers another way of obtaining a prolonged and augmented inspiration. If it is found that the tidal volume delivered by IPPB does not exceed the patient's spontaneous tidal volume, then IPPB should be considered unsuited for use in that patient.[25,34]
3. *Cycling rate*. The patient should always be encouraged to breathe as slowly as possible, and the therapist must work with most individuals to prevent a rapid cycling rate. The best treatment is usually achieved with slow deep breaths, 7 to 10 times per minute: Inspiration should last 2 to 4 seconds, followed by a pause for a further 2 seconds, after which expiration should take 2 to 4 seconds. A slowed breathing rate is essential if augmented tidal volumes are used, otherwise hyperventilation will result.
4. *Pressure*. Generally, any pressure can be used unless the prescribing physician stipulates that low pressure is required; reasons for this stipulation should be provided. Most patients require 10 to 15 cm H_2O pressure, whereas few require more than 20 cm H_2O.
5. *Flow*. The gas flow rate should be varied by the therapist according to the patient's need. Alterations of flow are often needed during the course of the treatment session. Therapists should use the lowest possible flow to ensure adequate tidal volume, without causing the patient to experience discomfort. This is where particular skill is needed in the administration of IPPB.
6. *Drugs*. The physician preferably should specify pharmacologic agents by name, dose, and frequency of administration. Protocols can incorporate prescribing information but must be worded carefully, since the appropriate dosage for individual patients is quite variable. In all cases the therapist should be aware of possible side-effects and adverse reactions to respiratory drugs, and these should be watched for during IPPB and treatment stopped prematurely if need be. The physician should be required to alter a specific prescription if the therapist finds that the patient cannot tolerate the prescribed drug or the dosage ordered.
7. *Humidity*. Generally, when IPPB is given to patients with airway disease, humidification of the gas should be provided. Although this is not essential, it is desirable in asthmatics and in cases of impaired mucokinesis. In practice, it is more convenient to aerosolize a bland solution (such as normal or half-normal saline) throughout the treatment. Sensitive patients may develop bronchospasm as a consequence of such therapy, and a prophylactic bronchodilator should be added to the solution for nebulization.
8. *Oxygen concentration*. Generally, IPPB should be given with room air, which may or may

not be humidified. However, oxygen-enriched air is preferable in hypoxic patients, particularly if the treatment is likely to cause a transient fall in Pa_{O_2}. Ideally, in such circumstances, 30% to 40% oxygen should be used.

9. *Time factor.* The therapy should last as short or as long a time as the therapist judges to be appropriate for each patient (*i.e.*, 5–30 minutes). In some patients, a few breaths of undiluted bronchodilator provides optimal therapy, and the IPPB session need last only a few minutes.
10. *Monitoring.* The therapist should usually check the heart rate and rhythm before, during, and after the IPPB session. In most cases, the therapist should auscultate the patient's back before and after the treatment. Before and several times during the treatment session the minute ventilation could be monitored, using a respirometer or a collection bag, to ensure that the tidal volume during IPPB is augmented.
11. *If adverse effects occur,* the IPPB should be stopped immediately and the physician advised of the need to revise the prescription.
12. *Record-keeping.* The therapist should record in detail the results of the IPPB session and suggest appropriate changes in the physician's prescription if need be. Periodically, a patient being treated for bronchospasm should have airflow and exhaled volume measured at the bedside to demonstrate that improvement is being produced by the IPPB aerosol treatment. Physicians are expected to read the notes of the therapist or nurse and to enter into the patient's record an assessment of the effects of the therapy.
13. *Automatic stop orders* should be applied after several days, so that the physician and therapist can evaluate the need for further therapy or for changes in management.

Although the perfect method of administering IPPB cannot be described, certain general comments can be made. If the patient is calm and cooperative and is breathing in a eupneic fashion, the therapist will have little difficulty in getting the patient to take a reasonable treatment. If the patient is breathing rapidly and is short of breath, however, IPPB may not be readily accepted, and indeed a useful treatment may be virtually impossible, especially if the patient is also confused and uncooperative. In such cases the therapist may have to spend a great deal of time soothing the patient and encouraging a calm, slow, spontaneous breathing pattern.

The machine will have to be introduced to the patient carefully and sympathetically. The therapist should select an appropriate mouthpiece, and the patient should try using it without the machine attached. Once the patient has accepted the mouthpiece and has shown willingness to cooperate, the therapist will have to use skill in determining an appropriate flow pattern for that patient. In the dyspneic subject, many respirator setting changes may have to be made until the patient considers the IPPB treatment acceptable.

As the treatment progresses, further changes will have to be made to attain an appropriate breathing pattern and tidal volume. Once the patient has learned to take a treatment, subsequent sessions should be simpler. If the patient remains recalcitrant, a mask may be needed, although it is less likely that such a "treatment" will result in any measurable benefit. Thus, if a mask is used, the patient will need to breathe through the mouth to obtain maximal aerosol benefits, and this optimal breathing pattern is not likely to be achieved.

Clearly, from this approach no IPPB treatment should be regarded as simply a matter of having a patient receive a series of positive pressure inspirations. The active participation of the therapist is essential, and numerous decisions must be made by the person supervising each treatment. The therapist should regard most sessions as treatments, but, if the patient is capable, the sessions should also incorporate some teaching. The patient must be encouraged to relax and to breathe deeply, and he should be taught how to cough effectively.

In those selected cases when domiciliary IPPB will be required later, the patient should be taught how to set up the respirator and to adjust the settings. The therapist may judge that a nose-clip should be used to obtain adequate inspired volumes, or a face mask to attain effective delivery of a suitable volume of gas. The therapist should consider the use of a retard cap to facilitate full expiration in patients with emphysema or bullous disease; however, the physician must be asked to authorize this form of therapy. The monitoring of expired volumes (using a respirometer or collection bag) will demonstrate the effectiveness of the IPPB and can be used as a guide to the advisability of using a retard cap. In all cases, however, the therapist should encourage slow expiration and should stress the value of pursed-lip breathing to the patient with obstructive airway disease.

IPPB must be considered a potentially valueless or even harmful form of therapy unless administered appropriately. Each patient's treatment should be evaluated to see what results are achieved, and at least evey few days during hospitalization bedside tests should be carried out to determine whether objective improvement can be documented. If no benefits can be demonstrated, then the use of IPPB cannot be justified, and the health care team should consider other ways of providing help for the patient. Ideally, there should never be a physician's order simply for "IPPB" q.i.d.," and, equally ideally, it may be appropriate for the physician to order "respiratory therapy consultation," thereby allowing the therapist to evaluate the patient and to draw up a comprehensive treatment plan that can be presented to the physician for authorization. In many hospitals, it would be apropriate for the respiratory therapist to fill out most of the details on an order sheet. The physician would then amend or complete the order, if necessary, and authorize the prescription by signing the sheet. In such cases the well-trained therapist will utilize IPPB as only one of the various components to be employed in any given respiratory therapy session.

REFERENCES

1. Baker JP: Magnitude of usage of intermittent positive pressure breathing. Am Rev Respir Dis 110, No. 6, Part 2:170, 1974
2. Barach AL, Martin T, Eckman M: Positive pressure respiration and its application to the treatment of acute pulmonary edema. Ann Intern Med 12:754, 1938
3. Bloomfield P et al: Comparison of salbutamol given intravenously and by intermittent positive-pressure breathing in life-threatening asthma. Br Med J 1:848, 1979
4. Braun SR, Smith RT, McCarthy TM et al: Evaluating the changing role of respiratory therapy services at two hospitals. JAMA 245:2033, 1981
5. Cherniack RM: Intermittent positive pressure breathing in management of chronic obstructive disease: Current state of the art. Am Rev Respir Dis 110, No. 6, Part 2:188, 1974
6. Cherniack RM, Svanhill E: Long-term use of intermittent positive-pressure breathing (IPPB) in chronic obstructive pulmonary disease. Am Rev Respir Dis 113:721, 1976
7. Curtis JK, Liska AP, Rasmussen HK et al: IPPB therapy in chronic obstructive pulmonary disease: An evaluation of long-term home treatment. JAMA 206:1037, 1968
8. Davis JT: The influence of intrathoracic pressure on fluid and electrolyte balance. Chest 62:118S, 1972
9. Fairley HB, Britt BA: The adequacy of the air-mix control in ventilators operated from an oxygen source. Can Med Assoc J 90:1394, 1964
10. Fouts JB, Brashear RE: Intermittent positive pressure breathing: A critical appraisal. Postgrad Med 59:103, 1976
11. Gazioglu K et al: Effect of isoproterenol on gas exchange during air and oxygen breathing in patients with asthma. Am J Med 50:185, 1971
12. Hughes RL: Do no harm—cheaply. Chest 77:582, 1980
12a. Intermittent Positive Pressure Breathing Trial Group: Intermittent positive pressure breathing therapy of chronic obstructive pulmonary diseases: A clinical trial. Ann Intern Med 99:612, 1983
13. Karetzky MS: Asthma mortality: An analysis of one year's experience, review of the literature and assessment of current modes of therapy. Medicine 54:471, 1975
14. Keighley JFH: Response to sympathomimetic aerosols of differing particle size in subjects with chronic bronchitis. Am Rev Respir Dis 98:879, 1968
15. Khambatta, HJ, Baratz RA: IPPB, plasma ADH, and urine flow in conscious man. J Appl Physiol 33:362, 1972
16. Lefcoe NM, Carter P: Intermittent positive-pressure breathing and chronic obstructive pulmonary disease. Can Med Assoc J 103:279, 1970
17. Lefcoe NM, Patterson MAM: Adjunct therapy in chronic obstructive pulmonary disease. Am J Med 54:343, 1973
18. Lieberman J: The appropriate use of mucolytic agents. Am J Med 49:1, 1970
19. Loehning R, Milai AS, Safar P: Intermittent positive pressure breathing therapy. In Safar P (ed): Respiratory Therapy. Philadelphia, FA Davis, 1965
20. Loke J, Anthonisen NR: Effect of intermittent positive breathing on steady state chronic obstructive pulmonary disease. Am Rev Respir Dis 110, No. 6, Part 2:178, 1974
21. Luisada AA: Pulmonary Edema in Man and Animals, p 98. St Louis, WH Green, 1970
22. McConnell DH, Maloney JV, Buckberg GD: Postoperative intermittent positive pressure breathing treatments. J Thorac Cardiovasc Surg 68:944, 1974
23. Mayock RL: IPPB is a useful modality in the treatment of chronic obstructive lung disease. In Ingelfinger FJ, Ebert RV, Finland M et al (eds): Controversy in Internal Medicine, 2nd ed. Philadelphia, WB Saunders, 1974
24. Miller RD, Hepper NGG: The dangers and limitations of IPPB in managing diseases affecting ventilation. In Ingelfinger FJ, Ebert RV, Finland M et al (eds): Controversy in Internal Medicine, 2nd ed. Philadelphia, WB Saunders, 1974
25. Morrison DR, Powers WE, Boocks RD: Volume-oriented IPPB: A report of six months' routine use. Respir Care 21:792, 1976
26. Motley HL: IPPB in severe pulmonary emphysema. Respir Ther 6:47, 1976
27. Motley HL et al: Observations on the use of positive pressure. J Aviation Med 18:417, 1947
28. Murray JF: Review of the state of the art of intermittent positive pressure breathing therapy. Am Rev Respir Dis 110, No. 6, Part 2:193, 1974
29. Murray JF: Indications for mechanical aids to assist lung inflation in medical patients. Am Rev Respir Dis 122, No. 5, Part 2:121, 1980
30. O'Donohue WJ: Maximum volume IPPB for the management of pulmonary atelectasis. Chest 76:683, 1979
31. Pierce AK: Assisted respiration. Annu Rev Med 20:431, 1969
32. Pierce AK (ed): Conference on the scientific basis of respiratory therapy. Temple University Conference Center at Sugarloaf, Pennsylvania. Am Rev Respir Dis 110, No. 6, Part 2: 1974

33. Pontoppidan, H: Mechanical aids to lung expansion in non-intubated surgical patients. Am Rev Respir Dis 122, No. 5, Part 2:109, 1980
34. Powers WE, Morrison DR: Evaluation of inspired volumes in postoperative patients receiving volume-oriented IPPB. Respir Care 23:39, 1978
35. Rau JL: Intermittent positive pressure breathing (IPPB). Crit Care Update 5:5, 1978
36. Respiratory Care Committee of the American Thoracic Society: Guidelines for the use of intermittent positive pressure breathing (IPPB). Respir Care 25:365, 1980
37. Schapira M, Daum S: Hemodynamics of the pulmonary circulation in patients on intermittent positive pressure breathing with a Bird respirator. Anesth Analg 53:31, 1974
38. Sheldon GP: Pressure breathing in chronic obstructive lung disease. Medicine 42:197, 1963
39. Smelzer TH, Barnett TB: Bronchodilator aerosol: Comparison of administration methods. JAMA 223:884, 1973
40. Sukumalchantra Y, Park SS, Williams MH: The effect of intermittent positive pressure breathing (IPPB) in acute ventilatory failure. Am Rev Respir Dis 92:885, 1965
41. Thornton JA, Darke CS, Herbert P: Intermittent positive pressure breathing (IPPB) in chronic respiratory disease. Anaesthesia 29:44, 1974
42. Torres A, Lyons HA, Emerson P: The effects of intermittent positive pressure breathing on the intrapulmonary distribution of inspired air. Am J Med 29:946, 1960
43. Webb HH, Tierney DF: Experimental pulmonary edema due to intermittent positive pressure ventilation with high inflation pressures. Protection by positive end-expiratory pressure. Am Rev Respir Dis 110:556, 1974
44. Welch MA et al: Methods of intermittent positive pressure breathing. Chest 78:463, 1980
45. Yanda RL: Quality control of IPPB therapy: A baseline study. Respir Care 18:33, 1973
46. Yanda RL: Quality control of inhalation therapy: The results of therapy, with and without control, and methods of developing such control, in a community hospital. Chest 66:61, 1974
47. Ziment I: Why are they saying bad things about IPPB? Respir Care 18:677, 1973
48. Ziment I: IPPB: Correct usage. Crit Care Update pp 18–23, August 1976

24

Mechanical Ventilation

Robert R. Kirby • Robert A. Smith • David A. Desautels

Early references to ventilatory support appear in the *Bible*. Although other references to artificially supported ventilation are found over succeeding centuries, one of the most popular appears in a monograph published in 1796, entitled "An Attempt at an Historical Survey of Life-Saving Measures for Drowning Persons and Information on the Best Means by which They Can Again be Brought Back to Life," by Herholdt and Rafn.[4] This reference discussed mouth-to-mouth ventilation and other mechanical or manual methods of moving air, including the insertion of the tip of a bellows-type apparatus into the victim's windpipe and rhythmical inflation of his lungs. Later, a publication by Emerson described positive pressure breathing for the treatment of congestive heart failure and pulmonary edema.[3] Modern ventilatory support techniques, however, are an outgrowth of the tank-type respirator introduced by Drinker and Shaw in 1929. Since then, new techniques and types of ventilation have appeared rapidly.

The first positive pressure ventilators were pressure-cycled or volume-cycled. The pressure-cycled ventilator was designed to terminate gas delivery when a predetermined pressure had been attained. Thus the volume of gas delivered to the patient was related directly to lung compliance and inversely to airway resistance. Any leaks in the system reduced the amount of volume delivered to the patient. With large gas leaks the ventilators remained in prolonged inspiration, since the pressure necessary for terminating flow could not be reached.

Operation of volume-cycled ventilators required selection of a desired volume, which was then delivered into the breathing circuit. However, no controls or alarms were built into early models of such ventilators to detect or to compensate for leaks in the system, and they could be disconnected accidently from the patient without any visual or audible signs.

The popularization of intermittent positive pressure breathing (IPPB) therapy in the 1950s and early 1960s aided the rapid development of numerous types of sophisticated mechanical ventilators, although the merits of IPPB therapy continue to be debated today (see Chap. 23). Physicians soon recognized that ventilators that provided IPPB had significant limitations during prolonged mechanical ventilation and generally were not suitable for long-term patient care.

Control of the inspired oxygen concentration was not possible initially. Many pressure-cycled ventilators had only two settings that allegedly could deliver 40% and 100% oxygen. However, decreased compliance or increased airway resistance, which caused rapidly increased system pressure, altered the exact concentration of oxygen delivered at any given time, leading to excessive inspired oxygen concentrations and possible pulmonary oxygen toxicity. Systems that diluted oxygen with room air, or mixed high-pressure sources of oxygen and compressed air in separate air–oxygen blenders, were subsequently introduced.

Early ventilators lacked the necessary components to provide humidification. Tenacious secretions and mucus plugs often resulted during ventilation with dry gas, and mucociliary activity was depressed. Daily bronchoscopy was sometimes needed in patients supported with mechanical ventilation to maintain the patency of their airways.

Subsequently, heated humidifiers that could produce up to 100% relative humidity at body temperature and high efficiency nebulizers became commercially available. However, the clinician frequently had no reliable means of recognizing or controlling the exact level of humidification delivered to a patient. Underhumidification of respiratory gases or the delivery of an excessive water load were both possible. A patient's airway also could be burned with superheated mist should a heating device malfunction.

Initially mechanical ventilators had crude adjustments for pressure and volume that could not be controlled precisely, and clinicians frequently recommended that patients be ventilated through an uncuffed tracheostomy tube to prevent excessive tidal volume delivery. The danger of aspiration of gastric contents with uncuffed endotracheal and tracheostomy tubes became widely recognized. Later, control of the volume and pressure delivered to patients improved. Since known tidal volumes or predictable cycling pressures were difficult or impossible to attain with an uncuffed tube, cuffed tracheal tubes began to be used during prolonged mechanical ventilation (see Chap. 21). More recently, implant-tested, low-pressure cuffed tubes have allowed prolonged orotracheal or nasotracheal intubation in lieu of tracheostomy.

Early ventilators assisted or controlled respiration, but it was uncommon to find both modes available in a single unit. Subsequently both assisted and controlled ventilation were often available. As technology improved, ventilators that operated with pressure-cycled, time-cycled, or volume-cycled mechanisms could also be adjusted to change the inspiratory and expiratory pressure and flow patterns, with variable gas flow rates thereby allowing selection of a pattern of ventilation that was most advantageous to the patient. This increased flexibility allowed gas flow to be adjusted to compensate for the patient's pulmonary lesion, thus improving the distribution of ventilation.

Indications for mechanical ventilation also changed. Early mechanical ventilators were used for patients who could not sustain spontaneous ventilation. Hypoxemia without carbon dioxide retention was treated by supplemental oxygen breathing rather than by mechanical ventilatory support.

As early as 1912, however, continuous positive airway pressure in spontaneously breathing patients undergoing thoracic surgical procedures was shown to improve ventilation and to decrease or eliminate cyanosis. By the 1930s, several reports attested to the efficacy of continuous positive-pressure breathing (CPPB), without mechanical ventilation, in treating pulmonary edema, pneumonia, and asthma. This therapy was later used successfully in respiratory distress syndrome of the newborn (hyaline membrane disease) by Gregory and his colleagues (continuous positive airway pressure [CPAP]).[5]

In 1969, positive end-expiratory pressure (PEEP) was combined with controlled mechanical ventilation and used to treat acute respiratory failure in adult patients (adult respiratory distress syndrome [ARDS]). Manipulation of airway pressure in this syndrome, characterized by hypoxemia, usually without carbon dioxide retention, improved ventilation/perfusion ($\dot{V}/\dot{Q}$) relationships and increased Pa_{O_2} at the same or lower concentrations of inspired oxygen (FI_{O_2}).

Intermittent mandatory ventilation (IMV) was introduced in 1971 (infants) and 1973 (adults) as a means of weaning patients from prolonged mechanical ventilatory support. Subsequently IMV evolved into a technique of primary ventilatory care, combining the advantages of spontaneous breathing with those of conventional mechanical ventilation. The addition of PEEP/CPAP to IMV allowed clinicians to attack the problems of hypoxemia and carbon dioxide retention individually in a way that was not possible with conventional ventilators. Synchronized intermittent mandatory ventilation (SIMV) combined spontaneous breathing with periodic assisted or patient-triggered mechanical cycling and prevented superimposing mechanical breaths on spontaneous ones. This technique, which was alleged to decrease the risk of pulmonary barotrauma in comparison to IMV, was incorporated into the design of some later mechanical ventilators.

Other recently introduced forms of treatment, such as inflation hold (inspiratory pause) and synchronous or asynchronous independent lung ventilation, represent not so much new techniques as modification of existing ones. Such is not the case with the latest form of mechanical support, high-frequency positive-pressure ventilation (HFPPV), also known as high-frequency jet ventilation (HFJV), high-frequency ventilation (HFV), and high-frequency oscillation

(HFO). Although HFV is not new, having been introduced in one form in the late 1960s in Sweden, it has only recently become popular in the United States. No other technique of mechanical ventilation has generated so much interest, excitement, and confusion as HFV, which incorporates physical principles differing as much from each other as conventional mechanical ventilation does from spontaneous breathing.

At the time of this writing, little is known about how and why HFV works, and few commercially produced, FDA-approved, primary high-frequency ventilators are available for purchase and use in adults. However, many investigators from the fields of medicine and engineering are engaged in research seeking to define the optimal characteristics of the technique, and such ventilators will soon be forthcoming.

CLASSIFICATION OF MECHANICAL VENTILATORS

Classification of mechanical ventilators depends on the proposed function. In simplest terms, a ventilator functions as a substitute for the bellows action of the thoracic cage and diaphragm. To perform this function, the ventilator activity may be divided into separate categories (Table 24-1 and Fig. 24-1).

1. Inspiratory phase
2. Changeover from inspiratory to expiratory phase
3. Expiratory phase
4. Changeover from expiratory to inspiratory phase

Classification of mechanical ventilators has become difficult as manufacturers, responding to the demand from physicians and respiratory therapists, have developed increasingly complex units.

INSPIRATORY PHASE

During inspiration, a positive pressure gradient causes gas to flow from the ventilator to the patient's lungs. Four factors to be considered during the inspiratory phase are listed below.

1. Gas flow rate
2. Gas volume delivered
3. Airway pressure
4. Alveolar pressure

Table 24-1. Ventilator Variables

INSPIRATORY PHASE
Flow generator
Constant
Nonconstant
Inflation hold
CHANGEOVER FROM INSPIRATORY PHASE TO EXPIRATORY PHASE
Time-cycled
Pressure-cycled
Volume-cycled
Flow-cycled
Secondary limit
EXPIRATORY PHASE
Retard pressure
Subambient pressure
Threshold pressure (PEEP, ZEEP, and so forth)
CHANGEOVER FROM EXPIRATORY PHASE TO INSPIRATORY PHASE
Assistor
Controller
Assistor-controller
Intermittent mandatory ventilation (IMV)
Intermittent demand ventilation
Synchronized intermittent mandatory ventilation (SIMV)

These variables are not independent of one another, and each will be affected by changes in the lungs, thorax, and connecting airways. A mechanical ventilator can maintain either constant gas flow or pressure, but not both at the same time. Therefore ventilators may be classified as flow generators or pressure generators, depending on which of these two variables is held most steady.

Flow Generators

Constant Flow Generator. Constant gas flow requires a high source pressure to maintain a large pressure gradient between the ventilator and patient. The effects of alterations in airway resistance and pulmonary compliance on gas delivery are thus minimized. To accomplish this goal safely, constant flow generators (Fig. 24-2) must have high internal resistance that protects the patient from the full impact of the pressure source.

An oxygen cylinder with an on–off switch between the cylinder and the patient's lungs is an ex-

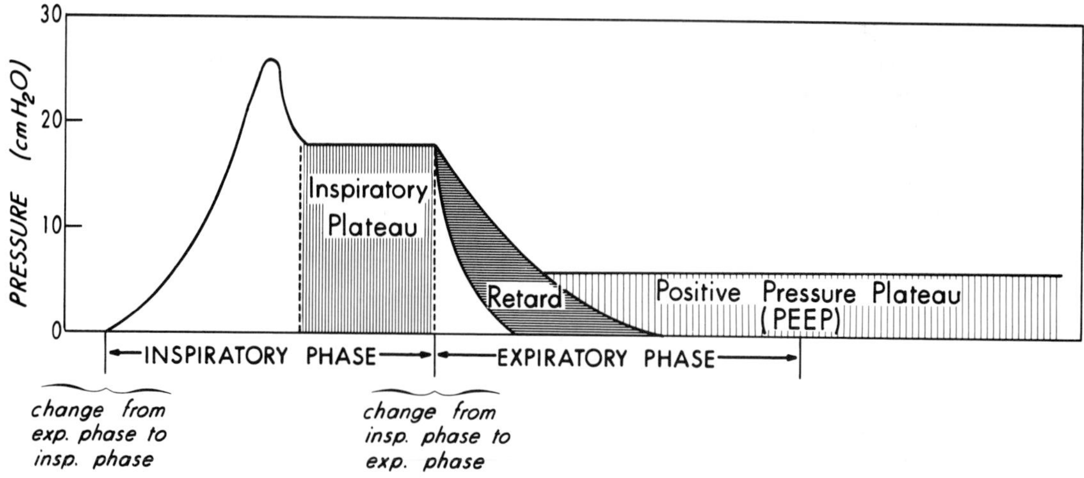

Fig. 24-1. Phases of the mechanical ventilator cycle with and without PEEP and retard.

ample of a constant flow generator. If a tidal volume of 500 ml were desired and the resistance of the cylinder valve was high enough to withstand a flow of 600 liters/min, the desired tidal volume would be achieved in an inspiratory duration of 0.05 second. Such a system is not practical from a clinical standpoint. However, a reducing valve and a sophisticated on–off switch would make this device more efficient and safer.

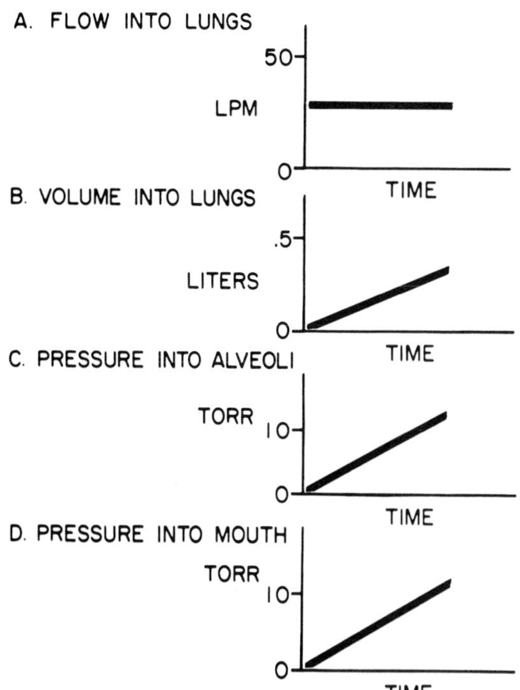

Fig. 24-2. Characteristics of a constant flow generator.

As the operating pressure of a constant flow generator is reduced, its characteristics become less and less "pure," and changes in the patient's resistance and compliance will alter the performance characteristics. If the operating pressure is reduced until it equals the pressure within the patient's lungs, the device in theory becomes a constant pressure generator, albeit an entirely ineffective one.

The difficulty in classifying ventilators as either constant flow or constant pressure generators is obvious. The two classifications form the extremes of an entire spectrum of performance, and most ventilators fall somewhere in between. Generally, if the flow rate remains relatively constant throughout the inspiratory phase while the pressure varies significantly, a ventilator is classified as a constant flow generator.

Various methods are used to develop constant gas flow in mechanical ventilators, including

1. high-pressure gas source with reducing valve;
2. compressor with or without a reducing valve;
3. blowers;
4. pressure transformers; and
5. gas injectors.

Injectors are not, strictly speaking, constant flow generators because they entrain varying amounts of auxiliary gas depending on the source pressure and downstream resistance. In the early and midportion of the inspiratory phase, gas flow is high and relatively constant; in the terminal phase, gas flow falls rapidly. Pressure is variable throughout.

Nonconstant Flow Generator. A ventilator is classified as a nonconstant flow generator (Fig. 24-3) when the flow rate changes but the flow pattern delivered to the patient is the same during each inspiration regardless of lung–thorax changes. The Emerson 3-PV ventilator is a nonconstant flow generator that provides a sine wave flow pattern by means of an eccentric cam and piston.

Pressure Generators

Constant Pressure Ventilator. A constant pressure generator (Fig. 24-4) maintains constant pressure in the patient-breathing circuit throughout inspiration, regardless of lung–thorax changes. It operates with low gas pressure and low internal resistance. Mapleson described a classic constant pressure generator as a combination bellows and weight.[6] As the weight pushes the bellows down, the pressure output remains constant. (The weight does not change.) Complete occlusion of the bellows outflow does not change the pressure or force per unit area.

Gas flow from a constant pressure generator decreases exponentially until the patient and ventilator system pressures equalize. The rate at which equilibrium is attained depends on the compliance and the resistance of both the patient and system, since the pressure differential is not as great in a constant pressure generator as it is in other types of ventilators. If patient compliance, C, is 0.05 liters/cm H_2O, ventilator resistance is 5 cm H_2O/liter/sec, and patient resistance is 5 cm H_2O/liter/sec, the following relationship holds.

1. Patient resistance + ventilator resistance = total resistance (R)

$$5 \text{ cm } H_2O\text{/liter/sec} + 5 \text{ cm } H_2O\text{/liter/sec} = 10 \text{ cm } H_2O\text{/liter/sec}$$

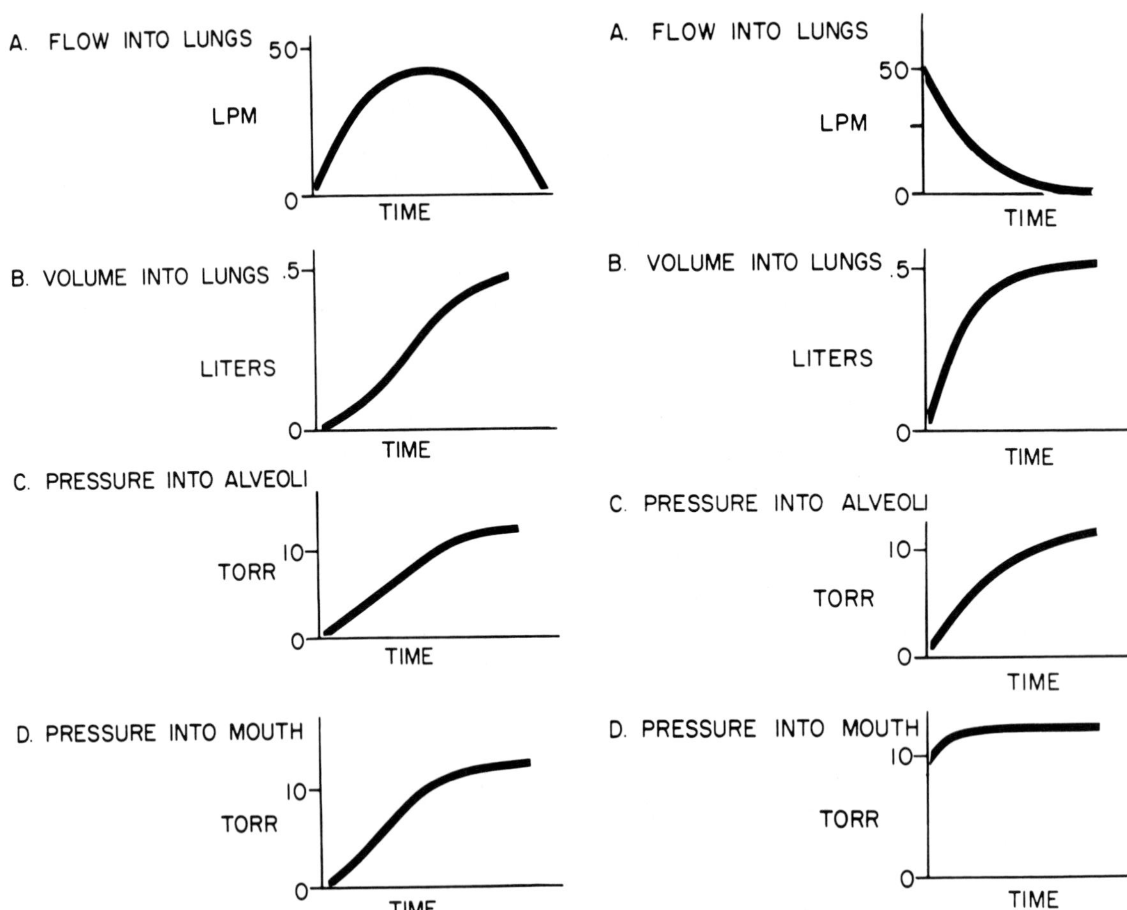

Fig. 24-3. Characteristics of a nonconstant flow generator.

Fig. 24-4. Characteristics of a constant pressure generator.

2. The resultant time constant (R × C) is

$$10 \text{ cm } H_2O/\text{liter/sec} \times 0.05 \text{ liters/cm } H_2O = 0.5 \text{ sec}$$

In 0.5 second (one time constant) 63% of the tidal volume will have been delivered, and, in 1.5 seconds, 95% will have been delivered. Because the approach of airway pressure to ventilator pressure is exponential, the two theoretically will never equalize and the pre-set tidal volume cannot be delivered quantitatively. Practically, this discrepancy is not important.

A constant pressure generator that employs pressure exceeding that which is necessary to deliver a desired tidal volume to the patient deviates from the "ideal" and attains characteristics of a constant flow generator.

Nonconstant Pressure Ventilator. A ventilator is classified as a nonconstant pressure generator (Fig. 24-5) if the pressure changes but the pressure *pattern* remains constant from breath to breath, regardless of changes in lung characteristics.

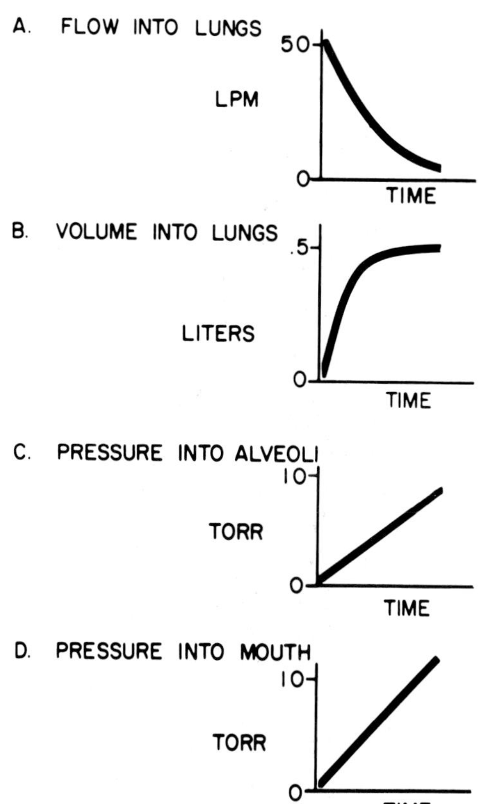

Fig. 24-5. Characteristics of a nonconstant pressure generator.

INFLATION HOLD (INSPIRATORY PLATEAU)

If strictly interpreted, an inflation hold should be considered part of the inspiratory phase, since the changeover from the inspiratory to the expiratory phase has not yet occurred (see Fig. 24-1). However, most ventilators that incorporate this mode into their design terminate gas flow during the inflation hold. We have elected, therefore, to separate inflation hold for purposes of classification. A few ventilators, such as the Baby Bird and Bird Mark VI, continue to deliver gas into the circuit throughout this period (and also during the expiratory phase); thus our decision is arbitrary. Once flow ceases, the delivered tidal volume within the patient's lungs is retained, and, theoretically, better distribution of gas to areas of low V/Q occurs. The duration of the inspiratory plateau usually is designated either in seconds or as a percentage of the total duration of the ventilatory cycle.

CHANGEOVER FROM INSPIRATORY TO EXPIRATORY PHASE

The changeover portion of the respiratory cycle is most familiar to clinicians. In 1958, Elam proposed that ventilators be classified into two primary categories: pressure-limited but volume-variable; and volume-limited but pressure-variable.[2] However, since leaks might develop within the ventilator circuit or other factors might alter the basic operational characteristics, Hunter proposed the terms " pressure preset" and volume pre-set." This classification eliminated the problem of determining whether the selected pressure or volume actually was delivered to the patient.

Mapleson introduced a third classification, which has become the most popular, and included the following categories.[6]

1. Time-cycled
2. Pressure-cycled
3. Volume-cycled
4. Flow-cycled

Table 24-2 lists the classifications of commonly used ventilators.

Time-Cycled Ventilators

Time-cycled ventilators terminate gas flow and change to the expiratory phase when a preselected interval has elapsed after the start of inspiration. At the designated time the exhalation valve opens (unless an inflation hold is used), and the delivered tidal volume is vented to the ambient atmosphere. If gas flow is constant and the time interval precisely controlled, tidal volume can be predicted according to the relationship

$$\text{volume} = \text{flow (volume/unit time)} \times \text{time}.$$

This volume, however, is delivered into the circuit, not the patient. Changes in airway resistance and pulmonary or chest wall compliance may alter gas delivery to the patient and cause changes in airway pressure from one breath to the next.

Table 24-2. Ventilator Classification

	INSPIRATORY PHASE					CHANGE FROM INSPIRATORY TO EXPIRATORY			EXPIRATORY PHASE			CHANGE FROM EXPIRATORY TO INSPIRATORY				
	Flow Generator		*Pressure Generator*													
VENTILATOR	*Constant*	*Nonconstant*	*Constant*	*Nonconstant*	*Inspiratory Plateau*	*Time-Cycled*	*Pressure-Cycled*	*Volume-Cycled*	*Retard Pressure*	*Subambient Pressure*	*PEEP/CPAP*	*Assistor*	*Controller*	*Assistor-Controller*	*IMV*	*SIMV*
BABYbird	X					X				X	X		2		X	
IMVbird		X				X			X	X	X		2		X	
Bird Mark 6	X	2	2		X		X		*		X	2	X	2	*	
Bear (Bourns) LS104–150	X						2	X			X	X	X	X	*	
Bear BP-200			X		X	X					X		X		X	
Bear 1	X	X			X		2	X			X		X	X		X
Bear 2	X	X			X	2	2	X			X		X	X		X
Bennett MA-1	X									*	*	X	X	X	*	
Bennett MA-2	X							X			X	X	X	X		X
Bennett MA-2+2	X							X			X	X	X	X		X
Chemtron Gill-1			X		X		2	X			X	X	X	X	X	
Emerson 3PV		X				X		2			*	*	X		X	
Emerson IMV		X				X		2			X		2		X	
Engström ER 300		X			X	X			X		X		X		2	
Engström ECS 2000		X			X	X				*	X		X	X		
Foregger 210	X				X	X	2				X		X	X	X	
Healthydyne	X					X					X		X		X	
Monaghan 225	X					X	X	X			X	X	X	X		X
Ohio 560	X				X			X	X	*	X		X	X		
Ohio 550		X						X			*		X	X		
Ohio CCV2	X				X	2				X		X	X	X	X	
Sechrist IV 100B	X					X				X	X		X		X	
Searle	X				X	2		X			X	X	X	X		X
Siemens 900B	X	X			X	X	2				X	X	X	X	X	
Siemens 900C	X	X	2		X	X					X		X			X
Veriflow CV 200	X					X					X	X	X	X		X
Veriflow CV 2000	X					X					X	X	X	X		X

*Optional. X = primary function; 2 = alternate method of adjustment.

In the United States, time-cycled ventilators have been used extensively to ventilate neonates. Several time-cycled ventilator models developed for older children and adults appear to be as versatile as volume-cycled ventilators in terms of pressure and flow capabilities.

Pressure-Cycled Ventilators

Pressure-cycled ventilators terminate the inspiratory phase when a preselected internal pressure has been achieved. The exhalation valve then opens, initiating the expiratory phase. If an inflation hold is used, expiration is delayed.

Tidal volume and the time of delivery will vary according to airway resistance, pulmonary and chest wall compliance, and integrity of the ventilator circuit. A significant decrease in the gas delivered to the patient may occur either because of leaks within the ventilator circuit or increased resistance in the circuit or the patient's airway. A large circuit leak prevents the buildup in pressure needed to terminate gas flow, but the gas does not reach the patient. In contrast, increased resistance, which may be caused by kinking of the circuit tubing or endotracheal tube or by mucus and secretions within the patient's airway, causes a rapid buildup in pressure, and premature cycling occurs before adequate tidal volume has been delivered. Some pressure-cycled ventilators, such as the Bird Mark 14, incorporate an auxiliary flow augmentation device. This mechanism is activated at a preselected time during the inspiratory phase so that even with significant leaks, tidal volume is maintained and cycling pressure reached.

Adjustment to changes in the patient's compliance and resistance is limited with pressure-cycled ventilators; therefore, these ventilators are not usually adapted for use in intensive care. A general feeling prevails that the pressure and flow characteristics of these machines are insufficient to meet the requirements of a patient with acute respiratory failure because a constant pattern of ventilation is difficult to achieve. However, some pressure-cycled ventilators, such as the Bird Mark 9 and 14, could provide pressure and flow equal to, or in excess of, that provided by most volume- or time-cycled ventilators currently available.

Pressure-cycled ventilators usually lack a system to deliver precisely controlled levels of oxygen and PEEP. They are used predominantly for IPPB and home therapy.

Volume-Cycled Ventilators

Volume-cycled ventilators terminate the inspiratory phase when a preselected volume of gas has been delivered. As with pressure- and time-cycled ventilators, if an inflation hold is used, the expiratory phase will be delayed. Current volume-cycled ventilators are manufactured with pressure-limiting valves, some fixed and others adjustable, that prevent excessive pressure from developing within the system if airway obstruction occurs. Without this pressure-limiting valve, excessive pressure may lead to pulmonary barotrauma.

Volume-cycled ventilators generally cannot compensate for a significant air leak and may not indicate its presence. Gas delivery from a piston stroke or compressible bellows (the most common mechanical devices used to deliver tidal volume) continues unabated, even if the patient is disconnected from the circuit. A leak usually is detected by monitoring the exhaled tidal volume. When the value measured is significantly less than that delivered by the ventilator, a leak is present.

Physicians have been led to believe that volume-cycled ventilators maintain constant tidal volume delivery to the patient regardless of changes in resistance and compliance. This alleged characteristic is largely responsible for the popularity of these devices in critical care settings. Actually the volume of gas received by the patient may vary with volume-cycled ventilators, often considerably. When the ventilator cycles, gas flows into the circuit and the patient. How much is distributed to each depends on their relative compliance. If the patient's compliance decreases, a larger percentage of the tidal volume is lost within the circuit (expansion of the tubing and compression within the humidifier or nebulizer, water traps, bellows or cylinder, connectors, and so forth). Conversely, if the patient's compliance improves, less gas is retained within the circuit.

The compliance/compression factor is variable, but a value of 4 ml/cm H_2O is representative. This means that 4 ml of gas is retained within the circuit for each cm H_2O of circuit pressure developed. In severe ARDS that requires high airway pressures to maintain adequate ventilation, several hundred mililiters of the total volume may be retained in the circuit rather than delivered to the patient (Fig. 24-6). Personnel monitoring the patient and ventilator may be unaware of this discrepancy, however, because a spirometer connected to the exhalation valve assem-

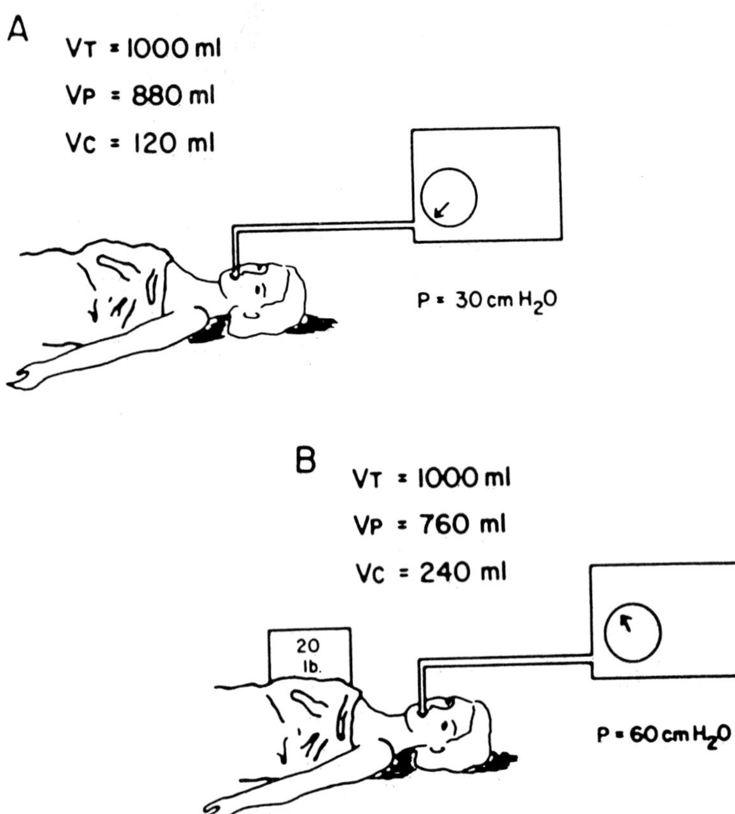

Fig. 24-6. Effect of changing patient compliance on ventilation. *(A)* A pressure of 30 cm H_2O delivers a tidal volume of 1000 ml, of which 880 ml reaches the patient and 120 ml is retained in the ventilator circuit. *(B)* The ventilator again delivers the 1000 ml tidal volume, but because of decreased patient compliance a pressure of 60 cm H_2O is needed, and only 760 ml reaches her, whereas 240 ml is lost to the circuit. In this example, circuit compliance/compression is 4 ml/cm H_2O. (V_T = total volume delivered by ventilator; V_P = patient volume; V_C = retained circuit volume; P = airway pressure).

bly records gas passing from both the patient and circuit. The sum of these is the volume that was delivered by the ventilator but not necessarily to the patient. The latter can be determined only if exhaled gas is collected between the patient's airway and the Y connector of the ventilator circuit, a technically difficult feat in some cases, or by interposing a respirometer in the same location.

Despite these problems, volume-cycled ventilators have proved popular in the ICU. They can provide high pressure and flow; oxygen delivery can be controlled accurately; the humidifiers are efficient; and, in many cases, they incorporate an alarm system to detect mechanical malfunctioning.

Flow-Cycled Ventilators

Flow-cycled ventilators terminate inspiration when gas flow falls below a critical level that is independent of airway pressure, tidal volume, or duration of inspiration. They are included here only for completeness, since they have no application in critical care. The best known example in the United States is the Bennett PR-2.

Secondary Limit

All commonly used mechanical ventilators have a maximum pressure capability. This limit may be incorporated into the basic design or added to the circuit in the form of a "pop-off" valve. Thus ventilators, whatever their primary cycling mechanism may be, are ultimately "pressure-limited" (whether or not they are also pressure-cycled). This feature is designed to protect the patient against possible excessive pressure buildup or tidal volume delivery that may occur inadvertently or through the carelessness of a respiratory care practitioner.

The pressure relief mechanism is adjustable in many ventilators, thereby adding to its protection effect. Commonly the relief pressure is set 5 to 10 cm H_2O higher than the pressure that is required to ventilate the patient. The primary time- or volume-cycling mechanism will then be operative, and slight to moderate decreases in compliance will be compensated for by the additional available pressure. Significant decreases in compliance or increases in resistance, or both, will cause a buildup in pressure that exceeds the limit that has been set. The relief assembly is then activated, and the excess gas flow and pressure, which might otherwise injure the patient, is vented from the circuit. An alarm usually sounds at the same time to alert persons caring for the patient that something has gone wrong.

In some ventilators it is possible to remove or inactivate the pressure limiting valve assembly and thereby develop a higher operational pressure. This temptation should be resisted because of the risk of injury to the patient and because ventilators generally are designed to operate efficiently within a preselected range of pressure.

EXPIRATORY PHASE

The expiratory phase begins when the exhalation valve opens. The valve may open immediately upon cessation of inspiration or later if an inflation hold is interposed. Ventilator modulation of expiratory events has assumed increasing importance.

Because exhalation usually is passive, a longer time is required than for inhalation. However, this ratio (I:E ratio) should be individualized, particularly when an inflation hold is deemed necessary.

Expiratory Retard

Observation of patients with chronic obstructive pulmonary disease (COPD), who use purse-lipped breathing apparently to prevent premature airway collapse and air trapping, has led to the design of systems that increase resistance or retardation to exhalation (see Fig. 24-1). More complete emptying of the lungs (decreased FRC) occurs, in contrast to PEEP, which is used characteristically to increase FRC. At the termination of expiratory retardation, airway pressure returns to ambient before the next cycle.

All ventilator circuits produce a certain amount of retardation because of the intrinsic resistance to flow of airway connectors, tubing, and the exhalation valve. The respiratory therapist must be aware of the normal expiratory flow pattern so that he can detect undesirable increases in retardation. The easiest method of detecting increased expiratory retardation is to note the rate at which the airway pressure manometer needle returns to baseline level from the peak following inflation. To be most accurate, one should measure the airway pressure as close as possible to the junction of the ventilator circuit and patient; otherwise, the pressure measurements may be altered by resistance of the ventilator, tubing, and so forth.

How important or desirable the use of expiratory retard is during mechanical ventilation of patients with COPD, acute asthmatic attacks, or the like is unknown. Some studies suggest that the importance attached to purse-lipped breathing has been exaggerated.

Subambient Pressure

The application of a subambient negative pressure to the ventilator circuit during the expiratory phase has been advocated primarily for two purposes: to decrease mean airway, and hence mean intrathoracic pressure, in order to enhance venous return and to improve cardiac output; and to offset the effects of excessive resistance that may result from an artificial airway. Reduction of circuit pressure in this way increases the pressure gradient across the tube from the patient end to the circuit end, and in theory should enhance expiratory gas flow. How much practical importance may be attached to this maneuver is unclear. The use of subambient pressure has fallen from favor because of the difficulty in determining whether the reduced pressure is transmitted to the patient side of the airway. If this occurs, airway collapse and air trapping, the opposite of what is desired, will occur.

Positive End-Expiratory Pressure (PEEP)

Application of positive pressure to the airway during the expiratory phase (see Fig. 24-1) is a mainstay in the treatment of ARDS. The effects of this therapy presumably prevent terminal airway and alveolar collapse and improve overall $\dot{V}/\dot{Q}$ ratios, although some regional $\dot{V}/\dot{Q}$ relationships may actually worsen. Improvement in pulmonary compliance and arterial oxygenation is often significant and may allow a reduction of FI_{O_2}, a desirable goal to prevent absorption atelectasis and pulmonary oxygen toxicity.

Various techniques are used to generate PEEP. A simple method allows patient exhalation through tubing, the distal end of which is under water. The level of PEEP depends on the depth to which the tubing has been submerged. With other systems, the ventilator activates a valve assembly during exhalation. The valve closes when the desired expiratory positive pressure is reached, and any gas that has not been exhaled is held within the lungs and ventilator circuit until the end of the cycle. In some cases the valve used to create PEEP also has a high internal resistance, which gives an expiratory retard effect. An elevated mean intrathoracic pressure above that produced by PEEP may result. This can be significant in reducing venous return in the patient with marginal intravascular volume or cardiovascular performance.

Before 1975, the recommended maximum level of PEEP was 10 to 15 cm H_2O; however, a significant number of patients with severe ARDS did not respond with improved oxygenation and decreased shunting at these levels. Subsequent reports attest to the fact that increased PEEP (40 cm H_2O or more) can be used in selected patients combined with IMV. A reduced mortality with no increase in ventilator related morbidity has been reported.

This therapy (termed "super PEEP" by some) requires meticulous cardiopulmonary monitoring, including pulmonary arterial catheterization. Since some ventilators cannot attain such pressure, it must be generated by special devices such as the Emerson water column PEEP-exhalation valve assembly.

High-level PEEP is indicated for a small percentage of patients. Most persons who require PEEP respond adequately to the earlier recommended levels. For those who do not, however, a willingness on the part of clinicians and respiratory therapists to apply more aggressive therapy may be life-saving.

CHANGEOVER FROM EXPIRATORY TO INSPIRATORY PHASE

Once the expiratory phase has been completed, a new inspiratory phase is initiated. This cycling may be performed either by the patient or by the ventilator.

Assist Ventilators

A ventilator that incorporates an assist (patient-triggered) mode must be equipped with a mechanism that detects the decrease in airway pressure caused by the patient's voluntary inspiratory activity. An adjustment control allows change of the pressure decrement (sensitivity) which triggers the inspiratory phase, thereby controlling the ventilator response time. Once the ventilator has initiated inspiration, it will deliver gas flow until the desired pressure, volume, or time limit has been reached. The ventilator assist mechanism may be electronic, magnetic, fluidic, or pneumatic.

Control Ventilators

Control ventilators cycle automatically at a rate selected by the operator. The adjustment usually is made by a knob calibrated in breaths per minute. The ventilator will cycle regardless of the patient's need or desire for a breath but guarantees a minimum level of minute ventilation in the apneic, sedated, or paralyzed patient as long as the ventilator-patient connection is intact and no air leaks are present. Not all ventilators have single controls that set respiratory frequency *per se*. In some, inspiratory or expiratory timers are available, or controls that vary inspiratory flow rate and expiratory time.

Assist-Control Ventilators

Assist-control ventilators may operate in either mode individually or in both simultaneously (*i.e.*, the ventilator will assist the patient's spontaneous respirations, and will also cycle itself should the patient stop breathing or breathe so weakly that the ventilator cannot function as an assistor).

Intermittent Mandatory Ventilatory (IMV)

Ventilators with IMV capability allow the patient to breathe spontaneously, usually through an independent gas supply, but periodically (at a preselected rate and volume) cycle to give a "mandated" breath. Thus a combination of spontaneous and controlled breaths is provided for the best overall pattern of ventilation in the individual patient. As with controlled ventilation, a minimum level of minute ventilation is provided. Various methods of administering IMV have been used, both "homemade" and factory installed. Most, however, operate with a gas reservoir directed into the inspiratory limb of the ventilator circuit through a unidirectional valve (Fig. 24-7). When the patient inspires, the valve opens, admitting gas from the reservoir; when the ventilator cycles, the valve closes, and gas flow proceeds normally. Gas provided for spontaneous breathing may flow either continuously or from a demand regulator that is activated by the patient.

INDICATIONS FOR MECHANICAL VENTILATION

The decision to institute mechanical ventilation is a serious one. Such therapy entails significant risks to the patient, and the potential benefits must be enough to justify these risks. Proper understanding of the ventilator, its limitations, and the physiological effects it may produce will limit the untoward responses and complications.

A useful categorization of the indications for mechanical ventilation takes into account whether the lungs are primarily involved in the disease process, secondarily affected by other organ dysfunction, or are normal but compromised because of failure to breathe. The therapeutic implications in each type of disorder are quite different, although entities such as flail chest encompass more than one abnormality.

FAILURE TO BREATHE

Failure to breathe may result from any disease process that involves the neuromuscular ventilatory axis. In the absence of pre-existing pulmonary disease, the lung function is not compromised. If ventilation is supported by mechanical techniques, alveolar–capillary gas exchange proceeds normally.

Nevertheless, secondary pulmonary involvement may occur. Patients who must be totally immobilized for long periods and require prolonged tracheal intubation or tracheostomy are increasingly susceptible to infection. They usually cannot mobilize their secretions or cough effectively. Frequent tracheal aspiration using aseptic techniques must be performed, and vigorous attempts should be made to provide good bronchial hygiene through postural drainage, change of position, and chest physiotherapy.

Neuromuscular Disease

Disease processes such as poliomyelitis, Guillain–Barré syndrome, myasthenia gravis, and organic phosphate poisoning produce respiratory insufficiency by preventing normal neuromuscular transmission and effector organ responses. Respiratory paralysis may develop gradually, and the patient will become unable to maintain normal alveolar ventilation. The deterioration of arterial blood gases (hypoxemia when the patient breathes air, and hypercarbia) is a direct result of hypoventilation and is not caused by functional disorder of the lungs.

Many of these conditions are potentially reversible; the primary problem from a mechanical ventilatory standpoint is that weeks, and often months, of support must be provided before the patient can once again maintain his own ventilation. Physicians and respiratory therapists involved in the treatment of these patients must provide meticulous airway care. The threat of traumatic damage to the trachea by either endotracheal or tracheostomy tubes and their occlusive cuffs increases with the duration of mechanical ventilation.

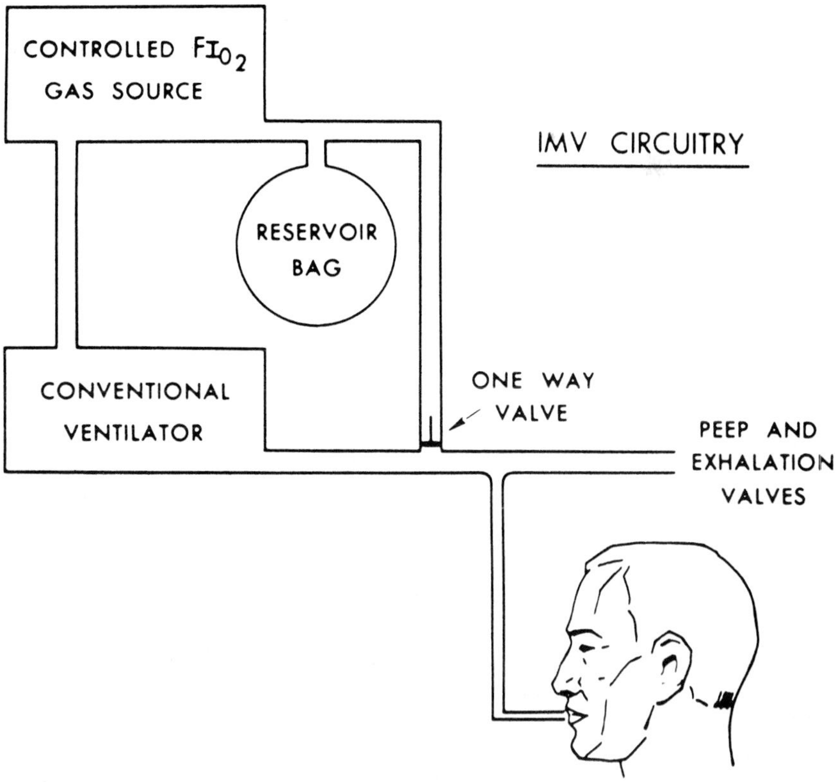

Fig. 24-7. IMV circuitry. A demand regulator is substituted for the reservoir bag in some commercially available systems. Spontaneous ventilation is supported from the bag or regulator, while controlled breaths delivered intermittently from the ventilator close the unidirectional valve and are directed to the patient. (Reproduced with permission from Kirby RR: IMV held satisfactory alternative to assisted, contolled ventilation. Clin Trends Anesthesiol *6*(4); Nov–Dec 1976)

Central Nervous System (CNS) Disease

Diseases that originate in the brain or spinal cord (*see* Chap. 34) are included as diseases of the CNS. Direct trauma that causes cerebral hemorrhage or transection of the spinal cord at a high cervical level is the most immediately life-threatening. If the patient survives the initial insult, however, prolonged mechanical ventilatory support, sometimes for the duration of his life, may be needed. A complication of brain trauma is neurogenic pulmonary edema, which may result from regional hypoxemia or hypoperfusion of the hypothalamic area at the base of the brain. Here an organic pulmonary lesion is superimposed on the functional derangement caused by the CNS lesion.

Other CNS disorders that lead to ventilatory abnormalities include bacterial and viral infectious processes such as meningoencephalitis and tetanus. These conditions often are associated with initial tachypnea and hyperventilation, but if respiratory arrest and convulsions ensue, mechanical ventilation may be needed for prolonged periods.

More perplexing and less common are primary CNS disorders that result in alveolar hypoventilation. These may be present in premature infants who have no detectable organic lung disease and who experience long apneic periods. Tactile stimulation may initiate and sustain ventilation, but, if not, mechanical ventilation is needed. In older chilren and adults with this problem, hypoventilation occurs with sleep; as long as the person is awake, ventilation appears to be normal. This syndrome (primary idiopathic alveolar hypoventilation, or Ondine's curse) thus far has no explanation. In particularly severe cases, however, tracheostomy and mechanical ventilation during the sleeping hours may be needed.

Finally, a number of disease processes of unknown etiologies progress slowly but eventually result in respiratory failure, including multiple sclerosis and amyotrophic lateral sclerosis. Clinical courses vary from patient to patient, but at present the long-term prognosis generally is not favorable.

Musculoskeletal Disease

The most common musculoskeletal derangement involves chest wall trauma with multiple rib fractures and subsequent disruption of ventilation (flail chest). In the past patients with this lesion required mechanical ventilation for 20 days or longer before ventilation occurred without flail. Recent evidence shows that the flail is not of primary significance, but rather the underlying pulmonary injury, and that the total period of mechanical ventilation can be shortened significantly or even eliminated. Other disease entities in this category include kyphoscoliosis, muscular dystrophies, and dermatomyositis.

DISORDERS OF PULMONARY GAS EXCHANGE

Pulmonary gas exchange disorders collectively account for the largest numbers of patients who require mechanical ventilation in neonatal, pediatric, and adult intensive care units. These disorders are characterized by primary pulmonary involvement rather than by extrapulmonary factors.

Respiratory Distress Syndrome of the Newborn (RDS)

RDS is associated primarily with prematurity of the newborn infant and is characterized by atelectasis, decreased FRC, right-to-left intrapulmonic shunting, hypoxemia, and CO_2 retention. Mortality figures before 1969 were as high as 80% in mechanically ventilated infants. However, since the introduction of PEEP/CPAP, used either alone or in conjunction with mechanical ventilation, survival has improved substantially. The subject is discussed in detail in Chapter 29.

Adult Respiratory Distress Syndrome (ARDS)

A large number of seemingly unrelated disease processes are included in ARDS. Pulmonary involvement, however, is similar, suggesting that the pathologic response of the lung to various noxious stimuli is limited. The disease characteristics of ARDS are similar to those of RDS. However, the Pa_{CO_2} usually is lower than normal. In fact, hypercapnia in a patient without chronic pulmonary disease is an ominous prognostic sign.

As in RDS, the signs and symptoms of ARDS frequently can be reversed with mechanical ventilation and PEEP. A clear-cut reduction in mortality, such as that seen in IRDS, has not been demonstrated probably because many patients with ARDS have multiple complicating problems (CNS damage, renal and hepatic failure, long-bone fractures, sepsis, hemorrhage, and cardiac disease, among others). This subject is discussed in detail in Chapter 36.

Cardiac Disease

Disorders of gas exchange occur with some cardiovascular diseases and secondarily affect pulmonary function. Any condition that leads to left-sided heart failure and significant elevation of left ventricular end-diastolic pressure can result in pulmonary edema and decreased arterial oxygenation. Mechanical ventilation may be used to improve oxygenation and impede venous return, thereby reversing cardiac dilatation and allowing the heart to contract more effectively.

If heart failure has been long-standing or severe, pulmonary hypertension will occur, and permanent structural changes lead to cor pulmonale. Mechanical ventilation may be needed, but the results are less dramatic and the prognosis is grave. This subject is discussed in detail in Chapter 32.

Table 24-3. Guidelines for Ventilatory Support in Adults with ARF*

DATUM	NORMAL RANGE	TRACHEAL INTUBATION AND VENTILATION INDICATED
MECHANICS		
Respiratory rate	12–20	>35
Vital capacity (ml/kg of body weight†)	65–75	<15
FEV_1 (ml/kg of body weight†)	50–60	<10
Inspiratory force (cm H_2O)	75–100	<25
OXYGENATION		
PaO_2 (mm Hg)	100–75 (air)	<70 (on mask O_2)
$P(A\text{-}aD_{O_2})^{1.0}$ (mm Hg)‡	25–65	>450
VENTILATION		
Pa_{CO_2} (mm Hg)	35–45	>55§
V_D/V_T	0.25–0.40	>0.60

(Reproduced with permission from Pontoppidan H, Geffin B, Lowenstein E: Acute respiratory failure in the adult. N Engl J Med 287:743, 1972)

*The trend of values is of utmost importance. The numerical guidelines should obviously not be adopted to the exclusion of clinical judgment. For example, a vital capacity below 15 ml/kg may prove sufficient provided the patient can still cough "effectively," if hypoxemia is prevented, as discussed in the text, and if hypercapnia is not progressive. However, such a patient needs frequent blood gas analyses and must be closely observed in a well-equipped, adequately staffed recovery room or intensive care unit.

†"Ideal" weight is used if weight appears grossly abnormal.

‡After 10 minutes of 100% oxygen.

§Except in patients with chronic hypercapnia.

Pulmonary Embolism

Venous thromboemboli and fat embolization often result in hypoxemia because of reflex bronchospasm, permeability changes in the alveolar–capillary membrane, and pulmonary microvascular hypertension. Mechanical ventilation with PEEP often is associated with marked improvement in oxygenation. This subject is discussed in Chapter 33.

Miscellaneous Disorders

Mechanical ventilation is indicated postoperatively in patients whose ventilation remains depressed from the residual effects of anesthetic agents or muscle relaxants. Support is maintained only until these effects have dissipated, and then may be discontinued rapidly.

Occasionally, mechanical ventilation is used in cases where the patient is at high risk of developing respiratory failure, although when the decision is made no direct evidence for failure is present. Prophylactic intervention with mechanical ventilation in an attempt to abort or prevent respiratory failure has many adherents, but little objective evidence supporting its use has been published.

CRITERIA FOR VENTILATORY SUPPORT

Various criteria have been suggested to ascertain when to begin mechanical ventilation[7] (Table 24-3). When pulmonary function tests are used as a guide either to initiate or to terminate mechanical ventilation, physicians must remember that many factors are involved in the individual tests themselves (Table 24-4). Few reasons can be advanced to ventilate a patient with chronic obstructive pulmonary disease solely on the basis of a Pa_{CO_2} of 70 torr if his normal Pa_{CO_2} is 60 to 70 torr. Conversely, an identical value in a previously healthy young adult suggests that ventilation should be supported. Each patient should be considered individually and laboratory measurements used as adjunctive aids that precede any decision to employ mechanical ventilation.

Table 24-4. Factors in Pulmonary Function Testing

- Baseline "normal" values for the individual patient
- Nature of the underlying disease process
- Patient understanding of the test procedure
- Patient cooperation and motivation
- Knowledge and skill of the person administering the tests

TECHNIQUES OF MECHANICAL VENTILATION

ASSISTED VENTILATION

Assisted (patient-triggered) ventilation (AV) is used to [1] deliver humidified gases and aerosols to patients with acute or chronic airway and parenchymal disease by IPPB; [2] provide ventilatory support for both adults and infants (particularly infants) with acute respiratory failure; and [3] wean patients from controlled mechanical ventilation (CMV) and initiate spontaneous respiratory activity (Fig. 24-8).

The arguments in support of this latter technique center primarily on the alleged normal physiologic aspects of such ventilation. Because the patient initiates the ventilator cycle, intrathoracic pressure decreases transiently before the mechanical respiratory phase, and venous return and cardiac output are enhanced. The patient sets his own ventilatory rate rather than being subjected to a superimposed, unsuitable pattern of ventilation. Theoretically, a more normal arterial *p*H and Pa_{CO_2} result. Finally periodic initiation of spontaneous ventilatory effort reinforces normal ventilatory activity by preventing "disuse" of the respiratory muscles.

No convincing evidence exists that assisted ventilation provides the cited advantages to a clinically significant degree. If an assist mechanism operates properly, it will respond instantaneously. When the ventilator cycles, the events that follow are identical to those in the "control" mode, and it is doubtful whether the above advantageous circulatory or respiratory effects ensue. On the other hand, if the assist mechanism is not functioning properly, the patient expends considerable effort attempting to breathe but cannot cycle the ventilator. He becomes agitated, hypoxic, hypercarbic, and "fights the ventilator." Controlled ventilation frequently is needed.

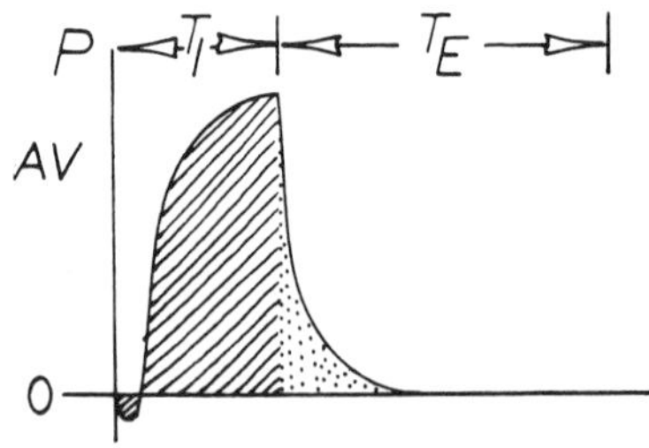

Fig. 24-8. Assisted (patient-triggered) ventilation (AV). An initial decrease in system pressure (P) results from the patient's spontaneous breathing effort. A sensing mechanism within the ventilator responds to the pressure decrement, and a mechanical cycle is initiated, producing gas flow and a positive pressure (T_I = inspiratory time; T_E = expiratory time). (Reproduced with permission from Eross B et al: Common ventilator modes: Terminology. In Kirby RR, Graybar GB (ed): Intermittent mandatory ventilation. Int Anesthesiol Clin *18*(2), 1980)

The effects of assisted ventilation on arterial *p*H and P_{CO_2} are not accurately ascertained without frequent arterial blood gas measurements. Underlying pulmonary abnormalities often increase a patient's minute ventilation to levels far above normal. Even though he is receiving assisted ventilation, his *p*H and Pa_{CO_2} may be abnormal.

The greatest difficulty with assisted ventilation is improper adjustment of the ventilator, leading to unreliability of many assist mechanisms. One frequently experiences situations in which the assist mode is so sensitive that the ventilator autocycles. In other instances it is so insensitive that the ventilator does not respond to the patient's inspiratory effort, and controlled ventilation must be used.

CONTROLLED VENTILATION

Controlled mechanical ventilation (CMV) (Fig. 24-9) is used in several clinical settings.

1. When apnea is present, either because of primary central nervous system dysfunction (e.g., severe brain trauma, spinal cord injuries, poliomyelitis) or because of drug overdosage, intentional sedation, or neuromuscular paralysis by drugs such as curare and pancuronium
2. As a backup (failsafe) for assisted ventilation, should the patient fail to sustain spontaneous ventilatory activity

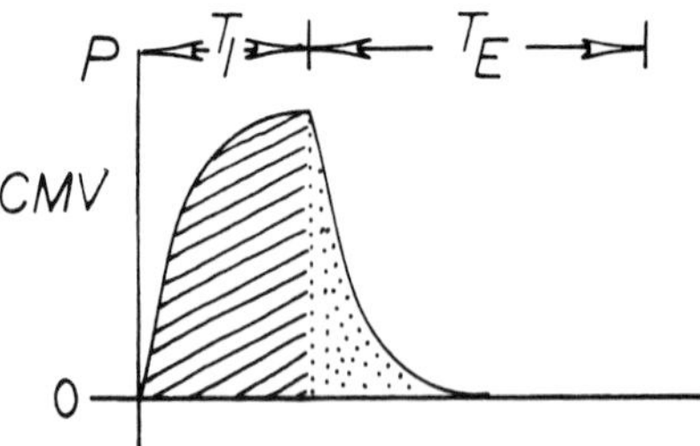

Fig. 24-9. Controlled ventilation (CMV). Ventilator cycling is automatic at a preselected rate. An initial pressure (P) decrement is not present. (Reproduced with permission from Eross B et al: Common ventilator modes: Terminology. In Kirby RR, Graybar GB (eds): Intermittent mandatory ventilation. Int Anesthesiol Clin *18*(2), 1980)

3. In conditions such as flail chest when spontaneous ventilatory effort is thought to be deleterious, and splinting of the chest wall is advocated
4. If therapy such as high-level PEEP makes the assist mode ineffective or of questionable reliability.

Generally, physicians and respiratory therapists use controlled mechanical ventilation when a certain level of ventilation must be "guaranteed" and when failure to supply this level of ventilation could be fatal. Most patients with severe respiratory insufficiency are initially treated with CMV to eliminate uncertainty as to the adequacy of support. However, certain aspects of ventilation peculiar to CMV must be understood by all persons who use it therapeutically.

When spontaneous ventilation is depressed by muscle paralysis or heavy sedation, accidental disconnection of the ventilator circuit may occur. The ventilator's alarm systems serve to decrease the possibility that such a disconnection will go unnoticed; nevertheless, such incidents are reported each year.

Often controlled ventilation is not facilitated by sedative or paralytic drugs, but rather by deliberately increased minute ventilation so that hyperventilation ensues and the Pa_{CO_2} falls below normal levels of 35 to 45 torr. As long as most patients are not hypoxemic, they will respond by becoming apneic, and their ventilation can then be controlled readily. Recent studies, however, suggest that the respiratory alkalemia induced by such techniques may be deleterious to the patient's overall physiological status (Table 24-5). Such therapy may exacerbate the primary condition, increasing the patient's need for mechanical ventilation.

Table 24-5. Adverse Effects of Respiratory Alkalemia

Decreased
Cardiac output
Cerebral blood flow
Pulmonary compliance
Serum potassium
Serum ionized calcium
Increased
Oxygen consumption
Airway resistance
Oxyhemoglobin affinity (transient)

Controlled ventilation does not guarantee that patients will not attempt to initiate spontaneous ventilation. In such instances the ventilator will not respond if it is used in a strictly control mode, and the ventilatory pattern becomes asynchronous: the patient attempts to take more breaths than the ventilator will provide. Failure to obtain a breath on demand leads to patient apprehension and may result in CO_2 retention.

The effects of CMV on cardiopulmonary function cannot be overlooked. Rapid controlled ventilation with large tidal volumes increases mean intrathoracic pressure, particularly when combined with PEEP, and venous return and cardiac output decrease. Thus cardiovascular function may be depressed both by respiratory alkalemia and by mechanical factors secondary to CMV.

INTERMITTENT MANDATORY VENTILATION (IMV)

In 1971 IMV (Fig. 24-10) was introduced to wean infants from mechanical ventilation. Later IMV was found to be similarly efficacious in adults. Further work has established that certain benefits are derived when IMV is used as a primary form of ventilatory support rather than solely as a weaning technique.

1. Conventional weaning techniques interpose periods in which the patient depends entirely

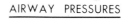

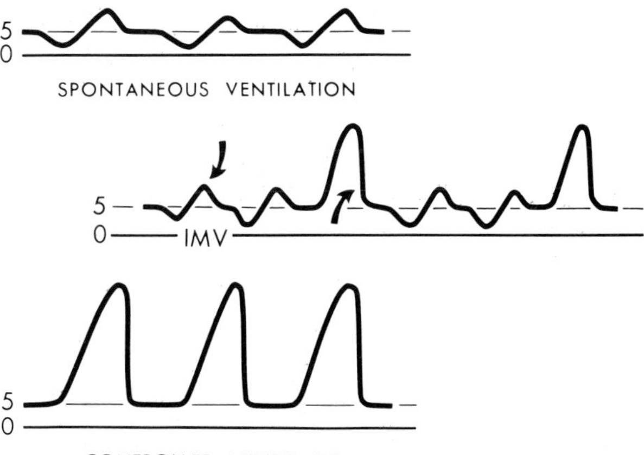

Fig. 24-10. IMV. A combination of both spontaneous and ventilator controlled ventilation can be delivered at any ratio. Lower mean airway and intrapleural pressures result, compared to controlled ventilation.

on the ventilator with periods in which he must breathe on his own. Such alternating support may be physiologically as well as psychologically unsound. Abrupt discontinuation of ventilation can produce anxiety and tachypnea, increase $\dot{V}O_2$, and ultimately result in a failure to wean. IMV allows a smooth transition from controlled to spontaneous ventilation by gradually slowing the ventilator rate as the patient assumes an increasing percentage of the total work of breathing. No other variables (e.g., tidal volume, FI_{O_2}, PEEP) need be changed.

2. Throughout the entire period of ventilation, the Pa_{CO_2} and pH are maintained relatively constant. Only enough ventilator support is given to maintain these arterial blood gas values within the range deemed appropriate for the individual patient. The patient is not forced to submit to a pattern of ventilation controlled by the ventilator; rather the ventilator augments the patient's own ventilatory effort to the degree necessary. Respiratory alkalemia is avoided without resorting to depressant drugs or added mechanical dead space. This is particularly important in patients with chronic obstructive pulmonary disease who suffer acutely superimposed respiratory failure and require mechanical ventilatory support. A very low IMV rate will return these patients' Pa_{CO_2} and pH levels toward their own "normal" values. The patient with a baseline, steady-state Pa_{CO_2} of 65 torr receives only enough IMV to achieve this level, rather than being controlled at levels of 35 to 45 torr, as previously customary.
3. Very high levels of PEEP may be used with IMV in contrast to the level that may be used successfully with CMV. *Mean* intrathoracic pressure is lower at any given level of expiratory positive pressure, and venous return is affected less deleteriously with IMV (Fig. 24-11). Patients who fail to respond to conventional therapy or who would otherwise have died or been consigned to extracorporeal membrane oxygenator support (ECMO) may be treated with PEEP as high as 30 to 40 torr, since the nonmandated breaths reduce the cardiovascular effects of positive pressure.
4. Drugs such as morphine are required only for pain and not to induce respiratory depression. Neuromuscular blocking drugs are seldom needed. Thus the dangers of profound hypoxemia are lessened, should the patient be disconnected from the ventilator accidentally.

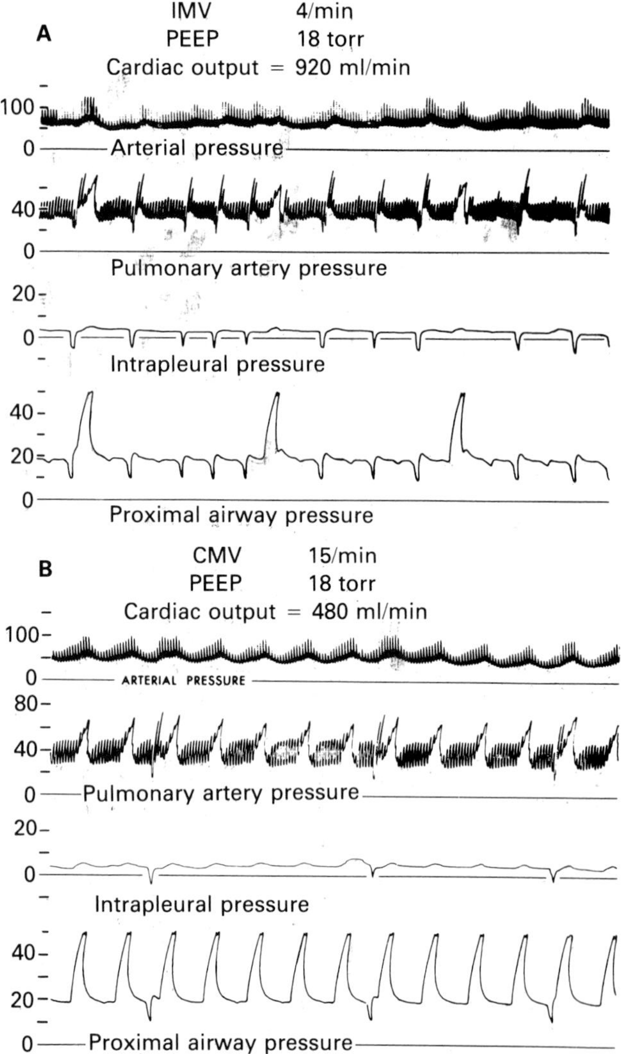

Fig. 24-11. Hemodynamic effects of IMV compared to CMV at increased PEEP. *(A)* Fewer mechanical cycles and maintenance of spontaneous breathing result in decreased intrapleural pressure, augmentation of venous return, and maintenance of blood pressure, stroke volume, and cardiac output. *(B)* CMV (with the exception of three spontaneous breaths) significantly compromises cardiovascular function. (Reproduced with permission from Kirby RR: Mechanical ventilation in acute ventilatory failure: Facts, fiction and fallacies. In Brunner EA et al (eds): Current Problems in Anesthesia and Critical Care Medicine. Copyright © 1977 by Year Book Medical Publishers, Chicago.

As with any system of ventilator support, certain potential disadvantages may be noted.

1. Many IMV devices are "homemade." Improper assembly, such as unidirectional valves installed backward, may result in total malfunction and can be disastrous to the patient if not detected immediately. This problem is less frequent in manufactured units that incorporate IMV. Valves that "stick" upon switchover to nonmandated mode are also an occasional problem.
2. If a patient who has previously needed a low IMV rate becomes apneic, his ventilation will not be supported adequately. IMV should be used only in those patients in whom CNS function is intact enough to facilitate regular spontaneous ventilatory effort. *The physican or respiratory therapist can be no less vigilant simply because the patient is receiving IMV!*
3. The delivery of a mandated breath from the ventilator just as the patient finishes spontaneous inspiration could lead to overdistension of the lung. Whether this concern is justified is debatable, particularly since a "sigh" mechanism has been used on many mechanical ventilators to achieve this very end: the delivery of a larger than normal tidal volume in the hope of preventing microatelectasis. However, newly designed IMV apparatuses are now available that deliver the mandated breath only at the beginning of the patient's spontaneous inspiration (SIMV).

The terminology applied to this modification of the basic IMV technique by the manufacturers of ventilators providing this option is *synchronized intermittent mandatory ventilation (SIMV)* or *intermittent demand ventilation (IDV)*. Although this concept is attractive theoretically, published evidence shows that it offers no advantage over conventional IMV. Further, the ventilator may fail to cycle appropriately, similar to the failure of certain assist mechanisms, a disturbing consideration.

HIGH-FREQUENCY VENTILATION (HFV)

High-frequency ventilation represents a significant departure from conventional mechanical ventilation. It is an oversimplification to consider the various mechanisms employed as though they were only slight modifications of a basic principle. As originally described, HFPPV did not differ as greatly from IPPV as is now supposed. Frequencies ranged from 60 to 100 cycles per minute (1–1.7 Hz), and tidal volume, although reduced, still exceeded calculated dead space. Of major significance was the reduction in peak and mean airway pressure and an associated decrease in transmitted pressure to the intrapleural space.

Subsequent development has increased the frequencies used up to 3000 per minute (50 Hz) in clinical use and up to 7200 per minute (120 Hz) in experimental animals. To achieve the higher frequencies, drive mechanisms incorporate rotary fixed orifices and amplifier-speaker assemblies. Tidal volume delivery is often considerably less than predicted dead space, and the mechanism by which alveolar ventilation is achieved is highly controversial.

The present and future roles of HFV are difficult to define. Experimental protocols have been hampered by the fact that existing high-frequency ventilators are available in small numbers and almost entirely in prototype form. Hence the characteristics of one system often have little resemblance to those of another, and large scale studies are difficult at best. Because of this limited availability, investigators cannot corroborate or refute the reported experimental and clinical findings of others. These same limitations have made it virtually impossible to define optimal frequencies, tidal volume, and pressure.

Many experimental studies have appeared in the published literature since 1978. However, clinical information has mostly been limited to case reports or series in which the small number of patients studied makes interpretation difficult. Nevertheless, most people involved in HFV research are optimistic that its proper role will eventually be defined and that the technique, in its many forms, will contribute significantly to reduced ventilator-related morbidity. In the meantime, if the studies of HFV do nothing more than elucidate mechanisms by which ventilation is possible under the operant conditions, the gain in knowledge will be substantial.

COMPLICATIONS OF MECHANICAL VENTILATION

PULMONARY BAROTRAUMA

Among the most significant complications of mechanical ventilation are the various forms of barotrauma, including

1. pulmonary interstitial emphysema;
2. pneumomediastinum;
3. pneumopericardium;
4. pneumoperitoneum and pneumoretroperitoneum;
5. tension pneumothorax; and
6. venous and arterial air embolism.

Current thought holds that the initiating event in "barotrauma" is overdistension of alveoli by either excessive pressure, volume, or both, with a resultant rupture of air into the perivascular sheaths and proximal dissection to the mediastinum. There it may rupture into the mediastinum or through the pleural reflections of the great vessels to the pericardium. Further dissection along the fascial planes into the subcutaneous tissues of the neck, head, thorax, and the rest of the body (subcutaneous emphysema) also occurs (*see* Fig. 14-25).

Except for vascular air embolism, which is often fatal (in massive cases it is instantaneously fatal), the most dangerous conditions are tension pneumothorax and pneumopericardium. In each case the venous return is reduced significantly, producing a fall in arterial blood pressure and in cardiac output. With tension pneumothorax, decreased ventilation is also present.

The incidence of barotrauma (primarily pneumothorax) with mechanical ventilation has been cited at 10% to 20%, although in infants an incidence as high as 30% has been reported. Even though PEEP would seem to increase the risk, this possibility has not been proved. Lowering the number of mechanical inflations per minute with IMV decreases mean intrathoracic pressure compared to techniques where ventilation is controlled and may also lower the incidence of barotrauma.

Control of inspiratory flow rates to achieve more uniform distribution of gas flow appears warranted to prevent gross overdistension of areas of high $\dot{V}/\dot{Q}$. It also seems prudent to use exhalation systems that produce a minimal amount of retardation to flow (unless more is specifically desired for a given patient) to further decrease the mean intrathoracic pressure.

The presence of subcutaneous emphysema, although not necessarily dangerous in itself, indicates the presence of barotrauma. Frequent physical examination to determine the adequacy of breath sounds bilaterally, constant monitoring of vital signs, and serial chest roentgenograms are all needed for early detection of complications of ventilator therapy. Personnel should be familiar with simple techniques to decompress a tension pneumothorax in emergencies. *Prophylactic* bilateral chest tube thoracostomies should not be performed in patients undergoing mechanical ventilation with PEEP. No published evidence has demonstrated the efficacy of such treatment.

CARDIOVASCULAR COMPLICATIONS

Any mechanism that increases intrathoracic pressure tends to reduce venous return and cardiac output. This observation was documented by Cournand and his associates in studies on intermittent positive pressure breathing.[1] Cournand's studies, however, were performed on animals and people with normal pulmonary structure and function. More recent studies suggest that in patients who have acute respiratory failure and whose lungs have decreased compliance, the depressant cardiovascular effects of mechanical ventilation and PEEP may be minimal unless the patient is hypovolemic. Much of the high airway pressure dissipates within the noncompliant lung before it can be transmitted to the great vessels within the intrapleural space.

The effects of PEEP can be minimized by infusing judicious amounts of blood, plasma expanders, and balanced electrolyte solutions to maintain or to expand the blood volume above normal. The depression of blood pressure and cardiac output by mechanical ventilation and PEEP can also be reduced markedly by IMV (*see* Fig. 24-11). Again, a low mean intrathoracic pressure resulting from fewer mechanical breaths and the patient's spontaneous breathing appears to be of paramount importance.

A major advantage of HFV may be reduced cardiovascular depressant effects compared to conventional ventilation. Tidal volume approaches, and in some instances is less than, calculated dead space, and peak and mean airway pressures are very low (at least in normal experimental subjects). Unfortunately these advantages may not be as great in patients with ARDS. Recent studies suggest that in order to improve Pa_{O_2}, mean airway pressure equal to that achieved with conventional ventilatory techniques is needed. The technique should be very useful in certain specific forms of respiratory insufficiency that at present are poorly managed by conventional methods, including bronchopleural-cutaneous fistula, malignant pulmonary interstitial emphysema, diaphragmatic hernia in the newborn, and acute exacerbations of COPD that require mechanical ventilatory support.

MISCELLANEOUS COMPLICATIONS

Many other complications associated with mechanical ventilation may occur, including pulmonary infection, airway obstruction, and tracheal damage from improper occlusive cuffs. Most of these problems can be minimized, if not eliminated, through careful attention by the physician, nurse, and respiratory therapist.

CHOICE OF A MECHANICAL VENTILATOR

Several factors should be considered before a mechanical ventilator is purchased, including the purpose for which it will be used, the experience of the people who will be using it, the ease of maintenance or repair, the initial cost, and its reliability and versatility (see Table 24-2).

In the past decade the number of sophisticated ventilators (and their cost) has increased substantially. Volume-cycled ventilators that can be used in an ICU which cost less than $6000 are rare. In some instances, the factors responsible for such high costs do not appear to offer sufficient improvement in care to justify the capital outlay.

Part of the difficulty in ventilator design has been that some manufacturers fail to heed the needs of patients, physicians, or respiratory therapists. Engineering masterpieces have been produced that were of little clinical usefulness. Performance characteristics in a laboratory frequently have little resemblance to those of the clinical setting! Recently, increasing cooperation has developed among manufacturers, their engineering staffs, and the physician consumer. Ventilators now meet the exacting physiological requirements of patients with acute and chronic respiratory disease more adequately than did those of the past.

The characteristics of an "ideal" ventilator are summarized in Table 24-6. At present no available device meets all suggested specifications, nor is it necessary that all ventilators should. A respiratory therapist primarily involved with IPPB therapy and routine postoperative ventilation has no need for the machine that can provide PEEP, IMV, high inspiratory pressures, and so forth. To spend money for such features is extravagant. On the other hand, a ventilator that will be used in an ICU to treat severely ill patients with acute respiratory failure should have most, if not all, of these features. No ventilator or ventilatory technique can provide optimal ventilation to all patients.

Table 24-6. Ideal Mechanical Ventilator

OPERATIONAL CHARACTERISTICS

- Volume or time-cycled
  - V_T = 10–200 ml (infants)
  - = 50–500 ml (children)
  - = 200–2000 ml (adults)
- Variable inspiratory flow rate (up to 150 liters/min for adult)
- Variable I:E ratio
- Peak inspiratory pressure limit
  - 60 torr (infants)
  - 100 torr (children, adults)
- Control, assist, and IMV modes available
- PEEP or CPAP up to at least 50 cm H_2O
  - (Ideal upper limit unknown at this time)
  - (Threshold rather than flow resistor)
- Frequency 0–60 breaths per minute (more for HFV)
- Inspiratory plateau up to 2 seconds
- Expiratory retard

ALARMS

- Minimum and maximum pressure in airway
- Oxygen concentration
- Inspiratory gas temperature
- Humidifier/nebulizer water level
- Electrical or pneumatic power failure

SERVO MECHANISMS (AUTOMATIC FEEDBACK CONTROL)

- F_IO_2 (flow and pressure independent)
- Inspiratory gas temperature
- Humidifier/nebulizer water level

MONITORS

- Airway pressure
- Frequency
- Tidal volume (patient)
- Inspiratory gas temperature (at patient airway)

Before purchase, one should use the ventilator for a trial period in the clinical setting. A reputable manufacturer confident of his product will comply with such a request. The purchase price of these intricate devices is too great to depend on advertising in brochures or journals or on exhibits using lung analogues at professional meetings.

The durability and the reliability of the ventilator are of paramount importance. Ease or availability of repair should be ascertained before purchase. Increased sophistication often is accompanied by increased fragility and "down time." Few consequences are more serious than those incidental to ventilator malfunction during the support of a critically ill patient.

The respiratory therapist should decide whether the features of the ventilator he contemplates purchasing are necessary or, at the least, desirable. For example, many ventilators provide a "sigh" mode to increase the delivered tidal volume at periodic intervals. At one time, periodic sighing was considered essential in prolonged ventilatory support. At present, however, many clinicians believe that sighs are not indicated when PEEP is used. Hence the sigh mechanism may well add a needless cost.

Finally, there is indeed a difference in mechanical ventilators. A rather trite observation has become popular in recent years to the effect that it is not the *ventilator* that is important but rather the *operator* of the ventilator. Certainly, nobody will dispute that it is essential to have a knowledgeable and skilled person determining how the ventilator is to be used. However, it is patently untrue to assert that any one mechanical ventilator is as good as another. If such were true, those who espouse this philosophy would use the least expensive, least complex ventilator available.

The problem facing the respiratory therapist is to catalog those features that he or she considers most important to provide a continuing high level of respiratory care and then to see which currently available model most closely meets those requirements.

FUNCTIONAL DESCRIPTION OF COMMON VENTILATORS

A systematic description of commonly used mechanical ventilators follows. Several are no longer commercially available in the United States (e.g. Gill-1, IMV-bird, Monaghan 560, Foregger 210, Searle VVA); however, we think that enough of each type are still being used to warrant inclusion.

BABYbird

Classification

The BABYbird ventilator (Fig. 24-12) is a pneumatically powered constant flow generator that is time-cycled. It can provide subambient, ambient, or positive expiratory pressures and can be used in control, IMV, or CPAP mode.

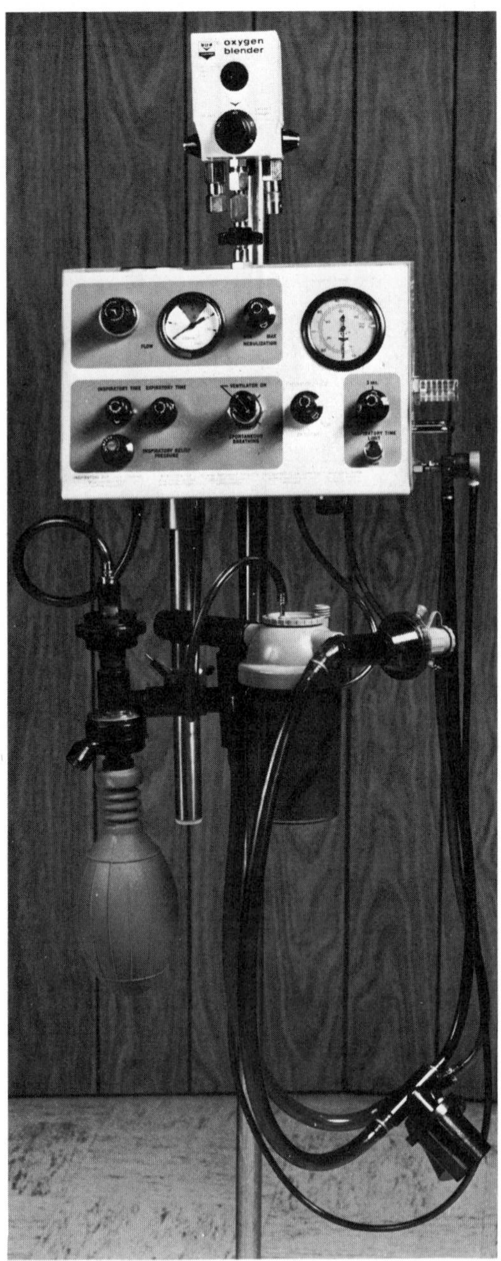

Fig. 24-12. BABYbird Ventilator, equipped with an oxygen blender.

Mechanism

The BABYbird is pneumatically operated and is powered by high-pressure air and oxygen mixed in the blender (A) to provide the desired $F_{I_{O_2}}$ (Fig. 24-13). This gas mixture is delivered into a source manifold where a low-pressure alarm (B) warns of any decreased pressure within the ventilator system. A flowmeter (D) delivers the flow (C) to the patient with the appropriate jet nubulization. The inspiratory breathing system also houses a pressure relief valve (E), which exhausts any pressure in the patient breathing circuit over 65 torr. This is the entire inspiratory circuit if the patient is breathing spontaneously. However, if the on–off control (F) is turned to IMV, a second circuit is activated. Gas pressure is delivered to the cycling mechanism (G), which has an inspiratory (H) and expiratory (I) timer to control the intermittent flow to two mechanisms, one during inspiration and one during expiration. During the expiratory phase, pressure may be delivered to a Venturi system (J), which provides an expiratory flow gradient. During the inspiratory phase, pressure is delivered through a restricting valve (K), which controls the downstream pressure to a second Venturi system (L). This system occludes the outflowing valve system (M) so that gas flow, no longer passing freely from the outflow valve, is delivered into the patient's lungs. A pressure gauge (N) measures the proximal airway pressure.

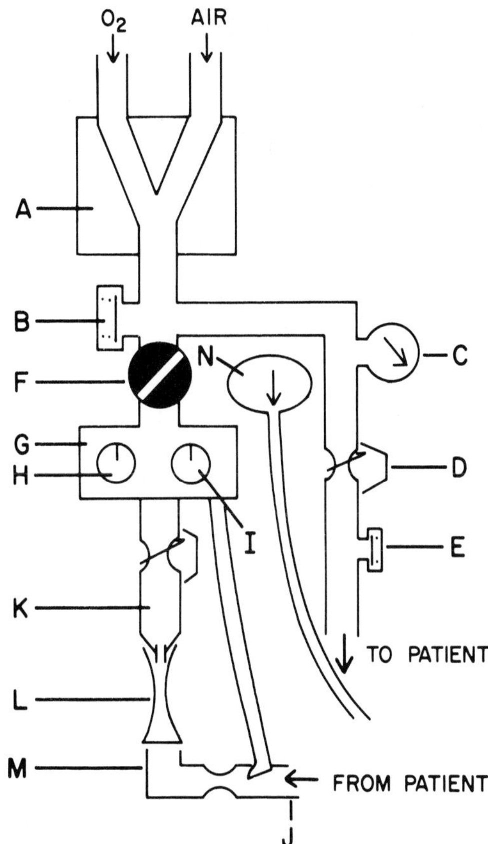

Fig. 24-13. Schematic diagram of the BABYbird Ventilator.

Operation

The BABYbird operates easily but occasionally is misunderstood because IMV is the primary mode of ventilation (Fig. 24-14). In simplest terms, gas that flows continuously through the ventilator circuit periodically is diverted to the patient by closure of the exhalation valve.

The operator connects the air and oxygen lines to 50 psi gas sources and selects the desired FI_{O_2}. Next, the flowmeter (A) is adjusted (B) between 0 and 30 liters/min according to the patient's needs. An arbitrary value, approximately twice the patient's predicted maximal inspiratory flow rate, is used initially. All flow from the ventilator is directed through the nebulizer; however, only part of it goes through the jet of the Venturi to produce particulate water. When the nebulization knob (C) is turned fully clockwise, a maximum of 12 liters/min will be delivered through the Venturi. As the nebulizer control is turned counterclockwise, less and less flow is directed through the nebulizer Venturi jet and more is directed into the supplemental gas port of the nebulizer, the auxiliary flow input receiver. This auxiliary flow line should not be occluded or inadvertently connected to the nebulizer Venturi.

If the patient is to breathe spontaneously, these are the only controls that need to be adjusted. If IMV mode is desired, the selector knob (D) is turned to IMV to activate the ventilator portion of the BABYbird. A suitable inspiratory time (0.4–2.5 sec) is set with the inspiratory time knob (E). *The duration of inspiration and the rate of flow determine the tidal volume delivered by the ventilator.* Selection of expiratory time with expiratory time control (F) allows respiratory frequencies of 1 to 100 breaths per minute.

The inspiratory relief pressure control (G) determines the pressure limit of the system. A mechanical peak inspiratory pressure relief valve set at 65 torr also is present. The expiratory flow gradient knob (I) reduces expiratory flow resistance by decreasing resistance to flow through the breathing circuit. This is accomplished by a Venturi proximal to the outflow valve. The operator can stop inspiration manually (K) or by a time-cycled mechanism (J).

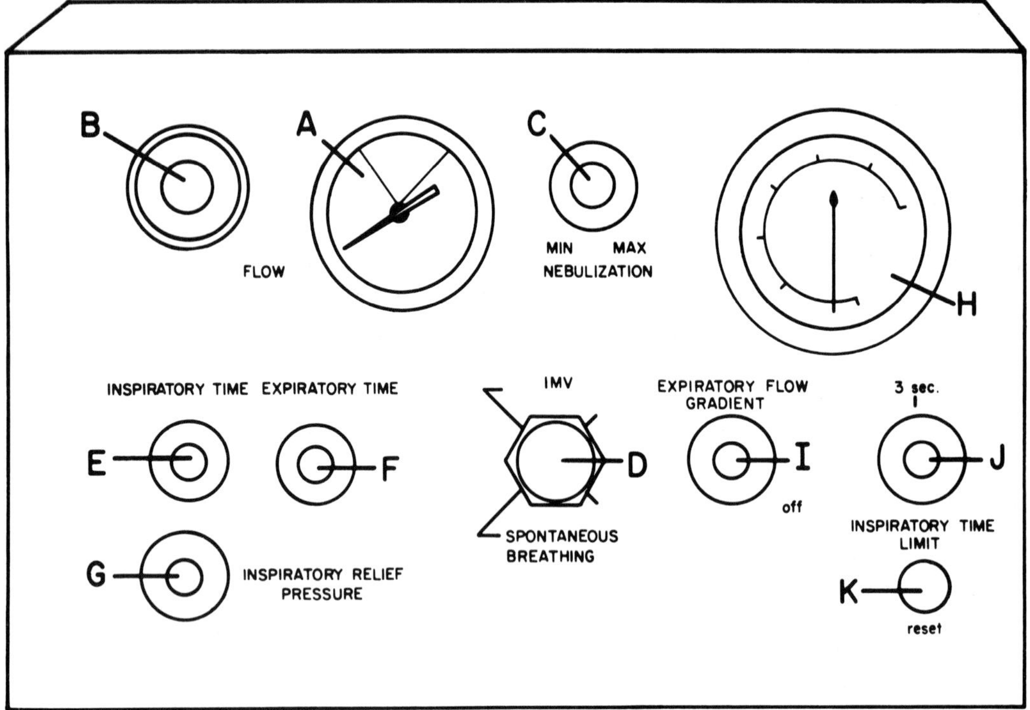

Fig. 24-14. Control panel of the BABYbird Ventilator.

PEEP or CPAP can be adjusted between 0 to 30 torr by a lever on the outflow valve. A test lung on the side of the BABYbird ventilator allows adjustment of these controls before the patient is connected to the breathing circuit. An additional safety device is the manual resuscitation bag attached to the lower part of the BABYbird ventilator. It can be used at any time to ventilate the patient.

Humidity

Humidity is provided by a Bird 500-cc inline nebulizer. (The output is described above.)

Cleaning and Sterilizing

The breathing circuit is easily accessible because of the quick disconnect features used in connecting the breathing system to the ventilator. However, washing is difficult because of many convolutions in the bonded shuttle valve assembly. Cold or gas sterilization of the permanent apparatus is necessary because no disposable circuit has been developed. This system is prone to contamination; therefore, breathing circuits must be changed at least daily and, in the case of problem patients, every 8 hours, if possible.

Accessories

No accessories are listed for this model.

Troubleshooting

The most common problem is leakage. Leaks may occur because of a faulty source gas supply system, because of loose connections in the breathing circuit, or because a part has been forgotten in reassembling the ventilator after it has been cleaned and sterilized. A decrease in line pressure will activate an oxygen-blender alarm if the pressure differential between oxygen and air exceeds 20 psi. If the alarm at the bottom of the ventilator is activated, the internal pressure of the ventilator has fallen below 45 psi or the inspiratory time is prolonged excessively. If the patient is not receiving adequate nebulization, the auxiliary and nebulizer lines may be crossed or inserted into the wrong ports.

If an undesirable residual positive-baseline pressure remains on the pressure gauge, the flow to the patient probably is too great for the breathing circuit. This baseline pressure can be eliminated by increasing the size of the breathing tubes, reducing the flow, or turning the expiratory flow gradient control counterclockwise until the indicated pressure returns to the level desired.

IMVbird

Classification

The IMVbird (Fig. 24-15) is a time-cycled, nonconstant flow generator with an adjustable inspiratory time, inspiratory flow rate, and inspiratory flow decelerator. During the expiratory phase, threshold positive pressure, subambient pressure, and retard capabilities are available. Controlled ventilation and IMV are the ventilatory modes featured.

Mechanism

The IMVbird (Fig. 24-16) is pneumatically powered by a high-flow oxygen blender *(A)*, which is serviced by a 50 psi source of air and oxygen delivered by a manually operated on–off master switch *(B)* to a demand flow accelerator servo *(C)*. As spontaneous inspiratory effort is initiated, the valve opens and provides accelerated gas flow to meet the patient's spontaneous inspiratory demand. The pressure-sensing port for the demand valve is at the proximal airway, which maximizes sensitivity and minimizes patient effort. Gas flow from *B* to the master cartridge *(D)* is metered to the timing circuit, which cycles the ventilator to inspiration or exhalation. The metering of gas from the master cartridge is regulated by the expiratory time *(E)* and the inspiratory time *(F)* con-

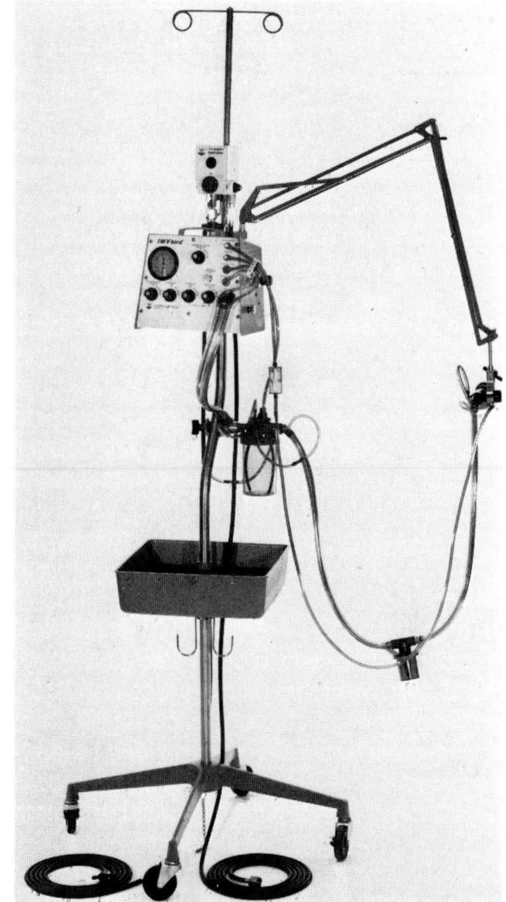

Fig. 24-15. IMVbird.

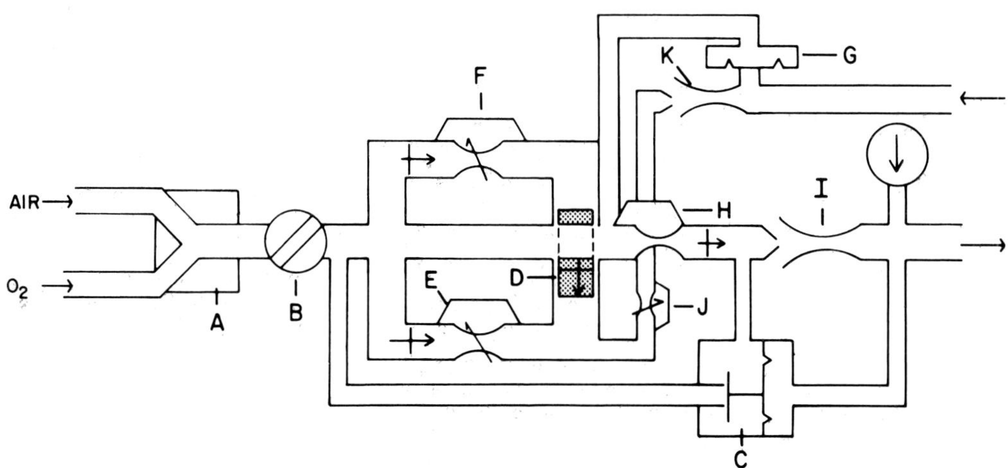

Fig. 24-16. Schematic diagram of the IMVbird.

trol knobs. When gas is bled away *(F)*, the master cartridge opens, initiating mechanical inspiration. The inspiratory phase is terminated when sufficient gas flow is metered through control E, closing the master cartridge and sequencing the ventilator into the exhalation phase.

During mechanical inspiration a portion of the gas is diverted to pressurize the exhalation valve *(G)*, facilitating the delivery of a mandatory breath. The inspiratory flow-rate metering valve *(H)* mediates flow during the controlled breath. The flow is directed into an injector *(I)*, which entrains gas from a reservoir of equal oxygen concentration, which is delivered into the inspiratory breathing circuit. The positive expiratory threshold pressure is adjusted with control *(J)* delivering gas to a Venturi system *(K)* during the mechanical expiratory phase. The spontaneous demand flow system is integrated with the end-expiratory pressure control mechanism by an automatic baseline compensator, which minimizes positive or negative deflections from the baseline airway pressure.

Operation

The oxygen blender is connected to 50 psi air and oxygen sources. As shown in Figure 24-17, the inspiratory flow-rate control knob *(A)* meters flow to the inspiratory breathing circuit which, in conjunction with the adjustable inspiratory time control *(B)*, sets a wide range of tidal volumes (80–3000 ml). The inspiratory timer increases the inspiratory time from 0.5 to 4 seconds as the control knob is rotated clockwise. A lockout circuit is provided to depressurize the exhalation valve automatically should the ventilator fail during the mechanical inspiratory phase. This internally adjustable mechanism is pre-set to terminate the mechanical inspiratory phase after 5 seconds.

The mechanical expiratory time interval is adjusted with control C. Clockwise rotation will increase the expiratory phase from 1 second to more than 3 minutes. This interval allows the patient to breathe spontaneously, and a wide range of IMV rates are possible. During the expiratory phase, the manual inspi-

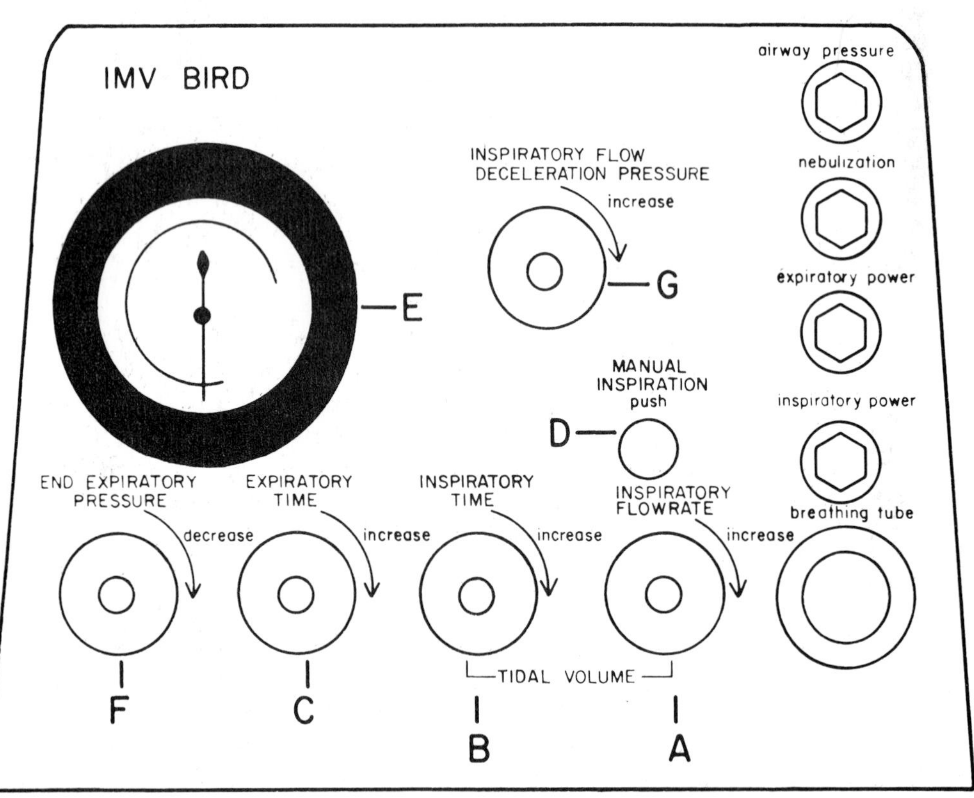

Fig. 24-17. Control panel of the IMVbird.

ration button (D) can be depressed to initiate a mandatory inspiration. If the button remains engaged, the ventilator will continue to deliver mechanical volume until the 5-second lockout mechanism terminates inspiration and dumps the tidal volume to ambient. Proximal airway pressure is monitored on the pressure gauge (E), which is calibrated in both cm H_2O and mm Hg. The end-expiratory pressure control (F) adjusts the amount of positive threshold pressure (0–40 cm H_2O pressure) desired during the expiratory phase.

The mechanical inspiratory flow pattern may be manipulated by adjusting the inspiratory flow deceleration pressure control (G), thus decreasing the flow rate at any preselected pressure between 20 and 75 cm H_2O. An internal overpressure governor provides a maximum pressure limit of 110 cm H_2O. Hose connections on the front panel are color-coded and indexed for the proper circuit connections.

Humidity

Humidity is provided by a dual-jet 500-ml Bird nebulizer. This nebulizer must be powered by a high-pressure source at a liter flow of 5 to 10/min. Nebulizer gas flow is included as part of the flow rate contributing to the mandatory tidal volume. An auxiliary nebulizer control on the side panel supplements total gas flow to the patient during spontaneous demand flow breathing. Condensation collects in the tubing, since the nebulizer is proximal to the breathing assembly; however, a water trap is provided on the loop of the circuit tubes.

Cleaning and Sterilizing

All patient breathing tubes, nebulizers, and parts that come in contact with moisture must be removed at least every 24 hours to avoid contaminating the patient by the breathing circuit. The equipment should be cold-sterilized or gas-autoclaved before repeated use.

Accessories

No accessories are listed for this model.

Troubleshooting

Leaks are a problem because of the large number of hose connections. The small high-pressure tubing connections are vital to the function of this ventilator, but leaks readily are found because of the high flow of escaping gas through a small orifice that makes an audible hiss. Internal leaks are uncommon.

BIRD MARK 6

Classification

The Bird Mark 6 ventilator (Fig. 24-18) is a pneumatic nonconstant flow generator with a biphasic flow pattern created by a flow accelerator. It is pressure-cycled with an optional inspiratory plateau. Neither retard nor PEEP is an integral part of the ventilator but can be added. The ventilator is primarily a controller, although it can be used with IMV-assisted ventilation.

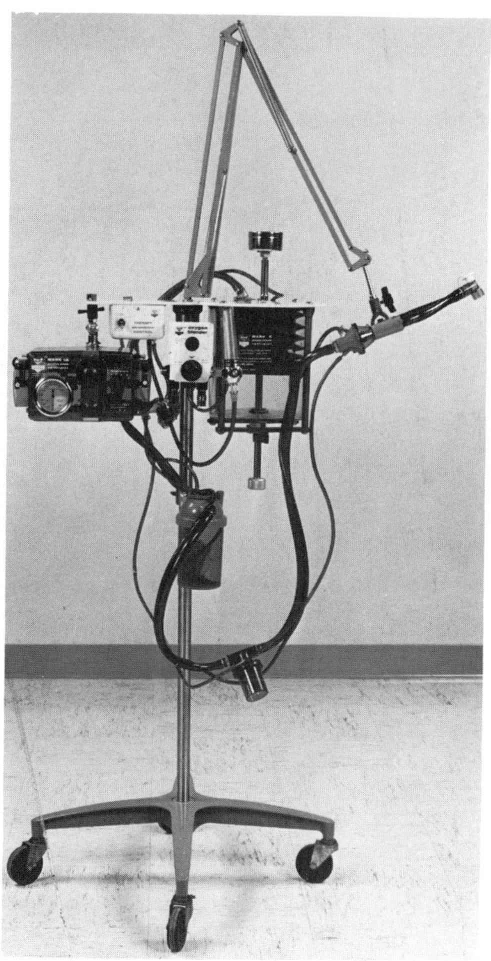

Fig. 24-18. Bird Mark 6 Ventilator shown with an oxygen blender and a Bird Mark 14 Serro Ventilator.

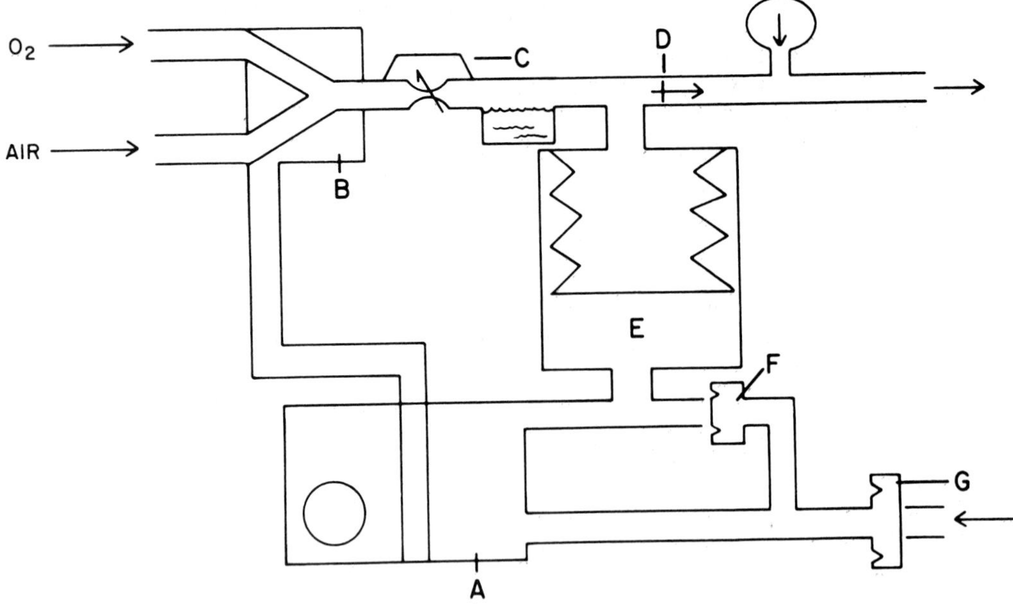

Fig. 24-19. Schematic diagram of the Bird Mark 6 Ventilator.

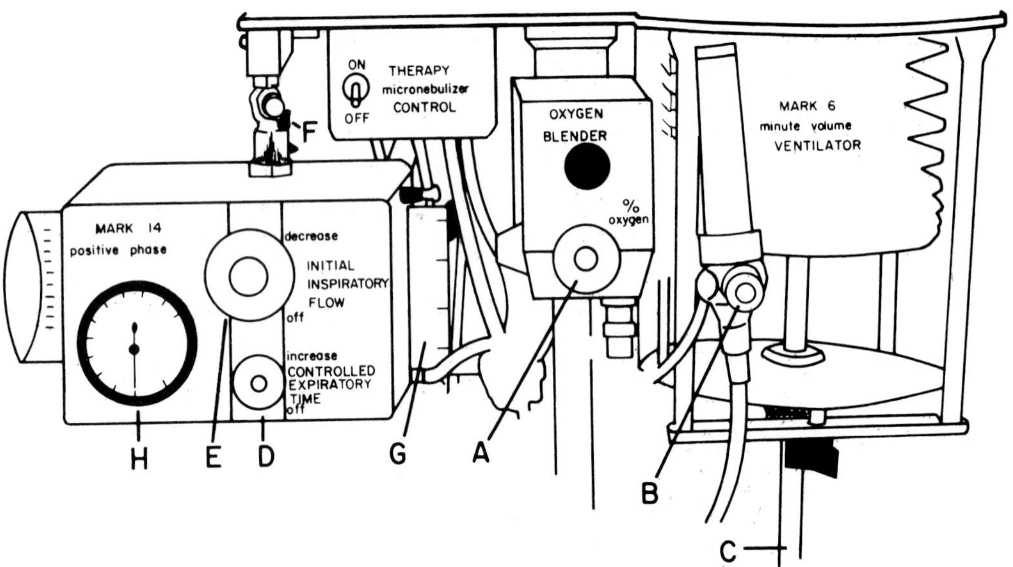

Fig. 24-20. Control panel and bellows assembly of the Bird Mark 6 Ventilator.

Mechanism

The ventilator is powered by a Bird Mark 14 servo ventilator* (A), which compresses a bellows (Fig. 24-19). Air and oxygen at 50 psi are mixed in a blender (B). Gas from the blender is delivered by a flowmeter (C), which determines the minute ventilation into the bellows assembly as the latter descends during exhalation. When the Mark 14 cycles on, the bellows assembly is pressurized, and gas from the bellows flows through a unidirectional valve (D) into the inspiratory limb of the breathing assembly.

Pressurization of the bellows occurs as the output of the Mark 14 is delivered into a plastic canister (E) that contains the bellows following closure of valve F. A second exhalation valve (G) simultaneously closes the patient circuit. When the Mark 14 cycles to the "off" position, pressure of valves F and G is released and the gas is exhausted from the canister and patient. Descent and refilling of the bellows follow to prepare for the next cycle.

Operation

The oxygen blender is connected to 50 psi sources of air and oxygen, and the appropriate oxygen concentration is selected (A) (Fig. 24-20). The desired minute volume is selected by the flowmeter (B). Tidal volume is determined by a position-adjustable shaft (C), which stops the bellows' descent at a specific volume. The cycling rate is adjusted by the expiratory timer control (D) on the Mark 14 ventilator, which adjusts expiratory time from 1.2 to 30 seconds, depending on the tidal volume and flowmeter settings. With inspiratory times from 0.6 to 6 seconds (depending on the tidal volume), a respiratory frequency range between 2 and 33 breaths per minute is possible. Inspiratory time is determined by the flow-rate adjustment (E) on the servo and the flow accelerator (F). These controls can be used simultaneously or sequentially, allowing a wide range of inspiratory flow patterns. If only the primary flow control (E) is used, the flow pattern is constant. If the flow accelerator is used, the flow is increased and the flow pattern becomes nonconstant and biphasic. A peak flow rate of 110 liters/min is possible.

*Other ventilators in the Bird Mark series may also be used. Depending on which ventilator is used, the ventilator may function as a constant or nonconstant flow generator, or a constant pressure generator.

The ventilator may be used in a pressure-limiting mode by adjusting the pressure setting (G). The pressure shown on the Mark 14 (H) is not the pressure at the patient's airway, but rather that required to compress the bellows. Elevation of the Mark 14 pressure limit will maintain the bellows in the uppermost position, thereby producing an inspiratory plateau.

Humidity

Humidity is provided by a 500-ml inline nebulizer activated by gas flow from the flowmeter. Because a major portion of this nebulized water is delivered into the bellows system, the bellows must be removed, cleaned, and sterilized with the breathing assembly at least once every 24 hours. Water particles that coalesce in the tubing system rain out into water traps, which must be maintained at the most dependent position of the breathing tubes.

Cleaning and Sterilizing

The patient breathing assembly, bellows, and nebulizer should be exchanged at least daily.

Accessories

Pressure relief valves are available.

Troubleshooting

Leaks are a major problem. The most common sites are at the bellows sealing gasket and at the nebulizer sealing ring. If no leaks are present in these areas, the bellows will remain in the uppermost position after the Mark 14 cycles and the flowmeter is turned off.

Another possible problem is the disconnection or unplugging of one of the many extraneous tubing connections, but these usually are identified easily by a hissing sound. Any other malfunctions probably will be in the Mark 14 servo unit. This ventilator is extremely reliable, however, and little difficulty should be experienced.

BEAR MEDICAL LS104–150

Classification

The LS104–150 infant ventilator (Fig. 24-21) is an electronic, piston-driven, constant flow generator. It is volume-cycled and may be used as an assistor, as-

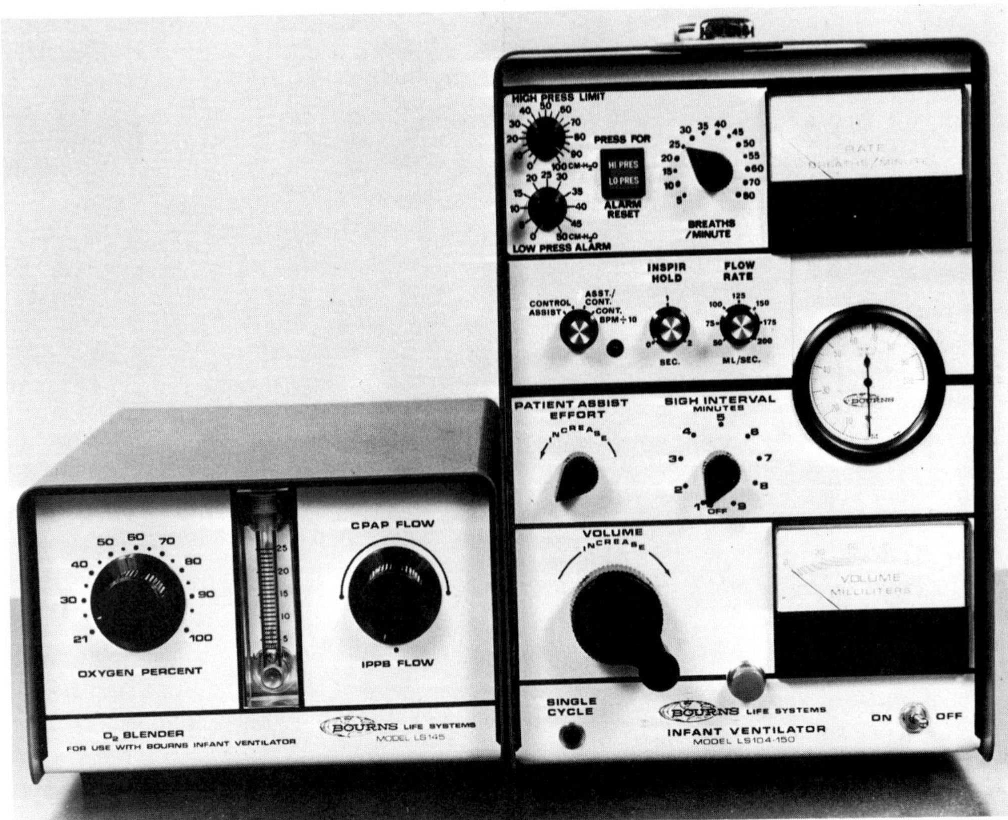

Fig. 24-21. Bourns LS104–150 Infant Ventilator.

sistor-controller, controller, or in an IMV mode. Positive pressure may be used during exhalation, and an inspiratory plateau capability is present.

Mechanism

High-pressure oxygen and air are delivered to a blending device (A), which mixes the oxygen concentration to the desired proportion (Fig. 24-22). This gas mixture is delivered at ambient pressure to a cylinder manifold (B) containing two unidirectional valves (C), which maintain proper gas flow direction, and an adjustable relief pressure valve (D). The piston (E) is attached to the walls of the cylinder by a rolling diaphragm (F). At the end of each inspiration, the piston returns to the pre-set volume, adjusted with a hand crank (G), by a reverse drive clutch. The piston will remain in the load position until the electronic unit (H) signals the forward clutch to engage the master gear (I) and move the piston at the rate set by the motor (J). Forward motion is signaled by the electronics unit in response to the rate control timer, the assist transducer, or the single breath button. Flow rate is controlled by the speed of the motor (J). Termination of inspiration and arming for the next inspiratory phase are signaled by magnetic reed switches when full piston motion has occurred. Ventilator system pressure is displayed on the pressure gauge (K).

Operation

Fifty psi oxygen and air connections are attached, and the ventilator mode (A) is selected (Fig. 24-23). If the ventilator is to be used on control or assist, the control is set to IPPB flow. However, if CPAP or IMV is to be used, the selector is set at CPAP flow and the flow adjusted on the flowmeter (B) to a rate adequate to exceed the patient's peak inspiratory flow rate. The oxygen concentration selector (C) sets the desired concentration. The ventilator should be turned on (D) 4

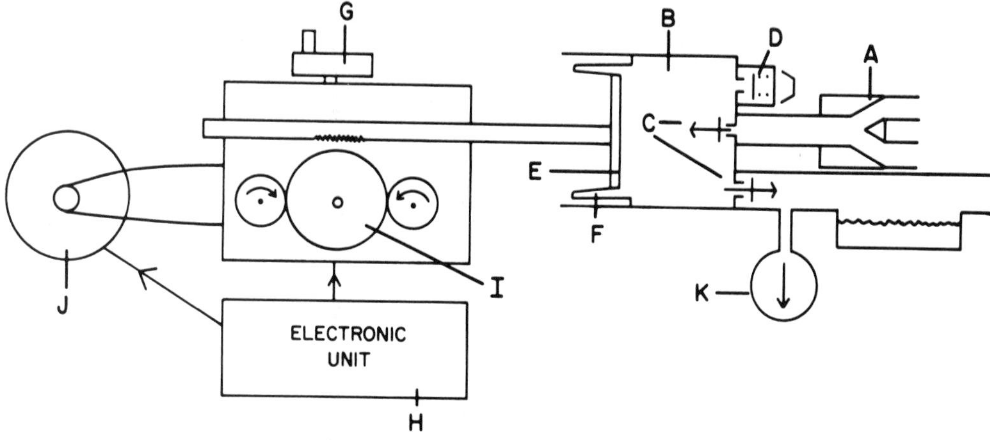

Fig. 24-22. Schematic diagram of the Bourns LS104–150 Ventilator.

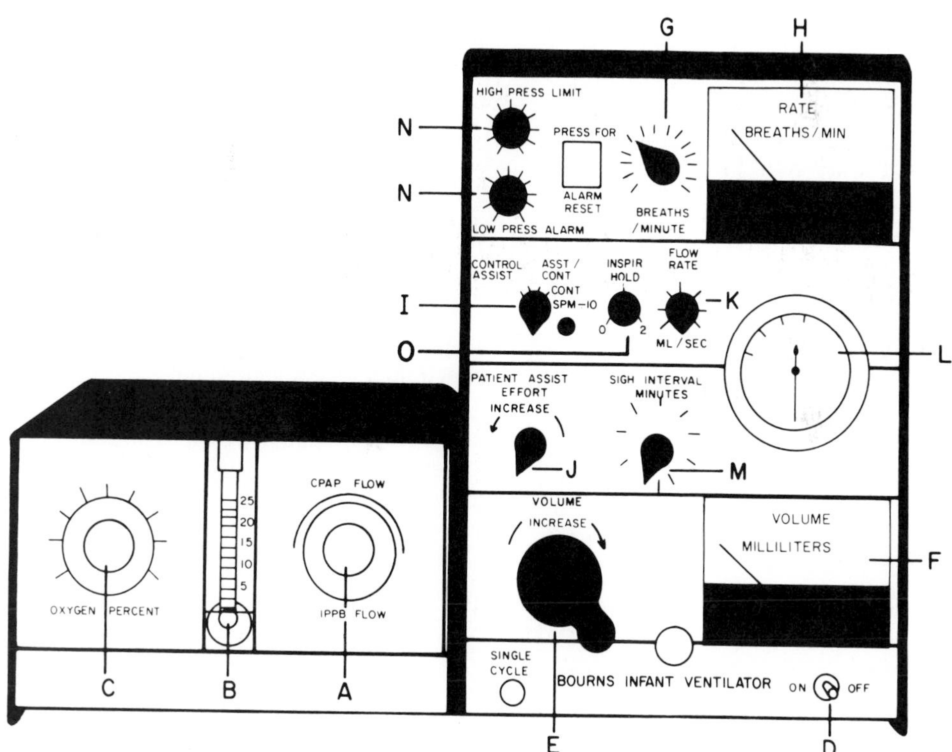

Fig. 24-23. Control panel of the Bourns LS104–150 Ventilator.

to 5 minutes before initiating ventilation (a "power on" indicator light will denote that the ventilator is on). Tidal volume is adjusted by turning the hand crank (E) until the desired volume (5–150 ml) is displayed on the volume meter (F). The compressibility factor for the Bourns ventilator is 0.3 to 0.45 ml/cm H_2O, depending on the type of nebulizer or humidifier and length of tubing. Breathing rate is adjusted by control G between 5 to 80 breaths per minute and read at H. The mode selector (I) determines the desired mode of operation. In the assist mode, if the assist rate is not maintained at 60% or more of the control rate (G), there will be a 10-second delay, and the control phase will take over for 5 seconds and then revert to assist. This selector mode will continue to cycle from assist to control as a safety measure as long as the patient's breathing rate is less than 60% of the set rate. An additional mode selection is available.

Sensitivity during assisted ventilation is adjusted by the patient assist effort control (J) and a sensitivity control at the rear of the ventilator. Sensitivity should be adjusted when the ventilator is connected to the patient. This ventilator is so sensitive that it may respond to changes in airway pressure caused by the infant's heartbeat. PEEP will not significantly change the sensitivity of the assist mode. An IMV mode is available.

Once the mode has been selected, the flow rate (K) is adjusted. This control is calibrated from 50 to 200 ml/sec. This flow rate is multiplied by 0.06 to find the flow in liters per minute.

Sigh volumes are achieved by two tidal volumes given in rapid succession. The interval between sigh breaths can be set between 1 to 9 minutes on control M. If no sigh breath is desired, the control can be switched off.

A range of 0 to 100 cm H_2O is available as a primary or secondary pressure limit for both normal tidal volume and sigh volume modes. When the pressure limit has been attained, the ventilator cycles to the expiratory phase unless the inspiratory hold (O) is activated. The pressure alarm system (N) has both high- and low-pressure adjustment knobs. The low-pressure alarm system indicates a disconnection or a leak in the ventilator system. A volume control for the audible alarm is available on the rear of the ventilator.

The low- and high-pressure alarms provide short pulses at the end of each inspiratory phase, whereas the apnea alarm sounds continuously until the ventilator changes from the assist mode to the control mode. The latter alarm operates only in the assist mode.

A single cycle button is available on the face of the ventilator so that the operator may trigger the ventilator whenever he wishes to instigate a breath manually.

Cleaning and Sterilizing

The ventilator breathing system is three-eighths inch ID tygon tubing, which is readily available in most hospitals. This system should be changed at least daily. Because the breathing system is divided into an inspiratory and expiratory system, gas flow is unidirectional; therefore, contamination of the exhalation valve should not contaminate the patient. The exhalation valve is relatively difficult to remove for sterilization except in-between patients.

Accessories

CPAP and IMV attachments, an ultrasonic nebulizer, a heated humidifier, extra ultrasonic nebulizer cups, a gas mixing box, an oxygen blender, a cart, and a tilt bed are available.

Troubleshooting

A significant leak will trigger the low-pressure alarm. This complex electronic ventilator should be repaired only by the manufacturer's representative or the factory itself.

Humidity

Two humidity options are available: a modified mistogen-heated humidifier or an ultrasonic nebulizer. Ventilator gas flow passes through the heated humidifier at the temperature selected by the clinician. Considerable water may condense in the ventilator tubing of this unit, and therefore the tubing must be cleared frequently to prevent occlusion and increased resistance to flow.

The ultrasonic nebulizer is an option. This unit has been modified to provide a lower than normal water output and should not be replaced by a conventional unit. Water condensation may also be significant with this nebulizer.

Distilled water, not saline, should be used to prevent corrosion.

BEAR MEDICAL SYSTEMS BP-200 INFANT VENTILATOR

Classification

The BP-200 is an electronically controlled, pneumatically powered, time-cycled constant flow generator (Fig. 24-24). It may be operated in either a CPAP or IMV/IPPB mode and can provide an inspiratory pressure plateau.

Mechanism

Air and oxygen, at 15 to 75 and 30 to 75 psi, respectively, are pressure equilibrated and mixed to desired FI_{O_2} (A) (Fig. 24-25). A continuous flow of blended gas is metered (B) into a calibrated Thorpe tube (not illustrated) and directed past a spring tension pressure relief valve (C). The gas is warmed and humidified (D) before it enters the breathing circuit. During mechanical inspiration a solenoid valve (E) closes, interrupting continuous flow vent, thus diverting gas into the infant's airway. During mechanical exhalation or CPAP, the patient breathes spontaneously from the continuous flow of gas. Gas flow may be opposed by a pressurized expiratory check-leaf valve (F). The amount of threshold expiratory generated depends on jet Venturi (G) flow metered by the PEEP/CPAP control (H).

Operation

Ventilator function and parameters are adjusted on a compact control panel (Fig. 24-26). A four-position control knob (A) serves as electrical power switch, alarm test, and ventilatory mode selector (IPPB/IMV or CPAP). In the alarm test position an audible alarm buzzer should sound. When CPAP is selected, the pneumatic and electrical alarm circuit is activated. If air or oxygen inlet pressure decreases below 15 or 30 psi, respectively, or an electrical power interruption occurs, an audible battery alarm is activated. If IPPB/IMV is selected, the ventilator will time cycle in addition to engaging the electronic and pneumatic power loss surveillance alarm system. When the mode selection is in any position but off, the amber-colored power light (B) is illuminated. Mechanical tidal volume is the result of an adjusted breathing rate (C) (range 1–150 breaths/min), I:E ratio control (D) (range 4:1 to 1:10), and continuous flow control (E) (range 0–20 liters/min). The continuous flow is indicated by means of a calibrated Thorpe tube (G). At low IMV rates the maximum inspiratory time control (F) (range

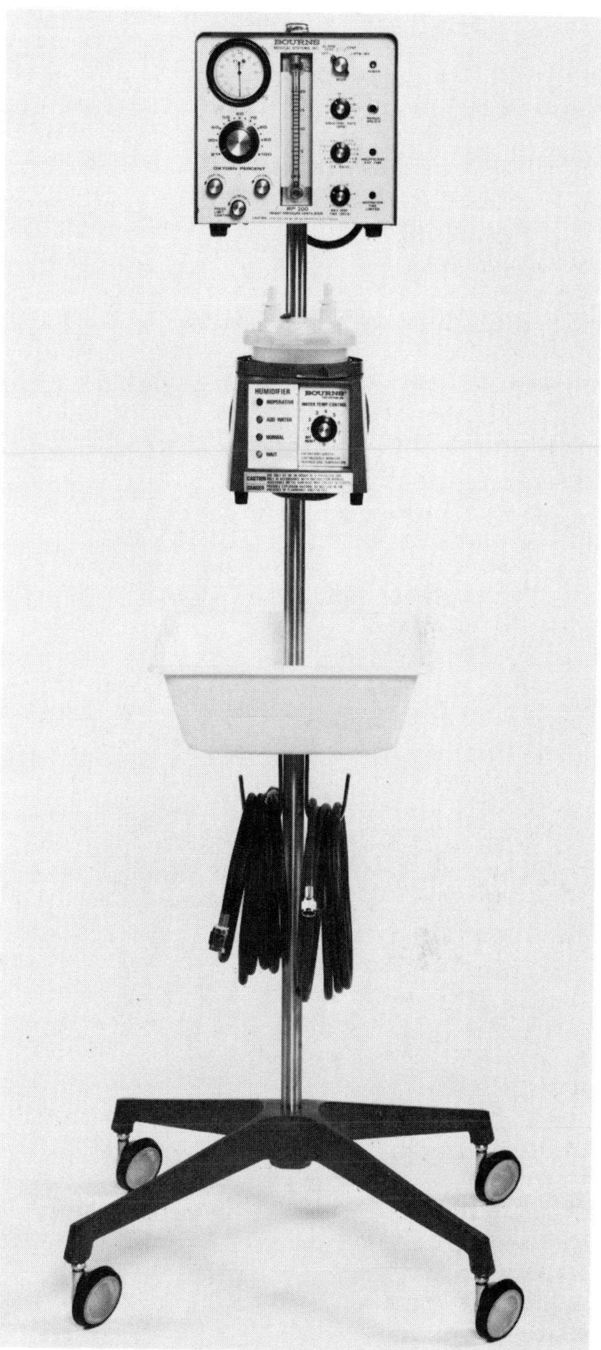

Fig. 24-24. Bourns BP 200 Infant Ventilator. (Courtesy of Bear Medical Systems)

0.1–3.0 sec.) may be used to override I:E control, obviating prolonged inspiratory time. When maximum inspiratory time has been reached, a red indicator light (H) illuminates. If the electronic timer allows

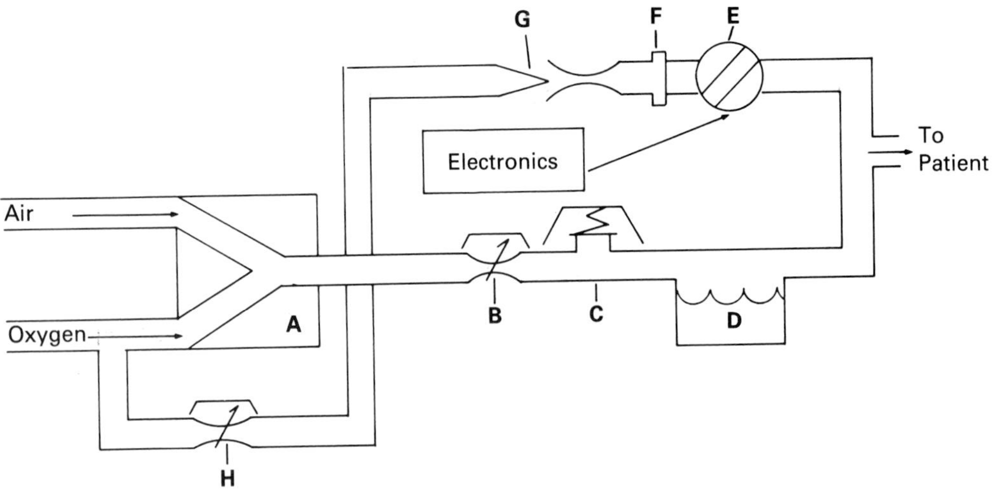

Fig. 24-25. Schematic diagram of the BP-200.

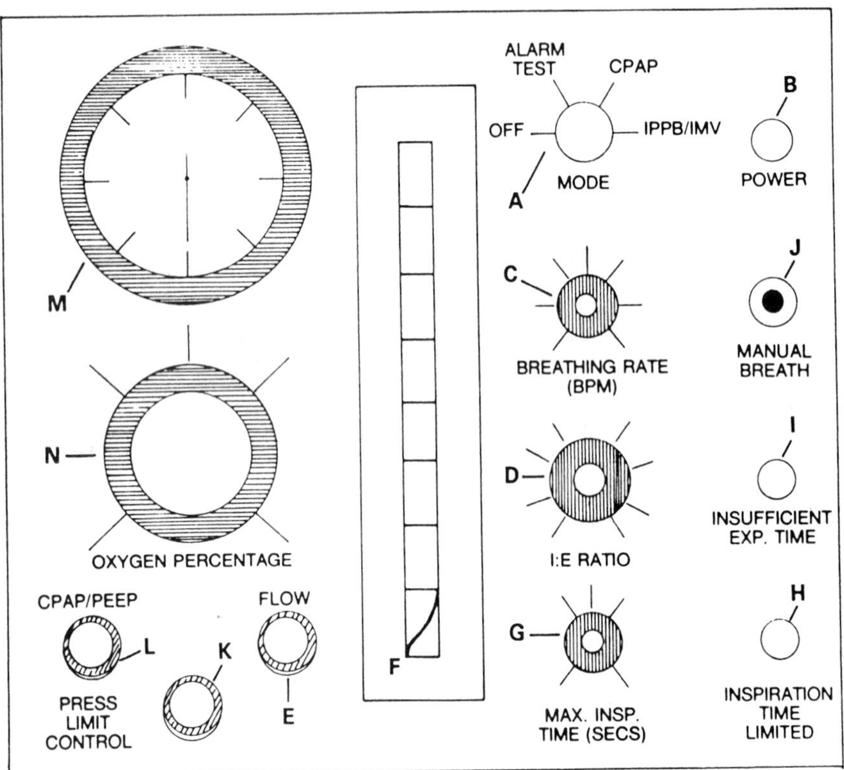

Fig. 24-26. Control panel of the BP-200.

adjusted mechanical expiratory times less than 0.22 to 0.28 seconds, a red insufficient expiratory time light (I) illuminates. A manual breath (J) may be administered only in the CPAP mode and is determined by ventilator settings similar to IMV/IPPB tidal volume.

Peak inspiratory (K) and threshold expiratory (L) pressure may be regulated from 12 cm H_2O at 2 liters/min to greater than 80 cm H_2O at 20 liters/min. and 0 to 20 cm H_2O at $\geq$ 45 psi O_2 inlet pressure, respectively. Each is adjusted by an uncalibrated control; consequently the pressure limit must be observed on an aneroid manometer (M) while the proximal airway connection is occluded. FI_{O_2} is adjustable (N) from 0.21 to 1.0.

Humidity

A 180-ml water reservoir heated humidifier with nine temperature control settings is provided. The humidifier assembly has four indicator lights: wait—reservoir temperature has not reached set level; normal—reservoir temperature is within 7°F of set value; add water—reservoir volume is low; and inoperative.

Cleaning and Sterilizing

The patient circuit should be changed at least every 24 hours. Tygon tubing, connectors, and humidifier may be sterilized by gas, liquid, or steam or pasteurized.

Accessories

Standard accessories include pedestal/pole mount, hose rack, air and oxygen hose assemblies, heated humidifier, and accessory tray.

Troubleshooting

The simplicity of this ventilator facilitates rapid recognition of problems. An audible alarm indicates either pneumatic or electrical power loss; if this occurs, gas inlet pressure gauges on the rear panel, the electrical connection, or the circuit breaker should be checked. Failure to develop circuit pressure during IPPB/IMV is usually caused by circuit leaks or a low pressure limit adjustment.

BEAR MEDICAL SYSTEMS BEAR 1 VOLUME VENTILATOR

Classification

The Bear 1 (Fig. 24-27) adult volume ventilator is an electronically controlled, pneumatically powered, modified constant flow generator. It is volume-cycled with assist-control, synchronized IMV, PEEP, and CPAP capabilities. The inspiratory phase may be extended by a plateau.

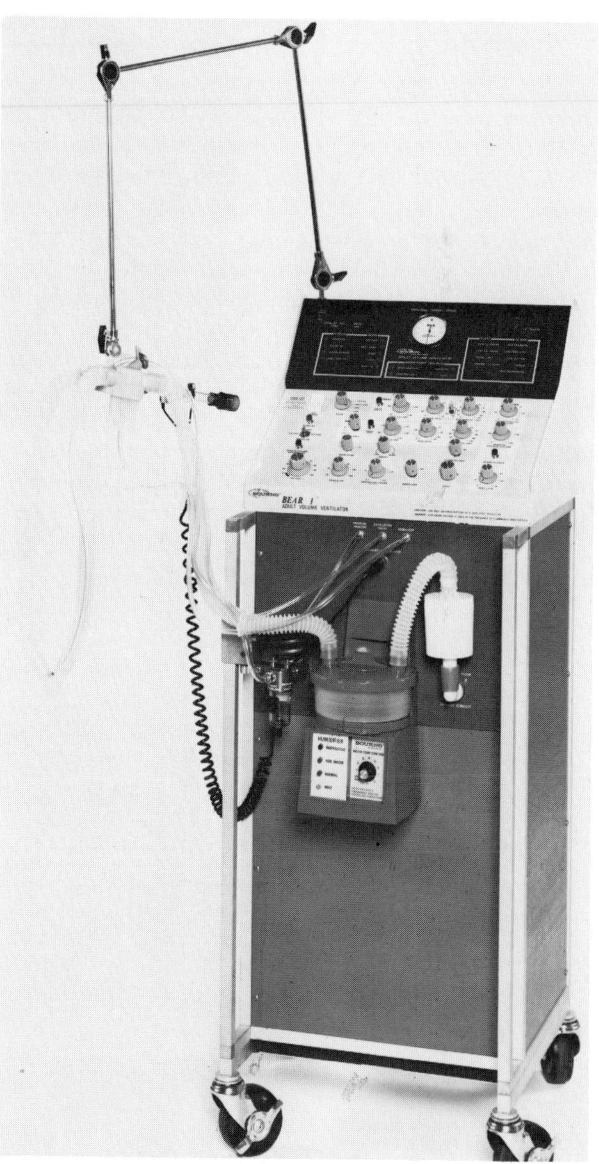

Fig. 24-27. Bear 1 Adult Volume Ventilator. (Courtesy of Bear Medical Systems)

Mechanism

The ventilator is powered by 30 to 100 psi sources of air and oxygen. If a malfunction causes reduced pressure of either of the gases, a crossover solenoid (A) is activated so that the remaining functional gas continues ventilator operation (Fig. 24-28). If the air pressure fails, a switchover valve (B) activates a compressor (C). This compressor also functions if the high-pressure line is not connected to an external source of compressed air. Both the air and oxygen pressure are matched in the system and delivered to a gas-blending device (D). This mixed gas then passes to a solenoid valve (E), which functions as the main on–off switch. Some gas also bypasses the main solenoid valve to perform other functions described below. From the main solenoid valve, the gas is adjusted through a set of two controls. The first (F) modifies the waveform delivered to the patient; the second (G) determines the peak flow rate. A vortex flow sensor (H) measures the volume of gas delivered to the patient. If the main solenoid-controlled time interval is not adequate to provide the preselected tidal volume, the flow transducer senses the discrepancy and signals the solenoid to remain open for an extended period until the volume has been delivered. An adjustable safety pop-off valve (I) limits the peak inspiratory pressure, and a subambient pressure valve (J) allows the patient to inspire room air if a ventilator malfunction occurs. Humidification is provided by a cascade heated humidifier (K).

A secondary system bypasses the main patient supply flow. This system provides gas for spontaneous breathing in the synchronized IMV (SIMV) mode of ventilation. A patient-sensing pressure line (L) controls gas flow from a demand valve (M). With SIMV the demand valve supplies gas flow to the patient distal to the main solenoid and waveform control valves. If the assist sensor (N) is activated, the IMV is synchronized with the patient's inspiratory effort, and the tidal volume is delivered through the main solenoid and flow modification valves. PEEP is adjusted by a PEEP control valve (O) and a Venturi (P), which pressurizes the exhalation valve (Q) during the expiratory phase.

Operation

The ventilator is connected to a 50 psi oxygen source and a 115 volt, 60 Hz electrical power source. If a 50 psi air source is available, the ventilator compressor system is bypassed. The type of ventilation desired is programmed by the mode selector knob (A) (Fig. 24-29). In the assist-control mode a built-in safety feature does not allow the patient to initiate a breath until at least 100 milliseconds after termination of the previous exhalation. If the patient becomes apneic, the ventilator will revert to a control mode at the frequency set on the normal rate control.

In the SIMV mode, gas flow increases as necessary to meet the patient's spontaneous ventilatory demand. When the appropriate time interval has

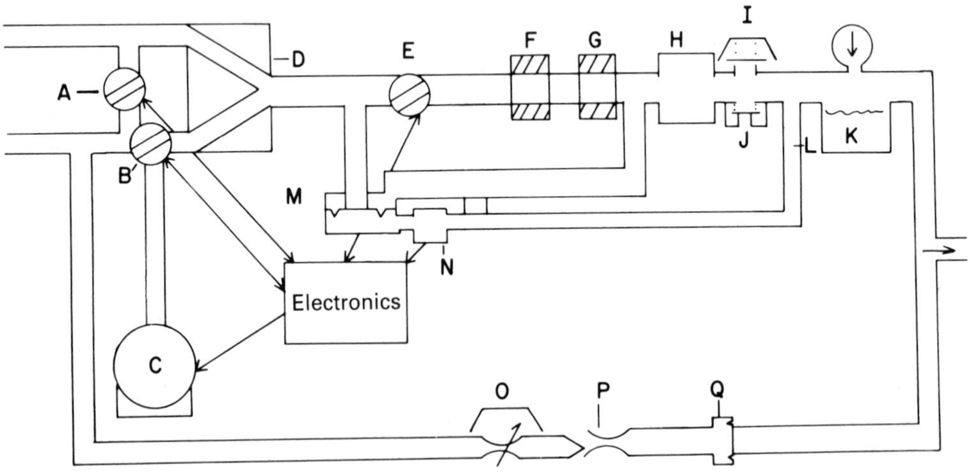

Fig. 24-28. Schematic diagram of the Bear 1.

elapsed, the IMV breath is delivered in response to (and synchronous with) the spontaneous effort.

The tidal volume control (B) is adjustable from 100 to 2000 ml. A rate control (C) has a normal range of 5 to 60 breaths per minute; however, a "divisible by 10" toggle switch extends the range from 0.5 to 60 breaths per minute. The lower rates are used for SIMV. The pressure control (D) adjusts the pressure limit from 0 to 100 cm H_2O. The ventilator may be placed on "standby" by depression of standby button E. In this mode the patient may breathe spontaneously. A standby light remains illuminated until 60 seconds have elapsed, at which time an audible alarm sounds.

Single or multiple sigh breaths (F) may be programmed. A separate sigh volume is selected (G) from 150 to 3000 ml and may be delivered from 2 to 60 times per hour (H). The sigh breath has a separate pressure limit (I) from 0 to 100 cm H_2O.

A minute volume accumulator (K) measures both ventilator and spontaneous breaths and displays them as exhaled minute volume. After 1 minute of display the indicator automatically reverts back to a tidal volume display. The inspiratory flow pattern is altered by a waveform control (L) that modifies the normal square wave flow pattern by decelerating or tapering the flow as inspiration continues and as pressure in the circuit increases. Inspiratory flow deceleration from 120 down to 40 liters/min is available.

The assist control (M) adjusts the degree of patient effort required to trigger the machine to the inspiratory phase and is adjustable from −0.5 to −10 cm H_2O. A ratio limit control (N) provides an audible alarm if the inspiratory to expiratory ratio is 1:1.

The oxygen percentage control (O) is adjustable from 21% to 100%. The inspiratory flow control (P) is adjustable from 20 to 120 liters/min. Spontaneous ventilation is not affected by this control. An inspiratory pause control (Q) delays the opening of the exhalation valve from 0 to 2 seconds. This delay is part of the inspiratory time and is therefore included in the I:E ratio calculation. If this control is used to generate I:E ratios, the I:E ratio limit control switch must be turned off.

A nebulizer control (R) activates the medication nebulizer. The PEEP control (S) adjusts PEEP from 0

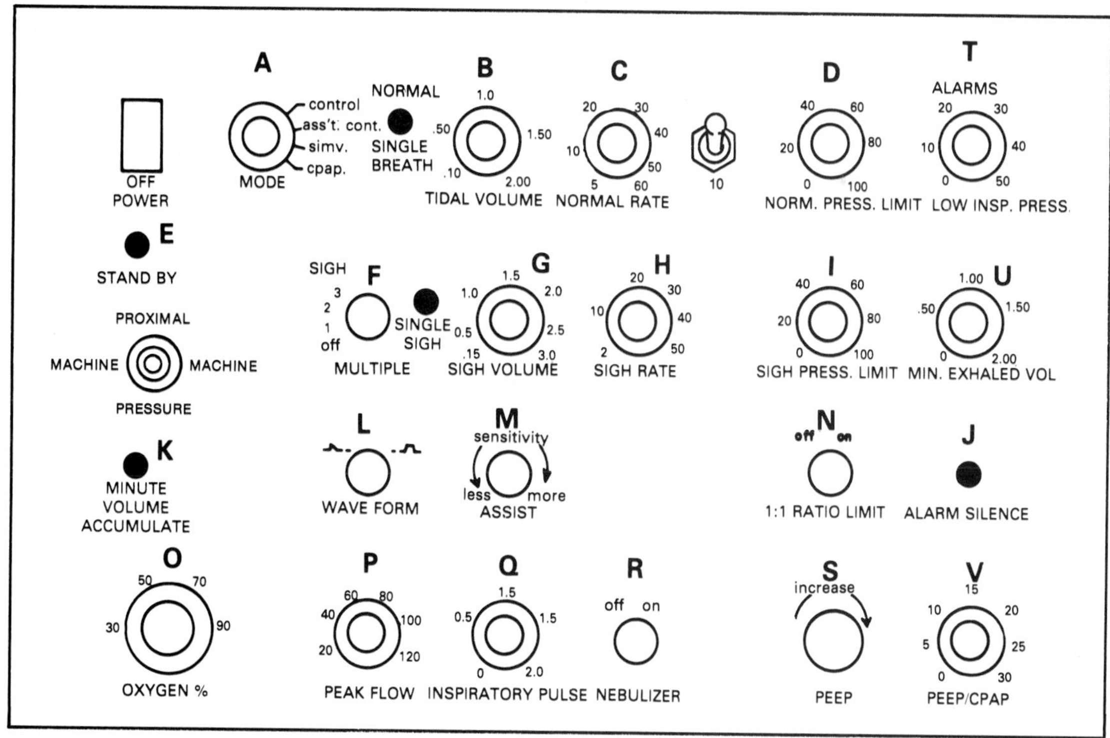

Fig. 24-29. Control panel of the Bear 1 Ventilator.

to 30 cm H_2O. This PEEP control is self-adjusting to compensate for minor leaks within the system.

The alarm systems have three controls on the main control panel. A low inspiratory pressure alarm (T) sets the lower limit of inspiratory positive pressure that must be generated by ventilator cycling. The minimum exhaled volume control (U) is adjustable from 0 to 2000 ml. If the exhaled volume is less than the volume indicated for three consecutive breaths, the alarm is activated. All alarms can be silenced for 60 seconds by depressing alarm silence button J. The PEEP/CPAP alarm (V) is adjustable from 0 to 30 cm H_2O. A visual and audible alarm is activated when the PEEP or CPAP level falls below the control setting. Multiple indicator and alarm lights are displayed on the upright ventilator panel, including pressure, exhaled volume, rate, and I:E ratio displays, as well as indicator lights for power-on, standby, alarm silence, nebulizer-on, control mode, assist/control mode, SIMV mode, CPAP mode, rate "divisible by 10," spontaneous breath, control breath, sigh breath, low oxygen pressure, low air pressure, pressure limit, inverse I:E ratio, low pressure, low PEEP/CPAP, low exhaled volume, apnea, and ventilator inoperative.

Humidity

Humidity is provided by a heated humidifier.

Cleaning and Sterilizing

Most parts of the patient breathing circuit may be disassembled, washed, and gas-autoclaved. However, the spirometer transducer crystals, bacteria filters, and particle filters should not be immersed in water or cold sterilants.

Troubleshooting

Troubleshooting is simplified by the 28 lights and monitors that indicate problems as they develop.

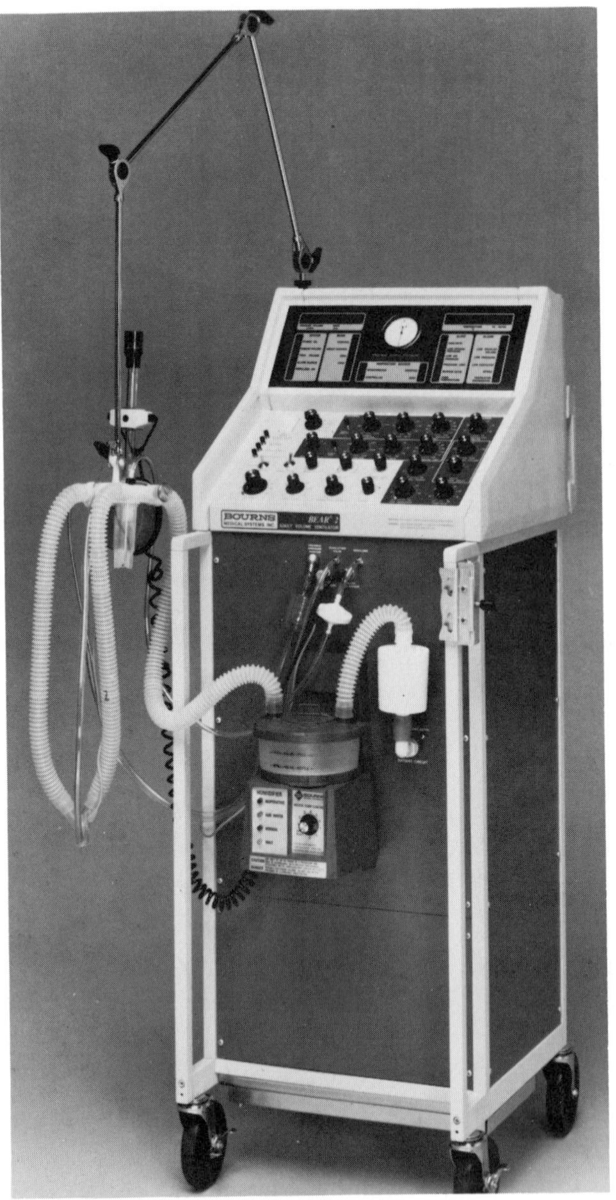

Fig. 24-30. Bear Medical Systems Bear 2 Adult Ventilator. (Courtesy of Bear Medical Systems)

BEAR MEDICAL SYSTEMS, BEAR 2 ADULT VOLUME VENTILATOR

Classification

The Bear 2 (Fig. 24-30) adult volume ventilator is an electronically controlled, pneumatically powered, modified constant flow generator. It is volume or pressure cycled unless inspiratory pause is used, then it is time-cycled. It has control, assist-control, synchronized IMV and CPAP capabilities.

Mechanism

The ventilator is powered by 30 to 100 psi sources of air and oxygen. If a malfunction causes reduced pressure of either gas, a crossover solenoid (A) is activated so that the remaining functional gas continues ventilator operation (Fig. 24-31). If the external air pressure fails or if internal air pressure falls below 9.5 psi, a switchover valve (B) activates a compressor (C). This compressor also functions if the high-pressure line is not connected to an external source of compressed air. Both the air and oxygen pressures are reduced to about 11 psi and mixed at calibrated rates as selected by the blender control (D). This mixed gas passes to a solenoid valve (E), which functions as the main on–off switch. Some gas also bypasses the main solenoid valve to perform other functions as controlled by the bypass solenoid valve (R).

A constant or decelerating (tapered) inspiratory flow pattern may be selected by a toggle switch (F), which regulates driving pressure to the peak flow control (G). In the square wave position, driving pressure is 3.0 psi, and ventilator outflow is equal to the peak flow adjustment. When flow taper is activated, driving pressure is reduced to 1.8 psi and inspiratory flow decelerates as circuit pressure increases. Flow will decelerate to 50% of the peak flow set at 120 cm H_2O back pressure to a minimum of 10 liters/min.

When the peak flow control valve (G) meters gas flow to the patient with the flow taper control set for square wave, there will be only a 15% drop in pressure shortly before termination of inspiration. Once the appropriate volume has passed through the flow transducer (H), a signal is sent via the electronic system to the main solenoid valve (E) to terminate inspiration unless the pressure limit control (I) has already cycled the ventilator to exhalation. Should an inspiratory pause be desired, the patient exhalation valve (Q) will remain closed for the extended pause period once the tidal volume has been delivered. It is during this phase that the ventilator is considered time-cycled. If all pneumatic and electronic systems fail, there is an antiasphyxiation valve (J) through which a spontaneously breathing patient may inspire. Humidification is provided by an adjustable heated humidifier (K).

A secondary system bypasses the main patient supply flow. This system provides gas for spontaneous breathing in synchronized IMV (SIMV) and CPAP modes. A patient-sensing pressure line (L) controls gas from a demand valve (M), which is activated in the assist-control, SIMV, and CPAP modes. The demand valve (M) system provides gas flow up to 120 liters/min distal to the main solenoid valve (E) and wave form control (F). If the assist sensor (N) is activated, the IMV is synchronized with the patient's inspiratory efforts, and the tidal volume is delivered through the main solenoid (E) and flow modification valves (F). PEEP is adjusted by the PEEP control valve (O) and a Venturi (P), which pressurizes the exhalation valve (Q) during the expiratory phase. The compensation chamber (S) adjusts the demand valve to the PEEP pressure and adjusts pressure on the exhalation valve during peak expiratory flow periods.

Operation

The ventilator is connected to a 50 psi oxygen source and a 115 volt, 60 Hz electrical power source. If a 50

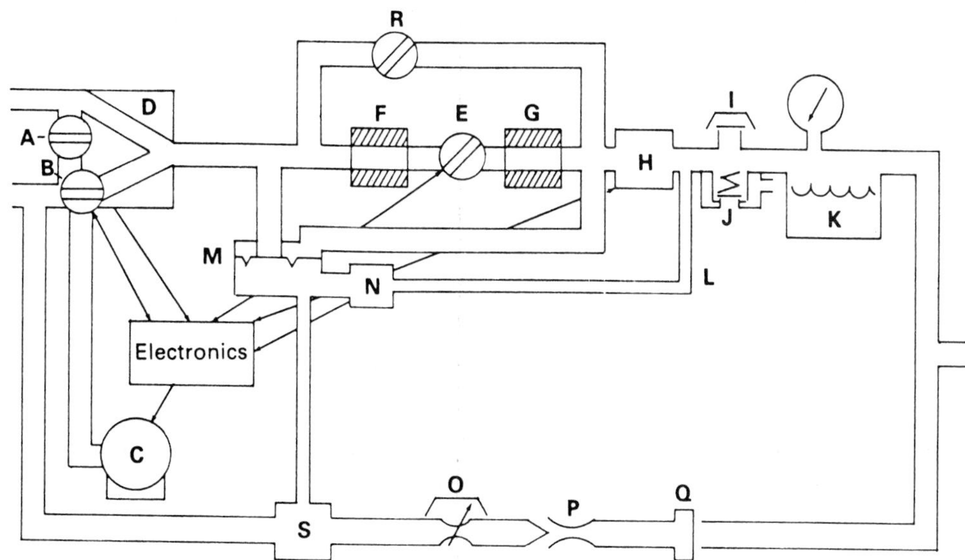

Fig. 24-31. Schematic diagram of Bear 2.

psi air source is available, the ventilator compressor system is bypassed. The type of ventilation desired is programmed by the mode selector knob (A) (Fig. 24-32). In the assist-control mode a built-in safety feature does not allow the patient to initiate a breath for at least 350 msec after termination of the previous exhalation. If the patient becomes apneic, the ventilator reverts to a control mode at the frequency set on the normal rate control (C).

In the SIMV and CPAP mode the patient breathes spontaneously, setting his rate, tidal volume, and peak flow up to a maximum of 120 liters/min. When a mandatory breath is delivered, all machine settings are met for tidal volume, peak flow, and so forth. Triggering the SIMV is accomplished by activating the assist-control sensitivity after the designated spontaneous breathing period has elapsed. Should the patient not trigger a breath, one cycling period elapses, then the ventilator switches to control mode. The detection delay (U) may alarm during this period if the expiratory time exceeds delay time and the patient is apneic.

The tidal volume control (B) is adjustable from 100 to 2000 ml. A rate control (C) has a normal range of 0.5 to 60 breaths per minute. The pressure control (D) adjusts the pressure limit from 0 to 120 cm H_2O.

Single or multiple sigh breaths (E) may be programmed. A separate sigh volume is selected (F) from 150 to 3000 ml and may be delivered 2 to 60 times per hour (G). The sigh breath has a separate pressure limit (H) from 0 to 120 cm H_2O.

The pressure may be measured from either the machine or a proximal tap. The pressure sensing selector (I) may be directed to sample either pressure. There will be some difference between the two pressures because of system and humidifier resistance. A constant 1 liter/min bleed in the proximal pressure measuring line prevents humidification buildup. A one-fourth inch tubing should be used to connect to the proximal tap. The wave form selector (J) may be used to deliver a square wave flow pattern in which the flow will decrease only 15% as the tidal volume is attained or a tapered flow pattern that reduces the flow by 50%. The flow taper cannot be used when the peak flow is set below 20 liters/min because the minimum flow is 10 liters/min. The nebulizer control (K) diverts a portion of the tidal volume through the nebulizer so that oxygen concentrations and tidal volumes are not altered during medication delivery. This nebulizer cannot be used if the peak flow (O) is set below 30 liters/min. The assist control (L) adjusts the degree of patient effort required to trigger the ma-

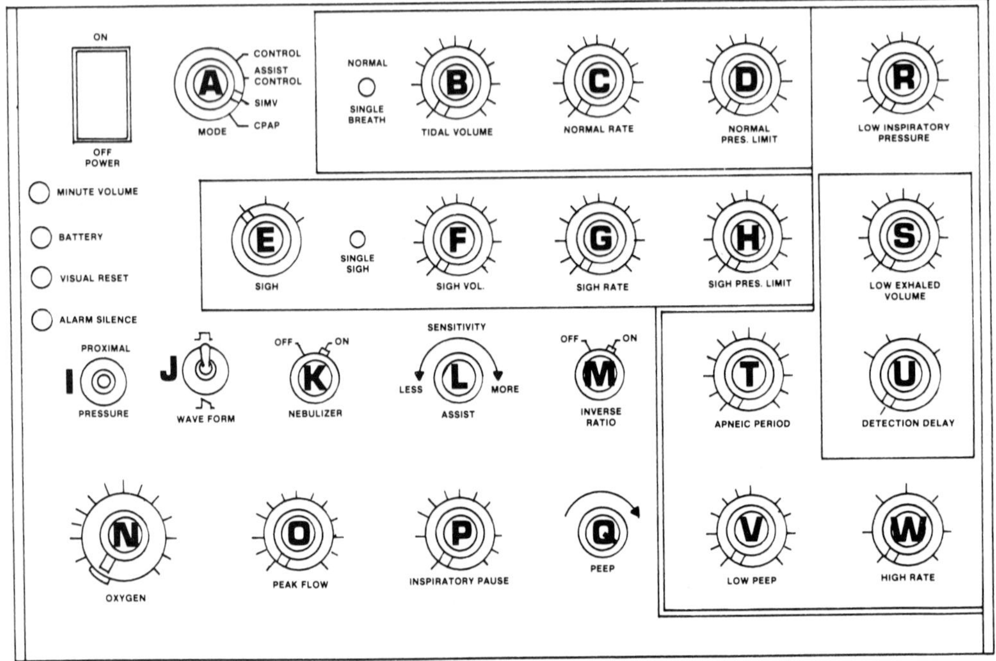

Fig. 24-32. Control panel of the Bear 2.

chine. This setting may be adjusted between −1 and −5 cm H_2O. Turning the control toward the "more" makes the system more sensitive both in the assist-control mode and spontaneous breathing mode. The volume of gas added to the system by the patient's inspiratory efforts will be added to the tidal volume as measured by the tidal volume flow tube. A ratio limit control (M) provides an audible alarm if the inspiratory or expiratory ratio exceeds 1:1 and inspiration is terminated. If this control is turned on, inverse I:E ratios may be attained. This control is inactivated in the assist-control and SIMV modes.

The oxygen percentage control (N) is adjustable from 21% to 100%. The peak flow control (O) is adjustable from 10 to 120 liters/min. This control does not affect the spontaneous inspiratory flow but will affect the flow taper if it is set below 20 liters/min and the nebulizer if it is set below 30 liters/min (*see* text). An inspiratory pause control (P) delays the opening of the exhalation valve once the tidal volume has been delivered from 0 to 2 seconds. Only in this configuration is this ventilator considered a time-cycled ventilator. This pause period is included in the inspiratory time and therefore should be considered when setting appropriate I:E ratios. The PEEP control (Q) can be set between 0 and 50 cm H_2O. The PEEP control can maintain its calibrated pressure with leaks up to 25 liters/min for 7 to 9 seconds. In the CPAP mode the patient breaths from the demand valve with flows up to 100 liters/min.

The alarm and monitoring systems have six adjustable controls on the face of the ventilator and multiple displays on the monitoring console. A low inspiratory pressure alarm (R) sets the lower limit of inspiratory positive pressure that must be generated by ventilator cycling. The minimum exhaled volume control (S) is adjustable from 0 to 2000 ml. If the exhaled volume is less than the volume indicated for the number of consecutive breaths indicated on the detection delay control (U), the alarm is activated. Once this alarm has been activated, it can be deactivated by one breath with the appropriate tidal volume. The apneic period alarm (T) is adjustable from 2 to 20 seconds; if the breath interval exceeds the alarm setting, the alarm will activate. The low PEEP/CPAP alarm (V) is adjustable from 0 to 50 cm H_2O; should the PEEP level fall below the level set, the alarm will activate. The high rate alarm (W), adjustable from 10 to 80 breaths per minute, is activated when respirations exceed the limit set. All alarms have corresponding lights that are activated on the display console to alert the therapist as to which alarm has been activated. Besides these indicator lights, there are LED displays for tidal volume, minute volume, rate, temperature, and I:E ratio. Should a "ventilator inoperative" display appear, the ventilator must be turned off to correct this alarm.

Signal outputs provided on the back of the ventilator allow remote nurse call, 9 VDC outlet for accessories, pressure signal output, and flow signal output.

Humidity

Humidity is provided by an adjustable heated humidifier with indicator lights that maintains the temperature within 7 degrees and indicates when the humidifier needs water or is inoperative. The flow resistance of the humidifier is 3.5 cm H_2O/liter/sec at the full line and 1.9 cm H_2O/liter/sec at the refill line. It requires 10 to 30 minutes to warm up to temperature.

Cleaning and Sterilizing

Most parts of the patient breathing circuit may be disassembled, washed, and gas-autoclaved; however, bacterial filters should not be wet if they are white. Blue filters may be used in a moist environment. Neither flow cables nor temperature probes should be sterilized in any way, merely wiped gently after each patient use with alcohol or germicide.

Troubleshooting

Troubleshooting is simplified by the 24 indicator lights and four LED displays on the monitoring console. This is coupled with a rather complete troubleshooting guide in the instruction manual available when purchasing this ventilator.

BENNETT MA-1

Classification

The Bennett MA-1 ventilator (Fig. 24-33) is an electrically powered, volume-cycled, constant flow generator that is secondarily pressure-cycled. Because of low driving pressure, in the face of low compliance it becomes a constant pressure ventilator. Expiratory retard and expiratory positive pressure are available. The MA-1 can function as an assistor, a controller, and an assistor-controller. IMV is available as an option.

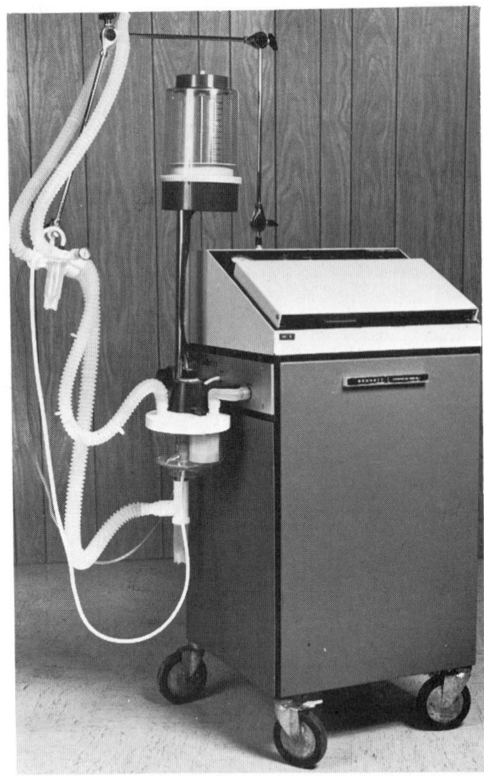

Fig. 24-33. Bennett MA-1 Ventilator.

Mechanism

Air is drawn into the MA-1 system (Fig. 24-34) through an air filter (A) to an oxygen blender (C) by the descending bellows. From a compressor (B), air is pumped into the power drive system, which causes the bellows to ascend. A solenoid valve (D) cycles the ventilator according to the logic of the electronic circuit, producing inspiratory and expiratory phases. The compressed gas passes through a Venturi (E), which boosts the flow. Distal to the Venturi booster is a peak-flow control knob (F), which regulates the inspiratory flow rate delivered to the patient by the rate of compression of the bellows. After passage by the flow-rate control, the gas bifurcates. The major flow goes into the bellows compression canister (G) through a one-way valve, whereas a secondary flow compresses a mushroom valve (H). The mushroom valve port exhausts the gas from the bellows compression chamber once inspiration has been completed.

In the patient intake circuit, air is drawn in through the bacteria filter (A) and delivered to a blending chamber (C), where it is mixed with oxygen to the correct proportions selected by the oxygen control knob (I). Oxygen flow to the blending chamber is controlled electronically and proportioned by an oxygen delivery bellows (J). The oxygen-air mixture then enters the bellows through a one-way valve as it begins its descent in expiration. When the bellows begins to ascend, a second one-way valve opens, and the bellows gas is discharged into the patient circuit. Pressure is monitored by the ventilator system pressure gauge (K) and is regulated by a pressure relief control (L). If the assist mode is used, the sensitivity is adjusted by control M. The patient system bifurcates, and pressure is delivered to the exhalation valve (N) to seal the system during inspiration. Gas to this mushroom valve can also be controlled independently if PEEP is desired.

Operation

The Bennett MA-1 ventilator is connected to an electrical power source of 115 volts, 60 Hz, and the power switch (A) is turned to "on" (Fig. 24-35). If oxygen is desired, the hose is plugged into a 50 psi oxygen outlet. The humidifier should be filled and adjusted to the proper temperature at least 20 minutes before use. If the ventilator is plugged into an electrical outlet, the humidifier will preheat when the switch is on standby. The ventilator sensitivity (B) is adjusted to that level desired if assisted ventilation is used. A desired peak flow (15–100 liters/min) is selected (C). Breathing ventilator rates from 1 to 60 are available (D). Tidal volumes up to 2200 ml are available by setting the normal volume control (E). The normal pressure limit control (F) then is adjusted to the desired limit. Pressure-cycled ventilation may also be used, but the pressure limit alarm (P) will sound at the termination of each inspiration unless it is silenced. The sigh pressure limit (G) and the sigh volume limit (H) function exactly as the normal pressure and volume limit controls do, but at greater pre-set intervals. The sigh is not additive to the normal breath and therefore has its own independent volume and pressure. Multiple sighs (up to three) may be administered at each interval selected (I). Manually controlled normal breaths or sighs may be administered by pushing the appropriate button (J).

Oxygen concentration is controlled from 21% to 100% (K). This control is fully adjustable within these ranges and accurate to within ±2.5%. This is a pneumatically powered control, and any high-pressure gas source will operate it. Thus careful attention to the oxygen connection is essential. The amount of expi-

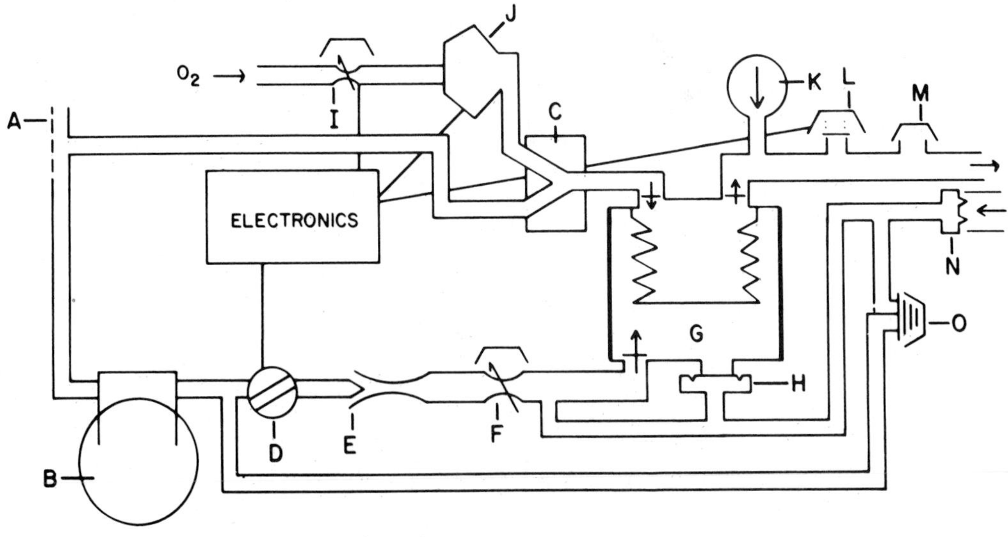

Fig. 24-34. Schematic diagram of the Bennett MA-1 Ventilator.

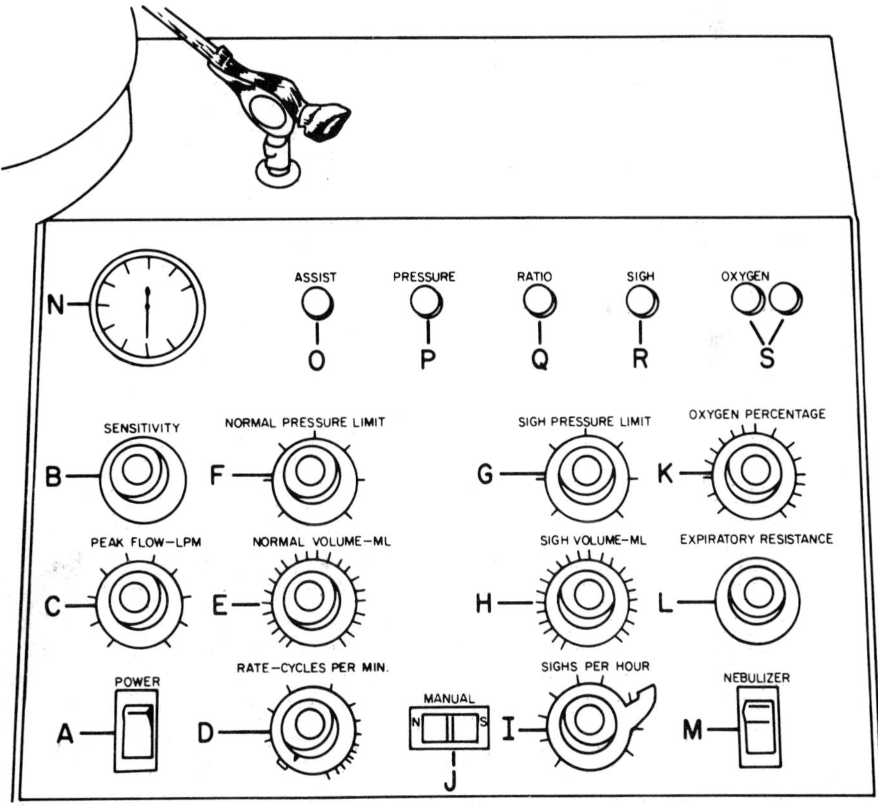

Fig. 24-35. Control panel of the Bennett MA-1 Ventilator.

ratory retard is controlled by the expiratory resistance control (L). Nebulization of medication is achieved by filling a nebulizer cup and activating switch M. PEEP is adjusted by an optional control on the side of the ventilator (adjustable between 0 and 10 cm H_2O pressure) and can be read on the ventilator system pressure gauge (N).

The monitoring and alarm systems have a panel of lights on the front of the ventilator that are tested by depressing the light to indicate whether the bulb is still functional. These alarm lights include an amber assist light (O), indicating that the patient has initiated the breath; a pressure light (P), which illuminates red whenever the pressure limit has been reached (an audible alarm accompanies this light to warn the operator that the pressure limit has been exceeded); a ratio light (Q), which is activated during controlled respiration if the I:E ratio is less than 1:1, thus indicating a need to alter the inspiratory flow rate or ventilator frequency*; a sigh light (R), which illuminates each time a sigh is administered; and an oxygen light system (S), consisting of two lights, one red and one green. When the ventilator is connected to a high-pressure gas source of any kind, the green light will light if an oxygen concentration greater than 21% has been selected. The red light will activate and an audible alarm will sound whenever a high-pressure gas source has not been connected to the ventilator and the oxygen control knob (K) is turned to some value other than 21%. An internal safety valve relieves at 85 cm H_2O pressure.

Humidity

Humidification is provided by a cascade humidifier. The water is heated by an element controlled by selecting one of a series of sequential numbers on a dial. A minimum of 20 minutes of warm-up is required. If the water level in the humidifier drops below the refill level, the heating element will no longer heat the water, and the humidity will fall considerably.

Cleaning and Sterilizing

Cleaning and sterilizing are performed by removing the external breathing system from the ventilator and cleaning and sterilizing it by standard procedures. If a Bennett spirometer is used, however, the electronic and pneumatic parts must not be washed.

*The ratio light is only functional during controlled ventilation and is inactivated by each "assist" breath.

Accessories

A PEEP control, a subambient pressure control, a temperature alarm, and an IMV conversion are available.

Troubleshooting

Because electronic components form a major part of this ventilator, most major malfunctions should be repaired by a manufacturer's representative.

If the ventilator will not develop pressure and no leaks are found in the system, the exhalation mushroom valve may be incompetent. A tear or hole in the mushroom valve can prevent satisfactory development of pressure. Also, a thermometer should be placed in the orifice provided or a leak will develop. If the ventilator is used without the spirometer, the spirometer outlet must be plugged for the ventilator to develop pressure. If the humidifier does not heat satisfactorily, the water level may be inadequate, the heating element may be burned out, or the safety switch may not be making contact with the humidifier cover. One of the most difficult leaks to find is that from a loose screw in the heating element housed in the humidifier cover. Another leak that is difficult to find is a disconnection of the bacteria filter inside the ventilator door.

BENNETT MA-2 VENTILATOR

Classification

The MA-2 ventilator (Fig. 24-36) is an electronically operated volume-cycled ventilator with a secondary pressure limit. Against zero backpressure, it is a constant flow generator. Mechanical inspiration is either controlled or patient triggered and may be terminated by a selected pressure limit or extended beyond the dynamic phase by a plateau. Threshold positive pressure may be added to the expiratory phase.

Mechanism

Pneumatic power (Fig. 24-37) is derived from either an external source of compressed air or when filtered (A) ambient air is drawn in and compressed internally (B). When an external source of compressed air ($\geq$ 35 psi) is used, a pressure switch (C) shuts down the internal compressor. If external source pressure decreases below 35 psi, the compressor is activated, providing uninterrupted pneumatic power.

During mechanical inspiration, a solenoid valve (E) opens, allowing passage of compressed air to

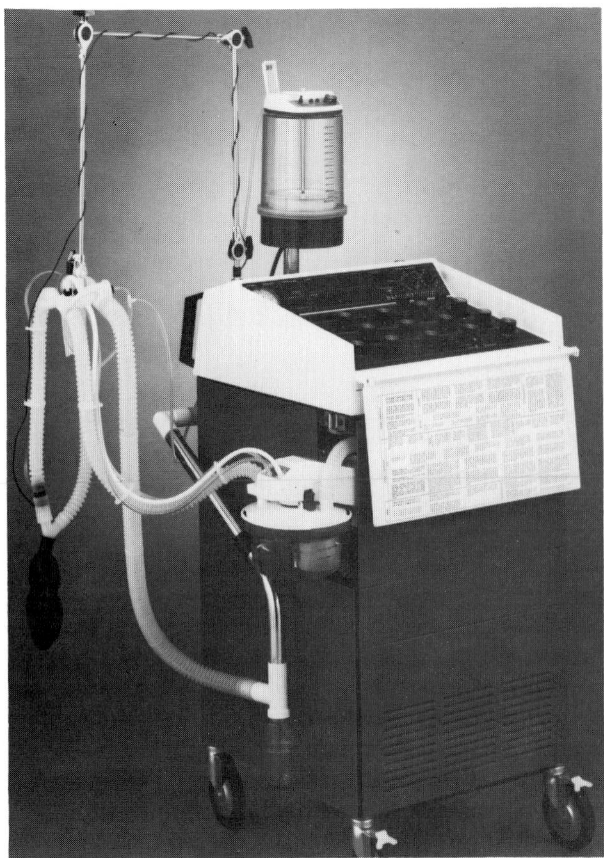

Fig. 24-36. Bennett MA-2 Ventilator.

power a Venturi (F). A peak flow control (G) regulates total flow (Venturi drive plus entrained gas) to the bellows canister (H). A small amount of gas is shunted to the canister depressurizing valve (I) and circuit exhalation valve (R). As gas enters the canister, the bellows is compressed, delivering volume (VT) to the inspiratory circuit containing a pressure relief valve (L), heated cascade humidifier (not illustrated), and sensors for detecting patient inspiratory (M) and expiratory (N) effort, loss of PEEP (O), and low inspiratory pressure (P). When the tidal volume (or pre-set pressure relief) has been reached, mechanical inspiration is terminated. The exhalation valve (R) and canister valve (I) are vented open, depressurizing the breathing circuit and canister, respectively. As canister pressure decreases, the bellows descends and fills with filtered ambient air (A) and oxygen (regulated by FI_{O_2} control [J]) via a proportioning system (D).

An oxygen accumulator (K) senses the internally regulated oxygen line pressure (1.8–2.1 cm H_2O). If the FI_{O_2} is set above 0.21 and this pressure exceeds 3 to 5 cm H_2O or falls below 1 cm H_2O, an audible and visual alarm is activated. Pressure, not FI_{O_2}, activates the alarm; therefore any compressed gas source could inadvertently be connected to the oxygen inlet. This possibility is somewhat reduced by the presence of a DISS oxygen inlet.

Operation

The MA-2 ventilator is powered by a 115 volt, 60 Hz electrical source. All electronic components (except humidifier heater) are activated when the power control knob (A) is turned on (Fig. 24-38). If the ventilator is connected to an electrical outlet, the humidifier heater may be turned on (B) and the temperature adjusted (C) independently of the main power control. This facilitates heating of the water reservoir before use.

Ventilatory mode is selected by depressing either SIMV/CPAP (D) or CMV (E) button. Normal mechanical inspiratory phase functions include the high-pressure limit (F), CMV/SIMV volume (G), CMV rate (H), peak flow (I), SIMV rate (J), and sensitivity (K).

In the SIMV or CMV mode, mechanical tidal volume (range minimal to 2200 ml) and peak inspiratory flow (range 20–125 liters/min) are adjusted by the SIMV/CMV volume and peak flow controls, respectively. Peak airway pressure is adjustable from 20 to 120 cm H_2O, with a depressible catch at 80 cm H_2O for safety. Separate ventilator cycling controls are provided for CMV rate (range 0–60 breaths/min). SIMV rate (low rate 0.3–3 breaths/min), and high rate (0–30 breaths/min). Inspiratory effort triggering, SIMV, and demand flow (spontaneous breathing in the SIMV and CPAP modes) is adjusted with the sensitivity control (range minus 10 cm H_2O to autocycling-uncalibrated). Once adjusted, the inspiratory effort necessary for a given ventilator response is not altered by changes in end-expiratory pressure. End-expiratory pressure (PEEP or CPAP) is adjustable from 0 to 45 cm H_2O by an uncalibrated knob (L).

In the CMV mode, dynamic mechanical inspiration may be extended (range 0–2 seconds) with the plateau control (M). When CMV inspiration is pressure cycled, no plateau occurs.

A manual inspiration (N) equivalent to the CMV/SIMV volume may be delivered during mechanical exhalation in any mode. After manual inspiration, the CMV and SIMV rate timer re-zeros. Mechanical inspiration may be terminated by depressing the manual exhalation button (O). Manual exhalation may be used in any mode and allows the bellows to refill completely.

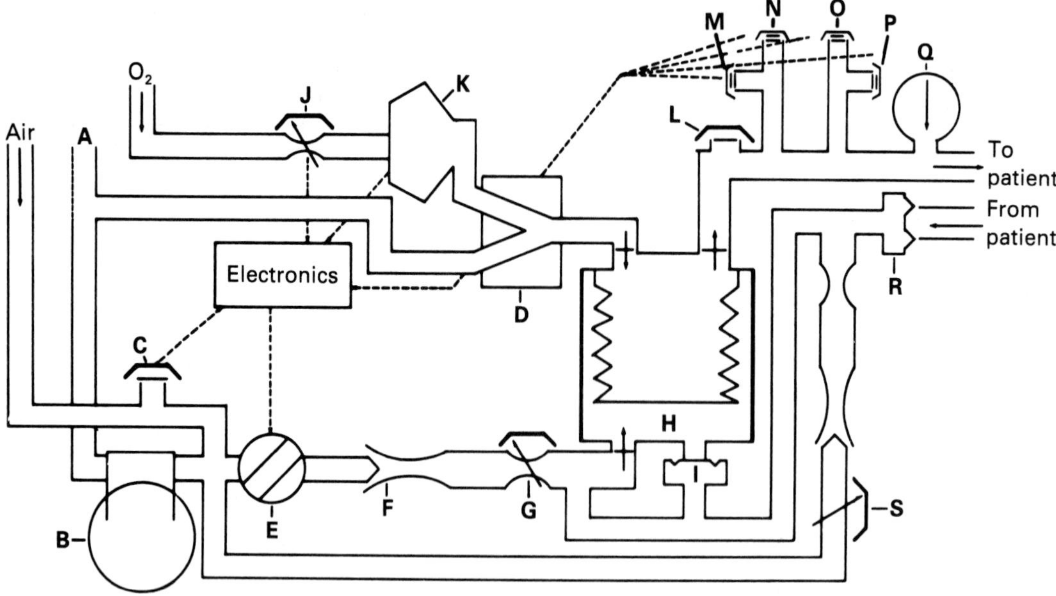

Fig. 24-37. Schematic diagram of the MA-2.

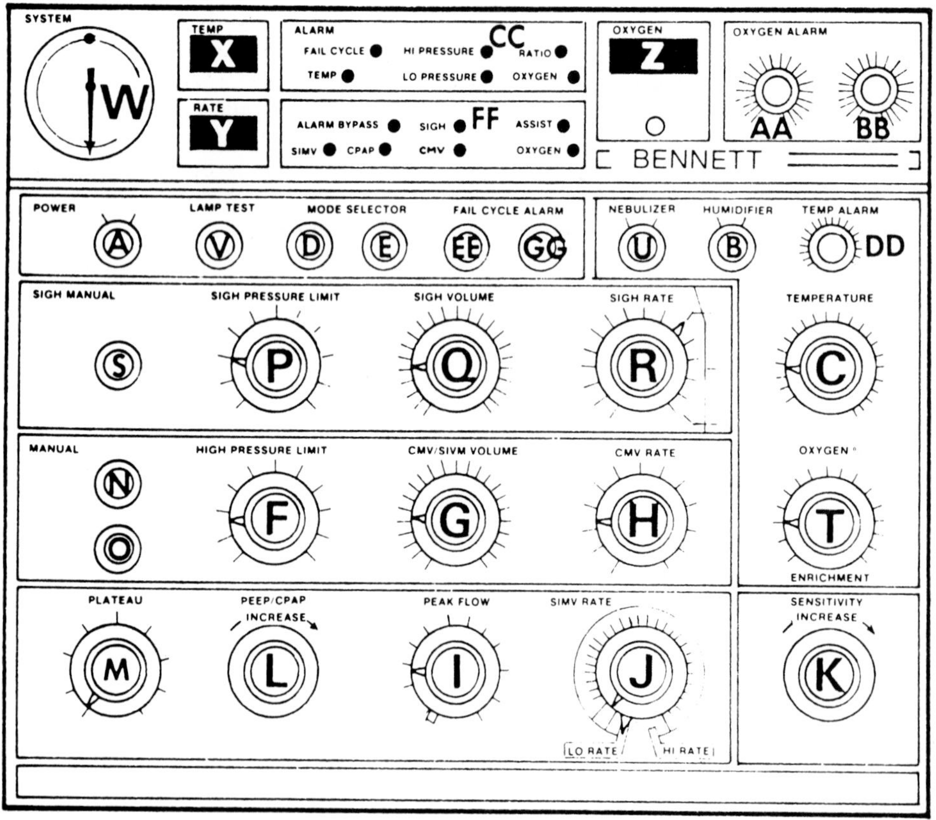

Fig. 24-38. Control panel for MA-2.

When "sighing" is desired, the following variables are adjusted: sigh pressure limit (P) (range 20–120 cm H_2O); sigh volume (Q) (range minimal to 2200 ml); and sigh rate (R) (range off, 1–15 cycles/hr) in multiples of one, two, or three breaths/cycle. A manual inspiration (S) equivalent to sigh volume may be delivered during manual exhalation in any mode. After a manual sigh inspiration, the rate timer resets at zero.

FI_{O_2} is regulated (range 0.21–1.0) by the oxygen percentage control (T). Aerosol therapy in conjunction with mechanical inspiration may be administered by filling the circuit medication cup and turning the nebulizer control (U) on.

Monitoring and alarm system are located primarily at the top of the control panel. The LED displays (temperature, rate, and oxygen percentage), mode indicator lights (SIMV, CPAP, CMV, oxygen, audio-alarm bypass, sigh, and assist), and visual alarm lights (temperature, low pressure, oxygen, fail to cycle, high pressure, and I:E ratio) are all illuminated by depressing the lamp test button (V).

Proximal airway pressure is indicated on an aneroid manometer (W) (range −10 to +120 cm H_2O). Manometer pressure may not correlate with the value set on high-pressure limit control. The indicated manometer pressure is generally lower because the peak pressure relief valve is proximal to flow resistance offered by the humidifier.

Proximal airway temperature is measured by a thermistor and displayed (X) in degrees Celsius. Total ventilatory rate (*i.e.*, mechanical and spontaneous) is indicated (Y) and updated every four breaths. An optional oxygen percent display (Z) that indicates the value measured by an oxygen sensor in the outflow circuit is available. A high (AA) and low (BB) oxygen limit may be set and, if reached, will activate an audible and visual alarm.

All alarm conditions activate an audible as well as a visual indication (CC). A fail to cycle alarm occurs when main power is on and 20 seconds elapse without either a ventilator inspiratory or an expiratory phase (e.g., spontaneous breath, SIMV, or CMV). It essentially functions as an apnea alarm. The high-pressure indicator is illuminated when peak inspiratory pressure is reached cycling the ventilator to exhalation. The ratio alarm is activated when inspiration exceeds 50% of total cycle time determined by CMV rate. It alarms throughout the inspiratory phase until the condition is corrected and functions only in the CMV mode.

The temperature alarm is activated if the proximal airway temperature exceeds the selected value (DD). A low-pressure alarm condition exists when the proximal airway pressure relative to baseline either does not increase at least 10 cm H_2O during SIMV or CMV or decreases 5 cm H_2O for more than 1 second. This alarm function detects leaks and patient disconnections. The oxygen indicator is illuminated when either the low or high limits are exceeded.

Audible alarms may be silenced for 2 minutes by depressing the bypass button (EE), which also illuminates the audio alarm bypass in the mode indicator section (FF). Audio alarms may be reset manually (GG) before elapsed bypass time. The ventilatory mode in progress (SIMV, CPAP, CMV, oxygen, sigh, assist) is indicated by appropriate illumination. The oxygen indicator is lighted when $FI_{O_2} > 0.21$. Any patient-triggered breath will illuminate the assist indicator.

An MA•2+2 has been commercially released for clinical use. Functionally it remains similar to the MA-2 except for three alterations. The low inspiratory pressure alarm is adjustable from 2 to 80 cm H_2O instead of a fixed 10 cm H_2O. A universal humidifier mount has been incorporated to accommodate either Cascade I or II or other commercially available humidifiers while retaining temperature display and adjustable alarms. The manual expiration control has been deleted because an automatic bellows reset system has been installed. This mechanism obviates the necessity for manual refilling of internal bellows in the face of exhaustive leaks on CPAP/PEEP or after transient disconnections. The conspicuous change is the control panel (Fig. 24-39).

Humidity

Humidification is provided by a Cascade humidifier. The water reservoir is heated by an element to maintain the proximal airway temperature selected by the temperature control knob.

Cleaning and Sterilizing

External breathing circuits should be changed at least every 24 hours. Between patients, the ventilator surface should be wiped with a disinfectant.

Accessories

An oxygen sensor, display, and high–low alarm are optional (discussed in Operation section).

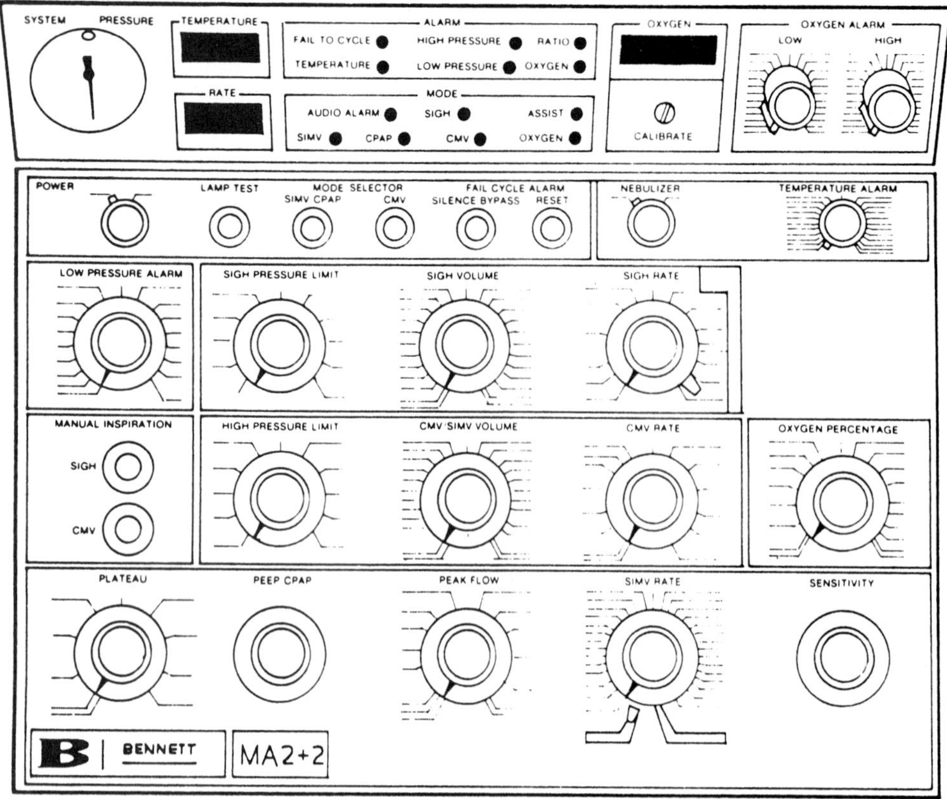

Fig. 24-39. Control panel of the MA•2 + 2.

Troubleshooting

If the ventilator will not develop pressure and no loose connections or leaks are found, the exhalation mushroom valve may be incompetent. Alarm condition troubleshooting is greatly enhanced by visual indications on the control panel.

CHEMTRON GILL-1

Classification

The Gill-1 ventilator (Fig. 24-40) can be classified as a constant pressure generator because gas delivery is controlled by gravity acting on a weighted piston and bellows. However, the great weight of the piston provides substantial flows that are not affected significantly by airway resistance; thus it more closely approximates a constant flow generator. An inspiratory plateau is available. It is volume-cycled with a secondary pressure limit backup, which can be used as the primary cycling mechanism if the controls are adjusted appropriately. Positive pressure plateaus are available during the expiratory phase. It is also an assistor, controller, assistor-controller, and IMV ventilator.

Mechanism

An electronic component package (A) controls the ventilator (Fig. 24-41). The piston delivery system is a weighted bellows (B) regulated by a series of electronically operated solenoid switches. The piston initially is pushed up by a pressurized gas source. Pressurized oxygen is delivered to a chamber (C) through an oxygen adjusting valve (D) and is mixed with ambient air. This mixture is delivered into a holding chamber (E) below the bellows, where the gas is held during expiration because the patient circuit-cycling solenoid (F) seals and isolates this area from the patient breathing system. When the ventilator inspiratory phase begins, the patient cycling solenoid (F) opens and the bellows weight delivers the tidal volume to the circuit. En route to the patient, the gas mixture passes a filter (G), an oxygen analyzer (H), and a heated humidifier (I). Pressure limit is adjusted

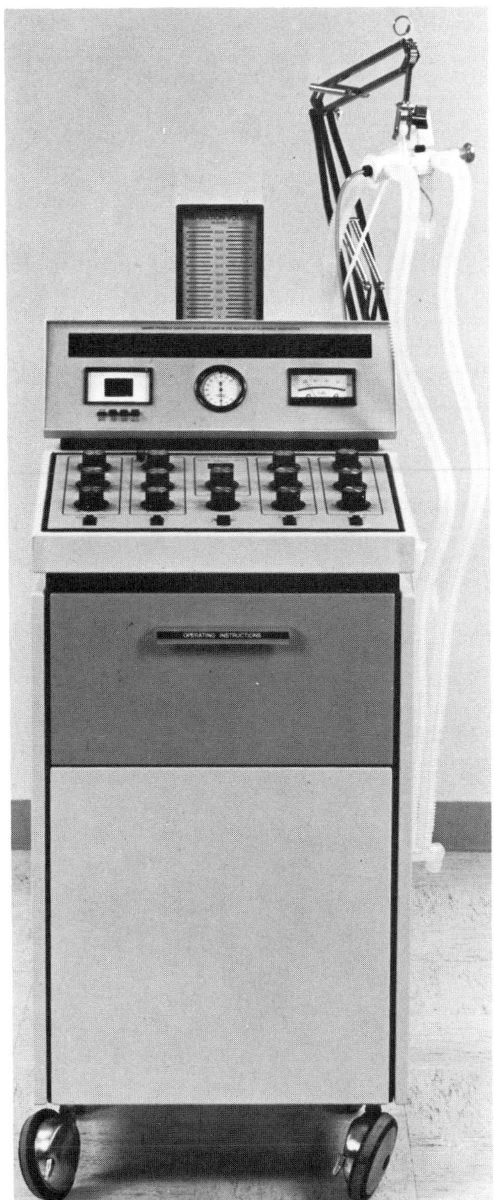

Fig. 24-40. Chemtron Gill-1 Ventilator.

by valve J, which ceases inspiration and begins expiration. A pressure gauge to monitor system pressure and an inspiratory effort adjustment (K) to transmit patient inspiratory effort to the electronic cycling mechanisms are available.

On the opposite side of the weighted piston are controls for the piston and exhalation valves. Once the piston is in position to deliver a tidal volume, gas must be displaced into the area above the piston or it will not descend. While drawing air in through a filter, a solenoid (L) cycles open, allowing gas to flow behind the piston so that it may drop during inspiration. Control M regulates the rate of fall, and hence the flow rate to the patient. A solenoid (N) locks out the bellows system during inspiration so that a pump can deliver pressure to the exhalation valve (P). This exhalation valve can also be pressurized through a looping circuit that adjusts PEEP by control Q. During the expiratory phase, solenoid N opens and the vacuum side of pump O develops a vacuum in chamber R to draw the piston back up to the desired displacement volume.

Operation

The main power switch is turned on and the respiratory rate (A) adjusted between 6 and 60 breaths per minute (Fig. 24-42). With the IMV modification, this rate can be lowered to one breath every 3 minutes. The respiratory rate is displayed digitally on the respiratory monitor (B). This display averages the breaths over a 30-second period. Some models have selector switches that also display inspiratory time, expiratory time, and the I:E ratio. Although the display range has a large differential range, the cycling modes themselves have the following capabilities: an inspiratory time of 0.1 to 5 seconds, an expiratory time of 0.5 to 9.9 seconds, and an I:E ratio of 1:1 to 1:100. Each variable can be displayed by pressing the appropriate selector button under the digital readout. Tidal volume is adjusted by the normal tidal volume control (C) between 150 and 2100 ml. The pressure relief control (D) can modify this volume between 20 and 100 cm H_2O. The time allocated to inspiration depends on the flow-rate control (E) with a range of 10 to 120 liters/min and inspiratory durations of 0.1 to 5 seconds. If the inspiratory time is prolonged, a light will signal to indicate an I:E ratio of greater than 1:1.

An inflation hold (F) can extend inspiration at peak inflation by 2 seconds. During the expiratory phase, both subambient and positive pressure plateaus may be adjusted by the end-expiratory pressure limit (G). This control can bring the expiratory phase to a subambient pressure of -15 cm H_2O as well as to a positive pressure of 50 cm H_2O. This control is infinitely variable within its range. Oxygen concentrations are selected with the oxygen percentage control (H) and monitored on the oxygen monitor (I). The response time of this monitor is 30 seconds; therefore, oxygen adjustments should be made slowly. Calibra-

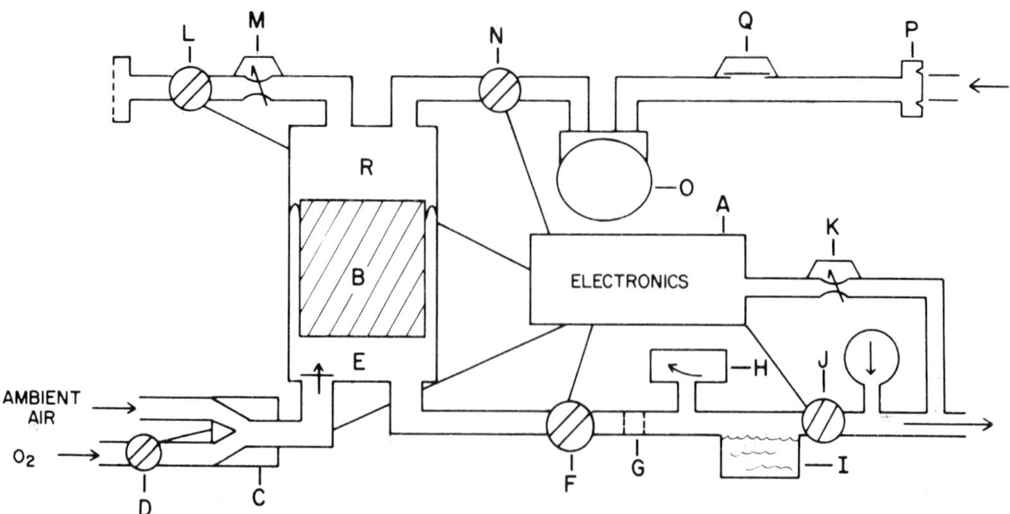

Fig. 24-41. Schematic diagram of the Chemtron Gill-1 Ventilator.

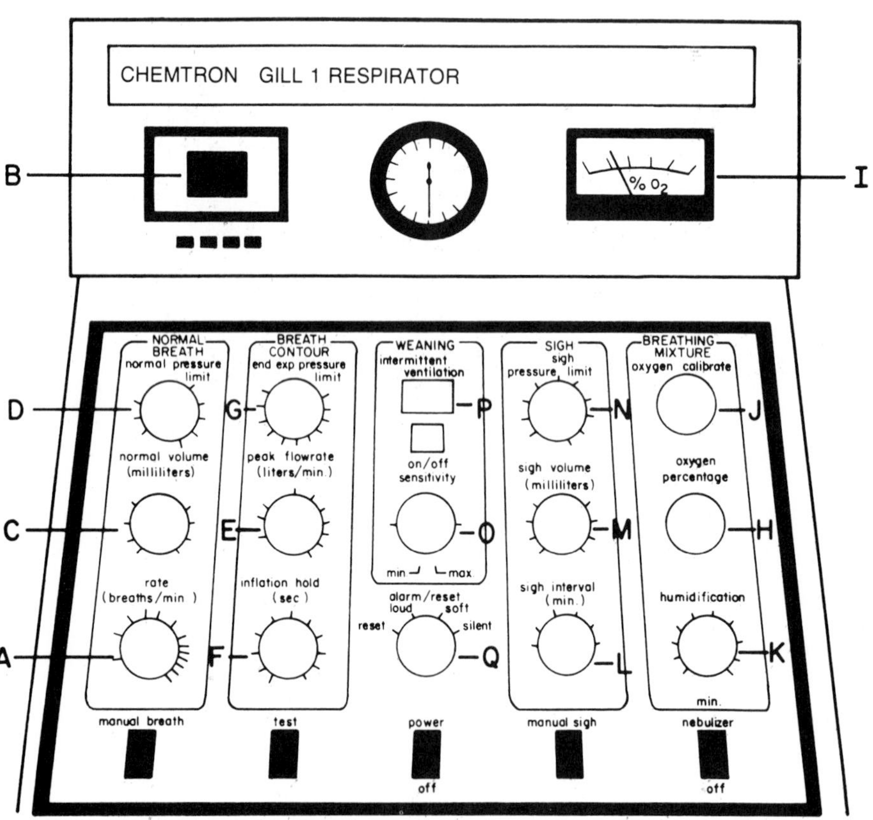

Fig. 24-42. Control panel of the Chemtron Gill-1 Ventilator.

tion of this oxygen monitor is performed with the oxygen calibration control (J) and a source of 100% oxygen at the oxygen sensor. Humidification is controlled by an adjustable heat control (K).

Sigh breaths are independent of the normal volume. The interval between sighs is adjusted at 2-minute increments up to 10 minutes by the sigh interval control (L), whereas the sigh volume and pressure limit are controlled by M and N, respectively. If assisted ventilation is desired, an effort control (O) is provided to adjust the amount of subambient pressure required to trigger the cycling mechanism. This control functions independently of the pressure plateau so that if PEEP is dialed into the system, the patient can still initiate an inspiration by decreasing pressure slightly below the PEEP pressure. If an IMV mode is selected, a timer (P) selects the total respiratory cycle time.

The alarm selector (Q) resets, softens, loudens, or silences the alarms. The alarm-competency control system monitors pressure limit, improper cycle, low pressure, power failure, control mode, assist mode, oxygen add, sigh mode, improper oxygen, I:E ratio, fill humidifier and alarms silent functions.

Humidity

Humidity is provided by a passive, heated humidifier that bubbles the ventilator gas mixture through heated water. A refill-sensing light indicates when the humidifier needs refilling.

Cleaning and Sterilizing

All inline bacteria filters and intake filters should be removed and replaced periodically to avoid diminution of flow. To function properly, the vacuum and pump motors need adequate circulating air.

The breathing assembly must be exchanged for a sterilized one at least every 24 hours. If a disposable breathing assembly is used, the nebulizer filter, pressure sensing line, thermometer, thermometer adapter, and pressure-sensing isolator should be retained.

Troubleshooting

If a power failure occurs, a battery-operated power failure light and audible alarm are triggered.

If the oxygen alarm is activated, line pressure is below 35 psi, the oxygen filter needs cleaning, or the oxygen line has been connected improperly.

The low-pressure alarm signals if the inspiratory pressure is no greater than 8 cm H_2O. The improper cycle alarm triggers if an improper I:E ratio has occurred for 20 seconds, if the ventilator has not cycled for 20 seconds, or if the pressure limit has occurred for 20 seconds.

Caution: Should the ventilator indicate it has delivered 2100 ml of volume, the piston may have dropped into the lower chamber. If this occurs, the ventilator should be removed and a service representative called.

EMERSON POSTOPERATIVE VENTILATOR-3PV

Classification

The Emerson 3PV (Fig. 24-43) is an electronic, time-cycled, nonconstant flow generator with secondary pressure-limit capability. It is used primarily as a con-

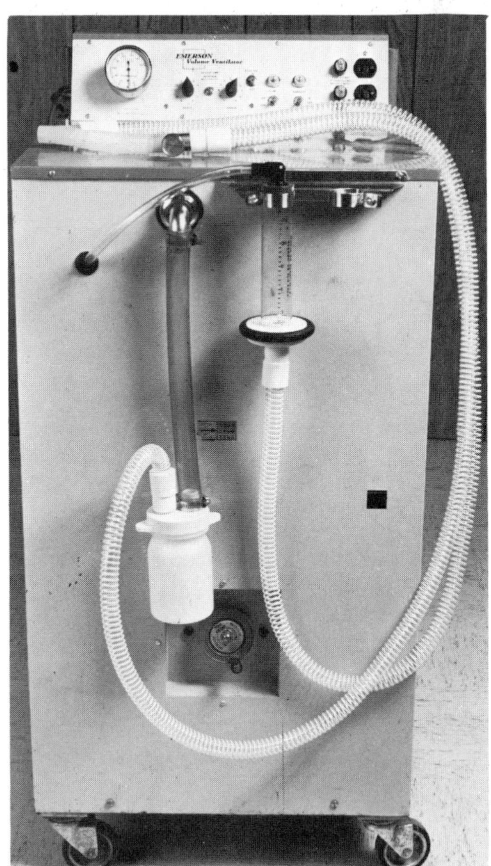

Fig. 24-43. Emerson Postoperative 3PV Ventilator.

troller, although an optional patient-triggering mechanism is available. Threshold expiratory pressure may be administered and the 3PV easily modified to provide IMV.

Mechanism

The 3PV is operated and powered electronically (Fig. 24-44). Ambient air drawn into a reservoir "trombone" (A) may be enriched with oxygen by means of an inlet nipple (B) to provide desired FI_{O_2}. As the piston (C) moves downward (negative displacement), reservoir gas is drawn into the chamber (E) via a unidirectional valve (D). Chamber displacement is determined by turning a crank handle (F), which regulates piston rod linkage (G). A cam (J) mounted on a pulley wheel is designed so that microswitch (H) is closed when the piston is at its downward terminus and open at maximum upward position. Inspiratory and expiratory time (I:E ratio) controls regulate a d.c. motor (K) and hence piston speed by means of a pulley (L) when the microswitch is closed and open, respectively. A second microswitch (H) phases the optional sigh mechanism.

During positive displacement, the piston (C) compresses chamber gas, creating sufficient pressure to close intake valve D, open outflow valve M, and close exhalation valve N. System pressure equalizes on both sides of the exhalation valve and is indicated on an aneroid manometer (O). Gas flow to the patient circuit is warmed and moistened by a passover humidifier (P). Peak pressure is limited by an adjustable relief valve (Q).

Operation

The ventilator is connected to a 115 volt, 60 Hz electrical outlet (Fig. 24-45). Sterile water is added to the humidifier and the filling port cap secured with the wrench provided. The humidifier heater is controlled by a three-position toggle switch (B): HI, OFF, and LO. Generally the HI (high) heating position is required to provide adequate humidification, especially when the continuous flow modification for IMV is used. Mechanical tidal volume is set by turning the hand crank and the value read on the volume indicator (low center and center of chassis). A two-position toggle switch (A) turns the piston drive motor on or off. In the ON position, inspiratory (C) and expiratory (D) time adjustments determine the ventilator cycling frequency. System pressure is indicated on an aneroid manometer (E).

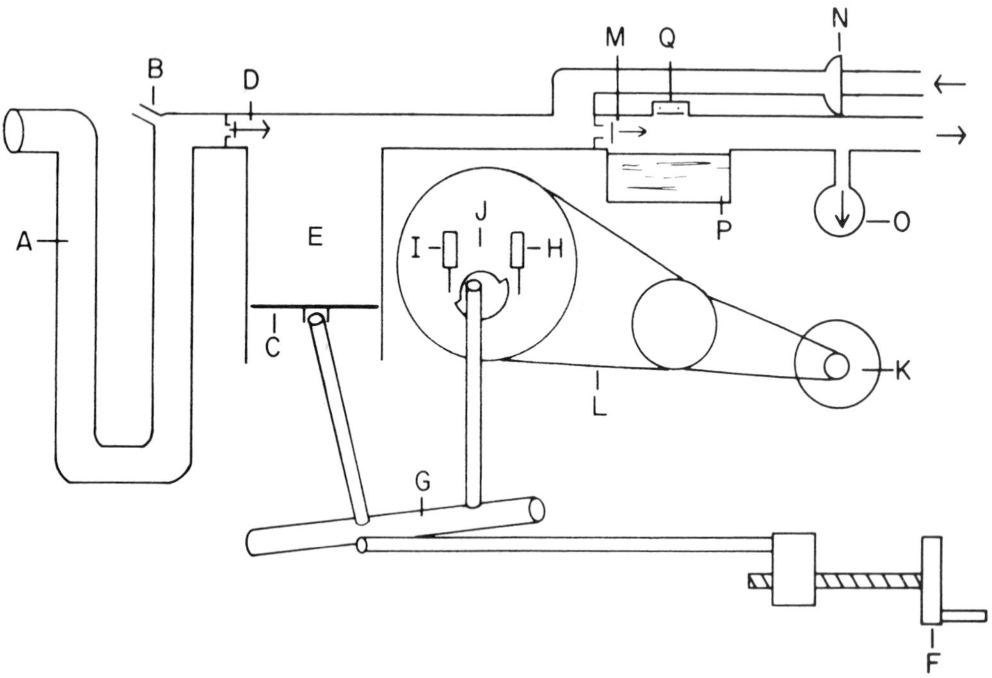

Fig. 24-44. Schematic diagram of the Emerson 3PV Volume Ventilator.

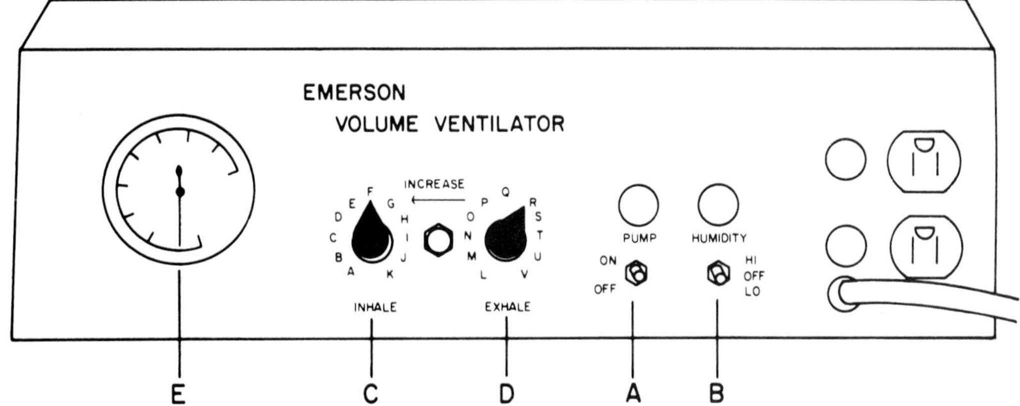

Fig. 24-45. Control panel of the Emerson 3PV Volume Ventilator.

Humidity

Humidification of inspired gas from the 3PV occurs by means of a converted pressure cooker mounted on a hot plate. It is a heated reservoir passover humidifier.

Cleaning and Sterilizing

The patient-breathing circuit should be changed at least every 24 hours. Copper mesh in the main outflow tube tends to minimize bacterial contamination. This mesh should be changed when it becomes discolored.

Accessories

Optional equipment includes a spirometer, respiratory alarm system, sigh attachment, patient trigger mechanism, and IMV modification.

Troubleshooting

Because of its functional design, the 3PV is a veritable workhorse. Potential system leaks may occur at welded seams (humidifier, especially) exhalation valve, water trap, and, rarely, the piston ring.

The electronic components of the newer models have caused few problems, with the possible exception of the turn-screw on the panel between the inspiratory and expiratory timing knobs. This control adjusts the ventilator to hospital voltage. It should be adjusted for the lowest projected voltage drop. Indiscriminate tampering with the turn-screw may result in malfunction.

EMERSON IMVentilator–3MV

Classification

The Emerson 3MV (Fig. 24-46) is an electronically powered, time-cycled, nonconstant flow generator with secondary pressure-limit capability. Inspiratory flow is similar to the positive phase of a sine wave pattern. It has a variable inspiratory time, and threshold expiratory pressure may be instituted. The 3MV is used primarily in an IMV mode, although it may be used as a controller.

Mechanism

Air and oxygen are mixed (A) to provide a desired FI_{O_2} for filling two 5-liter anesthesia bags (Fig. 24-47). One bag (B) serves as gas source for the mechanical tidal volume. The other (C) provides a reservoir of gas for spontaneous ventilation. Two pressure relief valves (D, E) prevent overdistension of the anesthesia bags.

During mechanical exhalation, gas from reservoir B is drawn into the cylinder (F) by the downward piston stroke. The cylinder displacement is regulated by a crank handle (J) connected to piston rod linkage (K). Displacement volume is calibrated in increments of 100 ml from 0 to 2200 ml. As the position terminates its downward motion, a microswitch (I) is closed by a rotating cam (H), initiating an electronic signal for mechanical inspiration. Power to the d.c. motor (G) is regulated by the inspiratory time control. An increased current flow accelerates motor speed, thus shortening inspiratory duration.

Mechanical inspiration is initiated when positive displacement of the piston occurs, forcing most cyl-

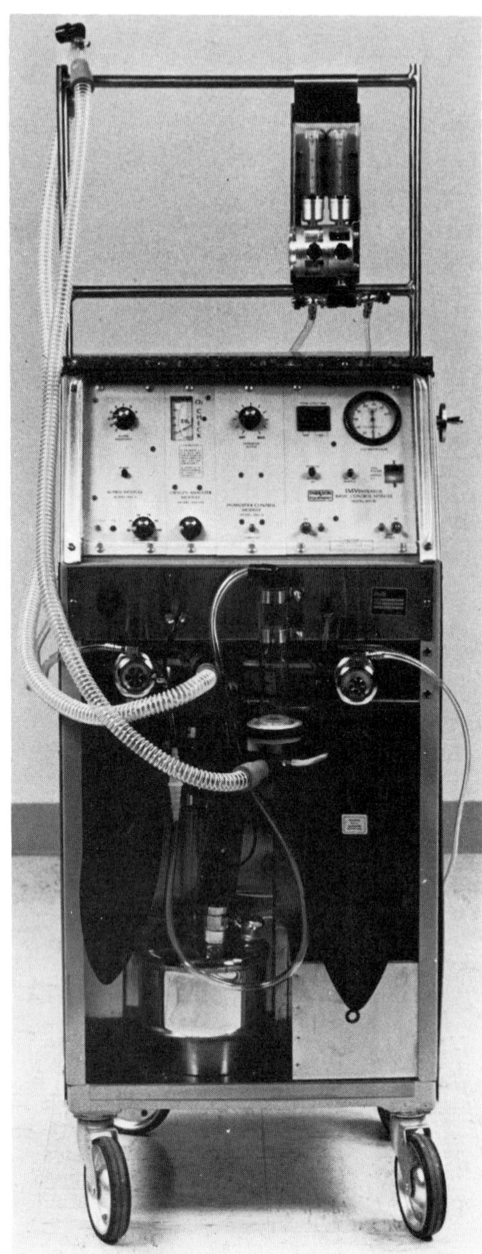

Fig. 24-46. Emerson IMVentilator.

inder gas through a passover heated humidifier (L) into the patient circuit. A small amount of gas is shunted to pressurize and close an exhalation valve (M), which may also be loaded with water to produce threshold expiratory pressure. System pressure increases simultaneously on each side of the exhalation valve and is indicated on an aneroid manometer (N). Maximum system pressure is adjustable by means of a relief valve (O) on the humidifier.

Operation

A modular control panel (Fig. 24-48) is provided to isolate functions, allow installation of various options, and facilitate repair service. The main power switch (A) activates all electronic functions except the piston motor. Heat to the humidifier is regulated by a humidifier output control (B). $F_{I_{O_2}}$ is adjusted by an air–oxygen blending device and is measured by an optional oxygen analyzer (C).

Mechanical ventilation frequency is determined by adjusting total cycle time (B) (range 0.2–22 breaths/min). Inspiratory duration, from 0.5 to 2.5 seconds, is selected with the inspiratory time control (E). Mechanical tidal volume is adjusted with a hand crank on the right side of the ventilator chassis and displayed on the panel in 100-ml intervals (F). The d.c. motor is activated by the pump switch (G). Once the mechanical tidal volume has been delivered, the volume pump light illuminates. A mechanical inspiration may be administered (when pump is on) by depressing an IMV manual button. An alarm module provides a sensitivity control (H), allowing adjustment to sense pressure. An audible alarm is activated when circuit pressure falls below the desired level (e.g., loss of CPAP or patient disconnect). A time delay may be engaged by depressing the button (I), deactivating the alarm for up to 120 seconds. The time delay allows tracheal suctioning or other procedures that require transient disconnection without an audible alarm.

Humidity

Humidification and warming of inspired gas are effected by a passover heated humidifier. A panel control regulates temperature.

Cleaning and Sterilizing

The patient circuit should be changed at least every 24 hours. Copper mesh in the main outflow tube tends to minimize bacterial contamination. This mesh should be changed when it becomes discolored.

Accessories

Optimal devices include warming control for heated breathing circuit, demand valve for IMV and CPAP,

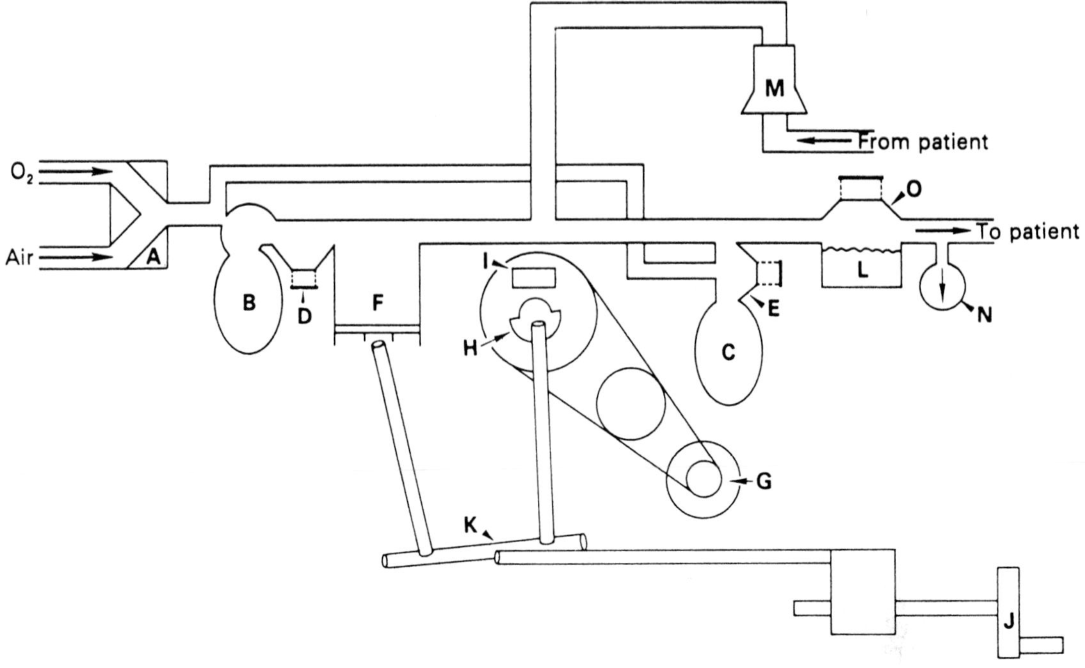

Fig. 24-47. Schematic diagram of Emerson IMV Ventilator.

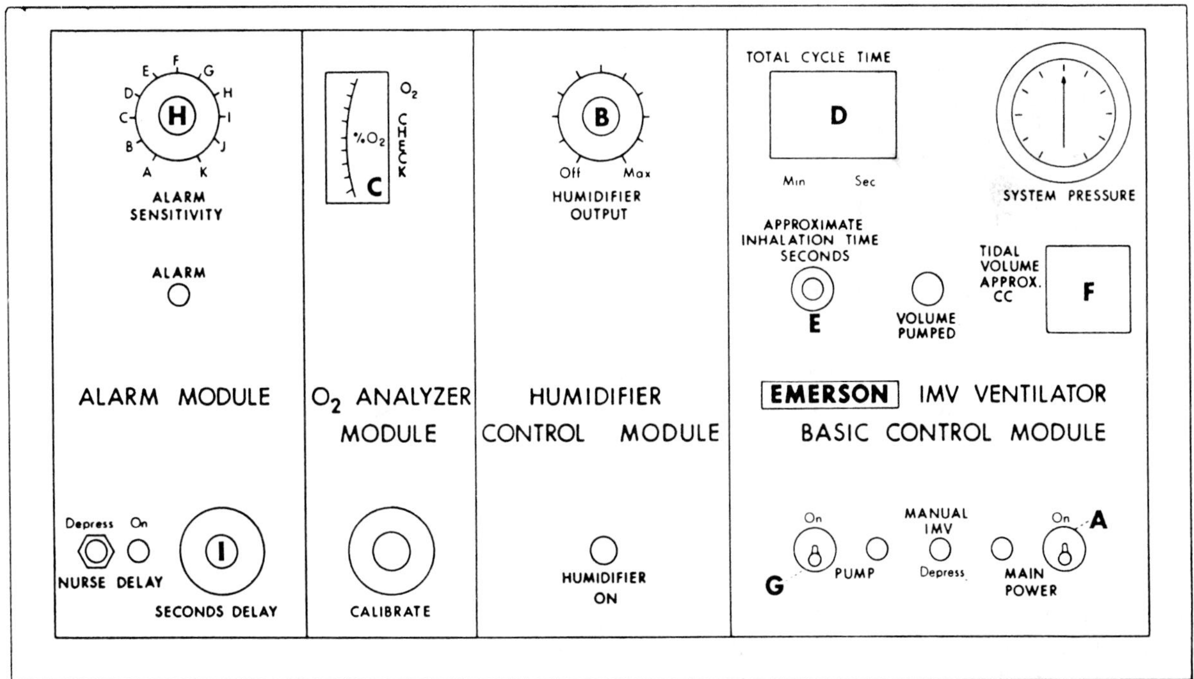

Fig. 24-48. Control panel of Emerson IMV Ventilator.

1000-cc cylinder, 500-cc cylinder, and oxygen analyzer module.

Troubleshooting

All connections must be tight and high-pressure leak proof. Few problems are encountered because of the practical design.

ENGSTRÖM ER 300

Classification

The Engström ER 300 (Fig. 24-49) is a time-cycled ventilator with secondary pressure relief. This ventilator is a controller with a valve that is adjustable to allow a modified IMV-spontaneous breathing pattern. PEEP and expiratory retard can be used.

Mechanism

A constant-speed AC motor (A) is linked to a variable-speed gearbox (B) (Fig. 24-50). The gear ratio selected determines the time allowed for the total respiratory cycle. The inspiratory portion of the respiratory cycle is determined by a pressure release valve that opens automatically after two thirds of the forward thrust of a piston has taken place. This portion of the total forward thrust of the piston corresponds to one third of the total cycle, leaving two thirds for the expiratory phase (1:2 I:E ratio). The piston is driven to the right of the cylinder (C) by a piston shaft attached eccentrically to a wheel, thereby providing a characteristic sine wave pressure pattern. This pressure is transmitted to an overpressure chamber (D), which contains a respiratory bag (E). En route to the overpressure chamber, excess gas is allowed to leak through an emptying pressure adjustment valve (F). This overpressure valve adjustment is set above the normal inspiratory pressure required to deliver the prescribed tidal volume. Excess pressure beyond the emptying pressure limit is vented to avoid high piston drive pressures.

Gas is delivered to the respiratory bag (E) by means of a mixing valve (G) through a dose valve (H), which controls the volume. The minute volume in conjunction with the frequency determines what the

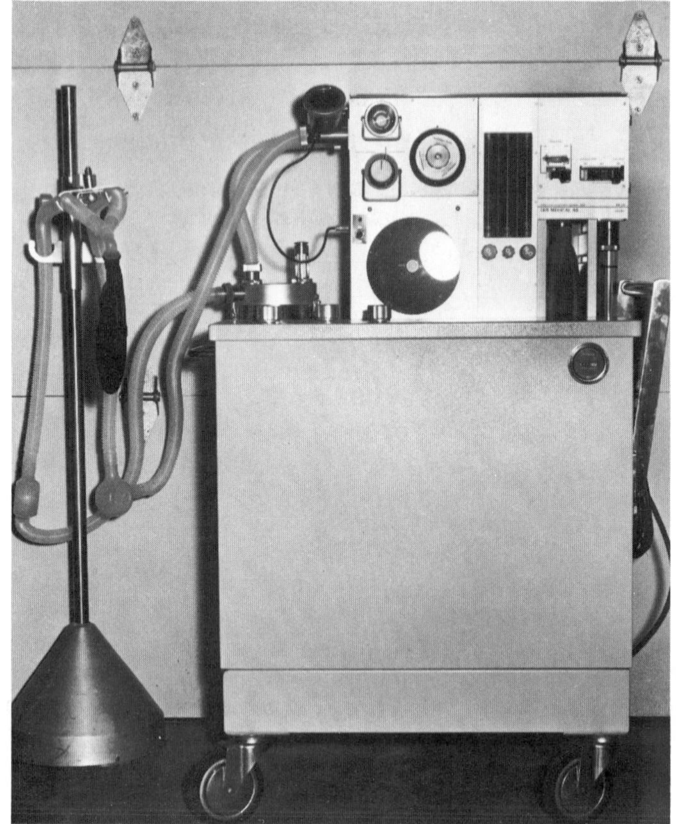

Fig. 24-49. Engström ER 300 Ventilator.

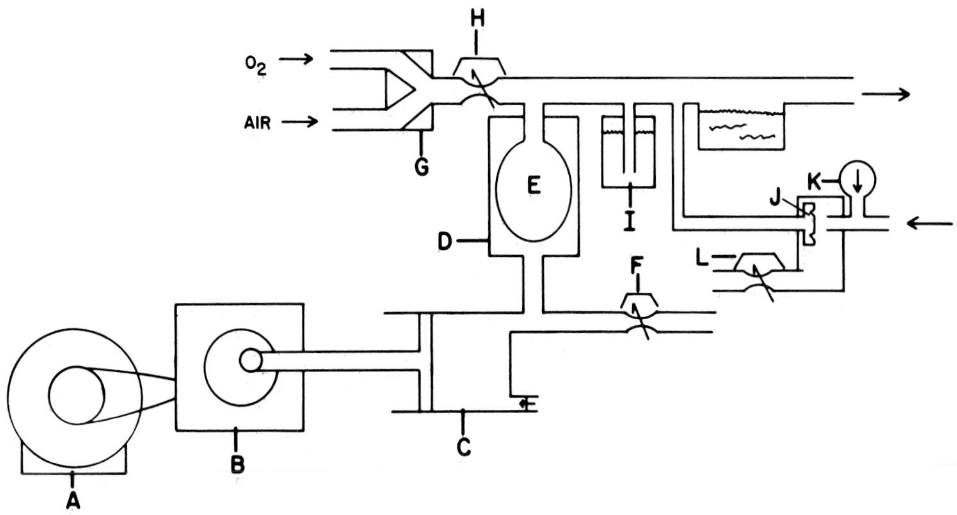

Fig. 24-50. Schematic diagram of Engström ER 300 Ventilator.

delivered tidal volume on each individual breath will be. Once the piston begins its stroke, the respiratory bag (E) is compressed by pressure in the overpressure chamber until the tidal volume has been delivered or the pressure limit reached on the adjustable safety valve (I). The gas is delivered to the patient through a heated humidifier. During the gas delivery, pressure is diverted to an exhalation valve (J) to provide a closed system. Pressure is measured by a gauge (K) on the expiratory limb. Exhaled gas from the exhalation valve passes through the end-expiratory pressure and expiratory resistance valve (L) and then to a spirometer.

Operation

An on–off switch (A) activates the electronic portion of the ventilator (Fig. 24-51). The respiratory frequency is adjusted to between 12 and 36 breaths per minute by the frequency control (B). Emptying pressure is adjusted to a value greater than the pressure required to ventilate the patient by the emptying pressure control (C). The level of the pressure differential controls the slope of the flow curve. If the emptying pressure is slightly greater than the pressure required to ventilate the patient, flow rates will be slow and volume delivery will require the entire inspiratory phase. However, if the emptying pressure is considerably higher than that required to ventilate the patient, the flow rate will increase, the volume will be delivered rapidly, and an inspiratory plateau will occur. The additional emptying pressure is not transmitted to the patient. Once the bag has collapsed, further gas delivery does not occur. A secondary pressure limit control (D) is available to adjust the inspiratory relief pressure to between 30 and 90 cm H_2O.

Gas concentrations to be delivered to the patient are controlled by a rotameter (E) for oxygen and by a dose meter (F), which automatically adjusts the amount of ambient air drawn into the ventilator. Minute volume is expressed in liters per minute and is the result of the combined oxygen and air mixtures. The number of breaths set on the frequency control sets the tidal volume.

Expiratory pressure and expiratory resistance are adjusted by controls (G). The patient pressure gauge has a physical contact alarm monitor built into the pressure gauge needle and face. This alarm can be turned on or off (H) at the front of the ventilator. When on, it provides visual and audible alarms.

Humidity

A heated humidifier provides up to 12 g of water per minute. It is a gas passover type with a filter serving as a wick to provide increased surface area. Inspiratory gas is heated by a heating plate at the base of the metal humidifier jar.

Cleaning and Sterilizing

Most parts of this ventilator can be autoclaved, with the exception of the spirometer, exhalation valve, and water lock container, which must be cold-sterilized. Exhalation valves and all removable parts should be changed every 24 hours.

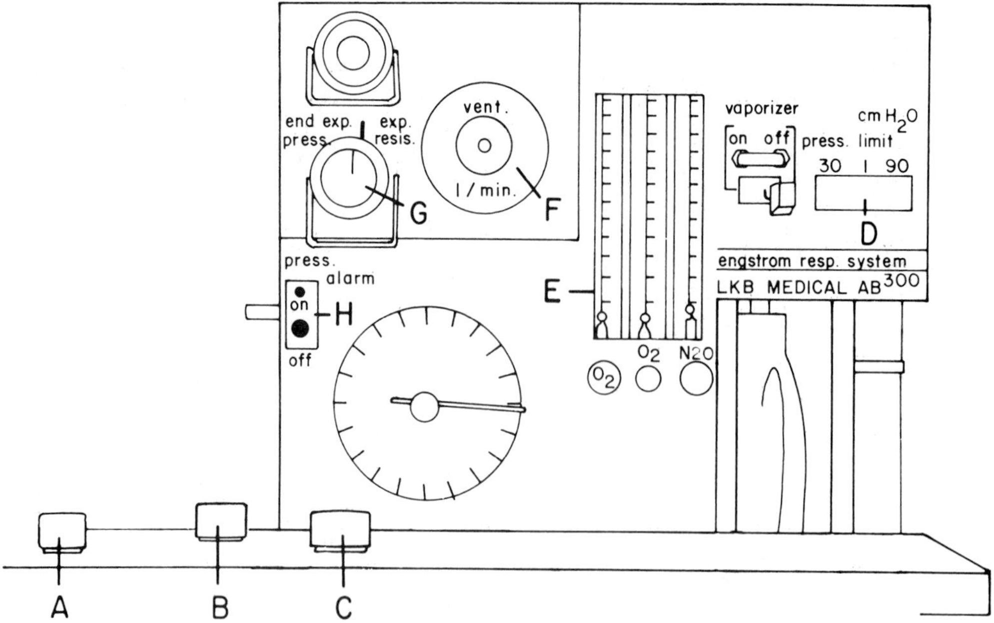

Fig. 24-51. Control panel of the Engström ER 300 Ventilator.

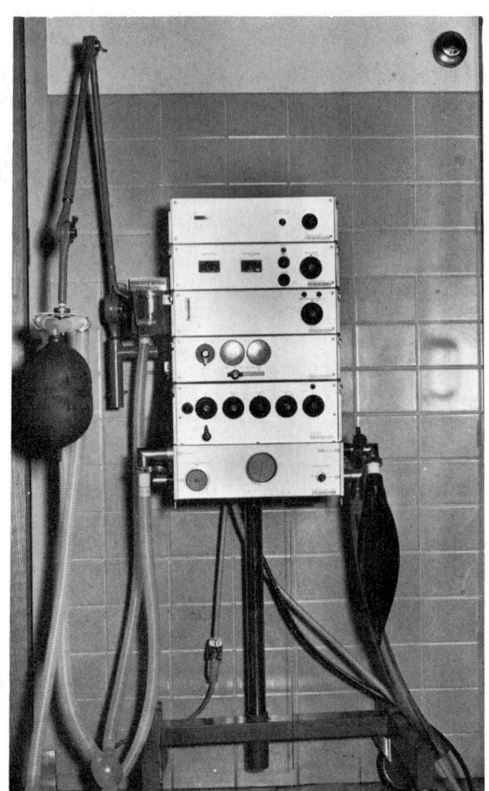

Fig. 24-52. Engström ECS 2000 Ventilator.

Accessories

Many different models of Engström ventilators are available. Outlets for subambient pressure ventilation are available, as are those for anesthesia models and fixed-frequency models.

Troubleshooting

Adjustment of emptying pressure is critical to ensure the desired tidal volume delivery. If power is disconnected accidentally, alarm systems give a continuous, audible signal, whereas an alarm signals intermittently when pressure is low or gas delivery inadequate for the minute volume setting.

Proper functioning of the expiratory valve can be confirmed by visually checking the relative movements of the pressure manometer and the spirometer. The spirometer needle should move only during the exhalation phase.

ENGSTRÖM ECS 2000

Classification

The Engström ECS 2000 ventilator (Fig. 24-52 is an electronically controlled, pneumatically powered, nonconstant flow generator. It is a time-cycled ventilator with secondary pressure-limiting capabilities and adjustable inspiratory plateau. PEEP and an optional subambient pressure attachment are available. This ventilator can serve as an assistor or assistor-controller.

Mechanism

Air and oxygen are delivered at pressures between 34 and 85 psi to a pressure regulator in the mixing unit (*A*), and then from the pressure regulator to a chamber (*B*), which is divided into two compartments (1 and 2) by a flexible membrane (*C*) (Fig. 24-53). An increasing power generator delivers pressure to compartment 1 after compartment 2 has been filled to the desired volume by a flow control (*D*). The selected gas volume in compartment 2 passes through a one-way valve to the patient. A pressure-limiting device (*E*) is adjustable to between 10 and 100 cm H_2O. The increasing power generator is regulated by the pneumatic and electronic control that monitors input pressures as well as compartment pressures, delivery time, and delivery flow. If the volume from compartment 2 is delivered sooner than the designated inspiratory time, the ventilator will provide an inspiratory plateau. The exhaled tidal volume is monitored by an expiratory pressure gauge and passes through an exhalation valve (*F*) and magnetic PEEP valve (*G*). This gas is then deposited into chamber 4 of the ventilatory monitoring chamber (*H*) because of back pressure from the outflow valve (*I*), whereas chamber 3 is at atmospheric pressure. During the next inspiration, a constant flow of gas is delivered into compartment 3, displacing the flexible membrane (*J*) until the volume of compartment 4 has been expelled.

Operation

The Engström ECS 2000 is a modular ventilator that can be arranged in various combinations as desired by the individual operator. Figure 24-54 shows the power supply (*A*), volume measurement (*B*), ultrasonic nebulizer (*C*), mixer (*D*), ventilator (*E*), and patient units (*F*). The power supply (*A*) provides 24 volts to the other modular units when the on–off switch (*G*) is on. This unit has a circuit breaker that can be reset by pressing the reset button if a malfunction occurs or if the current load exceeds 15 amps. An elapsed timer displays the number of hours the unit has been in operation.

The volume measurement component (*B*) provides a digital display of both the exhaled tidal (*H*) and minute volumes (*I*) in liters and liters per minute,

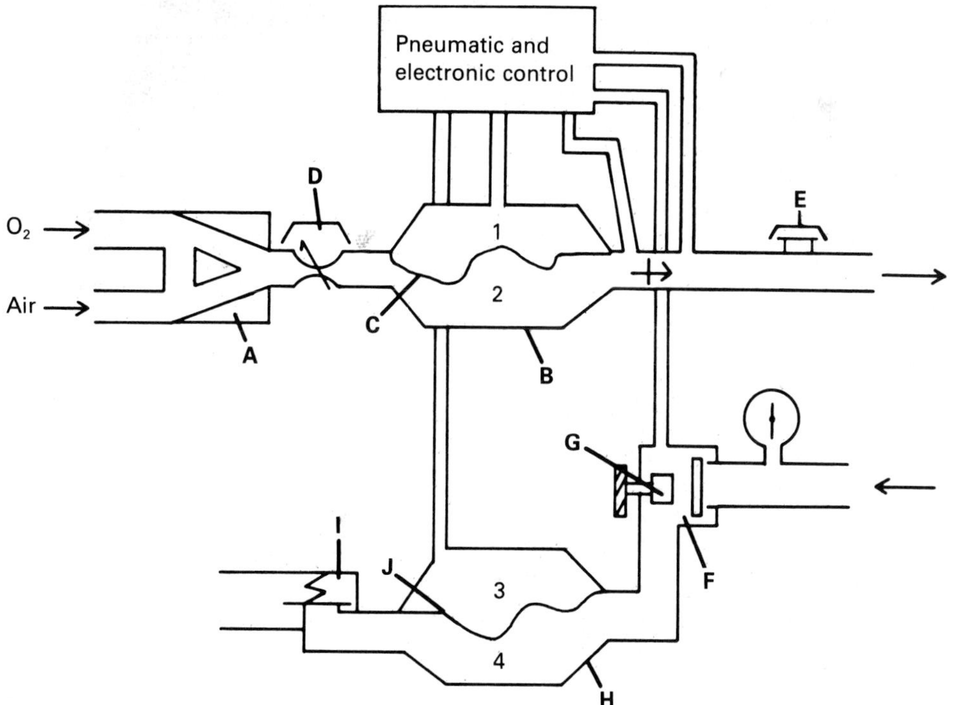

Fig. 24-53. Schematic diagram of Engström ECS 2000 Ventilator.

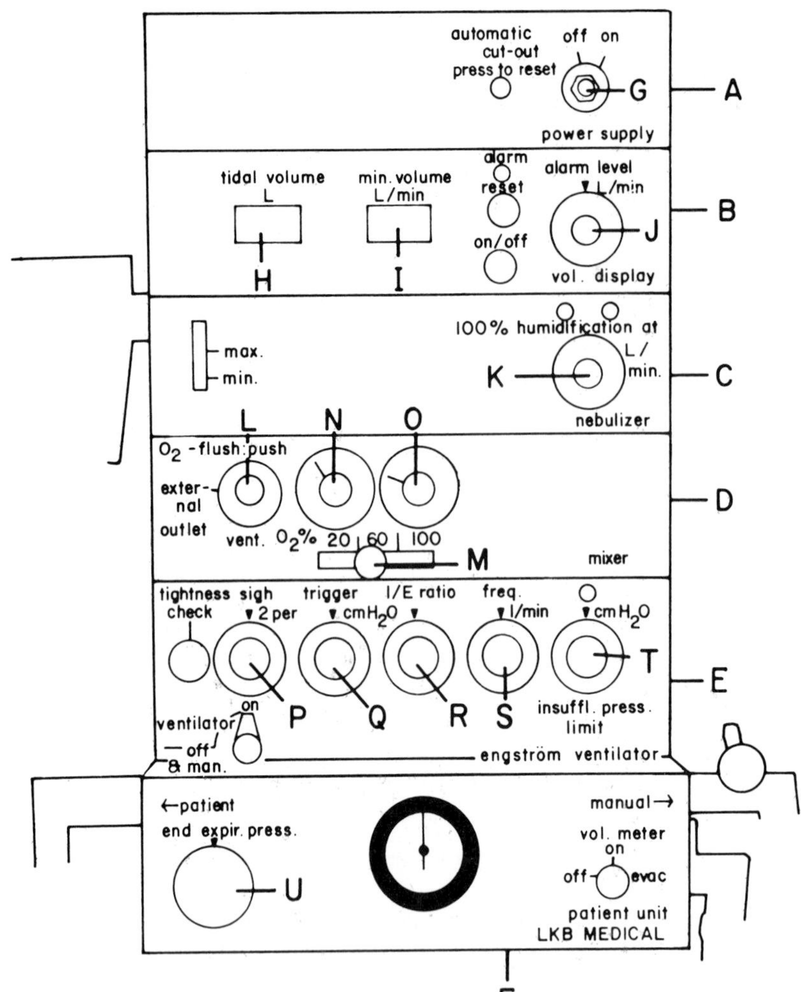

Fig. 24-54. Control panel of the Engström ECS 2000 Ventilator.

respectively. If a tidal volume is less than 100 ml, it is not displayed immediately but is averaged for 3 breaths. An alarm level (*J*) can be set to the desired minute volume. If the expired minute ventilation is below that selected, an audible and visual alarm will be activated. When reset, the alarm will remain off for 1 minute before sounding again. The alarm module is also activated during other component malfunctions, such as high pressure in the patient circuit; failures in the power supply, oxygen power, or air supply; or water level depletion. Besides energizing the volume measurement component alarm, these alarms activate additional alarms on their individual component to make isolating the malfunction easier. The on–off button on *B* controls only the volume measurement display and the expiratory gas volume and pressure alarm. Alarms originating in other modules are still activated by malfunctions of their particular component.

In the ultrasonic nebulizer module (*C*), 100% relative humidification is provided by adjustment of control *K* to the same minute volume as that indicated on the ventilator. If a relative humidity less than 100% is desired, control *K* is adjusted to the liter flow that will give the desired relative humidity. As an example, if 50% relative humidity is desired and the ventilator is set to deliver 10 liters/min, the nebulizer control is set on 5 liters/min. A water level indicator allows monitoring of fluid levels in the nebulizer, and alarm lights indicate when the water level is too low and the nebulizer is shut down.

The mixer module (*D*) has a selector control (*L*) to provide the desired gas mixture to an outlet at the side of the ventilator or to the ventilator itself. The selector control also has a button that provides 100% oxygen whenever it is depressed. A slider control (*M*) selects the oxygen concentration, whereas flowmeters display the delivered air flow (*N*) and oxygen flow

(O). Alarms are present for both high- and low-pressure gas sources.

On the ventilator module *(E)*, an on–off switch is provided. In the "off" position, manual inflation may be provided with the manual bag attachment. Periodic sighs can be delivered every one hundredth to four hundredth breath by control *P*. The sigh volume is twice the tidal volume. The sigh breath is delivered twice before recycling to the normal tidal volume. The ventilator sensitivity can be adjusted by the trigger control *(Q)* to between -1 and -20 cm H_2O for patient-assisted ventilation. In the assist mode the ventilator will pressure-cycle without any inspiratory plateau pressure. The I:E ratio *(R)* may be set to between 1:1 and 1:3, independent of the frequency of the respiratory cycle. Frequency of respiration is set by the frequency control *(S)* from 6 to 60 breaths per minute. Inflation pressure limit is set by control *T*. This control can be set from 10 to 100 cm H_2O. After airway pressure reaches this limit, flow delivery ceases and a light above insufflation pressure limit (T) is illuminated, indicating that the set tidal volume has not delivered during the designated inspiratory time. Accordingly, flow will continue until the full tidal volume has been delivered. If the inspiratory time is longer than required to deliver prescribed tidal volume, the inspiratory pressure will hold in a plateau phase until inspiration has been terminated.

The patient unit *(F)* has attachments for respiratory hose connections, exhalation valves, and directional valves to ventilate the patient manually. This unit is easily removed for cleaning and sterilizing. It also houses the valve *U*, which adjusts PEEP to between 0 and 10 cm H_2O.

Humidity

Humidity is provided by the ultrasonic nebulizer module, as described in the preceding section.

Cleaning and Sterilizing

The patient unit can be removed and disassembled for cleaning. All parts except the pressure manometer can be cleaned and steam-autoclaved. This treatment is also recommended for the ultrasonic nebulizer parts.

Accessories

Subambient pressure attachments and sigh mechanisms are options available on designated units.

Troubleshooting

Periodic volume measurements and general cleaning are recommended. If no leaks are found in the patient system but volume delivery is inadequate, the patient unit connection on the front of the ventilator should be checked. Also, the flexible membrane may be inverted if overpressurized, thereby stopping patient gas input. Finally, after the flexible membrane has been cleaned, it must not be reassembled upside down.

FOREGGER 210 VOLUME VENTILATOR

Classification

The Foregger 210 ventilator (Fig. 24-55) is an electronically and pneumatically powered constant flow generator with inspiratory plateau capability. It is time-cycled with control, assist-control, and IMV modes. PEEP and CPAP are available as standard features.

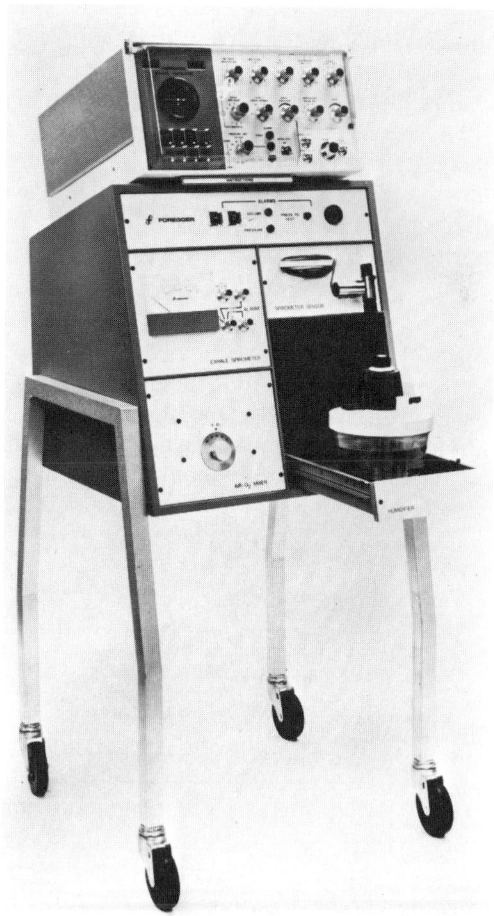

Fig. 24-55. Foregger 210 Volume Ventilator.

Mechanism

High-pressure air and oxygen are delivered to an internal blender *(A)* at 50 psi (Fig. 24-56). The mixed gas is then filtered *(B)*, regulated to 33 to 35 psi, and delivered to a series of electronically controlled solenoid valves. The IMV solenoid *(C)* is open during the ventilator expiratory phase to provide a continuous gas flow for spontaneous breathing. This flow of gas is adjusted by a flow control valve *(D)* in conjunction with a reservoir bag and IMV valve assembly to meet the patient's inspiratory demand.

The ventilator inspiratory timing solenoid *(E)* and flow control valve *(F)* determine the mechanical tidal volume. Closure of the exhalation valve *(O)* is effected by activation of the patient valve solenoid *(G)*. Metered expiratory threshold pressure (PEEP) is controlled by the PEEP solenoid *(H)*. A positive pressure limiting valve *(I)* and a fixed (-6 cm H_2O) "negative pressure" relief valve *(J)* limit the operational pressures in the patient circuit. The pressure-sensing module *(K)* monitors and transduces all pressure changes to the electronic control. Simultaneous visual monitoring is provided by the airway pressure gauge *(L)*. Gas flow is delivered to the patient through a passive-heated humidifier *(H)*, and flow to the circuit nebulizer *(P)* is provided by a nebulizer selector valve *(Q)*. A matched pair of flow resistors *(N)* provide the same flow to the patient circuit when the nebulizer selector valve is in the "on" or "off" position, thereby maintaining the preselected mechanical tidal volume.

Operation

The Foregger 210 is divided into upper control and lower console units (Fig. 24-57). Operation is effected by a series of 8 function selector switches *(A)* located beneath the pressure gauge in the control unit. Each selector switch is depressed independently to activate its individual function and remains depressed and illuminated as long as that function is used (except for the manual start switch that initiates the inspiratory phase).

The audio off selector switch *(A)* is depressed when audible alarm signals are not desired. While depressed, the switch is illuminated by a flashing light, and an audible chirping sound occurs at 5-second intervals.

The IMV switch *(A)* activates the IMV function, which is controlled by the IMV-rate *(B)* and IMV-flow knobs. IMV rate varies from 0 to 15 breaths per minute. Gas flow for the spontaneous breathing component of IMV is from 0.2 to 0.8 liters/sec (12–48 liters/min) and passes through a heated humidifier to a reservoir bag and IMV valve, thence to the patient. After the IMV switch has been depressed, sigh, assist, and inspiratory pause selector switches are automatically deactivated.

Mechanical minute volume delivered by the ventilator is determined by three controls. I:E ratio *(D)* and the inspiratory time *(E)* knobs regulate the entire respiratory cycle. Inspiration varies from 0.4 to 4.0 seconds. The ventilator rate is thus 4 to 75 breaths per minute in the control mode and is monitored digitally in the LED display (BPM) above the pressure gauge.

Tidal volume is the product of both inspiratory time *(E)* and inspiratory flow *(F)*, which varies from 0.2 to 2.0 liters/sec (12–120 liters/min). It is also displayed digitally above the pressure gauge.

The sigh switch *(A)* activates three controls *(G, H,* and *L)*. The sighs per hour knob *(G)* determines the sigh frequency of 4 to 15 sighs per hour in multiples of one to three. Sigh volume is set by the sigh percentage above normal knob *(H)*. This selector allows the operator to augment normal tidal volume by 25%, 50%, 75%, or 100% increments. Pressure-limiting of

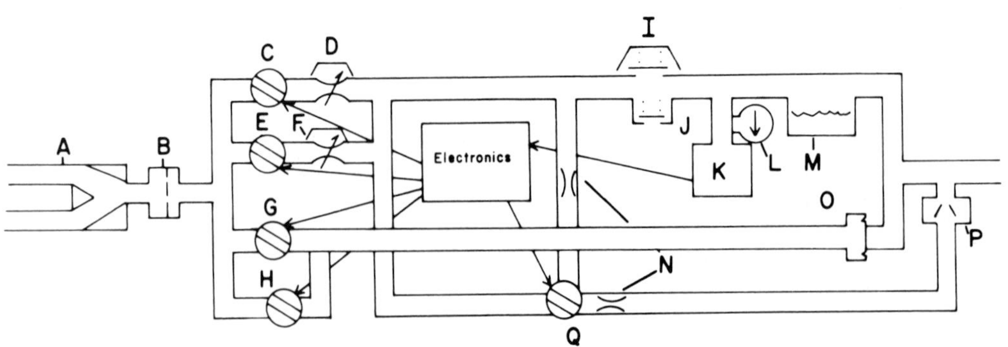

Fig. 24-56. Schematic diagram of the Foregger 210 Ventilator.

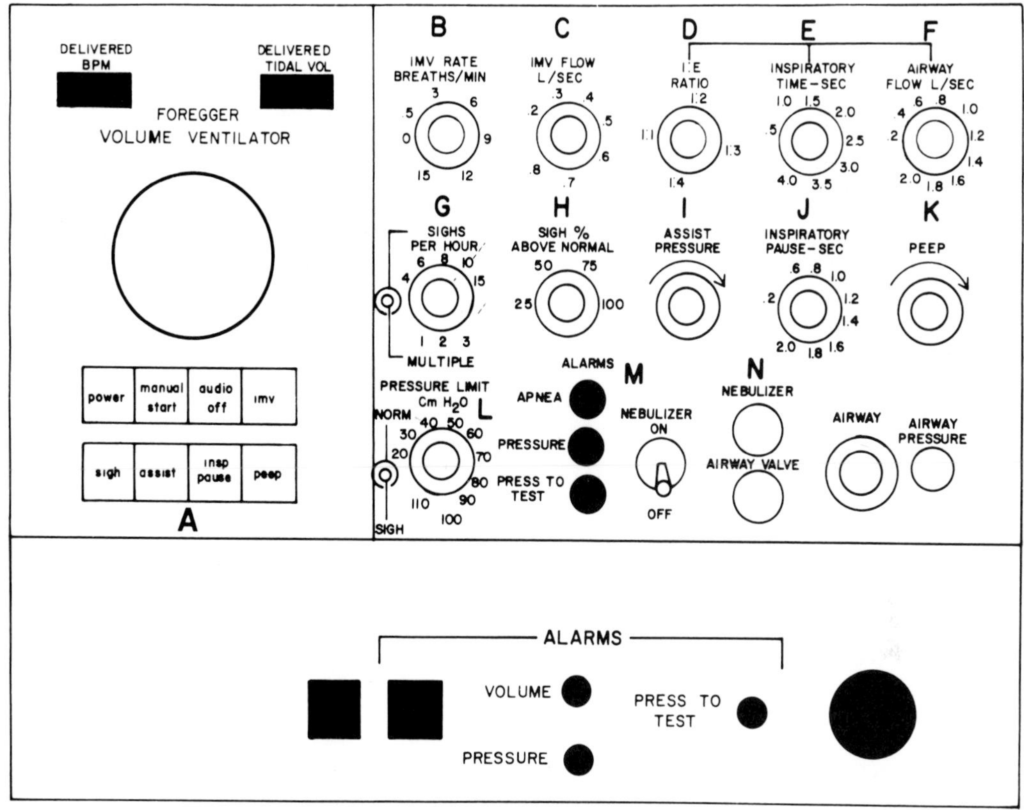

Fig. 24-57. Control panel of the Foregger 210 Ventilator.

the sigh volume is provided by the inner concentric knob on the pressure limit control *(L)*.

The assist switch *(A)* activates the assist pressure control *(I)*. This control determines the effort necessary to initiate patient-triggered mechanical inspiration. Clockwise adjustment increases sensitivity (decreases the required effort). Selection of an assist pressure slightly below PEEP allows assisted ventilation even at relatively high PEEP.

The inspiratory pause switch *(A)* activates the inspiratory pause (plateau) control *(J)*. This control prolongs inspiration from 0.2 to 2 seconds beyond the normal duration set by the inspiratory time control *(E)*.

The PEEP switch *(A)* activates the PEEP control *(K)*, which is adjustable between 2 and 35 cm H_2O. Clockwise rotation of *(K)* increases PEEP, which is monitored on the pressure manometer. PEEP discontinued, both the PEEP switch *(A)* and the PEEP control *(K)* must be turned off. Otherwise, if the PEEP switch is subsequently depressed, the previous level will be established.

The pressure limit control *(L)* is active whenever the ventilator is in operation. Its normal pressure limit range is 20 to 110 cm H_2O for both normal and sigh tidal volumes.

An apnea alarm *(M)* is illuminated when the airway pressure does not exceed an internally determined threshold, and a continuous audible alarm also sounds. The pressure alarm *(M)* lights and a continuous audible signal is generated when the pressure limit *(L)* is exceeded or if the control unit pressure drops below 20 psi. If pressure-cycled ventilation is used, the audible portion of this alarm can be silenced by depressing the audio-off selector switch *(A)*.

The press-to-test switch *(M)* provides an internal check of the integrity of the electronic components and entire alarm circuitry. When depressed, all lights and audible alarm signals are activated.

A nebulizer toggle switch *(N)* controls the operation of the medicament nebulizer. Tidal volume and FI_{O_2} are automatically maintained constant with or without the added nebulizer gas flow.

Humidity

Humidity should be provided by a heated cascade humidifier (shown as M in Fig. 24-56). However, a humidifier and patient circuit are not included with the ventilator.

Cleaning and Sterilizing

Air filters and spirometer sensors should not be steam-autoclaved. The spirometer sensor and the IMV valve may be cleaned and gas- or cold-sterilized, but they should not be disassembled.

Accessories

An air compressor is available.

Troubleshooting

The press-to-test switch evaluates the condition of the electronic components. If a malfunction should occur, modular circuit boards and other electrical components may be exchanged in the field by the company service representative for easy repair. External circuit breakers are provided on the unit to protect the unit from voltage overload; these should be checked whenever an electrical malfunction occurs.

HEALTHYDYNE INFANT VENTILATOR

Classification

The Healthdyne Infant Ventilator (Fig. 24-58) is a pneumatically operated, electronically controlled constant flow generator that is time-cycled. It can provide ambient or positive pressures on exhalation and can be used in control, IMV, or CPAP modes.

Mechanism

The Healthdyne Infant Ventilator requires a blender (A) (Fig. 24-59) external to the ventilator system, which provides the gas mixture desired at 30 to 60 psi; the gas supply is then split to the patient system and a control system. The patient system adjusts the gas flow by means of a flow meter system (B) before being humidified by a humidifier (C) of the operator's choice. The control system regulates (D) the system pressure to 30 psi before it passes through the maximum pressure control (E) and the CPAP control (F). Each of these controls regulates the inflation pressure to the exhalation valve, the maximum pressure control (E) during the inspiratory phase acting as a pressure limit and the CPAP control (F) during the expiratory phase. The electronic components control these controls and the cycling solenoid (G), which phases the ventilator from the inspiratory mode to expiratory.

Operation

The Healthdyne Infant Ventilator is simple to use and operate because of a computer (Fig. 24-60) attached to the top of the ventilator. This computer does not alter any function of the ventilator but does allow the operator to analyze the impact of ventilator settings before, during, and after a patient has been ventilated.

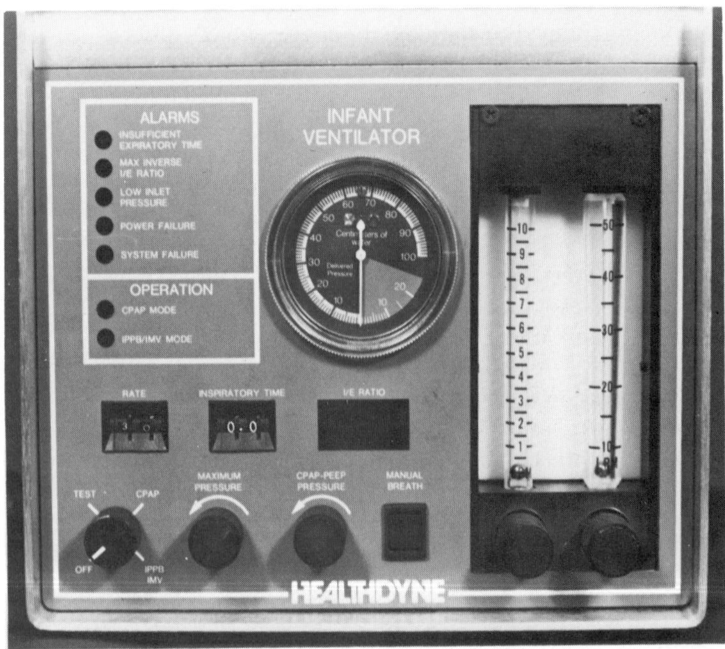

Fig. 24-58. Healthdyne Infant Ventilator. (Courtesy of Healthdyne Corporation)

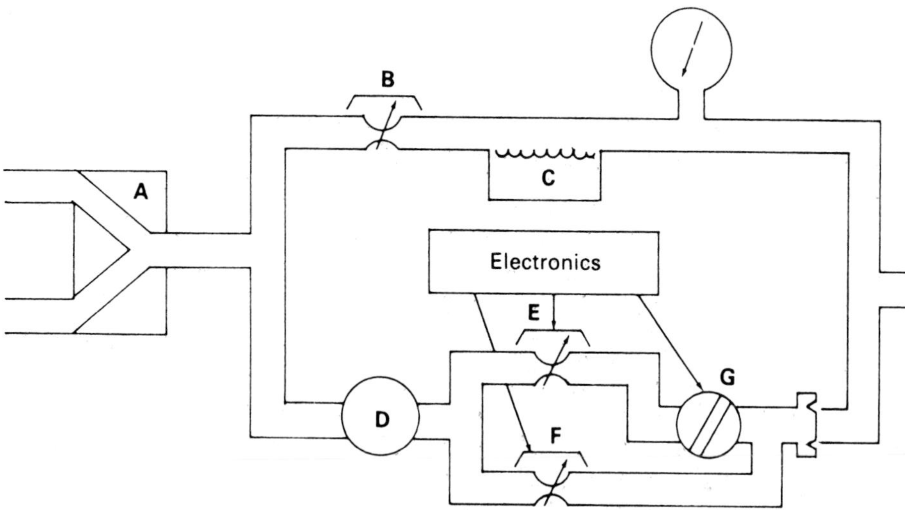

Fig. 24-59. Schematic diagram of Healthdyne Infant Ventilator.

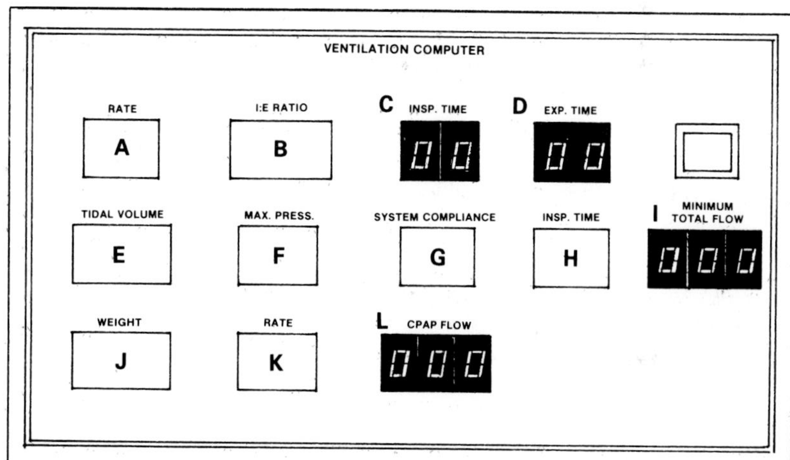

Fig. 24-60. Ventilation computer of Healthdyne Infant Ventilator.

Divided into three segments, the ventilation computer allows the operator to calculate inspiratory and expiratory time, IPPB/IMV flowrate, and CPAP flowrate.

The first segment requires that the rate (A) and I:E ratio (B) be set in order to determine the inspiratory (C) and expiratory (D) time. Once the appropriate values have been determined, they may be set on the face of the ventilator.

The second grouping of computer inputs determines the minimum required flow. Helpful in conserving gas, the required flow is calculated by dialing in either the appropriate tidal volume (E) or the maximum pressure (F). Whichever value is selected, the other must be set on zero. Should both values be dialed in, the computer will select the maximum pressure (F) value and disregard the tidal volume (E). The system compliance (G) may be calculated by multiplying the flow by the inspiratory time and dividing that value by the maximum pressure or estimating from values provided in the operator's manual. Next, the inspiratory time (H) is dialed in and the minimum total flow (I) noted. This flow is then dialed into the ventilator flow meters (M) with the corresponding inspiratory (O) and maximum pressure (R) (Fig. 24-61).

The third row of computer settings (see Fig. 24-60) is to set the normal CPAP flow (L) by dialing in the child's weight (J) in kilograms and the rate (K). The computer then provides the operator with the proper CPAP flow (L) setting.

The Ventilation Computer is *totally independent* of the ventilator controls. *What is set and read out on the computer does not adjust the ventilator.*

The ventilator control panel (see Fig. 24-61) has a flowmeter system (M) that adjusts the continuous

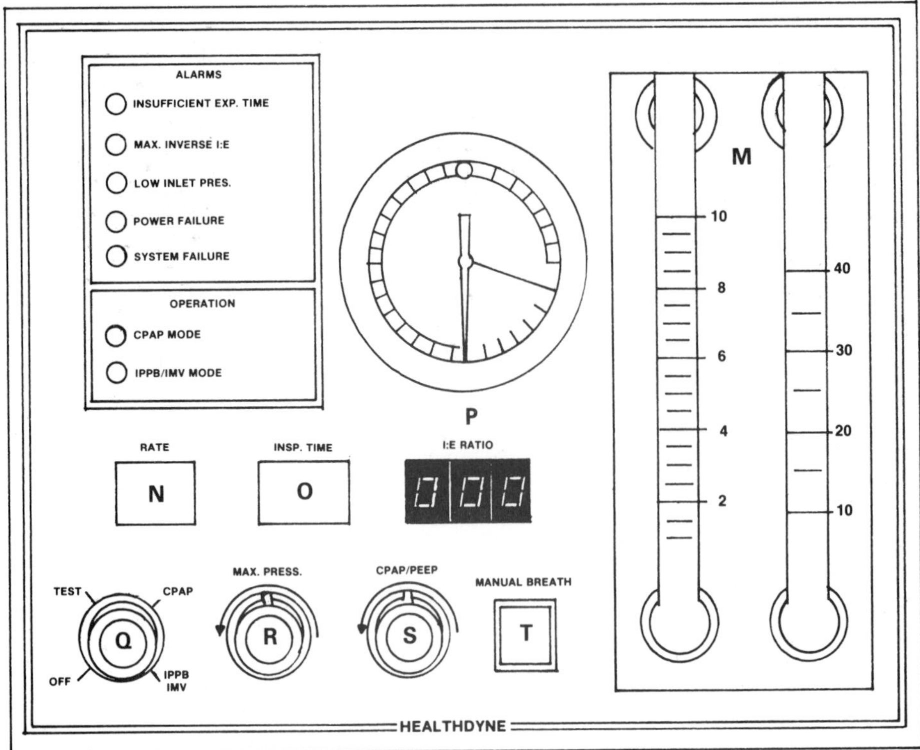

Fig. 24-61. Control panel of Healthdyne Infant Ventilator.

flow of gas to the patient. This flowmeter system has two flowmeters: one fine and one gross, which are additive. Should 22 liters/min be desired, 20 liters/min is adjusted on one flowmeter and two on the other. Neither of these flowmeters is back-pressure compensated. The rate (N) is then dialed in on the face of the ventilator between 1 and 150 breaths per minute. Completely independent, this control paces the ventilator at its set rate regardless of the I:E ratio. The inspiratory time control (O), adjustable from 0.1 to 4.9 seconds, is also independent. Because both the rate (N) and inspiratory time controls are independent, the I:E ratio display (P) completely depends on them. This allows inverse I:E ratio to that desired by the operator; however, since the inspiratory segment of the I:E ratio is fixed at one on the display, inverse I:E ratios are shown as fractions of one, such as 1:0.5 for a 2:1 ratio.

The mode selector (Q) has four selector positions: off, test, CPAP, and IPPB/IMV. In the test position, all displays should indicate "8", and an audible alarm will sound. If the power failure light does not light, its battery should be replaced. In the CPAP mode, the ventilator ignores all controls except the CPAP setting, flow settings, and manual breath push button (T). Because the manual breath push button (T) is active, all adjustments should be dialed to appropriate settings for a mechanical inflation. Should the manual breath button (T) be pushed, the inflation will go only to the maximum inflation pressure and pre-set inspiratory time. The IPPB/IMV mode allows the ventilator to provide mechanical breaths at prescribed intervals. The maximum pressure control (R) is adjustable from 0 to 100 cm H_2O. This control may also be used to establish an inspiratory hold if the pressure is limited to a designated level and the time-cycle has not yet terminated the inspiratory phase. CPAP/PEEP (S) may be adjustable from 0 to 20 cm H_2O in either the CPAP or IPPB/IMV modes.

Humidity

Humidity is provided by the humidifier of the operator's choosing.

Cleaning and Sterilizing

The simple patient breathing system is easily disconnected and cleaned. The unit itself should be wiped with a germicidal or bacteriocidal agent. The ventilator unit should not be gas sterilized.

Accessories

Accessories include power pac (for battery operation), pressure and rate monitors, and alarms.

Troubleshooting

A complex electronic ventilator, this unit should not be repaired in the field.

MONAGHAN 225

Classification

The Monaghan 225 (Fig. 24-62) is a volume-cycled constant flow generator. It can be operated with either a secondary pressure or time limit. Positive expiratory pressure is available, and it can be used as an assistor, controller or assistor-controller. Newer models offer SIMV.

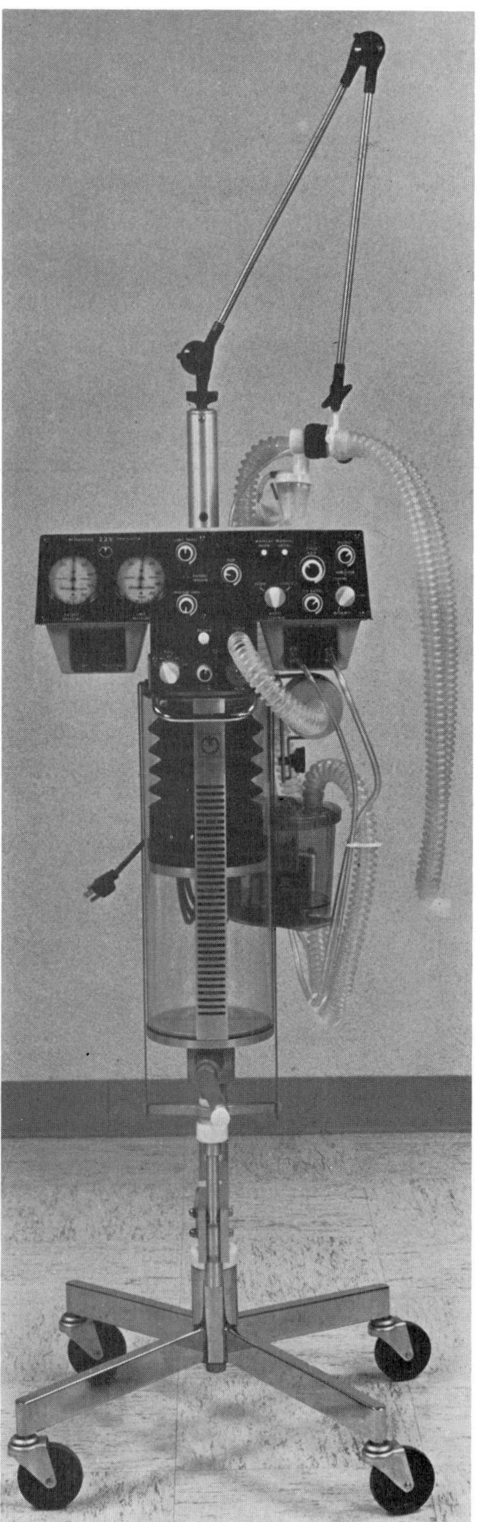

Fig. 24-62. Monaghan 225 Ventilator.

Mechanism

The Monaghan 225 is pneumatically operated with fluid logic and is powered by a 50 psi oxygen source (Fig. 24-63). Electrical power heats the humidifier. Oxygen is delivered to the main valve (A), which is programmed by the logic system to align the valve system properly. The fluidic control is adjusted by controls on the front panel of the ventilator to determine the respiratory phasing of the ventilator. The inspiratory time, pressure limit, patient trigger, and volume limit all have inputs and outputs from this programming center (B). Flow rate to the bellows chamber is controlled by the flow-rate control (C), which determines the rate at which the bellows is compressed.

Pressurization is developed in chamber D by this gas source when the fluidic OR gate (E) closes the mushroom valve (F). Simultaneous closure of the patient exhalation valve (G) is also accomplished by the fluidic OR gate. A mushroom valve (F) also serves as a safety pressure limit at 100 cm H_2O. Once inspiration has been completed, the oxygen that has compressed the bellows is exhausted through a control valve (H). This control delivers the amount of oxygen to be mixed with air brought in through a filter (I) to the prescribed oxygen concentration as determined by control H. After the bellows volume has been delivered to the patient, it is humidified and the pressure monitored. The system can be pressure-limited by an inspiratory pressure relief control (J). The pressure relief system, or gate, and main valve functions are controlled by the fluid logic system. Inspiratory effort can

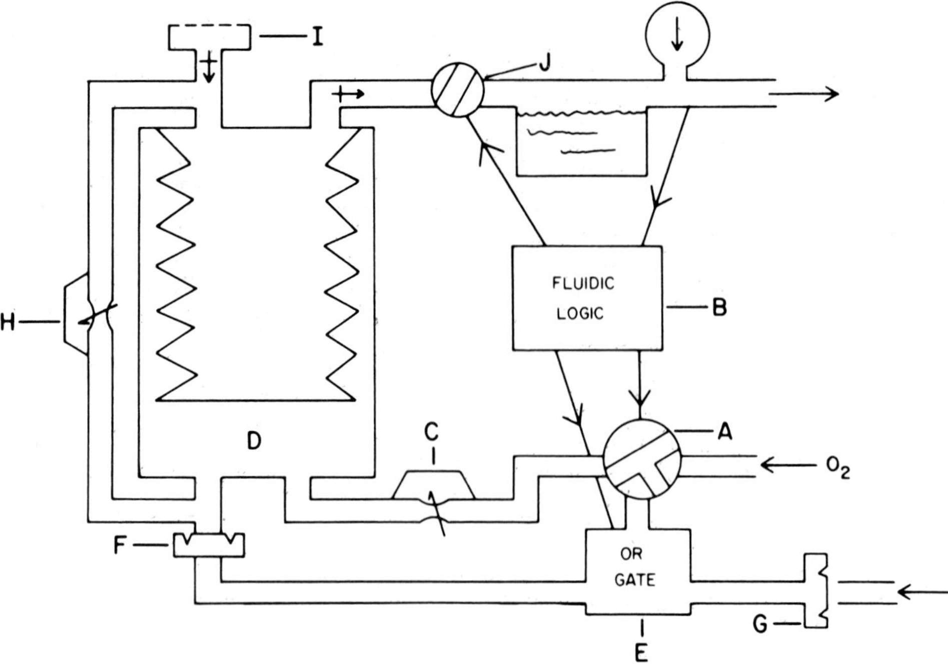

Fig. 24-63. Schematic diagram of the Monaghan 225 Ventilator.

also be programmed into the logic system and adjusted to allow for assisted breaths.

Operation

The Monaghan 225 is connected to a 50 psi oxygen source and the humidifier plugged into an electrical outlet at least 20 minutes before use (Fig. 24-64). The mode selector (A) is dialed appropriately and the rate set on the cycle rate (B). The cycle rate controls the expiratory time and has a range of 0.5 to 7.5 seconds. The I:E ratio control (C) regulates the inspiratory time between 0.5 and 1.88 seconds and the I:E ratio between 1:1 and 1:4. These two controls give a breathing rate range of 4 to 60 breaths per minute. Volume to be delivered (100–3300 ml) is determined by a hand crank located at the bottom of the bellows. Any attempt to deliver volumes below 100 ml may result in erratic volume delivery. The ventilator also can be pressure-limited by adjustment of the pressure limit control (D). The maximum pressure obtainable is 100 cm H_2O. The flow control (E) adjusts the rate of bellows compression. Peak flow of 100 liters/min against zero back pressure is possible.

If the mode selector has been turned either to the assist or to the assist-control mode, assisted ventilation is possible. The trigger sensitivity control (F) adjusts the amount of subambient pressure the patient must generate. When the patient has initiated an assisted breath, an indicator light will so inform the operator. A manual inspiratory start button (G) is also present. Manual depression of button H will abort tidal volume delivery. Pneumatic "lights" (I) indicate whether the tidal volume delivery has been terminated by time- or pressure-cycling. If neither of these lights flash, volume-cycling has occurred.

Oxygen concentration is selected by the percent of oxygen control (J). This gas mixer requires no high-pressure air source to deliver oxygen concentrations from 21% to 100%. PEEP up to 20 cm H_2O can be dialed by the PEEP control (K). Nebulization of medication can be provided by adjustment of switch (L).

Humidity

Humidity is provided by a unique passive-heated humidifier that utilizes the breathing assembly pressure changes to pump heated water from a large reservoir chamber into a smaller humidifying chamber. This smaller chamber decreases the resistance to the initiation of assisted ventilation. The amount of heat is thermostatically controlled at the humidifier, and condensation may occur in the tubing circuit.

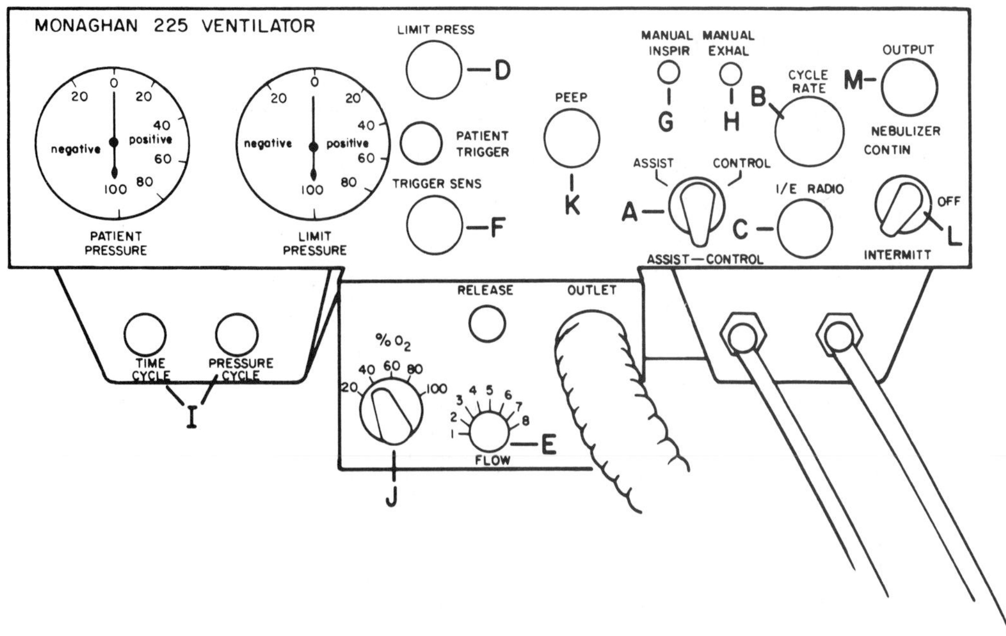

Fig. 24-64. Control panel of the Monaghan 225 Ventilator.

Cleaning and Sterilizing

The breathing assembly should be changed at least every 24 hours. It must be disassembled according to manufacturer's specifications and washed in mild detergents. The patient hose, manifold, exhalation diaphragm holder, and humidifier may be either cold-, gas-, or steam-autoclaved. Bacteria filters should also be sterilized by steam-autoclaving. The bellows assembly ordinarily does not need to be sterilized because it is inside the ventilator and is exposed only to the delivery gas.

Accessories

A ventilator monitor and an alarm system are available.

Troubleshooting

Fluid logic ventilators incorporate few moving parts; therefore, relatively trouble-free service should be expected. If the ventilator autocycles, the sensitivity may be too great or the PEEP control may be on. The PEEP control will autocycle the ventilator unless it is connected to a patient or test lung.

Improper oxygen delivery may result from the medication nebulizer being turned on, plugging of the air intake filter, or a hole in the bellows or bellows check-valve assembly. Erratic cycling and oxygen concentration delivery are expected if the tidal volume is set below 100 ml tidal volume; such attempts at low tidal volumes should be avoided.

OHIO 560

Classification

The Ohio 560 ventilator (Fig. 24-65) is an electronically powered, constant flow generator with inspiratory plateau capability. It is a volume-cycled ventilator with a secondary pressure limiting adjustment. During the expiratory phase, a positive pressure or an optional subambient pressure may be added. This ventilator can serve as a controller, or assistor-controller but cannot be used as a strict assistor alone because the expiratory timer cannot be turned off.

Mechanism

High-pressure oxygen delivered to a mixing chamber (A) is blended with air and then delivered to an accumulator bag (B) to provide the desired concentration (Fig. 24-66). This gas mixture is flow-directed by a series of unidirectional valves into two bellows (C and D). Bellows C provides a sigh volume that is ad-

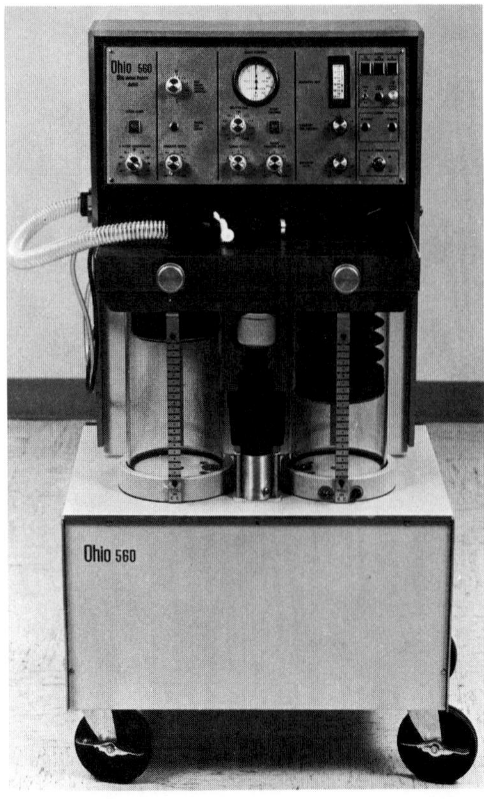

Fig. 24-65. Ohio 560 Ventilator.

ditive to the normal tidal volume bellows (D). The bellows is compressed for gas delivery by a turbine motor (E), which develops pressure in the bellows compression chambers (F). The cycling of this compression is governed by switch (G), which can be electronically controlled or can be opened by the patient for an assisted breath by tubing (H). Compression within the bellows chambers (F) is built by closing the mushroom exhaust valve (I). These exhaust valves prevent air from escaping during inspiration, then deflate and allow the compression chambers to exhaust during expiration. During inspiration, the patient expiration valve (J) is closed. The bellows contents are determined by controls that adjust displacement volume. As the bellows is compressed, gas passes through a control (K) that adjusts the flow rate, the inspiratory time, and the I:E ratio. The inspiratory relief pressure control (L) operates the secondary pressure limit.

Operation

The power switch (A) is turned on and the appropriate tidal volume (range 0–2000 ml) (B) selected (Fig. 24-67). The sigh breath, if desired, can also be selected by the deep-breath volume control (C). These volumes are additive. Inspiratory time is adjusted by the inspiratory flow control (D). Time allotted for the requisite volume delivery is determined by the flow rate. The maximal flow capability of this ventilator is 180 liters/min with 0 resistance and 100 liters/min against a 40 cm H_2O back pressure. The duration of expiration is controlled by the expiratory time control (E), which has a range of 0.5 to 7 seconds. A ventilator rate between 6 and 50 breaths per minute is possible. Time can be extended, however, into an inspiratory plateau. An inspiratory hold of 0.2 to 2 seconds is adjusted by the inflation hold control (F). Use of the inflation hold will alter the breathing rate.

The number of sighs is adjusted by the deep-breath interval control (G), which can be set from 0 to 10-minute intervals in 2-minute increments. A manual deep-breath button (H) is also present. Ventilator rate is displayed on a respiration rate monitor. If at any time the operator wishes to cycle the ventilator manually, he may do so by pressing the manual inflation button (I), which will immediately initiate a normal tidal volume. A manual exhalation button (J) will dump pressure in the patient circuit when depressed. If the patient initiates a breath, a patient-triggering light indicates an assisted respiration. Sensitivity is adjusted by the patient-triggering effort, knob K. The minimum effort required is 0.5 cm H_2O subambient pressure. Oxygen delivery is adjusted by control L.

A pressure relief control inside the table panel (not shown) can be set from 10 to 100 cm H_2O. Available alarms include the failure-to-cycle light (M), the low-pressure alarm (N), and the high-pressure alarm (O), each of which can be reset (P). The failure-to-cycle alarm will signal if the inspiratory phase extends beyond 8 seconds or if the expiratory phase exceeds 14 seconds. Once the problem has been corrected, the reset button is pushed. If the ventilator does not develop a pressure greater than 8 cm H_2O during normal cycling, the low-pressure alarm will signal. The high-pressure alarm signals that the pressure limit has been exceeded.

An expiratory plateau (0–15 cm H_2O) can be set by the PEEP control (Q). This pressure and inspiratory pressure are monitored on a pressure manometer labeled "Patient Resistance."

Humidity

Humidification is provided by an ultrasonic nebulizer with a 0 ≃ 3 ml/min output control (R). Only factory-supplied nebulizers should be substituted for this nebulizer.

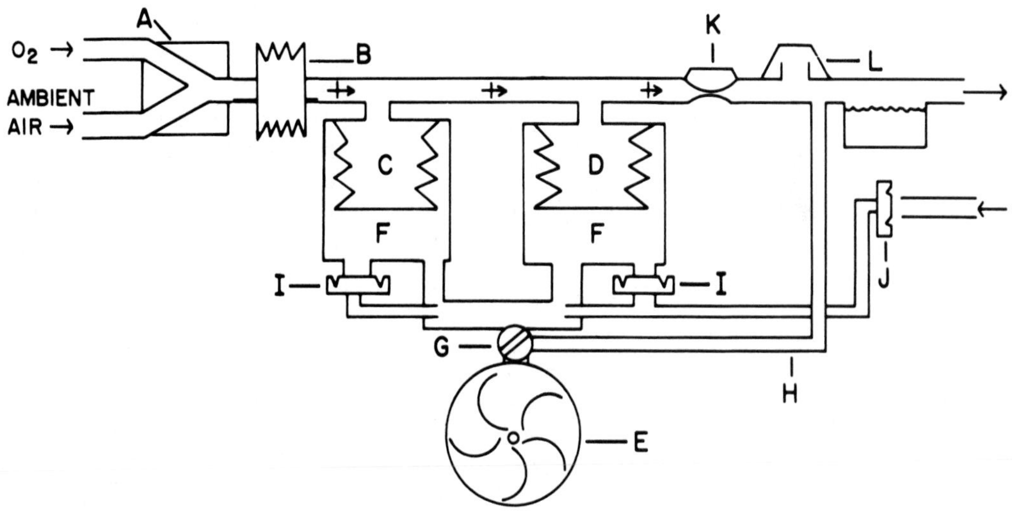

Fig. 24-66. Schematic diagram of the Ohio 560 Ventilator.

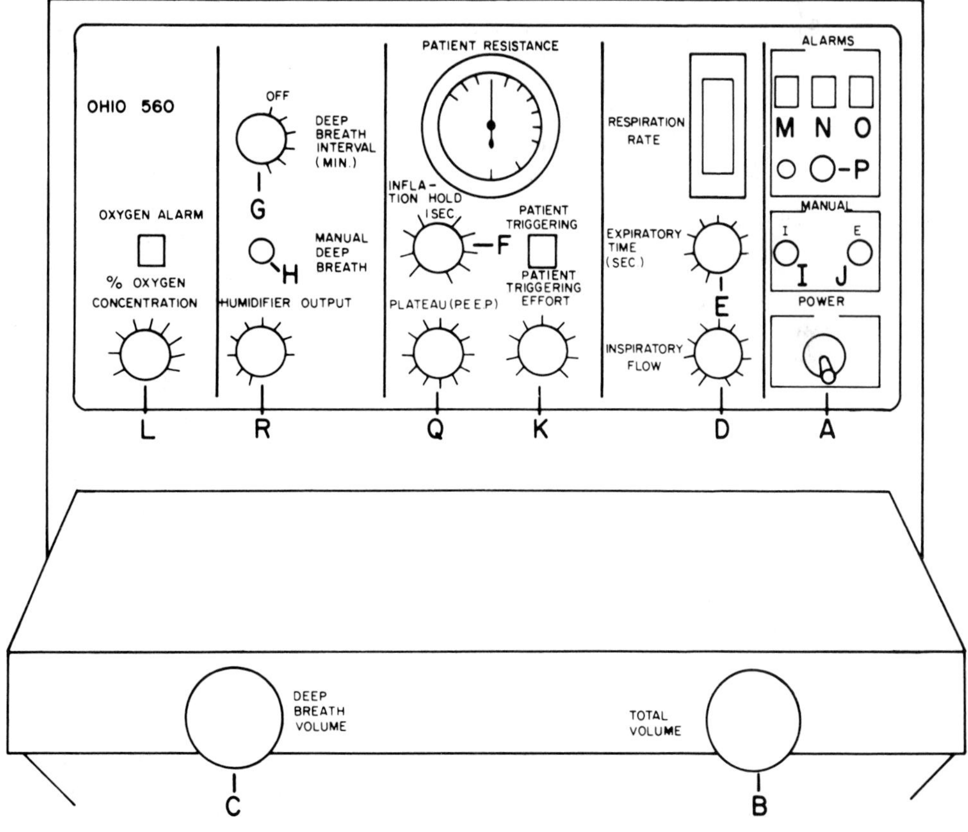

Fig. 24-67. Control panel of the Ohio 560 Ventilator.

Cleaning and Sterilizing

The breathing assembly, including the nebulizer, should be changed at least daily, and more often in problem patients. Observe normal precautions for cleaning and sterilizing plastics.

Accessories

A drug nebulizer and subambient pressure system are available.

Troubleshooting

The mushroom exhalation valve may be a source of leakage. It must seat and inflate properly. Dirty intake filters or leaks in the accumulation bag may be responsible for inappropriate oxygen concentrations. In earlier models, belt slippage on the turbine occurred frequently. If the ventilator ceases to deliver pressure, the belt drive may not be connected to the turbine inside the lower front panel of the ventilator.

OHIO 550

Classification

The Ohio 550 ventilator (Fig. 24-68) is a nonconstant flow generator that is volume-cycled, but a secondary pressure-limiting function that attaches to the patient circuit is available. Because of the low driving pressure, in the face of low compliance, this ventilator will become a constant pressure ventilator. Exhalation is passive, but the clinician has the option of developing expiratory positive pressure. This ventilator can serve as a controller or an assistor-controller.

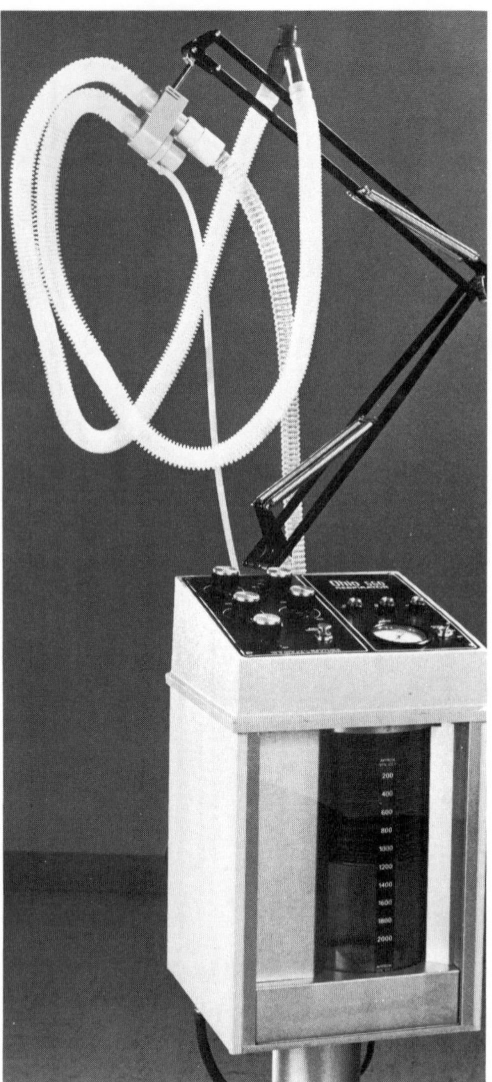

Fig. 24-68. Ohio 550 Ventilator.

Mechanism

This pneumatically powered ventilator (Fig. 24-69) is operated by a high-pressure oxygen source that blends ambient air in a gas-mixing device *(A)* and delivers the appropriate gas mixture through a unidirectional valve into the patient bellows system *(B)* to a second unidirectional valve, which ensures proper flow direction into the patient-breathing circuit. The pressure developed in the ventilator system is monitored on the pressure gauge *(C)*. The gas mixture passes through a bacteria filter *(D)*, through a humidifier and to the patient. Cyclic compression of the bellows is controlled by the integrated fluidic circuit. After pressure from the oxygen source develops, an interfacing valve *(E)* controls the on–off cycling of the ventilator system. As the powering gas is directed toward the compression canister *(F)*, it passes through a flow control *(G)* and a Venturi booster *(H)*, both of which combine to vary the inspiratory flow rate, the inspiratory time, and the I:E ratio. At the same time, the compression canister builds pressure for the beginning of inspiration. Pressure is also developing in the compression canister exhalation valve *(I)*. This exhalation mushroom valve will seal the compression canister so that inspiration can take place. Once inspiration has been completed, the pressure is released from this mushroom valve, and the gas used to compress the patient bellows system is exhausted from the compression canister. The bellows then refills with the appropriate gas mixture in preparation for the next

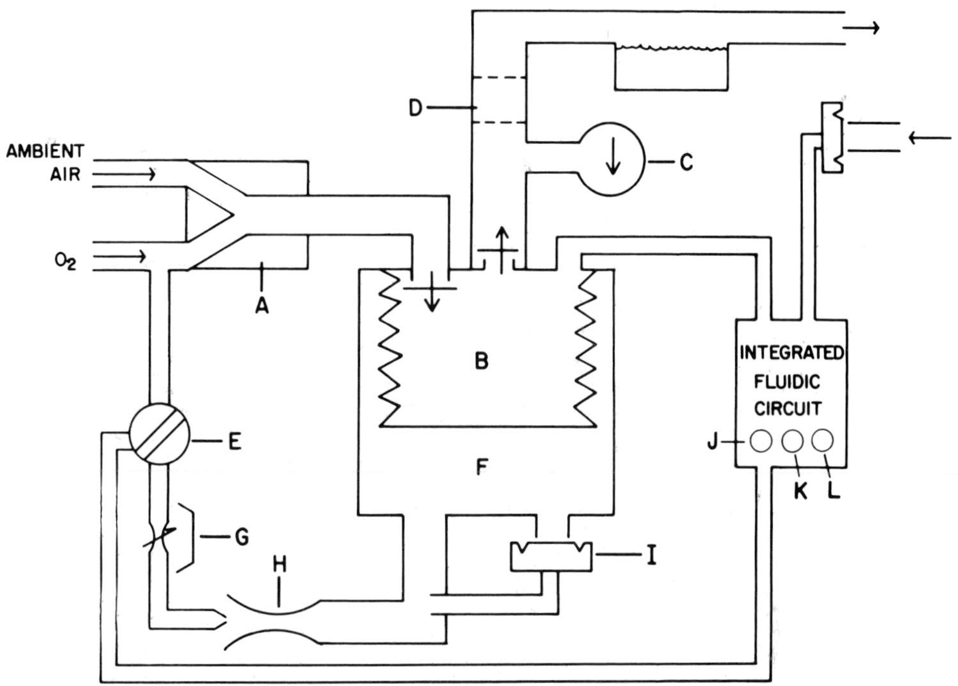

Fig. 24-69. Schematic diagram of the Ohio 550 Ventilator.

inspiration. The bellows volume displacement is adjusted by control *(J)*. The time the bellows will remain down before it begins the next inspiratory phase is determined by the integrated fluidic control, using the expiratory timer valve *(K)*. This control delays the beginning of inspiration by fluidic logic until the next control breath is to be delivered. If in the meantime, the patient wishes to initiate an assisted breath, he may do so, providing adequate sensitivity is provided by the patient-triggering effort control *(L)*.

Operation

The Ohio 550 ventilator is connected into a 50 psi source of the desired gas. Since this ventilator is pneumatically operated, variation in gas pressure can change the characteristics of the ventilator and the flow patterns it delivers. The ventilator is turned on by the pneumatic on–off switch *(A)* (Fig. 24-70). The tidal volume (200–2000 ml in 200-ml graduated increments) is selected with the tidal volume control *(B)*, which raises or lowers the bellows. The inspiratory flow rate that is adjusted by the inspiratory flow-rate control *(C)* is not calibrated throughout its range; it has only a minimum-to-maximum setting. Without back pressure, this control has a range of 30 to 90 liters/min. With 40 cm H_2O back pressure, the maximum flow rate is 60 liters/min. The breathing rate is adjusted by the expiratory time control *(D)*. This control is not calibrated over its scale. In the minimum position, the expiratory delay time is 1 second before a subsequent inspiration is initiated. The maximum setting of the expiratory time control is 17 seconds; however, since the logic system and alarm will not allow an expiratory phase longer than 15 seconds, the true maximum expiratory time is 15 seconds. The effort required to initiate an assisted breath is adjusted by the patient-triggering effort control *(E)*, which can be adjusted between 0.5 and 5 cm H_2O subambient pressure. A manual inspiration button *(F)* will initiate an inspiration and will continue to hold this inspiration as long as the button is depressed (up to 15 seconds). Oxygen concentration is selected by the oxygen concentration control *(G)* that mixes oxygen and ambient air—an advantage when compressed air is unavailable.

The alarm system can be turned on or off by the pneumatic toggle switch *(H)*. When light *(I)* is green, the patient has initiated the breath. This light does not have an accompanying audible signal.

The failure-to-cycle light *(J)* has an accompanying audible signal that can be canceled by the audible alarm switch *(H)*. The failure-to-cycle light will alarm if inspiration is held for longer than 5 seconds. Once

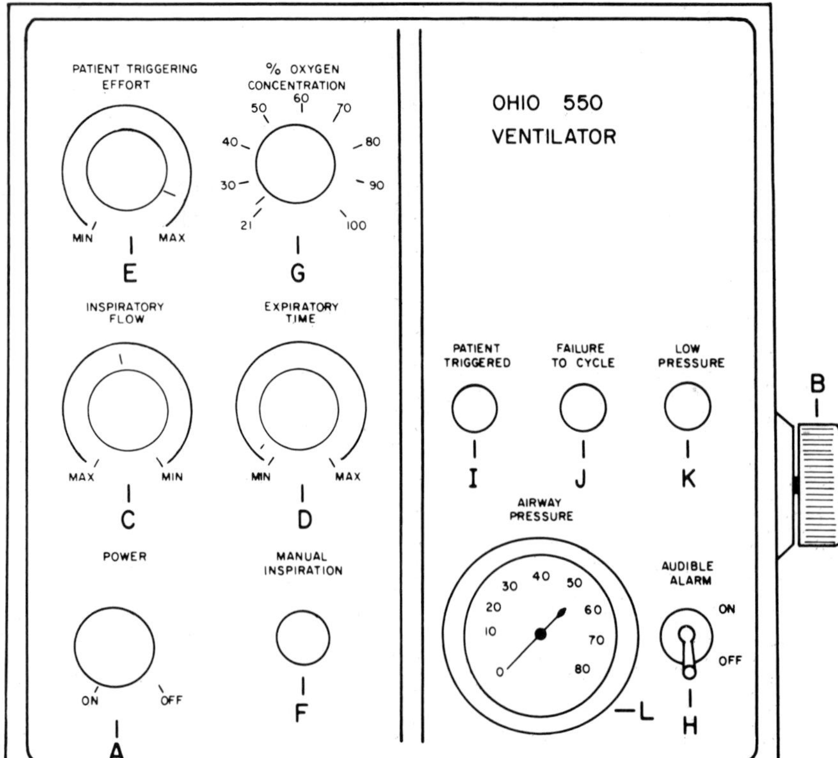

Fig. 24-70. Control panel of the Ohio 550 Ventilator.

this alarm has been initiated, the ventilator automatically will switch to the expiratory phase and dump the volume held in the system. This alarm will also be initiated if any expiratory phase is held for longer than 15 seconds. The low-pressure alarm *(K)* signals if a pressure no greater than 8 cm H_2O is developed for 15 seconds, thus signifying a possible leak, or disconnection. The ventilator system pressure monitor *(L)* indicates delivery pressures up to 70 cm H_2O. An optional pressure relief valve is available if secondary pressure limiting is desired. This pressure relief valve can be adjusted as low as 10 cm H_2O.

Humidity

Humidity for the Ohio 550 is provided by an electrically heated humidifier. It should be filled and plugged in at least 20 minutes before the appropriate humidification temperature needs to be reached. It must be adjusted to high temperatures at the humidifier so that airway temperature is as close as possible to body temperature. Gas temperature at the patient's airway should be monitored continuously. Condensation will occur in the breathing tubing as the gas cools en route to the patient's airway.

Cleaning and Sterilizing

With the exception of the thermometer and the bacteria filters, the entire patient-breathing system can be steam-autoclaved, gas-autoclaved, or cold-sterilized. The manufacturer's recommendations should be followed. The ventilator itself should not be steam-autoclaved.

Accessories

A PEEP attachment and a pressure relief valve are available.

Troubleshooting

If the air intake filter becomes plugged with dust or lint, the bellows will rise or fall slowly and erratically. Since the inlet and output attachments on the humidifier are of the same size, they may be reversed inadvertently. If this occurs, humidification will be reduced markedly.

OHIO CCV2 ADULT VENTILATOR

Classification

The Ohio CCV2 (Fig. 24-71) is an electronically powered, constant flow generator with inspiratory plateau capability. It is a volume-cycled ventilator with a secondary pressure limiting adjustment. It can also be considered a time-cycled ventilator in the inspiratory pause mode. During the expiratory phase, positive pressure is available for PEEP. This ventilator can serve as a controller, assist-controller, IMV, or synchronized IMV ventilator.

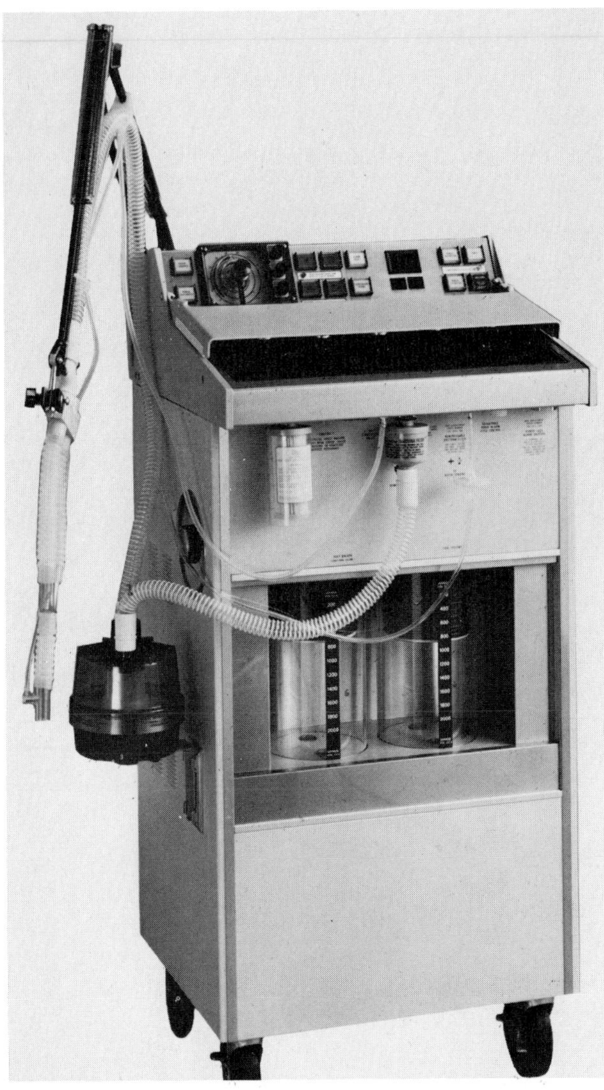

Fig. 24-71. Ohio CCV2 Adult Ventilator. (Courtesy of Ohio Medical Corporation)

Mechanism

High-pressure oxygen is delivered to a mixing chamber (A) (Fig. 24-72) where the high-pressure oxygen is reduced and mixed with low-pressure air, which has been drawn in by descending bellows (B) and (C). Simultaneously, gas is delivered to a bag (D) for spontaneous ventilation during IMV/SIMV. Compression of bellows (B) and (C) is accomplished when the electronics cycle the ventilator to inspiration.

Once inspiration has been initiated, the tidal volume actuator (E) compresses valve (G), allowing gas to flow into the canister (I) from the turbine via valve (H). This pressurization of the canister compresses the bellows (B) and delivers the tidal volume to the patient circuit. Should a sigh volume be desired, the deep breath actuator (F) cycles valves (G) and (H), and the deep breath bellows (C) and tidal bellows (B) volumes will be delivered. Control (J) regulates inspiratory flow rate. Inspired gas is warmed and moistened by a heated humidifier. When the tidal volume bellows (B) is being compressed, pressure is also delivered to close the exhalation valve (L) via tubing (N). Enroute to compressing the exhalation valve (L), a needle valve (M) is placed to control the escape of gas from the exhalation valve during the expiratory phase to control the level of PEEP.

Operation

The power switch (A) (Fig. 24-73) is turned on and the appropriate tidal volume (range 200–2000 ml) adjusted by the tidal volume bellows (B) to the measured volume desired. Should a sigh volume be needed, the deep breath bellows (C) should also be adjusted. This volume should be adjusted (range 200–2000 ml) so that it is added to the tidal volume breath on inspiration. If the deep breath option is selected, multiple deep breaths may be given by dialing control (D). The rate at which the deep breaths are delivered is determined by the deep breath interval control (E) and is available every 3 to 15 minutes. The inspiratory flow control (F) adjusts the flow rate from the bellows into the patient system. The flow rate is influenced by inspiratory back-pressure and as such is calibrated in letters rather than liters per minute. Under normal conditions, flows are available between 10 and 200 liters/min but diminish rapidly as the peak pressure

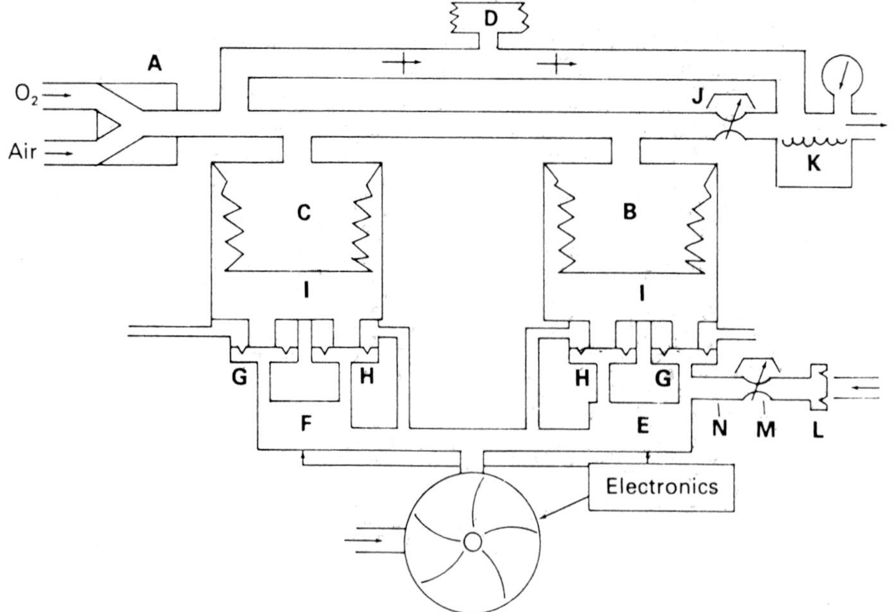

Fig. 24-72. Schematic diagram of Ohio CCV2 Ventilator.

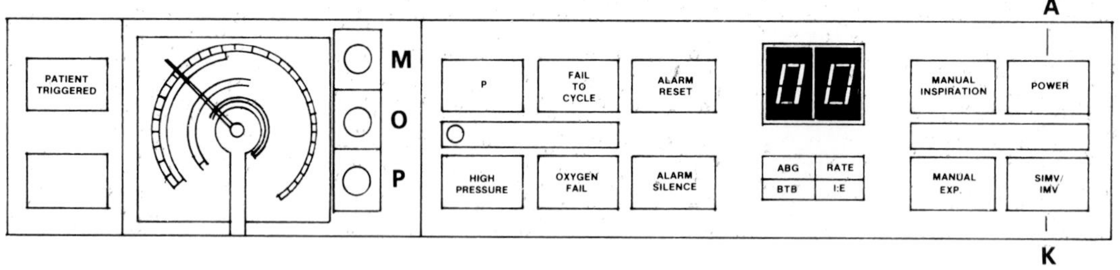

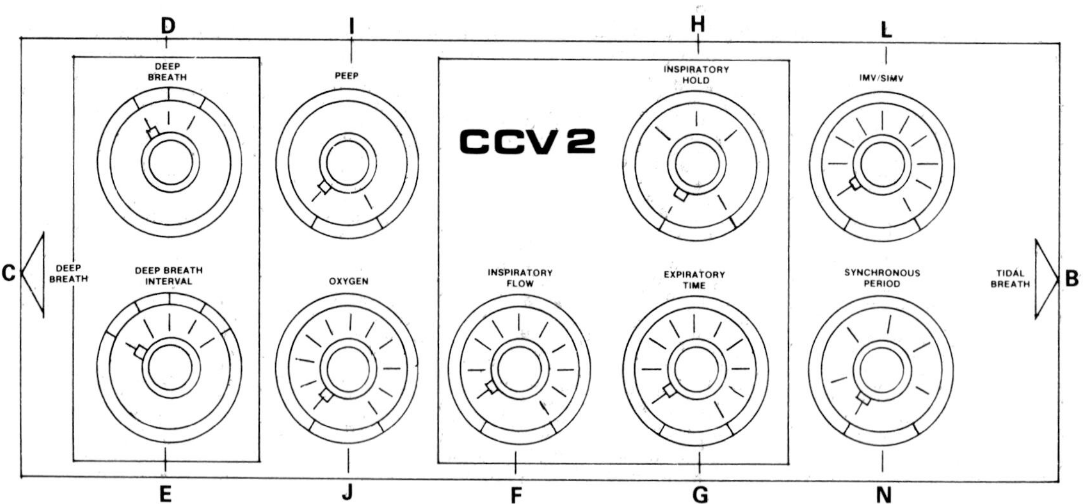

Fig. 24-73. Control panel of Ohio CCV2 Ventilator.

approaches 100 cm H_2O. The expiratory time (G) (range 0.1 to 10 sec) sets the rate at which the ventilator triggers in the control mode. This control does not function in the IMV/SIMV mode, but it has been suggested that the operator set a base rate should the ventilator revert to control. The inspiratory hold control (H) is adjusted from 0 to 2 seconds. During this pause period, the bellows remain at the full inspiration position and the ventilator is time-cycled.

Positive end-expiratory pressure (PEEP) may be adjusted to a maximum of 38 cm H_2O by the PEEP control (I). In control or assist-control the patient-trigger control (M) will need to be adjusted when the PEEP valve is. This is not so in the IMV/SIMV mode; in these modes the PEEP level automatically adjusts the patient-trigger level if CPAP is used. The oxygen control (J) is adjustable from 21% to 100%; however, the alarm system is only for the oxygen input to this system; oxygen concentrations still must be measured.

The IMV/SIMV control (K) turns the ventilator into the IMV/SIMV mode. Once this mode has been selected, the control for respiratory frequency is turned over to the IMV/SIMV minimum interval control (L). This control is adjustable from 10 to 120 seconds and beyond to infinity. The interval between breaths is set at the desired time period. Should IMV be desired, the synchronous period control (N) is adjusted to zero; then each time the minimal interval (L) time has elapsed, a mandatory breath is delivered at the settings already established on the face of the ventilator. If SIMV is desired, the synchronous period (N) is adjusted to a specific period to 10 seconds. After the minimal interval (L) time period has elapsed, the ventilator will wait the prescribed time for the patient to initiate a breath. Once this effort has been made, the ventilator will deliver the breath at the settings already prescribed on the face of the ventilator. If the patient does not meet the pressure differential dialed in on the differential pressure control (O) during his spontaneous or mechanical breathing, the ventilator will be forced out of the IMV/SIMV mode after 15 seconds and into the controlled mode. The differential pressure control (O) is adjustable between −10 and 50 cm H_2O. The high-pressure control (P) is adjustable from 30 to 100 cm H_2O and should be used only as an alarm; this control should not be used to pressure cycle the ventilator. Setting the alarm below the PEEP level or above 100 cm H_2O inactivates the alarm.

Humidity

Humidification is provided by a heated humidifier that bubbles the ventilation volume through the humidifier. A continuous flow (50 cc/min) of gas through the proximal sensing line keeps humidity out of the pressure sensing line.

Cleaning and Sterilizing

Parts may be liquid, gas, or steam autoclaved with caution. Ethylene oxide sterilants with excessive amounts of freon will "craze" delicate plastic items. The heater assembly should not be immersed; the proximal sensing tee should not be autoclaved; and disposable filters should be discarded.

Accessories

Many accessories are available, including oxygen monitors, gas proportionators, and CPAP kits.

Troubleshooting

The air intake for the turbines must be cleaned frequently to avoid damage to this ventilator, and the bellows must be examined frequently for leaks.

SECHRIST IV 100B INFANT VENTILATOR

Classification

The Sechrist IV 100B ventilator (Fig. 24-74) is a gas-powered, fluidic, and electonically operated modifiable constant flow generator that is time cycled. It can provide subambient, ambient, and positive pressure expiratory pressures and can be used for control, IMV, and CPAP.

Mechanism

The Sechrist IV 100B ventilator (Fig. 24-75) is basically a gas-blending device (A) with humidifier (B) that can occlude an exhalation valve (C) by means of an elaborate fluidic and microprocessor system. When an inspiration is desired, the micropressor signals the solenoid valve (D) to close; this develops back pressure through the fluidic unit (E), which in turn sends pressure to fluidic unit (F). Fluidic unit (F) provides a 12 psi pressure through only one of its legs to the inspiratory pressure control (G); gas continues to flow through various one-way valves and restricting orifices to the exhalation valve (C). The main flow of gas to the exhalation valve may be supplemented by additional gas from the wave form modifier (H). The wave form modifier, if fully open, opens and closes the exhalation valve abruptly, providing a square wave form pattern. Should the wave form modifier decrease the gas flow to the exhalation valve, the flow pattern will tend toward a sine wave flow pattern. During the expiratory phase the solenoid valve (D) is opened, and the normal route of gas flow is switched to the other leg of fluidic unit (E); this provides gas flow to the proximal airway tap as a purge to remove humidity, the negative pressure jet (I), and the expiratory pressure control (J). The expiratory pressure control (J) also provides gas flow to the exhalation valve in order to provide CPAP/PEEP when needed. A blender (K) is necessary to allow the fluidics to cycle.

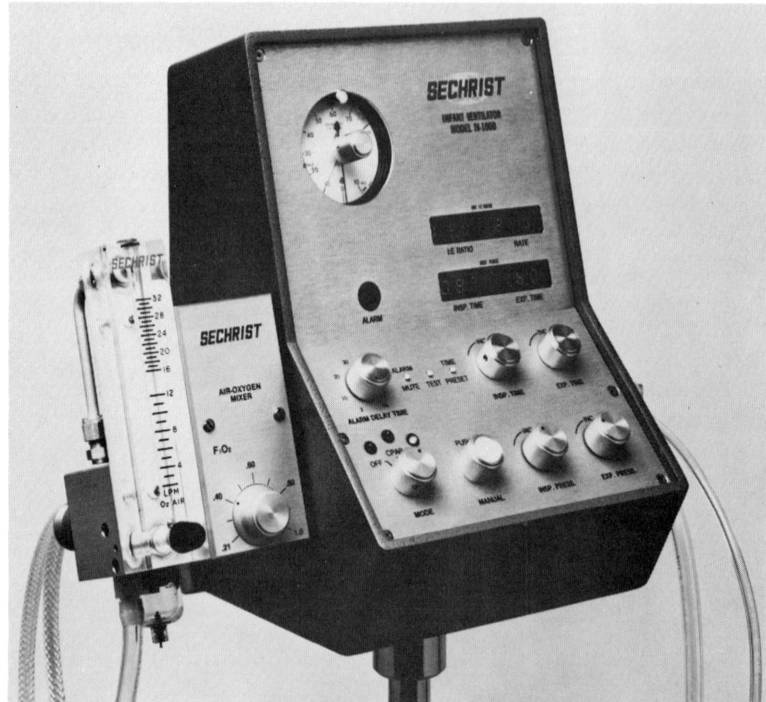

Fig. 24-74. Sechrist IV 100B Infant Ventilator. (Courtesy of Sechrist Corp.)

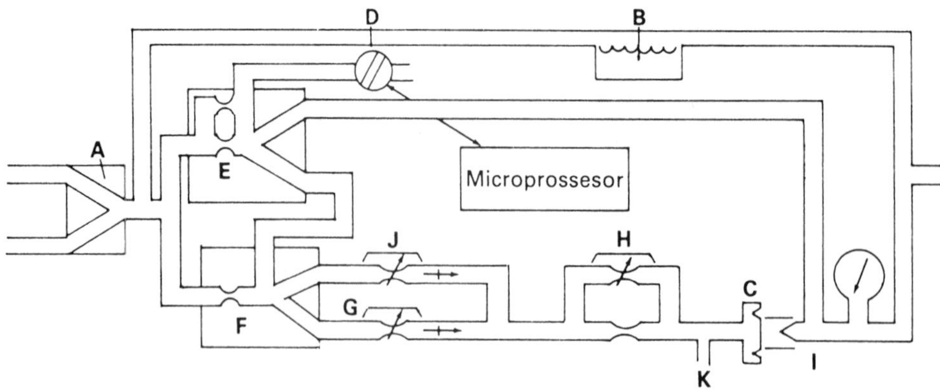

Fig. 24-75. Schematic diagram of the Sechrist IV 100B Infant Ventilator.

Operation

The Sechrist IV 100B ventilator (Fig. 24-76) is a compact neonatal ventilator that can easily be used for transport or long-term ventilation. Flow from the flow indicator (A) is blended in the air–oxygen mixer (B) to the desired concentration. The inspiratory time (C) is adjustable from 0.10 to 2.90 seconds. The time selected is indicated on the LED display for inspiratory time (D). This is a real time display of what the micoprocessor will use to match its time base generator against. Once the time base generator has indicated the time dialed on the inspiratory time control (C), the microprocessor terminates the inspiratory phase. The expiratory time control (E), which is adjustable from 0.2 to 60 seconds, and the expiratory time display (F) are similar to the inspiratory functions. Once the inspiratory time (C) and expiratory time (E) have been programmed into the unit, the microprocessor can calculate the I:E ratio (G) and rate (H), which is adjustable from 1 to 200 breaths per minute.

The inspiratory pressure limit (I) is adjustable from 7 to 70 cm H_2O, and the expiratory pressure (CPAP/PEEP) (J) is adjustable from −2 to 15 cm H_2O. A manual button (K) allows a single breath at any time. This breath will be limited to the inspiratory pressure limit (I) set but will continue as long as the button is held down. The mode selector switch (L) provides the choice of IMV or CPAP.

The alarm systems provided are delay time (M), which is adjustable from 3 to 60 seconds, and a low-pressure alarm (N). The low-pressure alarm functions by passing the patient airway pressure monitor needle through a light and sensing device that must be interrupted at frequent intervals. Should this light source not be interrupted for the period designated on the delay time (M) for reasons such as low airway pressure, leak, patient disconnection, failure to cycle, source gas failure, or power failure, the audible and visual (O) alarms will function. These alarms may be silenced for 25 seconds but will then alarm again.

This light (16 pounds) unit can be battery operated in order to be used on transport.

Humidity

Humidity is provided by any type of heated humidifier the operator chooses.

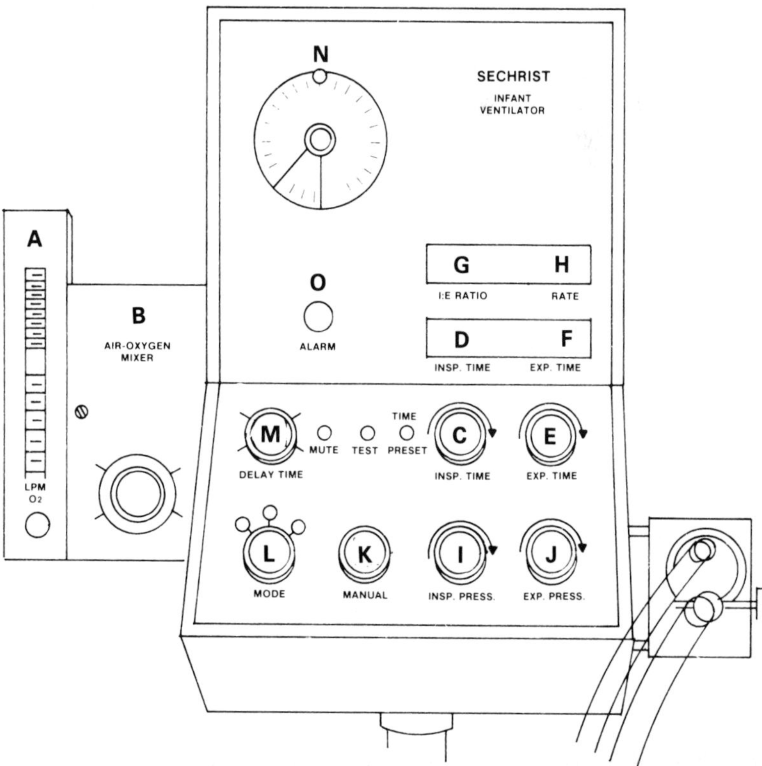

Fig. 24-76. Control panel of the Sechrist IV 100B Infant Ventilator.

Cleaning and Sterilizing

A simple patient-breathing circuit is used to keep the compressible volume small, and the exhalation valve is durable and easy to disassemble. Caution should be used in sterilizing this exhalation valve, however, because ethylene oxide may craze it and liquid sterilizing solutions may discolor it.

Troubleshooting

A comprehensive trouble-shooting chart is included in the operators manual to simplify even further this simple and durable machine.

SEARLE VVA

Classification

The Searle VVA (Fig. 24-77) is a modified constant flow generator and a volume-cycled ventilator with a secondary pressure limit. Positive expiratory pressure plateau is available. This ventilator can function as an assistor, controller, or assistor-controller.

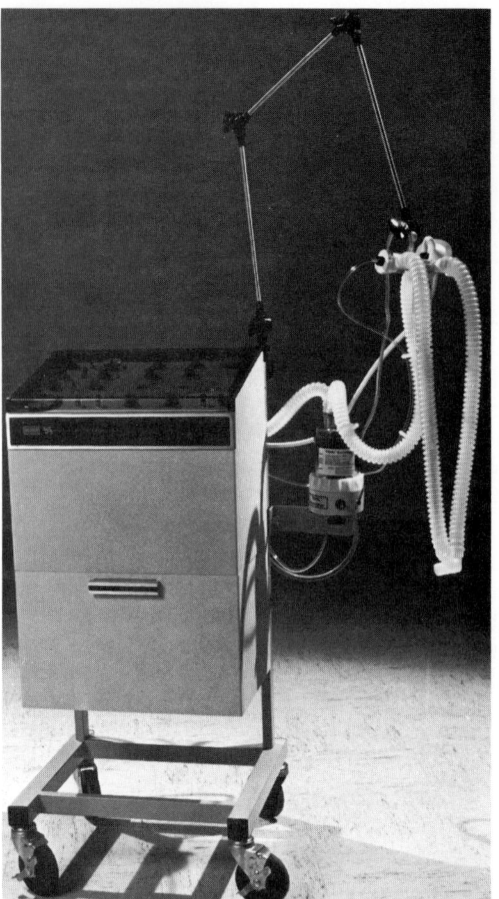

Fig. 24-77. Searle VVA Ventilator.

Mechanism

This ventilator is pneumatically and electronically operated (Fig. 24-78). A compressor *(A)* provides high-pressure air to mix with oxygen in the cylinder chamber. Two solenoid valves *(B)* operated by an electronic logic circuit open the air and oxygen systems for a prescribed time to obtain the desired oxygen concentration. The volume to be delivered is set by volume selector *C*, which adjusts the piston travel. Inspiration is initiated by a signal from the electronic control, and springs *(D)* compress the piston and rolling diaphragm. A solenoid *(E)* opens, and tidal volume is delivered. A flow control *(F)* responds to a signal from the pressure sensor *(G)*, and, depending on the back pressure, flow will increase or decrease to maintain set value. At the same time that inspiration is delivered to the patient, flow is provided to the exhalation valve *(H)*.

Operation

Power button *A* turns on the ventilator (Fig. 24-79). This button will remain lit as long as the power is on. The tidal volume is selected at 300 to 2200 ml with the tidal volume control *(B)*. Respiratory rate *(C)*, adjustable between 5 and 60 breaths per minute, is displayed on the respiratory rate monitor *(D)* and represents an average of the preceding 8 to 10 breaths. I:E ratios, between 1:0.9 and 1:9, are displayed on monitor *E*. If the ratio is less than 1:1 an alarm will warn the operator. Peak inspiratory flow rates, between 20 and 200 liters/min, are obtained by adjusting the flow-rate control *(F)*, and a sustained flow between 90 and 100 liters/min is possible with back pressures up to 100 cm H_2O. The flow-rate pattern can be altered from a square wave to a tapering flow by control *(G)*, which acts as an inspiratory time-delay flow modifier. Tapering from a square wave may be controlled at the completion of one half to two thirds of the inspiratory volume delivery, but the I:E ratio will also be altered. Once inspiration has been delivered, an inspiratory plateau can be held up to 3 seconds by the inflation hold control *(H)*. Oxygen concentration can be set between 21% and 100% by *(I)*. If the oxygen selector

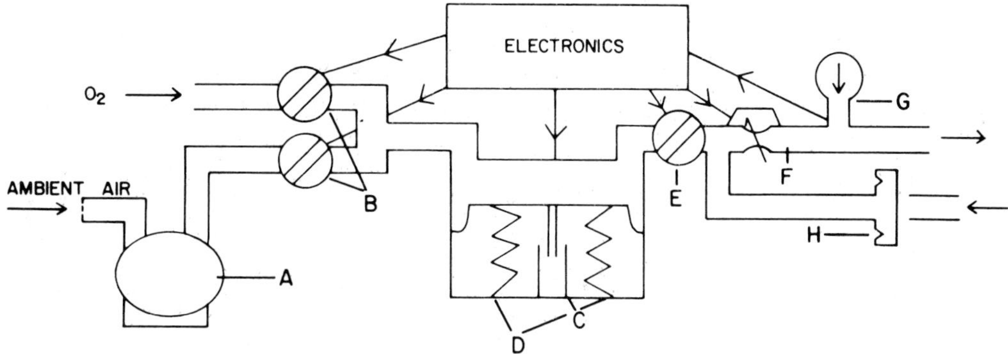

Fig. 24-78. Schematic diagram of the Searle VVA Ventilator.

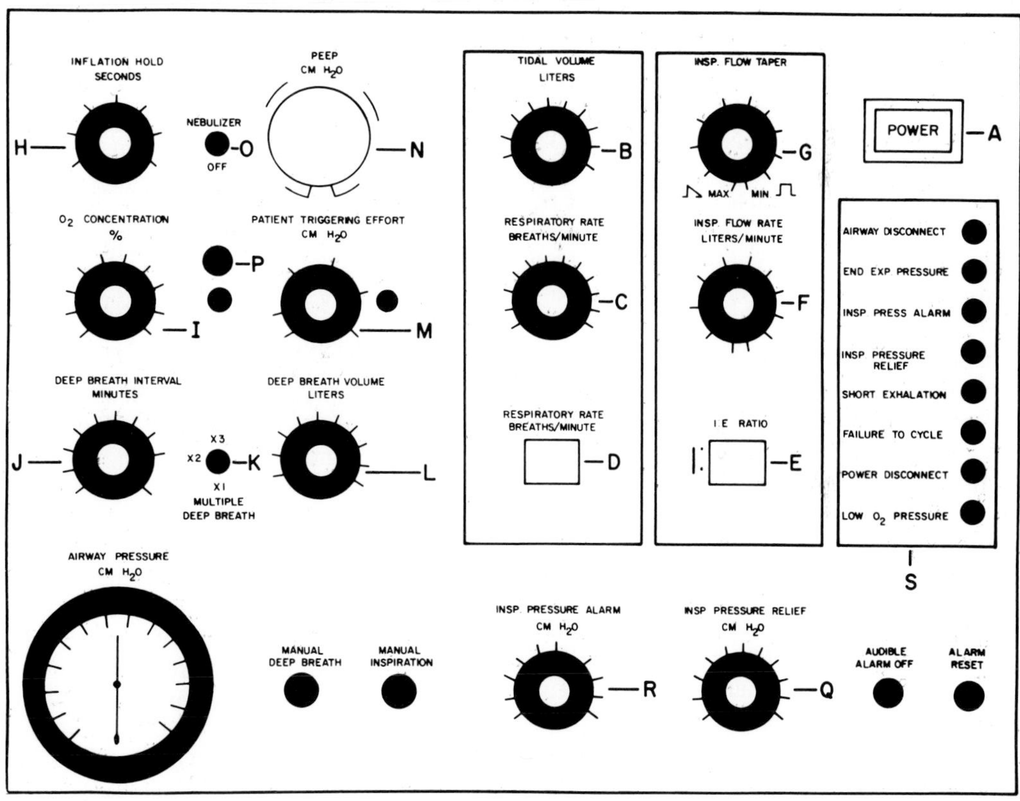

Fig. 24-79. Control panel of the Searle VVA Ventilator.

control is turned to the "off" position, the oxygen alarm system will not alarm if the oxygen power hose is not plugged in. Sigh breaths can be programmed at intervals of 1 to 10 minutes by the deep-breath interval control *(J)*, in multiples of 1, 2, or 3 breaths by switch *(K)*, and at a volume determined by the deep-breath volume control *(L)*. Patient-triggering effort *(M)* controls the level of subambient pressure needed to trigger "ventilator assist" and can be regulated between 0.2 and 20 cm H_2O. If this control is turned to the "off" position, the patient cannot cycle the ventilator to the assist mode. Sensitivity is retained as PEEP is increased by control *(N)*. PEEP is adjustable between 0 and 20 cm H_2O with locking positions at 5 and 10 cm H_2O.

A medication nebulizer can be used with nebulizer switch *(O)*. If the operator wishes to deliver 100% oxygen to the patient for 2 minutes, the normal oxygen mixing process can be bypassed by pressing the 100% oxygen button *(P)*. Normal and sigh breaths may be delivered by pressing appropriate buttons to deliver these tidal volumes out of sequence with the machine cycling mechanism. Both the normal and sigh breaths can be pressure-limited by the inspiratory pressure relief control *(Q)*. Adjustment of the inspiratory pressure alarm *(R)* at a value below the relief pressure warns of excessive pressure buildup. A series of alarms *(S)* indicates various malfunctions. These alarms may be silenced or reset as needed.

Humidity

The passive, heated humidifier utilizes a reusable heating base with a disposable humidifying element. The humidifying element is supplied with sterile distilled water via an I.V. bottle system. Water is delivered to a reservoir area for heating. Once the ventilator tidal volume has been delivered, water is pumped up into an open cell foam that acts as a wick to provide proper relative humidity to the patient. This humidifier system allegedly provides 90% relative humidity at minute volumes up to 40 liters/min. A flow arrangement maintains the proper water level in the humidifier from the i.v. system.

Cleaning and Sterilizing

The humidifier cartridge is only for one-time use and should be disposed of between each patient or every 24 hours. The remaining patient-breathing assembly should be removed and exchanged at least every 24 hours or more often as indicated.

Accessories

An IMV module (termed IDV by the manufacturer), a wedge spirometer, and a battery power pack are available.

Troubleshooting

This ventilator has an elaborate monitoring/alarm system for both close and remote use. Some of the alarm systems monitor airway disconnect, end-expiratory pressure, inspiratory pressure, inspiratory pressure relief, short exhalation, failure to cycle, power disconnect, and low oxygen pressure. Thus alterations in almost any performance characteristic will be displayed instantaneously.

SIEMENS-ELEMA SERVO VENTILATOR 900B

The Servo 900B (Fig. 24-80) is a time-cycled ventilator that may be operated as a constant, nonconstant, or decelerating flow generator. Mechanical inspiration may be controlled or patient triggered and extended beyond the dynamic phase as a plateau. During mechanical exhalation, flow retardation may be used.

Mechanism

The Servo 900B is electronically operated and pneumatically powered (Fig. 24-81). An air–oxygen blender (A) provides gas at the desired FI_{O_2}. Metered gas may be added by means of an auxiliary inlet (B). On demand, valve (C) opens, allowing blended gas into the pressurized concertina bag (D). The pressure is indicated on manometer (E) and generated by adjustable spring tension (F). During mechanical inspiration, gas from the concertina bag is delivered to the patient circuit by means of a servo system. The inspiratory servo mechanism comprises a flow transducer (G) and scissor valve (I) interfaced by an electronic control. Gas delivery is measured by the flow transducer and signaled to the electronic system, where it is integrated and compared to pre-set volume. The inspiratory scissor valve opening is instantaneously manipulated to provide proper flow to deliver the desired volume in the allotted time. Ventilator outflow pressure is measured by a transducer (J). Exhaled gas from the patient circuit passes through a flow transducer (K) and expiratory scissor valve (I) also interfaced with an electronic control (i.e., expiratory servo system). The signal from transducer (K) is fed to an electronic control for valve (I) adjustments based on the selected expiratory flow rate. Exhaled gas is vented through a unidirectional valve (M), where a threshold pressure device may be added.

Operation

Ventilator function and variables are adjusted and displayed on the control panel (Fig. 24-82). Instead of selecting a tidal volume directly, one adjusts a minute volume (A) (range 0.5–25 to 30 liters/min) and rate (B) (range 6–60 breaths/min). The inspiratory time (C) and pause time (D) are regulated as a percentage of total ventilatory cycle time and are cumulative. However, as a safety measure, if the I:E ratio exceeds 4:1, the pause time is automatically reduced. Inspiratory time is graduated in 15%, 20%, 25%, 33%, and 50% of the total respiratory cycle. Inspiratory pause time may be 0, 5%, 10%, 20%, and 30%, except in the IMV mode where it is omitted independently of the setting.

Spring tension on the concertina bag is regulated by a working pressure control (E) and is adjustable from 10 to 100 cm H_2O.

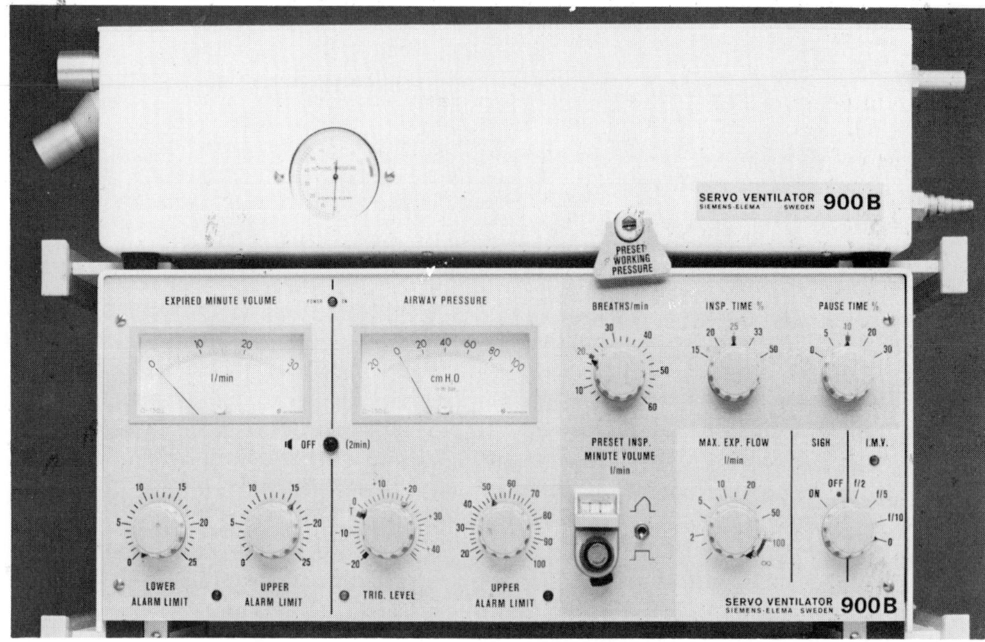

Fig. 24-80. Siemens-Elema Servo 900B Ventilator. (Courtesy of Siemens–Elema Corp.)

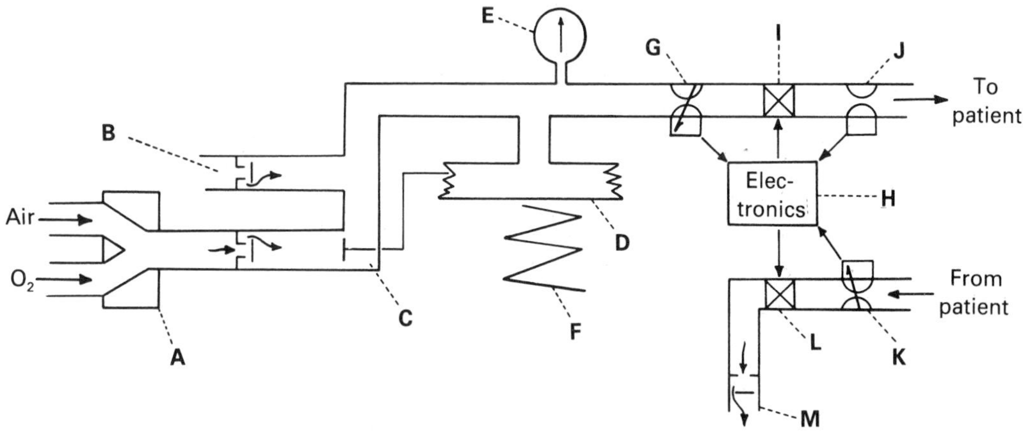

Fig. 24-81. Schematic diagram of Servo 900B Ventilator.

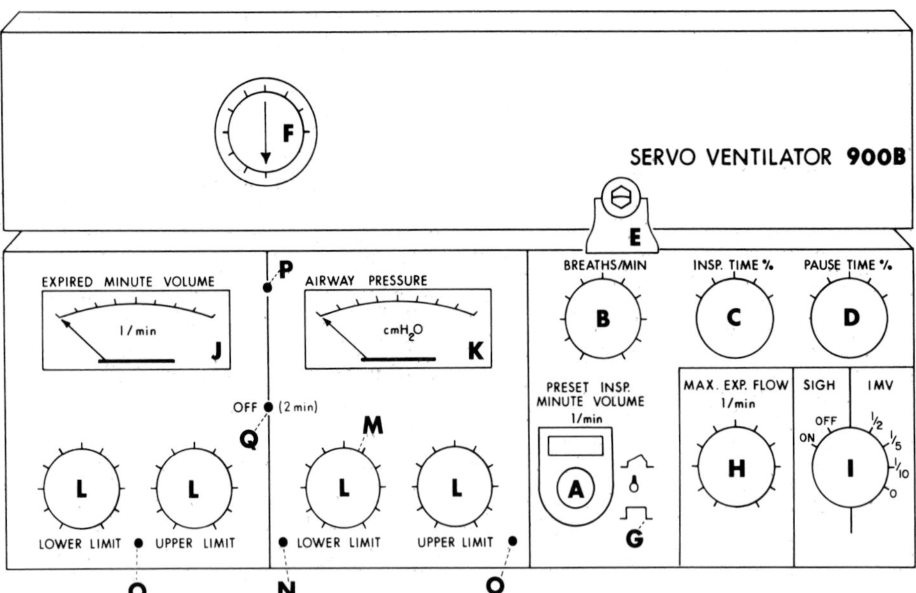

Fig. 24-82. Control panel of Servo 900B Ventilator.

Various inspiratory flow patterns are attainable with the Servo 900B. A toggle switch (G) allows selection of either a constant or accelerating inspiratory flow curve. In the IMV mode, the ventilator delivers a constant flow regardless of flow pattern selector setting. A decelerating flow pattern is achieved when working pressure is adjusted to a level equal to peak airway pressure. The expiratory flow pattern is adjustable (H) from 1.0 to infinity liters/min. Expiratory retard is added by decreasing maximum expiratory flow rate until the desired effect has been achieved (e.g., to prevent premature airway collapse). A deep breath (twice selected tidal volume) can be administered every 100 ventilatory cycles by placing the control knob (I) in the on-position.

IMV is activated by the sigh-IMV knob (I). IMV rates are adjusted by engaging various positions: f/2, f/5, f/10, and f/0 (*i.e.*, frequency of breaths/mins divided by 2, 5, 10, or 0). The 0 position is for CPAP therapy. When the IMV function is switched on, the patient may breathe spontaneously from the reservoir of gas in the concertina bag. A pressure transducer senses spontaneous effort, and electronics regulate demand flow by means of the inspiratory valve. When the patient begins spontaneous exhalation, the transducer senses above baseline pressure effecting inspiratory valve closure and expiratory valve opening. The IMV breath is synchronized with an inspiratory effort (SIMV).

Exhaled minute volume (combined spontaneous and mechanical) is displayed on an analogue meter (J). The airway pressure meter (K) has a range of −20 to 100 cm H_2O. Each meter has an upper and lower limit audible alarm except the lower-pressure limit. The lower-pressure limit knob (M) serves as inspiratory effort control for patient-triggered mechanical breaths and demand flow during spontaneous breathing. It must be adjusted to accommodate changes in baseline pressure (*i.e.*, CPAP). If the upper pressure limit has been reached, the ventilator automatically cycles to exhalation while activating an audible and visual alarm.

Indicator light (N) illuminates when the patient initiates either a mechanical or spontaneous breath. Light (O) illuminates and an audible alarm activates if the preselected pressure limit has been reached. Light P illuminates when the main electronic power is on. If an electrical power failure occurs or the ventilator becomes unplugged, light (P) will flash and an audible alarm will sound. Both are battery powered. All alarms may be silenced for 2 minutes by depressing button (Q).

Output from the inspiratory and expiratory flow transducer and pressure transducer may be recorded via cable connections on the rear panel. Recording flow patterns and airway pressure may facilitate ventilatory trend analysis.

Humidity

There is no standard humidifier for the Servo 900B. Various humidification systems will suffice; however, they should not require an additional gas source (e.g., jet nebulizers) because this would increase delivered minute volume. A Servo Humidifier 150 or 151 (depending on VT used) is available. It operates as a heat and moisture exchanger that requires no water reservoir or electrical power.

Cleaning and Sterilizing

The internal inspiratory circuit delivers dry, filtered gas; it may thus need cleaning only periodically. However, the expiratory system is generally moist, possibly contaminated, and should be sterilized between patients. The flow transducer should be soaked in 70% ethanol for about one hour, rinsed with distilled water, and steam autoclaved (150° F).

Accessories

Optional devices available include an air–oxygen blender, PEEP device, NEEP device, CO_2 analyzer, lung mechanics calculator (compliance, resistance), monitoring unit (minute volume, tidal volume; peak, pause, and mean airway pressure) and alarm unit (central monitoring of volume and pressure for up to six Servo ventilators).

Troubleshooting

Performance failures may be caused by internal system leaks in valve assemblies or the concertina bag. Valve system leaks are correctable but may be difficult to detect. When the rubber valves are inserted, twisting must be avoided to prevent unnecessary flow resistance. If the meter reads erroneously elevated minute volume, the flow transducer screen may have accumulated moisture.

SIEMENS-ELEMA SERVO VENTILATOR 900C

The Servo 900C (Fig. 24-83) is a time-cycled ventilator that may function as a constant, nonconstant, or decelerating flow generator or as a constant pressure generator. Mechanical inspiration is either controlled or patient activated and may be terminated by a selected pressure limit or extended beyond the dynamic phase by a plateau. Threshold positive pressure may be applied to the expiratory phase.

Mechanism

The Servo 900C is electronically operated and pneumatically powered (Fig. 24-84). An air–oxygen mixer

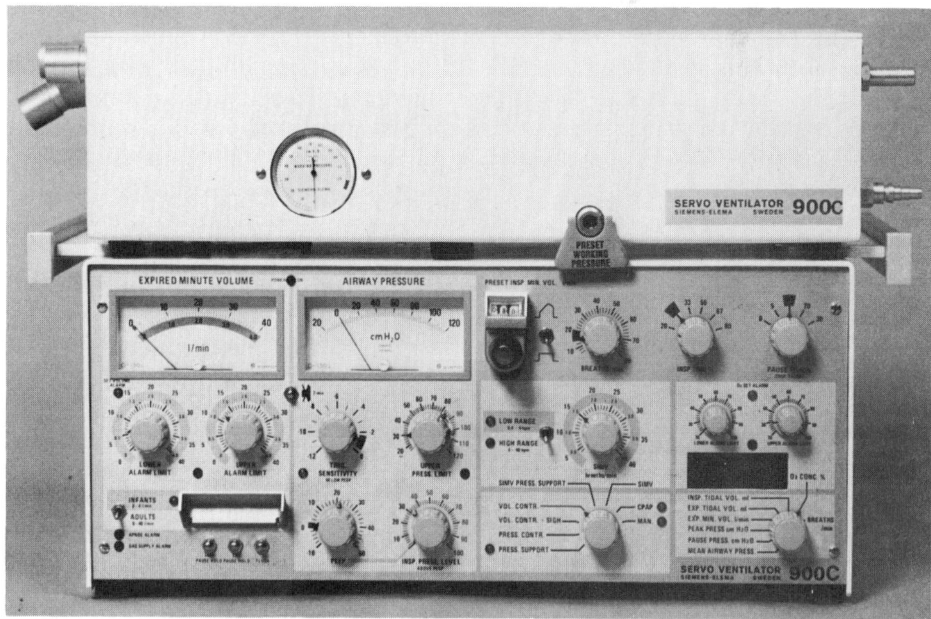

Fig. 24-83. Siemens–Elema Servo Ventilator 900C. (Courtesy of Siemens–Elema Corp.)

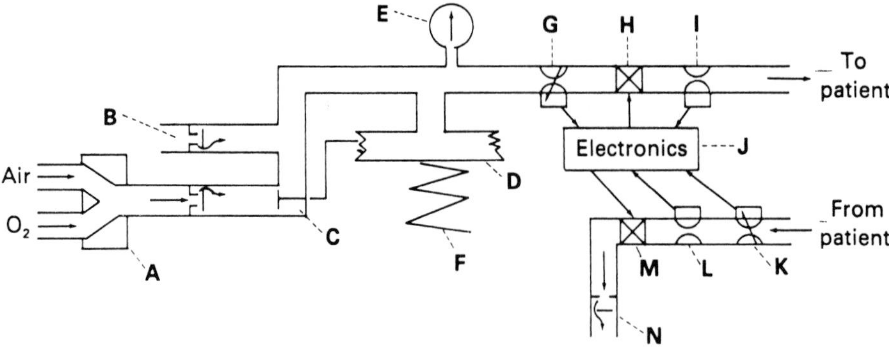

Fig. 24-84. Schematic diagram of Servo 900C Ventilator.

(A) provides gas at the prescribed FI_{O_2}. Metered gas may be added by means of an auxiliary inlet (B). On demand, a valve (C) opens, allowing mixed gas to flow by an oxygen sensor and through a bacterial filter (not illustrated) into a pressurized concertina bag (D). The pressure is indicated on manometer (E) and is generated by adjustable spring tension (F). During mechanical inspiration, gas from the concertina bag is directed into the patient circuit by means of an inspiratory servo system. The servo mechanism consists of a flow transducer (G), inspiratory valve (H), and pressure transducer (I) interfaced in a feedback loop to an electronic control (J). Gas delivery is measured by the flow transducer, whereupon it is integrated and referenced to the preselected volume by the electronic unit. Inspiratory valve opening is modulated, allowing appropriate flow to guarantee volume delivery in the allocated inspiratory time. In the pressure support mode (discussed later), the inspiratory pressure transducer signal is processed electronically and referenced to the set value maintained by inspiratory valve flow regulation. Exhaled gas enters the expiratory servo circuit, comprising a flow transducer (K), pressure transducer (L), and expiratory valve (M) interfaced in a feedback system with the electronics. During exhalation, the pressure transducer signal to the electronics is compared to the selected PEEP-level. The expiratory valve is modulated to obtain the desired end-expiratory pressure, which may be an ambient or a given PEEP. Exhaled gas is ultimately vented through a unidirectional valve (N).

Operation

Ventilator function and variables are adjusted and displayed on a compact control panel (Fig. 24-85). Mechanical tidal volume is the result of an adjusted minute volume (A) (range 0.5–40 liters/min) and rate (B) (range 5–120 breaths/min). The inspiratory time (C) and pause time (D) are regulated as a percentage of the total ventilatory cycle and are cumulative. If the inspiratory time exceeds 80% of the total ventilatory cycle, the pause time is automatically reduced. Inspiratory time is adjustable at 20%, 25%, 33%, 50%, 67% and 80% of the ventilatory cycle. There are five pause times: 0, 5%, 10%, 20% and 30%.

An accelerating or constant flow inspiratory pattern may be selected (E). A decelerating inspiratory flow pattern can be used by adjusting (F) the ventilator working pressure (G) to a level equal to, or slightly higher than, peak airway pressure.

The desired ventilatory modality is selected by an eight-position rotary knob (H). Ventilatory modes include pressure support, pressure control, volume controlled with periodic sigh, volume controlled, SIMV with pressure support, SIMV, CPAP, and manual.

Pressure supported ventilation (PRESS SUPPORT) provides an adjustable constant airway pressure during spontaneous breathing. If pressurized inspiration exceeds 80% of the breathing cycle, the inspiratory valve closes, and the exhalation valve vents pressure to a pre-set end-expiratory pressure level. The inspiratory pressure support is normally terminated when the inspiratory flow transducer measures little or no flow or the pressure transducer senses an excess value.

Pressure controlled (PRESS CONTR) ventilation provides a constant airway pressure during selected mechanical inspiratory time. This can be patient triggered or controlled. The constant pressure is maintained by the inspiratory servo feedback system (similar to INSP PRESS SUPPORT mode). Delivered mechanical tidal volume depends on inspiratory pressure, ventilatory rate, and inspiratory time.

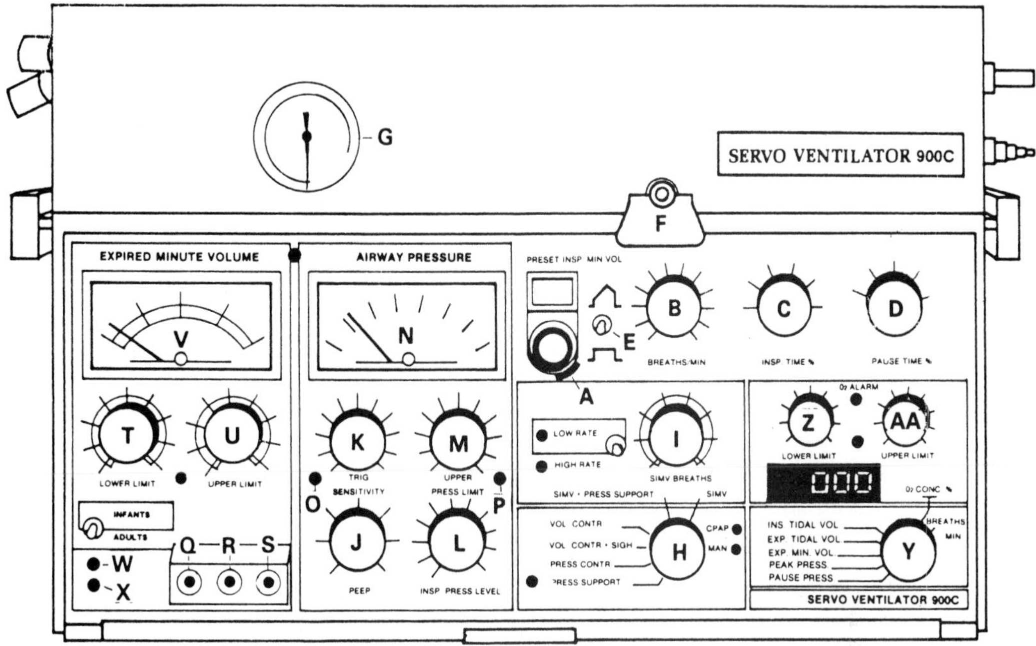

Fig. 24-85. Control panel of Servo 900C Ventilator.

Volume controlled and sigh (VOL CONTR + SIGH) mode provides consistent tidal volume delivery to the circuit with every hundredth breath being doubled in volume. The volume controlled (VOL CONTR) mode provides tidal ventilation without a sigh.

In the SIMV and pressure support (SIMV + PRESS SUPPORT) mode, the patient breathes spontaneously at a selected constant airway pressure and intermittently triggers a mechanical tidal volume. The SIMV rate is adjustable (I) in two ranges: low rate, 0.4 to 4/min and high rate, 4 to 40/min. While in the SIMV mode, spontaneous ventilation occurs at baseline (*i.e.*, ambient or end-expiratory) pressure. In the CPAP position, spontaneous ventilation at end-expiratory pressure is not augmented with any mechanical breaths.

The manual (MAN) mode is used in conjunction with an anesthesia bag and manual ventilation valve (accessory equipment) attached to the ventilator outflow port and connected to the inspiratory limb of the breathing circuit (e.g., anesthesia system). During manual inflation (bag compression), circuit pressure rises; when it reaches 4 cm H_2O the ventilator exhalation valve closes, diverting the compressed volume to the patient. During exhalation, as the circuit pressure decreases to less than 4 cm H_2O, the ventilator exhalation valve opens. When the circuit pressure is $\leq$ 2 cm H_2O demand flow from the ventilator refills the bag. The apnea alarm is deactivated while in MAN mode.

Airway pressure during mechanical or spontaneous breathing modes is manipulated by the following control knobs: PEEP (J), TRIG SENSITIVITY BELOW PEEP (K), INSP PRESS LEVEL ABOVE PEEP (L) AND UPPER PRESS LIMIT (M). The airway pressure (range −20 to 120 cm H_2O) is indicated on an analogue meter (N).

PEEP is adjustable from 0 to 50 cm H_2O with a safety catch at 20 cm H_2O. Another safety catch at 0 deters inadvertent NEEP (negative end-expiratory pressure; range 0–10 cm H_2O subatmospheric) when that optional function has been incorporated. Inspiratory effort (below PEEP) necessary for patient-triggered breaths is adjustable from 0 to 20 cm H_2O subatmospheric. Each patient-triggered breath activates an indicator light (O). During PRESS SUPPORT, PRESS CONTR, and SIMV + PRESS SUPPORT modes, the constant airway pressure above PEEP is adjustable from 0 to 100 cm H_2O, with a safety catch at 30 cm H_2O.

Peak airway pressure may be limited from 20 to 120 cm H_2O. When the upper pressure limit is exceeded, the ventilator cycles to exhalation while an audible and visual (P) alarm is activated.

A small hood located beneath the UPPER ALARM LIMIT encloses pushbuttons for the following functions: inspiratory pause hold (INSP PAUSE HOLD)

(Q), expiratory pause hold (EXP PAUSE HOLD) (R), and GAS CHANGE (S). Each function is activated for as long as the pushbutton is depressed. The INSP PAUSE HOLD may be used to enhance alveolar gas mixing to provide an accurate mean expired CO_2 analysis. Stable end-expiratory pressure measurements may be effected by extending exhalation via EXP PAUSE HOLD. To quickly change the patient's inspired gas mixture, the GAS CHANGE button is depressed, which rapidly "washes" the internal and external circuits with the "new" gas mixture.

A lower (T) and upper (U) limit for exhaled minute volume is adjustable in two ranges: infants, 0 to 4 liters/min and adults, 0 to 40 liters/min. When either the lower or upper limit has been reached, an audible and visual alarm is activated. The exhaled minute volume is displayed on an analogue meter (V).

If apnea occurs for more than 15 seconds, an audible and visual alarm (W) is activated. A visual and audible alarm occurs if the gas supply (X) fails to maintain adequate pressure in the concertina bag.

A digital readout of variables selected by an eight-position rotary knob (Y) facilitates documentation of mean airway pressure (MEAN AIRWAY PRESS cm H_2O), pause or inspiratory plateau pressure (PAUSE PRESS cm H_2O), peak airway pressure (PEAK PRESS cm H_2O), expired minute volume (EXP MIN VOL liters/min), expired tidal volume (EXP TIDAL VOL ml), inspired tidal volume (INSP TIDAL VOL ml), oxygen concentration (O_2 CONC %), oxygen concentration (O_2 CONC %), and breaths/min.

The lower (Z) and upper (AA) limits for FI_{O_2} are adjustable from 0.20 to 1.0. If either has been reached, an audible and visual alarm is activated.

Cleaning and Sterilizing

The internal inspiratory circuit delivers dry, filtered gas, and thus may need cleaning only periodically. However, the expiratory system is generally moist, possibly contaminated, and should be sterilized between patients. The flow transducer should be soaked in 70% ethanol for about 1 hour, rinsed with distilled water, and steam autoclaved (150° F).

Accessories

Optional devices available include an air–oxygen blender, NEEP device, CO_2 analyzer, lung mechanics calculator (compliance, resistance), monitoring unit (minute volume, tidal volume; peak, pause, and mean airway pressure), and alarm unit (central monitoring of volume and pressure for up to six Servo ventilators).

Troubleshooting

Performance failures may be caused by internal system leaks in valve assemblies or the concertina bag. Valve system leaks are correctable but may be difficult to detect. When the rubber valves are inserted, twisting must be avoided to prevent unnecessary flow resistance. If the meter reads erroneously elevated minute volume, the flow transducer screen may have accumulated moisture.

VERIFLO CV 200 AND CV 2000*

Classification

The CV 200 (Fig. 24-86) is a constant flow generator specifically designed for pediatric use. The CV 2000 is a constant flow generator for adults. Functioning primarily as time-cycled ventilators, these models have secondary pressure-limiting capabilities. Positive pressure plateaus are available on the expiratory phase. SIMV, assist, control, and assist-control modes are available.

Mechanism

The ventilators are pneumatically operated by 50 psi air and oxygen sources (Fig. 24-87). The gases are mixed in a mixing chamber (A), then switched (B) to either a continuous flow or ventilator control system. The continuous flow system provides gas for spontaneous breathing and PEEP. Flow control for this system is provided by an expiratory flow control (K). If the control mode switch (B) is turned to ventilator control, the remaining controls are activated. Integrating information from the inspiratory time control and the ratio control, the cycle generator (C) times the opening and closing of switch (D), which controls the inspiratory and expiratory phasing of the ventilator. This control will remain open and allow gas to flow to the patient at a rate controlled by the flow-rate control (E) for as long as the inspiratory time control is activated. Once inspiratory time has ceased, the I:E ratio control will prevent gas flow to the patient. Delay in the cycling of this generator during the expiratory phase can be implemented by an IMV timer (F), which extends the expiratory time to accommodate slower rates. The cycle generator is also influenced by the

*Subsequently became the McGaw CV 200 and CV 2000.

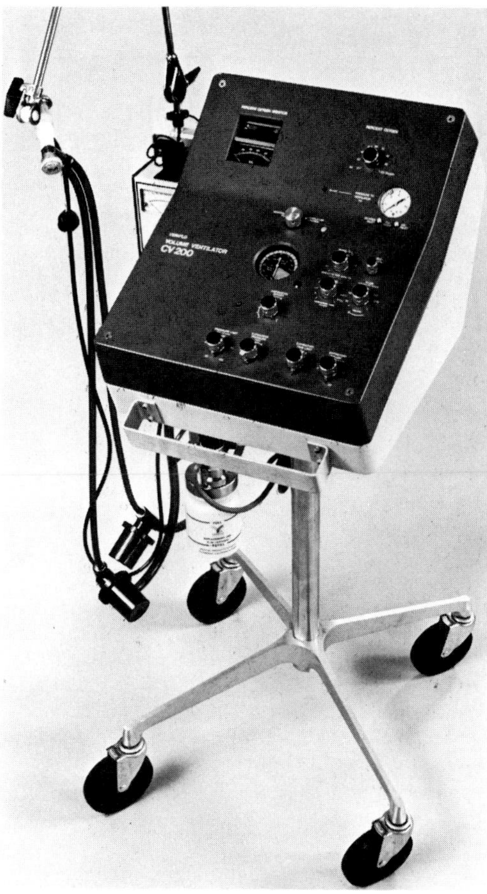

Fig. 24-86. CV 200 Ventilator.

sensor (G), which responds to patient inspiratory efforts and allows assisted ventilation according to the inspiratory effort control setting. Secondary pressure-limiting is controlled by the pressure limit control (H), which can be set between 20 and 100 cm H_2O. The gas passes through a one-way valve that isolates the two circuits, as well as a bacteria filter and humidifier. On the expiratory side of the system, a PEEP control (I) is connected to the expiratory valve system (J) of the ventilator.

Operation

Both air and oxygen delivered to the ventilator should be between 40 and 50 psi. The pressure of either of the operational gases can be monitored by the pressure gauge (A) (Fig. 24-88). This gauge selectively will monitor either of the two gases independently, depending on the button (B) depressed. If the pressure being delivered to the ventilator is inadequate, it can be adjusted by a turn-screw (C). Gas mixture is determined by the percent oxygen control (D) and monitored by the percent oxygen monitor (E). The ventilator is turned to continuous flow or control by the mode selector (F). In the continuous flow configuration, the patient breathes spontaneously without assistance or mandatory breaths from the ventilator. Once the selector has been turned to the control mode, IMV is implemented. In this mode the ventilator controls are activated and the remaining controls adjust the respiratory pattern. The inspiratory time can be adjusted by the inspiratory time control (G) between 0.3 to 3 seconds on the CV 200 and 0.4 to 4 seconds on the CV 2000. Once the inspiratory time has been selected, the respiratory rate is controlled by the I:E ratio. Turning the ratio TI/TE control (H) between 1:1 and 1:5 allows controlled ventilation, and between 1:1 and 1:infinity allows IMV. Tidal volume is altered by adjusting the inspiratory flow rate on the flow/volume control (I). This control is calibrated in milliliters per second, which equates to a flow range of between 1.8 and 16 liters/min on the CV 200 and between 12 and 100 liters/min on the CV 2000. If assisted ventilation is used, the amount of subambient pressure required to trigger the machine is set by the inspiratory effort control (J). The effort required can be adjusted between 0.5 and 8 cm H_2O subambient pressure. When 8 cm H_2O subambient pressure has been reached, the ventilator will initiate a controlled breath. If pressure-limiting is desired, the pressure limit control (K) adjusts from 20 to 100 cm H_2O.

The IMV interval (L) can extend the expiratory time toward infinity. When IMV is activated, expiratory flow must be provided. This expiratory flow (M) is available from 0 to 20 liters/min in the CV 200 and 0 to 30 liters/min in the CV 2000. PEEP is adjusted between 0 to 20 cm H_2O with the expiratory pressure control (N). Sigh breaths are available only by pressing button (O). This sigh breath provides a 50% increase in tidal volume.

Humidity

Humidity is provided by a heated humidifier.

Cleaning and Sterilizing

The patient breathing assembly should be exchanged at least daily.

Accessories

A respiratory monitor is available.

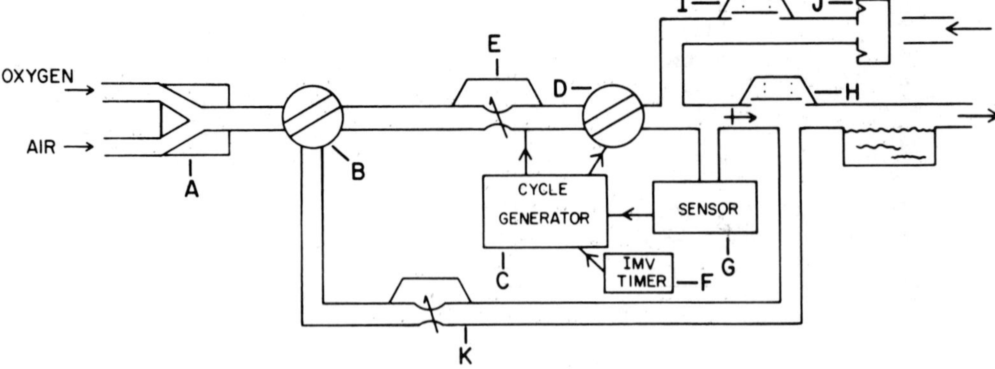

Fig. 24-87. Schematic diagram of the CV 200 Ventilator.

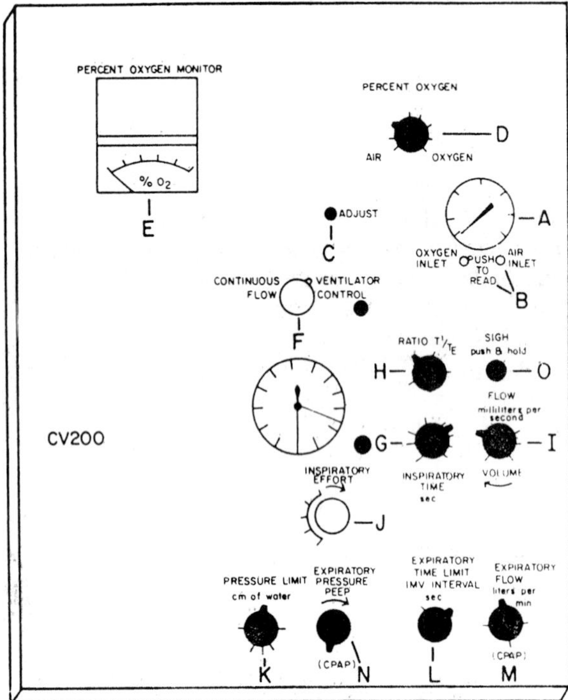

Fig. 24-88. Control panel of CV 200 Ventilator.

Troubleshooting

Slippage of knob controls may invalidate the calibration controlling flow and tidal volume. The calibration of these controls should therefore be checked frequently. The usual precautions for preventing leaks must be maintained.

APPENDIX

Ventilator compressible volume is that volume of a total ventilator system subject to increased pressure during inspiration. Determining the volume contained in the ventilator system from the piston or bellows to the exhalation valve by water displacement allows calculation of a compressibility factor for any particular ventilator. Once the total ventilator system volume has been determined, Boyle's law can be used to determine the particular compressibility factor. Manipulation of the formula is as follows.

$$\text{Boyle's law:}\quad P_1V_1 = P_2V_2 \tag{1}$$

$$V_2 = \frac{P_1V_1}{P_2}$$

Ventilator system volume is then broken down into system volume plus the adjusted ventilator tidal volume.

$$V_V + V_{T2} = \frac{P_1(V_V + V_{T1})}{P_2}$$

Further manipulation solves for the resultant tidal volume (2):

$$V_{T2} = \frac{P_1(V_V + V_{T1})}{P_2} - V_V \tag{2}$$

The formula for compressibility (3) is simply a determination of the amount of volume change per pressure increment change.

$$C = \frac{V_{T1} - V_{T2}}{P_2 - P_1} \tag{3}$$

Formula 2 is then substituted into 3 for further manipulation to a resultant formula 4, which is used to determine the compressibility factor for any particular ventilator in which the ventilator system volume is known.

$$C = V_{T_1} - \frac{\left[\dfrac{P_1(V_V + V_{T1}) - V_V}{P_2}\right]}{P_2 - P_1}$$

$$C = \frac{V_{T1}}{P_2 - P_1} - \left[\frac{P_1(V_V + V_{T1})}{P_2(P_2 - P_1)} - \frac{V_V}{P_2 - P_1}\right] \quad (4)$$

$$C = V_{T1} - \left[\frac{P_1(V_V + V_{T1}) - V_V(P_2)}{P_2(P_2 - P_1)}\right]$$

$$C = \frac{P_2(V_{T1}) - [P_1(V_V + V_{T1}) - V_V(P_2)]}{P_2(P_2 - P_1)}$$

where P_1 = absolute pressure in cm H_2O
P_2 = absolute pressure plus inspiratory pressure in cm H_2O
V_1 = ventilator system volume consisting of
V_v = ventilator system volume
V_{T_1} = prescribed volume change
V_2 = ventilator system volume consisting of
V_v = ventilator system volume
V_{T2} = actual volume delivered
C = compressibility factor

Example: If a ventilator with a system volume of 4200 ml delivers a prescribed tidal volume of 600 ml and it requires 20 cm H_2O to do this, what is the actual volume delivered to the patient, and what is the compressibility factor of this ventilator at this pressure?

$$C = \frac{P_2(V_{T1}) - [P_1(V_V + V_{T1}) - V_V(P_2)]}{P_2(P_2 - P_1)}$$

$$C = \frac{(1053.6 \text{ cm } H_2O)(600 \text{ ml}) - [1033.6 \text{ cm } H_2O\ (4200 \text{ ml} + 600 \text{ ml}) - 4200 \text{ ml}\ (1053.6 \text{ cm } H_2O)]}{1053.6 \text{ cm } H_2O\ (1053.6 \text{ cm } H_2O - 1033.6 \text{ cm } H_2O)}$$

$$= \frac{632160 - [1033.6(4800) - 4425120]}{1053.6(20)}$$

$$= \frac{632160 - 536160}{21072} = 4.56 \text{ ml/cm } H_2O$$

Compressibility factor = 4.56 ml/cm H_2O
Patient volume = 600 − (4.56)(20)
= 508.8 ml

Patient volume could also be found from formula 2 without use of the compressibility factor:

$$V_{T2} = \frac{P_1(V_V + V_{T1}) - V_V}{P_2}$$

$$= \frac{1033.6(4200 + 600)}{1053.6} - 4200$$

$$= \frac{1033.6(4800)}{1053.6} - 4200$$

$$= 4708.8 - 4200$$

$$= 508.8 \text{ ml}$$

The above examples are used only with nondistensible breathing assemblies, since increased distensibility will also increase the measured exhaled volume without the patient's receiving the tidal volume.

A more practical method for determining approximate ventilator compressible volume is to occlude the patient connection and deliver a prescribed ventilator volume into the closed circuit. It is important that the volume selected not cycle or pressure-limit the ventilator and that the entire volume be compressed in the circuit. Once the ventilator volume has been selected, the machine is triggered into the inspiratory phase and the system pressure noted. To eliminate leaks, the expired volume is measured to confirm the selected ventilator volume. The pressure noted is then divided into the volume selected to determine the approximate system compressible volume.

REFERENCES

1. Cournand A et al: Physiological studies of the effects of intermittent positive pressure breathing on cardiac output in man. Am J Physiol 152:162, 1948
2. Elam JO, Kerr JH, Janney CD: Performance of ventilators. Effect of changes in lung-thorax compliance. Anesthesiology 19:56, 1958
3. Emerson H: Artificial respiration in the treatment of edema of the lungs. Arch Intern Med 3:368, 1909
4. Herholdt JD, Rafn CG: An Attempt at an Historical Survey of Life-Saving Measures for Drowning Persons and Information on the Best Means by Which They Can be Brought Back to Life. Aarhus, Denmark, Stiftsbogtrykkeriet, 1960
5. Gregory GA et al: Treatment of the idiopathic respiratory distress syndrome with continuous positive airway pressure. N Engl J Med 284:1333, 1971
6. Mapleson WW: The effect of changes of lung characteristics on the functioning of automatic ventilators. Anaesthesia 17:300, 1962
7. Pontoppidan H, Geffin B, Lowenstein E: Acute respiratory failure in the adult. N Engl J Med 287:743, 1972

BIBLIOGRAPHY

General Texts

Avery ME, Fletcher BD, Williams R: The Lung and its Disorders in the Newborn Infant, 4th ed. Philadelphia, WB Saunders, 1981

Bendixen HH et al: Respiratory Care. St Louis, CV Mosby, 1965

Dobkin AB: Ventilators and Inhalation Therapy. Boston, Little, Brown, 1972

Egan D: Fundamentals of Respiratory Therapy, 3rd ed. St Louis, CV Mosby, 1982

Goldsmith JP, Karotkin EH: Assisted Ventilation in the Neonate. Philadelphia, WB Saunders, 1981

Grenard S: Introduction to Respiratory Therapy. Monsey, NY, Glenn Educational Medical Services, 1971

Grenard S et al: Advanced Study in Respiratory Therapy. Monsey, NY, Glenn Educational Medical Services, 1971

Heironimous T, Bageant RA: Mechanical Artificial Ventilation, 3rd ed. Springfield, IL, Charles C Thomas, 1977

Hunsinger DL et al: Respiratory Technology. Reston, VA, Prentice-Hall, 1973
Kirby RR: Design of mechanical ventilators. In Thebeault DW, Gregory GA (eds): Neonatal Pulmonary Care, pp 154–167. Menlo Park, CA, Addison–Wesley, 1979
Kirby RR: Intermittent mandatory ventilation. In Refresher Courses in Anesthesiology, pp 169–188. Philadelphia, JB Lippincott, 1979
Kirby RR, Desautels D, Model JH et al: Mechanical ventilation. In Respiratory Care, 1st ed, pp 583–663. Philadelphia, JB Lippincott, 1977
Kirby RR, Graybar GB (eds): Intermittent mandatory ventilation. In International Anesthesiology Clinics. Boston, Little, Brown, 1980
Mushin WW, Rendall–Baker L, Thompson PW et al: Automatic Ventilation of the Lungs. Oxford, Blackwell Scientific, 1980
Petty TL: Intensive and Rehabilitative Respiratory Care, 2nd ed. Philadelphia, Lea & Febiger, 1974
Safar P, Kunkel HG: Respiratory Therapy. Philadelphia, FA Davis, 1965
Shapiro BA: Clinical Application of Respiratory Care, pp 319–392; 439–459. Chicago, Yearbook, 1979
Smith RA: Respiratory care. In Miller RD (ed): Anesthesia, pp 1379–1434. New York, Churchill–Livingstone, 1981
Swyer PR: An assessment of artificial respiration in the newborn. In Lucey JF (ed): Problems of Neonatal Intensive Care Units, p 25. Columbus, OH, Ross Laboratories, 1969
Young J, Crocker D: Principles and Practice of Respiratory Therapy, 2nd ed. Chicago, Yearbook, 1976

Journals

Ashbaugh DG, Petty TL, Bigelow DB et al: Continuous positive pressure breathing (CPPB) in adult respiratory distress syndrome. J Thorac Cardiovasc Surg 57:31, 1969
Avery AE, Mörch ET, Benson DW: Critically crushed chests: A new method of treatment with continuous hyperventilation to produce alkalotic apnea and internal pneumatic stabilization. J Thorac Surg 32:291, 1956
Barach AL: Recent advances in inhalational treatment of cardiac and respiratory disease: Principles and methods. NY State J Med 37:1095, 1937
Barach AL, Bickerman HA, Petty TL: Perspectives in pressure breathing. Respir Care 20:627, 1975
Barach AL, Marin S, Eckman M: Positive pressure respiration and its application to the treatment of acute pulmonary edema. Ann Intern Med 12:754, 1938
Beach T, Miller E, Grenvik A: Hemodynamic response to discontinuance of mechanical ventilation. Crit Care Med 1:85, 1973
Bendixen HH, Bullwinkel B, Hedley–Whyte J et al: Atelectasis and shunting during spontaneous ventilation in anesthetized patients. Anesthesiology 25:297, 1964
Benjaminsson E, Klain M: Intraoperative dual-mode independent lung ventilation of a patient with bronchopleural fistula. Anesth Analg 60:118, 1981
Björk VO, Engström CE: The treatment of ventilatory insufficiency after pulmonary resection with tracheostomy and prolonged artificial ventilation. J Thorac Surg 30:356, 1955
Bland RD, Kim MH, Light MJ et al: High frequency mechanical ventilation in severe hyaline membrane disease: An alternative treatment? Crit Care Med 8:275, 1980
Bunnell S: The use of nitrous oxide and oxygen to maintain anesthesia and positive pressure for thoracic surgery. JAMA 58:835, 1912
Burgess WA, Anderson DE: Performance of respiratory expiratory valves. Am Hyg Assoc J 28:216, 1966
Carlon GC, Howland WS, Turnbull AD et al: Pulmonary venous admixture during mechanical ventilation and varying FIO_2 and PEEP. Crit Care Med 8:616, 1980
Carlon GC, Kahn RC, Howland WS et al: Clinical experience with high frequency jet ventilation. Crit Care Med 9:1, 1981
Cheney FW: The need for standards of performance. Anesthesiology 34:307, 1971
Civetta JM, Bron R, Gabel JC: A simple and effective method of employing spontaneous positive-pressure ventilation. J Thorac Cardiovasc Surg 63:312, 1972
Cullen P, Modell JH, Kirby RR et al: Treatment of flail chest—use of intermittent mandatory ventilation and positive end-expiratory pressure. Arch Surg 110:1099, 1975
de Lemos RA et al: Continuous positive airway pressure as an adjunct to mechanical ventilation in the newborn with respiratory distress syndrome. Anesth Analg 52:328, 1973
Downs JB, Klein EF, Desautels D et al: Intermittent mandatory ventilation: A new approach to weaning patients from mechanical ventilators. Chest 64:331, 1973
Elder JD et al: An evaluation of mechanical ventilating devices. Anesthesiology 24:95, 1963
Elsbert CA: Clinical experiences with intratracheal insufflation (Meltzer), with remarks upon the value of the method for thoracic surgery. JAMA 54:23, 1910
Engström C: Treatment of severe cases of respiratory paralysis by the Engström universal respirator. Br Med J 2:666, 1954
Epstein RA: The sensitivities and response times of ventilatory assistors. Anesthesiology 34:321, 1971
Fairley HB, Hunter DD: The performance of respirators used in the treatment of respiratory insufficiency. Can Med Assoc J 90:1397, 1964
Fleming WH, Bowen JC: A comparative evaluation of pressure-limited and volume-limited respirators for prolonged post-operative ventilatory support in combat casualties. Ann Surg 176:49, 1972
Froese AB, Bryan AC: Effects of anesthesia and paralysis on diaphragmatic mechanics in man. Anesthesiology 41:242, 1974
Froese AB, Bryan AC: Editorial: High frequency ventilation. Am Rev Resp Dis 123:249, 1981
Garg GP, Hunter JW, Adair DL: A simple modification of an adult volume ventilator for use with infants. Respir Care 20:246, 1975
Green NW, Janeway HH: Artificial respiration and intrathoracic esophageal surgery. JAMA 52:58, 1909
Greenbaum DM, Millen EJ, Eross B et al: Continuous positive airway pressure without tracheal intubation in spontaneously breathing patients. Chest 69:615, 1976
Greer JR, Donald I: A volume controlled patient-cycled respirator for adults. Br J Anaesth 30:32, 1958
Grogono AW, Sinopoli LM: A new classification system for intermittent positive pressure ventilators. Respir Care 19:199, 1974
Han HY, Lowe HJ: Humidification of inspired air. JAMA 205:303, 1968
Hillman KM, Barber JD: Asynchronous independent lung ventilation (AILV). Crit Care Med 8:390, 1980
Holaday DA, Rattenborg CC: Automatic lung ventilators. Anesthesiology 23:493, 1962
Hunter AR: The classification of respirators. Anaesthesia 16:231, 1961
Inkster JS, Pearson DT: Some infant ventilator systems. Br J Anaesth 39:667, 1967
Kirby RR: A new pediatric volume ventilator. Anesth Analg 50:533, 1971
Kirby RR: Intermittent mandatory ventilation in the neonate. Crit Care Med 5:18, 1977

Kirby RR: Mechanical ventilation of the newborn: Pitfalls and practice. Perinat Neonat 5:47, 1981

Kirby RR, Downs JB, Civetta JM et al: High level positive end-expiratory pressure (PEEP) in acute respiratory insufficiency. Chest 67:156, 1975

Kirby RR, Perry JC, Calderwood HW et al: Cardiorespiratory effects of high positive end-expiratory pressure. Anesthesiology 43:533, 1975

Kirby RR, Robison EJ, Schulz J et al: Continuous flow ventilation as an alternative to assisted or controlled ventilation in infants. Anesth Analg 51:871, 1972

Kumar A, Pontoppidan H, Falke KJ: Pulmonary barotrauma during mechanical ventilation. Crit Care Med 1:181, 1973

Kumar A et al: Continuous positive pressure ventilation in acute respiratory failure. N Engl J Med 283:1430, 1970

Lassen HCA: A preliminary report on the 1952 epidemic of poliomyelitis in Copenhagen with special reference to the treatment of acute respiratory insufficiency. Lancet 1:37, 1953

Lewinsohn GE et al: Control of inspired oxygen concentration in pressure cycled ventilators. JAMA 211:301, 1970

Lewis FR, Blaisdell FW, Schlobohm RM: Incidence and outcome of post-traumatic respiratory failure. Arch Surg 112:436, 1977

Llewellyn MA, Swyer PR: Assisted and controlled ventilation in the newborn period: Effect on oxygenaion. Br J Anaesth 43:926, 1971

Lohand L, Charabarti MK: The internal compliance of ventilators. Anaesthesia 26:414, 1971

Lutch JS, Murray JF: Continuous positive pressure ventilation: Effects on systemic oxygen transport and tissue oxygenation. Ann Intern Med 76:193, 1972

McPherson SP, et al: A circuit that combines ventilator weaning methods using continuous flow ventilation (CFV). Respir Care 20:261, 1975

Maloney JV, Derrick WS, Whittenberger JL: A device producing regulated assisted respiration. II. The prevention of hypoventilation and mediastinal motion during intrathoracic surgery. Anesthesiology 13:23, 1952

Maloney JV et al: Importance of negative pressure phase in mechanical respirators. JAMA 152:212, 1953

Matas R: Artificial respiration by direct intralaryngeal intubation with a modified O'Dwyer tube and a new graduated air pump, in its applications to medical and surgical practice. Am Med 3:97, 1902

Modell JH: Ventilation/perfusion changes during mechanical ventilation. Dis Chest 55:447, 1969

Musgrove AH: Controlled respiration in thoracic surgery: A new mechanical respirator. Anaesthesia 7:77, 1952

Nash G, Blennerhassett JB, Pontoppidan H: Pulmonary lesions associated with oxygen therapy and artificial ventilation. N Engl J Med 276:309, 1967

Norlander OP et al: Controlled ventilation in medical practice. Anaesthesia 16:285, 1961

Peslin RL: The physical properties of ventilators in the inspiratory phase. Anesthesiology 30:315, 1969

Petty TL: Editorial: IMV vs. IMC. Chest 67:630, 1975

Petty TL, Ashbaugh DG: The adult respiratory distress syndrome. Chest 60:233, 1971

Piergeorge AR: Modification of the Bennett MA-1 ventilator for intermittent mandatory ventilation. Respir Care 20:255, 1975

Pollack MM, Fields AI, Holbrook PR: Cardiopulmonary parameters during high PEEP in children. Crit Care Med 8:372, 1980

Pontoppidan H, Berry PR: Regulation of the inspired oxygen concentration during artificial ventilation. JAMA 201:290, 1967

Pontoppidan H, Geffin B, Lowenstein E: Acute respiratory failure in the adult. N Engl J Med 287:690, 1972

Popovitch J, O'Neal A, Deepak VIJ et al: Differential lung ventilation with a modified ventilator. Crit Care Med 9:490, 1981

Powers SR, Manual R, Neclerio M et al: Physiologic consequences of positive end-expiratory pressure (PEEP) ventilation. Ann Surg 178:265, 1973

Qvist J et al: Hemodynamic response to mechanical ventilation with PEEP: The effect of hypervolemia. Anesthesiology 42:45, 1975

Reynolds EOR: Effect of alterations in mechanical ventilator settings on pulmonary gas exchange in hyaline membrane disease. Arch Dis Child 46:152, 1971

Reynolds RN: A pulmonary ventilator for infants. Anesthesiology 25:712, 1965

Robbins L, Crocker D, Smith RM: Tidal volume losses of volume-limited ventilators. Anesth Analg 46:294, 1967

Rochford J, Welch RF, Winks DP: An electronic time-cycled respirator. Br J Anaesth 30:23, 1958

Rose DM, Downs JB, Heenan TJ: Temporal responses of functional residual capacity and oxygen tension to changes in PEEP. Crit Care Med 9:79, 1981

Simbrunner G, Gregory GA: Performance of neonatal ventilators: The effects of changes in resistance and compliance. Crit Care Med 9:509, 1981

Sjöstrand U: High-frequency positive pressure ventilation (HFPPV): A review. Crit Care Med 8:345, 1980

Sjöstrand U, Eriksson IA: High rates and low tidal volumes in mechanical ventilation—not just a matter of ventilatory frequency. Anesth Analg 59:567, 1980

Smith RA, Kirby RR, Civetta JM et al: Continuous positive airway pressure (CPAP) by face mask. Crit Care Med 8:483, 1980

Steir M, Ching N, Roberts ER: Pneumothorax complicating continuous ventilator support. J Thorac Cardiovasc Surg 67:17, 1974

Sugarman HJ, Rogers RM, Miller LD: Positive end-expiratory pressure (PEEP): Indications and physiologic considerations. Chest 62:86, 1972

Suter PM, Fairley HB, Isenberg MD: Optimum end-expiratory pressure in patients with acute pulmonary failure. N Engl J Med 292:284, 1975

Trimble C et al: Pathophysiologic role of hypocarbia in posttraumatic respiratory insufficiency. Am J Surg 122:633, 1971

Urban BJ, Weitzner SW: The Amsterdam infant ventilator and the Ayre T-piece in mechanical ventilation. Anesthesiology 40:423, 1974

Vidyasagar D, Pildes RS, Salem MR: Use of Amsterdam infant ventilator for continuous positive pressure breathing. Crit Care Med 2:89, 1974

Webb P, Troutman SJ, Annis JF: Comparison of three IPPB respirators on a mechanical lung analog. Inhalation Ther 15:112, 1970

Weigl J: Gas trapping in the respiratory system: An analytical study. Third International Conference on Neonatal Intensive Care. Alberta, Canada, August 30, 1973

Weill H, Williams TB, Burk RH: Laboratory and clinical evaluation of a new volume ventilator. Chest 67:14, 1975

25

Techniques of Ventilator Weaning

John E. Hodgkin • Laura S. Gray • George G. Burton

Weaning a patient from continuous ventilation is often a difficult, frustrating task. The weaning period is critical for the patient both physiologically and psychologically. Many such patients have marginal respiratory reserve, and determining whether the patient can maintain adequate alveolar ventilation with spontaneous breathing may be challenging to the respiratory care team. The weaning process ranges from the simple (as with a patient recovering from a drug overdose) to the complex (as in a patient with adult respiratory distress syndrome). If proper guidelines are followed, weaning need not be a risky experience for the patient.

FACTORS TO BE IMPROVED BEFORE WEANING

The patient's general condition must be evaluated and problems resolved or improved. A list of these general considerations follows.

GENERAL FACTORS WORTH IMPROVING BEFORE RESPIRATOR WEANING IS INITIATED

- Acid–base abnormalities (particularly metabolic alkalemia)
- Anemia
- Arrhythmias
- Caloric depletion
- Electrolyte abnormalities
- Exercise tolerance
- Fever
- Fluid balance
- Hyperglycemia
- Infection
- Protein loss
- Reduced cardiac output
- Renal failure
- Shock
- Sleep deprivation
- State of consciousness

The time to start thinking about weaning is at the onset of continuous ventilation. The respiratory care team should keep a daily record of variables that will indicate when weaning is, or is not, feasible (Fig. 25-1).

Acid–base abnormalities are commonly associated with the continuous ventilation period. Alkalemia of both respiratory and metabolic origin seems to be especially common and is physiologically troublesome. The normal compensatory mechanism for metabolic alkalemia involves alveolar hypoventilation, which not only produces hypoxemia but also leads to atelectasis with worsening ventilation/perfusion

Pt Name________________________ Age: _____ Height: _____ Sex: _____

Diagnosis: ________________________

	Date/Time	Date/Time	Date/Time
Correctable Parameters			
Hb-g.%			
Temp. F.			
Blood Pressure			
Electrolytes			
Chest X-ray			
Secretions			
Cardiac Output			
Arterial Blood Gases	pH____ $PaCO_2$____ HCO_3____ BE____ PaO_2____ SaO_2____ Vt____ Rate____ F_IO_2____	pH____ $PaCO_2$____ HCO_3____ BE____ PaO_2____ SaO_2____ Vt____ Rate____ F_IO_2____	pH____ $PaCO_2$____ HCO_3____ BE____ PaO_2____ SaO_2____ Vt____ Rate____ F_IO_2____
Tests			
$\dot{V}/\dot{Q}$ Matchup:			
V_D/V_T			
$P(A\text{-}a)O_2$ on 100% O_2			
Shunt			
Mechanical Ability:			
Maximal Inspiratory Pressure			
Vital Capacity			
Minute Ventilation and MVV			
FEV_1			

Fig. 25-1. Daily record of parameters that indicate when weaning is feasible.

match-up. Alkalemia also causes a leftward shift of the oxyhemoglobin dissociation curve, resulting in an increased hemoglobin affinity for oxygen and thus impaired delivery of oxygen to tissues.

Hyperventilation with resultant hypocapnia often occurs during continuous ventilation. Hypocapnia itself may produce ventilation/perfusion imbalance within the lung. Respiratory alkalemia, if prolonged, may be maximally compensated by renal mechanisms, with a decreased plasma bicarbonate. After spontaneous ventilation has been resumed, the Pa_{CO_2} may increase, resulting, with the decreased bicarbonate, in acidosis. This is particularly a problem in patients with chronic obstructive airway diseases who have chronic hypercapnia. It is worthwhile to review the patient's past medical records to ascertain his prerespiratory failure blood gas values, since the ultimate goal is achievement of these values. The "relative" hypocapnia, whether alkalemia is present or not, must be corrected before weaning is initiated because the patient with severe obstructive airway disease may not be able to maintain a value lower than his usual Pa_{CO_2} once spontaneous breathing has been initiated, and therefore may develop acute respiratory acidemia during the initial weaning attempt. However, the patient's Pa_{CO_2} before the present illness is not always known.

There are multiple determinants of systemic oxygen transport; however, frequently only the partial pressure of oxygen in the arterial blood (Pa_{O_2}) is considered. *Anemia* results in a decreased oxygen carrying capacity; thus generally a hemoglobin of at least 10 g/100 ml of blood is preferable for weaning. *Cardiac output* and blood pressure should be optimized to ensure adequate oxygen delivery to the tissues. Cardiac *arrhythmias* should be controlled because they may decrease the cardiac output, as well as being potentially life-threatening. Because of the life-threatening potential of arrhythmias, a cardiac monitor should be used on all patients during weaning.

Hypokalemia may cause myocardial irritability and thus must be corrected; it may also lead to metabolic alkalemia. The combination of hypoxemia, alkalemia, and hypokalemia strongly predisposes to arrhythmias. *Hyponatremia, hyperglycemia,* and *renal failure* should all be treated and restored to normal as far as possible before weaning is begun.

Caloric and protein depletion may occur over a period of mechanical ventilation in the patient being sustained solely by intravenous fluids. The patient will develop muscle wasting because of inactivity, and therefore proper nutrition and an exercise program should be started well in advance of anticipated weaning in the patient who has spent a prolonged period on the respirator.

Fever should be controlled because it increases oxygen consumption. Its presence often signifies *infection,* which also increases oxygen demand; thus both fever and infection should be eliminated, if possible, before weaning patients with minimal respiratory reserve.

Fluid balance can be critical, especially if borderline pulmonary edema is present. Continuous ventilation has been shown to promote fluid retention occasionally, which could further compromise the patient's respiratory reserve. This is particularly likely to occur in malnourished patients with a low colloid osmotic pressure secondary to *hypoalbuminemia.* Patients receiving inadequate fluids or diuretics may develop hypovolemia, which in turn can reduce the cardiac output and blood pressure. *Body weight* and *fluid intake and output* should be monitored carefully to prevent further compromise of the patient's reserve.

Sleep deprivation and *pain* are common in patients in the intensive care environment and interfere with the patient's ability to resume spontaneous ventilation. Narcotics and tranquilizer medication should be reduced or discontinued, if possible, to ensure alertness and to avoid respiratory center depression. However, a minimal analgesic dose is often useful in weaning the postoperative patient, since it dulls pain sufficiently to enable the patient to take deep breaths, optimizing alveolar ventilation and preventing atelectasis. Adequate rest enhances the patient's ability to cooperate; sedatives should therefore not be totally abandoned but used intelligently. Although most physicians would prefer the patient to be alert, conscious, and cooperative at the start of weaning, this is not always possible. In patients with severe head injuries or cerebral vascular accidents, *consciousness* may be slow in returning and may follow successful weaning by weeks or even months.

DETERMINATION OF ADEQUATE PULMONARY FUNCTION

One must determine whether the patient has the ventilatory capacity to maintain adequate spontaneous ventilation and oxygenation off the respirator. This evaluation can be divided into two categories of tests[2]: the patient's mechanical or neuromuscular ability to breathe; and the lungs' ability to oxygenate the arterial blood adequately (e.g., ventilation/perfusion equality, diffusion defect, or shunt). The variables listed below give the minimal values considered necessary to instigate the weaning process.

If the patient must be disconnected from the ventilator in order to perform the test, a standard procedure should be followed. First, while the patient is still connected to the ventilator, one should carefully explain the exact testing procedure and demonstrate the use of the equipment. Next, the patient should be allowed to practice the test to be performed. The test should then be repeated about three times, with the best effort being recorded. After each test, the patient should be placed back on the ventilator for about 30 seconds so that he does not become unnecessarily short of breath. The vital capacity, forced expiratory volume in 1 second (FEV_1), and peak inspiratory pressure can be tested without giving extra oxygen while off the ventilator. The maximal voluntary ventilation (MVV), however, requires additional oxygen.

PHYSIOLOGICAL PARAMETERS THAT SUGGEST RESPIRATOR WEANING IS FEASIBLE

TESTS OF MECHANICAL CAPABILITY

1. Peak inspiratory pressure	> -20 cm H_2O
2. Vital capacity	$>$ 10–15 ml/kg bw
3. Forced expiratory volume in one second	$>$ 10 ml/kg bw
4. Resting minute ventilation (can be doubled with a maximal voluntary ventilation maneuver)	$<$ 10 liters/min

TESTS OF OXYGENATION CAPABILITY

1. $P(A\text{-}a)_{O_2}$ on 100% O_2	$<$ 300–350 torr
2. Pa_{O_2} on 100% O_2	$>$ 300 torr
3. Pa_{O_2} on $\leq$ 40% O_2	$\geq$ 60 torr
4. Shunt fraction	$<$ 15%
5. Dead space/tidal volume	$<$ 0.55–0.6

The *peak inspiratory pressure* is measured by attaching an aneroid manometer (a pressure-measuring instrument) to the endotracheal or tracheostomy tube and then having the patient, after a maximal exhalation, inhale as forcefully as possible. Negative pressures greater than -20 cm H_2O suggest adequate inspiratory muscle strength to provide for sighs, as well as for the deep inhalations necessary for an effective cough.

The vital capacity (VC) can be measured easily with any instrument that measures expired volume (e.g., the Wright Respirometer). The patient is instructed to take a maximal inspiration and then exhale maximally. Serial vital capacity measurements are better indicators of respiratory reserve than is tidal volume or breathing frequency, and are particularly useful in following the status of patients with neuromuscular weakness (e.g., Guillain-Barré syndrome). The VC should be greater than 10 to 15 ml/kg body weight to be able to sigh deeply enough to avoid atelectasis.

The FEV_1 is considered by some to be a useful indicator of weaning ability in the COPD patient. The vital capacity may be nearly normal if the patient slowly exhales. However, airway collapse may occur with forced exhalation. An FEV_1 of at least 10 ml/kg body weight makes successful weaning more likely.

Although a patient may be able to deliver an acceptable vital capacity when removed from the respirator, the ability to sustain the muscular effort necessary for normal gas exchange is, of course, crucial. The MVV test, although criticized because of its great dependence on patient effort, is a test of this ability. The patient is a candidate for extubation if his spontaneous resting ventilation is less than 10 liters/min *and* if he can double the resting minute ventilation with an MVV maneuver.[4]

The *alveolar–arterial difference for oxygen* [$P(A\text{-}a)_{O_2}$] is an index of the lungs' ability to transfer oxygen from the inspired gas to the blood. A $P(A\text{-}a)_{O_2}$ of less than 300 to 350 torr or a Pa_{O_2} greater than 300 torr on 100% oxygen indicates adequate pulmonary oxygenation ability to allow weaning. However, since 100% oxygen predisposes to atelectasis, the use of 100% oxygen for the simple and sole purpose of checking the $P(A\text{-}a)_{O_2}$ should be avoided. If the Pa_{O_2} is at least 60 torr on a fractional inspired oxygen (FI_{O_2}) of 0.4 or less, the patient's ventilation/perfusion matchup, diffusing ability, and degree of shunt are acceptable to allow satisfactory weaning.

The presence of significant shunting clearly interferes with the ability to oxygenate the blood adequately. The most frequent cause of intrapulmonary shunting in respirator-dependent patients is airway obstruction secondary to accumulation of secretions, bronchospasm, or a combination of the two. These conditions are usually partially correctable by proper suctioning, use of bronchodilators, and vigorous chest physiotherapy. Shunts larger than 20% reportedly make successful weaning unlikely, with a shunt less than 15% being preferable. Generally, however, this measurement is not available, and even when it is, the effect of shunt on tissue oxygenation varies considerably with the hemoglobin, cardiac output, and a-vO_2 difference.

The physiological dead space/tidal volume ratio (VD/VT) is a measurement of that portion of each breath that does not participate in effective gas exchange. Improvement in intrapulmonary gas mixing is generally followed by a reduction in VD/VT. The VD/VT should be less than 0.55 to 0.6 to allow adequate oxygenation.

Some of these screening tests should be performed daily, with both the absolute value and trend being observed (*see* Fig. 25–1). Some patients will never achieve a "passing" score on all of the tests, but trends in the right direction can be a helpful indicator of weaning ability.

TECHNIQUES OF WEANING

Weaning a ventilator patient may involve one or a combination of two methods: T-piece trials of spontaneous breathing, or intermittent mandatory ventilation (IMV), which allows the patient to breathe spontaneously while receiving a specified, decreasing number of ventilator-delivered breaths per minute.

Psychological preparation is very important and must begin before the patient has been disconnected from the ventilator. The respiratory therapists and nurses in whom the patient has shown the most confidence should be used during the weaning process.

Before each weaning or testing period, the nurse or therapist should explain every detail of the procedure to the patient. He should be assured that he will not be left alone and may be returned to the ventilator at his request. Early in the weaning schedule someone should always be with the patient for reassurance, as well as to check the equipment for malfunction. Frequent encouragement is needed because the success of weaning depends largely on the attitude of, and effort exerted by, the patient. The need for psychological preparation appears to be directly proportional to the length of continuous ventilation. During the weaning period, setbacks are common, and the patient and staff must be prepared to accept this.

The goal of the T-piece method is to allow spontaneous ventilation while providing supplemental oxygen as needed. The tubing from the gas source attaches to the T-piece, which in turn is connected to the endotracheal tube. While the patient is receiving humidified oxygen by a T-tube system, care must be taken to prevent significant entrainment of room air. The application of a reservoir tubing distal to the patient's T-piece can prevent room air entrainment (Fig. 25-2). With a flow of at least 10 liters/min and a 120-cc reservoir tubing, one can usually maintain an FI_{O_2} up to 0.5 without difficulty.

The system's design should be simple. One-way valves, reservoir bags, and elaborate systems can be hazardous. Valves can be inadvertently placed in the system the wrong way, and reservoir bags can fill with water. If mechanical dead space is needed to raise the Pa_{CO_2} in a patient with marked hyperventilation, it should be added between the T-piece and the endotracheal or tracheostomy tube.

During periods of spontaneous breathing on the T-piece setup, the trach-tube cuff can be deflated, removing pressure from the tracheal mucosa and allowing gas to pass around, as well as through, the tube. The cuff should be left inflated if there is a significant risk of aspirating saliva or gastric contents. Obviously, the cuff must be inflated whenever ventilator-initiated breaths are being delivered.

Suctioning the patient just before and during a T-piece weaning trial may help clear the airway, resulting in a reduced work of breathing and improved gas exchange. It is useful to hyperoxygenate the patient before and after suctioning to prevent hypoxemia and subsequent deterioration. Hyperinflation should also be used after suctioning to reverse any suctioning-induced atelectasis.

Initially, spontaneous breathing may result in a decreased Pa_{O_2} level. Hypoventilation, with smaller

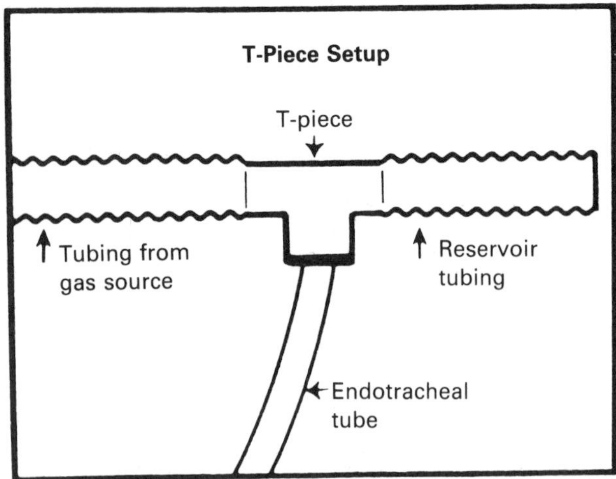

Fig. 25-2. Diagram of T-piece set-up. (Gray LS, Hodgkin JE: Ventilator Weaning. New York, Parke–Davis, 1981)

tidal volumes, and atelectasis, with resultant physiologic shunting, may occur. Therefore, the patient will initially need a higher inspired oxygen fraction while off the ventilator than while on it. Increasing the FI_{O_2} 0.1 above the ventilator setting is an acceptable rule of thumb to prevent hypoxemia from occurring. For example, if the FI_{O_2} is 0.3 on the respirator, the FI_{O_2} should be increased to 0.4 when initiating T-piece trials. However, one should remember that the patient with chronic carbon dioxide retention may need a hypoxic drive to breathe; thus routinely raising the FI_{O_2} in this type of patient may be hazardous.

Generally, T-piece trials should not be initiated until adequate oxygenation is present with a ventilator-delivered FI_{O_2} of 0.4 or less. This allows for an increased FI_{O_2} without running a significant risk of developing oxygen toxicity.

A sitting or semirecumbent position is usually best tolerated during the weaning procedure. The patient should be made as comfortable as possible before disconnecting him from the ventilator.

As mentioned earlier, an ECG monitor should be attached during the weaning process, since both early detection and early treatment of arrhythmias are essential.

After all the preliminary preparation has been completed, the actual weaning trial begins. A weaning flowsheet, as shown in Figure 25-3, is a useful way of charting the patient's progress. The initial values of pulse, blood pressure, and ECG are taken just before the patient is disconnected from the ventilator. The initial values for tidal volume and respiratory rate are taken during the first 2 minutes of the weaning trial.

Date/ Time	Pulse	Blood Pressure	Tidal Volume	Resp. Rate	EKG Rhythm	Exhaled CO_2	Total Time Off	F_IO_2	pH	PaO_2	$PaCO_2$	Tech. Comments

Fig. 25-3. Weaning flow-sheet.

Volume measurements are more accurate if one takes a cumulative volume and divides it by the respiratory rate to produce an average tidal volume. During the time the patient is disconnected from the ventilator, the tip of the respirator tubing should be placed in a clean plastic bag to prevent contamination.

The variables of pulse, blood pressure, tidal volume, and respiratory rate are checked every 5 minutes, and the patient is reconnected to the ventilator if any adverse effects occur (*see* below).

FACTORS THAT INDICATE PATIENT SHOULD BE RECONNECTED TO VENTILATOR

1. Blood pressure: rise or fall (generally 20 mm Hg systolic or 10 mm Hg diastolic)
2. Pulse: increase of 20/min or rate > 110/min
3. Respiratory rate: increase of 10/min or rate > 30/min
4. Tidal volume: < 250–300 ml (in adults)
5. Significant ECG change (e.g., dangerous arrhythmia)
6. $Pa_{O_2} < 60$ torr
7. $Pa_{CO_2} > 55$ torr
8. $pH < 7.35$

One may accept a lower Pa_{O_2} or *p*H, or both, and a higher Pa_{CO_2} in patients with chronic obstructive pulmonary disease. These precise values are guidelines only and may not be applicable in all patients. Perhaps the most important criterion for satisfactory weaning is assessment by the nurse, therapist, and physician of the patient and his clinical appearance. When the patient can tolerate being off the respirator for 30 minutes, the variables are checked thereafter every 15 minutes. Usually it is not useful to check arterial blood gases until the patient has been off the ventilator for about 15 to 20 minutes. The ability to monitor end-tidal P_{CO_2} allows for early detection of hyperventilation or hypoventilation, whereas ear oximetry and transcutaneous P_{O_2} electrodes allow continuous monitoring of the adequacy of blood oxygenation. These types of monitoring can lessen the need for arterial blood analysis and can quickly alert the patient care team to a deteriorating respiratory status.

During the early stages of weaning, a strict time limit is imposed, with 10 to 20 minutes per hour being a routine starting point. This limit is usually increased by increments of 5 to 15 minutes per hour if the patient tolerates it. These limits give the patient a goal to aim for, but, more importantly, they help prevent fatigue. During these early stages the patient may be reconnected to the ventilator at any time at his request. Arguing with a scared, dyspneic patient will not promote patient confidence or cooperation. When the patient tolerates 45 to 60 minutes of continuous weaning, one can usually increase the weaning increments quite rapidly. The patient often has minimal energy reserve, and attempting to wean through the night will be excessively fatiguing. Therefore, weaning through the night is initiated only when the patient can go through the day with only periodic intermittent positive pressure breathing (IPPB) treatments.

The second weaning technique, *intermittent mandatory ventilation* (IMV), has become increasingly popular.[1] IMV involves gradually reducing the number of ventilator-delivered breaths and using a technical setup that allows the patient to breathe spontaneously between ventilator-delivered breaths (*see* Fig. 24-10 and Fig. 25-4). Thus respirator support can be gradually withdrawn, allowing the patient to resume spontaneous ventilation slowly. If the ventilator is gradually withdrawn using IMV, time is provided for the kidneys to achieve metabolic compensation in the patient with chronic CO_2 retention.

There are various methods to achieve proper IMV. Many ventilators currently offer a convenient IMV mode. In this case, simple control adjustment can place the patient on an IMV mode. However, IMV need not be limited to "built-in" systems, it can also be achieved by attaching some basic respiratory equipment to a pressure or volume-limited ventilator.

If spontaneous effort is inadequate during IMV, the patient may develop acid–base and oxygenation disturbances as the frequency of the ventilator-delivered breaths is decreased. Close invasive or noninvasive monitoring of oxygenation and ventilation (Pa_{CO_2} or Ptc_{CO_2}) should be performed, as with the T-piece technique. Factors that indicate the need to reconnect the patient to the ventilator when using the T-piece technique would also, if present, suggest the need for more frequent mandated breaths with the IMV technique. Initially, the patient will still need rest periods with full ventilator support.

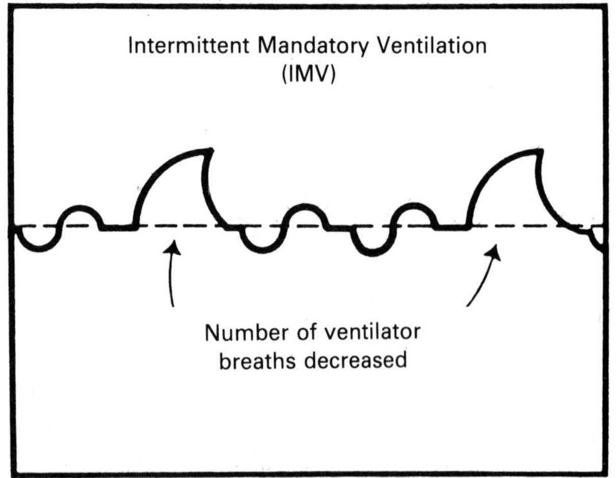

Fig. 25-4. Diagram of IMV (Gray LS, Hodgkin JE: Ventilator Weaning. New York, Parke–Davis, 1981)

A combination of IMV with continuous positive pressure breathing (CPPB) helps to maintain adequate oxygenation in patients with reduced lung compliance, for example, in those with adult respiratory distress syndrome (ARDS). The use of CPPB as weaning progresses helps to limit small airway and alveolar collapse.

Advantages of the T-piece weaning method include low cost and simplicity. The equipment is easily assembled, and there is little risk of problems from the equipment itself. The major disadvantage of the T-piece method is that it requires total maintenance of respiration by the patient. This represents an abrupt change from his previous ventilator dependence. Therefore the patient must be monitored very closely during T-piece trials of spontaneous breathing. Another disadvantage is the patient's *realization* that he will suddenly be breathing independently, which may be frightening.

A major advantage of the IMV weaning method is convenience. With the system set up in conjunction with a ventilator, simply changing the respirator rate alters the patient's weaning progression and the patient's safety is more readily ensured, since ventilator-delivered breaths continue at the IMV rate. By gradually decreasing the IMV rate, the best arterial P_{CO_2} the patient can achieve with spontaneous ventilation can be safely determined in those patients in whom the previous stable P_{CO_2} is unknown. The method is also less stressful from the patient's viewpoint owing to the gradual withdrawal of ventilator support.

One disadvantage of IMV is the higher cost. A ventilator remains in continual use with constant gas flow to meet the patient's demands, and a blender, although not required, is convenient for accurate FI_{O_2} adjustment. Another disadvantage of IMV is the potential for equipment error. The setup is relatively complex, requiring careful assembly and monitoring once applied. Additionally, IMV rates may provide inadequate stress to the respiratory muscles, so that muscle strength is not increased appropriately, whereas sustained low IMV rates, without rest periods, may lead to significant respiratory muscle fatigue and dysfunction.

Another potential disadvantage of IMV is that it may prolong the weaning process. With the graded reduction in ventilator rate, patients may remain intubated significantly longer than with the T-piece method.

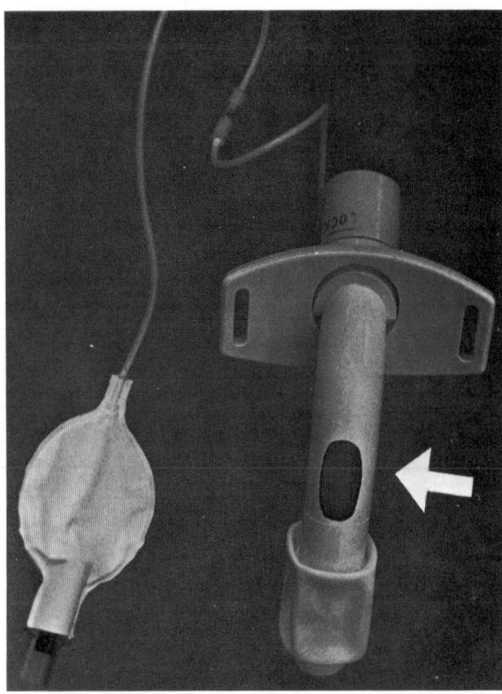

Fig. 25-5. Fenestrated tracheostomy tube.

It is important to remember during any weaning attempt that each patient is different and techniques should be individualized to meet his needs. Advantages and disadvantages are often subjective and vary with patient and institution.

In particularly difficult weaning cases, one might consider the use of a fenestrated tracheostomy tube (Fig. 25-5). With the cuff deflated and the inner cannula removed, the patient can breathe through the normal tube channel, through the fenestration in the posterior (superior) portion of the tube, and around the tube. This results in an increased inspired volume for the same amount of effort by reducing resistance to air flow. The site of the fenestration must be checked often, since occasionally the fenestration will be plugged by adjacent tissue. Before reconnecting the patient to the ventilator, the inner cannula must be reinserted and the cuff reinflated.

High-frequency ventilation has reportedly aided in weaning patients who have been difficult to wean conventionally.[3] This technique still requires further evaluation before it becomes routine.

By following a well-organized, comprehensive weaning approach, most patients can be successfully returned to spontaneous breathing. Weaning need not be a trial-and-error technique fraught with danger, but can be safely accomplished with proper expertise.

REFERENCES

1. Downs JB et al: Intermittent mandatory ventilation: A new approach to weaning patients from mechanical ventilation. Chest 64:331, 1973
2. Hodgkin JE, Bowser MA, Burton GG: Respirator weaning. Crit Care Med 2:96, 1974
3. Kalla R, Wald M, Klain M: Weaning of ventilator dependent patients by high frequency jet ventilation. Crit Care Med 9:162, 1981
4. Sahn SA, Lakshminarayan S: Bedside criteria for discontinuation of mechanical ventilation. Chest 63:1002, 1973

BIBLIOGRAPHY

Factors To Be Optimized Prior to Weaning

Feeley TW, Hedley–Whyte J: Current concepts: Weaning from controlled ventilation and oxygen. N Engl J Med 292:903, 1975

Hodgkin JE, Bowser MA, Burton GG: Respirator weaning. Crit Care Med 2:96, 1974

Lifschitz MD et al: Marked hypercapnia secondary to severe metabolic alkalosis. Ann Intern Med 77:405, 1972

Technique of Weaning

Bowser MA, Hodgkin JE, Burton GG: A systematic approach to ventilator weaning. Respir Care 20:958, 1975

Dalton BC et al: A method for supplemental oxygen administration during weaning from mechanical ventilation. Anesthesiology 33:452, 1970

Downs JB et al: Intermittent mandatory ventilation: A new approach to weaning patients from mechanical ventilators. Chest 64:331, 1973

Fell T, Cheney FW: Prevention of hypoxia during endotracheal suction. Ann Surg 174:24, 1971

Osborn JJ et al: Respiratory causes of "sudden unexplained arrhythmia" in post-thoracotomy patients. Surgery 69:24, 1971

Determination of Adequate Pulmonary Function

Bendixen HH et al: Respiratory Care. St Louis, CV Mosby, 1965

Pontoppidan H, Laver MB, Geffin B: Acute respiratory failure in the surgical patient. In Welch CE (ed): Advances in Surgery, Vol 4, p 163. Chicago, Yearbook, 1970

Sahn SA, Lakshminarayan S: Bedside criteria for discontinuation of mechanical ventilation. Chest 63:1002, 1973

26

Chest Physical Therapy and Related Procedures

Jacqueline Ryan Barrascout

By virtue of training and background, the professional physical therapist can be a valuable member of the acute care and rehabilitation teams that provide comprehensive care to patients with respiratory disease. Many of the concepts, skills, and techniques discussed within this chapter are not the exclusive "tools of the trade" of any one professional or technical discipline but should be studied, developed, and applied by various respiratory care team members, including respiratory therapists,[21] with the common goal of providing the best possible care at all times.

Physical therapy modalities have been applied in the care of respiratory disease for many years, particularly in England and elsewhere in Europe. General acceptance and use of physical therapy, particularly in acute care of the adult pulmonary patient and general care of neonates and children, have been slow to reach their full potential in the United States.

This chapter is intended to provide the physical therapist and other respiratory care workers with detailed information on clinical evaluation of the patient and with guidelines for developing physical therapy treatment plans for both short- and long-term use. The physical therapy skills and techniques needed for quality patient care during acute respiratory illness, preoperative and postoperative periods, subacute and chronic illness, and rehabilitation will also be presented.

PHYSICAL THERAPY EVALUATION

The therapist may begin treatment at the direction and guidance of a specific treatment referral, or may be asked to provide a consultation service and make treatment recommendations. In either case the patient and his records must be thoroughly evaluated so that the therapist may develop an optimal treatment plan.

GENERAL EVALUATION

A review of the chart should provide the therapist with information on the nature of the patient's problem, an assessment of the current status of his condition, and some insight into his prognosis and his physician's treatment goals. Of particular importance in the patient's record are blood gas studies, pulmonary function tests, radiographic findings, blood pressure records, cardiac status and history, medications administered, laboratory results such as hemoglobin, hematocrit, and sputum culture, and a review of any concomitant conditions that may affect the treatment plan.

During a bedside or outpatient physical therapy evaluation, the pulmonary patient is likely to be apprehensive and fearful of exertion and its resultant dyspnea. Until the patient can be reassured that his limitations are fully comprehended by the therapist, the efforts of the "exercise therapist" may be met with considerable apprehension and even resistance.

SPECIFIC EVALUATION

The specific physical therapy evaluation must be done to integrate and to correlate the physiological data related to the patient's pulmonary physiology and exercise stress testing, blood gases, and cardiac status with his actual ability to function in a given environment. Initially, the therapist will obtain much information from general observations and from an interview of the patient in the hospital or in an ambulatory treatment area.

When first meeting and greeting the patient, the therapist should note any apparent respiratory distress, the respiratory rate, and the apparent depth of respiration. Careful observation of speech patterns (such as the patient's breathing between every two or three words) will give the therapist a starting point for training.

Observation of the patient's habitually assumed postures often provides the initial clues to excessive use of the accessory muscles of respiration. Patients with long-standing pulmonary disease and those in acute distress sit, stand, walk, and position themselves in bed in classical postures (*see* Fig. 13-1). It is particularly important for the therapist to observe postures in which the upper extremities are used as support. Commonly, patients prop themselves up by placing their hands on their knees, resting their forearms on a bedside table or kitchen table, or stand leaning forward with their hands on their thighs or on a chair back, counter, sink, or other nearby object. The trunk is generally slightly flexed at the waist, shoulders internally rotated, elbows slightly flexed, and the palms of the hands rest on the supporting surface. Fixation of the shoulder girdle provides a mechanical advantage to the accessory muscles of respiration, and the flexion at the waist produces some upward pressure on the base of the diaphragm, improving gas exchange, as does forward bending of the head.

Other habitual postures, such as sleeping on the same side, should be noted for their implications about secretion retention and bronchial hygiene.

By means of an interview, the therapist can obtain an awareness of the patient's own attitudes about his illness, his understanding of his condition, and his motivation and expectations for therapy. It is common for the patient with chronic disease to be depressed and to express a "go away and leave me alone" attitude. It is most important that an atmosphere of hope and encouragement be established quickly. A few "instant successes" always help to gain the patient's trust and cooperation. If one can prove to the patient that he can tolerate more diverse and strenuous activities, his motivation and understanding of his treatment program will be enhanced.

The therapist will want to inquire about the patient's level of functioning before his current illness or exacerbation of preexisting chronic disease. As the patient describes his activities and those things that cause him distress, or ruefully reports those things that he has eliminated from his activities, patterns will begin to emerge. Upper extremity movements that require heavy work or are usually performed above shoulder level cause dyspnea and are generally avoided by the respiratory patient. Bending, squatting, and stooping, and movements of knee toward chest (many dressing and self-care activities) cause distress and are done reluctantly or avoided. It is useful to have the patient demonstrate, if feasible, an activity such as picking up a shoe from the floor if he has described limitations in squatting or bending activities. While he is bending or squatting, the therapist should observe the patient carefully for breath holding. If this occurs, a simple breathing control technique can solve the problem and create an "instant success" for motivational purposes.

The patient will often describe his ability to walk "at his own pace" in rather indefinite terms. He may perceive that he can walk six or eight blocks on the level, but in fact has not felt well enough to do so for several weeks or months. When possible and indicated, it is helpful to measure objectively the extent of ambulation and to monitor the patient's pulse, degree of dyspnea, and cyanosis (or blood gas values) in response to walking. This can be done as part of the actual physical evaluation.

Muscular Breathing Pattern

The observable muscular components of breathing involve the use of the diaphragm, intercostals, accessory cervicothoracic, and expiratory muscles. The therapist must observe and record the muscles used during each phase of respiration and compare this with a quiet, "normal breathing pattern" (*see* Chaps. 9 and 13). There is often a marked difference between habitual muscular use and the muscular pattern that can be observed when instructions and proprioceptive cues are given that call for alterations in the breathing pattern. In such cases breathing retraining may be indicated. The muscular pattern of breathing should be observed in the supine, sitting, standing, and ambulatory postures when feasible and comparative recording done. There are several different methods of recording breathing patterns but all are quite subjective. The presence or absence of pursed-lip breathing, the use of accessory respiratory muscles, and the contribution of the intercostal muscles and diaphragm should be observed and recorded.

Chest Wall Mobility

The maintenance of chest wall mobility is particularly important in postoperative cases, in patients whose neuromuscular dysfunction has resulted in impaired respiratory function, in spinal deformities, and in some collagen diseases (e.g., scleroderma or rheumatoid spondylitis).

Chest wall mobility can be measured by means of a nonstretchable tape measure or calipers. Actual end-expiratory and end-inspiratory measurements should be recorded, not only the actual excursion of expansion. Landmarks from which measurements were taken should also be recorded so that measurements will be reproducible. The xyphoid and its corresponding spinous process (T-11) posteriorly are commonly used landmarks. Another method of quickly observing and documenting chest wall mobility is for the therapist to place his hands on the patient's back with thumb tips approximated and aligned with a specific spinous process in the lower thoracic spine. The palm and fingers are placed in firm contact against the patient's posterior rib cage (Fig. 26-1). The therapist can then observe and measure chest wall mobility as his thumbs separate during the inspiratory movements of the chest wall. Similar techniques are useful for observing localized chest wall mobility and immobility.

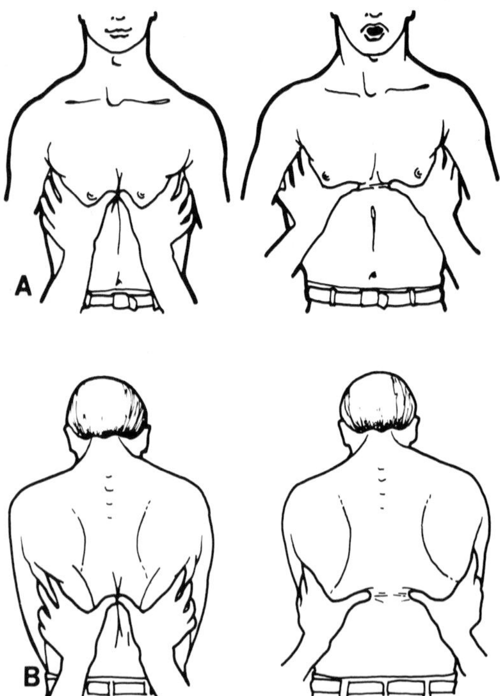

Fig. 26-1. Measurement of chest wall mobility: *(A)* anterior; *(B)* posterior. The figures to the left are in full expiration.

Cough

Just as patients have habitual muscular breathing patterns, they also have "cough habits." An evaluation of cough effectiveness should be done. The cough is a protective mechanism elicited by stimulation of the larynx, trachea, and larger bronchi. Afferent fibers of the vagus nerve carry impulses to the medullary cough center. The mechanism of an effective cough is divided into four parts: a deep inspiration, usually through the mouth; closure of both the epiglottis and the vocal cords shut tightly to keep air trapped in the chest; contraction of the abdominal muscles, causing them to push forcefully against the diaphragm (at the same time the other expiratory muscles also contract forcefully); and the vocal cords and the epiglottis opening suddenly, allowing the air that has been trapped to exit as an expiratory blast through the mouth. When the epiglottis and the vocal cords are closed and the above muscles contract, pressures within the thorax may exceed 100 mm Hg; the velocity of exhaled air (and sputum!) may exceed 100 miles/hr.

Serial coughing is more effective than paroxysms of wracking, explosive cough. With serial coughing the compression and expansion of the airways are thought to loosen secretions, which then are subjected to "misting" by the high linear velocity of cough-generated airflow. The therapist should observe and record the sequencing and effectiveness of the cough as carefully as possible. Several observations of spontaneous or induced coughing episodes are sometimes necessary to achieve this end.

Ambulatory Status

Ambulatory status should be evaluated from a respiratory viewpoint as well as from a general viewpoint of documenting distances attained in a given time and functional parameters, such as the ability to climb stairs and ramps. The physiological response to exertion should be recorded, including pulse rate change, recovery time, dyspnea, dyspnea recovery time, cyanosis or pallor, and any cough or wheezing initiated. Untoward effects of exercise should be noted.

Functional classifications of ambulatory status are widely used and help to define current levels, to project treatment goals, and to objectify changes. One such useful classification is described in Chapter 13.

Activities of Daily Living

Evaluation of the patient's ability to perform activities of daily living is a precise confirmation of the many observations made during the interview phase. A checklist of activities similar to the functinal evaluation forms used for many other chronic disabilities can be used here.

By asking pertinent questions and by observing performance, the therapist can pinpoint activities wherein the patient uses inefficient respiratory or other muscle mechanics, and can identify specific activities during which the patient is unable to coordinate breathing and gross body movement patterns. This information is valuable when assessing treatment program effectiveness because improvement in these functional parameters and the patient's increased perception of well-being are often the most tangible results of intensive treatment efforts. The need for instruction of the patient in work simplification techniques will become apparent in this phase of the evaluation.

Finally, the therapist should look at the overall strength, range of motion, and posture of his patient. Where other problems are present, specific muscle testing or goniometric measurements may be indicated. In patients with chronic pulmonary disease, the therapist may be assessing the end results of chronic inactivity, poor general fitness, and debility. The degree of physical fitness of the body that surrounds the impaired cardiopulmonary system can be either an asset or a detriment. Improved general fitness and efficiency should be a major goal in the treatment plan.

A kyphotic posture, tight anterior shoulder muscles, and a forward head position are frequently present as a result of chronic respiratory disease and aging. Neck muscle discomfort and "tension" in the neck and shoulder girdle are problems that commonly result. Limitation in trunk, shoulder, neck, or hip mobility may interfere with bronchial hygiene maneuvers and specific exercise programs, and these potential limitations must therefore be evaluated. Obesity, abdominal ptosis, spinal deformities, past surgeries, and rib or vertebral fractures can have significant implications for the success or failure of a treatment program.

At this point the information obtained from review of the medical records, the patient interview, and the findings of the specific physical therapy evaluation can be transformed into an individually tailored treatment plan. The selection of appropriate treatment techniques and practical treatment goals is a difficult task. The literature is replete with "evidence" supporting the claims of various treatment programs. How much improvement in life function is actually attainable? Many questions remain unanswered. The discipline of physical therapy, like medicine, has not always been able to deliver "hard data" that fully explain why certain treatment procedures are successful. Moreover, it does not discard procedures and modalities until they demonstrate their worthlessness by controlled studies over a reasonable time.

The following discussion of treatment goals and treatment techniques will be presented in light of both common clinical experience and, where possible, a critical review of what the literature does or does not reveal about these techniques.

BREATHING RETRAINING

OBJECTIVES

The objectives of breathing retraining techniques include the following:

1. To promote greater use of the diaphragm and decreased use of the upper rib cage and cervicothoracic accessory muscles
2. To increase proprioceptive awareness of the muscles of respiration and to suppress the tendency for hurried and gasping respiration
3. To provide the patient with tools with which he may better handle the distressful symptom of dyspnea
4. To identify and to provide a means by which inefficient and inappropriate muscle use can be diminished or eliminated (relaxation and biofeedback techniques)
5. To improve effectiveness of alveolar ventilation by increasing tidal volume, prolonging pulmonary emptying time, and hopefully improving intrapulmonary gas mixing and ventilation/perfusion relationships

6. To improve the strength and endurance of the inspiratory muscles
7. To improve the effectiveness of cough
8. To improve the delivery of therapeutic aerosols
9. To teach the patient to coordinate his breathing with body motions and activities of daily living
10. To relieve exertional dyspnea so that the patient can improve his physical fitness and general tolerance to activity.

PURSED-LIP BREATHING

Pursed-lip breathing is a technique often spontaneously adopted by patients with obstructive pulmonary disease. For those patients who do not do so intuitively, the technique should be taught (Fig. 26-2).

Pursed-lip breathing is easily learned and becomes a valuable tool for improving control of respiration and prolonging pulmonary emptying time. Using this technique, the patient learns to control rate and depth of breathing and often finds that by this conscious effort he can reduce his feeling of dyspnea and tendency toward panic.

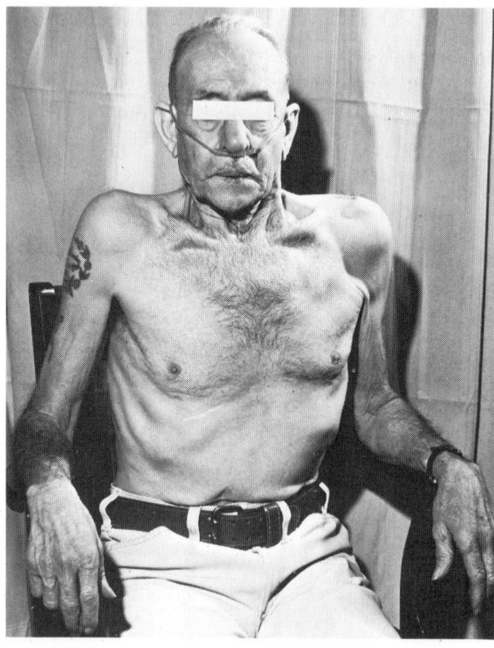

Fig. 26-2. Emphysematous patient demonstrating pursed-lip breathing.

The patient is instructed to inhale slowly and then to blow out slowly through pursed lips in a prolonged but relaxed manner. The expiratory phase would be at least twice as long as the inspiratory phase. Pursed-lip breathing is the first step in gaining control of dyspnea and in providing improved ventilation before voluntary coughing.

Mueller and Petty have demonstrated physiological benefits in the patient with obstructive pulmonary disease who breathes with pursed lips at rest.[18] Improved alveolar ventilation, reduced respiratory rate, and improved intrapulmonary $\dot{V}/\dot{Q}$ balance as indicated by a decreased alveolar–arterial oxygen gradient have been reported with this change in breathing pattern. However, simple, slow, deep breathing may have the same effects.[24] A major portion of the apparent effectiveness of the technique appears to derive from changes in rate and depth of respiration. Ingram and Schilder believed that the maneuver, a benefit of pursed-lip breathing, was a result of decreased airway pressure.[12] It was speculated that pursed-lip breathing might alter the "length:tension inappropriateness" of the respiratory musculature that is sensed by the patient as dyspnea.[11]

DIAPHRAGMATIC BREATHING

Historically, diaphragmatic breathing has been the major focus of breathing retraining routines. The altered position and resulting mechanical disadvantage of the diaphragm in the presence of chronic obstructive disease are apparent clinically and radiographically. The uniqueness of the diaphragm should be fully appreciated. It is primarily responsible for quiet breathing with the chest muscles probably used mostly for stabilization and prevention of distortion as the diaphragm contracts.[15] The diaphragm overcomes principally elastic and resistive forces rather than inertial loads. The fact that the diaphragm is under voluntary as well as involuntary control and must contract every few seconds without long periods of rest is also unique.[22]

Many patients with obstructive disease rely excessively on the cervicothoracic accessory muscles, although increased diaphragmatic use is potentially available and can be elicited when appropriate, well-understood, proprioceptive cues are given.

The strength of diaphragmatic contraction depends on muscle fiber length. Since inspiratory muscle fiber length is a function of lung volume, the greater the lung volume the shorter the resting fiber length of the inspiratory muscles, and thereafter the weaker their contractile force. Thus there is a theoretical advantage to breathe at or near FRC.[6]

EMG studies have confirmed that the supine and forward-leaning positions cause increased pressure against the diaghragm, improving its tension-length situation. This helps to explain the frequently observed forward-leaning habit pattern seen in the COPD patient.[22]

Quite recent studies provide much additional insight into the alteration of diaphragmatic functioning in COPD. It is generally agreed that inspiratory muscle weakness does occur and that this weakness may play a role in ventilatory failure. Sharp states that "ventilatory failure develops because the balance between respiratory mechanical impedances and the muscle power to overcome them has tipped in favor of the impedance and against the respiratory muscles."[22] Additionally respiratory muscle weakness and lack of respiratory muscle endurance play a significant role in limited exercise tolerance. EMG frequency spectrum analysis can reliably detect diaphragmatic fatigue, since it is well known that EMG frequencies shift downward toward lower frequencies as fatigue develops. These EMG fatigue patterns have been noted to precede incoordination of respiratory muscles as seen in irregularities in patterns of thoracoabdominal motion.[9]

Increased diaphragmatic breathing may improve the distribution of ventilation to the basal lung segments, but no such selective alterations have been demonstrated thus far. Miller, and later Gemimez, showed that diaphragmatic excursion might be increased and the use of accessory cervicothoracic muscles reduced with proper training.[8,17] The consensus of published studies is that the major benefits derived from diaphragmatic breathing training are reduced respiratory rate, increased tidal volume, increased alveolar ventilation, reduced functional residual capacity, and increased strength and endurance of the diaphragm.

To achieve improved diaphragmatic breathing and the physiological benefits just described, the therapist must first teach the patient where the diaphragm is located and how it moves and functions. Drawings, mirrors, and other visual aids will prove invaluable.

Training is begun with the patient in the position of greatest breathing comfort. The environment should be quiet and at a comfortable temperature. The therapist should place his hand immediately below the xiphoid process in the epigastric triangle. The patient is then asked to inhale and in so doing to lift the therapist's hand gently. One must observe for arching of the patient's back and abdominal protrusion; these maneuvers can be deceiving since they mimic the appearance of diaphragmatic breathing.

Many patients cannot perform diaphragmatic breathing initially. Some additional techniques will facilitate proprioceptive awareness. One such approach is to have the patient place his fingers firmly just below the xiphoid and to sniff quickly and strongly. In so doing, he should feel the epigastric area move outward against his fingers, thus reinforcing his awareness of diaphragmatic location and motion. The patient can then be instructed to sniff to initiate diaphragmatic motion and then continue to inhale in a deep, slow, controlled manner in place of the original sniffing maneuver.

Patients without significant orthopnea can be placed in a supine Trendelenburg position to facilitate diaphragmatic awareness and motion. This position uses the forces of gravity and the weight of the abdominal contents to produce increased curvature of the diaphragmatic dome, thus increasing the passive stretch applied to the diaphragm. The diaphragm responds to these imposed demands by contracting more strongly through the slightly increased arc of movement. Diaphragmatic breathing retraining can be initiated in this position and then progressed to more functional positions.

If attempts to achieve increased diaphragmatic breathing by epigastric cues result in excessive back arching and abdominal protrusion instead of the desired alteration in breathing pattern, it may be best to drop all reference to the "abdominal" diaphragmatic or epigastric component and to turn the patient's attention to lateral expansion maneuvers. With the therapist's hands placed firmly on the patient's lower lateral rib cage, the patient is instructed to inhale so that the ribs push outward against the therapist's hands. This maneuver will facilitate diaphragmatic as well as intercostal muscle activity. The patient should both feel and see the concomitant lateral expansion and epigastric rise.

If attempts to achieve diaphragmatic breathing appear to cause a decrease in the circumferential diameter of the lower chest wall (paradoxical retraction), one can be quite sure that the diaphragm is extremely low-lying and flattened. As a result the contraction of its fibers is in a more horizontal plane, thus causing the inward, paradoxical movement.

By placing one hand on the epigastric area and the other on the apical chest with thumb and index finger at the insertion of the sternocleidomastoid muscles, the patient can monitor the relative motion and

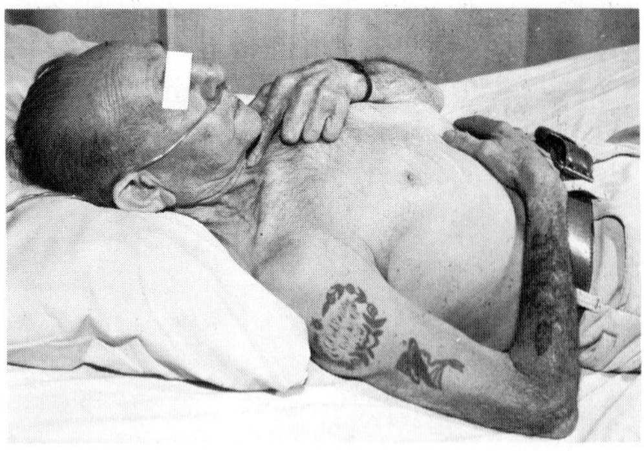

Fig. 26-3. Hand placement for monitoring of accessory muscle use.

tension of his own respiratory muscles (Fig. 26-3). This can be further reinforced by visual feedback, using a mirror.

The use of biofeedback techniques shows promise in enhancing breathing retraining procedures. EMG biofeedback surface electrodes can be placed to monitor excessive use of accessory muscles and inappropriate muscle tension. The patient consciously attempts to decrease the feedback signals being received from these unwanted and inefficient muscular components. Conversely electrodes are placed to pick up the activity of the diaphragm, and therefore reinforcement of the desired muscular breathing pattern is possible. Once increased awareness and use of the diaphragm have been achieved, the patient should be encouraged to practice diaphragmatic breathing while supine, sitting, standing, and walking.

Diaphragmatic weights (1–10 pound weights placed on the upper abdomen) have been used in breathing retraining programs. The rationale for this approach is based on the fact that diaphragmatic strength, like that of other skeletal muscles, should increase as a result of performing work against increased resistance. Additionally, diaphragmatic weights placed on the epigastric area provide an excellent proprioceptive cue. Judgment should be exercised in selecting the amount of weight used, remembering the proximity of major blood vessels.

Improved inspiratory muscle strength and endurance may well improve the patient's ability to handle the added restrictive load imposed by acute respiratory infection and may improve exercise performance. Inspiratory muscle training to enhance strength and endurance has been studied in quadriplegia, cystic fibrosis, and chronic obstructive pulmonary disease. In research animals such training has resulted in an increased mitochondrial density and an increased concentration of aerobic enzymes.[14]

In respiratory patients there is strong evidence that inspiratory muscle training (particularly of the diaphragm) is a valuable adjunct to the rehabilitation process and that it enhances exercise performance, particularly in patients who exhibit diaphragmatic fatigue patterns on EMG.[19]

SEGMENTAL BREATHING

Although little objective data support the concept of retraining selected (rib cage) muscles other than the diaphragm, some enthusiasm still persists for "segmental" breathing retraining.

Segmental breathing is taught to patients in an effort to promote or to maintain chest wall mobility. Segmental breathing is thought to be valuable when treating abdominal or thoracic surgery patients; neurologic diseases that affect the muscles of respiration; patients with musculoskeletal problems such as kyphosis, scoliosis, or arthritis involving the spine; and asthma and other obstructive pulmonary diseases.

The therapist teaches the patient to localize three or four areas of his chest wall: apical, middle, lateral basal, and posterior basal segments. The therapist places his hands firmly on the chest wall where increased muscular effort and expansion are desired. The patient is then asked to inhale and to expand the chest directly under the therapist's hands. Constant, but not overwhelming, pressure is maintained throughout inspiration, with a slight reduction of pressure as full inspiration is achieved.

Quiet, relaxed, and perhaps pursed-lip exhalation is then encouraged. The therapist may apply some gentle pressure at the end of expiration to encourage complete emptying. A slight, rapid compression followed by constant resistance during inspiration may facilitate this localized intercostal movement via the muscle spindle. It is clinically evident that selective alterations in localized chest wall movement can be achieved by segmental breathing techniques (Fig. 26-4).

Proper positioning of the patient is essential to achieve relaxation and to minimize the work of postural muscles while segmental breathing is being done. Relaxation of the cervicothoracic accessory muscles, spinal extensors, and abdominal muscles will allow better contraction of the intercostal muscles and diaphragm.

Logically, alterations in the relative shape of the chest wall should in turn alter the relative distribution of ventilation. However, no studies to date have demonstrated that voluntarily achieved changes in the shape of the chest wall have an effect on distribution

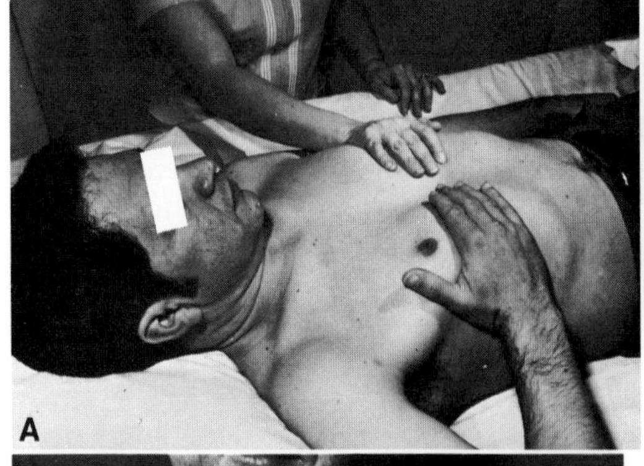

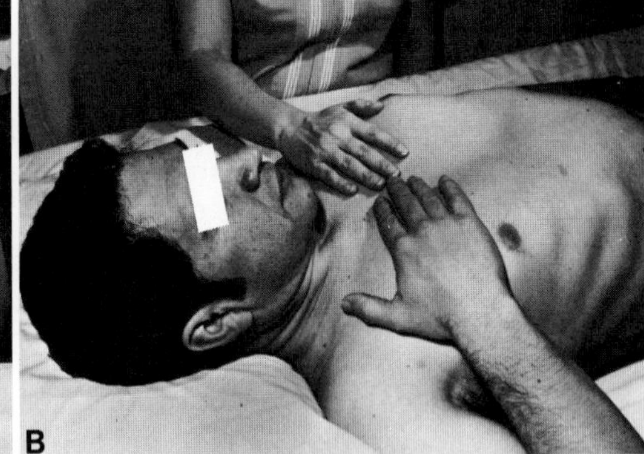

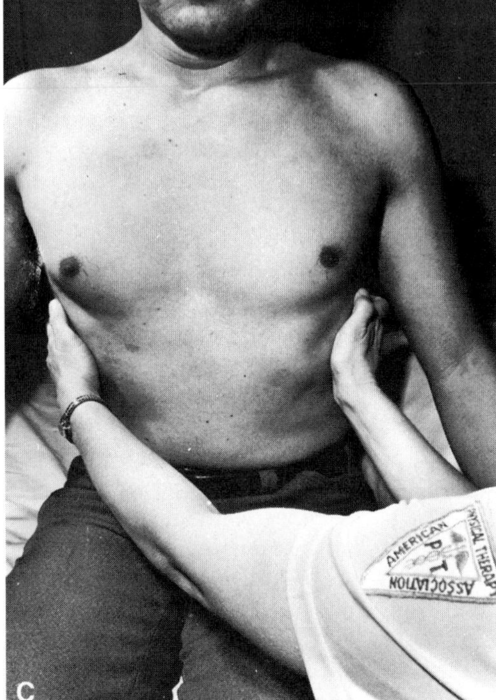

Fig. 26-4. Segmental breathing: *(A)* anterior base; *(B)* upper lobes; *(C)* lateral base.

of ventilation, although there is evidence that local distending pressure may be dependent on local chest wall geometry. Segmental breathing, however, is an excellent tool for maintaining chest wall mobility and for overcoming the fear of deep breathing and muscular protective splinting that occurs so often in the postoperative care period.

BREATHING AND MOVEMENT

The major goal of all aspects of breathing retraining is to allow the patient to achieve a higher level of function in his everyday living. Breathing retraining should therefore be ultimately applied in exercises that have direct application and carry-over to the individual's activities of daily living (ADL). The patient, whose self-care has become limited because of his dyspnea, must learn how to coordinate the demands of activities he desires with the proper and most efficient breathing pattern he has been taught. In the following discussion, we shall examine some of the more common ADL limitations and a systematic approach by which these problems can be eliminated, or at least minimized, by breathing retraining.

One begins this portion of training by reviewing the limitations in ADL and examples of breathing inefficiency that were identified in the initial evaluation. Bending, stooping, and squatting activities are often a source of fatigue and dyspnea for the patient. One of the most common problems is that of breath-holding while doing these activities. This can easily be demonstrated on a normal person as well. For the respiratory patient, however, this brief period without breathing leads to considerable dyspnea and discomfort. The therapist should instruct the patient to inhale before bending, and then to exhale through pursed lips as he bends. He should inhale again as he returns to the seated or upright position.

These maneuvers can be practiced beginning with early range of motion exercises in the acute care unit. The patient can learn to avoid breath-holding and to coordinate breathing with hip or trunk flexion or with strong abdominal muscle actions as he practices the simple Williams' lower back exercises, familiar to physical therapists. Expiration is gently paced so that expiration occurs as the knee comes toward the chest and returns to the resting position. Remember that hip flexion and abdominal stabilization of the pelvis occur isotonically and then eccentrically during this movement. Similarly coordinated motions include single straight leg raising, modified sit-ups, pelvic tilt exercises, trunk bending, and semisquats. Any activity that calls up actual abdominal muscular force or causes compression of the abdominal area by increasing the proximity of the knees to the chest should be coupled with expiration. The patient will find that previously difficult activities such as lower extremity dressing, washing feet and legs, and picking up objects from the floor become less distressful when these simple principles are followed.

Motions of the upper extremities create dyspnea in many respiratory patients. The patient who excessively relies on the accessory muscles for respiratory assistance supports himself on his arms in such a way as to gain maximum mechanical advantage of these accessory muscles. These "accessory" muscles of respiration are normally the prime movers of the neck and shoulder girdle; when the extremities are fixed (as the patient leans forward to support himself on his arms), these muscles literally pull on the chest wall. Although this position may lessen the feeling of dyspnea, it will severely limit his self-care activities. It is most difficult for a patient to brush his teeth or change clothes with his body weight leaning on his hands, arms, or elbows. The therapist must keep in mind that he cannot eliminate the patient's dependence on accessory muscles unless an alternative muscular pattern of breathing has been achieved. To free the muscles of the shoulders for functional activities, improved intercostal and diaphragmatic breathing training must come first.

Activities designed to improve coordination of arm movements and breathing are based on a few simple observations. Movements of the arms in forward flexion or abduction ending above the head will tend to elevate the entire chest and coordinate well with inspiration. Abduction movements done unilaterally or bilaterally also tend to promote chest expansion, whereas abduction toward or across the midline of the body tends to promote chest compression, or at least a return to an end-expiratory resting position.

Shoulder rotational activities have considerable functional carry-over and are easily analyzed as to their role in breathing. External rotation facilitates inspiration, and expiration will naturally follow after internal rotation has been done. The diagonal patterns of Knott and Voss can easily fit into this type of analysis.[13] Finally, movements such as lifting heavy objects should be performed during expiration, and breath-holding should be discouraged. Using these concepts, a program can be developed that is suitable for the acutely ill patient just beginning to cope with his environment, as well as for the moderately active, ambulatory care patient for whom both strengthening exercises and breathing coordination exercises may be indicated.

In summary, the therapist should examine the movements and muscles involved in a given functional activity and ascertain how they relate to the movements of the chest wall and abdomen during inspiration and expiration. The patient with respiratory disease must be seen as a victim of muscular mechanical disadvantage who needs to gain every possible advantage from proper and efficient coordination of his breathing efforts with those of his ADL.

POSTURAL DRAINAGE AND PERCUSSION

EFFICACY OF THE PROCEDURE

Hypersecretion and retention of sputum are frequently major problems in both acute and chronic pulmonary disorders. It is generally accepted that improved ejection of sputum from the lungs has a positive effect on the patient's course and sense of well-being. Postural drainage increases sputum volume when performed in appropriate patients using proper segmental positioning and percussion-vibration techniques, particularly in patients with cystic fibrosis, bronchiectasis, and lung abscess.[10]

The mechanism by which the therapeutic benefit of postural drainage is achieved is not clear, nor has it been adequately studied. Some believe that enhanced airway clearance occurs primarily in the larger, more central airways. However, evidence related to gas exchange (such as an improved arterial P_{O_2} and alveolar–arterial P_{O_2} difference) tends to support improvement in effective peripheral clearance as well. Pham and associates demonstrated temporary improvement in FEV_1 after postural drainage.[20]

Hypersecretion and retention of sputum occur for many reasons. A primary reason may be the basic nature of the underlying disease, as in chronic bronchitis, asthmatic bronchitis, pneumonia, cystic fibrosis, and bronchiectasis. In addition to the underlying disease process, the inability to cough effectively, which implies impairment of either the muscular pump force or the adequacy of air flow, or both, may be a major factor. The absence of the normal deep sigh mechanism, the tendency toward drying and crusting of secretions, or the presence of an endotracheal tube may also contribute to sputum retention. Mellins has shown that ciliary dyskinesia occurs in patients with cystic fibrosis when inflammation is superimposed.[16] This further supports the need for gravitational and mechanical assistance to improve sputum ejection. Mellins supports the efficacy of postural drainage procedures, stating that

> It is a common clinical observation that some forms of acute lung collapse in the young infant that are resistant to all other methods of treatment including IPPB dramatically respond to chest percussion and vibration by reinflation. This is especially true in the newly diagnosed infant with cystic fibrosis.

Similarly, it has been noted in some adults with bronchiectasis that cough is impaired by dynamic airway collapse, and thus postural drainage is indicated.

POSTURAL DRAINAGE TECHNIQUES

Before beginning the actual postural drainage procedure, the therapist should be aware of the diagnosis for which the procedure is being administered, the lung segments and lobes involved, the cardiac status of the patient, past thoracic or spinal surgeries, and the presence of osteoporosis or any structural abnormality of the chest wall and spine. Treatment should not be instituted without a close examination by the therapist of the unclothed part over which percussion and vibration are to be done.

When possible, one should view the roentgenograms or read the radiologist's report. The therapist should always auscultate before and after treatment so that charting may be more precise and the treatment procedure properly individualized to each patient's needs.

Postural drainage should begin with proper positioning for the uppermost involved pulmonary segment (Fig. 26-5, 26-6). This may be determined by auscultation or review of the roentgenograpic findings. With a chest that is "quiet to auscultation," it may be necessary to do a complete segment-by-segment procedure to make some clinical observations as to the major sites of obstruction. One might suspect that active percussion and vibration to the upper lobe segments are unnecessary, since these drain spontaneously in response to the upright posture. This concept is not consistent with the accepted drainage positions for two of the three upper lobe segments (see Fig. 26-6), and in clinical practice attention to upper lobe segments often results in marked sputum ejection. *Again, the areas to be treated should be selected on the basis of auscultation and roentgenographic findings.*

The positioning, percussion, and vibration should proceed through the potentially involved segments in such a way as to clear the segments and airways above before treating lower ones. Many patients who need postural drainage exhibit considerable dyspnea and tolerate almost any activity poorly. Accordingly, oxygen therapy may be needed during postural drainage and percussion therapy, as may supplemental bronchodilator therapy. The order of positioning should be such that movement and exertion on the patient's part are minimized. Thoughtful and orderly positioning will eliminate many side-to-side turns that are excessively fatiguing and may allow the patient to tolerate the procedure more successfully. Postural drainage procedures should not be performed immediately after the patient has eaten, since nausea and vomiting can occur during the treatment, with the possible occurrence of aspiration.

Percussion should be done with the cupped hand applied to the rib cage immediately over the pulmonary segment being drained (Fig. 26-7). The hand should make a "popping," hollow sound as it strikes the chest wall. The patient should not be able to feel the entire outline of the hand but should feel the air pocket within the hand. Percussion is done throughout inspiration and expiration. Vibration is performed during exhalation at the rate of about 30 to 50 cycles/sec. The time spent in percussion and postural drainage of each segment cannot be arbitrarily stated but must be determined by experience in each patient. Generally, if no increase in cough or expectoration occurs after 5 to 10 minutes, the therapist should proceed to another lobe or segment. Care should be taken to avoid percussing the sternum, spine or scapula, kidney area, abdomen, and the female breasts.

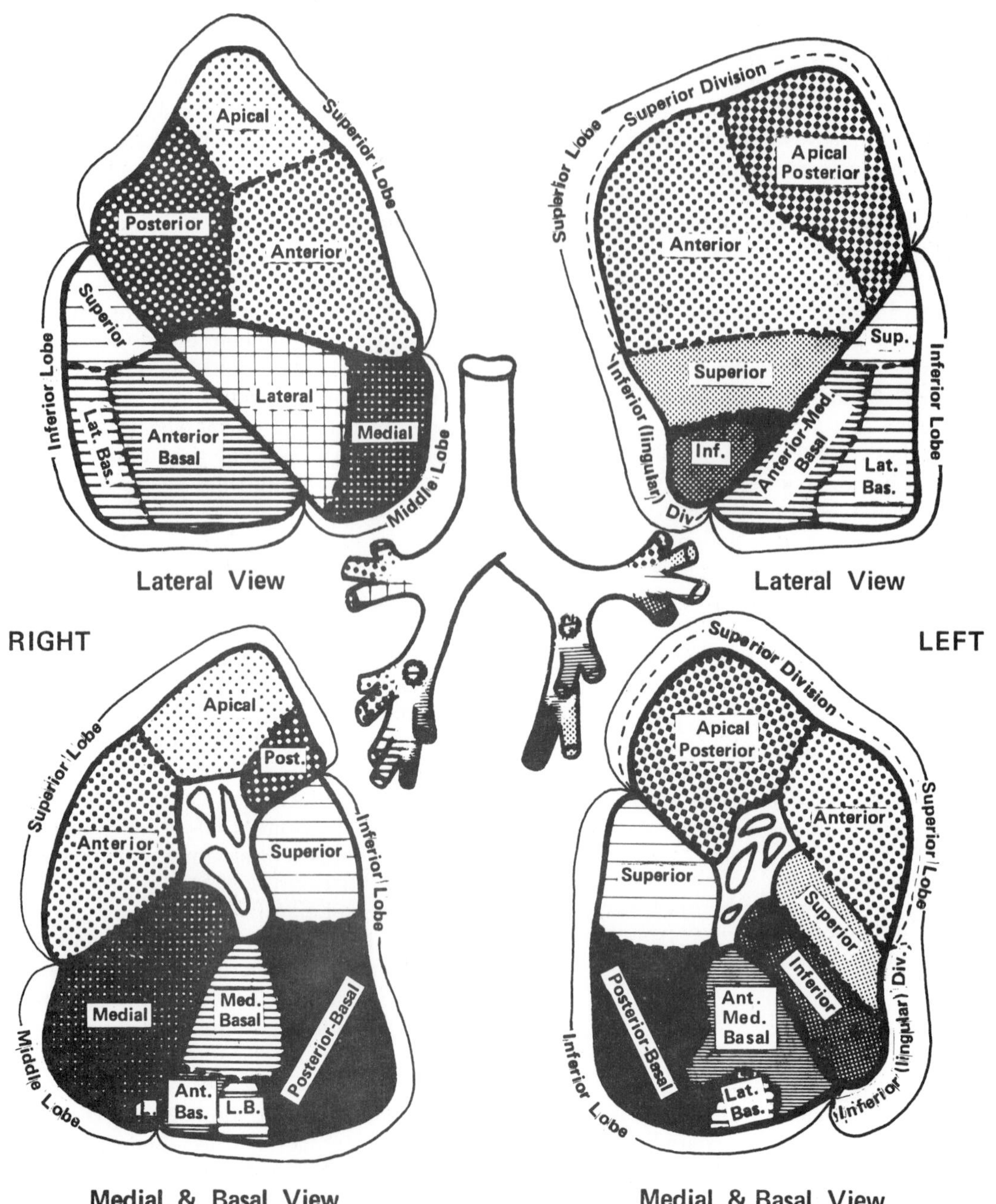

Fig. 26-5. The pulmonary segments.

Vibration is described as a strong, repetitive isometric contraction of shoulder and forearm. This should create effective vibration on the chest wall of an infant, but my clinical impression is that little, if any, effective vibration is achieved isometrically when treating an adult patient. Vibration is probably most effective when done by means of rapid, low-amplitude, repetitive flexion and extension of the elbow with pressure against the chest wall. Even greater benefit may be obtained when percussion is performed with mechanical vibration–percussion instruments, although caution must be used to avoid trauma to the soft tissues of the chest wall.

Special precautions must be taken when performing these procedures in patients who may develop hemoptysis from carcinoma, tuberculosis, lung abscess, or bronchiectasis. Care should also be taken in giving percussion to elderly or very fearful patients. Obviously, percussion and vibration must be modified for recent postoperative cases, avoiding the areas of recent surgery.

The method by which head-down positioning is achieved in the hospital or clinic setting varies greatly. Pillows, electric hospital beds with Trendelenburg positions, tilt tables, slant boards, bed jacks, bed blocks, wedge pillows, and electric rocking beds (polio respirators) are all used. Most therapists find that the use of pillows alone is cumbersome and inadequate for long-term home drainage procedures. If the patient is to continue postural drainage procedures at home, the specific treatment plan and method should be worked out in the institutional setting and its feasibility determined before discharge. It is unrealistic to expect most patients to be conscientious about home programs if they have to "invent the equipment" before doing the treatment procedure.

COUGH TRAINING

Adequate cough is perhaps the most vital factor in sputum management. The inability to cough effectively may mean the difference between adequate and inadequate air exchange, and thus cough stimulation and training are an essential part of patient care. Several factors may impair a patient's ability to cough, including muscular weakness resulting from neurologic or musculoskeletal disease or trauma, weakness secondary to muscular dysfunction as a result of prolonged respirator management, inflammation, and perhaps tracheal or laryngeal stenosis from intubation, pain caused by trauma or surgery, sedation, and structural abnormalities such as bronchiectasis, tracheobronchomegaly, or tracheomalacia.

The ineffective cough is usually highpitched and originates high in the throat and chest. A more effective cough sounds hollow and deep. Proper positioning, support, verbal cues, and stimulation techniques can improve cough effectiveness.

Nonproductive, hacking cough should be discouraged and appropriate measures taken to suppress the cough or to eliminate the source or irritation. The cough in response to obstruction by mucus or other material should be controlled and used effectively. I always discourage the first few hacking coughs that arise during postural drainage or breathing exercises. Patients need to become aware of the difference between "annoyance coughing" and coughing for the purpose of moving sputum. If asked, most patients can discern whether there is something in the upper airways that coughing is likely to dislodge. Pursed-lip breathing and sipping tepid water often reduce the irritation causing nonproductive hacking.

Posture clearly affects the ability to cough. When exertional dyspnea and pain are not limiting factors, the patient should be encouraged to cough in the sitting position. If possible, it is preferable to have the feet supported rather than dangling. The trunk should be flexed slightly forward. If it is not feasible to have the patient sit up, an alternative is to have the patient assume a sidelying position with the hips and knees in flexion. These positions are intended to improve muscular force effectiveness and to prevent muscular strains, particularly in the lower back.

Gentle cricoid cartilage pressure is sometimes effective in stimulating a cough effort. Bilateral manual vibration or quick compression of the lower lateral rib cage is also effective in stimulating cough. When voluntary cough initiation is present but the patient cannot generate the last bit of force needed to clear sputum from the upper airway, one may find it helpful to have the patient pinch his knees and upper thighs together strongly at the instant of his tussive effort. The increase in tension in the pelvic floor thus produced is often effective in generating enough additional flow and force to eject the stubbornly adherent sputum.

The effectiveness with which a person coughs basically depends on the muscular force generated and the velocity of air flow within the airways. Patients with relatively well-preserved flow rates will be able to cough using greater force and higher lung volumes, whereas patients with dynamic airway collapse and poor flow rates will do better coughing from a

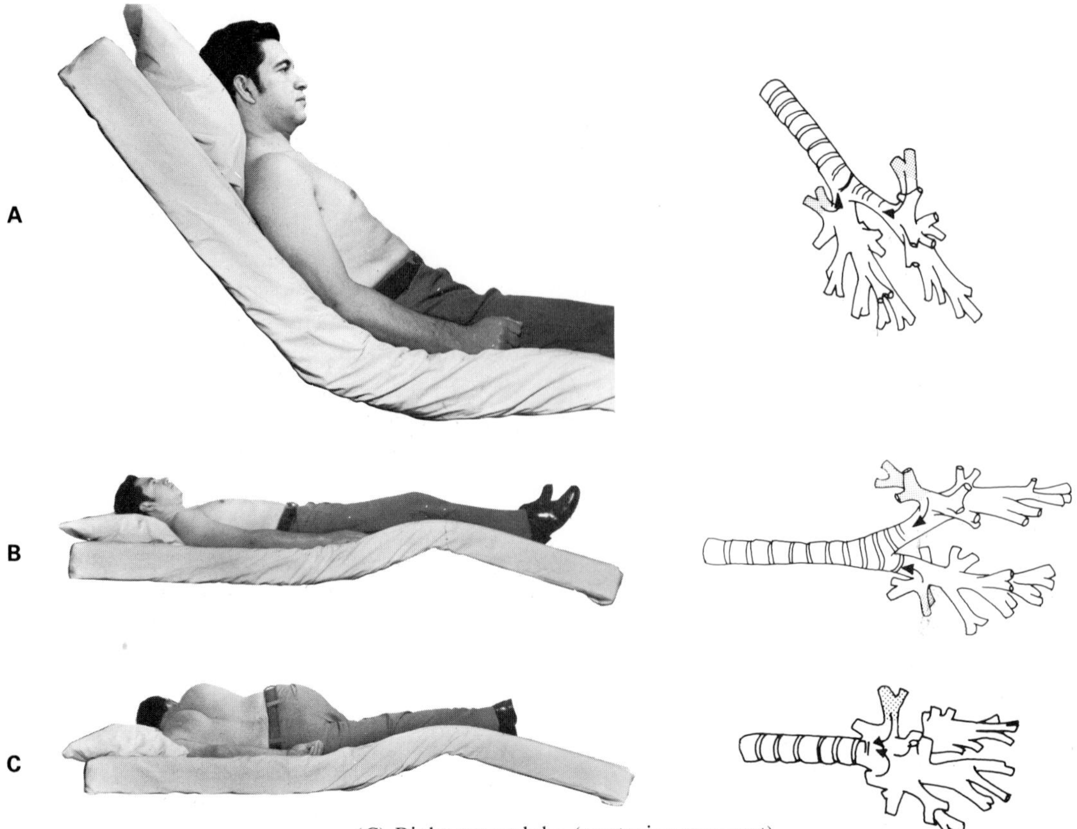

A

B

C

(*C*) Right upper lobe (posterior segment).

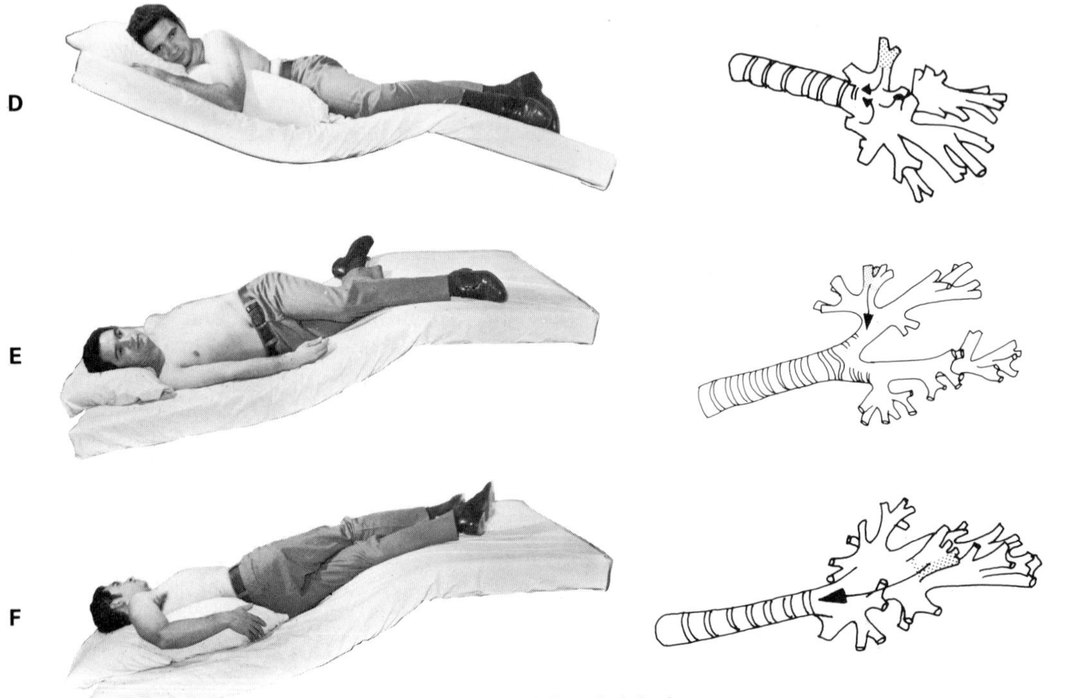

D

E

F

(*F*) Middle lobe of right lung.

Fig. 26-6. *See legend on the opposite page.*

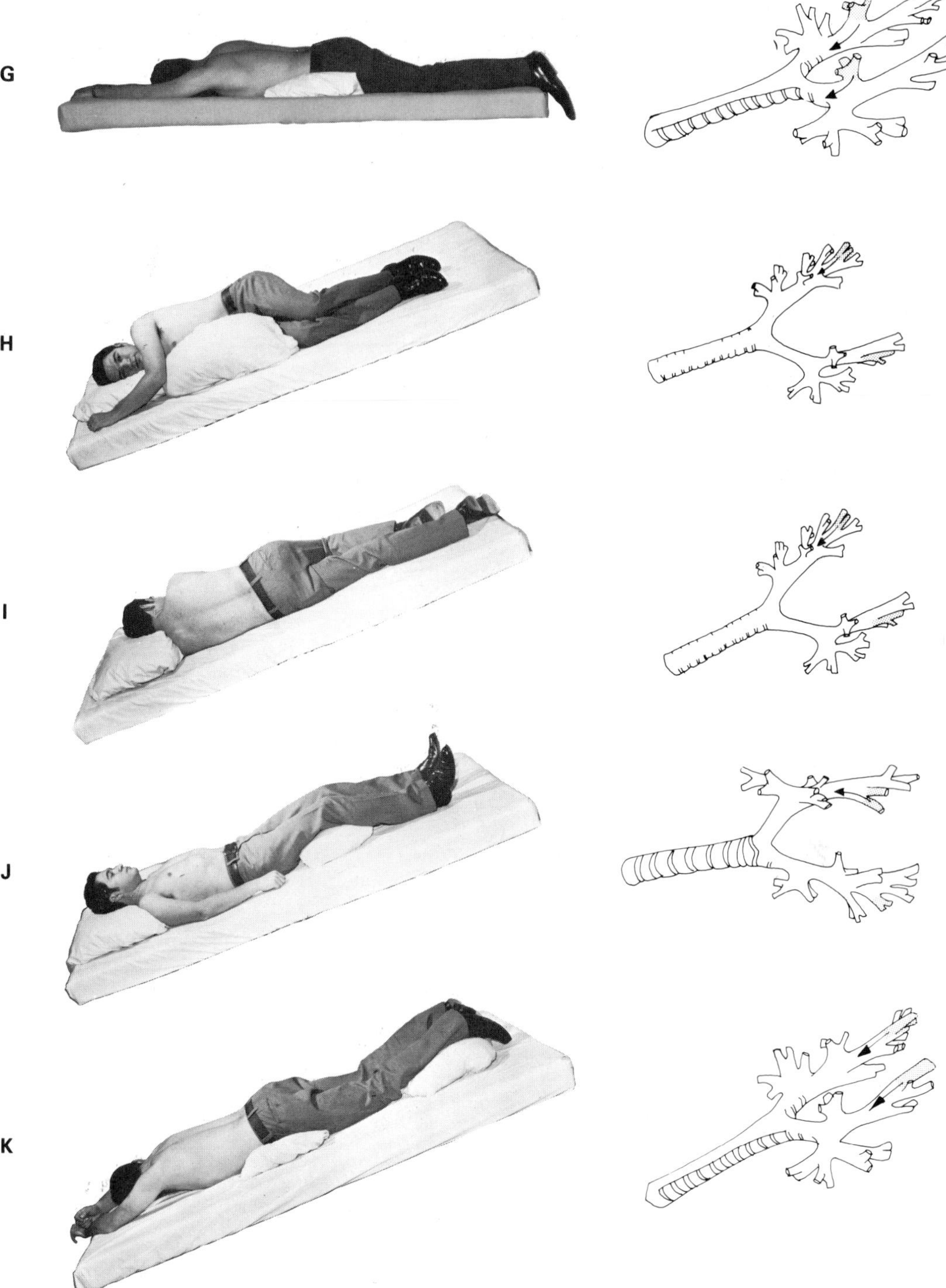

Fig. 26-6. Postural drainage positions for specific pulmonary segments. *(A)* Left and right upper lobes (apical segment). *(B)* Left and right upper lobes (anterior segments). *(C)* Right upper lobe (posterior segment). *(D)* Left upper lobe (posterior segment). *(E)* Left upper lobe (lingular segment). *(F)* Middle lobe of right lung. *(G)* Lower lobe (superior segment), patient lying prone with one pillow under abdomen. *(H)* Left lower lobe (lateral basal segment). *(I)* Left and right lower lobes (anterior basal segments). *(J)* Left and right lower lobes (anterior basal segments). *(K)* Left and right lower lobes (posterior basal segments).

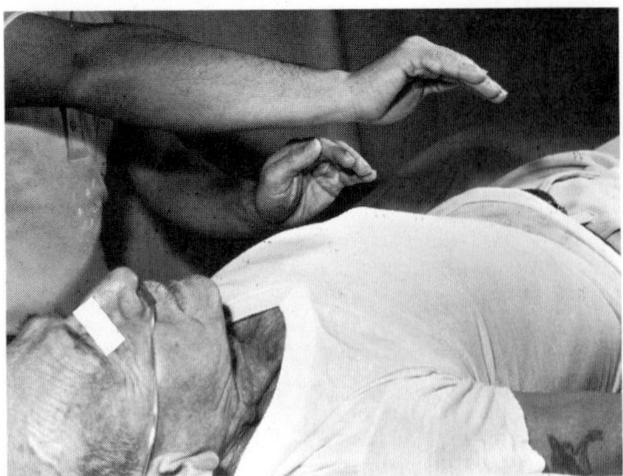

Fig. 26-7. Hand positioning for chest percussion.

midinspiratory position in a staccato rhythm at relatively lower velocities.

It is important that the patient understand that it is air pushing from behind the obstruction that moves it outward. As mentioned before, the therapist should discourage the initial impulse to cough. He should instruct the patient to take two or three deep breaths, followed by relaxed pursed-lip exhalations, and then to inspire to the appropriate depth in relationship to his tendency toward airway collapse, hold his breath very briefly, and then cough explosively, or in a staccato fashion as is individually appropriate. If cough is not productive, the patient should relax, control his dyspnea, improve ventilation by slow deep breathing with pursed-lip exhalation, and, if he still feels that the sputum is "ready," repeat the controlled cough effort.

The therapist should record the amount, color, viscosity, character, and origin (if obvious from segmental drainage position) of sputum ejected. Cough training for the postoperative patient will be discussed in a subsequent section.

PHYSICAL THERAPY ASPECTS OF PREOPERATIVE AND POSTOPERATIVE CARE

Postoperative pulmonary complications are not uncommon and may be extremely dangerous (see Chap. 37). All too commonly in this country, chest physical therapy modalities are used primarily in the postoperative phase or after a pulmonary complication has set in, rather than preoperatively as well.

Some conditions in which chest physical therapy plays an important role include lobectomy, segmental resection, pneumonectomy, thoracoplasty, surgical correction or pectus excavatum, open heart surgery via sternotomy or lateral thoracotomy, radial mastectomy, and upper abdominal surgery.

The goals of chest physical therapy in surgical patients are numerous and often uniquely suited to the therapist's skills. Further, these goals are achievable and generally validated by clinical research. Goals for treatment of the surgery patient include

1. maintaining adequate ventilation and preventing atelectasis;
2. providing adequate bronchial hygiene and preventing or minimizing postoperative pulmonary complications;
3. maintaining or regaining preoperative chest wall mobility;
4. assisting in regaining full expansion of remaining lung tissue;
5. maintaining or regaining mobility of shoulder, shoulder girdle, and spine;
6. preventing postural defects;
7. restoring exercise tolerance;
8. improving circulatory dynamics and venous return to prevent venous thrombosis and emboli; and
9. assisting the patient to return to the greatest possible ADL through general reconditioning efforts.

Thoren found roentgenographic evidence of postoperative atelectasis in 42% of a nontreated control group and 27% of a treatment group where postoperative physical therapy, including deep breathing exercises, was done. He found the incidence of atelectasis to be only 13% in a group treated preoperatively as well as postoperatively.[25]

Bartlett has discussed the physiological rationale of good postoperative respiratory care in Chapter 37. The therapist must use the often brief preoperative session to accomplish several objectives. A sense of rapport, confidence, and appropriate patient education must be developed. The patient should be aware of the site of the proposed incision and the possibility that postoperative pain will make some movements, coughing, and deep breathing difficult and painful. He should be reassured that the therapist will help the patient work through these problems.

Segmental breathing, diaphragmatic breathing, protective coughing, and necessary range of motion exercises should be taught to the patient before surgery so that use of these techniques can begin immediately after surgery. If the patient understands why he must do certain somewhat unpleasant activities, compliance and cooperation will be enhanced.

In the immediate postoperative period, the therapist must reevaluate the patient and review his medical record. Items of particular concern include status of lungs by auscultation and current x-rays; nature of equipment being used postoperatively, such as ventilators, chest tubes, and pumps; and general status variables such as pulse rate, temperature, respiratory rate, and blood pressure and blood gas data.

Treatment in the immediate postoperative period should be directed at the specific goals previously stated, using postural drainage, breathing retraining, and increased mobility and ADL retraining techniques, as previously discussed.

Postoperative coughing may engender both fear and pain. The patient should be positioned so as to minimize traction on the incision site. The therapist, or the patient, may place his hands firmly on either side of the incision to reduce such traction. The careful placement of pillows and flexion of the trunk against a pillow are also helpful.

To avoid forceful coughing, many patients spontaneously adopt a technique called "huffing." This is achieved by breathing in as deeply as possible and then using the expiratory muscles strongly, but without vocal cord closure. This results in a "breathy" forced expiration, as opposed to explosive coughing. In postoperative patients, huffing may be an effective alternative preliminary to coughing but is not an adequate substitute. This practice should be discouraged in patients with obstructive pulmonary disease.

RECONDITIONING EXERCISES

Patients with chronic lung disease are nearly always "out of shape" (physiologically unfit). They have been caught up in a cycle of events starting with dyspnea on exertion, decreased activity level, decreased physiological capacity to handle certain activities, further increase in exertional dyspnea, and finally, further decrease in activities attempted (Fig. 26-8).[1,7]

To appreciate fully the need for, and the value of, a reconditioning program, it is necessary to review some significant physiological concepts. The occurrence of marked physical deconditioning is a natural consequence of the specific physiological impairments inherent in the disease processes. Wasserman and Whipp summarized the problem well, stating that "one of the most disabling effects of heart and lung disease is the decreased maximal rate of oxygen transport and thus the capacity of work and exercise is reduced."[26] The inefficiency of the oxygen transport system in the patient with obstructive disease is seen in the low $\dot{V}O_2$ max levels achieved and the high heart rates for a given workload. The $\dot{V}O_2$ max is compromised secondary to respiratory muscle weakness, narrowed obstructed airways, and destroyed alveoli. In emphysema the increased nonelastic resistance of the lungs contributes to the low $\dot{V}O_2$ max and affects the patient's ability to sustain workloads. Impairment in pulmonary function variables, alteration in arterial blood gas values, impairment in cardiac variables, and alterations in hemodynamic responses such as pulmonary capillary hypertension, shunting, and cor pulmonale all provide the physiological basis for reduced physical work capacity.

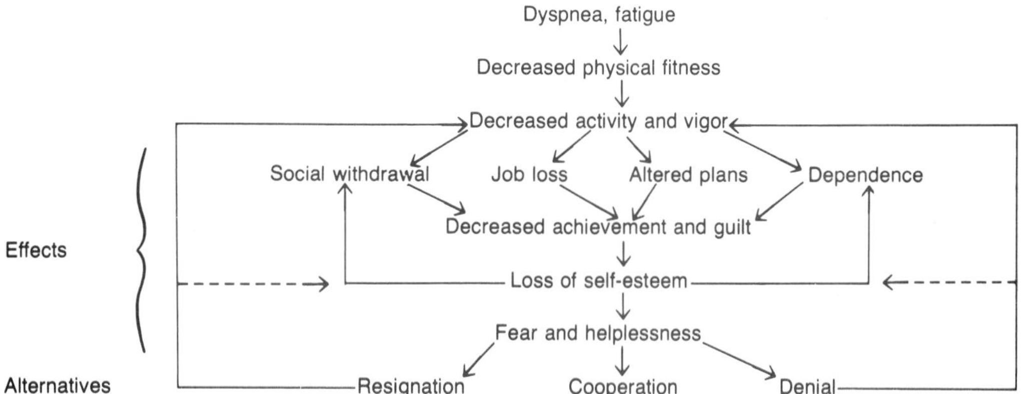

Fig. 26-8. Interaction of physiologic, psychologic, and social variables in patients with chronic pulmonary disease.

The respiratory quotient (RQ) (ratio of the quantity of CO_2 produced to the quantity of O_2 consumed) is also revealing. In normal persons and in patients with COPD, during exercise, as the value approaches R = 1.0, metabolism depends on an anaerobic process and exhaustion is near. Amsterdam states that patients with obstructive pulmonary disease reach exhaustion at RQ values far less than 1.0. This inability of the respiratory system to supply oxygen for aerobic processes is an important determinant of physical work capacity.[2]

Cardiopulmonary efficiency depends on adequately matched airflow and perfusion of blood through the pulmonary capillary bed, intact diffusion process, adequate hemoglobin as a biochemical transport mechanism, and, of course, adequate systemic circulation; left heart function sufficient to circulate oxygenated blood; and right heart function sufficient to distribute blood through open pulmonary capillaries.

The work of breathing is another significant factor that determines the patient's ability to exercise. About 20% of the work of breathing is required to overcome tissue resistance and 80% to overcome airway resistance. At high workloads the cost of ventilation may reach 10% of the total oxygen uptake in normal subjects. The increased airway resistance and decreased compliance inherent in obstructive disease greatly increase the work of breathing. Despite the documented increased work of breathing, oxygen consumption may be normal per unit of external work at submaximal levels, and this is probably achieved at the expense of work not reflected in oxygen uptake. High serum lactate levels suggest that an increased amount of work may be being done anaerobically.[23]

Graded physical fitness-endurance exercise programs are an essential part of overall comprehensive management of patients with pulmonary disease. This aspect of treatment is likely to result in changes that will be easily identified and appreciated by the patient, easily documented, and cost-effective.

Before the implementation of a fitness/endurance exercise program, an exercise evaluation should be done. This evaluation serves to define the patient's exercise tolerance and limiting factors that may not be present or apparent at rest. Pertinent data derived from such testing include the presence of hypoxemia (arterial desaturation), hypercapnia, abnormal blood pressure responses, abnormal heart rhythm, myocardial ischemia, exercise-induced heart failure, and exercise-induced bronchoconstriction.

The exercise evaluation also establishes a baseline from which training can begin and serves as a standard with which future progress can be compared. The use of actual gas samples or the use of nomograms to compute the percentage of predicted $\dot{V}O_2$ max achieved by the patient is also very helpful for evaluating the level of exercise tolerance and for comparison with future test results. This exercise evaluation, including rest and exercise arterial blood gas analysis, is usually performed by the pulmonary physician or other professional and technical personnel.

The physical therapist, as the exercise specialist of the health-care professions, is able to evaluate strength, muscular efficiency of motion, cardiorespiratory fitness, and functinal exercise needs and limitations of each patient. Age and concomitant medical problems may greatly influence the nature and magnitude of the reconditioning program. Conditions such as degenerative arthritis, orthopedic problems, diabetes, hypertension, and cardiac disease will influence the physical therapist's selection and modification of the exercise program.

The exercises will be designed first to accomplish short-term functional goals, such as the patient's achieving independence in self-care activities and sufficient ambulation endurance to meet the demands of his usual environment. Considerable physiological adaptation to exercise demands can be achieved by the patient with pulmonary disease. Buskirk defines physiological adaptation as "any property or response of an organism which favors survival in a stressful environment."[5] Graded exercise conditioning programs for patients with chronic obstructive lung disease undoubtedly improve their "quality of living," although improvement in pulmonary function variables *per se* usually does not occur, nor have studies shown a reduction is overall mortality as a result.

The long-term goal of a fitness-endurance reconditioning program can be defined in relatively precise physiological terms. A review of recent work in the field of exercise physiology is imperative for any respiratory care worker involved in pulmonary rehabilitation.[3,23] As a result of reconditioning exercise training, several physiological adaptations should occur: For a given submaximal workload, after exercise conditioning the heart rate will be lower, systolic blood pressure reduced, and blood flow through working muscles decreased, although muscular O_2 consumption is maintained, as reflected in the arteriovenous O_2 difference. Physical reconditioning produces an increased maximal skeletal blood flow for a given submaximal workload. There also may be an increased number of mitochondria and aerobic enzymes in the trained muscle as well as an improvement of the MVV and $\dot{V}O_2$ max as a result of reconditioning training.[4]

It is generally accepted that muscular and cardiorespiratory fitness, like strength, must (to some degree) be developed for specific tasks. Reconditioning exercises should include upper extremity and trunk activities along with lower extremity exercises such as walking and bicycling.

The previous discussion of exercises for coordination of breathing with functional movements provides the first stage of general reconditioning. These activities can be modified for use in the acute care unit and, when used with increasing resistance and repetition, are valuable for developing specific extremity and cardiorespiratory fitness. Again, exercises should facilitate respiratory control and discourage breath-holding with its potential for producing the Valsalva effect.

Before beginning a physical reconditioning program, one must review the results of the patient's pulmonary function tests, exercise blood gas studies, and his resting and exercise ECG. The need for supplemental oxygen during exercise training will have been assessed, as discussed previously.

The therapist can effectively use data related to the oxygen cost of various activities and work classification scales as a basis for selecting and intensifying the exercise program within the patient's physiological limitations, as defined by his blood gas values, pulmonary function, and cardiac responses (Tables 26-1, 26-2). Additionally, nomograms for predicting the $\dot{V}O_2$ of a given treadmill or bicycle ergometer workload are very useful.

The administration of supplemental oxygen to manage patients with COPD at rest and during exer-

Table 26-1. Physiological Variables in Various Degrees of Physical Exercise*

		Metabolic Rate		Ventilation					
Classification of Work	Pulse *rate/min*	$\dot{V}O_2$ *liters/min*	*Calories/ min*	*Volume* $\dot{V}_E$	*Rate f.*	RQ	Lactic Acid in Multiples of Resting Value	Metabolic Equivalents *mets*	Time That Work Can Be Sustained
Light									
Very light	80	0.5		10.0			Normal	2.5	
Mild	<100	0.5–1.0	<4	10–20	<14	0.85	Normal	2.5–5.0	Indefinite
Moderate	<120	1.0–1.5	<7.5	20–35	<15	0.85	Normal	5.0–7.5	8 hours daily on the job
Optimal	<140	1.5–2.0	<10	35–50	<16	0.90	1.5×	7.5–10.0	8 hours daily for a few weeks (seasonal work, military maneuvers)
Heavy									
Strenuous	<160	2.0–2.5	<12.5	50–65	<20	0.95	2×	10–12.5	4 hours, two or three times a week for a few weeks (special physical training)
Maximal	<180	2.5–3.0	<15	60–86	<25	1.0	5–6×	12.5–15	1 to 2 hours, occasionally (usually in competitive sports)
Severe									
Exhausting	180+	3.0	15+	85	30+	2.0+	6× or more	15.0	A few minutes, rarely

*(Adapted from Parmley LF Jr (ed): Proceedings of the National Workshop on Exercise in the Prevention, Evaluation, and Treatment of Heart Disease. S Car Med Assoc J 65:5, 1969)

Table 26-2. Work Equivalents of Various Activities for a 70-kg Person*

ACTIVITY	CALORIES/ MIN	METABOLIC EQUIV-ALENTS† *mets*	ACTIVITY	CALORIES/ MIN	METABOLIC EQUIV-ALENTS† *mets*
SELF-CARE			HOUSEWORK		
Rest, supine	1.0	1.0	Hand sewing	1.4	1.0
Sitting	1.2	1.0	Sweeping floor	1.7	1.5
Standing, relaxed	1.4	1.0	Machine sewing	1.8	1.5
Eating	1.4	1.0	Polishing furniture	2.4	2.0
Conversation	1.4	1.0	Peeling potatoes	2.9	2.5
Dressing, undressing	2.3	2.0	Scrubbing, standing	2.9	2.5
Washing hands, face	2.5	2.0	Washing small clothes	3.0	2.5
Bedside commode	3.6	3.0	Kneading dough	3.3	2.5
Walking, 2.5 mph	3.6	3.0	Scrubbing floors	3.6	3.0
Showering	4.2	3.5	Cleaning windows	3.7	3.0
Using bedpan	4.7	4.0	Making beds	3.9	3.0
Walking downstairs	5.2	4.5	Ironing, standing	4.2	3.5
Walking, 3.5 mph	5.6	5.5	Mopping	4.2	3.5
Propulsion, wheelchair	2.4	2.0	Wringing by hand	4.4	3.5
Ambulation, braces and crutches	8.0	6.5	Hanging wash	4.5	3.5
			Beating carpets	4.9	4.0
INDUSTRIAL			RECREATIONAL		
Watch repairing	1.6	1.5	Painting, sitting	2.0	1.5
Armature winding	2.2	2.0	Playing piano	2.5	2.0
Radio assembly	2.7	2.5	Driving car	2.8	2.0
Sewing at machine	2.9	2.5	Canoeing, 2.5 mph	3.0	2.5
Bricklaying	4.0	3.5	Horseback riding, slow	3.0	2.5
Plastering	4.1	3.5	Volleyball	3.0	2.5
Tractor ploughing	4.2	3.5	Bowling	4.4	3.5
Wheeling barrow (115 lb, 2.5 mph)	5.0	4.0	Cycling, 5.5 mph	4.5	3.5
			Golfing	5.0	4.0
Horse ploughing	5.9	5.0	Swimming, 20 yd/min	5.0	4.0
Carpentry	6.8	5.5	Dancing	5.5	4.5
Mowing lawn by hand	7.7	6.5	Gardening	5.6	4.5
Felling tree	8.0	6.5	Tennis	7.1	6.0
Shoveling	8.5	7.0	Trotting horse	8.0	6.5
Ascending stairs (17-lb load, 27 ft/min)	9.0	7.5	Spading	8.6	7.0
			Skiing	9.9	8.0
Planing	9.1	7.5	Squash	10.2	8.5
Tending furnace	10.2	8.5	Cycling, 13 mph	11.0	9.0
Ascending stairs (22-lb load, 54 ft/min)	16.2	13.5			

(Cardiac Reconditioning and Work Evaluation Units–Exercise Equivalents. Denver, Colorado Heart Association.)

*Note the surprisingly large energy expenditure of some activities of "early ambulation" (*e.g.,* showering, walking on crutches).

†The approximate resting energy expenditure.

cise began in the early 1950s. Although it is now a well-accepted therapeutic approach in selected patients, the exact mechanism responsible for the subjective and physical work tolerance improvements is not well understood, and a simplistic view of the correction of hypoxemia does not provide the total answer. It is generally accepted that the indications for ambulatory oxygen systems and long-term oxygen therapy include exercise-induced desaturation, overt cor pulmonale, substantial pulmonary hypertension, extreme exercise impairment, and impaired neuropsychiatric functioning in COPD.

When supplemental oxygen during exercise is administered in sufficient quantity to correct hypoxemia without an increase in the Pa_{CO_2}, there tends to be significant relief of exertional dyspnea, decreased heart rate and minute ventilation. A wide variety of portable oxygen systems are available.

Although the physiological mechanism responsible for the improvement in physical work capacity in these patients is not clearly understood, one's clinical experience quickly demonstrates that these improvements are easily documented and clinically significant with regard to an increase in the patient's overall functional level. The literature abounds with research and case studies describing the effects of physical reconditioning programs in patients with COPD. The most significant effects include increased maximal exercise level; improved neuromuscular coordination; heavier workloads that can be sustained for longer periods and frequently with less oxygen consumption; improved use of delivered oxygen; increased motivation; heightened sense of well-being and self-worth; and decreased heart rate, ventilation, O_2 consumption, and CO_2 production for a given workload.

Reconditioning exercise programs for the respiratory patient should follow the same basic principles as do those for patients with cardiac disease. Exercise should be graded and gradually progressed. Activities that require short bursts of energy are inappropriate; each exercise bout should include a warm-up phase, a work or stress phase, and a cool-out phase. Remember, the major goal is to increase exercise tolerance for functional living. The exercise format can use one or more of the traditional approaches such as continuous or interval training. The physical therapist must begin at the level appropriate to the patient's fitness/endurance status. Frequently the patient has such decreased specific muscle strength and endurance that the initial limiting factors to walking, treadmill walking, or bicycling are not cardiopulmonary symptoms but muscle fatigue and pain. An interval training approach using low- to moderate-intensity workloads is often the most appropriate. Therefore the use of 2- or 3-minute work phases followed by rest periods and repeated to tolerance provides a beginning point. Exercise time is increased as exercise tolerance improves, and eventually continuous exercise training can become the training mode.

The reconditioning process should include exercises for increasing strength and endurance of large muscle groups; upper extremities; trunk musculature; and the lower extremities. The integration and coordination of the patient's total program into his reconditioning routine must be carefully considered. It is essential that optimal timing of bronchial hygiene and the administration of medications, particularly bronchodilators, be achieved to gain maximum benefit from the exercise training sessions. Once an optimal pattern in terms of sequence and timing has been established, it should be communicated to the patient so that he will understand the interrelationships of the various aspects of his care and can follow through in his home program.

As part of the education of the patient, one must give him guidelines so that he may judge whether his home reconditioning program is adequate or whether he is overdoing or underdoing. Most patients tend to anticipate the onset of dyspnea and are concerned that dyspnea may be a signal that they are causing further damage to their lungs. It must be made clear that shortness of breath is an indication of the work of breathing and occurs in normal subjects as well as in patients with COPD. The patient should be taught to use breathing control techniques, as described previously, and to evaluate objectively his level of dyspnea and the time required for him to return to his resting level. It is also useful for the therapist to attempt to objectify the subjective reports from the patient that he is becoming short of breath during an exercise session. Use of a grading scale as described in Chapter 13 can provide a more quantified estimation of disability.

The patient who has participated in a supervised physical reconditioning program will have been evaluated about his heart rate, dyspnea, and blood pressure responses to given exercise workloads. This allows the physical therapist to give the patient physiologically based and safe guidelines on heart rate, walking speeds, grades, bicycling intensity, dyspnea, and length of exercise periods to be used in his ongoing home reconditioning program. It must also be made clear to the patient that he must carry out his reconditioning program at least every other day to maintain the physiological benefit.

The signs of poor physiological response to exercise are numerous and should be documented and reported to the referring physician.

1. Decline in heart rate with exercise
2. Failure of heart rate to increase appropriate to workload
3. Drop in, or failure of, systolic blood pressure to raise appropriately to workload
4. Significant increase in hypoxemia (e.g., cyanosis)
5. Significant retention of CO_2
6. Tachycardia inappropriate to workload, or development of cardiac arrhythmias
7. Tachypnea
8. Severe dyspnea
9. Severe diaphoresis
10. Dizziness
11. Decline in mental acuteness
12. Physical incoordination
13. Ataxia
14. Visual disturbances

The selection of equipment to use in a reconditioning program will depend on space, cost, and treatment philosophy. Therapists should avoid overdependence on treadmills and bicycles. These are excellent tools by which a safe, progressive, and well-documented exercise program can be provided, but there is not an absolute carry-over of activity levels achieved on a treadmill or bicycle with work performed on level grades or inclines, and exercise conditioning should include ample walking exercise in a home- and community-like environment while the patient is still in the hospital.

Frequently environmental factors such as cold, snow, rain, wind, and air pollution prohibit the patient's outdoor walking program. Alternatives such as stationary bicycling and the use of indoor shopping malls should be explored.

SUMMARY

Chest physical therapy is a challenging specialty area that requires the therapist to integrate various physiological, neuromuscular, and kinesiological parameters. There remains a tremendous need for clinical and physiological research so that optimal treatment may be intelligently applied to the vast population of respiratory patients.

REFERENCES

1. ACCP Scientific Committee Report: Pulmonary rehabilitation. Bull Am Coll Chest Physicians 14:35, 1975
2. Amsterdam EA: Exercise in Cardiovascular Health and Disease. New York, Yorke Medical Books, 1977
3. Astrand PO: Textbook of Work Physiology. New York, McGraw–Hill, 1970
4. Belman MJ: Ventilatory muscle training improves exercise capacity in C.O.P.D. patients. Am Rev Respir Dis 121:273, 1980
5. Buskirk E: Cardiovascular adaptation to physical effort in healthy men. In Naughton JP et al (eds): Exercise Testing and Exercise Training in Coronary Heart Disease. New York, Academic Press, 1973
6. Danon J, Sharp JT, Druz WS et al: Effects of increased functional residual capacity upon inspiratory muscle function. Am Rev Respir Dis 105:1017, 1972
7. Fishman DB, Petty TL: Physical, symptomatic, and psychological improvement in patients receiving comprehensive care for chronic airway obstruction. J Chronic Dis 24:775, 1971
8. Gimenez M: Exercise training with oxygen supply and directed breathing in patients with chronic airway obstruction. Respiration 37:157, 1979
9. Gross D: Electromyographic patterns of diaphragmatic fatigue. J Appl Physiol 46, No. 1:1, 1979
10. Hodgkin JE: The scientific status of chest physiotherapy. Respir Care 26:657, 1981
11. Howell JBL: Breathlessness in pulmonary disease. In Howell JBL, Campbell EJM (eds): Breathlessness. Oxford, Blackwell Scientific, 1966
12. Ingram RH, Schilder DP: The effects of pursed lip expiration on the pulmonary pressure-flow relationship in obstructive lung disease. Am Rev Respir Dis 96:381, 1967
13. Knott M, Voss DE: Proprioceptive Neuromuscular Facilitation: Patterns and Techniques. 2nd ed. New York, Harper & Row, 1968
14. Leiberman DA: Adaptation of guinea pig diaphragm muscle to aging and endurance training. Am J Physiol 222:556, 1972
15. Macklem PT: Respiratory muscles: The vital pump. Chest 78:5, 1980
16. Mellins RB: Pulmonary physiotherapy in the pediatric age group. Am Rev Respir Dis (Suppl), 110:137, 1974
17. Miller WF: A physiologic evaluation of the effects of diaphragmatic breathing training in patients with chronic pulmonary emphysema. Am J Med 17:471, 1954
18. Mueller RE, Petty TL, Filley GF: Ventilation and arterial blood gas changes induced by pursed lip breathing. J Appl Physiol 28:784, 1970
19. Pardy RL: The effects of inspiratory muscle training on exercise performance. Am Rev Respir Dis 123:426, 1981
20. Pham QT et al: Pulmonary function and rheologic status of bronchial secretions collected by spontaneous expectorations and after physiotherapy. Bull Physiopathol Respir 9:293, 1973
21. Shapiro BA: Chest physical therapy administered by respiratory therapists. Respir Care 26:655, 1981

22. Sharp JT: Respiratory muscles: A review of old and new concepts. Lung 157:185, 1980
23. Shuey CB: An evaluation of exercise tests in chronic obstructive lung disease. J Appl Physiol 27:256, 1969
24. Thoman RL, Stoker GL, Ross JC: The efficacy of pursed-lip breathing in patients with chronic obstructive pulmonary disease. Am Rev Respir Dis 93:100, 1966
25. Thoren L: Postoperative pulmonary complications: Observations on their prevention by means of physiotherapy. Acta Chir Scan 107:193, 1975
26. Wasserman K, Whipp BJ: Exercise physiology in health and disease. Am Rev Respir Dis 112:219, 1975

BIBLIOGRAPHY

General

Conference on the Scientific Basis of Respiratory Therapy. Am Rev Respir Dis 105:129, 1972

Gaskell DV, Webber BA: The Bromptom Hospital Guide to Chest Physiotherapy, 2nd ed. Oxford, Blackwell Scientific, 1974

Pulmonary Rehabilitation

Community resources for rehabilitation of patients with chronic obstructive pulmonary diseases and cor pulmonale. Report of Inter-Society Commission for Heart Disease Resources. Circulation 49:A1, May 1974

Hodgkin JE et al: Chronic obstructive airway diseases: Current concepts in diagnosis and comprehensive care. JAMA 232:1243, 1975

Petty TL: Pulmonary rehabilitation. Basics of RD 4, No. 1, September 1975 (available from the American Thoracic Society)

Self-Study Materials for Patients

Modrak M: Better Living and Breathing: A Manual for Patients. St Louis, CV Mosby, 1975

Petty TL, Nett LM: For Those Who Live and Breathe. A Manual for Patients with Emphysema and Chronic Bronchitis, 2nd ed. Springfield IL, Charles C Thomas, 1972

27

Pulmonary Rehabilitation

Alan R. Yee • John E. Hodgkin
Eileen G. Zorn • David L. McLean

Over the past several decades, the treatment of patients with chronic debilitating respiratory disease has become of increasing interest to pulmonary specialists. As understanding of the pathophysiology and treatment of pulmonary disease increased, it became evident that these patients could best be cared for by specialists with a knowledge of the unique problems of *chronically* ill pulmonary patients. Although some aspects of pulmonary rehabilitation may be useful for patients with various chronic respiratory diseases, rehabilitation is most helpful for those with chronic obstructive pulmonary disease (COPD)—for example, emphysema, chronic bronchitis, bronchial asthma, and bronchiectasis. Of concern is the control or alleviation of the symptoms and pathophysiological complications of respiratory impairment as well as teaching of the patient how to achieve optimal ability for carrying out activities of daily living.[26] Pulmonary rehabilitation should not be viewed as only a treatment of the patient with end-stage lung disease but as an important part of good care for all patients with impairment of function from pulmonary disease. It includes not only palliative care but also preventive medicine.

ECONOMIC IMPACT OF COPD

The cost of COPD is excessive in terms of lives affected as well as money spent. In the mid 1970s, about 14 million Americans were diagnosed as having COPD, and COPD accounted for about 10% of hospital admissions.[18] These patients had disease ranging in severity from mild to severe. The mortality rate was 19 per 100,000 population,[47] with COPD being fifth among the top 15 causes of death in adults (Table 27-1).[54]

In 1979, the Social Security Administration estimated that approximately 190,000 persons under the age of 65 had received disability benefits because of COPD. These payments totaled some $900 million. In addition, about 90,000 persons "disabled" from respiratory disease were removed from the disabled category because they had now reached the age of 65. Some $350 million was paid to these retired persons in 1979 from the Old Age and Survivor's Insurance Trust Fund.*

The economic impact from the care of patients with emphysema and chronic bronchitis was estimated in 1977 to total about $5.7 billion and for patients with asthma, $1.5 billion.[47]

Although one can obtain statistical data on the economic impact of COPD, the total cost of COPD to the patients themselves cannot be measured. The emotional, physical, and social losses that people experience must also be considered. If a person loses his

*Lerner P: Personal communication. Social Security Administration, 1980

Table 27-1. Death Rates for 15 Leading Causes of Death: United States, 1980[54]

RANK	CAUSE OF DEATH	DEATH RATE (PER 100,000)	PERCENTAGE OF TOTAL DEATHS
....	All causes	892.6	100.0
1	Diseases of heart	343.0	38.4
2	Malignant neoplasms, including neoplasms of lymphatic and hematopoietic tissues	186.3	20.9
3	Cerebrovascular diseases	76.6	8.6
4	Accidents and adverse effects	47.9	5.4
....	Motor vehicle accidents	24.4	2.7
....	All other accidents and adverse effects	23.5	2.6
5	Chronic obstructive pulmonary diseases and allied conditions	25.1	2.8
6	Pneumonia and influenza	23.7	2.7
7	Diabetes mellitus	15.4	1.7
8	Chronic liver disease and cirrhosis	14.1	1.6
9	Atherosclerosis	13.4	1.5
10	Suicide	12.7	1.4
11	Homicide and legal intervention	11.3	1.3
12	Certain conditions originating in the perinatal period	10.1	1.1
13	Nephritis, nephrotic syndrome, and nephrosis	7.8	0.9
14	Congenital anomalies	6.2	0.7
15	Septicemia	4.1	0.5
....	All other causes	94.9	10.6

job through dyspnea and is no longer the "breadwinner," there can also be a loss of self-respect and self-confidence. There is a potential lowering of ego strength when one changes from being a functioning, contributing member of society and the family to one who is dependent on others. This can often lead to depression and withdrawal, with further loss of self-respect. The effect this stress has on a person, his family, and friends can be much more significant than the actual loss in dollars and cents.

DEFINITION

The concept of rehabilitation is not new. In 1942, the Council on Rehabilitation defined rehabilitation "as the restoration of the individual to the fullest medical, mental, emotional, social, and vocational potential of which he/she is capable."

Pulmonary rehabilitation is not only concerned with control of symptoms and disease but also with promotion and maintenance of health. Rehabilitation is a process whereby a change in a patient hopefully reflects a movement toward health and an increased level of wellness.

Patients must understand their rehabilitative potential so that they have the information needed for decision-making. Rehabilitation helps the person to identify his "assets and liabilities" as well as his available avenues for change. Rehabilitation must have a purpose for each individual involved in the program.

The American College of Chest Physicians has adopted the following definition of pulmonary rehabilitation.

> An art of medical practice wherein an individually tailored multidisciplinary program is formulated, which, through accurate diagnosis, therapy, emotional support, and education, stabilizes or reverses both the physio- and psychopathology of pulmonary diseases and attempts to return the individual to the highest possible functional capacity allowed by his pulmonary handicap and overall life situation.[41]

As pointed out in the recent official American Thoracic Society Statement on Pulmonary Rehabilitation,[46] "in the broadest sense, pulmonary rehabilitation means providing good, comprehensive respiratory care for patients with pulmonary disease."

RESOURCES FOR DELIVERY OF A REHABILITATION PROGRAM

The number and type of personnel needed for a pulmonary rehabilitation program vary from one facility to another. To provide good rehabilitation, one does not necessarily have to be in a university setting or a large tertiary hospital. None of the resources discussed in this chapter is beyond that available to the clinician in private practice.

The key member of any rehabilitation team is, of course, the patient; the patient should be the focus of any rehabilitation program. It is the patient's understanding of his own disease and his individual goals that help modify how the program is administered. For each patient the rehabilitation program must be individualized, as consideration is given to such things as background, family situation, vocation, and level of education.

Some rehabilitation programs simply comprise a physician with a nurse or therapist. Others use a multidisciplinary team, which may include a physician, nurse, respiratory therapist, cardiopulmonary technologist, physical therapist, psychiatrist or psychologist, social worker, occupational therapist, vocational rehabilitation specialist, recreational therapist, dietician, and chaplain. Not all members of a multidisciplinary team will be needed for each patient, although their services should be available if needed. A physician in private practice can refer patients with specific needs to these individuals, if necessary. The services of one allied health area may be provided by another member of the team if the person is knowledgeable in that area. Table 27-2 lists the services that should be available for patients undergoing pulmonary rehabilitation, even though not all patients with COPD will need all these services.

A physician with a well-trained pulmonary nurse or therapist can be very effective. The quantity of allied health professionals is not important to the patient, but rather their dedication, knowledge, and concern. Multidisciplinary teams are particularly appropriate, however, if large numbers of patients are referred and for teaching or research purposes.[46]

Pulmonary rehabilitation programs may either be inpatient, outpatient, or a combination of both. Inpatient programs may last anywhere from 1 to 2 weeks, and they usually allow for intensive instruction, education, and exercise training in a controlled environment. They are particularly convenient for patients who live a great distance from the facility and those who are deteriorating rapidly. Outpatient programs generally cost less than half of most inpatient programs. They can be arranged around a patient's job responsibilities, but compliance with the program may be diminished because of less constant supervision. Some programs provide home care services for the respiratory patient, which can greatly assist with follow-up care. These services can be provided directly by the rehabilitation program itself or in cooperation with a local visiting nurses' association.

Table 27-2. Pulmonary Rehabilitation Services[46]

ESSENTIAL SERVICES

- Initial medical evaluation and care plan
- Patient education, evaluation, and program coordination
- Respiratory therapy techniques
- Physical therapy techniques, including exercise conditioning
- Daily performance evaluation
- Social service evaluation
- Nutritional evaluation

ADDITIONAL SERVICES

- Psychological evaluation
- Psychiatric evaluation
- Vocational evaluation

SEQUENCE OF CARE

An appropriate sequence of care should be followed for patients in a pulmonary rehabilitation program (Table 27-3).[13,46]

Several factors reportedly affect the ultimate success or lack thereof of a patient in a pulmonary rehabilitation program. For those COPD patients with moderate to moderately severe disease, the benefits of a rehabilitation program may be greater than in those with very mild or very severe disease. The presence of other coexisting disabling diseases such as heart disease, cancer, or severe arthritis may make a patient unable to obtain much benefit from a rehabilitation program. Some of the other factors that may affect the success of the rehabilitation program are the age of the patient, intelligence,[15] and occupation. Those patients with good family support and strong personal motivation[24] would probably have greater potential for success than would those who do not. With these multiple factors, the major consideration is whether the patient is symptomatic. It would therefore be very appropriate to consider any symptomatic COPD patient for pulmonary rehabilitation.

Table 27-3. Sequence of a Pulmonary Rehabilitation Program[46]

1. Patient selection
2. Initial evaluation
3. Determine goals
4. Outline components of a pulmonary rehabilitation program
5. Assessment of patient's progress
6. Long-term follow-up

INITIAL EVALUATION

The initial evaluation of a patient should include a thorough history and physical examination, chest x-ray, pulmonary function tests, an electrocardiogram, and, when indicated, arterial blood gas analysis, sputum examination, and blood theophylline levels.[46] This initial assessment helps to establish a baseline for determining a patient's response to treatment.

A psychosocial evaluation can assist health professionals in determining the patient's and family's attitudes about the disease. The psychosocial assessment should review such things as the patient's family and other relationships, financial status, and life-style. After this information has been collected, possible psychosocial problems can be ascertained. Psychological tests that assess such things as the impact of the illness on the patient, his moods and attitudes, and stress as measured by recent life changes may also be used to evaluate the patient.

It is critical that a psychosocial assessment be included in every examination of the patient with chronic lung disease since the disease is often characterized by anxiety, social withdrawal, and low self-esteem. These patients often need immediate attention to these problems with the same amount of concern as is directed to shortness of breath and bronchospasm.

DETERMINATION OF GOALS

Short- and long-term goals should be established after the initial evaluation. The goals established must be attainable and tailored to the level of impairment, extent of disease, patient's personality, physical ability, and life-style. The patient must be able to express his own expectations and, along with the respiratory rehabilitation group, establish reasonable goals.

The immediate goal of any program is to alleviate and to control acute symptoms in the patient. This may be accomplished primarily by medications. For the setting of long-range goals, the patient should be intimately involved. Long-range goals should include improving the patient's capacity to carry out activities of daily living with regard to his life-style and teaching him how to evaluate his episodes of dyspnea so that he may avoid or minimize them in the future. By understanding his disease process, the patient can lessen the frequency of exacerbations. The purpose of rehabilitation is to decrease reliance on others and to promote independence in the patient.

COMPONENTS OF A PULMONARY REHABILITATION PROGRAM

PATIENT EDUCATION

The goals of patient education include helping the patient gain better control of his symptoms, promoting health and wellness, and reducing anxiety.[38] A proper understanding of how a patient and his family relate to the disease and its limitations is helpful in educating the patient. Behavior that demonstrates a step toward improving or maintaining health should be rewarded. This positive reinforcement should encourage more desired behavior. Attainable goals should be the focus of the educational program. By successfully completing minimal skills initially, the patient will also gain more confidence to allow him to attempt more complicated behaviors later.

Some basic principles of learning that should be considered when implementing an educational program for patients include the following.

1. The capacity of the person being educated—for example, his educational background—must be established to help define the learner.
2. The intrinsically motivated person tends to learn better.
3. Learning is facilitated by reward.
4. People need practice in setting up goals for themselves. Without practice, their goal-setting may be too low or unrealistically high.
5. Active participation rather than passive reception encourages learning.
6. Material presented should be meaningful.
7. Individual learners need to have opportunity to practice skills.
8. The learner must understand what entails "good results" as well as what constitutes a "mistake."

9. Experience should be provided for the learner to apply his learning.
10. The learner should be able to discover relationships between what is learned and himself.
11. The individual learner should also have opportunities to test his recall of pertinent information.

The environment provided for the individual's learning should be an "open" one that encourages the asking of questions, enhances self-confidence, and fosters independence. Health education should be designed to promote *patient compliance* as much as possible. The educational material must explain the need for, as well as the importance of, compliance. Consideration should be given to misconceptions that the person already has learned, and efforts should be made to "unlearn" these misconceptions early in the educational process.

A problem common to the treatment of many chronic diseases is the failure of patients to adhere to regimens known to be beneficial. One reason is the discouraging prospect of lifelong adherence to a regimen, or lifelong change in previously established behavior patterns or life-styles. Davis estimated, in 1966, that about 30% to 35% of patients fail to follow medical recommendations.[16]

Researchers have explored reasons for noncompliant, as well as for compliant, behavior. Contradictory data have emerged, and, as yet, many questions have not been fully answered. Until a clearer picture develops regarding the factors that influence compliance, we should continue measuring compliance with the "tools" available—serum drug levels, pill counts, keeping appointments, and patient reports—and wait for information to emerge that will help us become more effective. Common sense suggests that continuity in care may help eliminate factors that contribute to noncompliance. Evaluation of the possible causes of the noncompliant act should be accomplished in an effort to remove as many distracting items as possible so that the patient can be free to follow a path to optimal health and well-being.

Several components of the Health Belief Model[48] are thought to affect one's compliance.

1. The individual's belief in his susceptibility to the disease
2. His feelings about the severity of the disease
3. The person's understanding of benefits of the treatment program
4. The patient's understanding of certain "clues" to action that make the individual aware of his health beliefs and need to act
5. His belief in the value of good health

GENERAL

An important factor in the general management of a patient with COPD is the avoidance of smoking.[11] There has been some evidence that the course of COPD may be altered if the patient with very early airway obstruction stops smoking.[21] Encouraging the patient to stop smoking should be an integral part of any treatment program. Many times it takes more than just an encouraging word from the physician to help a patient stop smoking; there are many different types of smokers,[24] and the physician should work with the patient to help him find the smoking cessation technique best suited for him. Assistance from an individual's family in helping him to quit smoking should be used whenever possible.

Patients should avoid air pollution and other inhaled irritants as much as possible. Persons with respiratory tract infections should be avoided whenever possible. Large crowds should be avoided when respiratory infections are prevalent. Consideration should be given to such environmental factors as temperature, humidity, and altitude.

Extremes of temperature and humidity can aggravate airway obstruction. The use of air conditioners, humidifiers, and filtering systems may be helpful. High altitude can cause significant lowering of the Pa_{O_2}. Commercial airliners are pressurized at the equivalent of 5000 to 8000 feet elevation and may also cause serious hypoxemia. Adequate hydration should be maintained in an attempt to liquefy airway secretions. An influenza immunization should be given yearly, whereas present recommendations call for pneumococcal vaccine only once in a lifetime.

MEDICATIONS

Medications are an important component in the treatment program for patients with COPD. Medications are useful in achieving the short-range goal of relieving symptoms but should be combined with other therapeutic modalities as part of a comprehensive respiratory care program. With the large amount of medications given to COPD patients, care must be taken to avoid cross-reactions. One should also schedule medications and other treatments so that they do not disrupt the patient's life-style. It is important to coordinate activities of daily living, including exercise, with the patient's medication program. Inhaling bronchodilator a few minutes before activity may improve the patient's ability to be active by reversing or preventing bronchospasm.

Of the several categories of medications commonly used in respiratory patients, most commonly used are the bronchodilators. There are two major types: the methylxanthines and the sympathomimetic preparations. Prescribing the long-acting anhydrous theophylline preparations maintains constant blood levels, with the additional advantage of less frequent administration. The therapeutic theophylline blood level is 10 to 20 μg/ml. Beta sympathomimetic agents are available for use by both the oral and aerosol routes, with the beta-2 type agents being preferred. Parenteral sympathomimetic preparations and methylxanthines are usually reserved for hospitalized patients with an exacerbation of their lung disease.

Broad-spectrum antibiotics (ampicillin, amoxicillin, tetracycline, trimethoprim–sulfamethoxazole) are used during episodes of acute bronchitis. Corticosteroids can be given either orally or by aerosolized preparation and are indicated in patients with intermittent bronchospasm whose symptoms are not controlled by bronchodilators. Other medications that are sometimes useful in patients with COPD include diuretics, cromolyn sodium, psychopharmacologic agents (Table 27-4), and digitalis. When used appropriately, these drugs are all very helpful; they do, however, have side-effects that may lead to worsening of the patient's condition if not used appropriately. Chapters 20 and 31 discuss the use of medications in patients with respiratory disease.

RESPIRATORY THERAPY MODALITIES

Respiratory therapy provides several modalities of benefit for the patient with obstructive lung disease, including aerosol therapy, intermittent positive pressure breathing, and oxygen therapy.

Inhalation of bronchodilators is particularly effective because it results in a quick response with minimal systemic side-effects as compared with the oral route. Aerosolization of bronchodilators may be accomplished by inexpensive cartridge inhalers, hand-bulb nebulizers, or compressor pump nebulizers. Intermittent positive pressure breathing is also used for aerosolization of bronchodilators, although there are little data that it works more effectively than other methods available for aerosolization of bronchodilators. The NIH collaborative study comparing IPPB and compressor nebulizers in outpatients with COPD[27] did not demonstrate any advantage for IPPB therapy. Although aerosolization of bland mist is sometimes used in patients with thick secretions, there is little evidence of its efficacy in the liquification of lower airway secretions.

When low-flow oxygen is used in COPD patients who have prominent hypoxemia, there is improvement in psychological testing, motor coordination, exercise tolerance, and sleep patterns.[7,8,33] One report suggests that supplemental oxygen for at least 15 hours a day may delay the onset of pulmonary hypertension and cor pulmonale in the COPD patient.[51] In the recently concluded NIH cooperative Nocturnal Oxygen Therapy Trial, 203 patients with COPD with either a Pa_{O_2} of 55 mm Hg or less or a Pa_{O_2} of less than 60 mm Hg plus either polycythemia or evidence of cor pulmonale were randomly allocated to continuous oxygen therapy or 12-hour nocturnal oxygen therapy. The results show that mortality in the nocturnal oxygen therapy group after at least 12 months of follow-up was nearly twice that seen in the continuous oxygen therapy group.[14]

Although the use of low-flow oxygen is important in patients with COPD, increasing the Pa_{O_2} above 60 mm Hg may remove the hypoxic drive and lead to increased hypoventilation and a worsening of respiratory acidosis when the patient also has concomitant chronic CO_2 retention.

Basically three oxygen systems are available for home use. Metal cylinders that store gaseous oxygen at high pressures come in various sizes. A large "H" cylinder can be used as a stationary oxygen source (Fig. 27-1), and various small cylinders are available for portable use (Fig. 27-2). Some small cylinders come with adaptors so the patient can easily refill them from the large cylinder.

Liquid oxygen systems have the advantage of occupying less space than does gaseous oxygen, when comparing equivalent deliverable volumes. One can store, for example, 860 times as much liquid oxygen in the same amount of space as gaseous oxygen. Liquid systems come with portable "walkers" that are lightweight and can be refilled easily from the main reservoir (Fig. 27-3).

Recently, oxygen concentrators have become available (Fig. 27-4). Oxygen concentrators use a compressor that draws room air through a molecular sieve, filtering out most of the nitrogen molecules and "leaving behind" high-concentration (about 95%) oxygen. A flowmeter and oxygen humidifier similar to those used with cylinders and liquid oxygen systems are

(Text continues on p. 690)

Table 27-4. Psychopharmacologic Agents Used in Patients with Chronic Obstructive Pulmonary Disease

SPECIFIC MEDICATION	INDICATIONS	SPECIAL PROPERTIES	USUAL DAILY DOSE (ORAL) *mg*	DAILY DOSE IN MODERATE TO SEVERE COPD (ORAL) *mg*
ANXIOLYTIC AGENTS (Minor Tranquilizers)*				
Benzodiazepines				
Chlordiazepoxide (Librium)	Anxiety that is impending specific behaviors such as sleep, exercise, social interactions. Some cases of insomnia.	Poor absorption by the intramuscular route. For many the drug of choice in alcohol withdrawal.	10–200	10–100
Diazepam (Valium)	Same as for chlordiazepoxide	Poor absorption by the intramuscular route. Good muscular relaxant.	5–50	5–10
Clorazepate (Tranxene)	Same as for chlordiazepoxide.	Wide dose selection.	3.75–45	3.75–15
Glycerol Derivatives				
Meprobamate (Miltown, Equanil)	Not recommended. If used, same as chlordiazepoxide.	May have low safety factor with overdose as compared to other anxiolytic agents.	400–1600	200–800

Diphenylmethane Derivatives				
Hydroxyzine (Atarax, Vistaril)	Same as for chlordiazepoxide.	Antihistamine. Low abuse potential compared with other anxiolytic agents. Atropine-like side-effects.	25–200	10–100

(Dudley DL, Glaser EM, Jorgenson B et al: Psychosocial concomitants to rehabilitation in chronic obstructive pulmonary disease. Chest 77:677, 1980)

*Barbiturates produce unacceptable central nervous system depression, sedation, dependency, and addiction risk and have a low safety margin compared to the medications listed above, with the exception of meprobamate. For all anxiolytics listed, drowsiness or lack of attention may make operation of machinery dangerous. This is particularly so during initial treatment. Selected patients may need the usual daily dose. Respiratory depression with aggravation or onset of hypoxia and hypercarbia is always a possible complication when anxiolytic agents are used in patients with COPD.

Common Side-Effects	Precautions With	Contraindications
• Drowsiness • Ataxia • Confusion • Slurred speech • Headache • Dizziness • Impaired visual accommodation • Dependency • Dry mouth • Difficulty handling secretions	• Glaucoma • Anticoagulants • Renal impairment • Respiratory depression • Hepatic impairment • Pregnancy • Withdraw slowly when used long-term to avoid problems such as convulsions • Breast-feeding mothers—medication may be transferred via milk • May occasionally produce paradoxical rage or anxiety or depression	• Hypersensitivity • Porphyria (do not use meprobamate) • Comatose states • Severe dependency or addiction

(continued)

Table 27-4. *(Continued)*

SPECIFIC MEDICATION	INDICATIONS	SPECIAL PROPERTIES	USUAL DAILY DOSE (ORAL) *mg*	DAILY DOSE IN MODERATE TO SEVERE COPD (ORAL) *mg*
NEUROLEPTICS (Major Tranquilizers)*				
Phenothiazines				
Thioridazine (Mellaril)	Same as for chlorpromazine. When anticholinergic activity and sedation are desired.	Strongly anticholinergic compared to other neuroleptics on this chart. Inhibition of ejaculation. Pigmented retinitis in daily doses over 800 mg.	50–800	5–200
Chlorpromazine (Thorazine)	Hyperactive behavior in association with schizophrenia, mania, or other definable psychiatric disease. Need to attenuate disturbing sensory stimuli. When sedation is desirable.	Sedating.	50–2000	5–200
Fluphenazine (Prolixin)	Same as for chlorpromazine with less sedation.	Available in depot form (Prolixin Decanoate or Enanthate), which can be administered to patients who are unreliable or who prefer the convenience of not taking daily medications.	2–20 (oral) Depot form 12.5 to 75 mg every 1 to 3 weeks intramuscular injection.	1–10 (oral) Depot form 6.25 to 37.5 mg every 1 to 3 weeks intramuscular injection.
Dihydrolindolones				
Molindone (Mobane)	Same as for chlorpromazine.	Apparent low cardiovascular toxicity as compared with chlorpromazine. Does not block guanethidine. Little or no experience with the drug in COPD.	30–100	10–30

Thiothanxenes				
Thiothixene (Navane)	Same as for chlorpromazine.	Low anticholinergic activity. May have significant antidepressant effect.	5–80	2–20
Butyrophenones				
Haloperidol (Haldol)	Same as for chlorpromazine. When sedation and cardiovascular side-effects need to be avoided.	The least sedating neuroleptic. The most likely to produce Parkinson-type symptoms. Low cardiovascular toxicity. Low anticholinergic activity.	2–40	1–10

*As one moves from thioridazine to haloperidol, extrapyramidal symptoms increase, and, moving backward, alpha adrenergic blocking, allergic responses, sedation, atropine-like effects, seizures, and orthostatic hypotension generally increase. For all neuroleptics listed, drowsiness or lack of attention may make operation of machinery dangerous. This is particularly so during initial treatment. Selected patients may need the usual daily dose. Respiratory depression with aggravation or onset of hypoxia and hypercarbia is always a possible complication when neuroleptics are used in patients with COPD.

Neuroleptics generally can alter sexual function and drive. Each medication in this class can produce specific types of problems. For example, thioridazine *may* contribute to delayed or inhibited ejaculation and chlorpromazine *may* contribute to a simple reduction in sexual drive. On the other hand, both *may* increase sexual drive and performance in specific patients. In addition, sexual dysfunction is so common in patients who need to be treated with neuroleptics that it is often difficult to know what the cause of the change in sexual function is secondary to.

Common Side-Effects	Precautions With	Contraindications
• Blurred vision • Dysuria • Constipation • Nasal congestion • Postural hypotension • Photosensitivity • Drowsiness • Fatigue • Weight gain • Extrapyramidal side-effects • Respiratory depression • Potential difficulty handling secretions	• Seizures • Depression • Pregnancy • Respiratory disease • Cardiac disease • Respiratory depression • May reverse the hypertensive action of medications such as epinephrine and block the antihypertensive effect of guanethidine	• Comatose states • Central nervous system depression • Bone marrow depression • Subcortical brain damage • Seriously impaired liver function • Hypersensitivity • Uncontrolled epilepsy • Severe retarded depression

(continued)

Table 27-4. ***(Continued)***

SPECIFIC MEDICATION	INDICATIONS	SPECIAL PROPERTIES	USUAL DAILY DOSE (ORAL) *mg*	DAILY DOSE IN MODERATE TO SEVERE COPD (ORAL) *mg*
TRICYCLIC ANTIDEPRESSANTS*				
Amitriptyline (Elavil)	Agitated depression or prophylactic treatment of panic attacks.	Strongly anticholinergic. Strongly sedating. Reportedly high incidence of cardiac complications. Administer near bedtime.	50–300	10–100
Doxepin (Adapin or Sinequan)	Same as amitriptyline plus severe insomnia.	Compared with amitriptyline, it is moderately anticholinergic but equally sedating. Low cardiac toxicity. Little or no effect on respiratory center. Unlikely to inhibit guanethidine in doses under 150 mg. Administer near bedtime.	50–300	10–100
Imipramine (Presamine or Tofranil)	Depression that falls between the agitated and retarded categories. Prophylactic treatment of panic attacks.	Moderately anticholinergic. May be sedating. Potential cardiac complications. Administer near bedtime or during the day depending on degree of sedation.	50–300	10–100
Despiramine (Pertofrane, Norpramin)	Same as imipramine.	Weakly anticholinergic compared to amitriptyline. Tends to be more activating than imipramine. Lower incidence of potential cardiac complications compared to imipramine. Gradually administer during the day unless sedating effect predominates.	50–200	10–100

Protriptyline (Vivactil)	Retarded depression or depression associated with loss of energy.	Moderately anticholinergic. Potential cardiac complications. May be used in combination with amitriptyline or doxepin. Give the sedating antidepressant for sleep and protriptyline in the morning for energy. Administer in the morning and at noon. Activating effect should be apparent in hours.	5–60	2.5–20

*As one goes from amitriptyline to protriptyline, initial activation effect generally increases. Initial effects should be distinguished from the antidepressant effect that will follow in days. Initial sedation or activation is present in hours. However, initial effect is therapeutic and demonstrates to the patient that the condition is responsive to medications. Generally avoid giving a sedating antidepressant during the day or to a patient with a retarded depression. The initial sedation may incapacitate the patient and lead to noncompliance with therapy.

For all antidepressants listed, drowsiness or lack of attention may make operation of machinery dangerous. This is particularly so during initial treatment.

A beneficial side-effect of these medications in patients with COPD may be mild bronchodilation. Selected patients may need the usual daily dose.

Common Side-Effects	Precautions With	Contraindications
• Dry mouth • Potential difficulty handling secretions • Blurred vision • Constipation • Nausea • Heartburn • Hypotension • Weight gain	• Urinary retention • Cardiovascular disorders • Narrow-angle glaucoma • Organic brain syndrome • Schizophrenia • Mania • Convulsive disorders • Thyroid disease • Pregnancy • Potentiation of sympathomimetic amines • Blocking guanethidine	• Acute myocardial infarction • Hypersensitivity • Acute schizophrenia • Mania • Monoamine oxidase inhibitors

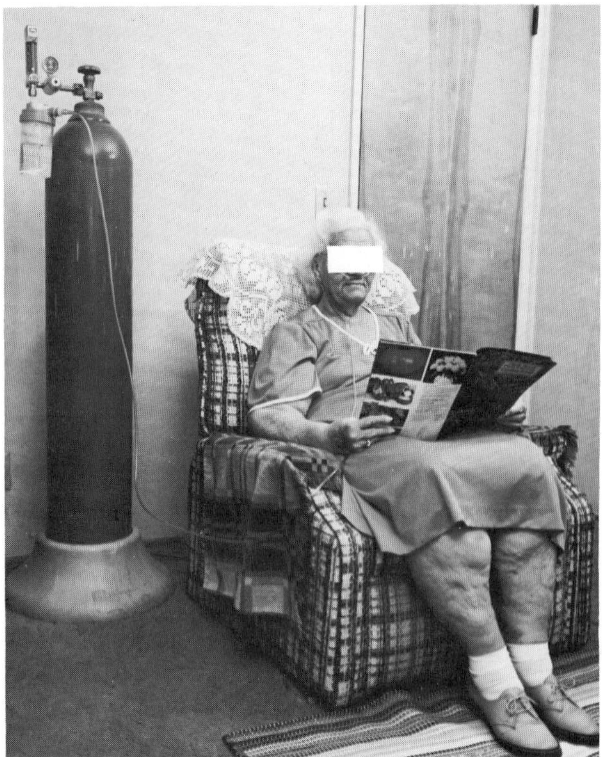

Fig. 27-1. Use of an "H" oxygen cylinder as a stationary oxygen source.

attached to the concentrator, so that the amount of oxygen prescribed by the physician can be easily delivered to the patient through a cannula or oxygen mask. Oxygen concentrations operate by electricity and resemble pieces of furniture. Patients using oxygen concentrators continuously must have a backup oxygen cylinder in the event of electrical failure and may also need a portable oxygen cylinder when away from their home supply.

The system that best meets the needs of the patient is the system that should be prescribed, but certain additional factors should be considered in selecting the home oxygen system. Cost is a major concern, and one that involves both the patient and third-party insurance carrier. For example, if the patient requires oxygen at the rate of 1 liter/min only while sleeping, neither the liquid oxygen system nor the oxygen concentrator should be considered. The liquid system is not appropriate because, at the low temperature at which liquid oxygen is stored (−300° F), the oxygen molecules at the top of the liquid are continually converting from the liquid to the gas phase, resulting in a pressure build-up. This excess pressure leads to venting of gas, resulting in wasted oxygen. This happens when the excess is not used continuously. The oxygen concentrator flat-rate monthly rental charge is higher than the cost of the three or four cylinders of high-pressure oxygen the patient would need per month at the liter flow mentioned in the example. The oxygen concentrator is cost-effective only when the monthly cost of gaseous oxygen equals or exceeds the cost of the concentrator. In such cases, Medicare and other third-party carriers will instruct the oxygen supplier to provide an oxygen concentrator for the patient.

Liquid oxygen is probably the most expensive home oxygen available, but it is also very convenient because the "reservoir" lasts longer than the large gaseous oxygen cylinders and comes with a "walker" that the patient or family members can easily refill from the reservoir. The walker also lasts longer than E-cylinders or other small cylinders and can be easily carried, allowing the patient to remain away from home for longer periods.

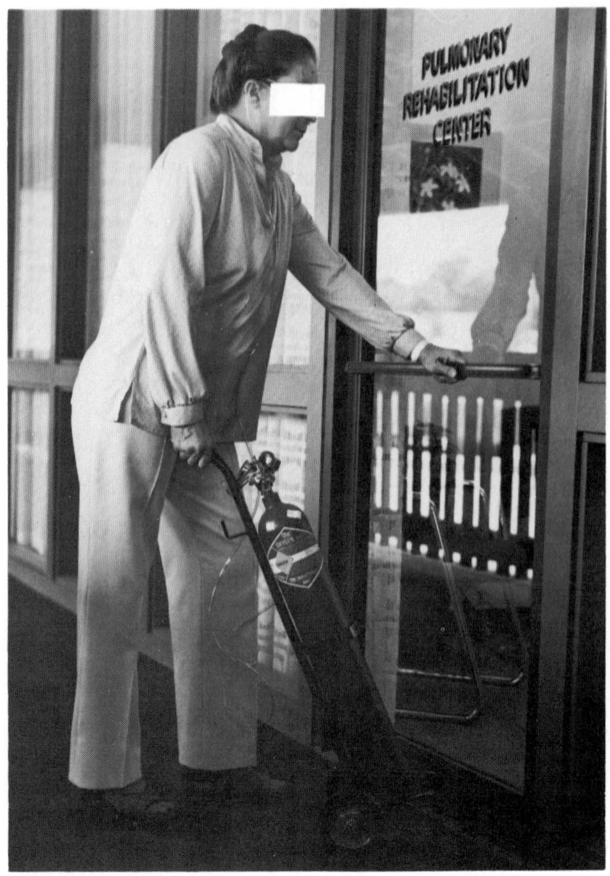

Fig. 27-2. Use of an "E" oxygen cylinder as a portable oxygen source.

PHYSICAL THERAPY AND EXERCISE RECONDITIONING

Physical therapy techniques used in respiratory rehabilitation programs include relaxation techniques, breathing retraining, chest percussion, bronchial drainage techniques, and exercise conditioning. These techniques have been discussed in Chapter 26.

Relaxation techniques have been used to help the patient control anxiety, agitation, and fear. Stress can exacerbate and aggravate existing physical and psychological symptoms. For patients with COPD, the sensation of dyspnea can create tension and fear. Relaxation techniques include biofeedback, transcendental meditation, or simply listening to soothing music in a quiet environment.

Breathing retraining, another physical therapy modality, has these goals:[24] to help control dyspnea through a relaxed pattern of slow breathing, and to increase alveolar ventilation in an attempt to improve or to maintain adequate gas exchange.

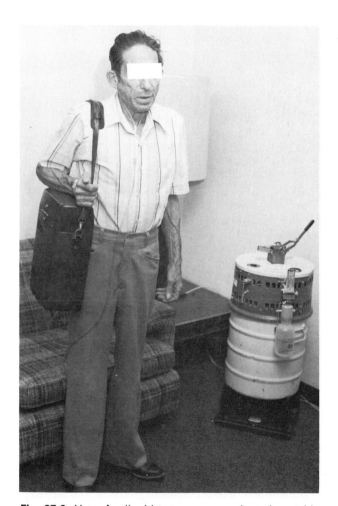

Fig. 27-3. Use of a liquid oxygen reservoir and portable walker unit as an oxygen source.

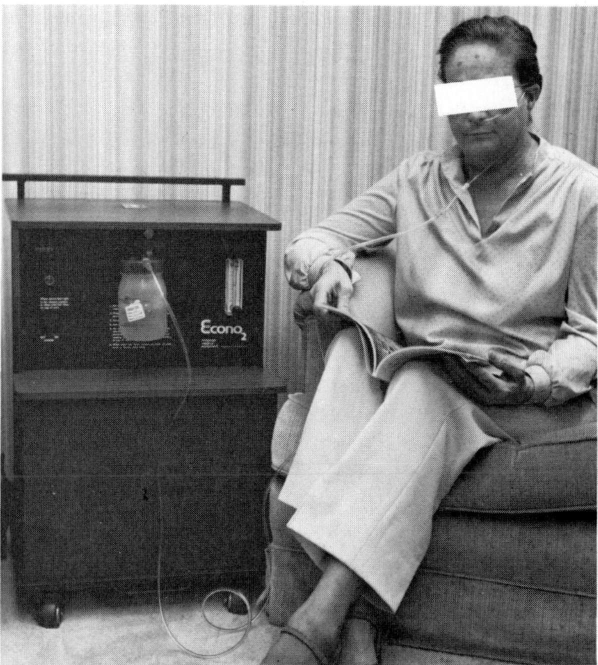

Fig. 27-4. An oxygen concentrator for home use.

The use of pursed lips along with "abdominal–diaphragmatic breathing" is the breathing technique most commonly used to reduce the respiratory rate and improve respiratory muscle coordination. With this technique, the patient inhales deeply with the abdominal muscles relaxed and then exhales through pursed lips, augmented by abdominal muscle contraction. While improved ventilation, reduced respiratory rate, and decreased alveolar-arterial oxygen gradients have been reported in patients using this breathing pattern,[36,53] similar blood gas improvements have occurred with slow deep breathing alone.[35] For many patients, however, these breathing techniques help relieve dyspnea.

Respiratory muscle strength and endurance may be enhanced by voluntary normocapnic hyperpnea[5,31] as well as by periodic breathing through a high-resistance device.[39] Patients with cystic fibrosis have achieved the same increase in ventilatory muscle function by participating in a 4-week physical activity training program at a summer camp that included intensive swimming and canoeing.[31]

Chest percussion and bronchial drainage techniques can improve clearance of secretions in those COPD patients with excessive amounts of secretions who are unable to clear their airways spontaneously because of an inability to take a deep breath or to cough effectively or because of tenacious sputum.[29] This technique should be reserved for those COPD patients who chronically expectorate greater than 30 cc of sputum daily.[37]

Patients with COPD generally lack activity and exercise endurance. Dyspnea and fatigue are the usual limiting factors in exercising COPD patients. Many patients reduce their physical activity dramatically to avoid this discomfort. This results in a worsening condition and leads to a cycle of increasing deconditioning. The physiological effects of exercise and its benefits in this patient population have been described in many reports.[4,6,24,50,55,56]

If an objective evaluation such as an incremental exercise stress test documents an impaired ability to exercise, an exercise prescription should be considered. There are four parts to a prescription: the mode of exercise; the intensity; the duration; and the frequency. Modes of exercise that could be selected include walking, swimming, and riding a bicycle. The mode selected for the patient should be the one that the patient prefers. Generally, to improve exercise tolerance significantly, one needs to exercise at an intensity of 60% to 80% of the maximal oxygen consumption (about 70–85% of the achievable maximal heart rate).[23,45] Patients with significant COPD may be unable to achieve this level of intensity immediately and need to start out exercising at a lower level. The important thing is to increase the intensity of exercise gradually to achieve improved conditioning. The exercise session should last at least 20 to 30 minutes with the patient exercising at least three to four times per week.[1,23,45]

When exercise is performed regularly, the patient usually gains an increased tolerance for dyspnea, has an improved appetite, and demonstrates an increased physical capability with resultant improvement in quality of life. The use of an ear oximeter to monitor oxygen saturation is a noninvasive, reliable way of evaluating blood oxygen levels during the exercise period. In patients with significant hypoxemia that limits exercise ability, supplemental oxygen may allow patients to participate in an exercise conditioning program and thus improve their level of activity.[3,9,42,44,52]

ACTIVITIES OF DAILY LIVING EVALUATION

Occupational and physical therapists can help evaluate a patient's activities of daily living. They can outline various energy-saving maneuvers to assist the patient in carrying out desired activities. Adaptive devices can be prescribed for patients to help them avoid excessive exertion when picking objects up from the floor, dressing, or bathing.

NUTRITIONAL EVALUATION

Although there is no specific diet for patients with COPD, they should be given dietary instructions to meet their needs. A dietician can make recommendations following a nutritional evaluation. Some general recommendations can be made about dietary patterns, such as avoidance of an increased amount of fluids during a meal, which can cause bloating. Patients with decreased appetite related to dyspnea, abdominal fullness from air swallowing, or nausea from medications should use a high protein diet with multiple small feedings throughout the day rather than two or three large meals. Nutritional supplements may be useful in patients with a poor appetite. The use of oxygen during meals may help hypoxemic patients to eat more comfortably. Often these patients have concomitant disease—for example, cardiovascular problems that would require other special dietary instructions.

PSYCHOSOCIAL REHABILITATION

Psychosocial rehabilitation focuses on the patient's reaction to COPD, how to handle the illness and its effects on daily life.[17,24] It deals with the patient's work, social, recreational, interpersonal and family relationships, and sex. The COPD patient's sexual activity and how he feels about it are basic components of his identity and ego strength and affect how he relates to his spouse. Psychotherapy and psychopharmacologic agents should be considered for those patients not responding satisfactorily to usual attempts by the physician and team members to help with their emotional problems.

Although counseling and strong supportive care are mainstays in dealing with psychiatric disorders in patients with COPD, psychopharmacologic agents are sometimes used as adjuncts to controlling the emotional disorder. Agents to treat anxiety should be used only on a short-term basis, since long-term use can lead to significant habituation. Diazepam and hydroxyzine are relatively safe anxiolytic agents; they can, however, result in undesirable side-effects such as drowsiness, dizziness, and confusion. A potential problem with the use of tranquilizers is sedation and potentiation of depression.

When anxiety and depression coexist, the symptoms of anxiety often mask the depression. If the anxiety alone is treated, the depression may worsen significantly. When selecting an antidepressant agent, one should ascertain the need for a sedating effect versus an activating effect.[17] Doxepin is an excellent medication for agitated, depressed patients because it can reduce or eliminate agitation in addition to its antidepressant effect. Protriptyline is a good antidepressant for depressed patients with low drive and motivation. Imipramine falls between doxepin and protriptyline and would be particularly useful when neither sedation nor activation is needed. Doxepin should be administered near bedtime to assist with sleep, whereas morning administration of protriptyline promotes daytime energy. For a more complete listing of psychopharmacologic agents, see Table 27-4.

VOCATIONAL REHABILITATION

The basic goal of rehabilitation is to return the patient with COPD to society as a self-sufficient, useful member. Once a patient's activity level has been optimized after a rehabilitation program, one should evaluate his potential for vocational restoration. A patient may be able to return to his previous employment or to the same occupational field in a different job or location. Sometimes a patient may need to be retrained in another field.[34]

Successful vocational rehabilitation is difficult to achieve in patients with COPD. Factors that can hinder successful vocational rehabilitation include a recent significant change in life-style, evidence of rapid clinical deterioration, major personality change, alcoholism, and inability to mobilize psychological and social assets.[30] Level of intelligence is also a factor in vocational options.[15] Other factors that lessen vocational rehabilitation potential include advanced age, the progressive nature of the disease, and limitations in the ability of the patient with respiratory impairment to retrain.[24] A proper approach to disability/impairment evaluation is essential when attempting to determine a patient's ability to work.[19]

ASSESSMENT OF PATIENT'S PROGRESS

The respiratory rehabilitation program should be continuously assessed and reassessed while a patient is in the program and after his discharge from the program. This allows for any necessary modifications to the program, as well as an evaluation of its overall effectiveness. The patient's program must change as he does.

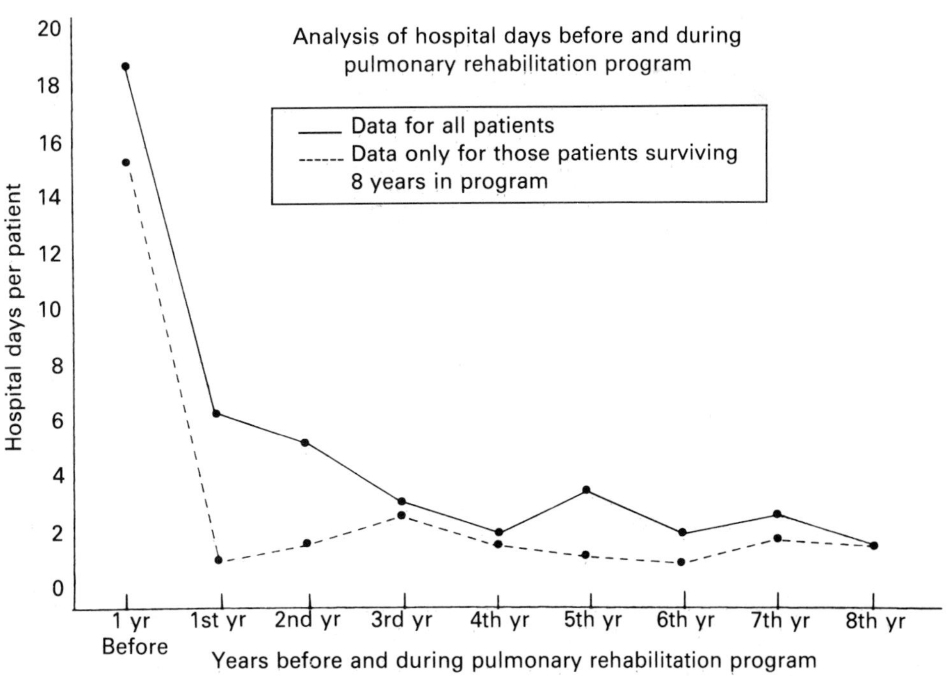

Fig. 27-5. Analysis of hospital days before and during a pulmonary rehabilitation program. (Data from the Loma Linda University Medical Center Pulmonary Rehabilitation Program)

LONG-TERM FOLLOW-UP

Once the patient has completed a rehabilitation program, follow-up treatment is generally resumed by the primary care physician. The rehabilitation team may work with the primary care physician in continuing to assess the patient in helping to modify the patient's program as his condition changes.

BENEFITS OF PULMONARY REHABILITATION

Benefits reported include an improved quality of life and enhanced ability to carry out daily activities.[22,24,32,40,49] Patients have achieved a significant reduction in their symptoms,[20,24] anxiety, depression, and somatic concerns with an associated improvement in ego strength.[2,17,20] The number of hospital days required per patient per year has been significantly reduced,[12,28] and some patients have been able to continue or to return to gainful employment.[22,30,43] An improvement in exercise tolerance has already been discussed.

Patients with COPD undergoing pulmonary rehabilitation at Loma Linda University Medical Center have required significantly fewer days of hospitalization as compared to the year before going through the program.[12] Although one may suggest that the reduction in hospital days noted simply reflects death of the sickest patients during the first years of follow-up, leaving the healthier patients toward the end, the number of hospital days required for those patients surviving only for the full 8 years is virtually identical (Fig. 27-5). Obviously, this marked reduction in hospitalization results in a significant cost-saving.

Although no improvement in survival or slowing of the deterioration of respiratory function has been documented in most reports, it is hoped that by implementing the components of comprehensive respiratory care discussed in this chapter in patients with relatively mild obstructive airway disease, one may, in fact, be able to alter the course of the disease favorably.

Pulmonary rehabilitation is not something that happens *TO* a patient but *WITH* a patient. It allows a patient to return to as normal a life as possible. This is accomplished through a combination of medications, education, training, and other modalities of a comprehensive respiratory care program. No one aspect of the program is more important than another, and each program must be individualized to fit a patient's needs.

REFERENCES

1. Adams WC, McHenry MM, Bernauer EM: Long-term physiologic adaptions to exercise with special reference to performance and cardiorespiratory function in health and disease. In Amsterdam EA, Wilmore JH, Demaria AN (eds): Exercise in Cardiovascular Health and Disease. New York, Yorke Medical Books, 1977
2. Agle DP, Baum GL, Chester EH et al: Multidiscipline treatment of chronic pulmonary insufficiency: Psychologic aspects of rehabilitation. Psychosom Med 35:41, 1973
3. Barach AL: Ambulatory oxygen therapy: Oxygen inhalation at home and out-of-doors. Dis Chest 35:229, 1959
4. Bass H, Whitcomb JF, Forman R: Exercise training: Therapy for patients with chronic obstructive pulmonary disease. Chest 57:116, 1970
5. Belman MJ, Mittman C: Ventilatory muscle training improves exercise capacity in chronic obstructive pulmonary disease patients. Am Rev Respir Dis 121:273, 1980
6. Belman MJ, Wasserman K: Exercise training and testing in patients with chronic obstructive pulmonary disease. Basics of RD 10, No. 2, November 1981 (available from the American Thoracic Society)
7. Block AJ: Low-flow oxygen therapy, treatment of the ambulant outpatient. Am Rev Respir Dis (Suppl)110:71, 1974
8. Block AJ, Castel JR, Keitt AS: Chronic oxygen therapy: Treatment of chronic obstructive pulmonary disease at sea level. Chest 65:279, 1974
9. Bradley BL, Garner AE, Billiu D et al: Oxygen-assisted exercise in chronic obstructive lung disease: The effect on exercise capacity and arterial blood gas tensions. Am Rev Respir Dis 118:239, 1978
10. Browning RJ, Olsen AM: The functional gastrointestinal disorders of pulmonary emphysema. Proc Staff Meet Mayo Clin 36:537, 1961
11. Buist AS, Sexton GJ, Nagy JM et al: The effect of smoking cessation and modification on lung function. Am Rev Respir Dis 114:115, 1976
12. Burton GG, Gee G, Hodgkin JE et al: Cost effectiveness studies in respiratory care: An overview and some possible early solutions. Hospitals 49:61, 1975
13. California Thoracic Society guidelines for pulmonary rehabilitation. A statement by the CTS Respiratory Care Assembly (newsletter). Respiratory Care Assembly of California Thoracic Society 8, No. 1, September 1979
14. Continuous or nocturnal oxygen therapy in hypoxemic chronic obstructive lung disease: A clinical trial. Ann Intern Med 93:391, 1980
15. Daughton DM, Fox AJ, Kass I et al: Physiological-intellectual components of rehabilitation success in patients with chronic obstructive pulmonary disease (COPD). J Chronic Dis 32:405, 1979
16. Davis MS: Variations in patients' compliance with doctors' orders: Analysis of congruence between survey responses and results of empirical investigations. J Med Educ 41:1037, November 1966
17. Dudley DL, Glaser EM, Jorgenson B et al: Psychosocial concomitants to rehabilitation in chronic obstructive pulmonary disease. Chest 77:413, 544, 677, 1980
18. Epidemiology of Respiratory Diseases Task Force Report: State of Knowledge, Problems and Needs, p 84. U.S. Department of Health and Human Services Publ No. 81–2019. Bethesda, National Heart, Lung, and Blood Institute, October 1980
19. Evaluation of impairment/disability secondary to respiratory disease. Report of the ALA/ATS Component Committee on Disability Criteria. ATS News 7, No. 3:20, 1981

20. Fishman DB, Petty TL: Physical, symptomatic, and psychological improvement in patients receiving comprehensive care for chronic airway obstruction. J Chronic Dis 24:775, 1971
21. Fletcher C, Peto R, Tinker C et al: The Natural History of Chronic Bronchitis and Emphysema. Oxford, Oxford University Press, 1976
22. Haas A, Cardon H: Rehabilitation in chronic obstructive pulmonary disease: A five-year study of 252 male patients. Med Clin North Am 53:593, 1969
23. Hellerstein HK, Hirsch EZ, Ader R et al: Principles of exercise prescription for normals and cardiac subjects. In Naughton J, Hellerstein HK (eds): Exercise Testing and Exercise Training in Coronary Heart Disease. New York, Academic Press, 1973
24. Hodgkin JE (ed): Chronic Obstructive Pulmonary Disease: Current Concepts in Diagnosis and Comprehensive Care. Park Ridge, IL, American College of Chest Physicians, 1979
25. Hodgkin JE: Pulmonary rehabilitation. In Simmons DH (ed): Current Pulmonology, Vol 3. New York, John Wiley & Sons, 1981
26. Hodgkin JE, Balchum OJ, Kass I et al: Chronic obstructive airway diseases: Current concepts in diagnosis and comprehensive care. JAMA 232:1243, 1975
27. Hodgkin JE, Zorn EG: Intermittent positive pressure breathing (IPPB) in the outpatient management of chronic obstructive pulmonary disease: Description of the NIH clinical trial. Respir Care 26:1095, 1981
28. Hudson LD, Tyler ML, Petty TL: Hospitalization needs during an outpatient rehabilitation program for severe chronic airway obstruction. Chest 70:606, 1976
29. Jones NL: Physical therapy–present state of the art. Am Rev Respir Dis (Suppl)110:132, 1974
30. Kass I, Dyksterhuis JE, Rubin H et al: Correlation of psychophysiological variables with vocational rehabilitation; outcome in chronic obstructive pulmonary disease patients. Chest 67:433, 1975
31. Keens TG, Krastins IRB, Wannamaker EM et al: Ventilatory muscle endurance training in normal subjects and patients with cystic fibrosis. Am Rev Respir Dis 116:853, 1977
32. Kimbel P, Kaplan AS, Alkalay I et al: An in-hospital program for rehabilitation of patients with chronic obstructive pulmonary disease. Chest (Suppl)60:6S, 1971
33. Levine BE, Bigelow DB, Hamstra RD et al: The role of long-term continuous oxygen administration in patients with chronic airway obstruction with hypoxemia. Ann Intern Med 66:639, 1967
34. Matzen RN: Vocational rehabilitation: The culmination of physical reconditioning. Chest (Suppl)60:21S, 1971
35. Motley HL: Effects of slow deep breathing on blood gas exchange in emphysema. Am Rev Respir Dis 88:484, 1963
36. Mueller RE, Petty TL, Filley GF: Ventilation and arterial blood gas changes induced by pursed lip breathing. J Appl Physiol 28:784, 1970
37. Murray JF: The ketchup-bottle method. N Engl J Med 300:1155, 1979
38. Nield M: The effect of health teaching on the anxiety level of patients with chronic obstructive lung disease. Nurs Res 20:537, 1971
39. Pardy RL, Rivington RN, Despas PJ et al: Inspiratory muscle training compared with physiotherapy inpatients with chronic airflow limitation. Am Rev Respir Dis 123:421, 1981
40. Petty TL: Ambulatory care for emphysema and chronic bronchitis. Chest 58:441, 1970
41. Petty TL: Pulmonary rehabilitation. Basics of RD, 4:1. New York, American Thoracic Society, 1975
42. Petty TL, Finigan MM: Clinical evaluation of prolonged ambulatory oxygen therapy in chronic airway obstruction. Am J Med 45:242, 1968
43. Petty TL, MacIlroy ER, Swergert MA et al: Chronic airway obstruction, respiratory insufficiency, and gainful employment. Arch Environ Health 21:71, 1970
44. Pierce AK, Paez PN, Miller WF: Exercise therapy with the aid of a portable oxygen supply in patients with emphysema. Am Rev Respir Dis 91:653, 1965
45. Pollock ML: The qualification of endurance training programs. In Wilmore JH (ed): Exercise and Sports Science Reviews. New York, Academic Press, 1973
46. Pulmonary rehabilitation. Official statement of the American Thoracic Society Executive Committee. Am Rev Respir Dis 124:663, 1981
47. Respiratory Diseases Task Force Report on Prevention, Control, Education, p 84. U.S. Department of Health, Education, and Welfare Publ No. (NIH) 77–1248. Bethesda, National Heart, Lung & Blood Institute, March 1977
48. Respiratory Diseases Task Force Report on Prevention, Control, Education, p 133. U.S. Department of Health, Education, and Welfare Publ No. (NIH) 77–1248. Bethesda, National Heart, Lung & Blood Institute, March 1977
49. Shapiro BA, Vostinak–Foley E, Hamilton BB et al: Rehabilitation in chronic obstructive pulmonary disease: A two-year prospective study. Respir Care 22:1045, 1977
50. Shephard RJ: Exercise and chronic obstructive lung disease. Exerc Sport Sci Rev 4:263, 1976
51. Stark RD, Finnegan P, Bishop JM: Daily requirement of oxygen to reverse pulmonary hypertension in patients with chronic bronchitis. Br Med J 3:724, 1972
52. Stein DA, Bradley BL, Miller WC: Mechanisms of oxygen effects on exercise in patients with chronic obstructive pulmonary disease. Chest 81:6, 1982
53. Thoman RL, Stoker GL, Ross JC: The efficacy of pursed-lip breathing in patients with chronic obstructive pulmonary disease. Am Rev Respir Dis 93:100, 1966
54. U.S. Department of Health and Human Services: Monthly Vital Statistics Report. 29, No. 13:5, September 17, 1981
55. Wasserman K, Whipp BJ: Exercise physiology in health and disease. Am Rev Respir Dis 112:219, 1975
56. Woolf CR, Suero JT: Alterations in lung mechanics and gas exchange following training in chronic obstructive lung disease. Dis Chest 55:37, 1969

SUGGESTED BIBLIOGRAPHY FOR GENERAL READING

Hodgkin JE (ed): Chronic Obstructive Pulmonary Disease: Current Concepts in Diagnosis and Comprehensive Care. Park Ridge, IL, American College of Chest Physicians, 1979

Hodgkin JE: Pulmonary rehabilitation. In Simmons D (ed): Current Pulmonology, Vol 3. New York, John Wiley & Sons, 1981

Lertzman MM, Cherniack RM: Rehabilitation of patients with chronic obstructive pulmonary disease. Am Rev Respir Dis 114:1145, 1976

Petty TL (ed): Chronic Obstructive Pulmonary Disease. New York, Marcel Dekker, 1978

Petty TL: Pulmonary rehabilitation. Basics of RD. New York, American Thoracic Society, 1975

Pulmonary rehabilitation. Official statement of the American Thoracic Society. Am Rev Respir Dis 124:663, 1981

Section Three

RESPIRATORY CARE IN CRITICAL ILLNESSES

28

Problems Unique to the Delivery of Respiratory Care in Infants and Children

Mary Ann Fletcher

Delivery of respiratory care to patients in the pediatric age group presents several unique problems that relate to size, to physical and intellectual maturation, and to diseases specific to neonates, infants, and children. On the one hand, these problems create therapeutic difficulties that necessitate special equipment and precautions. On the other hand, they help to make respiratory care of younger patients more interesting and challenging.

The most obvious problem is size. Although some husky adolescents are physically adults, most pediatric patients who need respiratory care are small. In intensive care nurseries, most respiratory care hours are spent caring for premature infants weighing less than 3 lb.

Compared to adults, the thoracic volume of a child is small, and the airways are narrow and short. The trachea of a term neonate is 3.5 mm to 4 mm in diameter and 4 cm in length from the larynx to the carina. In contrast, the trachea of an adult is 10 mm to 14 mm in diameter and 13 cm in length. Not only does the small size of the lung and airways necessitate specially designed equipment, but also, importantly, it affects pulmonary mechanics and the response of airways to disease.

The smaller airway in infants has greater resistance than in adults. Normal airway resistance during mouth breathing in an infant is about 7 cm H_2O/liter/sec, whereas in an adult it is about 0.5 to 1.5 cm H_2O/liter/sec.

Any decrease in diameter of the narrow infant airway will effect a much greater increase in airway resistance than will the same decrease in a larger adult airway. For example, if the 4-mm trachea in a neonate develops circumferential submucosal edema of 1 mm thickness, the airway diameter decreases by 50% from 4 mm to 2 mm. Additionally, decreasing the diameter of an airway that is already narrow may change a relatively laminar airflow pattern to one of increased turbulence, further increasing airway resistance and the work of breathing. In comparison, the same 1 mm of circumferential edema in an *adult* trachea would have far less effect on airway resistance, decreasing an airway of 14 mm by only 15%. It is clear why diseases that decrease airway diameter by edema or bronchospasm create more respiratory distress in a small infant than these same changes would cause in an adult.

Differences in size are even more obvious when one compares lung volumes. Tidal volume may be as little as 5 ml in a small premature neonate and more than 500 ml in an adult. The anatomical dead space, although maintaining a roughly constant ratio of 1 ml/lb, varies from 2 ml in a neonate to more than 150 ml in an adult. The dead space to tidal volume *ratio* remains essentially the same for all ages despite the large volume changes.

When compared to the adult chest, the supporting structures of neonates and young children are poorly developed and weak. The ribs are more cartilaginous and flexible, and the accessory respiratory muscles are poorly developed. The cartilage that provides support for conducting airways does not extend as far circumferentially and is thinner. Because of these structural differences, the airway and thorax in the neonate-pediatric age group do not sustain pressure differences well and collapse easily.

Equipment that is to be used for pediatric patients has to be specifically designed for their size. It is no less appropriate to put a 4-mm internal diameter endotracheal tube into an adult than it is to ventilate an infant with a device designed for an adult. Improperly sized equipment may do more harm than good. In summary, effective respiratory therapy demands consideration of individual differences and requirements.

OXYGEN THERAPY

SPECIAL CONSIDERATIONS, INDICATIONS, AND PRECAUTIONS

There are few respiratory diseases in pediatrics where administration of *oxygen for hypoxemia* is contraindicated. However, many infants and children with a chronically low Pa_{O_2} have adequate tissue oxygen levels to maintain normal body functions without tachycardia and lactic acidemia.[2] Importantly, they tolerate hypoxemia and develop normally because they have developed compensatory mechanisms, such as increased levels of hemoglobin, decreased hemoglobin–oxygen affinity, increased and redistributed cardiac output, and decreased oxygen consumption. Only when there is added stress such as fever, surgery, or respiratory infection that overwhelms the compensatory mechanisms is there a need for oxygen therapy. Children with cystic fibrosis, for example, generally adapt remarkably well to chronic hypoxemia except when faced with pneumonia. Similarly, children with cardiac lesions involving right-to-left intracardiac shunting benefit little from oxygen therapy unless there is superimposed pulmonary hypertension or disease. In neonates and infants, it is rarely necessary or efficacious to allow hypoxemia for maintenance of respiratory drive. In fact, in premature infants the administration of oxygen decreases apnea and increases the ventilatory response to carbon dioxide.

Although there are few contraindications to oxygen properly used, there are important precautions in its administration. As in any aged patient, oxygen should be considered a drug that has proper doses and routes of administration for maximum benefit, minimum toxicity, and reasonable cost-effectiveness.

Oxygen must be warmed and humidified. Cold air increases oxygen consumption in a neonate even when delivered only to its face. Air or gas mixtures that are too warm induce apnea and raise body temperature. The ideal temperature is 1 to 2 degrees below neutral thermal environment for oxygen therapy in neonates.* It should be about 2 degrees below normal body temperature when delivered directly into the lower airway through an endotracheal tube or tracheostomy. An oxygen-enriched environment may be 5 to 8 degrees below neutral thermal environment for an older child with a croup syndrome or fever but should not be so cold that he shivers.

METHODS OF DELIVERING OXYGEN TO NEONATES AND SMALL INFANTS

The most direct method of delivering oxygen is through an *endotracheal tube*. Rarely should an oral or nasal tracheal tube be left to atmospheric pressure; instead it should remain connected to low levels of continuous distending airway pressure to replace physiological respiratory resistance lost with the artificial airway. The administration of oxygen alone is not sufficient reason for intubation unless there is also a need for an airway or positive pressure ventilation.

Nasal catheters are acceptable routes for oxygen administration in small patients when low flow and low concentrations are sufficient.[3,4] Use of this route is particularly helpful in infants with chronic requirements of less than 30% oxygen, such as in infants during the long recovery period of bronchopulmonary dysplasia. These infants are better able to tolerate the swings in FI_{O_2} that occur with entrainment of room air on crying or displacement than are infants in the acute phase of illness or with highly reactive pulmonary blood flow. The catheter allows greater mobility and normalization of activity, interaction, and feeding.

*Neutral thermal environment is that environmental temperature at which the body has to expend the least energy to maintain its proper temperature. This temperature depends on body weight, metabolic rate, activity, and age. It is highest for the small, premature neonate, where it is close to core temperature, and decreases until early childhood, when adult values are assumed.

A nasal catheter may be adapted from a suction or feeding tube or 2.5-mm endotracheal tube. Tolerance is better when the tube is within the nose to the level just above the uvula and the flow rate is 0.5 liter/min or less.[3]

Alternatively, commercial nasal cannulas can be modified by cutting off the prongs at their base, leaving a wide hole in the tubing. Higher flows of 1 to 3 liters/min may be needed to counteract room air entrainment. Monitoring cardiovascular response and Ptc_{O_2} levels help determine the lowest effective flow and FI_{O_2}.

When fairly precise control of oxygen is essential and mobility is less important, the *oxygen head hood* is the most effective means of administration to small infants who are not intubated. The hoods come in various sizes, so that one can select appropriately for the infant's size and minute ventilation. The infant should not slide through the neck opening, nor should the opening constrict the neck. Flow into the hood should be just high enough to maintain the desired oxygen concentration while preventing carbon dioxide accumulation, generally at least three times the minute ventilation, and yet keep noise contamination as low as possible. One particular source of head hood noise is the to-and-fro motion of water collecting in the tubing from a humidified oxygen source. This "water hammer" effect can be quite loud; thus there should be frequent emptying of the connection tubing.

The hood should be clear plexiglass for visibility and fitted with a device for monitoring the temperature within. In cases where an external light source such as phototherapy (for hyperbilirubinemia) is over a hood, a greenhouse effect may allow overheating of the environment.

When necessary to remove or to open the hood for procedures, there must be an appropriate alternative oxygen source, usually through a mask, until the concentration is again stable. Oxygen monitors should be near the infant's airway within the hood to reflect the actual inspired concentration.

Face masks specifically designed for neonates and infants allow oxygen administration for short, specific periods of time. The masks must be soft enough to allow a tight fit without pressure. They should cover both the mouth and nose but not the eyes.

The most frequent use of masks for oxygen therapy is during positive pressure breathing with a bag or during removal from a head hood for the performance of procedures. A mask is also useful for administration of aerosolized medications and humidity as well as for intermittent application of continuous positive airway pressure. Because prolonged applications of masks for oxygen therapy and CPAP have too many side-effects, nasal tubes have largely replaced them.

Oxygen can be delivered to an infant in an *incubator*. Most incubators are equipped with air inlets that prevent the FI_{O_2} from exceeding 0.40 unless the inlets are closed. Generally it is inefficient and imprecise to attempt to maintain a high ambient oxygen concentration in the entire incubator. Every time the portholes are opened for nursing care, the oxygen content drops rapidly. High flow rates are needed to maintain higher concentrations of oxygen. An accurate FI_{O_2} is also difficult to establish. The following disadvantages of aerosolizing moisture to the whole incubator should be noted.

1. Fogging of the incubator interferes with visibility of the infant.
2. Soaking of the infant's bed and clothing may occur.
3. An environment is provided for growth of gram-negative organisms.

It is more efficient to use a hood within an incubator if the infant needs oxygen concentrations of 30% to 40% to avoid the disadvantages of nebulized mist in the entire incubator. This is particularly true if frequent nursing care that will disrupt the microenvironment is needed.

METHODS OF DELIVERING OXYGEN TO OLDER CHILDREN

Administration of oxygen to older children is more challenging than to the infant who is relatively more passive. *Nasal cannulas* and catheters may prove too irritating to the nasal mucosa. Modifications of the cannula with low flows are most accepted. Children tolerate *masks* poorly because the presence of something held over the mouth when there is respiratory distress often creates a feeling of helplessness and suffocation. Masks must be soft and dry to prevent irritation.

Hoods that are appropriately sized may be used, although they are poorly tolerated by other than young infants. They create too much of a sense of confinement; most children are too active to stay in them.

Croup tents generally are better tolerated. They may cover the entire child or just his head and chest.

They should be as small as possible for efficiency and kept closed at the bottom to prevent leakage of the heavier, cold oxygen. The maximum FI_{O_2} that can be achieved in such units is about 0.60.

The environmental temperature within oxygen tents must be closely monitored. Ice added to the cooling chamber will help to keep the temperature in a comfortable range (about 6–7°F below room temperature) and provides an effective means of cooling a febrile child. If the ice melts and is not replaced, the temperature within the tent may increase uncomfortably and raise the body temperature. At the same time, the convection currents that force cooled oxygen to concentrate below warm air will be lost, and the ambient oxygen concentration will decrease.

Oxygen delivered directly into an *endotracheal tube or tracheostomy* must be carefully humidified and warmed. It should be 2 degrees below body temperature. Any droplets that form on the inlet tubing should be kept from running into the airway. The tubing that leads to the airway should be properly supported to prevent undue stress on the airway.

MONITORING OXYGEN THERAPY

Oxygen therapy in pediatric patients may be both beneficial in the treatment of hypoxemia and harmful to the developing lung, eyes, and immature brain. Whereas some patients demonstrate remarkable resistance to pulmonary toxicity from oxygen, others, particularly when oxygen therapy is associated with positive pressure ventilation, develop chronic pulmonary changes such as bronchopulmonary dysplasia.

Oxygen therapy in premature infants is, in some instances, both life-saving and harmful. The normal vascular development of the premature eye is disturbed when vasoconstriction and vasodilation are associated with changes in retinal artery Pa_{O_2}. The resultant abnormal vascular development leads to various degrees of scarring, retinal detachment, and blindness (retinopathy of prematurity or *retrolental fibroplasia*). Although infants can develop retinopathy without receiving oxygen therapy, most cases are associated with prolonged oxygen therapy.

Changes in Pa_{O_2} as well as in Pa_{CO_2} may also affect cerebral blood flow and contribute to intracranial hemorrhage, a serious cause of neurologic sequelae for premature infants. Hyperoxemia has been associated with pathology in specific areas of the brain (pontosubicular necrosis).[1] In some cases, this condition is the direct effect of inspired oxygen or its toxic radical, whereas in others the damage depends on the blood oxygen level. In all cases where oxygen is used, it must be monitored so that only enough is consistently given to maintain tissue levels in the *nonhypoxic* range. For premature infants, tissue oxygen delivery may be adequate with central Pa_{O_2}'s of 50 torr to 65 torr, whereas larger infants and children may have symptoms, acidosis, and pulmonary hypertension if their level is not kept in the 70 torr to 90 torr range.

Oxygen monitoring, therefore, entails measuring and precisely controlling FI_{O_2} as well as blood levels. Documentation of inspired oxygen concentration is essential on a regular, frequent basis: hourly and whenever there is a change in patient status or in oxygen therapy being given.

The use of continuous intraarterial oxygen saturation catheters and of transcutaneous oxygen electrodes has allowed much more precise control over blood oxygen levels. The transcutaneous probes are especially accurate in pediatric patients and allow continuous noninvasive monitoring.

HUMIDITY THERAPY

While all oxygen or air under positive pressure must be properly humidified, humidity itself is often a therapeutic tool. It prevents drying of mucous membranes and secretions. It also decreases the insensible water loss that occurs at an increased rate when respiratory distress causes hyperventilation. Whereas excessive amounts of aerosols delivered directly into the airway may cause fluid overload and literally drown a patient, leading to circulating volume overload and hyponatremia, proper humidity keeps secretions liquid and aids in their removal from airways. Thick secretions may encrust on an artificial airway, increasing airway resistance and the work of breathing, and may produce complete airway obstruction.

The effectiveness of aerosol therapy is determined by the size of the particles produced, their density, and the method by which they are delivered. For practical purposes, the smaller the major airways, the smaller the particles must be to prevent deposition on the proximal mucous membranes before they reach the trachea. Generally, if liquefaction of thick tracheal secretions is the objective of therapy, particles must be less than 6 μm in diameter and concentrated in a dense fog.

If water vapor is needed to prevent airway dryness or excessive fluid loss, simple humidification of inspired air, without nebulization of fluid particles, may be all that is needed. Care must be taken to prevent excessive humidification with droplet formation in artificial airways. Not only may too much liquid be delivered to the patient, but also his airway diameter may be compromised.

Humidity therapy may benefit the small infant, in whom high surface area to body mass ratios means proportionately high transcutaneous water losses. In these cases, warmed moisturized air circulating over the body in an enclosed hood, incubator, or tent can decrease insensible water loss and caloric waste from evaporative heat loss.

The methods for delivering humidity are the same as those for delivering oxygen: hood, tents, masks, and endotracheal tubes. Care should be taken to avoid loss of patient visibility in dense humidity environments. Electronic monitoring helps in following the patient but cannot completely replace direct observation.

ACHIEVING PATIENT COOPERATION

Delivery of effective respiratory therapy usually requires patient cooperation. The inability of many pediatric patients to cooperate in the same manner as adults poses a challenge to persons charged with delivering respiratory care. When approached correctly, however, amazing degrees of cooperation are possible from infants and children of all ages. Frequently, young children can serve as models of ideal cooperation for recalcitrant adults!

A prerequisite for achieving cooperation is a positive attitude toward the patient. Children are particularly sensitive to detecting hostility or other negative attitudes. They respond in kind to genuine warmth and friendliness. A child needs to believe that the therapist sincerely enjoys being with him; that he is there to make him feel better; that he will not smother him with his masks and machines; and that he will not put him into a tent, leave, and forget about him. These feelings may come more from attitude and silent communication than from what is said aloud.

Positive communication often comes subconsciously by touch, tone of voice, and facial expressions. Even neonates respond positively to stroking, speaking softly, and cuddling. A feeling of impatience or a sensation of being bothered should never be communicated to the child.

Simple acts—such as brushing a young girl's hair, or that of her doll, while she does her own nebulization treatment, or rocking an infant during and after bronchial drainage—are effective. Taking a few extra minutes to play or communicate without rushing through a treatment often *saves* more minutes than it wastes.

When introducing oneself or a new treatment to a child, one should explain carefully the purpose of the equipment and procedures. One has to know at what level his patient functions and must speak to him in language that he understands. Young children relate to their toys, which often can be used to demonstrate what will be done. The best model is another child who is known to be cooperative.

Since fears of suffocation often accompany the use of masks or other restrictive equipment, children need to understand that their use will in fact make them more comfortable. Showing children pictures of astronauts in "hoods," pilots with "masks," and deep-sea divers with "mouthpieces" may help to convince them to accept respiratory treatment. Seeing themselves in a mirror assures them that they look like a model.

To assure children that a treatment will make them feel better, one must ensure that the equipment is appropriately sized and applied as comfortably as possible. An infant or child should never be forced to lie down while a mask is pressed into his face, covering his airway. He is much more likely to accept therapy when he is held in a lap or when his back is supported against the therapist's chest.

When intermittent positive pressure breathing is introduced, it should be started at very low pressures, until the child gets used to the strange feeling and learns to coordinate his breathing with that of the machine.

Communication is especially important when a child is on assisted or controlled ventilation. Since he cannot talk, he relies on eye contact or touching. Just having someone there is reassuring. Even when a child is semicomatose or heavily sedated, he may have some awareness of his environment and still needs affection and communication.

DISEASES SPECIFIC TO PEDIATRICS

The problems presented by respiratory diseases that are specific to neonatal and pediatric patients are discussed in Chapters 29 and 30. Some of them occur only in neonates or young children because of the immaturity of their pulmonary system. Others, which were previously limited to young children, are now seen in those surviving to adulthood because of more

The diaphragm develops during gestational week 7. The major portion arises from a ventral mesodermal septum contributed by the abdominal organs. The lat-

effective therapy. All require appropriate respiratory care designed for the disease *and* the patient.

REFERENCES

1. Ahdab–Barmada M, Moosy J, Painter M: Pontosubicular necrosis and hyperoxemia. Pediatrics 66:840, 1980
2. Bland R: Special considerations in oxygen therapy for infants and children. Am Rev Respir Dis 122:45, 1980
3. Guilfoile T, Dabe K: Nasal catheter oxygen therapy for infants. Respir Care 26:35, 1981
4. Pinney M, Cotton E: Home management of bronchopulmonary dysplasia. Pediatrics 58:856, 1976

BIBLIOGRAPHY

Burgess W, Chernick V: Respiratory Therapy in Newborn Infants and Children. New York, Thieme–Stratton, 1982

Kendig E Jr, Chernick V (eds): Disorders of the Respiratory Tract in Children, 3rd ed. Philadelphia, WB Saunders, 1977

Lough M, Doershuk C, Stern R: Pediatric Respiratory Therapy, 2nd ed. Chicago, Yearbook, 1979

Lough M, Williams T, Rawson J: Newborn Respiratory Care. Chicago, Yearbook, 1979

Shoemaker W, Vidyasagar D (eds): Transcutaneous O_2 and CO_2 monitoring of the adult and neonate. Crit Care Med 9:689, 1981

Thibeault D, Gregory G: Neonatal Pulmonary Care. Menlo Park, Addison–Wesley, 1979

29

Respiratory Distress Syndrome and Other Respiratory Diseases in Neonates

Mary Ann Fletcher

FETAL LUNG DEVELOPMENT

ANATOMICAL CONSIDERATIONS

The pathophysiology of many respiratory problems in neonates depends largely on what stage of anatomical and biochemical development the cardiopulmonary system has reached at the time of birth. Perinatal factors such as asphyxia, acidosis, infection, and anemia further influence the infant's pulmonary response to stress or disease. The anticipation, diagnosis, and treatment of respiratory dysfunction, much of which is preventive, require understanding of fetal and postnatal development and of the changes that occur with birth.

The development of the respiratory structures begins by day 24 of gestation. At that time the endodermal cell layer is a longitudinal tube. The primitive lung begins as a ventral outpouching of the tube. At days 26 to 28 the bronchial tree begins to develop by a series of asymmetric dichotomous branchings of the primitive lung bud. The branching continues until week 26, when the bronchial tree from glottis to terminal bronchioles has developed. The asymmetric branching results in segmental differences in the number of conducting airways. The shorter upper segmental airways are completed by week 14, whereas the lower segmental airways continue their divisions until week 16. Cartilage continues to appear until the 24th week.[10]

The development of the respiratory bronchioles occurs after week 16 and continues until about 2 months postnatally. Respiratory tissue begins to develop between weeks 24 and 26 as saccular structures form off the respiratory bronchioles. At birth the number (24,000,000) and size of alveoli are small compared to those seen a few weeks later.[12]

Two main types of pneumocytes line the alveoli. Type I cells are flattened and nonvacuolated, appearing like connective tissue. They cover 95% of the alveolar surface area.[27] Type II pneumocytes are vacuolated and contain lysosomes that are apparent storage sites of surfactant.[2]

Type II cells appear capable of differentiating into type I cells but not the reverse.[22] The ability of the lung to recover from damage depends partly on the ability of the type II cell to repopulate the alveolus with type I cells.[9] The type II cell can synthesize, store, and release surface active phospholipids.[5] Synthesis occurs in the endoplasmic reticulum and storage in the lamellar inclusion bodies.[15] These inclusions appear as early as 20 weeks' gestation.[25]

The development of the pulmonary blood supply parallels that of the bronchi and alveoli. It is not until weeks 25 to 26 that the capillary network provides sufficient alveolar–capillary surface area to allow extrauterine gas exchange.

The diaphragm develops during gestational week 7. The major portion arises from a ventral mesodermal septum contributed by the abdominal organs. The lateral portion of the diaphragm comes from the pleuroperitoneal membranes and from the thoracic musculature.

Mucous glands and goblet cells are the major sources of tracheobronchial secretions. They develop anatomically and functionally between weeks 12 and 26 and weeks 13 and 32, respectively. In contrast, smooth muscle found throughout the pulmonary system develops only in the last few weeks of gestation, the major development taking place postnatally.[16]

Cartilage starts to develop from early mesodermal cells by week 4 of gestation, and distinct rings are visible in the trachea by week 7. Although maturation of cartilage continues postnatally, the number of cartilage generations is established by week 24. Immature cartilage provides significantly less circumferential support than it does in adult conducting airways. Its relative weakness plays a contributing role in disease pathophysiology and symptoms.

Connective tissue of the lung is also incompletely developed at birth. Only a small amount of elastic tissue is present in the neonatal lung, but little, if any, further development of collagen occurs postnatally.[36] Lymphatics appear by 70 days and are well-developed at birth. These channels are a major route for clearance of lung fluid with initial lung aeration.

BIOCHEMICAL CONSIDERATIONS

The fetal lung is metabolically active during its anatomical development. It synthesizes and secretes two particularly important materials: lung fluid and surface active phospholipids.

Lung fluid appears to be an ultrafiltrate of blood that undergoes selective reabsorption and secretion in the lung.[32,41] It flows out of the trachea at an estimated rate of about 2 ml/kg/hr, where it is either swallowed or added to amniotic fluid.[30] Its contribution to amniotic fluid volume is far less than that from placental or renal sources, but abnormal deglutition, as in esophageal atresia, and decreased production, as in some types of pulmonary hypoplasia, will be associated with polyhydramnios and oligohydramnios, respectively.

Lung fluid is important in prenatal development, particularly in establishing total lung volume. It helps maintain the fetal lung at its apparent functional residual capacity. In conditions where the production of lung fluid is less than normal or there is excessive loss or turnover of fluid, pulmonary hypoplasia may result in lung volume that is inadequate to support the infant after birth.

The fetal lung also synthesizes, stores, and secretes surfactant. Surfactant is a complex of several materials that together provide the maximum surface tension reducing activity. The most important component is lecithin, dipalmitoyl phosphatidylcholine (DPPC), synthesized primarily by a choline incorporation pathway involving several enzymes found in lung that are inducible but rate limited for production.[26]

Although lamellar inclusions containing surfactant are visible in the type II cell even in the first half of gestation, the major production and release occurs during the last few weeks. Normally during the 34th to 35th week there is a surge in the amount of DPPC released into lung fluid and thence into amniotic fluid. Its appearance in adequate quantities signifies that the alveoli will most likely remain air filled after birth. Measurement in amniotic fluid of DPPC and other stabilizing phospholipids such as phosphatidyl glycerol (PG) allows antenatal assessment of biochemical maturity. The lecithin/sphingomyelin (L/S) ratio correlates fairly reliably to the presence of pulmonary surfactant. The finding of phosphatidyl glycerol further confirms that there will be stable surfactant and biochemically mature lungs.

The function of surfactant is to counteract the natural tendency of the alveolus to collapse on expiration. According to the *Laplace relationship*, the pressure exerted by alveolar surface tension* increases as the size of the sphere decreases. Thus, on expiration, the alveolus would collapse if surfactant were not present to decrease the surface tension.

FUNCTIONAL CHANGES AT BIRTH

At birth the lung must change from an organ that has been relatively inactive physiologically to one that can support respiration and numerous complex metabolic functions. The transition must occur success-

*Alveolar surface tension is a phenomenon occurring at the interface between the liquid alveolar lining layer and the air above it. The difference in cohesive attraction between the molecules of water in the hypophase beneath the surface as compared to that among the loosely aggregated molecules of air above results in a net downward and inward "pull," a variable measurable in dynes/cm. In pure water this is 72 dynes/cm, which accounts for the ability to float needles, razor blades, and other "inappropriately" dense substances on the surface of a container of water as long as soap or other detergents that break water cohesiveness (and lower its surface tension) are not added.

fully within minutes after birth if a neonate is to survive.

During labor and a natural birth descent through the vaginal canal, the contracting uterus and tight pelvis compress the thorax, expelling lung fluid from the upper airways. During the next few hours after birth, the fluid clears further from the trachea into the oropharynx, where it is either swallowed or expelled by sneezing. Fluid in the more distal airways and alveoli clears through the lymphatics. Normal respiratory excursions, crying, and grunting facilitate the clearance, whereas inadequate surfactant and noncompliant lung disease delay removal. Failure or delay in clearing excess fluid, caused when there is no thoracic compression during birth or when maternal analgesics inhibit the neonate's respiratory excursions, results in respiratory distress, usually transient but occasionally moderately severe (see Retained Lung Fluid, p. 723).

If thoracic compression and recoil do not occur, not only will there be more residual lung fluid, but also there will be a need for greater negative pressure to establish the first breath. Normally with the first few breaths both the tidal volume and functional residual capacity establish volumes close to their expected range. By the third or fourth extrauterine breath, only 20 cm H_2O negative pressure results in appropriate tidal volumes (see Fig. 9-3). As soon as lung fluid clears, surfactant is able to stabilize the alveolus and allow low pressure ventilation.

Just as the lung makes a dramatic transition from fluid to air filled, the circulatory system undergoes major changes. In the fetus the main source of oxygenation and nutrition is the placenta. The vascular resistance of the placenta is low, whereas that of the fetal pulmonary bed is high. Because the ductus arteriosus between the aorta and pulmonary artery is open, 90% of the blood that comes from the right ventricle crosses the ductus into the low-resistance systemic-placental circulation, and only 10% enters the pulmonary circulation. There is further intracardiac shunting across the foramen ovale. Well-oxygenated blood from the lower body and placental circulation crosses the foramen ovale to the left side of the heart and flows preferentially to the developing brain.

At birth the important factors in changing the fetal circulation to that of extrauterine life are lung expansion and shift to an air-filled organ, the loss of low-resistance placental circulation, and increased Pa_{O_2}. With aeration, pulmonary vascular resistance drops dramatically, whereas that of the systemic circulation rises with clamping of the umbilical cord. In response to the increased Pa_{O_2}, the ductus constricts and inhibits blood flow across it. The blood leaving the right ventricle no longer shunts through the ductus arteriosus but now perfuses the alveolar capillaries, where extrauterine respiration occurs. Because of the increased blood return from the pulmonary veins to the left atrium, the foramen ovale also closes functionally.

Difficulty in adaptation to the extrauterine circulation occurs when the lung fails to change from the fluid-filled to the air-filled state or if other factors prevent the normal postnatal fall in pulmonary vascular resistance. Likewise, if the systemic vascular resistance fails to rise (either because of shock in the infant owing to blood loss, hypothermia, or asphyxia), the circulation may continue to shunt via a patent ductus arteriosus. Further, certain developmental defects that require shunting in the cardiovascular system may not allow a normal transition to the expected extrauterine circulation.

POSTNATAL GROWTH

After birth, both the anteroposterior and transthoracic chest diameters increase, primarily because respiratory structures (respiratory bronchioles, alveolar ducts, and alveoli) increase in size as well as in numbers. Respiratory bronchioles have established their adult pattern by 2 months, whereas the alveolar ducts and sacs continue to develop throughout childhood.[7] The nonrespiratory tissues all have a significant degree of postnatal growth, primarily in mass and strength of the supporting structures.

NEONATAL RESUSCITATION: ASSISTED TRANSITION

The first respiratory problem of neonatal life may occur during the period when the newborn must abandon his dependence on placental respiration and change to full reliance on an independent, air-breathing pulmonary system. As we have seen, the infant requires muscle strength sufficient to create negative intrathoracic pressures up to 80 cm H_2O for the first breath or two. His airway must be patent to allow exchange of air for fluid. His heart must be capable of increasing pulmonary blood flow to about ten times what it had been before the onset of breathing only a few beats earlier. He must be capable of maintaining his own body temperature. If the infant lacks any of these required abilities, immediate assistance is needed for successful transition.

ANTICIPATION

The best guarantee for a good resuscitation is *anticipation* (i.e., anticipation of which infant will likely need assistance, what personnel should be present, and what equipment and medications should be ready for resuscitation). If a hospital cannot meet all the anticipated needs, then proper planning means transferring the mother for delivery to a hospital that can.

To some extent, virtually all infants are at risk at the time of birth. Unfortunately, there are unpredictable cases who, despite appropriate prenatal care and apparently uncomplicated gestations and deliveries, may still have initial depression or congenital anomalies that make transition complicated or impossible. There are some warning signs in maternal, pregnancy, and labor histories that alert us to those infants at higher risk for transitional difficulties. Recognition of these factors (listed below) allows appropriate anticipation and preparation.

MATERNAL FACTORS THAT DETERMINE THE HIGH-RISK INFANT

General

- No prenatal care
- Maternal age (<16 or >40)
- Fetal weight (too high or too low)
- Low socioeconomic class

Medical History

- Diabetes mellitus
- Cardiovascular disease (especially hypertension or vascular disease)
- Pulmonary disease (asthma)
- Renal disease
- Neurologic disease (seizure disorders, myasthenia gravis)
- Anemia, thrombocytopenia
- Infection
- Endocrine disease
- Drug addiction
- Collagen disease
- Rh-sensitization
- Smoking history

Pregnancy History

- Previous pregnancies
- Lengths of gestations (too long or too short)
- Birth asphyxia or trauma
- Previous cesarean section
- Early neonatal deaths

Present Pregnancy

- Toxemia
- Bleeding
- Multiple gestation
- Polyhydramnios or oligohydramnios
- Meconium staining of amniotic fluid
- Fetal presentation
- Prolonged rupture of membranes
- Medications
- Abnormal fetal heart pattern
- Fetal acidosis (pH < 7.20)
- Cesarean section

An increasing number of diagnostic tools are now clinically available that help to detect a fetus likely to have difficulty at birth. These include echosonography to detect size, position, and gross anomalies of the fetus and placenta; fetal breathing movements and activity; fetal heart rate response with movement and contractions; and endocrine analysis for placental well-being.

Since means for evaluating the fetus during labor are now readily available through fetal heart rate monitoring and intrauterine fetal scalp blood sampling, one can be more certain of detecting a baby likely to be depressed at birth as a result of birth asphyxia. A distressed fetus may demonstrate persistent bradycardia secondary to cord compression or fetal ECG patterns suggestive of placental insufficiency. In addition, the fetus may have a scalp blood *p*H that is less than 7.20 or one that is falling with successive samplings before delivery. The person charged with the transitional care of an infant should know if there have been any of these warning signs before birth in order to anticipate a need for resuscitation.

FETAL HEART RATE PATTERNS THAT SUGGEST NEONATAL INTRAUTERINE DISTRESS

- Persistent tachycardia in the absence of maternal fever (>160 beats/min)
- Persistent bradycardia (<120 beats/min)
- Loss of beat-to-beat variability not attributable to maternal medication (i.e., variability not returning with fetal stimulation)
- Late-onset cardiac rate deceleration (placental insufficiency)
- Variable cardiac rate deceleration that is severe (<60 beats/min) or prolonged (cord compression)

EQUIPMENT PREPARATION

Each delivery room should have all the equipment that may be needed for any kind of resuscitation. The resuscitation area should be no more than a few feet from the delivery site. Recommendations for equipment and medications for a resuscitation cart are listed below. This equipment should be simple, neatly organized, up-to-date, and in working order to maintain its usability. The delivery room resuscitation cart should include tools for clearing and providing an airway, a means for delivering warm, moist oxygen under controlled positive pressure ventilation, medications to counteract drug depression or metabolic abnormalities, and a method of maintaining controlled infant warmth.

Pressure valve resuscitators, such as the Elder valve, should not be used because control of the inspiratory pressure is not specific enough, the oxygen is cold and dry, and one cannot obtain a reliable indication of lung compliance when using such devices.

It is critical that there be a means of keeping the infant warm during the resuscitation. Delivery rooms are comfortably cool for the obstetrician but potentially disastrous for the neonate who, born wet, moves from a controlled intrauterine climate to one that requires intrinsic heat production or supply of extrinsic heat. The infants most likely to require more than routine resuscitation are those most poorly equipped to maintain their body temperature. Any of the radiant heat warmers available today generally are adequate for providing a satisfactory temperature for the infant.

DELIVERY ROOM EQUIPMENT FOR RESUSCITATION OF THE NEWBORN

- Warming bed
- Suction devices
    - Bulb syringes
    - DeLee traps
    - Catheters 5, 8, 10F
- Oral airway: 000, 00, 0
- Endotracheal tubes: 2.5, 3.0, 3.5
- Laryngoscope handle
    - Blades: Miller type 0 and 1
    - Extra bulbs and batteries
- Masks: Sizes 0–4
- Self-inflating bag: 0.5–1 liter size
- Anesthesia bag: 0.5 liter size
    - Manometer for airway pressure
- Warmed, humidified oxygen source with a blender
- Medications
    - Naloxone hydrochloride (Narcan)
    - Sterile water for injection
    - Sodium chloride for injection
    - Sodium bicarbonate: 1/2 mEq/ml
    - Epinephrine: 1:10,000
    - D-50-W: dilute 2:3 for D-20-W
    - Heparin
- Alcohol wipes
- Iodophore solution
- Syringes: 1, 3, 5, 20 ml
- Catheter trays: Equipped for arterial or umbilical venous line placement
- Dextrostix; hematocrit tubes; laboratory tubes; blood gas syringes

RECOGNITION OF THE DISTRESSED NEONATE

When a baby is born, persons in attendance must assess the condition in a rapid, comprehensive manner. Although it is easy to distinguish the normal infant who merely needs drying from the severely depressed infant who needs immediate intubation and cardiac massage, intermediate situations may be less obvious.

A set of graded observations, devised by Dr. Virginia Apgar, provides a means of standardizing the assessment and serves to identify most infants who need assistance. The modified scoring system, the *Apgar score*, is presented in Table 29-1. Values ordinarily are assigned specifically at 1 and 5 minutes as part of the conventional standardization, but the organized assessment may be made throughout the infant's transitional period as long as any distress is noted.

A number of general observations and conclusions can be made in the first 15 seconds while the infant's delivery is being completed, his mouth and nose suctioned, and his umbilical cord clamped. If the muscle tone is good and there is a reaction to the suctioning and handling, the need for vigorous resuscitation is unlikely to arise. Generally, an infant with an Apgar score of 7 or more will need only oral and nasal clearing and drying of skin unless his condition changes and Apgar score falls. If an infant is floppy and unresponsive, aggressive resuscitation almost certainly will be needed. If the infant is small and obviously premature, he is more likely to have a low Apgar score and require assistance.

Table 29-1. Apgar Score System*

	SCORE		
SIGN	*0*	*1*	*2*
Heart rate	Absent	Below 100	Over 100
Respiratory effort	Absent	Weak, irregular	Good, crying
Muscle tone	Flaccid	Some flexion of extremities	Active motion well flexed
Reflex irritability (response to suctioning)	No response	Grimace	Cry, cough, or sneeze
Color	Blue, pale	Body pink, extremities blue	Completely pink

*The condition of the newborn infant is expressed as a score that is the sum of five numbers obtained from the above variables. The numbers should be determined at 1 and 5 minutes after birth and thereafter until the baby is stable. Possible scores range from 0 to 10. The predictive value of this scoring system as an indicator of neonatal outcome is excellent. (Apgar V: Proposal for a new method of evaluation of the newborn infant. Anesth Analg 32:260, 1953; Apgar V et al: Evaluation of the newborn infant—second report. JAMA 168:1985, 1958)

PERSONNEL PREPARATION

When a high-risk or distressed fetus is identified, all persons who will help with his transitional care should be aware of his potential problems. Physicians and nurses can prepare mentally and physically for the procedures and equipment they may use. If respiratory problems are expected, as in a premature infant with pulmonary immaturity, the respiratory therapist can prepare the needed equipment ahead of time. The radiology department can ready the appropriate technicians and equipment. The blood bank can prepare for rapid assistance should exchange transfusion be necessary. With a coordinated team, precious minutes are gained when the neonate needs them most.

RESUSCITATION TECHNIQUES

As with any resuscitation, the first step in assisting respiration in the infant at birth is to clear the airway. The obstetrician usually does this as the head is delivered, but the infant may require repeated suctioning after delivery. The mouth is cleared first to prevent aspiration of the oropharyngeal contents, and then the nose is suctioned.

The safest instrument for suctioning is a bulb syringe. If a catheter is needed for deeper suctioning, it should be inserted carefully because significant bradycardia or perforation of the trachea may occur. If there are copious secretions, one should allow recovery between suctionings, using supplemental oxygen as indicated. Prolonged, persistent suctioning may cause bradycardia and subsequent apnea. When the trachea contains thick or particulate meconium or blood, it must be cleared completely, even *if* bradycardia develops during the procedure.

While suctioning is being done, the infant's body is dried, which stimulates the infant to cry. If further resuscitation is anticipated, the infant should be placed in a suitable controlled-heat environment.

Assessment of the infant is made during delivery and during the initial suctioning and the drying procedures. If the Apgar score is 3 or less on immediate evaluation, the infant will require intubation and positive pressure ventilation. If there is a rapid return in heart rate and respiratory effort, ventilation should be continued to assist the infant's own efforts until resuscitation has been completed. If there is no immediate response to ventilatory assistance and the endotracheal tube is correctly positioned with no apparent air leak, an umbilical catheter should be placed for administration of dilute sodium bicarbonate, 1 to 3 mEq/kg over several minutes. A plasma expander should be given only if there has been blood loss or the blood pressure is low.

If there is depression due to maternal analgesics for labor pains, naloxone hydrochloride (Narcan) may be given at 0.01 mg/kg. It should not be given if there has been maternal drug abuse to prevent initiation of withdrawal. If the depression results from inhalation of anesthesia, barbiturates, or magnesium sulfate, assisted ventilation is indicated until the depressant effect is no longer present.

If the Apgar score is between 4 and 6, warmed oxygen or intermittent assistance in ventilation with bag and mask may be given. If color and tone rapidly improve, oxygen administration may be continued until the infant's color is satisfactory. If the response is poor, one should consider intubation and use of the previously mentioned medications.

VENTILATION BY BAG AND MASK OR BAG AND TUBE

The distressed neonate needs positive pressure ventilation when alveolar ventilation is inadequate or respiratory effort insufficient. While hand ventilating, one can assess the adequacy initially by observing chest wall excursions. If the infant fails to make strong initial inspiratory *and* expiratory efforts, especially in cases where thoracic compression and recoil are limited, he may require higher initial pressures and take longer to achieve a normal functional residual capacity.[45] With normal lungs and proper tube position (*i.e.*, not in a mainstem bronchus), the requisite inflating pressures should drop quickly. It is appropriate to ventilate at frequencies up to 60/min to 80/min when hypercarbia and acidosis are present. Thirty to 40 breaths/min suffice in the absence of lung disease and asphyxia.

On occasion, simple application of continuous positive pressure of 4 to 6 cm H_2O by mask will stimulate a deeper respiratory effort in the absence of marked prematurity, asphyxia, or drug depression.

INTUBATION OF THE NEONATE

There are two general reasons for intubation in the neonate: removal of material from the trachea and provision of a guaranteed airway. The first indication often occurs in the delivery room after an infant has been delivered through thick or particulate meconium or has aspirated blood. In such instances, *orotracheal* intubation comes *before any other measures* of resuscitation. Later, intubation for removal of secretions may be needed in infants who cannot cough normally or when airway secretions are excessive or thickened.

The second general indication for intubation is the need for an airway to bypass an obstruction or as a route for positive pressure ventilation acutely during resuscitation. In an emergency, intubation should be by the oral route. For prolonged intubation in larger infants, some physicians prefer nasal intubations because of presumed increased stability and oral access. Contrary to popular belief, however, there may, in fact, *not* be significantly fewer extubations with the nasal route because flexion and rotation of the neck are the major causes of tube displacement.

Regardless of preferred route, care in fixation and monitoring for endotracheal tube position is essential. The total length of the tube within the trachea is only 2 cm to 4 cm; thus displacement into a bronchus or out of the trachea is the most frequent complication. Keeping the infant's head in the same sagittal plane as the body without extension or flexion helps maintain a stable tube position within the trachea.

Regardless of route, the tube should be constructed of a clear, nonbiologically active material; have a nontapered shape; be cut to minimize dead space; and be appropriately sized to the infant. One need not use the largest tube that will fit to prevent leak, since such tubes will produce more laryngeal and subglottic trauma (see Table 29-2 for suggested sizes.) A helpful relationship for emergency sizing of length is that for a 1000-g infant, the distance from lip to lip of tube is about 7 cm; for a 2000-g infant, 8 cm; and for a 3000 g infant, 9 cm.[42]

In preparation for intubation, one must carefully monitor the infant's status. One should position the infant flat on a bed without extending the neck, as one would in older patients. Because the larynx is rela-

Table 29-2. Selection of Endotracheal Tubes in Infants

		LENGTH WITHOUT CONNECTOR	
WEIGHT OF INFANT *g*	ID *mm*	*Nasotracheal Tube cm*	*Orotracheal Tube cm*
500–1000	2.5	8.0	6–7.0
1001–1400	3.0	8.5	
1401–1900		9.0	
1901–2200		9.5	7–8.0
2201–2600		10.0	
2601–3000	3.5	10.5	8–9.0
3001–3400		11.0	
3401–3700		11.5	
3701–4100		12.0	9–10.0
4101–4500	4.0	12.5	
>4500		13.0	

*ID = internal diameter.

tively higher in neonates, visualization is possible without neck extension, which narrows the laryngeal opening and makes passing the tube more difficult.

The oropharynx should be suctioned carefully, applying oxygen and ventilation as required by the infant's condition. Using a free forefinger, one next opens the infant's mouth and passes the laryngoscope blade atraumatically along the left side of the mouth to the level of the vallecula. While pulling on the blade to open the mouth further, one should pivot the blade on the back of the tongue and pass the tube along the other side of the mouth, not in the curve of the laryngoscope blade. Under full visualization, one passes the tube just through the glottis. Tube position can be assessed by auscultation and chest movement. The tube is then carefully fixed. Throughout the procedure, one must be certain that the infant receives enough oxygen, and one must stop and ventilate with a mask if bradycardia occurs.

NEONATAL RESPIRATORY DISTRESS SYNDROME

Respiratory distress syndrome (RDS) or hyaline membrane disease (HMD) represents the major respiratory problem in neonatal intensive care units. It is difficult to determine the worldwide incidence of RDS because its occurrence relates most specifically to the incidence of prematurity, which, in turn, is affected by many factors, including race, multiplicity of gestation, nutrition, and quality of medical care.

With improved perinatal care, both incidence and mortality have decreased, even though statistics now include lower birth weights and younger gestations. In perinatal centers in the United States, RDS currently occurs in only 10% to 15% of premature infants who weigh less than 2.5 kg at birth.[18] Still about 7000 deaths per year occur where RDS is the major illness, but in many cases intracranial hemorrhage and other complications of marked prematurity are the primary terminal events.

RDS affects premature infants primarily of less than 35 weeks' gestation. Although it does occur in older infants, there are usually complicating factors such as uncontrolled maternal diabetes or perinatal asphyxic episodes, particularly those related to fetal blood loss and hypoperfusion. There is a male-to-female case preponderance that exceeds the expected male-to-female neonatal ratio. There are also racial and familial tendencies distinct from gestational age but probably related to environment.[37]

CLINICAL PRESENTATION

The infant with classical RDS becomes symptomatic in the delivery suite. He frequently has a low Apgar score and needs some form of transitional resuscitation. For him, each breath requires an extraordinary respiratory effort. He is tachypneic. His alae nasi flare. His suprasternal, intercostal, and substernal muscles retract. His sternocleidomastoids contract as he uses his accessory muscles of respiration. With expiration, the infant emits an audible grunt against a closed glottis and may develop a short, whining expiratory cry.

His chest may have an increased anteroposterior diameter although his functional residual capacity is low. His diaphragm descends strongly with inspiration; as the diaphragm descends, the abdomen balloons out and the chest wall retracts (paradoxical respiration). The distressed infant becomes cyanotic in room air. His skin appears pale and dusky and frequently edematous. His urine output is low. The infant often is "floppy" and becomes more and more motionless, except for his respiratory effort. He requires increasing quantities of exogenous heat to keep his body temperature normal.

With progression of the disease, he may become even more tachypneic. His respiratory pattern may become paradoxical or demonstrate jerking inspiratory effort ("cog-wheeling"). He may develop apnea and may lose the normal beat-to-beat variability in heart rate. If symptoms progress rapidly without any stabilization or without response to appropriate therapy, the infant will die.

Each of these symptoms in the untreated infant reflects a physiological process during the course of RDS. With progressive atelectasis owing to inadequate synthesis of surface-active material, the amount of negative intrathoracic pressure needed to expand the lung with each inspiration remains high after birth and increases as the disease progresses. The chest shape and nasal flaring reflect the use of accessory muscles of respiration. The intercostal attachments and xiphisternal cartilage are poorly fixed and the ribs highly cartilaginous. As such, they are more compliant than the lung parenchyma, and they retract with inspiratory effort. The diaphragm performs the major work of ventilation. As it contracts, the diaphragm causes bulging of the abdominal contents against the weak rectus abdominis muscles. Grunting or whining reflects the effort to maintain increased intrathoracic pressure in order to prevent alveolar collapse on expiration. Cyanosis reflects hypoxemia from an increasingly large alveolar–arterial oxygen gradient as atelectasis progresses. The "cog-wheeling" pattern of respiration reflects carbon dioxide retention. Dusky skin color is associated with poor peripheral perfusion secondary to decreased cardiac output and progressive acidosis. Edema and poor urine output result from poor renal perfusion and decreased plasma oncotic pressure because of the low plasma proteins. A worsening metabolic acidosis from inadequate perfusion and a respiratory acidosis from insufficient ventilation develop.

The infant may fatigue and then become less responsive. He may actually appear to be in *less* respiratory distress because he is incapable of the great effort required to produce gas exchange. The heart rate becomes fixed because of loss of neural regulation of its variability. These last two findings are especially ominous and often signal impending death.

CLINICAL COURSE

The findings outlined previously depict the untreated infant or the infant who fails to respond to therapy. The progression of symptoms may be rapid, leading to death of the infant within a few hours of birth, or may be more gradual over the first 24 to 48 hours. If there are no associated complications, the infant who will recover stabilizes after about 36 hours and then gradually starts to improve by 72 hours. His requirements for assisted ventilation or CPAP or for oxygen may persist for as long as 1 or 2 weeks. Tachypnea, retractions, and flaring may persist for several weeks but generally resolve slowly as the infant continues to improve.

ROENTGENOGRAPHIC FINDINGS

The *serial* roentgenograms of an infant with RDS are diagnostic. The classic appearance in the untreated baby is that of reticulogranular infiltrates distributed throughout the lung fields, causing the appearance of "frosted glass" (Fig. 29-1). This appearance is due to alveolar atelectasis interspersed with overdistended aerated bronchioles and alveolar ducts and does *not* reflect the presence of hyaline membranes.

The earliest roentgenograms may appear relatively normal despite clinical symptoms. Rarely, there may be evidence of overdistention with the ribs in a horizontal position and increased anteroposterior diameter of the chest. More classically there is some loss of lung volume even very early. With progressive atelectasis, granularity increases and air bronchograms become more evident. Alternatively, in the first hours

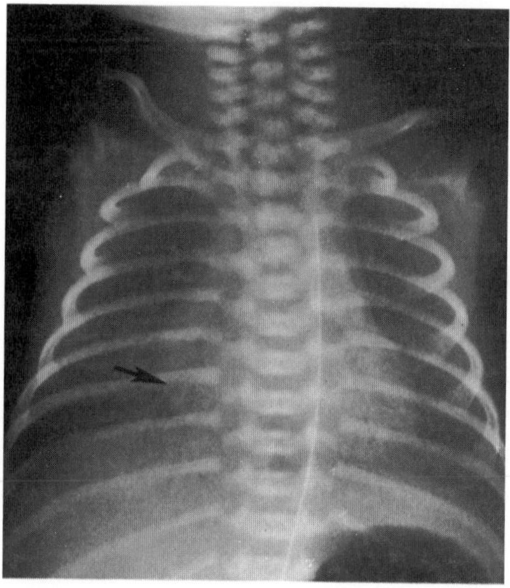

Fig. 29-1. Hyaline membrane disease (neonatal respiratory distress syndrome). Typical reticulogranular densities are diffusely distributed through both lung fields. Air bronchograms can be seen in the right lower lobe *(arrow)*.

after birth, the granularity may be almost obscured because of retention of lung fluid or because the depressed infant fails to establish initial lung expansion. After lung fluid has been cleared, however, classic granularity appears. Because the earliest roentgenograms may not be diagnostic, films at about 4 to 6 hours of age are more helpful in establishing the radiologic diagnosis of RDS.

Therapy with continuous positive airway pressure (CPAP) modifies the appearance of the roentgenogram, decreasing the confluence of the granularity. One may mistakenly infer significant improvement from the appearance of films taken before the institution of distending airway pressure. Roentgenographic changes may indicate that the pressure has decreased the amount of atelectasis, but they do not reflect progression or regression of RDS itself.

Gradually progressive consolidation reflects worsening of the disease process whose pathologic correlate is near-total atelectasis. In contrast, the more abrupt onset of total roentgenographic opacity, the "white-out," is associated with pulmonary edema of noncardiac origin (primarily secondary to an acute intracranial hemorrhage) or with massive bilateral pulmonary hemorrhage (Fig. 29-2B). These complications correlate with simultaneous worsening of the patient.

The roentgenographic resolution of uncomplicated RDS lags behind clinical improvement, al-

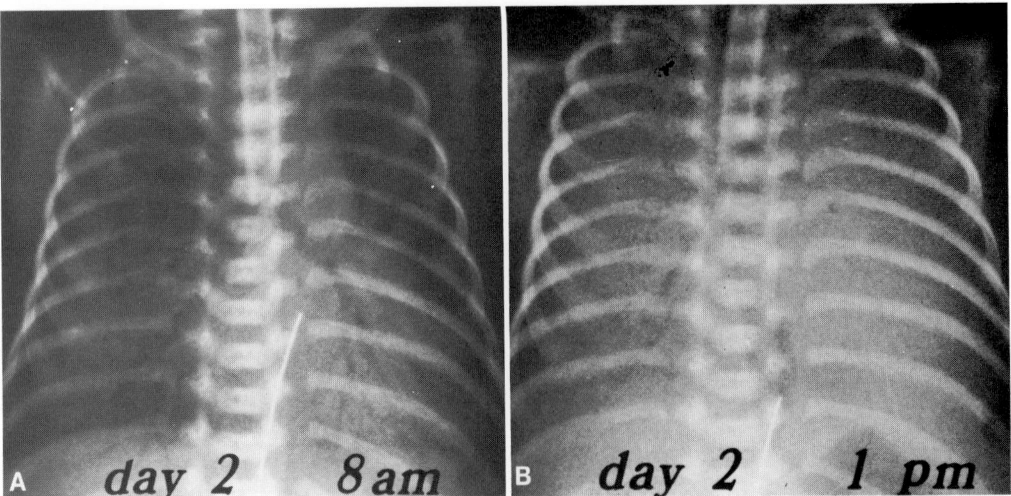

Fig. 29-2. *(A)* Chest roentgenogram of a 2-day-old premature infant with clearing hyaline membrane disease. Note the early upper lobe clearing compared to the lower lobes. *(B)* The same infant 5 hours later. Sudden reopacification of the lungs has occurred due to pulmonary hemorrhage. Large amounts of blood were suctioned from the endotracheal tube. Postmortem examination disclosed massive bilateral pulmonary hemorrhage.

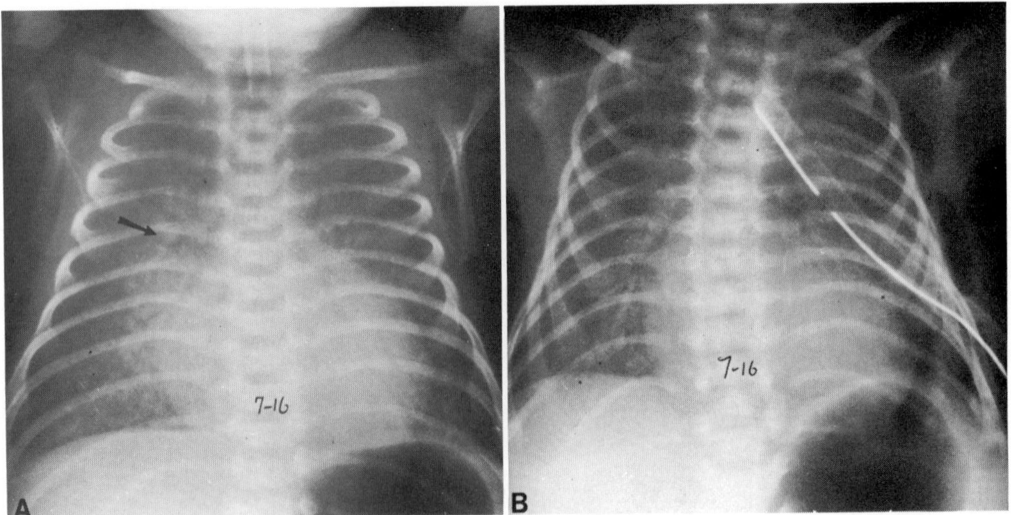

Fig. 29-3. *(A)* Recovering hyaline membrane disease with patent ductus arteriosus. There is evidence of roentgenographic improvement in hyaline membrane disease with less alveolar atelectasis, but there is increased pulmonary vascularity consistent with a left-to-right shunt through the ductus arteriosus. Clinical signs were consistent with a large patent ductus arteriosus (arrow points to enlarged pulmonary vessel). *(B)* This film of the same patient was taken immediately after ligation of a large patent ductus arteriosus. There is decreased pulmonary vascularity and heart size.

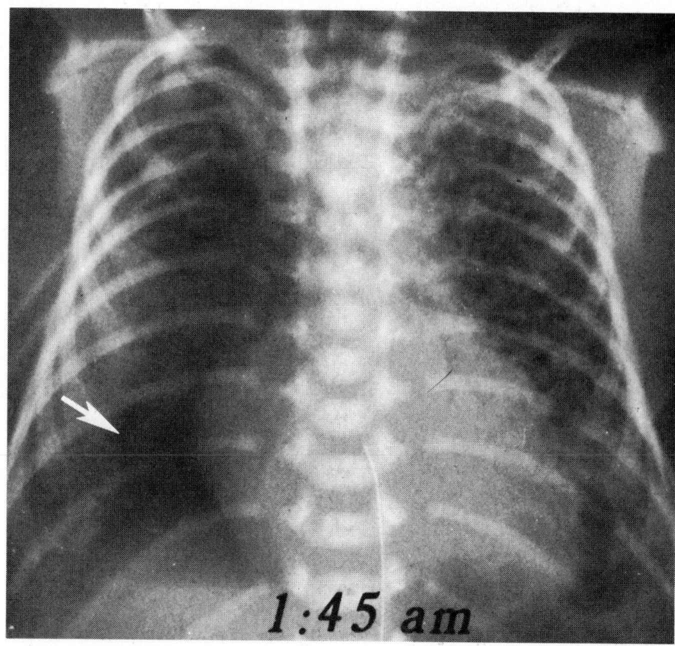

Fig. 29-4. Pneumothorax and interstitial emphysema. Pneumothorax on the right with chest tube in place. Note accumulation of air anteriorly and medially *(arrow)* because of noncompliance of the lungs and inability to collapse concentrically. Interstitial pulmonary emphysema involves the left lung; a left pneumothorax occurred shortly after this film had been taken.

though it may predict imminent improvement. Resolution with decreasing granularity occurs first in the upper lobes (Fig. 29-2A). In contrast, many complications associated with RDS appear on the roentgenogram before they can be distinguished reliably by clinical observation. Pneumonia or aspiration causes a patchy or focal pattern of increased consolidation. Pulmonary edema resulting from cardiovascular overload is demonstrated as cardiomegaly and vascular engorgement. The appearance of "shunt vessels," indicating an increased flow in the tortuous pulmonary vessels seen on end in the hilar areas, is associated with the left-to-right shunting across a patent ductus arteriosus (Fig. 29-3). Extraalveolar air collections such as interstitial emphysema, silent pneumothorax, and pneumomediastinum may appear on x-ray before any recognized clinical signs (Figs. 29-4 and 29-5). Pseudocysts, representing alveolar ruptures that remain within the pulmonary parenchyma, are detectable only on roentgenograms.

When interpreted along with the clinical evidence, roentgenograms play an invaluable role in the diagnosis and management of RDS.

PATHOLOGY

The pathologic findings in infants who die from RDS are variable and depend on the interval between death and autopsy and on the type of therapy given before death, but they usually are generalized and severe. The lungs appear liverlike, airless, and deep red because of atelectasis. They sink when immersed in water.

Histologic examination reveals marked atelectasis, making the alveolar spaces virtually indistinguishable (Fig. 29-6). The terminal bronchioles and alveolar ducts are dilated. The epithelium appears damaged, with necrosis and sloughing. If hyaline membranes are present, they appear as an eosinophilic lining of aerated portions of the terminal bronchioles or alveolar ducts. The lymphatics are markedly dilated. Leukocytes appear if the infant has lived more than 24 hours. Macrophages that ingest the fragmented membrane appear by 72 hours of life. Cellular proliferation of the epithelium, indicating bronchiolar repair, usually appears by the same time. Hemorrhage into alveoli may be present in some areas or may be generalized but is not invariably present.

On examination by electron microscopy, the membrane has the characteristics of fibrin with cellular debris. Type II epithelial cells are increased in number in proportion to the time of survival and contain abundant inclusion bodies. Evidence of damage to the epithelial cells is present.

Many complications of RDS often are present. Interstitial emphysema may appear as tiny blebs on the

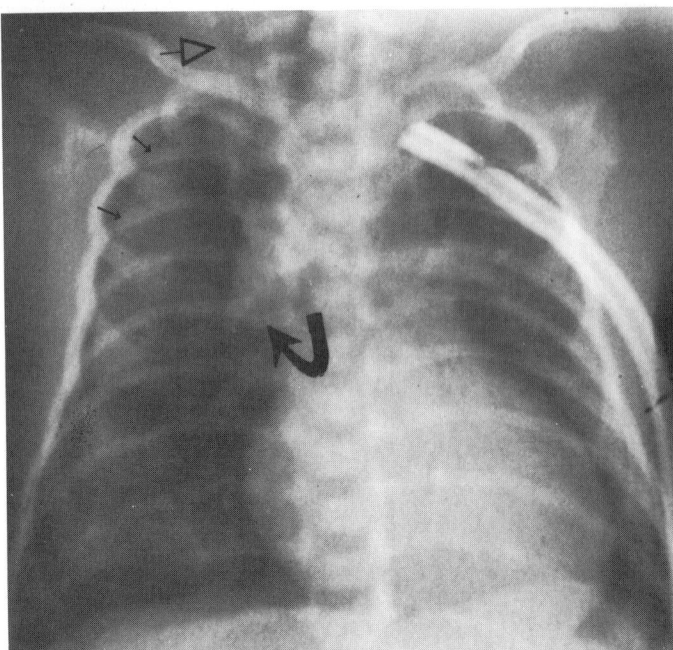

Fig. 29-5. Pneumothorax, pneumomediastinum, and subcutaneous emphysema. There is a pneumothorax on the right *(small arrows)* as well as a pneumomediastinum. Note the elevation of the thymus with air in the mediastinum producing the "spinnaker sail sign" *(large arrow).* Air has dissected from the mediastinum into the soft tissues of the neck *(open arrow).*

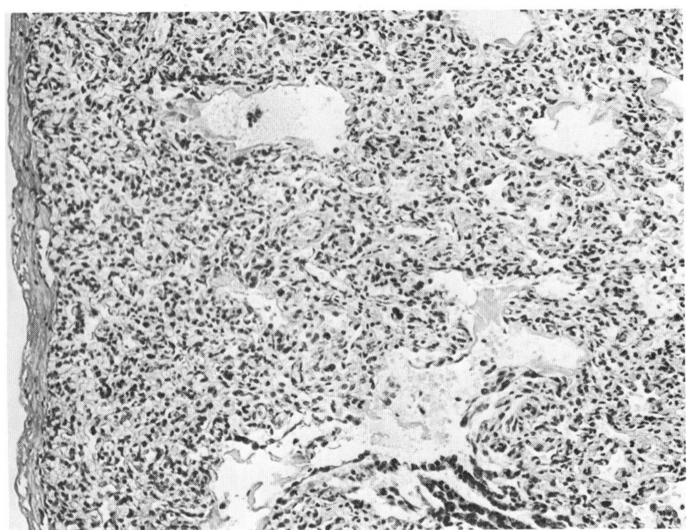

Fig. 29-6. Photomicrograph (×160) showing a peripheral portion of lung of a 1-day-old premature infant who died of hyaline membrane disease. Most air spaces are collapsed, particularly the alveoli. In the remaining ducts, protein precipitate and typical gray hyaline membrane are deposited at the periphery. There is simultaneous degeneration of some of the terminal bronchial epithelium. (Courtesy of Kurt Benirschke, M.D.)

pleural surface, or there may be other more extensive air collections in the pleural cavity or mediastinum. Pneumonia may cause a marked inflammatory response separate from that resulting from alveolar necrosis and repair.

The heart is dilated, particularly the right atrium and ventricle. The ductus arteriosus is widely patent. The liver is congested and has numerous sinusoidal infarcts, as well as fatty changes in the hepatocytes. The adrenals are smaller than normal for age. There may be microscopic or gross hemorrhages in the intestines and kidneys. In a series reported by Ambrus and coworkers, 67% of infants dying with RDS had intracranial hemorrhages, and 53% had hemorrhages in the lungs or other viscera. 1) Intracranial hemorrhage most often is located in the periventricular and intraventricular areas but also may be present in subdural or subarachnoid areas or within the brain tissue itself. It may be microscopic and show evidence of healing, or it may be massive and appear more acute.

LABORATORY FINDINGS IN RDS

Changes in blood chemistries in infants with RDS primarily depend on the extent of poor peripheral perfusion and anoxia that develop: There are no predictable biochemical changes. If the secondary phenomena are prevented or treated quickly, many chemical changes need not develop. Some alterations reflect poor perfusion and hypoxia: namely, lactic acidosis, elevated blood urea nitrogen, and hyperkalemia. There is a striking correlation between severity of RDS and low serum proteins and edema at birth. Anemia invariably is present from iatrogenic and accumulated blood losses as well as from prematurity. Hypocalcemia and hypoglycemia reflect the premature infant's inability to mobilize enough stores to keep up with body demands.

Arterial blood gases again often reflect treatment as well as response to accompanying stress. Progressive hypoxemia is the first and only consistent hallmark of RDS. Hypercarbia in the earliest stages more often represents inadequate respiratory drive because of hypoxemia, hypothermia, hypoglycemia, drug depression, or asphyxia than it does a pulmonary shunt directly related to RDS. One should consider a cause other than uncomplicated RDS if the Pa_{CO_2} is more abnormal than the Pa_{O_2}.

Newborns with RDS have reduced surfactant activity with immature lecithin/sphingomyelin (L/S) ratios of their tracheal or amniotic fluid aspirates.

Often metabolic acidosis occurs secondary to perinatal asphyxia, poor renal and peripheral perfusion, anemia, and tissue hypoxia. The immature and poorly perfused kidney does not handle metabolic acidosis well. As carbon dioxide accumulates, respiratory acidosis adds to the acid–base imbalance.

The degree of aberration of the blood gases is proportional to the severity of the disease process. Lack of response to appropriate treatment may be prognostic, but proper treatment requires recognition of the significance of each change and correlation with the clinical situation. For instance, a carbon dioxide tension of 40 torr may be normal for a newborn infant breathing at a rate of 40 to 50/min, but in an infant breathing at a rate of 80 to 110/min it reflects poor carbon dioxide excretion and inadequate compensation for metabolic acidosis.

Many infants with RDS manifest abnormalities in coagulation factors. Although values for "normal" prematures tend to reflect some degree of coagulation defect compared to older infants, those infants with the most severe symptoms from shock and hypoxia may have aberrations significant enough to contribute to or to cause a bleeding diathesis. The primary defects are in the vitamin-K-dependent factors produced in the liver. Some infants develop defects consistent with intravascular coagulation and consumption of platelets that are not attributable to sepsis or to thrombus formation particularly around catheters or at other bleeding sites.

TREATMENT

The treatment of RDS is directed at three general areas. The first is treatment directed at reversing or preventing the effects of the abnormal physiological changes in the lung: progressive diffuse alveolar atelectasis that results in an increased oxygen gradient and $\dot{V}/\dot{Q}$ abnormalities. The second area is directed at preventing and reversing the side-effects of asphyxia and poor perfusion: metabolic acidosis, poor renal output, edema with decreased circulatory volume, upset thermal homeostasis, abnormal electrolytes, and hypoglycemia. The final area includes all the complications involved in the course and treatment of the general disease process: infection, pulmonary air leaks, pulmonary edema/hemorrhage, bronchopulmonary dysplasia, patent ductus arteriosus, heart failure, bleeding diathesis, intracranial hemorrhage, anemia, retinal oxygen damage, hyperbilirubinemia, nutrition, and all the possible complications from the use of indwelling catheters and endotracheal tubes.

General Care

One of the most important basics in caring for all neonates and particularly small premature infants with lung disease is the need to provide an appropriate environmental temperature. Biochemical maintenance of body temperature involves oxygen consumption and by itself may cause hypoxemia and tissue hypoxia with acidosis. There is also tremendous use of calories so that up to 25% to 50% of an infant's daily intake may be wasted in temperature maintenance. *Airway temperature* requiring humidifier-heaters that reliably maintain the inspired gases at 35° to 36°C and 100% humidity must be carefully controlled. Additionally, the internal environment may have added humidity to decrease evaporative heat loss. Heat shields and blankets minimize convective, conductive, and radiant heat loss.

Fluid management of premature infants with RDS has radically changed in recent years. Because there is generally poor perfusion and renal output with metabolic acidosis, the tendency has been to infuse more fluid, particularly as part of delivery room resuscitation, to increase circulating volume. Unfortunately much of this fluid seems to shift fairly quickly to extravascular spaces, entering lung parenchyma and increasing peripheral edema. Although there has been initial improvement in most of these infants after fluid infusions, there may also be some relationship to later development of heart failure owing to patent ductus arteriosus, bronchopulmonary dysplasia, and intracranial hemorrhage. There now is emphasis to giving fluid, particularly blood transfusions, over more prolonged intervals to avoid the wide swings in vascular pressure that accompany bolus infusions and to limit total daily intake while using medications to improve renal blood flow. Effective ventilation with settings that optimally maintain functional residual capacity and tidal volume at close to normal volumes seems to be one of the most effective ways of assisting the blood pressure and circulation.

Continuous monitoring of blood gases transcutaneously (Ptc_{O_2}) allows earlier detection of tissue hypoxia and poor perfusion. Earlier correction results in more overall stability for the infant.

When metabolic acidosis does develop despite normal temperature, appropriate fluid intake, and ventilation and there is bicarbonate deficit, slow infusions of sodium bicarbonate are indicated. Bicarbonate is not indicated when acidosis results from carbon dioxide retention or when there is other remedial etiology. Generally when the pH is less than 7.20 or has been progressively worsening despite other corrective measures, bicarbonate will benefit the infant unless there is also hypernatremia. Rapid infusions of sodium bicarbonate with rapid changes in osmolality may be associated with intracranial hemorrhage as well as hypernatremia, hypokalemia, and hypocalcemia.

Hypoglycemia will occur in virtually all sick prematurely born infants unless there is a continuous infusion of glucose at 4 to 6 mg/kg/min. Similarly, hyperglycemia may develop despite previously "homeostatic" infusion rates, often indicating the onset of sepsis, intracranial hemorrhage, or some other complication.

Infants with RDS are not orally fed until there has been significant stabilization and apparent normal perfusion of the intestinal tract. Because the risk of regurgitation and aspiration is high in premature infants while on artificial ventilation or CPAP, most institutions delay initiating early gastric feedings. Poor intestinal perfusion relates to the development of necrotizing enterocolitis; concurrent parenteral nutrition allows low volume and slow rates of feeding.

During early stabilization, the use of continuous intraarterial oxygen saturation and transcutaneous monitoring in conjunction with arterial Pa_{O_2} monitoring allows more constant assessment and shortens the time between appropriate changes in therapy. Capillary blood gases are unreliable in the early stages of HMD, and intermittent arterial sampling portrays only a glimpse of the actual clinical situation.

Generally, when Pa_{O_2} by intermittent sampling is greater than 150 torr, one should decrease the FI_{O_2} by up to 0.20 and resample in 20 minutes. If the Pa_{O_2} is between 100 and 150, the FI_{O_2} should be decreased by 0.10 and for 85 to 100, by 0.05. When the infant is particularly labile, as when there is pulmonary hypertension or if he is disturbed by handling and procedures, one should decrease the FI_{O_2} more gradually. It is important to avoid wide swings in FI_{O_2}, high or low.

The periods in a noncomplicated course of RDS when oxygen regulation requires most adjustments are institution of oxygen therapy; institution of mechanical respiratory support; changes in airway pressure delivered; and onset of the diuretic phase of the illness.

Treatment with Increased Ambient Oxygen Concentrations

The primary defect of RDS is hypoxia. As long as a distressed infant is vigorous, with good respiratory effort and no evidence of an impending complication or respiratory insufficiency by blood gas analysis, an elevated ambient oxygen concentration may be all the respiratory support needed. Because there is a need for precise control of FI_{O_2}, blended, warmed, and humidified oxygen in an appropriate head hood is the most effective means of supplying the specific oxygen needs as determined by direct blood gas analysis or by transcutaneous monitoring. Regulating the FI_{O_2} to maintain the infant's Pa_{O_2} at the desired levels requires a good blender as well as a delivery system that does not have significant air leaks.

Generally, a Pa_{O_2} of 50 to 65 torr precludes tissue hypoxia in smaller infants, but it may be necessary to maintain the Pa_{O_2} at slightly higher levels in bigger babies if they show any evidence of pulmonary hypertension or tissue hypoxia. In these infants, in particular, keeping the Pa_{O_2} at 65 to 75 torr may correct metabolic acidosis secondary to tissue hypoxia. Oxygen saturation and oxygen content will vary enough over this portion of the oxygen dissociation curve so that slight measurable changes in Pa_{O_2} may produce a significant difference in oxygen delivery to the tissues.

Treatment with Distending Airway Pressure

The most effective treatment for the progressive atelectasis of RDS involves use of continuous distending pressure to improve the pattern of ventilation by preventing further atelectasis and recruiting collapsed alveoli.

Continuous positive airway pressure (CPAP) seems to provide airway stability and perhaps prevents alveolar collapse on expiration. Ideally, it should also prevent the development of alveolar collapse adjacent to overdistended (high compliance) alveolar areas.

CPAP alone is most effective in vigorous infants who weigh more than 1200 g who do not have significant retention of carbon dioxide. At the proper levels of CPAP, improvement in respiratory excursions occurs, usually with less grunting, slower rates, and apparently less work of breathing. At excessive levels, there is effectively an increase in dead space leading to carbon dioxide retention, as well as interference with cardiac output leading to both respiratory and metabolic acidoses.

The most direct method of delivering CPAP is through an endotracheal tube. Regulation of the proper levels of pressure is very important because there is direct airway transmission of pressure. Endotracheal CPAP is also used as a preextubation step in weaning from mechanical ventilation.

The most clinically useful method of delivering CPAP is through nasal prongs or a nasopharyngeal tube. The advantages of this method are that the infant still has glottic control so that, if necessary, by grunting he can generate even more expiratory pressure. Likewise, because all the pressure is not directly transmitted to the airway, some excess pressure and flow can be "popped off" through the mouth. Thus there is a slightly greater, and therefore safer, range of therapeutic effect when the pressure is directed above the glottis rather than directly into the trachea.

The easiest way to apply nasal CPAP is with commercially available nasal CPAP cannulae (Fig. 29-7) or by cutting an endotracheal tube about 2 cm shorter

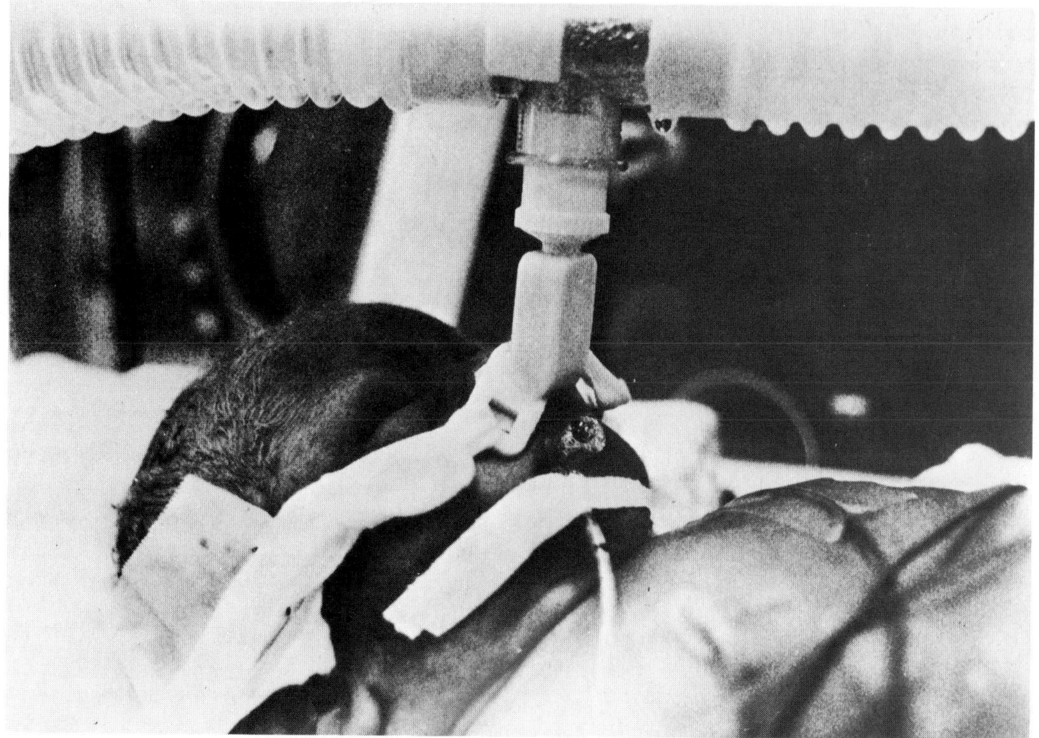

Fig. 29-7. Use of the nasal CPAP cannula (*see* text). (Reproduced by permission of Sherwood Medical Industries)

than the infant's calculated lip to glottic length (¾ nose to ear distance). The tube appears better tolerated in larger infants when it ends at the level of the uvula and neither irritates the pharynx nor allows high rates of gas flow to go past the nasal mucosa. Because exhaled humidity is not recaptured through nasopharyngeal tubes, higher humidification is needed than for the short nasal prongs or an endotracheal tube. It is necessary to confirm patency frequently, since crusting with gradual occlusion causes carbon dioxide retention and hypoxia that may be misinterpreted as worsening patient condition.

The initial levels of CPAP are 4 to 6 cm H_2O. One can determine the appropriate level for nasal CPAP by slowly increasing the level every 5 minutes until grunting stops and there is an increase in Ptc_{O_2} or Pa_{O_2}. If after improved oxygenation there is an increase in metabolic acidosis or in carbon dioxide, a decrease of a few cm H_2O pressure may normalize the blood gases. Larger infants who remain vigorous with good respiratory effort may respond positively to levels as high as 12 cm H_2O, whereas smaller infants tend to tire and need ventilation if not improved at levels of 8 cm H_2O.

When CPAP is at the level most effective for a particular infant, the oxygen requirements should stop increasing and stabilize or drop to a lower level than was required before initiation of the pressure. If the oxygen requirements continue to increase, the reasons may be inadequate levels of distending pressure, levels are too high with resultant impedance of circulating blood, inspired gas temperature too low, tube occlusion, development of a complication, or incorrect diagnosis.

One can see a fairly consistent response to therapy with CPAP when there are no complications and the pressure levels are correct for the infant. The FI_{O_2} requirement should be down to at least 0.6 after 6 hours of CPAP and to 0.5 by 12 to 24 hours after initiation of pressure.

There are no universal criteria for starting CPAP. Generally, however, when an infant has findings compatible with RDS and thus is expected to have progressive loss of alveolar volume and increased work of breathing, early institution of CPAP, particularly by nasal tube or prongs, may slow the atelectatic progression. If response to early CPAP is positive, there appears to be far less energy expenditure, oxygen consumption, carbon dioxide production, and acidosis with a shorter overall course than if the infant breathes spontaneously until he has high oxygen requirements and carbon dioxide retention before initiation of CPAP.

The following general criteria help determine what type of respiratory support is appropriate for an infant with RDS.

1. Indications for increased FI_{O_2} without pressure or assisted ventilation
   - Good respiratory effort
   - No CO_2 retention
   - Ability to maintain Pa_{O_2} at 50 torr on an FI_{O_2} of 0.5 or less
   - No tension pneumothorax
2. Indications for continuous distending airway pressure without assisted ventilation
   - No significant CO_2 retention (Pa_{CO_2} less than 60–65 torr)
   - pH of 7.25 or above
   - Inability to maintain Pa_{O_2} at 50 torr on an FI_{O_2} of less than 0.5
   - No apnea (unless apnea is secondary to primary alveolar hypoventilation or patent ductus arteriosus)
   - Diffusely decreased pulmonary compliance or collapsed distal airway disease only
   - Pulmonary edema secondary to patent ductus arteriosus
3. Indications for continuous ventilation with positive end-expiratory pressure (PEEP)*
   - Apnea (use 2–3 cm H_2O PEEP)
   - Shock (low PEEP)
   - Acidosis (progressive or resistant while attempting to maintain pH above 7.25)
   - $Pa_{CO_2} \geq 65$ torr or rapidly increasing Pa_{O_2} of 50 torr on an FI_{O_2} of 0.8
   - Status epilepticus with respiratory insufficiency

CPAP is especially important in weaning the infant from ventilatory support. Generally by 72 hours, simultaneous with or shortly after the infant begins a diuresis and his total urine output approximates or exceeds his intake, his requirements for oxygen and pressure decrease. When he requires an FI_{O_2} of 0.35 to 0.40, he should tolerate lowering CPAP or PEEP. Before extubation after mechanical ventilation, he may stay on endotracheal CPAP of 2 to 4 cm for a few hours. Up to 48 hours of nasal CPAP postextubation may be needed if there is significant glottic edema or if there is a poor cry indicating abnormal closure of the glottis. Using nasal CPAP postextubation allows both deposition of humidity and aerosolized medi-

*PEEP is added only in conditions of diffusely decreased pulmonary compliance or collapsed distal airway disease, or in pulmonary edema secondary to patent ductus arteriosus.

cations close to the glottis and aids in preventing the frequent postextubation complication of lobar atelectasis.

Treatment with Controlled Mechanical Ventilation

When an infant requires mechanical ventilation, two basic types of ventilators are available: pressure controlled/time-cycled or volume controlled/flow regulated. Use of pressure controlled/time-cycled machines has largely replaced the volume controlled machines in the care of infants with noncompliant lungs. Even one of the most commonly used infant volume machines, the Bourns LS104-150, is often modified to act as a pressure controlled machine by controlling the master pop-off pressure valve, increasing the stroke volume and slowing the stroke velocity with decreased flows. This type of use is mechanically hard on the machine but does allow pressure controlling. Use of pressure regulated machines with longer inspiratory times allows for use of lower PEEP and peak inspiratory pressures. Although use of truly reversed inspiratory/expiratory ratios at very low pressures is rare, changes of inspiratory time between 0.3 to 0.75 seconds instead of changing FI_{O_2} and peak pressures provide more control over mean airway pressure (MAP) and the shape of the pressure curve. For instance, shortening the inspiratory time without decreasing the peak pressure cuts the MAP and is sometimes effective in reversing the changes in interstitial emphysema. In contrast, an infant who seems to require more pressure and FI_{O_2} because of progressive atelectasis may respond significantly to increasing inspiratory time from 0.5 to 0.7 seconds; thus there is less need to increase peak pressure or FI_{O_2}.

When initiating mechanical ventilation after intubation, one should ventilate an infant by hand with controlled pressure, PEEP, and FI_{O_2} long enough to relax the patient, to reverse pulmonary hypertension by hyperventilation, if necessary, and to expand as many areas of atelectasis as possible. When done properly, hand ventilation *before* starting mechanical support allows use of lower machine pressures and shortens the time to stabilization. Appropriate initial settings on pressure machines if lungs are noncompliant are rates of 25 to 35, peak inspiratory pressure of 25 cm H_2O, PEEP of 5, and inspiratory time of 0.5 seconds. When settings are appropriate for any infant, the following should be observed.

1. Infant relaxes and allows machine to do most of the ventilation. Auscultation reveals breath sounds by machine *as effective* as infant's own breath sounds.
2. Chest excursions are appropriate: machine-generated about equal to spontaneous respiratory excursions.
3. Reversal of metabolic acidemia.
4. Improved perfusion.
5. Pa_{CO_2} in 40 to 50 torr range.
6. FI_{O_2} stabilizes at 0.50 to 0.60 within a few hours.

If there is an increasing FI_{O_2} requirement, one should check for a complication. If there is none, inspiratory time should be increased, rather than FI_{O_2} or peak pressure. If there is carbon dioxide retention as well as an increasing oxygen requirement, if the patient is fighting the ventilator, or if there is an increasing metabolic acidosis, tidal volume should be increased by increasing the peak pressure. If carbon dioxide retention persists, the ventilator frequency should be increased. As the pulmonary mechanics change during the course of RDS, so too will the ventilator requirements. Most rapid changes occur initially until the stabilization plateau phase and during recovery.

Ventilator Weaning

When an infant's requirements for oxygen have decreased and pulmonary compliance has improved enough to decrease the work of breathing, weaning from the ventilator may be started. The infant may be weaned from the ventilator to CPAP when blood oxygenation is acceptable with an FI_{O_2} less than 0.4, providing that there is no retention of carbon dioxide.

There are several ways to wean infants from full ventilatory support. The first is to decrease the ventilator rate by 5 to 10 breaths per minute until a rate of less than 5 per minute has been achieved. Small infants who weigh less than 1200 g may need continued weaning to 1 to 2 breaths/min, with the ventilator in effect giving "sighing" breaths.

Alternatively, when the rate is 5 to 10/min, the infant is placed on spontaneous ventilation with supplemental oxygen for 10 minutes and then ventilated for 1 to 2 hours. If he has tolerated spontaneous ventilation, the period of controlled ventilation is decreased progressively. When the time on the ventilator is down to 5 minutes, the infant may be left on spontaneous ventilation, with careful observation to assure that this is tolerated. Again the machine acts as a sighing instrument and allows the infant to rest.

Extubation

Extubation of any infant should be planned so that personnel attending him will be able to give careful observation during the following hours. After chest physiotherapy has been given and the infant thoroughly suctioned, the infant's lungs are hyperinflated slightly with oxygen-enriched air. The tube is removed during applied inspiration. The infant is then placed in humidified oxygen with an FI_{O_2} 10% higher than before extubation. Blood gas levels are monitored carefully to assure appropriate oxygen levels and to detect carbon dioxide retention.

If an infant has been on the ventilator or intubated for longer than 48 to 72 hours and if there is a weak or hoarse cry on extubation, nasal CPAP is appropriate to help maintain airway breathing and to prevent atelectasis. Immediately after extubation, one can use nebulized epinephrine (racemic epinephrine 2.25%, 0.25 ml in 3-ml saline) and Decadron (0.5 to 1 mg) to prevent and decrease glottic edema. The heart rate should be monitored to determine total dose for the epinephrine and to stop the treatment or decrease the dose if tachycardia develops. The epinephrine alone is repeated every 2 to 4 hours for up to 48 hours until glottic edema has resolved. Small infants may develop hyperglycemia because of systemic absorption of epinephrine. After extubation and until the lungs appear normal, a planned regimen of postural drainage and chest physiotherapy directed particularly at drainage of the upper lobes with cough simulation, sighing, and deep suctioning will prevent many postextubation pulmonary complications. Both efficacy and stress from the treatment must be continually reassessed. Application of 6 to 8 cm of CPAP by a lightly held mask *during* the physiotherapy and sighing with an inflation hold after suctioning are especially beneficial in infants who weigh less than 1500 to 1800 g. If there is stress during the procedure, increasing the FI_{O_2} or modifying the most stressful component may relieve the symptoms.

PROGNOSIS

A number of clinical observations may be predictive of outcome for an infant who receives appropriate treatment. Earlier scoring systems for prediction had been devised before good ventilatory assistance was readily available and, as such, are not as valid for infants treated by modern methods. The predictive observations vary from those easily discernible by the clinician to those requiring refined laboratory techniques. No score is assigned from weighing these additive factors, but they do suggest an overall prognosis in the face of appropriate therapy. Two of the more reliable early signs of imminent clinical improvement are onset of diuresis with decreased peripheral edema, and increased production of clear tracheal secretions. Simultaneously, or shortly thereafter, oxygen requirements start to fall. Factors predictive of outcome when optimum treatment is given are listed below.

FACTORS THAT SUGGEST A GOOD PROGNOSIS IN HYALINE MEMBRANE DISEASE*

- No associated birth asphyxia: Apgar scores > 5 at 1 min; > 7 at 5 min
- Good beat-to-beat variability in heart rate prenatally and postnatally
- Blood pressure easily maintained: stabilized within first 6 to 12 hours. Good urine output maintained
- Infant remains vigorous throughout
    - Interest in pacifier
    - Eyes-open appearance
- Decreasing oxygen requirement after institution of therapy
    - Decreased grunting when placed in oxygen
    - FI_{O_2} leveling at 0.55 to 0.60 within 6 hours after starting CPAP
    - Improvement in lung compliance with therapy (CPAP)
- pH above 7.25 without alkalinizing agent or assisted ventilation
- Pa_{CO_2} less than 60 torr; normal with assisted ventilation
- Infant starts producing tracheal secretions
    - Presence of surface-active phospholipids such as lecithin in tracheal secretions, especially phosphatidyl glycerol
    - Reappearance during treatment
- Diuresis after 36 hours. Output equals or exceeds 80% of intake
- No major complications such as CNS hemorrhage, patent ductus arteriosus, necrotizing enterocolitis, pneumonia, or unresolved pneumothorax

*The sooner these clinical factors appear, the better the prognosis and the shorter the course.

FACTORS THAT SUGGEST A POOR PROGNOSIS IN HYALINE MEMBRANE DISEASE*

- Birth asphyxia: Apgar scores
  $\leq$ 2 at 1 min; $\leq$ 4 at 5 min
- No beat-to-beat variability in heart rate
  - Lack of return of beat-to-beat variability after 24 hours of age
- Failure to maintain stable blood pressure (poor perfusion)
  - Poor urine output
  - Lactic acidosis
  - pH < 7.25 despite reasonable alkalinizing agents, volume expansion (or ventilation)
  - Elevation of serum K^+
- Increasing oxygen requirements
  - Failure to decrease FI_{O_2} to 0.55 to 0.60 within 6 to 12 hours after CPAP or PEEP has been started
  - Persistently elevated Pa_{CO_2} despite ventilation
- Persistent pulmonary hypertension
  - Right-to-left shunting across ductus
  - Failure to close foramen ovale
  - Persistent cardiomegaly
- Decreasing lung compliance despite appropriate CPAP or ventilation
- Low serum proteins (< 4.0 g/dl)
- Failure to produce tracheal secretions
  - No return of surface-active lecithins, especially phosphatidyl glycerol
- Serious complications
  - Clotting disorders
  - Nonexpandable pneumothorax
  - Pneumopericardium
  - Pneumonia
  - Pulmonary hemorrhage
- Neurologically depressed with evidence of CNS hemorrhage
  - Recurrence of apnea
- Sepsis

*These factors are especially ominous when present after 36 hours of vigorous and appropriate therapy.

RETAINED LUNG FLUID

The symptom complex of transient tachypnea of the newborn (TTN) resulting from retention of fetal lung fluid was first described as a distinct entity by Avery and coworkers in 1966.[3] It is also known as type II respiratory distress syndrome and transient respiratory distress of the newborn. The original patients described were all term infants with tachypnea but without grunting or significant retractions. Since the original description, there has been more awareness of the wide range of clinical symptoms caused by retained lung fluid, either as an isolated finding or complicating other neonatal pulmonary conditions.

TTN may occur in term or preterm infants. There is often a history of delivery by cesarean section without labor, maternal bleeding, prolapsed umbilical cord, diabetes, or maternal medication with meperidine (Demerol). In other cases, however, the obstetric history may be completely normal.

The specific syndrome of TTN occurs without other pulmonary disease, but retention of lung fluid occurs more often with pulmonary disease that inhibits its resorption, particularly when the respiratory distress syndrome is complicated by recurrent aspirations (often owing to congenital esophageal or tracheoesophageal abnormalities). In these diseases the retained lung fluid may complicate the early clinical course. Thus the diagnosis of TTN *per se* is one of exclusion.

CLINICAL PRESENTATION

The infant with TTN may present with a normal Apgar score, but often there is mild depression at birth followed by respiratory distress. Although there may be grunting and retractions, most infants demonstrate only tachypnea (to 120 respirations/min) and nasal flaring. There may be metabolic acidosis secondary to birth asphyxia and hypoxia or some degree of respiratory acidosis, but most infants compensate adequately. Arterial oxygen desaturation usually is mild and corrects with 30% to 40% oxygen. Most symptoms clear within 24 to 48 hours, although mild tachypnea may persist for several more days. Systemic hypoperfusion is rarely a problem unless associated with significant birth asphyxia or other complications. Occasional infants demonstrate severe respiratory embarrassment and require assisted ventilation for respiratory failure in the absence of any other complicating disease.

Infants with TTN have normal surfactant activity with mature lecithin/sphingomyelin (L/S) ratios of their tracheal or amniotic fluid aspirates.

ROENTGENOGRAPHIC PRESENTATION

Chest roentgenograms are diagnostic of retained lung fluid but may correlate poorly with the degree of clin-

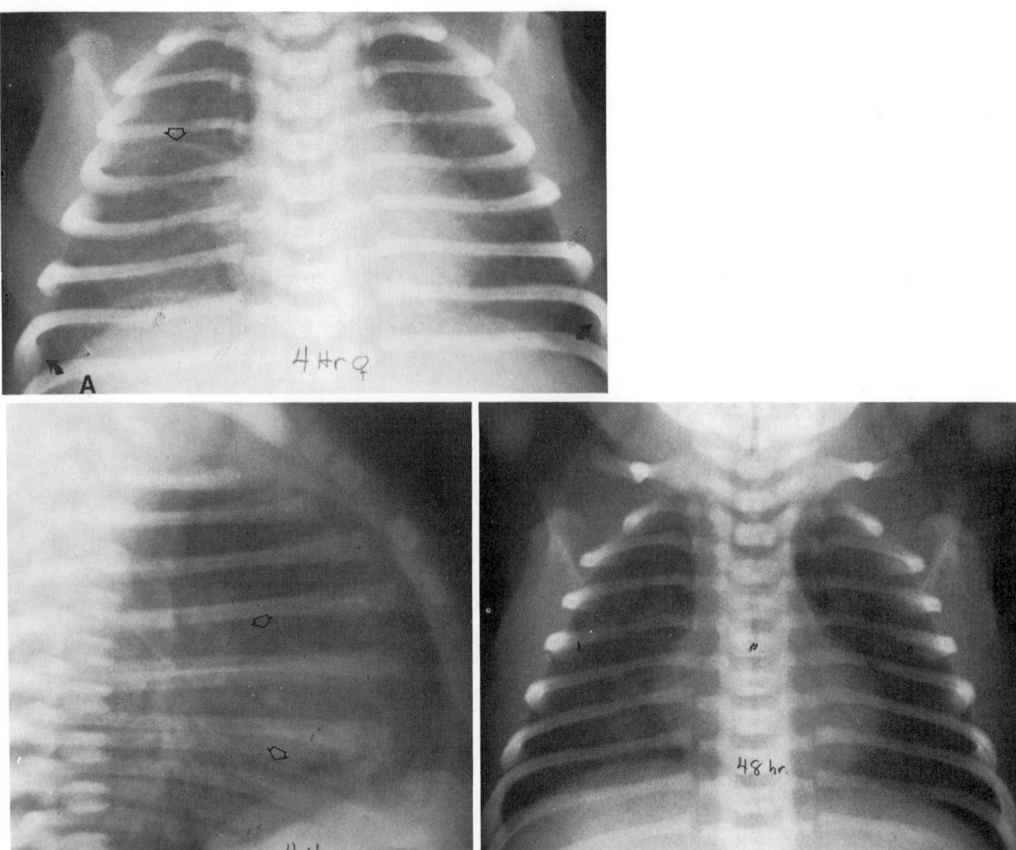

Fig. 29-8. *(A)* Retained lung fluid. Anteroposterior chest roentgenogram of a 4-hour-old baby with tachypnea. There is a small effusion bilaterally *(arrows)* and fluid in the fissures *(open arrow)*. Diffuse bilateral perihilar haze is due to distended pulmonary veins and lymphatics. *(B)* Lateral view of the same baby at 4 hours. Open arrows show fluid in fissures. *(C)* The same patient at 48 hours. The effusions and fluid in the fissures have disappeared, as has the diffuse bilateral haze. The patient had a normal respiratory rate at this time.

ical severity (Fig. 29-8). Early in the course, x-ray films may show extensive alveolar edema, but often there are only prominent ill-defined vascular markings compatible with engorged lymphatics. These findings are associated with accentuation of interlobar septa and with pleural effusions. There may be uniform hyperexpansion, flattened diaphragms, and bulging intercostal spaces. These latter findings may persist for a week after the symptoms are no longer present.

Although chest films indicate retention of lung fluid, they are not diagnostic of TTN by themselves. Early films of infants with respiratory distress syndrome also often show retention of lung fluid that obscures the typical pattern of fine granularity. As the lung fluid resorbs, the pattern appears.

TREATMENT

The treatment of TTN is primarily supportive with warmed humidified oxygen by hood as needed. Despite the occasional infant who needs very high inspired oxygen concentrations, respiratory assistance such as CPAP or IPPB is rarely needed unless there are associated complications. The retention of fluid may be unilateral, especially in the dependent lung; thus the infant's position should be changed regularly. As soon as the tachypnea subsides (usually below 60–70 respirations/min), oral feedings may be given. Before that, intravenous or gavaged feedings should be given. Long-term follow-up studies indicate no permanent pulmonary residual damage.

BRONCHOPULMONARY DYSPLASIA (BPD)

One of the complications of therapy of lung disease in neonates is the development of a chronic pulmonary condition known as bronchopulmonary dysplasia (BPD). The symptom complex, first described by Northway and coworkers in 1967, was thought to be secondary to prolonged exposure to elevated oxygen concentrations.[31] The disease and clinical symptoms most likely result from a combination of oxygen toxicity and positive pressure ventilation. The critical duration and quantity of each factor seem to vary from patient to patient. There appears to be a direct relation to the degree of prematurity of the lungs, but not necessarily to the severity of the primary pulmonary problem. It is most common in babies with RDS. Because the survival from RDS is now improved, more cases of BPD are appearing. There may not be an actual increase in the incidence,[44] but as case recognition improves there is an apparent increase in the diagnosis. Reported cases of BPD do relate to the degree of immaturity and overall survival from RDS. Centers with a large number of survivors of less than 1000 g birth weight report BPD in at least 20% of those infants.[47]

Symptoms have appeared in infants exposed to environments with elevated oxygen over prolonged periods without assisted ventilation as well as in infants administered positive pressure ventilation with only a moderately elevated FI_{O_2}. The three factors—pressure, oxygen, and time—appear to act synergistically.[35]

In years past, continuous negative pressure was used in the treatment of RDS. BPD appeared to be less severe in infants treated with continuous negative pressure. Institutions that used continuous negative pressure for therapy reported a lack of BPD in their patients so treated, whereas infants in the same nurseries who need positive pressure assistance may develop the findings.[40] The infants on positive pressure may represent more serious RDS. Some of these patients treated with continuous negative pressure do, however, show evidence of pulmonary fibrosis on long-term roentgenographic follow-up, which may be a less dramatic manifestation of the same process. The decreased incidence of full-blown disease is nonetheless real. Berg and coworkers reported a significant decrease in the incidence of BPD when PEEP was used with IPPB compared to IPPB alone (17.2% versus 36.2%) and no incidence in 42 patients treated with CPAP alone.[6] Infants treated with CPAP alone are also at lower risk to develop BPD.

CLINICAL PRESENTATION

The classic picture of BPD is that of a premature infant with some initial form of pulmonary compromise, most typically RDS, who requires assisted ventilation and who then does not demonstrate the expected clinical improvement over a prolonged course. Notably there is not the expected diuretic phase with mobilization of peripheral and pulmonary edema fluid. There often is delay in recovery and a persistent need for ventilation because of failure and shunting across a persistently patent ductus arteriosus. Unlike the infant who follows the expected course, there may be failure to initiate appropriate surfactant release because of excessive damage to the alveolar cells. Normally, tracheal aspirates begin to show the presence of surfactant at about the same time as diuresis and recovery begins. Infants who develop BPD do not show the same increase in tracheal fluid and do not release measurable diphosphatidyl choline or phosphatidyl glycerol.

Many of the infants who develop BPD have evidence of pulmonary air leaks and uneven ventilation throughout their early course of RDS. They will have interstitial emphysema leading to pneumothoraces, recurrent atelectases, most notably of the right upper lobe,[28] and emphysema of the lower lobes.

Severe respiratory insufficiency persists for days to weeks, leading to one of several courses, including progressive pulmonary failure and demise, chronic pulmonary insufficiency, or gradual recovery. Frequently, the outcome becomes evident only after many weeks of assisted ventilation.

Recovery from BPD requires repair of damaged lung tissue. If ventilation pressure and oxygen requirements progressively decrease and the infant demonstrates good weight gain, his lung has a chance to repair itself to such an extent that it can function remarkably well. Long-term follow-up of survivors of severe bronchopulmonary dysplasia reveals persistence of airway obstruction on testing and bronchial hyperreactivity with recurrent episodes of nonatopic wheezing.[39] Some respond to therapy with bronchodilators. Considering the initial extensive damage to the lungs, there is remarkable repair and compensation, leaving little long-term debilitation after recovery.

ROENTGENOGRAPHIC FINDINGS

Four stages of bronchopulmonary dysplasia may be seen on chest roentgenograms (Fig. 29-9).[30]

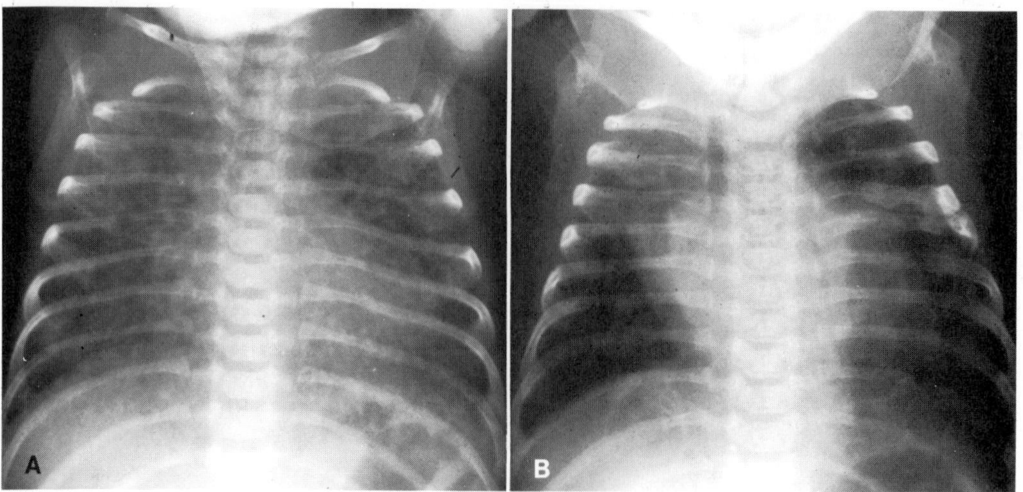

Fig. 29-9. *(A)* Bronchopulmonary dysplasia in a 2-month-old child with severe hyaline membrane disease and prolonged oxygen and ventilator therapy. Bilateral diffuse interstitial fibrosis and cystic change are present, consistent with stage IV bronchopulmonary dysplasia of Northway (*see* text). *(B)* Bronchopulmonary dysplasia in a 2½-month-old patient who had severe hyaline membrane disease, prolonged ventilator and oxygen therapy, and ligation for persistent patent ductus arteriosus. There is now advanced bronchopulmonary dysplasia with areas of cystic overexpansion of the lower lobes and considerable interstitial fibrosis, not well seen because of the marked cystic changes. The heart is enlarged because of cor pulmonale.

- Stage I: clinically and radiologically classic hyaline membrane disease
- Stage II: continued oxygen requirement with roentgenographic opacification of both lung fields
- Stage III: clinical improvement, with areas of rounded radiolucency throughout the lung fields alternating with areas of adjacent atelectasis, exhibiting a "spongelike" appearance
- Stage IV: persistent oxygen dependence with diffuse rales, associated with increasing size of cystic areas

Retrospectively, these stages are much more easily discerned than they are during a patient's clinical progression. Frequently not until the third week of disease can one detect characteristic roentgenographic changes. Stage I is the expected appearance of RDS. Stage II is virtually indistinguishable from any complete alveolar consolidation process, as in untreated, worsening RDS, massive pulmonary edema, hemorrhage, or pneumonia. Any of these complications of RDS could be expected during the same time period. Additionally the high incidence of pulmonary air leaks and patent ductus arteriosus obscures the radiologic appearance.

When compared to autopsy findings, the radiologic staging correlates in less than 50% of cases, with the pathologic changes more advanced than radiologically evident.[14,33]

PATHOLOGY

Based on autopsies of infants with RDS treated with high oxygen concentrations and positive pressure ventilation, Tsai and coworkers have described the pathologic sequence in the development of bronchopulmonary dysplasia.[43] In their series there were two general phases: The acute phase was seen after at least 20 hours of oxygen therapy and was superimposed on the classic changes of RDS. It was characterized by an exudative reaction with focal necrosis of respiratory mucosa, squamous metaplasia of tracheal and bronchial mucosa, and an intrabronchial exudate with necrotic mucosal cells. The alveoli and alveolar ducts were filled with an exudate composed of edema fluid, fibrin, occasional desquamated alveolar cells, and basophilic debris.

The proliferative phase, present after at least 50 hours of oxygen therapy, involved thickened septa with fibroblastic proliferation and formation of collagen and elastic fibers. This progressed to local areas of emphysematous alveoli alternating with coalescent alveoli and interstitial fibrosis. Some showed further progression to a fibroproliferative obliterative bronchiolitis with cystic bronchiectasis.

TREATMENT

The major thrust of treatment in infants at risk for BPD should be preventive. Because there is a high correlation between the occurrence of complications in RDS and the development of BPD, the most effective prevention may be to direct intensive efforts at preventing the complications—namely, air leaks, congestive heart failure from PDA, or iatrogenic fluid overload. Secondary should be strict attention to ventilator management; intervening before marked and less reversible changes occur; determining the most beneficial, least damaging inflating pressure for each patient; and weaning as quickly as possible.

When an infant appears to be developing BPD, most of the therapy is supportive, since recovery occurs only after a prolonged period and involves essentially reconstruction and regrowth of the lung. Good nutrition is essential. The ability of an infant with BPD to maintain an anabolic state and demonstrate solid weight gain is a good prognostic sign indicating that excessive caloric expenditure for the work of breathing is not stealing calories from growth.

Also essential is good pulmonary hygiene. The lungs in BPD are particularly prone to atelectasis and infection. Virtually every potential natural pulmonary defense is disrupted; thus there is a need for complete assistance in secretion production and mobilization, airway maintenance, and asepsis. The tendency toward recurrent atelectasis of the upper lobes, with emphysema of the lower lobes, requires that the infant be in an upright drainage position for part of his daily positioning cycle even when on the ventilator.

Because the lung parenchyma in BPD has excess interstitial fluid, the use of diuretics benefits some infants. Others respond to cessation of intravenous lipid infusion.

Lack of response to therapy leads to progressive discrepancies of both perfusion and ventilation. Terminal events are intractable cor pulmonale, infection, and progressive respiratory failure.

PULMONARY DYSMATURITY (WILSON-MIKITY SYNDROME)

In 1960, Wilson and Mikity described five premature infants who demonstrated a previously unrecognized syndrome with distinct clinical and roentgenographic patterns.[46] The symptom complex consists of progressive respiratory distress in previously well, premature infants whose chest roentgenograms showed diffuse cystic emphysema. Since then the syndrome has been recognized as a distinct entity whose etiology is obscure but which possibly reflects the immaturity of the pulmonary supporting structures.

The true incidence of this syndrome is unknown. In a large series by Hodgman and coworkers in 1969, the disease was recognized in 1 of every 90 infants weighing between 1 kg and 1.5 kg.[20] As general supportive care for tiny premature infants has improved their overall survival rate, there should have been an increased incidence in this diagnosis, but this has not been the case. It may be that current therapy is preventing the development of the full symptom complex or that there is overlap with the diagnosis of BPD.

ETIOLOGY

The etiology of pulmonary dysmaturity is undetermined. There seems to be an unequal rate of maturation in different areas of the lung with delay in alveolar development in less distended areas and overdistention in other areas further advanced.[4]

An alternative theory centers more on airway immaturity.[11] The more premature the lung, the greater the degree of distensibility or collapse of the tracheobronchial tree because of immaturity of the supporting structures (*see* Lung Development earlier in chapter). With expiration, the transpulmonary pressures developed by the premature infant easily could collapse small airways, with subsequent hyperexpansion of adjacent and more distal airways and alveoli.

CLINICAL PRESENTATION

The typical clinical pattern affects small premature infants weighing less than 1500 g. These infants are born after the expected obstetric complications associated with premature delivery (*i.e.*, maternal hemorrhage, toxemia, infection, and premature rupture of membranes). The babies tend to have lower Apgar scores than normal but usually do not require aggressive resuscitation. In the first 24 to 48 hours, they may be asymptomatic or demonstrate respiratory distress owing to mild hyaline membrane disease or retained lung fluid, from which they recover. Respiratory symptoms recur by 1 to 3 weeks of age, after a period without clinically evident pulmonary distress. There is then a gradual onset of intermittent tachypnea, retractions, and cyanosis that increases in severity over the next 2 to 4 weeks. By 4 to 8 weeks, symptoms are at their worst, with varying degrees of respiratory insufficiency. If recovery occurs, the symptoms disappear over the next 3 to 24 months. The mortality is from 2.5% to 60% in these patients, although other primary diseases may precipitate death. Some patients have persistent patent ductus arteriosus, although its occurrence may be no more frequent than the general incidence in the same gestational age group.

ROENTGENOGRAPHIC FINDINGS

The roentgenographic sequence in pulmonary dysmaturity is diagnostic when related to the clinical history (Fig. 29-10). At the onset of symptoms, the chest film may be normal but more often is surprisingly abnormal in comparison to the clinical severity. Initially there are coarse, streaky infiltrates alternating with small cystic areas distributed throughout both lung fields. After 1 to 5 months, the cysts at the lung bases enlarge and coalesce. The lungs become hyperexpanded, and the diaphragms are flat. The upper lobes continue to demonstrate the infiltrates after the lower lobes clear. Gradually the hyperexpansion abates. The roentgenograms return to normal by 3 to 24 months after the symptoms have resolved.

PULMONARY FUNCTION STUDIES

Pulmonary function studies have been limited but suggest decreased lung compliance, a reduced functional residual capacity with normal crying vital capacity, an increased expiratory airway resistance, and increased oxygen consumption with increased work of breathing. The blood gases demonstrate an elevated Pa_{CO_2} (50–70 torr) with hypoxemia and variable degrees of right-to-left shunting.

Follow-up studies at 8 to 10 years suggest continued focal differences in compliance and resistance of terminal lung units with different rates of emptying from adjacent lung units.[13] The physiological changes correlate well with autopsy findings.

PATHOLOGY

The pathologic examination correlates with the roentgenographic picture. Grossly, the lungs demonstrate uneven patterns of foci of hyperaeration alternating with areas of atelectasis or normal lung. The microscopic appearance is related directly to the degree of prematurity and the expected anatomy for gestational age and does not have any specific diagnostic appearance. Pulmonary fibrosis is not prominent unless there is associated cardiac disease, particularly PDA. It is distinguishable microscopically from bronchopulmonary dysplasia by the absence of significant cellular changes.

THERAPY

Therapy for pulmonary dysmaturity primarily is supportive. In view of a natural history of a return to normal pulmonary function upon survival, the support should be aggressive if respiratory assistance is needed. Antibiotics are not indicated unless there is an acute infection. Steroids or other medical regimens have no role. Theoretically, very low levels of continuous positive or negative transthoracic pressure (2–4 cm H_2O) may be useful in providing even ventilation by prevention of bronchiolar collapse; however, this has not been tested clinically once the diagnosis has been established.

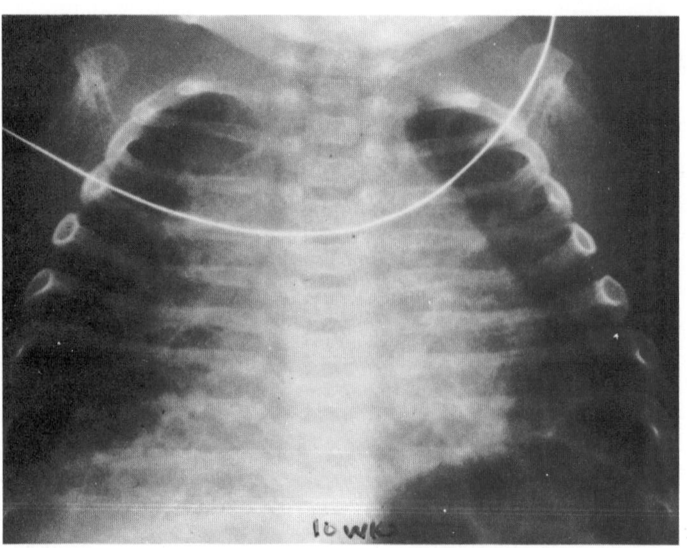

Fig. 29-10. The Wilson–Mikity syndrome. This 10-week-old child received less than 40% oxygen for 1 day. Endotracheal intubation or positive pressure ventilation was never performed. At 6 weeks the chest roentgenogram shows bilateral hyperaeration and cystic changes indistinguishable from bronchopulmonary dysplasia. The heart is enlarged secondary to cor pulmonale. At postmortem examination the lungs had changes typical of the Wilson–Mikity syndrome with no evidence of bronchopulmonary dysplasia.

PULMONARY HEMORRHAGE

Hemorrhage into lung occurs more frequently in neonates than in any other age group. On autopsy some degree of hemorrhage usually exists in association with other acute lung diseases, most particularly infection, RDS, or aspiration syndrome. It may not have been clinically significant. Massive pulmonary hemorrhage involving at least two lobes of the lung is less frequent but more often life-threatening.

Before the advent of modern perinatal care when there was less attention to prevention of hypothermia and asphyxia, massive hemorrhage occurred in as many as 17.8% of autopsied infants or in 11% of all infants weighing less than 2.5 kg at birth.[17] Although the incidence now is considerably lower, massive pulmonary hemorrhage still causes significant morbidity in intensive care nurseries.

Although massive pulmonary hemorrhage rarely presents as an apparently isolated process, it most often accompanies postasphyxial brain edema; intraventricular hemorrhage; lung disease where cellular damage or atelectasis predominate; left ventricular failure; or bleeding diatheses. It has been associated with rare metabolic abnormalities, notably congenital hyperammonemia.

CLINICAL PRESENTATION

The clinical presentation of pulmonary hemorrhage depends on the rapidity with which hemorrhage develops and is related to whatever primary disease the infant has. The classic picture is that of an already distressed infant who deteriorates further, developing a significant metabolic acidosis with intermittent bradycardia and gasping respirations or frank apnea. Effluent that appears to be primarily blood wells from the trachea; the skin becomes dusky and cyanotic; and the blood pressure falls. If the infant is on a volume-regulated ventilator, the peak airway pressure required for that volume increases. Frequently, there are simultaneous clinical signs of coagulopathy with oozing of umbilical blood, hematuria, or frank gastrointestinal bleeding. Usually in the presence of these signs there is associated laboratory evidence of coagulation defects but not necessarily disseminated intravascular coagulation. If pulmonary hemorrhage is the first evidence of bleeding, the coagulation studies may be normal initially but then become abnormal with progression of acidosis, hypoxemia, and shock.

The amount of bleeding initially may appear to be mild, especially if the infant is on CPAP or a ventilator. It may cause no obvious worsening of clinical symptoms, although there is more often a need for increased oxygen and pressure to maintain the infant's status.

Frequently, signs of intracranial hemorrhage precede the massive pulmonary hemorrhage. The infant becomes apneic and floppy or demonstrates decerebrate posturing, rarely with clonic–tonic seizuring. His fontanelle bulges and his hematocrit drops. His blood gases indicate a profound metabolic acidemia with incorrectable hypoxemia, although the carbon dioxide tension may be decreased easily with ventilation until a pulmonary hemorrhage develops.

PATHOLOGY

Analysis of the tracheal effluent usually shows a lower hematocrit and protein content than does the patient's blood, but the molecular size of the effluent protein suggests a plasma filtrate. The concentration of blood may increase with a progressing hemorrhage but never becomes pure blood.

On autopsy, hemorrhage may be evident throughout the lung parenchyma. Avery states that interstitial hemorrhage occurs most frequently in infants who die in the first day of life, whereas alveolar hemorrhage is more common if the infant dies later.[2] The primary disease, such as HMD, asphyxia, pneumonia, or aspiration, may also be identified at autopsy.

ETIOLOGY

There are probably multiple causes of pulmonary hemorrhage. In many cases the effluent is primarily pulmonary edema that becomes hemorrhagic because of easy rupture of pulmonary capillaries. The finding of hemorrhagic pulmonary edema seems especially true in neurogenic rather than cardiogenic edema—namely, in asphyxia and intracranial hemorrhaging.

Some cases of hemorrhage appear directly related to pulmonary parenchymal damage, as in meconium aspiration and necrotizing pneumonias. When the primary disease is RDS and there is alveolar atelectasis with distal airway collapse, absorption of inspired oxygen may leave a relative vacuum that increases transcapillary forces against an already low oncotic pressure because of decreased serum proteins. Animal studies have reproduced hemorrhagic atelectasis pathologically similar to that found in infants with RDS.[23]

Associated factors that may contribute to the process frequently are present in the infant who develops pulmonary hemorrhage. Many patients have been on assisted positive pressure ventilation or on increased ambient oxygen, which may damage alveoli and their capillaries. A number of patients demonstrate abnormal coagulation factors, not necessarily disseminated intravascular coagulopathies, but decreased production of hepatic clotting factors associated with asphyxia or passive congestion.

None of these factors is consistently present, nor does any appear to be of primary importance, but all may contribute to the hemorrhage once the initiating factor has started.

ROENTGENOGRAPHIC FINDINGS

The roentgenographic picture may range from complete alveolar–bronchiolar filling, giving a "white-out" appearance, to localized consolidation in one lobe or segment (*see* Fig. 29-2b). It is the rapidity with which radiologic changes in consolidation appear and disappear on treatment that suggests the diagnosis of hemorrhagic edema as opposed to infection.

TREATMENT

Most reports describe a high mortality with pulmonary hemorrhage; when it is associated with intracranial hemorrhage, the fatality rate is very high. If associated metabolic, neurologic, hematologic, or pulmonary conditions respond to therapy, there is a far better chance of survival from pulmonary hemorrhage.

The treatment of pulmonary hemorrhage depends on early diagnosis and aggressive intervention to stop advancement of the process. Immediate blood transfusion is indicated if there is hypovolemic shock. If the hemorrhage appears to result from congestive heart failure and left ventricular overload, decreasing the plasma volume may be of some benefit. Exchange transfusion is occasionally beneficial, whereas therapy with heparin is not.

Maintenance of a patent airway is paramount. If the infant is not already intubated, this should be done immediately. To maintain airway patency, high humidity in inspired gases is essential. Suctioning has to be *minimal* because the negative pressure induced in the airway may aggravate the hemorrhage.

The most important treatment of massive pulmonary hemorrhage is *continuous airway pressure.* Levels of PEEP considerably above those routinely used in treating RDS may be necessary. Increasing the pressure to 8 to 10 cm H_2O PEEP may dramatically stop a heavy effluent. Because dropping the pressure just 1 cm or 2 cm or stopping pressure during suctioning allows the bleeding to start, the high pressure often must remain until there is radiologic evidence of improvement. Ventilation with controlled pressure (square wave patterns) is more beneficial than ventilation with volume-controlled machines (*see* therapy section for RDS).

PULMONARY EDEMA

In neonates, pulmonary edema so often leads to pulmonary hemorrhage that it should be considered simultaneously. In the absence of primary lung disease, pulmonary edema presents as it does in adults. It may remain interstitial or advance to alveolar flooding as well. The most frequently seen cases of pulmonary edema occur in the premature infant who develops left-to-right shunting across a patent ductus arteriosus. Other cases are associated with congenital or acquired cardiac disease where there is elevated left ventricular pressure: hypoplastic left heart syndrome, aortic outflow tract obstruction, coarctation, asphyxic myocardiopathy, or massive vascular volume overload.

Treatment depends on the cause. Rapid diagnosis of congenital cardiac anomalies for proper surgical or medical intervention is essential. As volume overload is usually, but not always, present, diuresis is important. Low levels of PEEP or CPAP are effective when shunt congestion is primary.

PNEUMONIA

Pneumonia is a relatively common respiratory problem in the neonate and is the most frequent serious infection. The pneumonia may be congenital or acquired postnatally. If the infection is acquired *in utero*, it usually is due to direct aspiration of infected amniotic fluid. This type of pneumonia is caused by gram-negative coliforms, *Pseudomonas*, or *Proteus*.

The group B beta-hemolytic streptococcus causes sepsis and pneumonia that may appear at, or shortly after, birth, particularly in cases of prematurity after prolonged rupture of membranes. There is a very high maternal carrier rate of this organism, but infection of the infant with an overwhelming sepsis is unpredictable. The radiographic picture is virtually indistinguishable from HMD, and in many cases both processes occur simultaneously.

Frequently pneumonia acquired *in utero* is associated with maternal genitourinary tract infections, prolonged rupture of membranes, amnionitis, premature labor, or any intrauterine distress that predisposes to gasping respirations before or during delivery. The clinical findings of a low Apgar score plus chorioamnionitis especially indicate probable congenital pneumonia. This association requires an immediate evaluation of the newborn infant and his placenta in the delivery room.

Evidence of chorioamnionitis may be found by gross examination of the placenta for odor and cloudiness over the vessels on the fetal placental surface, as well as by touch preparations after stripping the amnion and staining with Wright's or Gram's stain and by frozen sections of the cord for the presence of polymorphonuclear leukocytes. Presence of significant numbers of live polymorphonuclear white cells in the gastric content within the first half hour of life may be helpful *when coupled* with other clinical information.

Hematogenous spread from the placenta appears to be the route of infection for toxoplasmosis, cytomegalovirus, Coxsackie virus, *Listeria monocytogenes*, tuberculosis, *Candida* species, and syphilis. Hematogenous spread may be associated with diffuse multisystem involvement, including sepsis, meningitis, hepatosplenomegaly, and bone changes on the roentgenogram. The gross and microscopic examination of the placenta may suggest the nature of the infection, since many of these agents cause specific placental changes.

Pneumonias acquired *in utero* are multilobar and frequently are associated with widespread infection and abscess formation. The infants have respiratory distress at birth. Early treatment with broad-spectrum antibiotics or specific antibiotics based on culture results, humidified air, and postural drainage with good tracheal toilet are indicated. If arterial blood gases indicate hypoxemia, oxygen therapy with careful monitoring should be provided. If respiratory failure ensues, appropriate assisted ventilation may be lifesaving.

Pneumonias acquired postnatally are usually due to organisms that inhabit skin, primarily staphylococci or streptococci, or to viral agents. The pneumonia may secondarily be due to seeding from any bacteremia or from contaminated respiratory equipment, most usually by *Pseudomonas* or *Serratia marcescens*. When the cause of infection is *Streptococcus*, frequently omphalitis or skin pustules are associated with fulminant septicemia. Pneumonia resulting from *Staphylococcus* also may be associated with skin lesions but may appear later in an asymptomatic nasal carrier. Most often the neonate presents from home with fever, lethargy, and tachypnea at 3 to 4 weeks of age. *Staphylococcus*, *E. coli*, and *Klebsiella* pneumonias especially are associated with the development of pneumatoceles and subsequent pneumothoraces. Specific antibiotic therapy should be based on culture results.

Parainfluenza viruses I and III and respiratory syncytial viruses have caused epidemics of pneumonia in nurseries. With no specific antiviral treatment against them, therapy is supportive, although efforts must be directed toward preventing epidemic spread.

Pneumonia is a complication of other primary respiratory diseases, especially RDS and aspiration of meconium or blood. Pneumonia resulting from postnatal aspiration is common in infants with tracheoesophageal fistulas, and pharyngeal incoordination in premature infants or those born with low Apgar scores or in infants with apnea and seizures.

ASPIRATION SYNDROMES

The normal fetus moves 1 ml to 5 ml of amniotic fluid in and out of its upper airways with periodic respiratory movements. When the fetus is stressed by an asphyxiating insult, it may make deep inspiratory gasps and aspirate amniotic fluid deeply into its airways. If the fetus is not born immediately after such a stress but recovers from the insult, the fluid is cleared out of the trachea by normal mucosal ciliary action.

The fetal lung tends to cleanse itself when it functions normally. Although squamous cells of aspirated amniotic fluid are present in autopsied lungs of infants dying intrapartum or shortly thereafter, normal amniotic fluid by itself is not harmful.

Respiratory distress results from aspiration of amniotic fluid that contains thick or particulate meconium, blood, or bacteria.

Aspiration occurs *in utero*, but even more important may be aspiration that occurs at the time of delivery. With the chest recoil that occurs after delivery of the thorax, any material present in the oropharynx may be drawn into the trachea. Suctioning the oropharynx before delivering the thorax removes that material and prevents aspiration at the time of delivery.

MECONIUM ASPIRATION

Associated with intrapartum stress is the passage of meconium into the amniotic fluid. About 8% to 10% of all term infants have some degree of meconium staining in the amniotic fluid at birth. Truly premature infants of less than 36 weeks' gestation rarely pass meconium. At greatest risk for meconium passage and aspiration at birth are postterm and postmature infants. These infants have a smaller volume of amniotic fluid to dilute any meconium that is passed. Their placentas have little vascular reserve to withstand blood flow changes during uterine contractions, thus predisposing the fetuses to hypoxic stress during their frequently prolonged labors.

Meconium is the content of the fetal bowel. It comprises swallowed amniotic fluid components that have not been digested, desquamated cells and enzymes from the fetal intestinal tract, and bile components, but primarily it is composed of mucopolysaccharides with little fat and no protein. Meconium is sterile. That which has been recently passed by a fetus because of acute stress may be undiluted by amniotic fluid, whereupon it is dark green, thick, and tenacious, or may be particulate after some dilution. When meconium has been passed some time earlier and diluted or partially metabolized, the fluid is yellowish and thin with small or absent particles.

The respiratory distress that results from meconium aspiration is due to acute obstruction of small airways. If the main airways remain obstructed and initial lung expansion is impossible, the infant's demise may be rapid. More often the infant can exert sufficient intrathoracic pressure to move the meconium plugs peripherally. Studies with tantalum in puppies have demonstrated that meconium is cleared from the major airways *peripherally* within 1 hour after instillation.

CLINICAL PRESENTATION

The infant who suffers from meconium aspiration often is postmature and is born through "pea-soup" meconium after some period of intrauterine distress. He has a low Apgar score with gasping respirations. From birth the infant is tachypneic, with grunting, retractions, flaring of alae nasi, and cyanosis proportionate to the degree of aspiration. There may be an increased anteroposterior diameter of the chest and intercostal bulging, especially if any degree of pneumothorax develops. The peak of distress occurs within the first 24 hours. If the infant needs assisted ventilation because of respiratory failure, the prognosis is poor.

Some infants who have had significant birth asphyxia develop progressive hypoxemia, hypocarbia, and a metabolic acidosis with poor peripheral perfusion. The severity of their symptoms seems far disproportionate to their roentgenographic findings. These infants appear to have severe pulmonary hypertension with marked ventilation/perfusion inequality. They usually respond poorly to increased ambient oxygen or to routine assisted ventilation.

ROENTGENOGRAPHIC PRESENTATION

The classic roentgenographic manifestations of meconium aspiration are focal or generalized areas of diminished aeration. These foci are patchy or confluent (Fig. 29-11). Consolidation may be unilateral or bilateral with no specific predilection for any lobe of lung. There is almost always evidence of air trapping. Pulmonary air leaks occur in about 10% of infants born in stained amniotic fluid, whereas 20% or more of those infants with symptoms of meconium aspiration will develop pulmonary air leaks. In the roentgenograms of infants showing consolidation or atelectasis, there often is thickening of the minor fissure from pleural fluid or evidence of pleural fluid in the costophrenic sulci.

The roentgenographic appearance of meconium aspiration is easily distinguished from that of RDS or transient tachypnea of the newborn, but the pulmonary changes are not distinguished as easily from

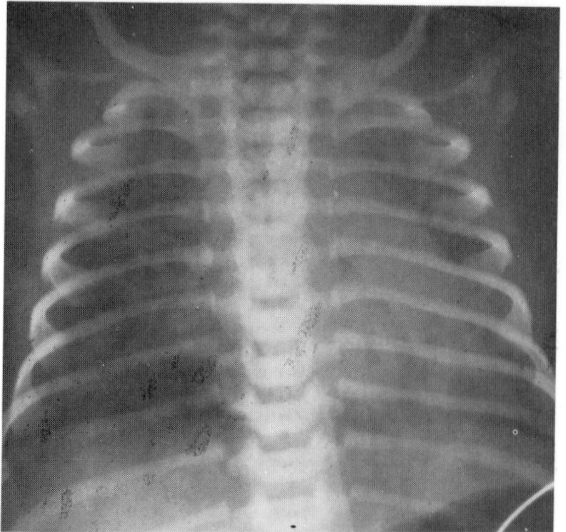

Fig. 29-11. Meconium aspiration. A term baby with a large amount of thick meconium suctioned from the trachea under direct visualization. There are bilateral patchy densities because of widespread focal atelectasis. Hyperaeration, not evident on this roentgenogram, developed 2 days later, followed by a pneumothorax. The infant recovered after 1 week of intensive respiratory care.

those seen in pulmonary hemorrhage or with intrapartum pneumonia. Distinction of these entities must be made clinically.

THERAPY

Successful management of infants who pass meconium during their intrapartum period depends on aggressive therapy aimed at prevention of aspiration. It is important to recognize the significance of meconium passage and to alleviate fetal distress before delivery whenever possible.

Because most of the aspiration occurs as the thorax recoils, completely clearing the oropharynx before delivering the thorax is the *most effective* means of preventing aspiration.

At delivery, the fetal condition should be rapidly assessed, as described earlier. All infants born through thick or particulate meconium should have direct tracheal intubation and suctioning. Since a large-bore suction catheter is needed, it is easiest to intubate with an orotracheal tube of appropriate size, using the operator's own mouth suction filtered through a mask that covers the mouth. Suctioning should be continued until the obstructing particulate material has been removed. Only then may positive pressure ventilation be applied. Usually the infant will have gasped before suctioning has been completed. Positive pressure ventilation should never be applied before suctioning has been performed!

Infants born through thin or watery meconium-stained fluid rarely have severe aspiration syndrome even though a large amount of fluid may be aspirated. Direct tracheal suctioning should be performed in these infants as their clinical condition indicates, but it is not necessarily routine if the fluid is not "pea soup," if it does not contain particles, and if there has been thorough suctioning before delivery.

Meconium may be present in the trachea even though it is not seen in the oropharynx! For this reason direct tracheal suctioning should be performed on all infants born through thick or particulate meconium, whether or not it is present in the oropharynx. There is strong evidence in favor of an aggressive approach to suctioning done properly in the delivery room. There is a lower incidence of symptoms and of pneumothorax in hospitals where all such infants are suctioned as compared to hospitals where positive pressure is applied before suctioning has been completed or only when thick meconium is found in the oropharynx.

Any infant with symptoms of aspiration should be observed closely for deterioration. Humidified, warmed oxygen should be given as indicated by hypoxemia on blood gas analysis. Pulmonary physiotherapy with postural drainage and suctioning should be performed especially frequently during the first 8 hours. Assisted ventilation for respiratory failure should be used if indicated. Antibiotics should be given to the infant because meconium may enhance bacterial growth.

The infant who shows rapid progression of clinical symptoms or who manifests signs of severe pulmonary hypertension with ventilation/perfusion inequality needs an even more aggressive approach to management. When clinical distress is excessive in relation to severity of aspiration radiographically or when there is a continually increasing requirement for oxygen, prompt respiratory and medical intervention is needed.

It is important to document blood gases at both the preductal (right radial) and postductal levels to determine if there is transductal right-to-left shunting. There may be intrapulmonary and intracardiac shunting as well, demonstrable by echocardiography. If there is evidence of pulmonary hypotension, it is often necessary to maintain a condition of hyperventilation such that the Pa_{CO_2} remains between 25 to 30 torr and Pa_{O_2} between 80 and 100 torr to increase pulmonary blood flow. Additionally, drug-induced paralysis may be necessary to allow mechanical control. If vascular volume and systemic perfusion are adequate, tolazoline (Priscoline) infusions may increase pulmonary blood flow. Given at a dose of 2 to 4 mg/kg/hr, tolazoline decreases pulmonary and systemic vascular resistance. Wrapping the extremities with elastic bandage prevents most of the systemic hypotension associated with both paralysis and tolazoline. Since gastrointestinal hemorrhage is a side-effect of tolazoline, antacid or local antihistaminic therapy prevents most of the severe cases of hemorrhage. Maintenance of high levels of inspired oxygen, high minute ventilation, and medications may be necessary for several weeks before recovery occurs.

If the infant develops hyperviscosity (*i.e.*, hematocrit of 70% or more), a partial exchange transfusion to help decrease the viscosity of the blood, and thus decrease the pulmonary vascular resistance, is indicated. Similarly transfusion to increase oxygen carrying capacity is necessary when anemia develops.

Air leaks require evacuation if they cause significant symptoms. Small air leaks will resorb spontaneously when the infant is placed in 100% oxygen for 2 to 3 hours. If the air leak causes respiratory embarrassment, it should be evacuated promptly by the methods described in the section on Pulmonary Air Leaks.

OTHER ASPIRATION SYNDROMES

Occasionally a baby is exposed to amniotic fluid contaminated with blood either of fetal or of maternal origin. Aspiration of this blood may cause severe respiratory symptoms similar to those of meconium aspiration. In addition signs of asphyxia are associated with loss of blood into the amniotic fluid. If the blood is of fetal origin, hypovolemia may occur from acute blood loss. Pulmonary hemorrhage is a frequent sequel to the aspiration of maternal blood.

Treatment of aspiration of hemorrhagic amniotic fluid is similar to that described for aspiration of meconium. Strict attention must be paid to possible consequences of any asphyxic insult, and particularly to an acute blood loss by the fetus. The prognosis for aspiration of hemorrhagic amniotic fluid may be poor.

PULMONARY AIR LEAKS

INTERSTITIAL PULMONARY EMPHYSEMA (PIE)

Unlike respiratory conditions in older patients, a frequent complication of respiratory distress in the neonate is the abnormal collection of extrapulmonary air. Although air may accumulate in various locations, the basic pathogenesis is the same for each. With excessive distending airway pressures from either a highly negative intrathoracic pressure or an exogenously applied positive airway pressure, the overstretched alveoli rupture, and air escapes into the interstitium. Because the neonatal lung has poorly developed routes for collateral ventilation, it is especially susceptible to alveolar rupture. With the movement of the lung, air travels further into the interstitium. It dissects along perivascular spaces until it ruptures into the pleural cavity or into the mediastinum or pericardium, where it accumulates. Air that has not yet reached an extraparenchymal cavity is known as interstitial pulmonary emphysema. The typical appearance most often is seen with HMD, especially when the infant is receiving high positive pressure ventilation.

On roentgenogram, the hyperlucencies representing the tiny air accumulations appear ovoid, or short, and streaky (see Fig. 29-4). They do not follow bronchial markings but appear "darker" than do air bronchograms. The interstitial emphysema pattern may be general or localized to one segment, unilateral or bilateral, depending on its stage of development.

The significance of interstitial emphysema is twofold. First, the entrapped air markedly decreases pulmonary compliance. Second, rupture of air into the mediastinum or pleural space adjacent to the involved area is imminent unless the progression of dissection is stopped.

If the infant is on CPAP, decreasing the pressure and increasing the FI_{O_2} may halt progression. If the infant is on intermittent positive pressure ventilation, lowering the pressures and inspiratory time while increasing frequency appears to be the most effective approach. When emphysema is severe, hand ventilation at rates of 100 to 120/min with very low pressures over several hours may be life-saving.[29]

When interstitial emphysema is unilateral, there are several possible approaches all directed at decreasing ventilation to the affected areas.[8] Selective intubation and ventilation of the unaffected lung allow collapse of the affected lung for several hours. Selective intubation of the right mainstem bronchus is far easier than that of the left.

Splinting the affected side sometimes helps by allowing more ventilation of the nonsplinted side. Heavy bandaging of the hemithorax and positioning with the abnormal, bandaged side dependent provides significant splinting of the compliant neonatal chest.

PNEUMOTHORAX

If the air ruptures into the pleural space, a pneumothorax develops. The symptoms depend on the amount of air accumulated, whether the air is accumulating under pressure, and on the extent of lung collapse. In RDS, the lung's stiffness may prevent complete collapse with accumulation of the large volumes of air that might be expected with a more compliant lung. What appears to be a small volume on the roentgenogram may, however, cause significant ventilatory insufficiency, especially in smaller infants who lack any pulmonary reserve. Additionally, because anteroposterior radiographs are taken with the infant supine, air layered anteriorly may not appear as radiolucent with a radiopaque, nonaerated lung collapsed behind it.

Spontaneous pneumothorax occurs in as many as 1% of normal deliveries. It is especially common in infants with HMD disease or aspiration syndromes or in those requiring resuscitation who are treated with artificial ventilation using high peak airway pressures. It is almost twice as common when IPPB with PEEP is used as when IPPB is used alone.[6]

As air accumulates in the pleural space, the infant develops increasing tachypnea, often with grunting. He frequently becomes noticeably agitated. In cases of tension pneumothorax, the chest on the affected side becomes squared and the intercostal spaces may bulge. The breath sounds are tubular but, because they are well-conducted from the opposite side, may be described as "good." After a brief rise the blood pressure falls, and metabolic acidosis develops if peripheral perfusion becomes inadequate. If the air leak continues, a significant collapse of lung and accumulation of air under pressure result. Such a bronchopleural fistula becomes even more dangerous because it may cause a significant shift of mediastinal structures to the opposite side. Thus it may be helpful to mark an X over the point of maximal cardiac impulse in any infant at risk to develop a pneumothorax as a reference point to detect a possible shift in mediastinal structures. Diagnosis may be made by transillumination of the chest with a fiberoptic bright but cool light source.[24]

The cardinal roentgenographic signs of pneumothorax include collapse of the lung with loss of the lung markings at the periphery and an expanded pleural space. If a tension pneumothorax is present, there may also be a shift of the heart and the mediastinum to the contralateral side, a flaring of the intercostal spaces with bulging of the parietal pleura, and compression or inversion of the ipsilateral hemidiaphragm (see Figs. 29-4 and 29-5).

IF RDS is present, the degree of lung collapse is not easily determined on roentgenogram. The affected lung may appear to "float" in the pleural air as the air accumulates in the nondependent portion of the chest. At first glance, the side with the pneumothorax may appear to be clearer than the opposite side because of overlying air and seemingly little collapse of the lung toward the mediastinum. A cross-table lateral view of the chest reveals air collection but is usually not necessary for diagnosis. Sometimes the air may accumulate medially, floating the lung away from the mediastinum and appearing to be within the mediastinal space. The distinction may be made on decubitus films by repositioning the infant to move the air up from the mediastinum or by collecting air along the costophrenic angle, sharply defining it.

Many spontaneous pneumothoraces do not require evacuation. They respond to an increased inspired oxygen concentration, which facilitates resorption. If the primary lung problem is RDS, severe pneumonia, or other diseases characterized by little pulmonary reserve and progressive unequal ventilation, almost any air accumulation should be evacuated.

Evacuation of the air accumulation, when indicated, should be done as quickly as possible, since an infant severely compromised by pneumothorax may decompensate very rapidly. While the equipment is being prepared and the skin made antiseptic for a more permanent tube placement, temporary evacuation can be done easily and safely with a small angiocatheter connected to a three-way stopcock and syringe, inserted at the fifth intercostal space in the anterior axillary line.

If air accumulation continues especially during positive pressure ventilation, management of chest tubes is slightly different than it is in adults, where larger tubes are used. It may be necessary to use higher suction pressures because the smaller tube diameter requires more pressure differential to allow enough flow to evacuate rapid air reaccumulation. The evacuation portals on the tube should be anterior if the infant is kept supine. The tube remains in place until there is no evidence of air leak. Because the intrathoracic volume taken up by the chest tube is proportionately large in tiny babies, removal often is necessary before spontaneous ventilation succeeds.

PNEUMOMEDIASTINUM

Pneumomediastinum occurs in the same infants who are at risk to develop pneumothorax. Although the symptoms of spontaneous pneumomediastinum may be subtle and go undetected, the incidence on random x-ray examination is less than that of spontaneous pneumothorax. Clinically the accumulation of mediastinal air may cause a sternal bulge that will be obvious as an increased anteroposterior diameter. The air may dissect into the soft tissue of the neck to cause swelling and crepitation, although less frequently than it does in adults. Despite the fact that the neonate's conducting airways collapse under less external pressure than do mature airways, the primary difficulty caused by pneumomediastinum is compression of major vessels. This prevents return of blood to the heart, causing a decrease in cardiac output and systemic and pulmonary hypoperfusion.

The roentgenographic presentation of pneumomediastinum in the newborn is an accumulation of air anterior to the heart on the lateral film or elevation of the thymus away from the cardiac silhouette in the anteroposterior or lateral projection (*see* Fig. 29-5). Air may be visualized extending to the soft tissues of the neck.

By itself, pneumomediastinum rarely requires treatment. However, if there appears to be progressive accumulation and intrathoracic dissection or in light of worsening pulmonary disease, evacuation may provide significant relief.

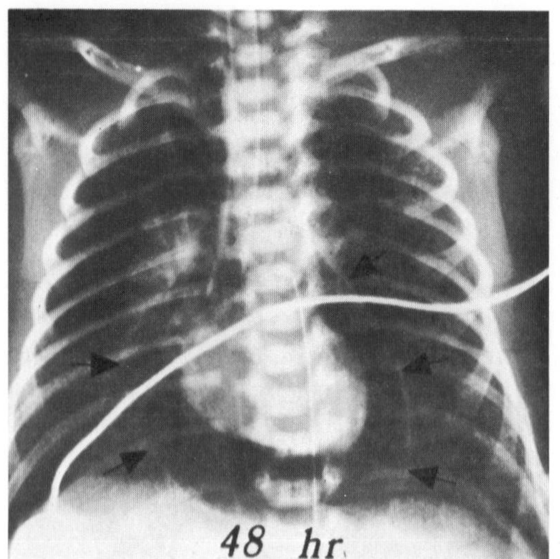

Fig. 29-12. Pneumopericardium. Air completely encircles the heart and is causing tamponade. Even though the endotracheal tube is down the right mainstem bronchus, no perforation of the tracheobronchial tree was present at postmortem examination.

PNEUMOPERICARDIUM

Despite the relative frequency of pulmonary air leaks in neonates, accumulation of air in the pericardial space is very uncommon. Since it may be life-threatening, however, it must be recognized and treated when indicated. Most cases have occurred in infants receiving assisted ventilation or who have required vigorous resuscitation.

The clinical findings depend on the amount of tamponade caused by air collecting within the pericardial sac. When the air is sufficient to restrict cardiac action, tachycardia, muffled heart sounds, and a decreased pulse pressure are observed. Sometimes the heart sounds are "absent" although there are still peripheral pulses. Once an infant manifests signs of tamponade from pneumopericardium, clinical deterioration is rapid unless the air is removed promptly.

On x-ray film air surrounding the heart and outlining the great vessels may be seen. The accumulation of air in the pericardium can be distinguished from that in the mediastinum by the former's circumferential location and its failure to extend into the soft tissues of the neck (Fig. 29-12).

If the infant develops a pneumopericardium while receiving high-pressure ventilation, the mortality rate is significantly higher than if the pneumopericardium is spontaneous. Those cases associated with infection carry an extremely high mortality.[48]

If evacuation is required to relieve tamponade, the air may be removed by inserting a tube (an angiocatheter) at the infracostal space adjacent to the left margin of the xiphoid and directing it dorsally and cephalad while aspirating. The ECG should be monitored for evidence of myocardial irritability, indicating needle contact with the myocardium.

PERIODIC BREATHING AND APNEA

Although the RDS is the most severe respiratory disease in preterm infants, the problems of periodic breathing and apnea are far more frequent. Periodic breathing is characterized by groups of breaths interrupted by intervals of apnea lasting longer than 3 seconds. A periodic breathing pattern is often a prelude to apnea, with resultant severe hypoxemia and bradycardia. If not reversed, such apneic episodes may be fatal. Although the infant may start breathing without any assistance, the apneic premature infant often needs stimulation and positive pressure ventilation if the apnea is not reversed quickly.

Periodic breathing usually appears after the first few days of life. It is more common and pronounced in smaller infants of lower gestational age. Most neonates breathe periodically, primarily during rapid eye movement (REM) sleep, as do adults and older infants. During REM sleep there is a depression in ventilation. In premature infants 90% of the sleep cycle is REM, whereas it occurs during 50% of sleep in the full-term neonate and 20% of adult sleep cycles. Thus, because the length of time spent in REM sleep composes a large proportion of time in the more premature infant, the likelihood of periodic breathing also increases.

Babies that breathe periodically have a lower respiratory minute volume, alveolar ventilation, and frequency. They have lower partial pressures of alveolar and arterial oxygen as well as higher partial pressures of alveolar and arterial carbon dioxide. The serum bicarbonate values are similar to adult values but are higher than in regular-breathing term infants.

Periodic breathing disappears upon stimulation, when the ambient air has a slightly increased percentage of carbon dioxide (2–4%), or when the FI_{O_2} is increased. Frequently an FI_{O_2} of 0.23 to 0.25 is effective in decreasing apneic episodes and in creating a more regular breathing pattern. The mechanism for this is unclear. Continuous negative pressure or continuous positive airway pressure is also effective in decreasing periodic breathing.

The primary medical treatment of apnea of prematurity is regular low doses of xanthine derivatives, caffeine, or theophylline. Caffeine is the apparent active end-product of theophylline and has an extended and unpredictable half-life in neonates, making measurement of serum levels mandatory.

Apnea not associated with periodic breathing or REM sleep usually is a sign of disease that may be in almost any organ-system in the neonate. It may be iatrogenically induced by a thermal environment that is inappropriate for that particular infant. An infant accustomed to one environmental temperature that is suddenly changed several degrees may respond with apnea. Central nervous system hemorrhage, edema, and infection routinely present as apnea, as may generalized sepsis, pneumonia, a patent ductus arteriosus, hypoglycemia, or drug depression.

Because apnea may be merely a symptom of more serious disease, all other possible etiologies should be excluded or treated before assuming it to be associated with periodic breathing and treating it as such.

Although most infants who demonstrate apnea gradually outgrow the episodes in both frequency and severity, there is a higher incidence of infant deaths from apparent sleep apnea or the sudden infant death syndrome (SIDS) after discharge. If testing during deep sleep reveals persistent abnormality of breathing pattern, home monitoring may be indicated.

ESOPHAGEAL ATRESIA AND TRACHEOESOPHAGEAL FISTULA

Esophageal atresia (EA) with or without tracheoesophageal fistula (TEF) is a congenital anomaly that may present as respiratory distress in the neonate. It may be associated with other anomalies, primarily those involving the cardiovascular and musculoskeletal systems. The incidence of TEF may be as high as 1:3000 deliveries.[21]

At least seven variations of anatomical presentation of EA and TEF reflect abnormal separation of the pulmonary system from the gastrointestinal tract early in gestation. The most frequent form, occurring in 85% of cases, combines esophageal atresia with a distal tracheoesophageal fistula (Fig. 29-13a). In this configuration, there is a blind and often dilated esophagus proximally and a short and narrow esophagus distally that connects to the trachea. The next most frequent combination is esophageal atresia without fistulous connection to the trachea (Fig. 29-13b). Other variations are rare (Fig. 29-13c, d, e).

The diagnosis of EA comes with the observation of excessive salivation and inability to control secretions or feedings in an otherwise normal neonate. If a radiopaque catheter is passed into the esophagus, it cannot pass the normal distance. There is no "rush" over the epigastrium during auscultation when air is injected through the catheter. The abdomen may be scaphoid if there is no tracheoesophageal fistula to allow air entry into the gut. When an endotracheal tube is placed, the stomach distends with positive pressure ventilation if the fistula is below the ET tube orifice.

On chest roentgenogram a dilated proximal pouch or coiled catheter within the pouch may be seen (Fig. 29-14). Radiopaque material sometimes is instilled to outline the pouch (Fig. 29-15). Lipid contrast solutions are probably more irritating than is dilute barium, but, because any contrast material may be aspirated and cause a reaction, its use should be avoided. Endoscopy with instillation of a nonirritating dye into the nonvisualized esophagus or trachea may disclose the site of the fistula when the dye enters the visualized area. The use of contrast materials and dyes in the neonate is discouraged unless a precise diagnosis depends on the information that might be found. Complications from these procedures do not warrant their use if they are not essential in the evaluation.

The successful treatment of EA or TEF depends partly on early surgical intervention to prevent recurrent aspiration pneumonias. Surgery may require staged procedures to create an adequate airway and esophagus as the child grows. Before surgery and for the first 48 hours postoperatively, infants are nursed prone with head elevated to reduce the chance of aspiration and to aid in clearing the lobar atelectasis that is frequent. The esophageal pouch is kept clear of secretions with sump drainage. Feedings may also be given through a gastrostomy that provides de-

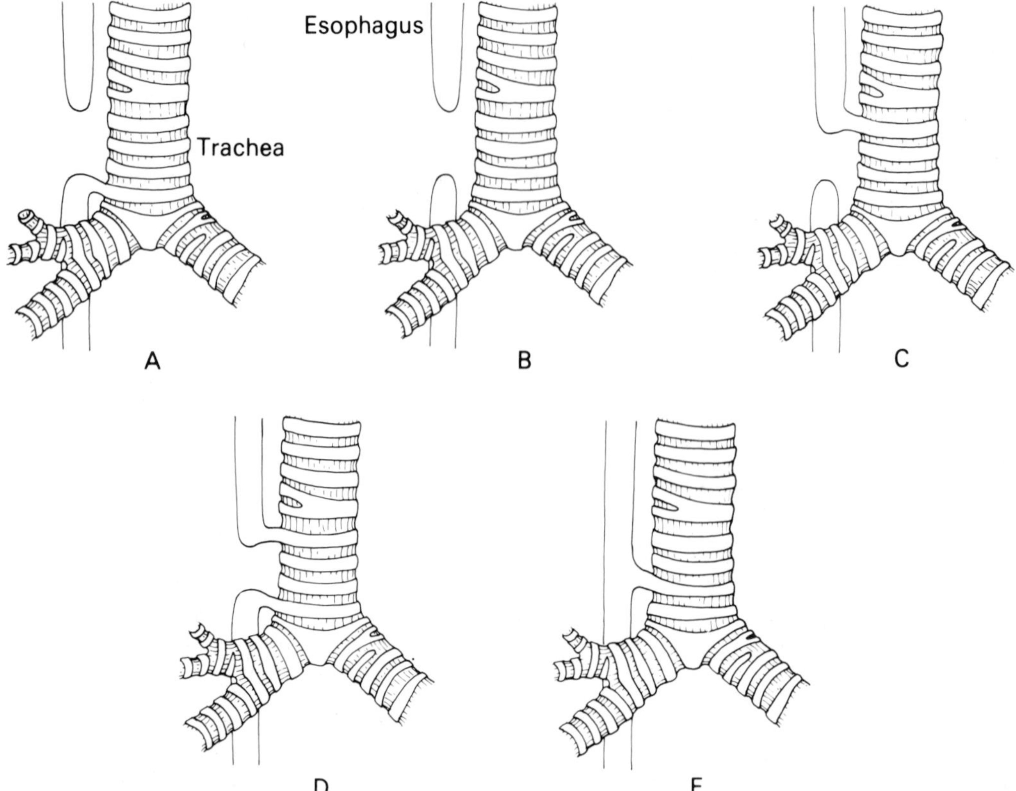

Fig. 29-13. Variations of esophageal atresia and tracheoesophageal fistulas (*see* text).

compression of the stomach contents. Care must be taken to avoid placing the esophagus under tension after its anastomosis. Vigorous physiotherapy usually is delayed until the third postoperative day to allow adequate wound closure.

One of the postoperative complications of TEF is the reformation of fistulas and strictures of trachea and esophagus. Multiple procedures may be needed over a long course.

DIAPHRAGMATIC HERNIA

The diaphragm is formed by contributions from several different sources early in gestation (see section on Fetal Lung Development). If a portion contributed by any one of these structures is incomplete or if the continuity of the diaphragm is lost during gestation, there may be free communication between the abdominal and thoracic cavities, resulting in a diaphragmatic hernia. The most common site for such a communication is the posterolateral portion of the diaphragm at the foramen of Bochdalek. The left side is involved at least five times more often than the right side, but, rarely, both sides may be involved. Occasionally, a hernia may involve the foramen of Morgagni in the substernal area. In these cases the hernia is more often on the right side and allows portions of the liver and intestine to locate adjacent to the heart in the anterior mediastinum. Although a hernia through the foramen of Morgagni may be recognized at birth, it usually presents later, often as an asymptomatic, mediastinal mass on a roentgenogram obtained for other reasons.

A diaphragmatic hernia through the foramen of Bochdalek may also be asymptomatic throughout infancy if it is small or does not involve a constant volume of abdominal contents herniating into the pleural space. If there is a large communication or if a significant volume of bowel has become entrapped early in gestation, severe, life-threatening symptoms occur immediately after birth. These symptoms result from compression of developing lung tissue. If the compression has been constant for a prolonged period *in utero*, the development of the lung is disrupted such that there may be fewer airway divisions than

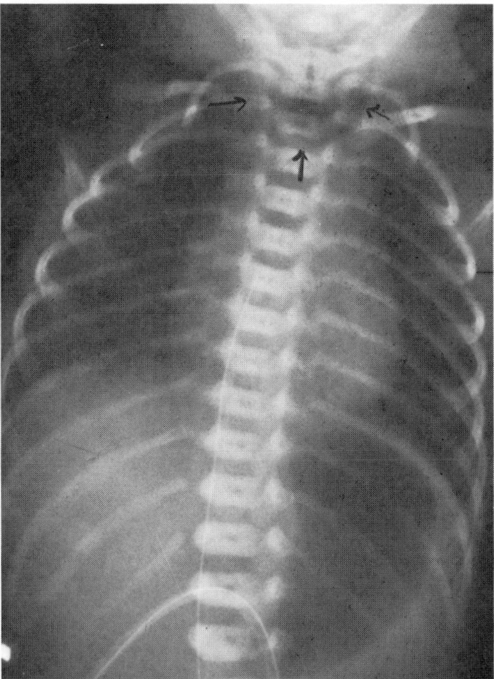

Fig. 29-14. Esophageal atresia with tracheoesophageal fistula. The chest film shows air in the dilated, atretic upper esophageal pouch. No aspiration pneumonia is noted as yet. Air in the stomach denotes the presence of a distal tracheoesophageal fistula.

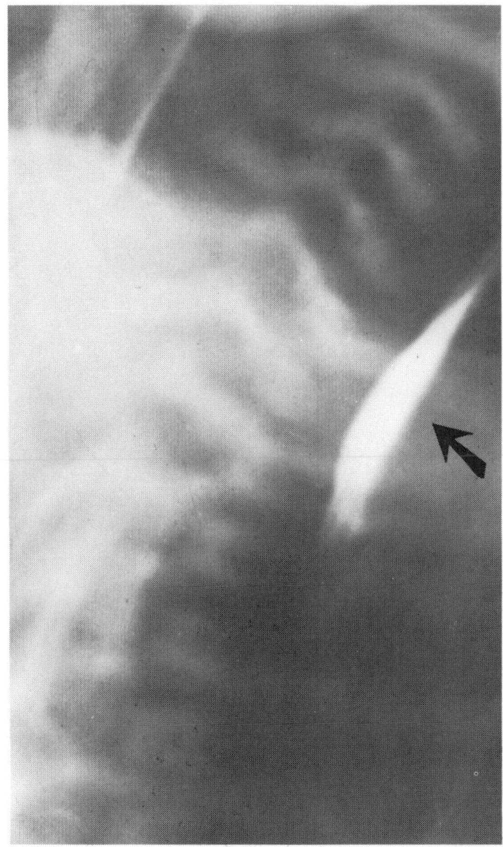

Fig. 29-15. Lateral view of esophageal atresia. There is a minute amount of contrast material *(arrow)* in the atretic upper esophageal pouch.

normal. The lung on the affected side is grossly hypoplastic, as expected. In addition, the lung on the opposite ("normal") side is hypoplastic and demonstrates a maturation arrest that may be evident only when the number of divisions are determined microscopically. The pulmonary arteries throughout the lung are more muscular than is appropriate for their size or developmental age.

The result of these combined abnormalities is severe respiratory insufficiency as soon as air breathing begins. The infant may have a good Apgar score at 1 minute, but it deteriorates with each successive breath. The chest appears distended while the abdomen initially is scaphoid. Resuscitation with positive pressure ventilation seems only to make the infant worse. If the hernia is on the left, the heart tones are shifted to the right side, with absence of breath sounds over the left chest. There is dullness to percussion over the side where the bowel is located, but only rarely are bowel sounds heard. Either because of vigorous resuscitation attempts with elevated positive pressures or because of the infant's own respiratory efforts, tension pneumothoraces develop very rapidly on *either* side. As the intestines distend with air, the respiratory compromise increases because of further compression of the lung.

The diagnosis should be suspected immediately based on the presenting physical findings, but the chest and abdominal radiographs are usually definite (Fig. 29-16). A radiopaque catheter should be placed into the esophagus as far as it will easily advance and a chest roentgenogram obtained. If the stomach is herniated, the catheter will be seen coiled in the thorax. Occasionally, if the herniation is relatively small, the bowel pattern in the chest is difficult to distinguish from the pneumatoceles of staphylococcal pneumonia or from congenital cystic lung disease.

The treatment of diaphragmatic hernia depends on its rapid recognition and surgical correction. It is essential to relieve the pressure that the displaced abdominal contents put on the lung and heart as quickly as possible. Continuous aspiration of the stomach contents should be started immediately. The trachea

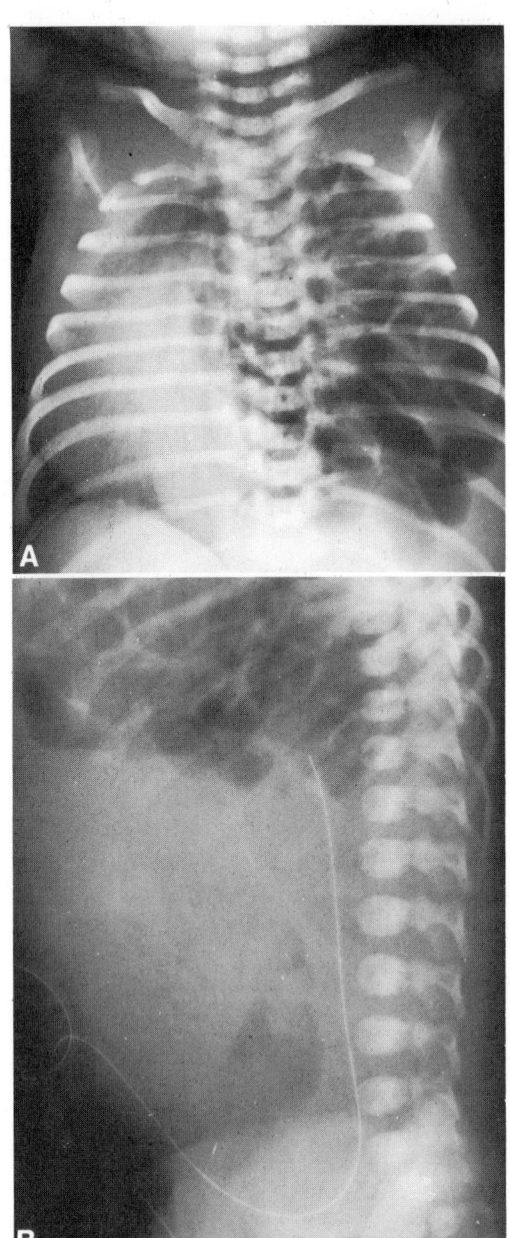

Fig. 29-16. *(A)* Anteroposterior view of a diaphragmatic hernia. This full-term newborn had respiratory distress from birth. Heart tones were heard on the right. Note the multiple loops of bowel in the left pleural space with herniation of the heart and mediastinum toward the right. *(B)* Lateral view of the same diaphragmatic hernia. Physical examination of the abdomen disclosed scaphoid configuration. The only air below the level of the diaphragm is in the stomach. Note the multiple loops of small bowel in the chest.

should be intubated to prevent further distention of bowel by swallowed air and to control ventilation.

Temperature should be carefully maintained. A catheter should be placed in the umbilical artery. Pneumothoraces are evacuated as soon as they develop.

Although the successful reconstruction of the diaphragm primarily depends on the skill of the surgeon and what remnants of muscle remain, the overall outcome depends on the nature of the functional lung tissue available. Although the number of alveoli in the functioning lung is apparently adequate, the major problem arises from the severe pulmonary hypertension that develops. Immediately postoperatively, ventilatory insufficiency may be associated with a nonreexpanded lung and pneumothoraces. After a few hours, although ventilation may be adequate, perfusion becomes inadequate because of markedly elevated pulmonary artery pressures. Occasionally, infusion of high doses of arterial vasodilators such as tolazoline have been successful in maintaining the infant until the pulmonary hypertension subsides. Hyperventilation and alkalinization help in reversing the hypertension. The perfusion/ventilation inequality persists for 36 to 72 hours, or more. If the pulmonary vasculature remains responsive to medical therapy and severe hypoxemia does not develop, the postoperative prognosis is excellent, although the course may be very stormy.

RESPIRATORY DISTRESS OWING TO NONPULMONARY CAUSES

The diagnosis of respiratory distress primarily owing to nonpulmonary problems in the neonate is not always obvious. Symptoms caused by disease with pulmonary system origin must be distinguished from those arising in the cardiac, central nervous, or neuromuscular systems. Most frequently, the distinction is between pulmonary or cardiac origin. The history (obviously short-term) and the physical examination provide the primary tools for diagnosis. Generally, if the symptoms reflect pulmonary disease, there is tachypnea accompanied by flaring of the alae nasi, chest wall retractions, and grunting. Tachypnea with deep cyanosis but without retractions suggests cardiac origin. If the respirations are ataxic, too shallow, or abnormally deep, CNS origin is likely.

In neonates, laboratory tools available to distinguish between respiratory and cardiac disease are not as helpful as they are in adults. The ECG most often is normal or only mildly abnormal in all respiratory problems as well as in most cardiac problems. The chest roentgenogram is helpful in experienced hands but may appear within normal limits despite severe disease in some cases. The echocardiogram is particularly useful for distinguishing cardiac diseases.

One of the more helpful available tools, when used properly, is the *oxygen challenge test*, where there is a comparison of response to room air and 100% oxygen over a short time. Use of indwelling catheters or transcutaneous oxygen electrodes shortens the test duration; thus the time of high oxygen exposure may be very brief. The steps and conclusions throughout the challenge test are presented in Figure 29-17. There is some overlap in response between cardiac and pulmonary etiologies, particularly when there are elements of pulmonary hypertension and systemic hypotension. Additionally any infant may have both cardiac and respiratory disease. However, when interpreted with other available information, the test may aid in distinguishing cardiac from pulmonary disease.

RESPIRATORY DISTRESS OWING TO PATENT DUCTUS ARTERIOSUS

One of the cardiovascular conditions that causes respiratory difficulty in the neonate is persistence of a patent ductus arteriosus (PDA). Normally the ductus arteriosus closes functionally in the first day of life and anatomically in the first month of life. The ductus remains open longer in the small premature infant, where it may be as wide as the aorta and can carry a large volume of blood from a high- to a low-resistance system. When pulmonary vascular resistance is high, as it is *in utero* or in pulmonary diseases such as RDS, the ductus shunts blood from the pulmonary artery to the aorta (right-to-left shunting), bypassing the pulmonary vascular bed and causing hypoxemia in the blood that supplies the lower extremities. If systemic resistance is higher than pulmonary resistance, as it is in extrauterine life, blood shunts from the systemic to the pulmonary system (left to right), increasing pulmonary blood flow and flooding the lungs. When the two systems have balanced vascular resistance, there is no shunting across the ductus, although it remains open.

In a premature infant with respiratory distress syndrome, pulmonary vascular resistance is relatively high and, during the most severe period of respiratory distress syndrome, is nearly equal to systemic resistance. Thus, although the ductus arteriosus remains open, little or no blood is shunted across the vessel because the resistances are similar on the two sides. As the pulmonary disease improves, pulmonary vascular resistance decreases, allowing shunting from systemic to pulmonary circulation. The lung fields and pulmonary vascular bed flood with the increased load, causing pulmonary edema, decreased pulmonary compliance, and an increased alveolar–arterial oxygen difference.

Physical examination reveals a very active precordium with visible axillary pulses and bounding peripheral pulses on palpation, reflecting a widened pulse pressure. A short, soft, systolic murmur is heard over the precordium. (The intensity of the murmur is related inversely to the size of the shunt.) Hepatomegaly, peripheral edema, and poor urine output may develop with congestive heart failure. The blood gases reflect metabolic acidemia, hypoxemia, and hypercapnia. The chest roentgenograms indicate increased vascularity of pulmonary vessels, edema, and cardiomegaly (*see* Fig. 29-3). Echocardiograms suggest increased volume to the left atrium proportional to the amount of pulmonary shunting.

The most definitive treatment of PDA is surgical ligation. Although the procedure itself in experienced hands is relatively benign, there are many potential complications associated with major surgery in neonates. One of the most serious consequences of ligation is the effect of abrupt changes in cerebral blood flow and pressure, potentially contributing to intracranial hemorrhaging in smaller premature infants. Other complications include serious side-effects of loss of thermal homeostasis and arterial blood gas fluctuations.

In selected infants, use of a prostaglandin synthetase inhibitor, indomethacin, accomplishes medical ligation of the ductus. Indomethacin is not effective in all infants, particularly the smallest and often sickest, and medical closure may not be permanent. Additionally indomethacin has serious side-effects that necessitate careful dosing and attention to the potential problems of bleeding, intestinal perforation, and renal failure.

Even though an ideal goal in the treatment of PDA is early closure in order to shorten ventilator and ox-

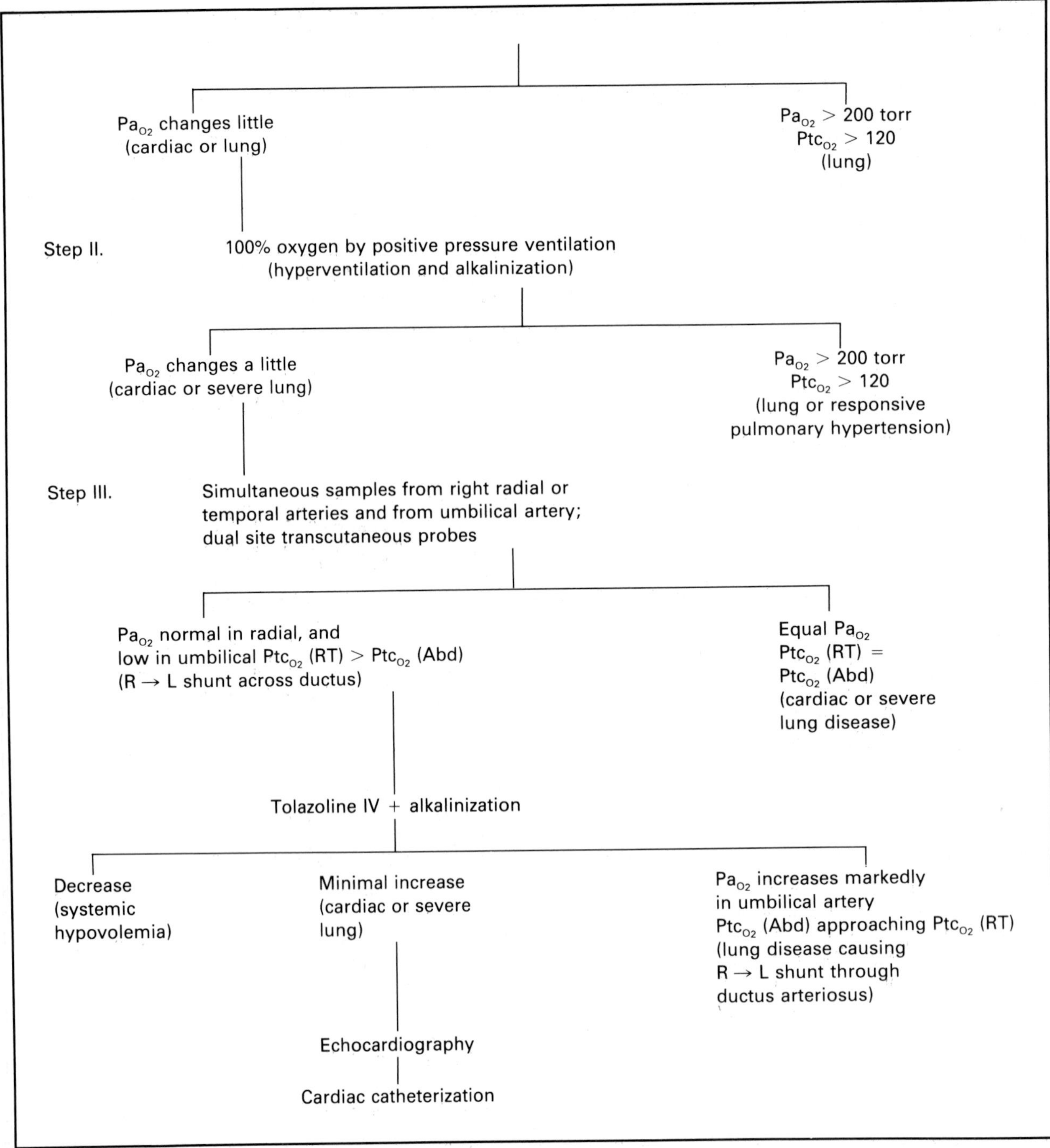

Fig. 29-17. "Oxygen challenge test" for distinguishing cardiac versus respiratory disease. Ptc_{O_2} (RT) = transcutaneous oxygen probe over right thorax (preductal); Ptc_{O_2} (Abd) = probe over abdomen (postductal).

ygen therapy, the side-effects in achieving that goal may outweigh the benefits.

A PDA also can cause symptoms in the neonate who does not have primary respiratory disease. Typically the ductus begins to shunt during the first week of life when natural resolution of prenatal pulmonary hypertension occurs. A PDA in such a case causes apnea, poor feeding, tachypnea, bounding pulses, inappropriate weight curves, and abnormal chest roentgenograms. Hepatomegaly and edema also may develop. Aggressive medical management using diuretics and indomethacin frequently is successful. Continuous positive airway pressure reverses pulmonary edema if it is not too severe. If restriction of fluids needs to be so severe that growth is prevented or if the infant requires assisted ventilation, and if indomethacin is unsuccessful or contraindicated, surgical ligation of the ductus should be done as soon as feasible.

RESPIRATORY DISTRESS OWING TO PERSISTENT FETAL CIRCULATION

The high pulmonary vascular resistance present at birth usually falls as the ventilated lungs fill with air and the PDA closes. In certain situations, however, persistent, high pulmonary vascular pressure is unyielding, even with minimal pulmonary parenchymal disease. Right-to-left shunting remains present. The cause for this is not known, although Siassi and coworkers have associated it with prenatal events of hypoxia and maternal hypotension.[38]

It is becoming increasingly evident that the unusually reactive pulmonary vasculature plays a significant role in many respiratory conditions in neonates. Changes in pulmonary blood flow may be relatively abrupt, with shunting across a patent ductus, the foramen ovale, or intrapulmonary vessels.

Two modes of therapy are helpful in treating pulmonary hyperventilation whether as an isolated condition or in the presence of lung disease: First is mechanical ventilation to control the Pa_{CO_2} at 25 to 30 torr while maintaining Pa_{O_2} at 80 to 100 torr with as steady a state as possible;[34] second is the use of the vasodilator tolazoline to encourage pulmonary blood flow.[19]

Despite the very critical condition of infants with pulmonary hypertension, as long as there is responsiveness to medical and respiratory therapy in the absence of other debilitating complications, the prognosis for complete recovery is excellent.

RESPIRATORY DISTRESS DUE TO HEMODYNAMIC ABNORMALITIES

Respiratory distress may occur in the neonate as the result of either too much or too little circulating blood volume. The most frequent reason for vascular overload is excessive placental transfusion or cord stripping at the time of delivery. The overload causes congestive heart failure, hepatomegaly, and pulmonary edema, with delayed absorption of normal lung fluid. Although the symptoms, primarily tachypnea, resolve spontaneously if the overload is not too great, diuresis or phlebotomy may be necessary if the pulmonary edema causes severe symptoms.

An inadequate circulating blood volume also causes respiratory distress. In hypovolemic shock or septic shock, pulmonary capillary integrity is lost, leading to alveolar edema with an increased alveolar–arterial oxygen difference. Simultaneously there is a metabolic acidosis, which causes the infant to try to compensate with hyperventilation. If metabolic acidosis is too severe or if there are conditions present that depress respiratory drive, such as drugs or hypoglycemia, the infant may in fact hypoventilate, be cyanotic, and be unable to compensate for the metabolic acidosis.

Polycythemia with or without increased blood volume increases blood viscosity when the hematocrit reaches a critical level between 65% and 70%. With increased blood viscosity, significant sludging of blood, an increased cardiac work load, hypoxemia, and hypoglycemia occur. Fetal red blood cells are less flexible than cells with adult hemoglobin and contribute to sludging in small vessels. The extraordinarily high rate of glycolysis in fetal erythrocytes helps cause hypoglycemia. Hyperviscosity affects both the cardiovascular and central nervous systems and causes respiratory distress from heart failure, pulmonary edema, CNS hypoxia, or hypoglycemia. If the hematocrit exceeds 65% after the first 3 or 4 hours of life, the baby should have a partial exchange transfusion with saline or plasma to lower the hematocrit and the viscosity.

Severe anemia *in utero* may cause significant respiratory distress at birth because of hypoxia, either from inadequate oxygen carrying capacity or from congestive heart failure, as in the case of *hydrops fetalis* resulting from severe Rh incompatibility. Immediate correction of the low hemoglobin levels by packed cell transfusion followed by exchange transfusion after initial stabilization is life-saving.

RESPIRATORY DISTRESS OWING TO NEUROLOGIC DISEASE

Changes in patterns of ventilation are often the primary sign of intracranial disease processes in the newborn infant. The acute onset of apnea heralds the onset of an intracranial bleed or increased intracranial pressure. Because many neurologic signs are "soft" in the neonate and "normal" is only narrowly distinguished from "abnormal," the onset of apnea may be one of the few signs that can be documented accurately. Apnea may represent seizure activity. If a CNS insult does not cause complete apnea, it may cause hypoventilation associated with floppiness or overt seizures, the onset of metabolic acidosis, or bradycardia. Less commonly, there may be more misleading symptoms of respiratory distress with hyperpnea, grunting, and a whining cry in the absence of flaring of the alae nasi, retractions, or cyanosis. Initially, the blood pH is normal or alkalotic from hyperventilation, but a metabolic acidosis develops if the CNS insult continues and causes circulatory insufficiency. Persistent pulmonary hypertension is sometimes documented in these cases, but the mechanism is unclear. Often there is a history of birth trauma or precipitous delivery, especially in very large babies or in premature infants. The spinal fluid may be hemorrhagic, reflecting a subarachnoid bleed or it may indicate CNS irritation from a bacterial or viral meningitis. Chest films are most often normal or may reflect mild cardiomegaly.

Therapy is supportive until the etiology of the CNS irritation is determined and then is specifically directed toward the cause, when possible. CNS insults such as meningitis or intracranial hemorrhage sufficient to cause significant respiratory symptoms usually carry a poor prognosis. In comparison, the prognosis for CNS insult resulting from generalized edema is much better, especially if the symptoms appear early during the course and do not persist beyond the first few days.

Congenital malformations of the central nervous system may present at birth with respiratory distress. Most notable is the *Arnold–Chiari* deformity, where there may be bilateral paralysis of vocal cords with stridor and upper airway obstruction. Spontaneous paralysis of one or both vocal cords also occurs in the absence of other illness or abnormalities.

Phrenic Nerve Paralysis

Respiratory distress owing to paralysis of the phrenic nerve (supplying the diaphragm) occurs primarily as the result of birth trauma in large babies and can present in an otherwise normal infant. More often the nerve paresis is associated with a palsy of the brachial plexus, causing weakness in the ipsilateral arm.

The infant may demonstrate little distress aside from a rapid respiratory rate. If atelectasis and pneumonia develop on the affected side, cyanosis, grunting, and flaring may appear. The cry may be weak and occasionally hoarse from an associated recurrent laryngeal nerve paresis. On physical examination decreased movement of the affected side is evident, or there may be paradoxical excursions of the two sides. The thorax and abdomen on the normal side will expand with inspiration, whereas the poorly fixed rib cage on the affected side either may not move or may actually decrease in apparent volume with inspiration. If the accessory muscles are used, the ribs will be pulled up with inspiration, but if there is an associated brachial palsy there will be unilateral retractions of the affected side.

Treatment depends on the extent of the respiratory compromise caused by the paralysis. If there is respiratory insufficiency, assisted ventilation is necessary. Often continuous negative pressure ventilation at low pressure is adequate and is preferable to positive pressure ventilation for prolonged periods. Nasal CPAP helps prevent loss of lung volume. Careful attention to prevention of aspiration and atelectasis is essential. If the phrenic nerve is avulsed, recovery is slow and may never be complete. If the injury is due to nerve edema without separation, the recovery is more rapid and usually complete.

RESPIRATORY DISTRESS DUE TO MUSCULOSKELETAL ABNORMALITIES

Weakness of the muscles of respiration sufficient to cause respiratory distress is associated with generalized muscular weakness. The infant is floppy, with poor respiratory effort, although he may appear neurologically intact, alert, and responsive. The most frequent condition that presents in the neonatal period is myasthenia gravis. *Transient neonatal myasthenia gravis* affects about 10% to 15% of offspring of affected mothers. This is an immunologic disorder in the mother in which an antibody attacks the acetylcholine receptor protein, interfering with neuromuscular transmission and causing muscle weakness. The maternal antibody crosses the placenta and acts in the fetus and newborn until naturally destroyed. More rarely the infant may himself have persistent myasthenia. If the level of antibody activity is high enough, the infant presents with muscular weakness that leads to respiratory insufficiency. Therapy includes neostigmine, exchange transfusion, and ventilatory support.

In all congenital neuromuscular or central neural abnormalities where there is respiratory embarrassment, the approach to therapy follows the same principles: postural drainage, cough simulation, sighing; airway maintenance with intubation and tracheostomy as needed; and ventilatory support as indicated by blood gases and examination.

RESPIRATORY DISTRESS OWING TO MISCELLANEOUS CAUSES

Infants with *metabolic acidosis* present with hyperpnea or tachypnea and floppiness. Although grunting may be present, there are few other signs of pulmonary disease, such as flaring, retractions, or cyanosis. As acidosis progresses, hyperpnea may change to hypoventilation, particularly in premature infants. Metabolic acidosis may reflect an inadequate circulating blood volume (e.g., hypovolemic shock secondary to acute blood loss at delivery or acute dehydration from diarrhea) or septic shock from either a bacterial or viral infection. If acidosis is more chronic, it usually reflects renal disease, particularly ones associated with inability to conserve bicarbonate.

Rarely, inspiratory stridor reflecting respiratory distress due to laryngospasm may accompany severe *hypocalcemia*. *Hypoglycemia* often causes hypoventilation, leading to complete apnea, particularly in premature infants. *Hypothermia* may induce hypoventilation or hyperpnea with grunting. If profound hypothermia is reversed at a rate faster than approximately 1°C/hr, apnea may develop from CNS edema associated with rewarming.

REFERENCES

1. Ambrus CM et al: Studies on hyaline membrane disease. 1. The fibrinolysin system in pathogenesis and therapy. Pediatrics 32:10, 1963
2. Avery ME, Fletcher BD, Williams RG: The lung and its disorders in the newborn infant. In Shaffer AJ, Markowitz M (eds): Major Problems in Clinical Pediatrics, Vol 1. Philadelphia, WB Saunders, 1981
3. Avery ME, Gatewood OB, Brumley G: Transient tachypnea of newborn. Am J Dis Child 111:380, 1966
4. Baghdassarian O, Avery ME, Neuhauser EBD: A form of pulmonary insufficiency in premature infants? Pulmonary dysmaturity. Am J Roentgenol 89:1020, 1963
5. Batenburg JJ, Van Golde MG: Formation of pulmonary surfactant in whole lung and in isolated type II alveolar cells. In Scarpelli EM, Cosmi EV (eds): Reviews in Perinatal Medicine, Vol 3. New York, Raven Press, 1979
6. Berg TJ et al: Bronchopulmonary dysplasia and lung rupture in hyaline membrane disease: Influence of continuing distending pressure. Pediatrics 55:51, 1975
7. Boyden EA, Tompsett DH: The changing patterns in the developing lungs of infants. Acta Anat 61:164, 1965
8. Brooks JG et al: Selective bronchial intubation for the treatment of severe localized pulmonary interstitial emphysema in newborn infants. J Pediatr 91:648, 1977
9. Brumley GW et al: Whole and disaturated lung phosphatidylcholine in cortisol-treated, intrauterine growth-retarded and twin control lambs at different gestational ages. Biol Neonate 31:155, 1977
10. Bucher U, Reid L: Development of the intrasegmental bronchial tree: The pattern of branching and development of cartilage at various stages of intrauterine life. Thorax 16:207, 1961
11. Burnard ED et al: Pulmonary insufficiency in prematurity. Austr Paediatr J 1:12, 1965
12. Charnock E, Doershuk CF: Developmental aspects of the human lung. Pediatr Clin North Am 20:275, 1973
13. Coates AL et al: Long-term pulmonary sequelae of the Wilson-Mikity syndrome. J Pediatr 92:247, 1978
14. Edwards DK, Colby TV, Northway WH: Radiologic-pathologic correlation in bronchopulmonary dysplasia. J Pediatr 95:834, 1979
15. Engle MJ, VanGolde MG, Wertz K: Transfers of phospholipids between subcellular fractions of the lung. FEBS Lett 82:277, 1978
16. Engle S: The structure of the respiratory tissue in the newly born. Acta Anat 19:353, 1953
17. Esterly JR, Oppenheimer EH: Massive pulmonary hemorrhage in newborn. 1. Pathologic considerations. J Pediatr 69:3, 1966
18. Farrell PM, Wood RE: Epidemiology of hyaline membrane disease in the United States: Analysis of national mortality statistics. Pediatrics 58:167, 1976
19. Goetzman BW et al: Neonatal hypoxia and pulmonary vasospasm: Response to tolazoline. J Pediatr 89:617, 1976
20. Hodgeman JE et al: Chronic respiratory distress in the premature infant (Wilson-Mikity syndrome). Pediatrics 44:179, 1969
21. Humphrey GH, Hogg BM, Ferrer J: Congenital atresia of esophagus. J Thorac Surg 32:332, 1956
22. Kauffman SL: Kinetics of alveolar epithelial hyperplasia of lungs of mice exposed to urethane. I. Quantitative analysis of cell population. Lab Invest 30:170, 1974
23. Kotas RV et al: A new model for neonatal pulmonary hemorrhage research. Pediatr Res 9:161, 1975
24. Kuhns LR et al: Diagnosis of pneumothorax and pneumomediastinum in the neonate by transillumination. Pediatrics 56:335, 1975
25. Lauweryns JM: "Hyaline membrane disease" in newborn infants. Macroscopic, radiographic, and light and electron microscopic studies. Hum Pathol 1:175, 1970
26. Mason RJ: Lipid metabolism. In Crystal RG (ed): The Biochemical Basis of Pulmonary Function. New York, Marcel Dekker, 1976
27. Meyrick B, Reid LM: Ultrastructure of alveolar lining and its development. In Hodson WA (ed): Development of the Lung. New York, Marcel Dekker, 1977
28. Moylan FMB, Shannon DC: Preferential distribution of lobar emphysema and atelectasis in bronchopulmonary dysplasia. Pediatrics 63:130, 1979
29. Ng KPK, Easa D: Management of interstitial emphysema by high-frequency low positive-pressure hand ventilation in the neonate. J Pediatr 95:117, 1979

30. Normand ICS et al: Permeability of lung capillaries and alveoli to non-electrolytes in the foetal lamb. J Physiol 219:303, 1971
31. Northway WH Jr, Rosan RC, Porter DY: Pulmonary disease following respiratory therapy of hyaline-membrane disease: Bronchopulmonary dysplasia. N Engl J Med 276:357, 1967
32. Olver RE, Strang LB: Ion fluxes across the pulmonary epithelium and secretion of lung liquid in the foetal lamb. J Physiol 241:327, 1974
33. Oppermann HC et al: Bronchopulmonary dysplasia in premature infants—radiological and pathological correlation. Pediatr Radiol 5:137, 1977
34. Peckham GP, Fox WW: Physiologic factors affecting pulmonary artery pressure in infants with persistent pulmonary hypertension. J Pediatr 93:1005, 1978
35. Philip AGS: Oxygen plus pressure plus time: The etiology of bronchopulmonary dysplasia. Pediatrics 55:44, 1975
36. Pierce JA, Hocott JB: Studies on the collagen and elastin content of the human lung. J Clin Invest 39:8, 1960
37. Ross S, Naeye RL: Racial and environmental influences on fetal lung maturation. Pediatrics 68:790, 1981
38. Siassi B et al: Persistent pulmonary vascular obstruction in newborn infants. J Pediatr 78:610, 1971
39. Smyth JA et al: Pulmonary function and bronchial hyperreactivity in long-term survivors of bronchopulmonary dysplasia. Pediatrics 68:336, 1981
40. Stern L: The role of respiration in the etiology and pathogenesis of bronchopulmonary dysplasia. J Pediatr 95:867, 1979
41. Strang LB: Uptake of liquid from the lungs at the start of breathing. In DeReuck AVS, Porter R (eds): Ciba Foundation Symposium: Development of the Lung. London, J & A Churchill, 1967
42. Tochen M: Orotracheal intubation in the newborn infant: A method for determining depth of tube insertion. J Pediatr 95:1050, 1979
43. Tsai SH et al: Bronchopulmonary dysplasia associated with oxygen therapy in infants with respiratory distress syndrome. Radiology 105:107, 1972
44. Truog WE, Prueitt JL, Woodrum DE: Unchanged incidence of bronchopulmonary dysplasia in survivors of hyaline membrane disease. J Pediatr 92:261, 1978
45. Vyas H, Milner AD, Hopkin IE: Intrathoracic pressure and volume changes during the spontaneous onset of respiration in babies born by cesarean section and by vaginal delivery. J Pediatr 99:787, 1981
46. Wilson MG, Mikity VG: A new form of respiratory disease in premature infants. Am J Dis Child 99:489, 1960
47. Wung JT et al: Changing incidence of bronchopulmonary dysplasia. J Pediatr 85:845, 1979
48. Yeh TF, Vidyasagar D, Pildes RS: Neonatal pneumopericardium. Pediatrics 54:429, 1974

BIBLIOGRAPHY

Fetal Lung Development

Avery ME: In pursuit of understanding the first breath. Am Rev Respir Dis 100:295, 1969

Boyden EA, Tompsett DH: The changing patterns in the developing lungs of infants. Acta Anat 61:164, 1965

Charnock EL, Doershuk CF: Developmental aspects of the human lung. Pediatr Clin North Am 20:275, 1973

Engle S: The structure of the respiratory tissue in the newly born. Acta Anat 19:353, 1953

Landing BH, Dixon LG: Congenital malformations of genetic disorders of the respiratory tract. Am Rev Respir Dis 120:151, 1979

Pierce JA, Hocott JB: Studies on the collagen and elastin content of the human lung. J Clin Invest 39:8, 1960

Respiratory Distress Syndrome

Bancalari E, Garcia OL, Jesse MJ: Effects of continuous negative pressure on lung mechanics in idiopathic respiratory distress syndrome. Pediatrics 51:485, 1973

Bryan MH et al: Pulmonary function studies during the first year of life in infants recovering from the respiratory distress syndrome. Pediatrics 52:169, 1973

Farrel PM, Avery ME: Hyaline membrane disease—state of the art. Am Rev Respir Dis 111:657, 1975

Frank L, Autor AP, Roberts RJ: Oxygen therapy and hyaline membrane disease: The effect of hyperoxia on pulmonary superoxide dismutase activity and the mediating role of plasma or serum. J Pediatr 90:105, 1977

Graven SN, Opitz JM, Harrison M: The respiratory distress syndrome: Risk factors related to maternal factors. Am J Obstet Gynecol 96:969, 1966

Gregory GA, Kitterman J, Phibbs R et al: Treatment of idiopathic respiratory distress syndrome with continuous positive airway pressure. N Engl J Med 284:1333, 1971

Krauss AN et al: Vital capacity in premature infants. Am Rev Respir Dis 108:1361, 1973

Notter RH, Shapiro DL: Lung surfactant in an era of replacement therapy. Pediatrics 68:781, 1981

Orme RLE et al: Effective pulmonary blood flow in preterm infants with and without respiratory distress: A simple bedside method using nitrous oxide. Pediatrics 52:179, 1973

Reynolds EOR: Methods of mechanical ventilation for hyaline membrane disease. Proc Roy Soc Med 67:10, 1974

Reynolds EOR, Taghizadeh A: Improved prognosis of infants mechanically ventilated for hyaline membrane disease. Arch Dis Child 49:505, 1974

Rhodes PG, Hall RT: Continuous positive airway pressure delivered by face mask in infants with the idiopathic respiratory distress syndrome: A controlled study. Pediatrics 52:1, 1973

Ross S, Naeye RL: Racial and environmental influences on fetal lung maturation. Pediatrics 68:790, 1981

Taeusch HW Jr: New directions in the management of RDS. Hosp Pract 10:53, 1975

Retained Lung Fluid

Avery ME, Gatewood OB, Brumley G: Transient tachypnea of newborn. Am J Dis Child 111:380, 1966

Steele RW, Copeland GA: Delayed resorption of pulmonary alveolar fluid in the neonate. Radiology 103:637, 1972

Sundell H et al: Studies on infants with type II respiratory distress syndrome. J Pediatr 78:754, 1971

Swischuk LE: Transient respiratory distress of the newborn (TRDN): A temporary disturbance of a normal phenomenon. Am J Roentgenol Radium Ther Nucl Med 108:557, 1970

Bronchopulmonary Dysplasia

Banerjee CK, Girling DJ, Wigglesworth JS: Pulmonary fibroplasia in newborn babies treated with oxygen and artificial ventilation. Arch Dis Child 47:509, 1972

Bonikos DS et al: Bronchopulmonary dysplasia: The pulmonary

pathologic sequel of necrotizing bronchiolitis and pulmonary fibrosis. Hum Pathol 7:643, 1976

Brown ER et al: Bronchopulmonary dysplasia: Possible relationship to pulmonary edema. J Pediatr 92:982, 1978

Division of Lung Diseases: National Heart, Lung and Blood Institute, National Institute of Health: Workshop on bronchopulmonary dysplasia. J Pediatr 95:815, 1979

Kapanci Y, Kaplan HP: Pathogenesis and reversibility of the pulmonary lesions of oxygen toxicity in monkeys. II. Ultrastructural and morphometric studies. Lab Invest 20:101, 1969

Mikity VG, Taber P: Complications in the treatment of respiratory distress syndrome: Bronchopulmonary dysplasia, oxygen toxicity and Wilson-Mikity syndrome. Pediatr Clin North Am 20:419, 1973

Moylan FMB et al: Edema of the pulmonary interstitium in infants and children. Pediatrics 55:783, 1975

Moylan FMB, Shannon DC: Preferential distribution of lobar emphysema and atelectasis in bronchopulmonary dysplasia. Pediatrics 63:130, 1979

Nickerson BG, Taussig LM: Family history of asthma in infants with bronchopulmonary dysplasia. Pediatrics 65:1140, 1980

Rhodes PG, Hall RT, Leonidas JC: Chronic pulmonary disease in neonates with assisted ventilation. Pediatrics 55:788, 1975

Smyth JS et al: Pulmonary function and bronchial hyperreactivity in long-term survivors of bronchopulmonary dysplasia. Pediatrics 68:336, 1981

Pulmonary Dysmaturity

Burnard ED et al: Pulmonary insufficiency in prematurity. Aust Paediatr J 1:12, 1965

Coates AL, Bergsteinsson H, Desmond K et al: Long-term pulmonary sequelae of the Wilson-Mikity syndrome. J Pediatr 92:247, 1978

Hodgeman JE et al: Chronic respiratory distress in the premature infant. Wilson-Mikity syndrome. Pediatrics 44:179, 1969

Jacob J, Edwards D, Gluck L: Early-onset sepsis and pneumonia observed as respiratory distress syndrome. Assessment of lung maturity. Am J Dis Child 134:766, 1980

Wilson MG, Mikity VG: A new form of respiratory distress in premature infants. Am J Dis Child 99:489, 1960

Pulmonary Hemorrhage

Cole VA et al: Pathogenesis of hemorrhagic pulmonary edema and massive pulmonary hemorrhage in the newborn. Pediatrics 51:175, 1973

Fedrick J, Butler N: Certain causes of neonatal death. IV. Massive pulmonary hemorrhage. Biol Neonate 18:243, 1971

Kotas RV et al: A new model for neonatal pulmonary hemorrhage research. Pediatr Res 9:161, 1975

Sheffield LJ et al: Massive pulmonary hemorrhage as a presenting feature in congenital hyperammonemia. J Pediatr 88:450, 1976

Pneumonia

Brook I, Martin WJ, Feingold SM: Neonatal pneumonia caused by members of the Bacteroides fragilis group. Clin Pediatr 19:541, 1980

Naeye RL, Dellinger WS, Blanc WA: Fetal and maternal features of antenatal bacterial infections. J Pediatr 79:733, 1971

Speer M, Rosan RC, Rudolph AJ: Hemophilus influenzae infection in the neonate mimicking respiratory distress syndrome. J Pediatr 93:295, 1978

Meconium Aspiration

Brown B, Gleicher N: Intrauterine meconium aspiration. Obstet Gynecol 57:26, 1981

Bryan CS: Enhancement of bacterial infection by meconium. Johns Hopkins Med J 121:9, 1967

Burke–Strickland M, Edwards NB: Meconium aspiration in the newborn. Minn Med 56:1031, 1973

Carson BS et al: Combined obstetric and pediatric approach to prevent meconium aspiration syndrome. Am J Obstet Gynecol 126:712, 1976

Fox WW et al: The therapeutic application of end-expiratory pressure in the meconium aspiration syndrome. Pediatrics 56:214, 1975

Gooding CA, Gregory GA: Roentgenographic analysis of meconium aspiration of the newborn. Radiology 100:131, 1971

Gooding CA et al: An experimental model for the study of meconium aspiration of the newborn. Radiology 100:137, 1971

Gregory GA et al: Meconium aspiration in infants—a prospective study. J Pediatr 85:848, 1974

Marshall R et al: Meconium aspiration syndrome. Am J Obstet Gynecol 131:672, 1978

Ting P, Brady JP: Tracheal suction in meconium aspiration. Am J Obstet Gynecol 122:767, 1975

Vidyasagar D et al: Assisted ventilation in infants with meconium aspiration syndrome. Pediatrics 56:208, 1975

Yeh TF et al: Hydrocortisone therapy in meconium aspiration syndrome: A controlled study. J Pediatr 90:140, 1977

Pulmonary Air Leaks

Anderson KD, Chandra R: Pneumothorax secondary to perforation of sequential bronchi by suction catheters. J Pediatr Surg 11:687, 1976

Boer HR, Andrews BF: Spontaneous pneumothorax in the neonate. South Med J 70:841, 1977

Chernick V, Reed MH: Pneumothorax and chylothorax in the neonatal period. J Pediatr 76:624, 1970

Fletcher B: Medial herniation of the parietal pleura: A useful sign of pneumothorax in supine neonates. Am J Roentgenol 130:469, 1978

Moessinger AC, Driscoll JM Jr, Wigger HJ: High incidence of lung perforation by chest tube in neonatal pneumothorax. J Pediatr 92:635, 1978

Monin P, Vert P: Pneumothorax. Clin Perinatol 5:335, 1978

Ng KPK, Easa D: Management of interstitial emphysema by high-frequency low positive pressure hand ventilation in the neonate. J Pediatr 95:117, 1979

Ogata ES et al: Pneumothorax in the respiratory distress syndrome: Incidence and effect on vital signs, blood gases and pH. Pediatrics 58:177, 1976

Pomerance JJ et al: Pneumopericardium complicating respiratory distress syndrome: Role of conservative management. J Pediatr 84:883, 1974

Rothberg AD, Marks KH, Maisels MJ: Understanding the pleurevac. Pediatrics 67:482, 1981

Varano LA, Maisels MJ: Pneumopericardium in the newborn: Diagnosis and pathogenesis. Pediatrics 53:941, 1974

Wyman ML, Kuhns LR: Accuracy of transillumination in the recognition of pneumothorax and pneumomediastinum in the neonate. Clin Pediatr 16:323, 1977

Yeh TF, Vidyasagar D, Pildes RS: Neonatal pneumopericardium. Pediatrics 54:429, 1974

Apnea and Periodic Breathing

Aranda JV et al: Efficacy of caffeine in treatment of apnea in the low birth weight infant. Pediatrics 61:528, 1978

Kattwinkel J: Neonatal apnea: Pathogenesis and therapy. J Pediatr 90:342, 1977

Naeye RL: Neonatal apnea: Underlying disorders. Pediatrics 63:8, 1979

Rigatto H, Brady JP: Periodic breathing and apnea in preterm infants. I. Evidence for hypoventilation possibly due to central respiratory depression. Pediatrics 50:202, 1972

Rigatto H, Brady JP: Periodic breathing and apnea in preterm infants. II. Hypoxia as a primary event. Pediatrics 50:219, 1972

Esophageal Atresia and Tracheoesophageal Fistula

Berdon WE et al: Plain film detection of right aortic arch in infants with esophageal atresia and tracheoesophageal fistula. J Pediatr Surg 14:436, 1979

Humphries GH, Hogg BM, Ferrer J: Congenital atresia of the esophagus. J Thorac Surg 32:332, 1956

Jolley SG et al: Patterns of gastroesophageal reflux in children following repair of esophageal atresia and distal tracheoesophageal fistula. J Pediatr Surg 15:857, 1980

Koop CE, Schnaufer L, Broennie AM: Esophageal atresia and tracheoesophageal fistula: Supportive measures that affect survival. Pediatrics 54:558, 1974

Milligan DWA, Levison H: Lung function in children following repair of tracheoesophageal fistula. J Pediatr 95:24, 1979

Parker AF, Christie DL, Cahill JL: Incidence and significance of gastroesophageal atresia and tracheoesophageal fistula and the need for anti-reflux procedures. J Pediatr Surg 14:5, 1979

Rickham PP: Infants with esophageal atresia weighing under 3 pounds. J Pediatr Surg 16:595, 1981

Smith WL, Franken EA, Smith JA: Pneumoesophagus as a sign of H type tracheoesophageal fistula. Pediatrics 58:907, 1976

Diaphragmatic Hernia

Bloss RS, Aranda JV, Beardmore HE: Vasodilator response and prediction of survival in congenital diaphragmatic hernia. J Pediatr Surg 16:118, 1981

Cohen D, Reid IS: Recurrent diaphragmatic hernia. J Pediatr Surg 16:42, 1981

Harrison MR et al: Congenital diaphragmatic hernia: The hidden mortality. J Pediatr Surg 13:227, 1978

Srouji MN, Buck B, Downes JJ: Congenital diaphragmatic hernia: Deleterious effects of pulmonary interstitial emphysema and tension extrapulmonary air. J Pediatr Surg 16:15, 1981

Reid IS, Hutcherson RJ: Long-term follow-up patients with congenital diaphragmatic hernia. J Pediatr Surg 11:939, 1976

Wohl MEB et al: The lung following repair of congenital diaphragmatic hernia. J Pediatr 90:405, 1977

Diaphragmatic Paralysis

Aldrich TK, Herman JH, Rochester DF: Bilateral diaphragmatic paralysis in the newborn infant. J Pediatr 97:988, 1980

Greene W, L'Heureux P, Hunt CE: Paralysis of the diaphragm. Am J Dis Child 129:1402, 1975

Haller JS Jr et al: Management of diaphragmatic paralysis in infants with special emphasis on selection of patients for operative plication. J Pediatr Surg 14:779, 1979

Muller N et al: The consequences of diaphragmatic muscle fatigue in the newborn infant. J Pediatr 95:793, 1979

Schwartz MZ, Fuller RM: Plication of the diaphragm for symptomatic phrenic nerve paralysis. J Pediatr Surg 13:259, 1978

30

Intensive Care of Asthma, Cystic Fibrosis, and Other Pediatric Respiratory Diseases

Mary Ann Fletcher

ASTHMA

Asthma is the most common serious respiratory condition of childhood. Mortality from asthma is very low, yet there is high morbidity in terms of hospital days, office visits, days lost from school, interference with normal childhood and family activities, and growth, making effective treatment of asthma an important pediatric goal.

Asthma occurs characteristically as episodes of bronchial narrowing, causing signs and symptoms of lower airway obstruction: cough, prolonged expiration, and wheezing. The degree of airway obstruction may be so mild that a patient is troubled only by an irritative, nonproductive cough or dyspnea on exertion; in contrast, the obstruction may be marked enough to cause severe hypoxemia and respiratory failure. Attacks and symptoms may be intermittent with functionally normal pulmonary status between attacks, or they may be fairly continuous with exacerbations leading to frequent hospitalizations and general debilitation because of chronically compromised pulmonary function.

INCIDENCE

The incidence and prevalence of childhood asthma are impossible to establish with accuracy because there is such wide variation in how the disease presents and is diagnosed. Since all that wheezes is not asthma, and all asthmatic episodes need not have audible wheezing, surveys using wheezing episodes as the basis for diagnosis will be inaccurate. The diagnoses of chronic bronchitis and bronchiolitis overlap, further confusing statistics.[44] Numerous reviews are available that attempt to define the scope of childhood asthma.[9,22,34]

More than 50% of children with asthma have symptoms during the first 2 years of life.[34] In younger children, mucosal edema and secretions predominate over bronchospasm, making their attacks less responsive to therapy with bronchodilators and therefore often underdiagnosed as classic asthmatic attacks.

PULMONARY PATHOPHYSIOLOGY

The primary abnormality of asthma is widespread airway narrowing, which causes obstruction to airflow. As bronchospasm persists, airway obstruction worsens with mucosal edema and mucus plugging. There are associated pulmonary abnormalities: changes in lung volume, compliance, and breathing patterns and use of the accessory respiratory muscles (Fig. 30-1).

The narrowing of airways in asthma is diffuse but uneven, so that there is overventilation of some alveoli with decreased ventilation in others. The un-

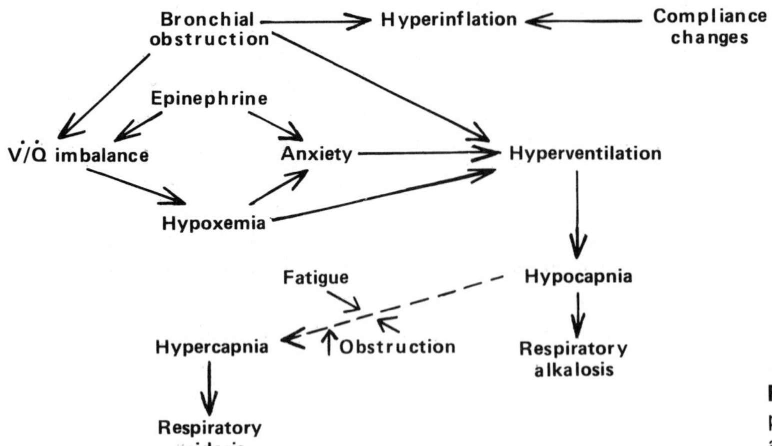

Fig. 30-1. Acute asthma: respiratory pathophysiology. (Leffert F: The management of acute severe asthma. J Pediatr 96:1, 1980)

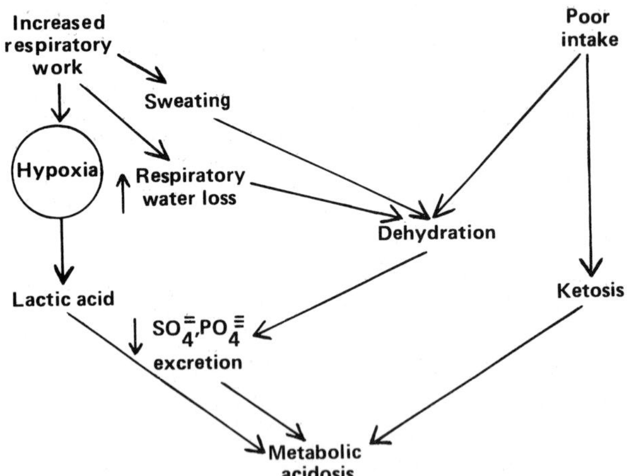

Fig. 30-2. Acute asthma: metabolic pathophysiology. (Leffert F: The management of acute severe asthma. J Pediatr 96:1, 1980)

equal distribution of ventilation leads to ventilation/perfusion ($\dot{V}/\dot{Q}$) abnormalities and *hypoxemia* early during the course. Conditions of stress or sympathomimetic medications that adversely affect alveolar perfusion may cause even more hypoxemia. This negative result of sympathomimetics on altering pulmonary circulation is usually transient until the desired effect on decreasing airway constriction improves ventilation in excess of impaired perfusion. In response to hypoxemia, anxiety, and metabolic derangements is increased respiratory drive leading to hypocapnia and *respiratory alkalosis*. If obstruction progresses or the child fatigues, hypercapnia leads to *respiratory acidosis* and respiratory failure.

METABOLIC ALTERATIONS

Metabolic changes occur during acute episodes of asthma (Fig. 30-2). These derangements result from both the marked increase in the work of breathing and the usual decrease in liquid and caloric intake by the child in respiratory distress. Because of increased water losses through sweating and tachypnea as well as decreased intake of fluids, the child easily becomes dehydrated, with poor renal perfusion and impaired excretion of organic acids. If tissue hypoxia is present, lactic acid accumulates. Poor caloric intake leads to breakdown of body fats and production of ketones. The accumulation of organic acids, lactate, and ketones leads to *metabolic acidosis*. As long as hyperventilation is sufficient to maintain a respiratory alkalosis, there is compensation for the base deficit with normalization of the arterial *p*H. When the P_{CO_2} "normalizes" and increases as respiratory failure ensues, there may be rapid decompensation with a *combined respiratory and metabolic acidosis.*

ETIOLOGY

The mechanism for initiating bronchospasm in asthma is unclear. Current thinking on the etiology of asthma is discussed in Chapter 31. Asthma may be induced by exercise. This stimulus is especially common as a precipitating factor in acute attacks in older children and young adults after episodes of vigorous steady exercise (e.g., running for 5–10 min). Exercise-induced bronchospasm occurs in most asthmatic children. The bronchospasm generally worsens after the exercise has stopped. The bronchospasm has been shown to be a reflex response to large airway cooling from the hyperventilation during exercise. The wheezing can usually be prevented by sympathomimetics, theophylline, and cromolyn sodium but usually not by anticholinergics such as atropine.

Attacks often follow emotionally charged encounters and may be used intentionally to gain sympathy or to strike out at a person, causing emotional distress. They may, however, be an unconscious result of emotional unrest as well. There are several mechanisms by which emotional upset could stimulate bronchoconstriction. Hyperventilation leads to a low Pa_{CO_2}, which itself may cause bronchoconstriction. Sudden inspiration stimulates irritant receptors of the lung, initiating reflex bronchoconstriction.

In younger children, more of the severe asthma attacks are associated with infections, primarily with the respiratory viruses normally prevalent in each age group. Antecedent symptoms include malaise, fever, or coryza. Asthma induced by viral infections may be due to an allergic response to the virus, a decreased threshold for stimulation of the irritant receptors of the airways by the respiratory mucosal infection, or an alteration of bronchomotor tone and secretion volume and viscosity controlled by the autonomic nervous system. In children with a family history of allergies, the first asthma attack often is preceded by viral bronchiolitis and is followed by recurrent episodes of asthma.[5]

Many patients develop bronchoconstriction when exposed to cold air, dust, air pollution, or cigarette smoke. The same irritants may cause bronchoconstriction in normal persons but in asthmatics cause reaction at a much lower level of exposure.

For a more complete discussion of theories on the pathogenesis of asthma, the articles by Boushey and Leffert are recommended.[1,28]

CLINICAL FEATURES

Physical findings in a child with an acute attack of asthma depend on several factors: First is the influence of psychological forces on how the child and parent perceive the respiratory stress. Some children exhibit extreme anxiety over relatively mild aberrations in their pulmonary function, whereas others appear hardly bothered by severe physiological stress. Denial of symptoms by either child or parent leads to delays in seeking appropriate treatment. The chronicity of pulmonary derangement is also important. If an acute attack occurs in an already debilitated patient with chronic asthma, the physical changes differ from those of a child completely symptom free between attacks.

At the beginning of an attack, when bronchial edema is mild, the only symptom may be a dry, hacking, irritative cough. Usually wheezing with mild prolongation of expiration is present on auscultation.

If an attack progresses, the cough often becomes more rattling in quality and productive of sputum. The patient becomes short of breath with labored respirations and audible wheezing. He speaks in short sentences or phrases, preferring to remain silent and concentrate his effort on breathing. He sits forward with his hands on his knees, his arms braced, his shoulders held high, and his chest distended with little movement. There are retractions of the suprasternal notch and intercostal spaces.

Acute attacks in children breathing at high lung volumes provoke many of the signs commonly associated with chronic obstructive airway diseases in adults: dyspnea, wheeze, coarse rales, prolonged expiration, scalene muscle contraction, supraclavicular retraction, and contraction of the sternocleidomastoid muscles. When compared to objective pulmonary function studies in children with acute attacks, the most significant correlation of severity is with contractions of the *sternocleidomastoid muscles*.[7]

As bronchospasm progresses toward more complete obstruction, there may be so little air movement that breath sounds and rales become inaudible. Coughing is virtually impossible. Respirations become shallow and rapid, the pulse increases, and pallor and cyanosis become marked. The patient becomes lethargic and unresponsive. Asphyxia is imminent unless the process is reversed.

In many cases the pulse is rapid and often thready. In the most severe cases, the pulse may be paradoxical with an accentuation of the diminished pressure on inspiration.* This finding, primarily owing to decreased right atrial filling on inspiration, ap-

*A pulse is said to be "paradoxical" when the systolic blood pressure during inspiration is more than 10 mm Hg below that during expiration. The pulse pressure normally drops no more than 5 to 10 mm Hg during inspiration. Because the pulmonary vascular bed normally increases in volume with inspiration, the left ventricular output decreases slightly during inspiration. With severe airway obstruction, right atrial filling is limited because of decreased compliance from lung overdistention and mediastinal stretching. This results in decreased right ventricular output, less volume through the pulmonary vascular bed returning to the left heart, and thus a further decrease in systemic pulse pressure.

pears to develop when there is a significant increase in the functional residual capacity along with high intra-alveolar pressures. ECG changes of right axis deviation are usually present when a paradoxical pulse develops.

The term "*status asthmaticus*" denotes a point in the clinical course of asthma when bronchospasm is no longer readily reversed by bronchodilators. The exact point at which nonresponsiveness occurs in any patient depends on a number of factors. Although some patients are in "status asthmaticus" almost as soon as any symptoms appear, they are more likely to develop it as delay between onset of symptoms and administration of effective medications grows longer. Patients on continuous, high-dose therapy regimens who present with symptoms in the emergency room are more likely to be in "status" than ones who have been on no medication or on low doses of intermittent seasonal medication. Children with concurrent respiratory infections are more likely to be unresponsive than those who are not infected.

PULMONARY FUNCTION TESTS

The effect of an acute asthmatic attack on pulmonary function tests is principally due to a change in airway resistance. Increased resistance results in decreased flow rates. The forced expiratory vital capacity is decreased. Static lung compliance is usually normal but may be increased during an acute attack. The functional residual capacity is elevated. The total lung capacity (TLC) may be increased as a result of severe air trapping. Pulmonary function often improves after inhalation of a bronchodilator, indicating a reversibility of the obstruction. During a symptom-free interval, the pulmonary function study findings may be completely normal. In many children with asymptomatic asthma, however, there are persistent abnormalities.

The most useful laboratory procedure for evaluating the child with asthma is the spirogram, particularly with a paper tracing to document cooperation and to provide a graphic demonstration of results of treatment to parents and the child. The most useful measurements are the FVC and FEV_1. More sophisticated measurements are needed only when there are complications or other possible diagnoses.

PATHOLOGY

Pathologic examination of lungs in "status asthmaticus" suggests three principal mechanisms that increase airway resistance: mucosal edema, accumulation of secretions, and bronchospasm. The airway walls are thickened from an increase in bronchial smooth muscle, enlarged bronchial mucous glands, and increased numbers of goblet cells, as well as mucosal and submucosal edema. The lumina contain cellular debris, inflammatory exudate, and mucus plugs. On autopsy after fatal asthma, the lungs invariably are extremely overinflated with emphysematous blebs and varying degrees of atelectasis.

The sputum in asthma is fairly characteristic. The mucus is often in stringy casts that retain the shape of their bronchiolar origins (Curschmann's spirals). Even when there is some degree of infection, the casts tend to maintain their shape for several hours. The sputum contains mucus, eosinophils, and polymorphonuclear cells.

ROENTGENOGRAPHIC FINDINGS

The most common abnormality on chest roentgenograms in children with asthma is hyperinflation. Extreme hyperinflation with flattening of the diaphragms or tenting at the costal insertions, herniation of the lung anteriorly and posteriorly, and bowing of the sternum reflect the marked air-trapping associated with severe status asthmaticus (Fig. 30-3).

About 25% of chest x-ray films obtained in hospitalized children with asthma will have evidence of infiltrates or pneumomediastinum. Although the presence of an infiltrate does not correlate with clinical severity, the presence of pulmonary air leaks relates directly to severity of disease. Pneumomediastinum occurs more frequently in older patients.[11] In asthmatics younger than 6 years of age, the pneumomediastinum rarely dissects into the neck, whereas in older children the air invariably dissects into cervical and axillary subcutaneous tissues. The extent of air distribution directly relates to clinical severity (*see* Fig. 30-3D).

A higher percentage of infiltrates is found on chest roentgenograms of children younger than 6 years of age. Infiltrates typically are perihilar and interstitial, varying from merely increased bronchovascular markings to diffuse peribronchial pneumonia. As often as not, infiltrates are associated with atelectasis, particularly in the right middle lobe. Recurrence of right middle lobe atelectasis in any one patient is unusual (*see* Fig. 30-3D) unless disease occurs in or around the right middle lobe bronchus (the so-called right middle lobe syndrome). This syndrome may arise from lymphadenopathy associated with pulmonary tuberculosis.

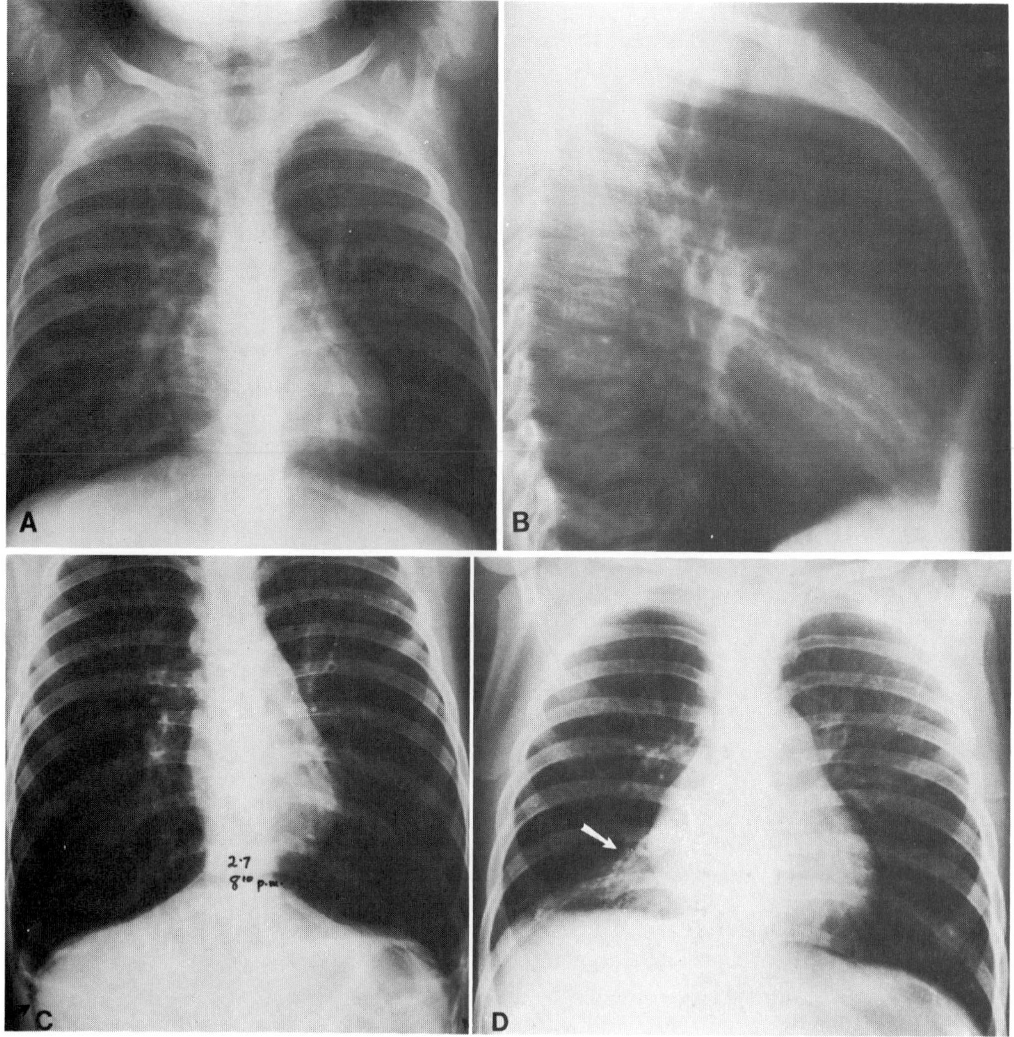

Fig. 30-3. *(A)* Anteroposterior chest roentgenogram during status asthmaticus in a 6-year-old. There is hyperaeration with flattening of the hemidiaphragms. *(B)* Lateral view of the same patient. There is marked anterior bowing of the sternum with flattened diaphragms. *(C)* Later admission of the same patient for status asthmaticus requiring endotracheal intubation. There is spontaneous subcutaneous emphysema in the supraclavicular and lower cervical areas that has dissected around the chest wall and between the muscles of the upper abdomen *(arrows)*. The pulmonary air leaks developed before the start of positive pressure ventilation. There is extreme hyperaeration with secondary microcardia. *(D)* Subsequent admission of the same patient. The right lower lobe is partially collapsed secondary to mucus plugging *(arrow)*.

TREATMENT

Any treatment plan for asthma has to take into account the fact that asthma is variable in its range of severity and in the functional impact that similar pathophysiological changes have on different people and on their families.

It is not always necessary or desirable to have such intensive therapy as may be needed to keep a child *completely* symptom free. On the other hand, neither should mild symptoms that herald more severe attacks be ignored, causing delay in the start of therapy in earlier, more reversible stages. How intensive a treatment plan needs to be depends partly on response to therapy. Asthma in many children is so mild that a few moments of rest will abort an attack. At the other extreme, asthma may be so severe that symptoms are always present and any exacerbation is life-threatening.

Acute asthma should be regarded as potentially life-threatening if not treated appropriately, and thus should be considered a medical emergency. The earlier that appropriate treatment is given, the less medication will be needed, the less heroic the treatment must be, and the more likely a quick response will occur.

Long-Term Management

Therapy of asthma is both short-term and long-term. The goal of long-term therapy is to allow a child to attend school regularly and to participate in active play with his peers so that his illness does not interfere with his physical, social, or intellectual growth and development. If this goal is met, neither his illness nor the treatment of it will keep him from achieving normal development and enjoying the normal activities of childhood. Long-term therapy for asthma includes identifying and avoiding precipitating factors whenever possible and reasonable.

If asthma is caused by a specific allergen (e.g., dander from the family dog), the value of removing the allergen (and the dog) is obvious, although considered with great resistance by family members. If precipitating causes center around emotional upset, therapy directed at such problems may be helpful.

If seasonal allergens cause episodes only during time of exposure, seasonal therapy may be all that is needed. Many physicians use desensitization therapy for the most common allergens. When properly used, this therapy may be beneficial. The use of desensitization therapy should be reserved until other conservative methods of therapy have been tried, and then only after appropriate allergy testing.

A number of environmental manipulations may be beneficial. A home visit by a nurse trained in environmental control is helpful. The family can be instructed on what *reasonable* measures they can take to make the home, particularly the patient's bedroom, less likely to contain high quantities of dust, mold, and pollens. Proper humidity and clean air filters, washable curtains, spreads, blankets and rugs, and dusting of shelves and furniture can decrease the quantity of allergen that challenges a patient. On occasion the home environment is so inappropriate on a physical or psychosocial basis that consideration should be given to placing the child in a temporarily sheltered environment. Some older children benefit from breathing exercises, which are designed to relieve shortness of breath and abort attacks that may be induced by exercise or anxiety and to avoid improper breathing patterns that worsen airway obstruction during any attack.*

Although preventing a child from participating in play or sports is not reasonable, directing him toward activities that have less tendency to cause bronchospasm may be helpful. Swimming and bicycling, for example, are less likely to cause bronchospasm than is running; however, important factors include the intensity of the exercise and environmental temperature.

Medical therapy as part of long-term treatment may involve inhaled or oral bronchodilators, decongestants, steroids, and agents that block allergic reactions. There are hundreds of products on the market, available over the counter or by prescription, that are promoted as being effective against asthma. Only a few basic compounds, however, if used properly, compose the essential armamentarium.

Although some of the most heavily advertised therapeutic aids are pocket nebulizers, their role in treating asthma in children is extremely controversial. Young children often cannot coordinate the deep inhalation necessary and may swallow most of any dose administered. Older children may become dependent on the quick relief inhalation offers and delay seeking proper medical assistance until an attack has progressed beyond the reversible stage. If cartridge inhalers are used, the patient should be cautioned against overusing them. The principal uses of inhaled sympathomimetics in chronic asthma are in the prevention of exercise-induced asthma or for rapid reversal of acute wheezing attacks during school or social occasions.[30]

The basic drug in managing chronic asthma is theophylline. It is currently available in three oral dosage forms: tablets, liquid, and slow-release capsules. Because a constant serum level of 10 to 20 μg/ml is the therapeutic goal, the sustained release forms that enable twice daily dosage are the most effective in achieving patient compliance.[19] Many compounds on the market are combinations of theophylline or its

*Booklets written for the child to help him institute and maintain correct breathing patterns are available through the American Academy of Pediatrics, P.O. Box 1034, Evanston, IL 60204.

derivative, aminophylline, a sympathomimetic (e.g., ephedrine), and a sedative (phenobarbital or hydroxyzine). Theophylline is the most effective ingredient in these compounds, but it is often not as effective in the levels provided in fixed compounds as it is when used alone and titrated to higher levels.[47] Combinations of theophylline and ephedrine in standard ratios are significantly less effective in decreasing symptoms and improving pulmonary function test findings than is theophylline alone in higher doses. Of importance, the addition of ephedrine *increases* the frequency of adverse effects. Therapy using these combination compounds is now rarely indicated.

The dose of theophylline (as aminophylline) that is effective is determined by starting at low oral doses (e.g., 4–6 mg/kg or less every 6 hours) and gradually increasing the dose until symptoms have been controlled. The tremor and tachycardia that are frequent at higher doses often subside after about 1 week of continued administration. Any evidence of central nervous system effect, such as convulsions or disorientation, or of gastrointestinal intolerance, such as pain, anorexia, or nausea and vomiting, are indications to reduce the dose. In children, average serum theophylline levels in the range of 13 μg/ml and 9 μg/ml are achieved at 2 and 4 hours, respectively, after a single oral dose of about 8.1 mg/kg of aminophylline. These levels are highly effective in controlling symptoms for most children.[47]

Oral adrenergic drugs such as terbutaline and metaproterenol act principally on β-2 sympathomimetic receptor sites, resulting in smooth muscle relaxation. These drugs may act synergistically or additively with theophylline. There may be some development of tolerance when used chronically; thus whether they should be used in the chronic oral treatment of asthma must be individualized to each patient. These drugs are especially effective as inhalants and may be indicated in selected cases as noted above.

Steroids are used as an adjunct to other forms of long-term treatment if satisfactory control has not been achieved despite good therapeutic doses of bronchodilators. Ideally, these are given as alternate-day doses to prevent adrenal suppression and to decrease other systemic side-effects. Initially, however, the daily dose of prednisone necessary to achieve control is established. This may be 1 mg/kg/day of prednisone; good control has to be achieved before attempts to switch to alternate-day therapy will be successful. If alternate-day doses are tolerated, the amount is gradually tapered until a minimum effective dose has been reached. A decrease of a few milligrams is made every 2 weeks only if good control remains. If symptoms recur, it is necessary to go to a dose higher than the previous level to regain control. Some children will not tolerate alternate-day doses, developing symptoms on the day without corticosteroids.

Only steroids that cause adrenal suppression for less than 24 hours, such as prednisone, prednisolone, or methylprednisolone, should be used in alternate-day therapy to allow endogenous production during intervening days. Triamcinolone, betamethasone, and dexamethasone suppress the adrenal cortex for up to 3 days, and thus are inappropriate for alternate-day use.

Occasionally a temporary period of continuous-day therapy will be necessary to help a child through an acute febrile illness, gastroenteritis, or operation. In these instances the previous alternate-day dose can usually be resumed without difficulty after the acute problem is over.

Beclomethasone dipropionate is effective as an aerosol. It is rapidly deactivated in plasma, and thus has minimal systemic effects.[20] Beclomethasone is clearly preferable to daily oral steroid therapy but, because of higher cost, may not be preferable to effective alternate-day oral prednisone therapy. It is not as useful in acute exacerbations of symptoms or in young children unable to take metered aerosol inhalants properly.

Cromolyn is useful in treating chronic asthma as a preventive measure when attacks are not allergen precipitated—therefore, principally in exercise-induced asthma. Because there are virtually no side-effects other than cough or nasal congestion, it is unique among asthma medications. Cromolyn is relatively expensive and is ineffective during acute episodes, and thus its use is limited to prevention.[15]

Antihistamines have been thought to be contraindicated in patients with asthma because of their drying properties. If there are associated symptoms of allergic rhinitis in an asthmatic child, their judicious use may be warranted and advantageous.

Antibiotics are used in asthma only when there is evidence of an acute bacterial infection. Originally most hospitalizations for asthma associated with infection were thought to be bacterial; thus antibiotics were used for virtually all patients with "status asthmaticus." More recent evidence suggests that most of these infections are viral and that "prophylactic" use of antibiotics in status asthmaticus is not indicated.

If there is evidence of bacterial infection, it should be treated with the appropriate antibiotic.

Short-Term Therapy: Acute Asthma

When a patient presents with an acute episode of asthma, he requires emergency evaluation so that proper treatment can be given. Initial evaluation establishes a fairly precise estimate of the clinical condition and determines what therapy is needed. It also provides a baseline for following the response to that therapy.

Although the history obtained at this time is brief, it is important to ascertain the following.

1. *Duration of symptoms:* any known precipitating factors such as infection, emotional upset, and exposure to known allergen
2. *Medications:* the time and amount of the last doses of all medications, particularly aminophylline, corticosteroids, epinephrine, or adrenergic inhalants
3. *State of hydration:* fluid intake, estimated urine output, vomiting, diarrhea, fever, and previous weight
4. *Evidence of concurrent infection:* fever, sore throat, earache, and illness in other family members
5. *Previous patterns of asthma attacks:* presence of complications such as subcutaneous or interstitial emphysema, pneumothorax, respiratory failure, and recurrent right middle lobe atelectasis, as well as what the patient considers to be the most effective medications or therapy helping his attacks.

Patients and parents often understate the duration of symptoms and severity of previous episodes, but their comments about the course and response should be considered in selecting a treatment plan.

While the pertinent history is being obtained, the patient is examined for signs helpful in determining his immediate clinical status. After therapy has been initiated, there is more time for a complete history and examination. Of importance in the initial examination are the following.

1. *General status:* fatigue, obtundation, anxiety
2. *Vital signs:* height and weight, heart and respiratory rates, blood pressures during inspiration and expiration to detect pulsus paradoxicus
3. *Skin:* color for cyanosis, pallor, turgor, presence of subcutaneous emphysema in axillae or neck, and moisture of mucous membranes
4. *Chest:* assessment of anteroposterior diameter, symmetry, and quality of breath sounds; presence of wheezing; rales; inspiratory:expiratory ratio; retractions; and use of accessory muscles, particularly the sternocleidomastoid muscles
5. *Eyegrounds:* for presence of papilledema (may indicate carbon dioxide retention)
6. Any other area referred to for pain or specific symptoms

A clinical scoring system is helpful in assessing the condition of the patient and his response to therapy. It should be used in conjunction *with* other forms of information such as arterial blood gases and pulmonary function studies. It is particularly useful in that it does not require a cooperative patient, it is noninvasive, and it can be done frequently and in a matter of seconds. There are two similar scoring systems: the "Clinical Asthma Evaluation Score" and the "Pulmonary Index." These are summarized in Tables 30-1 and 30-2.

In some cases that present to the emergency room or physician's office, the initial evaluation suggests that there may be a good response to epinephrine. On the other hand, the history, physical examination, and

Table 30-1. Clinical Asthma Evaluation Score*

	0	1	2
Pa_{O_2}, *torr*	70–100 in air	70–100 in air	70 in 40% O_2
Cyanosis	None	In air	In 40% O_2
Inspiratory breath sounds	Normal	Unequal	Decreased to absent
Accessory muscles used	None	Moderate	Maximal
Expiratory wheezing	None	Moderate	Marked
Cerebral function	Normal	Depressed or agitated	Coma

*A score of 5 or more is thought to indicate impending respiratory failure. A score of 7 or more with an arterial carbon dioxide tension (Pa_{CO_2}) of 65 torr indicates existing respiratory failure. (Wood DW, Downes JJ, Lecks HI: A clinical scoring system for the diagnosis of respiratory failure. Am J Dis Child 123:227, 1972)

Table 30-2. Pulmonary Index (Simplified Bronchiolitis Score)*

	NORMAL (0)	MILD (1)	MODERATE (2)	SEVERE (3)
Respiratory rate	40/min or less	40–50/min	50–60/min	60+/min
Wheezing	None	Wheezes	Throughout expiration	In both inspiration and expiration
Inspiratory–expiratory ratio	≥5/2	5/3–5/4	1/1	<1/1
Accessory muscle use	None	Equivocal	2+	4+

*The scores from the four categories are added to obtain the pulmonary index. Normal = 0 to 1; mild = 2 to 5; moderate = 6 to 11; severe = 12 to 16. (Modified from Dabbous IA, Tkachyk JS, Stamm SJ: A double-blind study on the effects of corticosteroids in the treatment of bronchiolitis. Pediatrics 37:477, 1966)

clinical score might suggest that the patient is in status asthmaticus and will not likely respond for more than a short period, if at all. The patient that is likely to get complete clearing of bronchospasm from a course of epinephrine injections is one who has had mild symptoms for a brief period, who has no evidence of a simultaneous respiratory infection, who has not recently been on medication or only on very low doses, who is well hydrated, who has had brief exposure to a known single allergen, or who has had excellent lasting response to epinephrine injections.

The dose of 1:1000 aqueous epinephrine is 0.01 ml/kg up to 0.3 ml total dose, subcutaneously, repeated in 15 to 20 minutes twice. If there is going to be good bronchodilatation from epinephrine, it will be evident after the first dose, within 15 minutes. It is rarely necessary to give a third dose. Between doses the patient should be given clear fluids to drink and should be kept at rest.

The use of epinephrine is particularly hazardous if there is evidence of any of the following.

1. Obtundation, respiratory decompensation, respiratory acidosis, or papilledema
2. Cardiac decompensation or arrhythmias
3. Severe dehydration with metabolic acidosis
4. After a long-acting epinephrine preparation has been administered in the previous 4 to 6 hours
5. Evidence of theophylline toxicity.

Terbutaline may be used as an alternative to epinephrine. In concentrations of 1 mg/ml, doses of 0.01 ml/kg (up to 0.3 ml), it appears to have greater potency and longer duration than does epinephrine.[39] The same precautions for use apply.

Theophylline is the principal drug for acute attacks of asthma. In some cases where an attack is induced by a specific and temporary allergen exposure, epinephrine or an inhaled adrenergic agent may stop the attack completely. More often when a patient presents, ongoing bronchospasm will require initiation or augmentation of sustained bronchodilator therapy. For mild attacks, and when tolerated, oral theophylline in a loading dose of 5 to 7.5 mg/kg in a quick-acting form will achieve a therapeutic level. Liquid oral preparations may also be given rectally with reliable absorption, although aminophylline suppositories should never be used. Oral theophylline is continued for at least 24 hours after the acute symptoms have gone.

Status Asthmaticus: In-Hospital Therapy

As soon as status asthmaticus is diagnosed, arrangements for emergency admission should be made. While this is effected, therapy can be started and the following laboratory studies obtained: a chest roentgenogram, primarily as a baseline in the event of further deterioration*; arterial blood gases; and admission chemistries such as CBC, electrolytes, urinalysis, and cultures, when indicated.

*Chest roentgenograms should always be double-checked for evidence of causes of wheezing and airway obstruction other than asthma (e.g., foreign bodies).

General Supportive Measures. The value of a calm, quiet environment that also involves careful observation cannot be overstressed in providing important rest to the asthmatic child. Comforting explanations of therapy and diagnostic procedures are important, as is reassurance that something will be done quickly to improve the symptoms.

Intravenous Fluids. In status asthmaticus, medications are given intravenously for at least the first 24 hours or until the patient can resume a good oral intake. Almost all children "in status" will have some degree of dehydration. If there is no evidence of cardiac decompensation, the patient needs replacement fluids for his estimated degree of dehydration as well as maintenance fluids. The extent of dehydration is estimated from weight loss, elevation of BUN, serum sodium, osmolality, hematocrit, decreased skin turgor or dry mucous membranes, thirst, decreased urine output, and urine specific gravity. Because the estimation often is made on subjective findings, replacement fluids are often overestimated and periodically reassessed on the basis of objective data to assure their appropriateness and effect. There is no indication to "push" fluids ahead of replacement and maintenance requirements, since there may be a tendency to develop pulmonary edema.

The following regimen may be initiated with frequent reevaluation as to efficacy.

1. In the *first hour* 10 to 15 ml/kg of 5% glucose in normal saline is infused. If the state of dehydration is severe, this may be continued a second hour.
2. In the *next 24 hours*, maintenance of intravenous fluids at 50 to 60 ml/kg/24 hr should be continued. The type of infusate should be determined by serum electrolyte measurements.

Intravenous Medications. *Buffers.* If metabolic acidosis is present, buffers are usually given to improve the pH when it is less than 7.30 or when the base deficit is greater than 5 mEq/liter. The dose of sodium bicarbonate is based on body weight and base deficit. For a conservative 25% correction,

$$0.5\ [\text{body weight (kg)} \times \text{base deficit (mEq/liter)} \times 0.3] = \text{mEq bicarbonate.}$$

The buffer is given as a slow infusion over several minutes. Although it may temporarily increase the Pa_{CO_2}, there is greater responsivenes to medications that decrease bronchospasm, and thus Pa_{CO_2} will usually decrease after the acidosis has been corrected. Buffer is not given to correct a *respiratory* acidosis.

Table 30-3. Theophylline Dose for Short-Term Therapy of Acute Symptoms When Serum Concentrations Will Not Be Monitored

AGE	DOSE* *mg/kg*	FREQUENCY
6–16 wk	3	Every 8 hr
17–29 wk	4	Every 8 hr
30–51 wk	4	Every 6 hr
52 wk–9 yr	5	Every 6 hr
9–16 yr	4	Every 6 hr
>16 yr	4	Every 8 hr

(Weinberger M: Management of asthma—a correction. Pediatrics 69:663, 1982 [Copyright American Academy of Pediatrics, 1982])
*Use ideal body weight for obese patients. Initial loading dose of 5 to 7.4 mg/kg should be given to attain therapeutic serum concentrations rapidly if no prior theophylline has been taken.

Bronchodilators. Between 5 and 7 mg/kg of aminophylline (approximately 85% theophylline) is given as a loading dose if the patient has not received any in the previous 6 to 8 hours. Lower doses may be given if oral theophylline has been taken recently.

After a loading dose, a constant infusion of aminophylline will maintain the serum level in the safe therapeutic range. Although serum levels should be monitored, the doses illustrated in Table 30-3 should be used if serum concentrations of theophylline have *not* been monitored.[32] Doses are reduced by 50% if there is fever, liver disease, heart failure, or symptoms of toxicity. If improvement in symptoms and pulmonary function studies is demonstrated with the lower doses, they should be used, but if response is poor, larger doses should be used while monitoring clinical evidence of toxicity and serum theophylline levels.

Adrenocorticosteroids. Pierson and coworkers recommend in *all* patients with status asthmaticus the use of i.v. betamethasone, 0.3 mg/kg, given as a stat dose because of its higher levels of unbound, and therefore pharmacologically active, corticosteroid.[37] This is followed by a continuous i.v. infusion of 0.3 mg/kg/24 hr. Alternatively, they recommend hydrocortisone hemisuccinate with a 7 mg/kg stat dose followed by 7 mg/kg/24 hr by continuous infusion.

Chai and Newcomb recommend 20 to 40 mg of methylprednisolone (Solu-Medrol), or 100 mg of hydrocortisone hemisuccinate (Solu-Cortef) every 6 hours because adrenal suppression is less with these agents.[3] Corticosteroids used for 5 days or less do not require tapering before cessation. Steroids should not be withheld from a patient in "status" while waiting to see if he gets better without them.

Antibiotics. If there is evidence of bacterial infection, such as pneumonia, otitis media, or purulent pharyngitis, appropriate antibiotics should be given.

Respiratory Therapy. *Oxygen.* All patients with status asthmaticus require supplemental humidified oxygen. Hypoxemia is invariably present in acute asthma; thus oxygen is always a basic part of therapy. The desired concentration of oxygen should be determined by measuring the arterial Po_2. Nasal cannulas are appropriate when hypoxemia is mild, but close-fitting masks are needed when higher $F_{I_{O_2}}$'s are essential.

Aerosolized Sympathomimetics. Several sympathomimetics are available and appropriate for use in children with status asthmaticus. The doses recommended vary depending on how the treatment is administered, and thus how much of the medication actually reaches the tracheal mucosa. In most cases, the maximum amount is given that does *not* cause tachycardia. A compressor device for nebulization with oxygen is the method of choice for most patients.[32] IPPB is usually not used to administer these drugs because, in some, it may worsen bronchospasm.

When a child can cooperate and coordinate his respiratory efforts, a Y-tube in the oxygen line delivers medications when the tube has been occluded. While the Y-tube is closed, the child inhales as deeply as possible and then holds his inspiration. This deep inhalation is repeated for a total of ten breaths. Up to ten additional inhalations may be taken if there is no tachycardia beyond 150 beats/min.[29]

If the child cannot coordinate the breathing, the Y-tube can be kept occluded for constant nebulization until all medication is gone. Isoetharine, metaproterenol, racemic epinephrine, and, most recently, terbutaline are also effectively used by aerosol inhalation.

Efficacy of aerosol treatments is monitored by subjective improvement and, more precisely, by bedside spirometry to compare FEV_1 before and after treatment. Isoproterenol may decrease the arterial Po_2 despite improvement in FEV_1. This effect is most dramatic in those patients who have the greatest improvement in FEV_1 after treatment. Most of the negative effect is eliminated with simultaneous oxygen administration.

Mucolytics as aerosols are rarely needed in uncomplicated asthma and are not recommended because they may, in fact, precipitate bronchospasm.

Bronchial Drainage. Frequently, after inhaled bronchodilator therapy, coughing is induced and secretions are mobilized. Chest physiotherapy and bronchial drainage may assist in clearing these secretions if they do not tire the patient or increase his work of breathing.

After each treatment, the therapist should help the child perform his breathing exercises. Reassurance from an understanding therapist who can assist him in proper breathing will do much to shorten the duration of the attack and to increase the efficacy of the medications.

If there is good response, parenteral therapy is continued for the first 24 hours and is tapered over the next 24 hours while switching to oral medications. The frequency of inhaled bronchodilators is decreased and put on a p.r.n. basis as soon as possible. As soon as oral medications are tolerated and inhaled bronchodilators are no longer needed for good clinical control, the patient may be discharged on oral medications. If there is a complicating infection or if there is a persistence of symptoms, discharge should not be rushed.

RESPIRATORY FAILURE

With prompt, vigorous treatment, most cases of status asthmaticus can be controlled and life-threatening respiratory failure prevented. Occasionally, late in an attack, a patient presents in respiratory failure before any therapy can be given, or he deteriorates despite appropriate management. This may occur because of the presence of complicating infection or pulmonary air leak but often occurs without evident complications.

Recognition of impending respiratory failure requires continuous observation of all patients with asthma. Lack of response to therapy or deterioration is suggested by the following.

1. Evidence of less air exchange: decreasing breath sounds, decreasing I:E ratio, maximal effort of all muscles of respiration with marked retractions, cyanosis

2. Evidence of CNS deterioration: agitation, disorientation, irrationality, obtundation, coma, decreased response to pain, muscle weakness.
3. Evidence of cardiac decompensation: increasing tachycardia not attributable to medications, gallop rhythm, right ventricular strain on ECG, pulsus paradoxus, tender hepatomegaly, poor peripheral perfusion
4. Exhaustion
5. Papilledema
6. Deteriorating pulmonary function test findings indicating increasing airway resistance and air trapping
7. Arterial blood gases: Pa_{CO_2} above 55 torr, Pa_{CO_2} steadily rising in a tiring patient, Pa_{O_2} less than 50 torr on 50% oxygen, or persistent metabolic acidosis

Downes and Wood have used isoproterenol infusions in children who have evidence of poor response to therapy or respiratory failure.[10] When following the children with continuous cardiac monitoring, precise infusion rates, intensive nursing care, and indwelling arterial lines for continuous blood gas analysis, Downes and Wood were able to avoid artificial ventilation in 19 of 20 children.

Isoproterenol is infused at an initial rate of about 0.1 μg/kg/min with the concentration of infusate from 2 to 10 μg/ml, depending on the hourly volume of fluid required by the patient. The dosage is increased by 0.1 μg/kg/min every 15 minutes until there is improvement (a reduction of Pa_{CO_2} by 10% or more from preinfusion level) or tachycardia (heart rate exceeding 190 beats/min). Blood gases are monitored at 15- to 30-minute intervals during the first 2 to 3 hours of infusion and every 2 to 6 hours thereafter. If the Pa_{CO_2} increases by 10% over the lowest Pa_{CO_2} obtained during infusion or if there is deterioration in clinical score (see Table 30-2), the dose is increased. When the Pa_{CO_2} remains below 45 torr with a clinical score below 4 at a dose of 0.1 μg/kg/min, the infusion is stopped. Aminophylline and steroids are continued during and after the infusion of isoproterenol.

The advantage of using isoproterenol is its short half-life of less than 5 minutes compared to that of aminophylline (about 3 hours). It can be titrated safely to effect a response and be rapidly decreased if toxicity occurs. Because of its cardiovascular effects, it requires precise administration. Isoproterenol cannot be used in patients with evidence of cardiac outflow obstruction (e.g., aortic stenosis) or pulmonary hypertension.

Complications are less frequently seen in children than in adults when isoproterenol is properly used and the patient closely monitored. However, ventricular tachycardia that is not dose-related and hypoxemia have been reported.

Mechanical ventilation is indicated if deterioration continues despite intravenous isoproterenol, if toxicity to isoproterenol develops before improvement is seen, or if the patient's condition is too critical to allow delaying assisted ventilation.

Ventilators are used to increase alveolar ventilation, to afford rest to a tired and exhausted patient, and to decrease the oxygen cost of breathing. Ventilation should be provided by a volume-controlled respirator.

Muscle relaxants or sedation with respiratory depressants may be necessary. Soleymani and coworkers recommend the use of morphine at 1 mg/4.5 kg of body weight, repeated every 5 to 10 minutes until effective ventilation and improved aeration have been accomplished.[40] Maximal respiratory depression occurs within approximately 7 minutes after morphine has been given intravenously. This dose appears helpful in attaining a level of sedation to allow controlled respiration by the mechanical ventilator.

Alternatively, total muscle paralysis may be used with curare-like drugs (e.g., pancuronium bromide, Pavulon). Because the patient may still be alert while totally paralyzed, sedation should also be given. If he is not totally sedated, continued reassurance should be given and care taken to make his surroundings as pleasant and relaxing as possible.

During controlled ventilation, intravenous medications are continued. Postural drainage and endotracheal suctioning must be done frequently, along with hourly position changes. Mechanical ventilation is continued until satisfactory improvement in airway resistance has been demonstrated.

The importance of communicating with the patient, no matter how young, during all stages of asthma cannot be overemphasized. Keeping his confidence in himself and in those caring for him is essential. Although status asthmaticus is one of the most challenging medical problems, intelligent, aggressive, and sympathetic management should provide uniformly positive results.

CYSTIC FIBROSIS

Cystic fibrosis (CF, mucoviscidosis) is the most common cause of severe, chronic respiratory disease in children and adolescents. Before the availability of modern therapy, most of its victims died from bronchopneumonia or malnutrition. In the 1930s CF was recognized as an entity, although it was thought that the pancreas was the single major organ involved. Most cases were diagnosed correctly only at autopsy. In the 1950s it was recognized that CF was, in fact, a generalized disorder affecting virtually all the exocrine glands. When the sweat test became available in 1954, the clinical diagnosis was made much more frequently. The average life expectancy in the 1950s for a child with CF was only 4 years. Recently, with the use of antibiotics and enzymes as well as better understanding of the disease, survival has improved dramatically. By 1976, the median survival was reported at 19 years of age with many more patients surviving well into adulthood.[8] Along with prolonged survival have come the concomitant social and economic problems associated with all chronic diseases, problems that must be considered in optimal treatment of the total entity.[16]

INCIDENCE

Cystic fibrosis is the most frequently lethal genetic disease among white children, being inherited as an autosomal recessive trait. It has been recognized in most population groups but is primarily a disease of whites, where its incidence is estimated at between 1:1000 and 1:3500 live births. Genetic carriers may represent 3% to 5% of the population. In blacks, the incidence is far lower, estimated at 1:17000, but there is a significant underdiagnosis or delay in proper testing in large black populations, so that the true incidence is probably higher than recognized.[21] There is no sex difference in incidence.

PATHOGENESIS AND PULMONARY PATHOPHYSIOLOGY

The basic biochemical, cellular, or subcellular defect of CF is still unknown and may be multifactorial. The disease gives rise to several problems, seemingly unrelated, which include abnormal physical and chemical behavior of the mucous secretions of different types of glands. These result in glandular orifice obstruction, a consistent elevation of sodium and chloride in sweat, an increase in several organic and enzymatic constituents as well as in calcium and phosphorus levels in submaxillary saliva, and suspected abnormalities in autonomic nervous system function supplying the organs involved.

A number of recent observations about these abnormalities are of interest, but, because a detailed discussion of all the proposed defects is beyond the scope of this chapter, they can only be summarized. There is a "ciliary dyskinesis factor" in the serum of patients with CF that inhibits ciliary motion in experimental animal models. There is another factor in saliva or sweat that inhibits sodium reabsorption in the parotid glands of rats. Calcium in high concentrations precipitates the glycoproteins of certain secretions (e.g., saliva). Because calcium is present in higher than normal concentrations in the saliva of patients with CF, it may cause precipitation of glycoproteins, and thus a change in the character of the secretions.

Although the etiology of the abnormal secretions produced by the submucous glands in lungs of persons with CF is unknown, its effects on the pathophysiology of pulmonary disease are better understood. The principal respiratory difficulty in CF consists of failure to clear bronchial secretions, leading to progressive obstruction and distal atelectasis. Secondary bronchial infection follows. The bronchial wall eventually is affected, and bronchiolectasis and bronchiectasis appear. Mucoid impaction of the bronchi, consisting of accumulation of viscous mucus in one or more bronchi, results in their obstruction and progressive dilatation. Because of collateral ventilation, overinflation of the lungs develops if the mucoid impaction is not removed.

Infections with *Pseudomonas aeruginosa*, *Staphylococcus aureus*, and other microorganisms are the primary cause of parenchymal lung damage in CF. A review of concepts regarding the pathogenesis of pulmonary infections by the various organisms in CF is available.[33]

PATHOLOGY

The chemical composition of the products of all the exocrine glands is abnormal, but there are no significant histologic changes in the glands themselves. Although the mucus-producing glands may be dilated from retained viscous secretions, the cells of the glands themselves are histologically normal.

The pancreas demonstrates specific changes early in the disease, but in the advanced stages the lesions are not diagnostic of CF. The changes in the pancreas are not fixed but evolve gradually. Characteristically, there is dilatation of the ducts and secretory acini forming cysts filled with concretions, fibrosis, and leukocytic infiltrate. Involvement may be mild or generalized. As the lesions progress, there is almost total replacement of the entire pancreas by fat and fibrosis.

Changes in the liver are analogous to those in the pancreas with focal obstructive changes from mucus plugs that contain bile. There may be significant changes in the liver before hepatic dysfunction is biochemically evident. In less than 5% of cases will there be enough change to cause clinical symptoms of portal vein obstruction with hypersplenism or esophageal varices.

The reproductive system is anatomically normal in the female but is uniformly abnormal in the male with CF. The structures that develop embryologically from the wolffian ducts, the body of the epididymis, the vas deferens, and seminal vesicle fail to develop normally. There is a high incidence of inguinal hernia, hydroceles, and undescended testes. The size of the testes is normal or small, but the secondary sex characteristics are normal, as is sexual function. The ejaculate has reduced volume and is aspermatic, although sperm is produced.

The most frequent reason for death is chronic pulmonary infection. The earliest pulmonary lesion is partial or complete plugging of small bronchioles by viscid secretions and edema. As infection with its resulting inflammation sets in, there is further decrease in the airway diameter. This gives rise to obstructive hyperinflation, bronchiolectasis, bronchiectasis, and pneumonia. Bronchospasm occurs in some, but not all, cases.[35]

At autopsy the trachea and bronchi are filled with mucopurulent material. The thorax is rounded, and the lungs are emphysematous. There are pleural adhesions, congestion, blebs, and pneumonic consolidations or abscesses with adjacent areas of atelectasis. There is also marked lymphadenopathy.

The upper respiratory tract is rarely normal. Chronic sinusitis occurs in most patients. Nasal polyps occur in about 10% of patients. These polyps may be bilateral, multiple, and recurrent. Other pathologic findings may be the result of malnutrition, particularly from deficiencies of fat-soluble vitamins.

DIAGNOSIS

The diagnosis of CF is established by two positive sweat tests and either the objective evidence of typical pancreatic and pulmonary involvement or a family history of CF.

Because of the great variation in severity and expression of the disease, CF should not be eliminated as a possible etiology for respiratory symptoms because a patient looks healthy. Cystic fibrosis is suggested when the following clinical situations arise: intestinal obstruction of the newborn infant, failure to thrive, "celiac" syndrome, rectal prolapse, malabsorption, chronic or recurrent symptoms of the upper or lower respiratory tract (including nasal polyps), chronic sinusitis, cirrhosis of the liver, portal hypertension, "heat stroke," and even male sterility.

Ninety percent of patients with CF show symptoms involving the upper and lower respiratory tract at some time. These symptoms may be a chronic cough, recurrent wheezing in infancy, recurrent pneumonitis, bronchitis, atelectasis, nasal polyposis, chronic sinusitis, empyema, or bronchiectasis.

Eighty percent demonstrate evidence of pancreatic insufficiency. They may show failure to thrive, despite a relatively good appetite, with bulky and foul-smelling bowel movements, a protuberant abdomen, recurrent rectal prolapse, meconium ileus (as a newborn infant) or fecal impaction (as an older child), bleeding due to vitamin K deficiency, edema due to low serum proteins, or "milk allergy."

The most reliable test for the diagnosis of CF is the quantitative analysis of the *sweat chloride and sodium*. The test is performed in four steps: stimulation of local sweat glands; collection of the specimen; quantitative analysis for chloride and sodium; and interpretation of the results.

The major method of stimulating the sweat glands is through pilocarpine iontophoresis. An electric current of 2.5 to 3.0 milliamperes for 5 to 10 minutes drives the pilocarpine into the skin. The drug may also be injected directly into the test site. The specimen is collected from the forearm, trunk, or thigh, avoiding the palms, forehead, and axillae. The specimen is absorbed onto preweighed gauze or filter paper or into a micropipette for 30 minutes. The weight or volume is then measured. The content of the sodium is determined by flame photometry and the chloride content by titration. The sodium and chloride concentrations should be within 10% to 15% of each other for reliability. The uncontaminated sample must be adequate in volume; the larger the sample, the more reliable the result. In reliable laboratories that do this test regularly, the finding of a sweat sodium concentration above 60 mEq/liter or a chloride above 70 mEq/liter is consistent with the diagnosis of CF. Table 30-4 gives the expected values in children with CF and in control subjects. Although other laboratories and some clinical cases do have borderline values, most cases are readily distinguished by this test. Some factors that may affect the results of the

Table 30-4. Normal Sweat Sodium, Chloride, and Potassium Values for Cystic Fibrosis (CF) Patients and Control Subjects

	CF PATIENTS			CONTROL SUBJECTS		
	Sodium	*Chloride*	*Potassium*	*Sodium*	*Chloride*	*Potassium*
	←———		*mEq/liter*			———→
Mean	111.190	115.330	22.930	28.154	28.025	10.339
SD	11.987	12.112	2.488	6.079	6.048	2.365
n	252	252	252	252	252	252
Minimum	75.4	78.6	13.8	15.9	7.7	6.0
Maximum	144.6	148.2	29.6	45.9	43.4	16.9

(Shwachman H et al: The sweat test: Sodium and chloride values. J Pediatr 98:577, 1981)

sweat test and that need to be considered in interpreting the results are listed below.

In the first weeks of life, normal infants tend to have elevated sweat electrolyte values that gradually return to normal. After puberty, the mean values increase. Elevated values of sweat electrolytes may be found in patients with adrenal insufficiency, ectodermal dysplasia, malnutrition, diabetes insipidus, glycogen storage disease, and allergic disease. The elevation in these diseases, however, is not consistent in repeated testing; symptoms and family history help distinguish the diseases. Some families tend to have higher values without any history of CF. Salt loading increases the values, whereas repeated stimulation of the sweat glands in the same area decreases the amount of sweat and electrolytes.

SWEAT TEST: FACTORS INFLUENCING LEVEL OF ELECTROLYTES

- The Patient
  - Nature of the disease
  - Genetic stock
  - Age
  - Sex: no difference noted in childhood; adult females sweat less than males with heat stimulation
  - Individual variation: noted on repeated testing; may be of considerable magnitude in some persons
  - Condition of patient: dehydration, circulatory failure, respiratory distress, hypothyroidism, malnutrition, edema, adrenal insufficiency, and so forth
  - Diet, especially salt intake
  - Time of day and season of year
  - Exhaustion of glands
  - Acclimatization
  - Activity of patient
  - Effect of drugs
  - Unknown or unrecognized factors
- Sweat Induction and Collection
  - Heat versus drug or combination
  - Environment and body temperature; humidity and effect of evaporation
  - Rate of sweating
  - Duration of sweat period
  - Area of body
  - Total body sweat versus local collection
- Drug Used and Application
  - Pilocarpine, furosemide, mecholyl
  - Method of application of drug: ID injection or by iontophoresis
- Analytical Factors
  - Size of sample
  - Weight determined in analytical balance by weighing sweat absorbed on gauze pads, cotton, filter paper
  - Volume measured directly with volumetric pipette
  - Method of determining chloride: semiquantitative, electrometric, titrimetric, polarographic
  - Flame-photometric analysis for sodium and potassium
  - Dilution factor
  - Contamination
  - Technical: personnel factor

(Guide to Diagnosis and Management of Cystic Fibrosis. Atlanta, National Cystic Fibrosis Research Foundation, 1971)

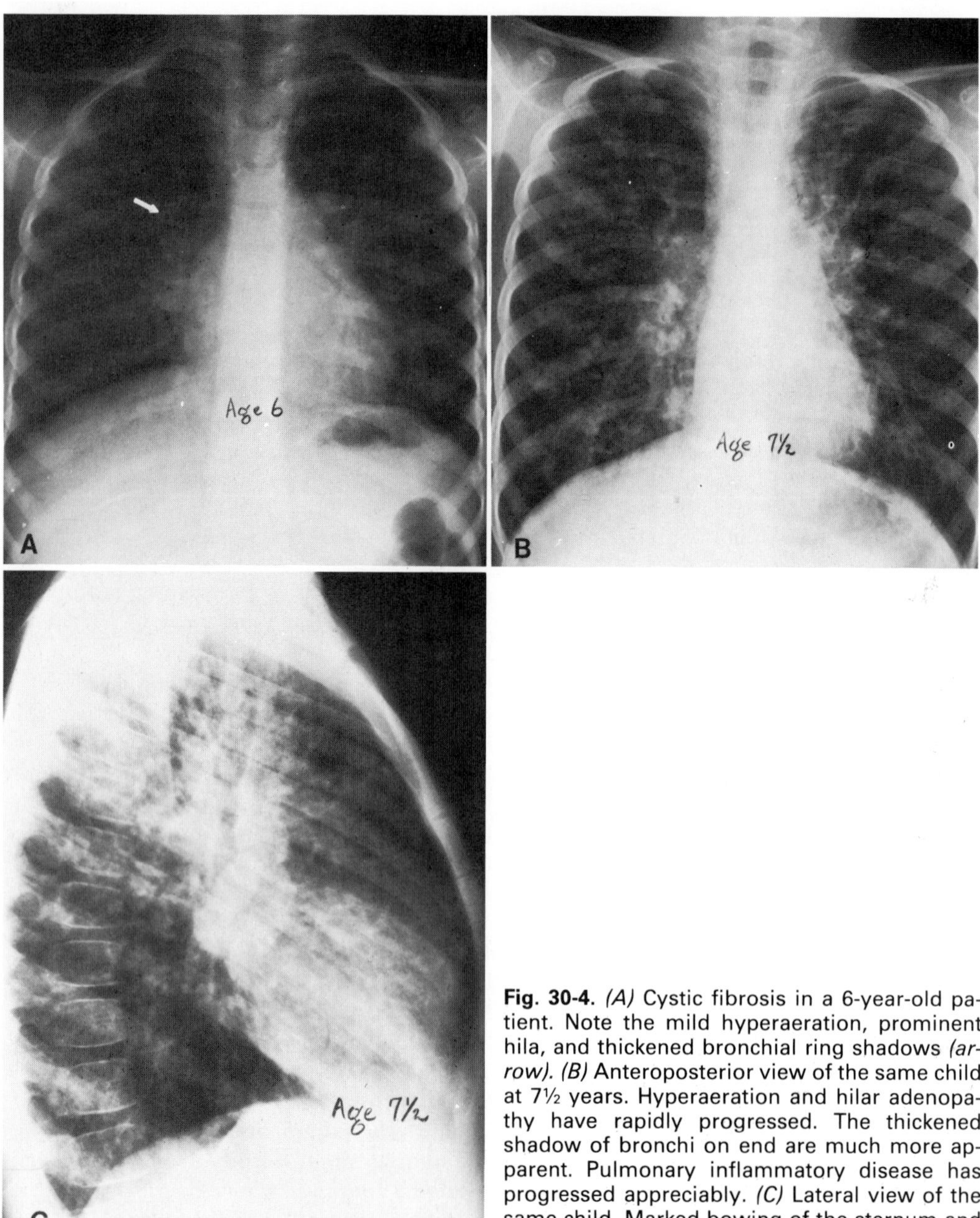

Fig. 30-4. *(A)* Cystic fibrosis in a 6-year-old patient. Note the mild hyperaeration, prominent hila, and thickened bronchial ring shadows *(arrow). (B)* Anteroposterior view of the same child at 7½ years. Hyperaeration and hilar adenopathy have rapidly progressed. The thickened shadow of bronchi on end are much more apparent. Pulmonary inflammatory disease has progressed appreciably. *(C)* Lateral view of the same child. Marked bowing of the sternum and hilar adenopathy are present.

Analysis of nail clippings or hair for electrolytes is reliable in 90% or more of young children but is too cumbersome for widescale screening. Meconium, the first excrement of a neonate, may be tested for albumin by a simple dipstick method, but this test has not proved reliable. The presence of albumin suggests pancreatic insufficiency, most likely owing to CF, and indicates the need for further investigation with sweat analysis and family history.

Pancreatic function should be tested in all patients suspected of having CF, although the test is not essential to diagnose CF. The most direct results are obtained by analysis of duodenal aspirate before and after intravenous secretin stimulation. The duodenal aspirate will have increased viscosity, decreased volume, low pH, and decreased bicarbonate concentration. The pancreatic enzymes will be decreased in proportion to the degree of pancreatic involvement.

All enzymes, or selected ones, may be involved. Whereas 15% of patients have adequate enzyme activity, 85% may have complete pancreatic insufficiency. Indirect analysis may be done by testing the stools for trypsin activity. Analysis of other stool components is of value when used in fat and protein balance studies and is especially helpful in determining the effectiveness of enzyme therapy.

ROENTGENOGRAPHIC FINDINGS

Chest roentgenograms are helpful in both the diagnosis and management of patients with CF (Fig. 30-4). The earliest changes seen in infancy are recurrent lobar atelectases, especially in the right upper lobe or migratory to various lobes. Early in the course there are changes of generalized obstructive disease with iregular aeration, patchy atelectasis, and mild hyperinflation. The bronchi are thickened when seen on end.

As the disease progresses, there is an increase in overinflation with flattening of the diaphragms, increased anteroposterior diameter with sternal bowing, pulmonary radiolucency, and a narrow cardiac silhouette. There may be scattered areas of infiltration and segmental or lobar atelectasis. The peribronchial markings increase, causing further thickening of bronchi on end. There may be marked enlargement of the perihilar nodes. Complications such as pneumothorax, abscess, or empyema may be seen.

The chest roentgenogram is helpful in evaluating patients. A scoring system that relates well to pulmonary function tests and to clinical scoring systems is shown in Table 30-5, with its correlation to the Shwachman score shown in Figure 30-5.

CLINICAL FEATURES

The mortality of CF is particularly high in the first year of life and is primarily the result of pulmonary complications now that the surgical management of meconium ileus is more satisfactory. If, however, extensive bowel resection is needed because of meconium ileus and bowel atresia, prolonged periods of hyperalimentation and marginal nutrition still contribute significant mortality. Respiratory distress may develop in infants with or without the development of lobar atelectasis. The clinical course is characterized by a bronchiolitis-like syndrome with secondary chronic obstructive pulmonary disease. There is marked respiratory distress, coughing, wheezing, poor air exchange, cyanosis, and hypoxemia in the absence of fever. Because of pancreatic insufficiency, feeding is difficult, with malnutrition and failure to thrive.

The primary difficulty in diagnosing CF in infants younger than 6 months of age is that often there is no family history of CF. Their symptoms are indistinguishable from those of bronchiolitis. Infants may develop their pulmonary problems early because viral bronchiolitis becomes secondarily infected by bacteria or because they handle viral infection poorly, owing to inability of the airways to maintain adequate hygiene. Because of the similarity between CF and viral bronchiolitis, the diagnosis is usually delayed for weeks or months while the respiratory disease progresses. Associated with prolonged respiratory distress is the development of malnutrition that goes unsuccessfully treated because its etiology is not recognized.

If a patient with CF survives early respiratory infections, he may first present as a young child with failure to thrive despite the presence of a good appetite. His history indicates frequent respiratory infections and chronic wheezing and coughing. Often he has been treated as an "allergic" child because of his respiratory symptoms. Unlike an allergic child, however, he has an exceptionally good appetite, even when having respiratory symptoms.

The clinical course in CF is determined primarily by the extent of pulmonary involvement and the development of pulmonary complications. In all patients with CF there are recurrent bouts of acute bronchopulmonary infection owing to *Pseudomonas aeruginosa*. These episodes consist of fever (usually low-grade), anorexia, lethargy, tachypnea, dyspnea, and an increased sputum production. Rales are almost always present, as are an elevated white blood cell count and acute infiltrative changes on roentgenographic examination. The vital capacity and the peak expiratory flow rate consistently are below established normal levels for the patient.

If these infectious episodes respond quickly to treatment, the parenchymal damage caused by infection is minimized, and there is a return to previous levels of pulmonary function. If the infections are prolonged, too frequent, untreated, or unresponsive, the course is one of more rapid deterioration to end-stage pulmonary disease. Pulmonary complications such as abscess, pneumothorax, and cor pulmonale accelerate the deterioration.

Although empyema is rare in older patients with CF, staphylococcal empyema may be the presenting illness in infants with CF. The incidence of empyema in all patients with CF is reportedly between 2% and

Table 30-5. Roentgenogram Scoring System*

CATEGORY	DEFINITION	SCORING
Air trapping	Generalized pulmonary overdistention presented as sternal bowing, depression of diaphragms, or thoracic kyphosis	0 = Absent 1, 2, 3, 4 = Increasing severity†
Linear markings	Line densities owing to prominence of bronchi; may be seen as parallel line densities, sometimes branching, or as "end-on" circular densities with thickening of bronchial wall	0 = Absent 1, 2, 3, 4 = Increasing severity†
Nodular-cystic lesions	Multiple, discrete, small, rounded densities, 0.5 cm in diameter or larger, with either radiopaque or radiolucent centers (does not refer to irregular linear markings); *confluent nodules not classified as large lesions*	0 = Absent 1, 2, 3, 4 = Increasing severity†
Large lesions	Segmental or lobar atelectasis or consolidation; includes acute pneumonia	0 = Absent 3 = Segmental or lobar atelectasis 5 = Multiple atelectasis
General severity	Impression of overall severity of changes on roentgenogram	0 = Absent 1, 2, 3, 4 = Increasing severity 5 = Complications (*e.g.,* cardiac enlargement, pneumothorax)

(Brasfield D et al: The chest roentgenogram in cystic fibrosis: A new scoring system. Pediatrics 63:24, 1979 [Copyright American Academy of Pediatrics, 1979])

*Total score = 25 − total demerit points.

†Score of 4 is most severe.

5%, with most cases occurring in patients younger than 1 year of age. Patients with cystic fibrosis with empyema constitute 3% to 7% of all patients hospitalized with empyema, with most of the cases due to *Staphylococcus.*[42]

COMPLICATIONS

The usual course of cystic fibrosis involves the development of various complications. Because many of these are expected, it is difficult to distinguish a feature of the disease from a complication *per se.* Some features of CF require prolonged survival before they are likely to develop, and therefore tend to be features of CF as seen in older children or young adults (e.g., diabetes mellitus or biliary cirrhosis), whereas other complications present only in infancy (e.g., meconium ileus, intestinal atresia, and empyema). Others may develop at any time throughout the entire course. Table 30-6 lists the features of CF which may develop in any patient, even when receiving optimum therapy.

PULMONARY FUNCTION ABNORMALITIES

The initial pulmonary signs of CF occur in the small airways. These changes are difficult to detect clini-

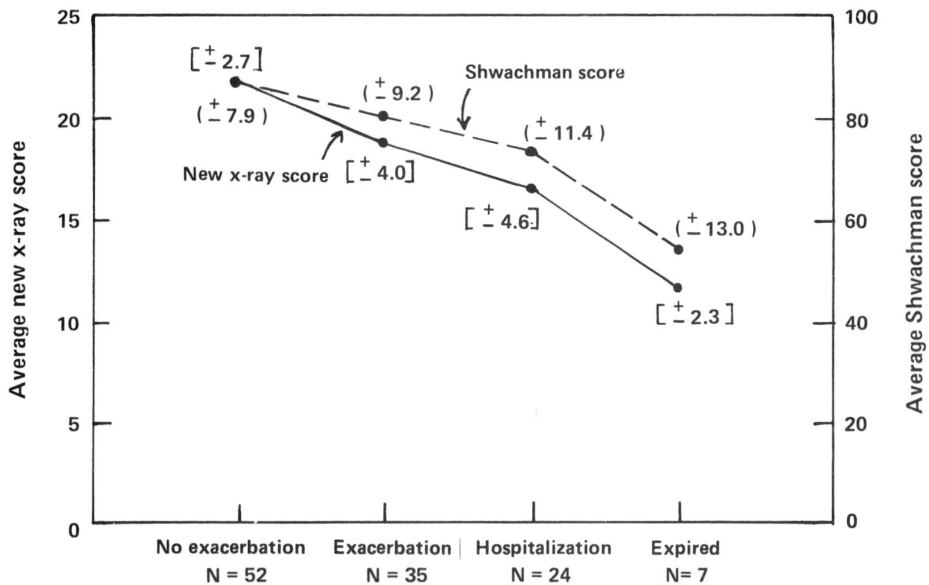

Fig. 30-5. Relationship between average roentgenogram score, average total Shwachman score, and pulmonary exacerbations, hospitalizations, and death. N = numbers of patients; [±1 SD] = 1 SD of roentgenogram score; (±1 SD) = 1 SD of total Shwachman score. (Brasfield D et al: The chest roentgenogram in cystic fibrosis: A new scoring system. Pediatrics 63:24, 1979. (Copyright American Academy of Pediatrics, 1979)

cally and roentgenographically until they have progressed. Unfortunately, the first abnormalities that can be tested by refined pulmonary function tests require cooperation that is not possible in younger patients with CF.

The first change in pulmonary mechanics is a decreasing dynamic compliance with increasing respiratory rate. This is measured by relating changes in lung volume to corresponding changes in transpulmonary pressure during tidal breathing at various frequencies of respiration. In the absence of any other abnormality, this change suggests maldistribution of ventilation, probably owing to disease in small airways. The maximal expiratory flow-volume curve is probably the easiest test of respiratory mechanics to detect early changes in the airways in CF and to follow the progress of disease.[25] Forced expiratory flow rates progressively decrease as obstruction progresses.

Uneven ventilation in early CF results in a decreased Pa_{O_2} with normal or slightly decreased Pa_{CO_2}. Some studies suggest that blood gas abnormalities occur before any other easily obtained parameter of lung function becomes abnormal.[24]

Obstruction tends to produce an increased functional residual capacity, a decreased expiratory reserve volume, and a proportionately greater increase in residual volume (RV). No change or a small increase in total lung capacity (TLC) may occur. Increase in residual volume is a very useful index of severity of CF when it is measured by body plethysmograph.

The relationship of the observed RV to the observed TLC results in a ratio that provides a more sensitive indication of change than does the RV alone. The ratio is markedly increased with severe obstruction.

EVALUATION OF CLINICAL STATUS AND PROGNOSIS

In the past 3 decades the prognosis for patients with CF has improved considerably. Today about 20% of all patients with CF are 15 years of age or older, with males averaging a longer survival than females. The most important determinants affecting prognosis appear to be early diagnosis when there are symptoms, delayed onset of symptoms, and the availability of specialized treatment facilities.

Because the disease varies in its severity, the prognosis for each person depends on the progression of pulmonary symptoms and the complications the patient develops. The length of time before diagnosis and institution of therapy determines to some extent the amount of pulmonary damage that occurs. Thus

Table 30-6. Complications of Cystic Fibrosis*

COMPLICATIONS	RESPIRATORY	MUSCULOSKELETAL	GASTROINTESTINAL	NUTRITIONAL	GROWTH AND DEVELOPMENT	CARDIAC	OTHER
Common	Emphysema, atelectasis, bronchiectasis, sinusitis, nasal polyposis (10–15%), hemoptysis—mild	Clubbing	Intestinal obstruction: meconium ileus (10–15%), atresia, fecal impaction. Inguinal hernia, biliary cirrhosis (5%), carbohydrate intolerance	Failure to thrive	Growth retardation, delayed sexual development	RVH on ECG	Male sterility
Occasional	Hemoptysis—massive, abscess formation	Osteoporosis	Diabetes mellitus (requiring insulin), duodenitis, pancreatitis, rectal prolapse, portal hypertension	Vitamin deficiency: vitamin K (bleeding), vitamin A, vitamin E		Cor pulmonale, pulmonary hypertension	
Rare	Pneumothorax, empyema (2–5%)	Osteomyelitis, osteoarthropathy (not clubbing)	Intussusception, pancreatic calcification, ascites, pneumatosis intestinalis, hypersplenism	Hypoproteinemia, edema, anemia secondary to low iron-binding protein	Gynecomastia	Myocardial fibrosis	Ocular changes, salt depletion, parotitis, hypergammaglobulinemia, anemia secondary to blood loss

*Figures in parentheses represent percentage of occurrence.

Table 30-7. System of Clinical Evaluation of Patients with Cystic Fibrosis

GRADING	POINTS	GENERAL ACTIVITY	PHYSICAL EXAMINATION	NUTRITION	X-RAY FINDINGS
Excellent (86–100)	25	Full normal activity; plays ball, goes to school regularly, and so forth	Normal; no cough; pulse and respirations normal; clear lungs; good posture	Maintains weight and height above 25th percentile; well-formed stools, almost normal; good muscle mass and tone	Clear lung fields
Good (71–85)	20	Lacks endurance and tires at end of day; good school attendance	Resting pulse and respirations normal; rare coughing or clearing of throat; no clubbing; clear lungs; minimal emphysema	Weight and height at approximately 15th to 20th percentile; stools slightly abnormal; fair muscle tone and mass	Minimal accentuation of bronchovascular markings; early emphysema
Mild (56–70)	15	May rest voluntarily during day; tires easily after exertion; fair school attendance	Occasional cough, perhaps in morning upon rising; respirations slightly elevated; mild emphysema; coarse breath sounds; rarely localized rales; early clubbing	Weight and height above 3rd percentile; stools usually abnormal, large and poorly formed; very little, if any, abdominal distention; poor muscle tone with reduced muscle mass	Mild emphysema with patchy atelectasis; increased bronchovascular markings
Moderate (41–55)	10	Home teacher; dyspneic after short walk; rests a great deal	Frequent cough; usually productive; chest retraction; moderate emphysema; may have chest deformity; rales usually present; clubbing 2 to 3+	Weight and height below 3rd percentile; poorly formed, bulky, fatty, offensive stools; flabby muscles and reduced mass; abdominal distention mild to moderate	Moderate emphysema; widespread areas of atelectasis with superimposed areas of infection; minimal bronchiectasis
Severe (40 or below)	5	Orthopneic, confined to bed or chair	Severe coughing spells; tachypnea with tachycardia and extensive pulmonary changes; may show signs of right-sided cardiac failure; clubbing 3 to 4+	Malnutrition marked; large, protuberant abdomen; rectal prolapse, large, foul, frequent, fatty bowel movements	Extensive changes with pulmonary obstructive phenomena and infection; lobar atelectasis and bronchiectasis

(Shwachman H, Kulczycki LL: Long-term study of 105 patients with cystic fibrosis. Am J Dis Child 96:6, 1958)

those infants who have a family history for the disease and are tested and diagnosed before 3 months of age have a much better chance of surviving to 20 years of age than do those that are diagnosed later, after prolonged, untreated respiratory illnesses or with prolonged malnutrition.

A number of scoring systems have been devised to provide the physician and family with some indication of the severity of disease and the expected response to therapy. The first one that has been widely used was developed by Shwachman and Kulczycki in 1958.[38] Table 30-7 summarizes their criteria and eval-

Table 30-8. Scoring System for Evaluation of Status in Cystic Fibrosis

STATUS		MAXIMUM POINTS*
Pulmonary		17
X-ray:		
Minimal accentuation of pulmonary markings	1–3	
Increased pulmonary markings; mild overaeration, atelectasis, or mucous plugging	4–6	
Moderate overaeration, fibrosis, atelectasis, or mucous plugging; early cyst formation	7–10	
Severe overaeration; extensive fibrosis and cyst formation, pulmonary obstruction, bronchiectasis	11–13	
Acute infiltrate	1–4	
Pulmonary function tests:		17
Vital capacity (VC) less than 90% predicted	1	
less than 80% predicted	3	
less than 70% predicted	5	
less than 60% predicted	7	
less than 50% predicted	9	
FEV_1 less than 70% of total VC	1	
less than 66% of total VC	2	
less than 58% of total VC	4	
less than 50% of total VC	6	
less than 42% of total VC	8	
Pulmonary exacerbation requiring intensive therapy:		5
Past 3 months	5	
Past year	3	
Pneumothorax:		5
Past 6 months or recurrent	5	
Ever	3	
Hemoptysis (omit if none since pulmonary surgery)		7
Massive: past 6 months	7	
more than 6 months ago	4	
Small amount in past year	1–3	
Pulmonary surgery (any resection)	2–7	7
Cor pulmonale	3–5	5
Physical examination of lungs	1–9	9
Sputum production or cough	1–3	3
Total pulmonary:		75
General		
Weight:		6
Poor appetite	1–2	
Less than third percentile	2	
Loss of more than 2 kg in past 3 months	2	
Loss of more than 5 kg in past year or significant decline from growth curve	4	
Activity:		10
Tires easily; unable to work or attend school	1–6	
Dyspnea after one flight or at rest	1–5	
Attitude:		9
Follows instructions or takes medications unreliably	1–6	
Depressed philosophy of cystic fibrosis	1–3	
Total general:		25
Total points deducted:		100
Final Score (100 minus points deducted)		

(Taussig LM *et al*: A new prognostic score and clinical evaluation system for cystic fibrosis. J. Pediatr 82:380, 1973)

*Maximum points that can be deducted for a given category.

uation. Their system was devised before newer therapeutic measures improved the prognosis and provided a longer life expectancy, during which time more complications would be encountered and treated.

The system of Shwachman and Kulczycki gives too much weight to nutritional status in view of more recent evidence that pulmonary function and roentgenographic changes are more helpful indicators. Their category of "general activity" is probably indirect evidence of pulmonary status.

A system presented by Taussig and associates has been used to determine response to therapy as well as general prognosis.[43] Maximum emphasis is placed on roentgenographic changes, pulmonary function tests, and occurrence of complications. This scoring system is presented in Table 30-8. Using this system, Taussig and coworkers have been able to predict 3- or 6-year mortality rates with a high degree of accuracy (Table 30-9). Not included in this scoring system are the important prognostic signs of arterial blood gases that are early indicators of pulmonary disease. No scoring system is perfect, but the Taussig system is the most comprehensive, considering available therapy. The scores should be assessed with each acute exacerbation to evaluate the efficacy of therapy, and every 6 months to determine general status. The results may be discussed with parents and the patient as appropriate.

THERAPY

Because the causative factors of cystic fibrosis are unknown, there is no specific treatment. Enough is known about the general pathogenesis to allow a rational approach to problems as, or before, they are encountered.

The first step in treatment involves establishing a general therapy plan for the patient. Often the patient is acutely ill when he is diagnosed as having CF, and initial therapy is directed toward controlling the problems, usually pulmonary.

As soon as possible after diagnosis, even while the illness is being controlled, the family is instructed about CF and what role each member will take in the care of the patient. A great deal of encouragement, education, and support is needed for both the patient and the family. They need to know that a team of personnel experienced in the problems of CF, including a physician, a respiratory therapist, a nutritionist, and a family service counselor, will help them through all aspects of the disease.

Table 30-9. Mortality Rates for Cystic Fibrosis Patients Evaluated by Scoring System*

SCORE	PERCENTAGE DYING	
	Within 3 yr	*Within 6 yr*
91–100	0 (0/11)	0 (0/5)
81–91	5 (2/39)	15 (3/20)
71–80	13 (3/23)	33 (4/12)
61–70	25 (4/16)	88 (7/8)
51–60	67 (6/9)	100 (7/7)
<50	100 (11/11)	100 (11/11)

*Numbers in parentheses indicate actual numbers of patients dying per numbers of patients evaluated within that category. (Taussig LM *et al*: A new prognostic score and clinical evaluation system for cystic fibrosis. J. Pediatr 82:380, 1973)

Although the degree to which any system is involved varies with each patient, the major problems that require treatment are bronchiolar and bronchial obstruction, pulmonary infection, and pancreatic insufficiency with associated nutritional deficiencies.

The most important treatment for the pulmonary system in CF involves the establishment and maintenance of *good pulmonary hygiene*. Because secretions are so viscid and the normal mechanisms for pulmonary hygiene are impaired in CF, there is a tendency for obstruction followed by infection in the smaller airways. Tenacious secretions collect and stimulate bronchospasm, edema, and, eventually, infection that causes further obstruction, setting up a destructive cycle. Eventually, if not broken, the cycle leads to irreversible pulmonary damage.

The methods available to break the cycle and to prevent pulmonary damage include nebulization, expectorants and bronchodilators, bronchial drainage and chest physiotherapy, intermittent positive pressure breathing, antibiotics, and certain environmental controls. Use of most of these methods is widely accepted, but the efficacy of others, particularly those involving nebulization therapy and IPPB, is controversial.

Aerosol and Humidity Therapy

Mist Tents. Mist tents have traditionally been used to humidify inspired air and to deposit particulate water in the respiratory tract. There are individual preferences as to when mist tents should be used, if at all. Usually they are reserved for use by children with significant pulmonary involvement, although there are arguments for using them prophylactically.

Mist tents are generally used only when the patient is sleeping but may be used for up to 18 hours a day when symptoms have increased during an exacerbation. Many patients subjectively report both increased ease in clearing secretions and more restful sleep because of decreased cough paroxysms. Some comparative studies, however, report no improvement or even slightly decreased ventilatory function in patients sleeping in tents that use plain water, as compared to ventilatory function in patients sleeping outside a tent.[36] A study of matched patients over an 18-month period has shown no change in the progressive loss of pulmonary function whether in a nocturnal mist tent or not.[2]

If mist tent therapy is started, copious mucus may be hydrated and loosened, aggravating airway obstruction if not cleared. Careful postural drainage to assist in clearing the secretions is essential. Whether pneumatic nebulizers or ultrasonic nebulizers are used, they must provide adequate water output to create a dense mist and suitable particle size (0.8–3.0 μm). The solutions used may be propylene glycol (10%) in distilled water, or one-quarter or one-half normal saline.

Complications from the use of mist tents generally result from improper care of the equipment. Unless extreme caution is used, home and institutional nebulization equipment harbors *Pseudomonas aeruginosa*, *Escherichia coli*, and *Serratia marcescens*. All solutions must be sterile and the equipment properly cleaned as often as necessary to prevent heavy colonization. Regular inspection of home equipment should be part of the total care plan for each patient.

Rarely, skin maceration and infection occur after prolonged use of a tent. This situation arises when proper skin hygiene is neglected in a sick person. Some patients develop bronchospasm or cough paroxysms from propylene glycol or from more concentrated solutions of saline, but, generally, properly applied mist therapy is well tolerated.

An important consideration is the loss of social contact that surrounds the use of tents. If the isolation incurred is more traumatic to the child than the benefits warrant, its use should be reconsidered. Most children accept the tent at night if it improves their sleep. In contrast, if a child seeks the isolation of the tent because of depression from his illness, the basic problem needs to be recognized and handled appropriately.

Aerosol Therapy. Aerosols are used prophylactically or therapeutically either in the hospital or as part of a home care program. They are used to liquefy tenacious secretions that cause coughing spells, to relieve bronchospasm, to decongest bronchial mucosa, and to combat bacterial infection. The agents used in CF as bronchodilators, decongestants, or mucolytics have been discussed in Chapter 20.

Frequently, combinations of agents are used to provide both decongestion and liquefaction. If bronchospasm occurs spontaneously or as the result of treatment with an agent, a bronchodilator may be added to the combination. Mucolytic agents such as N-acetylcysteine usually are reserved for use in more severely affected patients because of their higher costs. In some patients, warmed saline as an aerosol is effective in inducing sputum.

Because of individualized responses to various agents, it is sensible to use those that are the most effective for each patient, are the most reasonable in cost, and, at the same time, have the fewest adverse effects. The efficacy of all these agents should be evaluated by repeatedly measuring pulmonary function before, during, and after fair clinical trials.

Expectorants and Bronchodilators

Occasionally bronchodilators are helpful as adjuncts to other aerosol medications, particularly when there is evidence of bronchospasm. Theophylline, alone or in combination, is the most frequently used systemic bronchodilator. As in asthma, doses should be titrated to avoid toxic side-effects. Combinations of theophylline and ephedrine are often poorly tolerated, with the development of tachycardia, irritability, and hyperactivity, whereas theophylline alone is well tolerated. There is little indication for the sedatives that are added to many of the standard combination preparations containing ephedrine.

The systemic expectorants are usually used on a short-term basis. The two most commonly used systemic expectorants are iodides and glyceryl guaiacolate. The iodide preparations are likely to cause hypersensitivity or hypothyroidism if used excessively and are not recommended. The efficacy of these expectorant drugs is in question. Water is the best and safest expectorant.

Intermittent positive pressure breathing may be used on a short-term basis in patients with bronchospasm and increased bronchial secretions. It should not be used when there is significant air trapping and danger of pneumothorax. Pulmonary function should be measured before and after therapy. If there is evidence of increased air trapping by an increased FRC after IPPB, it should not be used in that patient. Nebulization of bland or pharmacologically active aerosol, without positive pressure, having the patient hold his breath at end-inspiration, is effective in older children (Table 30-10).

Bronchial Drainage

Chest physiotherapy with postural drainage and percussion-vibration is one of the most important phases in a treatment plan for maintaining good pulmonary hygiene. Because it is time-consuming and sometimes uncomfortable, its importance has to be emphasized repeatedly to the patient and his family (see Chap. 26). Although mist tents, aerosols, and oral fluids liquefy bronchial secretions, their effect is wasted if the secretions are not mobilized and removed. Good chest physiotherapy and thorough postural drainage provide this essential assistance. The areas to be emphasized are determined by chest roentgenograms and careful segmental auscultation, particularly when there is localized disease. Drainage should be done before meals, particularly in the early morning after sleep. It should be done thoroughly two times a day prophylactically and more often when there is an acute exacerbation. The chest physiotherapy that accompanies bronchial drainage should include deep breathing, assisted coughing, thoracic squeezing, and vibration.

Antibiotics

Although vigorous efforts at maintaining good pulmonary hygiene decrease bronchial obstruction and minimize the chance of infection, the usual course of CF is marked by repeated acute and chronic bronchopulmonary infections. Early recognition and aggressive treatment of infection are essential to prevent as much pulmonary damage as possible.

Fever, anorexia, and tachypnea, along with a change in the quantity or character of sputum, suggest the presence of acute infection. Pulmonary function studies will indicate deterioration below previously established levels. Chest x-ray films might show evidence of acute infiltrates, and cultures of the sputum reveal heavier growths. Chronic infection is more subtle in its manifestations but is suggested by failure of pulmonary function to improve after appropriate treatment of acute infection, failure to thrive, persistent lethargy, low-grade fever, and copious purulent sputum.

Selection of antibiotics for the treatment of bronchopulmonary infections is based on known sensitivities of the organisms present in sputum. More important, however, is the patient response to an antibiotic regimen. If an infection is detected early enough and the patient is not too toxic, oral antibiotics in high doses may be effective. Not infrequently, the high doses required orally are not tolerated (e.g., they cause gastrointestinal disturbances). Parenteral antibiotics are then necessary.

Intramuscular antibiotics are rarely used because of the large, irritating doses needed. Intravenous administration is the most satisfactory route to assure therapeutic blood levels. Intravenous medications may be given on an outpatient basis by the patient or parent through an indwelling venous line, usually a small "butterfly" needle connected to a heparin lock. The technique allows continued mobility for the patient, which is important for both his pulmonary hygiene and morale.

If the patient fails to respond to oral antibiotics or to parenteral antibiotics as an outpatient, hospital admission is indicated for more extensive therapy. In addition to parenteral antibiotics, intensive chest physiotherapy, postural drainage, and nebulization therapy are given during hospitalization.

Antibiotics may be given by aerosol as an adjunct to oral or parenteral antibiotics.[23] Administration by aerosol allows higher doses than are possible by other routes because less of the drug is absorbed systemically. A bronchodilator should be aerosolized with the antibiotic, since the antibiotic alone may precipitate bronchospasm. Aerosolization of antibiotics without oral or parenteral drug therapy is inadequate treatment for pneumonia; however, as an adjunct to systemic antimicrobials, such treatment may be helpful in reducing bacterial colonization (and, perhaps, infection) in patients with persistent or recurrent pneumonias, bronchitis, or bronchiectatic states.

Because infection is so important in the progression of pulmonary disease, much attention has been directed at preventing these changes by eliminating or decreasing the usual sputum colonization with continuous antibiotics. Although there are now more controlled studies, the efficacy of prophylactic or continuous antibiotics is still highly controversial.[18,33]

Table 30–10. Agents Used for Intermittent Aerosol Therapy in Patients with Cystic Fibrosis

GENERIC NAME (TRADE NAME)	HOW SUPPLIED	RECOMMENDED DOSAGE SCHEDULE (ROUTES OF ADMINISTRATION)	REMARKS AND CAUTION
Bronchodilators			
Isoproterenol (Isuprel)	60 ml; 10 ml bottle. 1:200 dilution	0.2–0.5 ml in 2 ml solution 2–3 times daily (aerosol)	Occasional tachycardia and headache noted owing to excessive use. Frequently mixed with phenylephrine or N-acetylcysteine
Racemic epinephrine as hydrochloride (Vaponefrin)	2.2% solution in vials of 7.5, 15, and 30 ml	4–10 drops in 2 ml of water (aerosol)	Frequently mixed with phenylephrine or propylene glycol. If solution turns brown, do not use it
Decongestant			
Phenylephrine HCl (Neosynephrine)	0.125%	2 ml 3 times daily (aerosol)	
Mucolytic agents			
Pancreatic dornase deoxyribonuclease extracted from beef pancreas (Dornavac)	100,000 units per vial with 2 ml of sterile diluent	50,000 units in 2 ml diluent twice a day (aerosol); 100,000 units in 2 ml diluent and 2 ml distilled water (IBI)*	No side-effect has been observed, but occasional sensitivity has been reported
Streptodornase (SD) Streptokinase (SK) (Varidase)	5,000 units SD per vial 20,000 units SK	10,000 units in 2 ml volume 2 times daily (aerosol)	Allergic reactions are rare
N-Acetylcysteine (Mucomyst) (Respaire)	20% 10 ml 30 ml vial 10% or 20% in 10, 30 ml vial	2 ml of 20% solution 2–3 times daily (aerosol); 3–4% 10 ml (IBI); 4% 50 ml (BL)†	Large amounts of secretions after treatment Bad side-effects rare. Occasional rhinorrhea, stomatitis. Bronchospasm, occasional. Often used with a bronchodilator
Propylene glycol	Made up to 3% to 10% solution by adding distilled water	2 ml 2–4 times daily (aerosol)	Frequently mixed with isoproterenol
Sodium bicarbonate	Made up to 3.7% solution by adding distilled water	2 ml 2–3 times daily (aerosol); 50–100 ml (BL)	Large mucoid molecular chains tend to break at high *p*H. Stimulates mucus flow
L-arginine	L-arginine 0.9 g. Arginine HCl 15.0 g plus distilled water 300 ml	2 ml 2–3 times daily (aerosol)	Breaks hydrogen bonds, detergent, binds metal ions

(Modified from Guide to Drug Therapy in Patients with Cystic Fibrosis. Atlanta, National Cystic Fibrosis Research Foundation, 1974)

*IBI = intrabronchial instillation.

†BL = bronchial lavage.

Bronchial Lavage

Occasionally, special procedures for clearing secretions from bronchi are indicated. If segmental disease persists despite an optimal therapy regimen, suctioning and localized lavage with a mucolytic agent and antibiotic under direct bronchoscopic visualization may be helpful.

Saline lavage of more than one segment for diffuse progressive pulmonary involvement is more hazardous because it requires general anesthesia and often causes a worsening of pulmonary function for several days after the procedure.

Atelectasis resolves as often after intensification of appropriate medical and respiratory therapy as it does after bronchoscopy with or without lavage. Thus there seems to be little role for the potentially hazardous procedure.[41]

Pancreatic Insufficiency

The patient with CF typically has an appetite that seems good despite his chronic pulmonary disease when he is not suffering from severe pulmonary insufficiency or serious infection. Maintenance of good pulmonary hygiene and control of pulmonary infection are essential prerequisites for maintaining good nutrition.

Despite a good appetite, the patient with CF will fail to thrive and will become malnourished if the malabsorption he suffers because of pancreatic insufficiency is not corrected. Replacement of pancreatic enzymes and a proper diet help to provide the nutrition required for good growth and development.

Diet should include larger than normal amounts of carbohydrate and protein, with a decreased proportion of fats. There should be an increase in calories of 50% to 100% above the normal requirements for age and weight, with two to two and one-half times the amount of proteins. The amount of fat ingested should be regulated by the degree of fat intolerance. Fats should not be eliminated from the diet entirely because fats are essential for balanced nutrition. Children with CF quickly learn to regulate their own diet to avoid foods they do not tolerate well, so as to avert symptoms of abdominal cramping, bloating, and increased stooling. Because these symptoms may be rather severe and because there are fewer calories available in the low fat diet, the actual intake in children with CF is less than their calculated daily requirement.[4]

All patients with CF require increased amounts of both water and fat-soluble vitamins. Cheilosis, superficial crusted fissures in the corners of the mouth, is frequently seen in patients with CF and indicates a need for riboflavin. Infants and patients with biliary cirrhosis or any evidence of hypoprothrombinemia require increased vitamin K. Commercially available vitamin preparations with additional vitamins A and E should be given daily.

Pancreatic enzymes are given with meals to most patients with CF to improve digestion and absorption of fat, protein, and fat-soluble vitamins. The type and dose used are determined by response of the patient in weight gain or in decreased fat malabsorption. The dosage is increased if symptoms of fat intolerance are present: light, mushy stools; rectal seepage of oil; or rectal prolapse. Pancreatic enzymes may cause anorexia or gastrointestinal distress if used in excess or if taken at inappropriate times. If a proper balance between fat intake and enzyme dose cannot be determined by subjective manipulation, balance studies of fat and protein intake and stool output may be necessary to achieve adequate regulation. Occasionally, allergy to pork protein in the commercial enzymes may necessitate use of beef enzyme extracts. *Oral enzymatic therapy does not affect the pulmonary component of CF.*

The careful follow-up of a patient's growth during childhood, or weight maintenance after full growth has been achieved, provides a most important parameter of the efficacy of both pulmonary and nutritional therapy. Failure to gain weight or weight loss should be thoroughly investigated with reevaluation of the total treatment program. An excellent review of the problems of malnutrition in CF is available.[4]

INFLAMMATORY UPPER AIRWAY OBSTRUCTION

Obstruction of the upper airway leading to acute and life-threatening respiratory distress is primarily a problem of early childhood. Obstructions may result from congenital malformations, foreign bodies, and allergic reactions but are most frequently associated with fairly specific viral or bacterial infections that result in acute inflammatory edema. The manifestations, and therefore the disease classifications, depend on what area of the airway is most affected. When the swelling is principally in the area above the larynx, involving the epiglottis and hypopharynx, the infection is *supraglottitis* or *epiglottitis*. When the disease is at or below the larynx, the inflammation causes *laryngitis, laryngotracheitis,* or *laryngotracheobronchitis*. "Croup" *per se* is not a disease but a description of the symptom complex that involves the harsh barking cough and hoarseness associated with upper airway inflammation.

Inflammatory edema severe enough to cause respiratory embarrassment is a disease of infants and young children for several reasons. First is their particular susceptibility on first exposure to the viruses most frequently involved. More important, however, are the anatomic differences of their larynges as compared to those of older children. The laryngeal airway is smaller in diameter and surface area in younger age groups and, as such, is more rapidly compromised by edema or spasm. In addition, the mucous membrane lining the vocal folds and epiglottis is more loosely attached and has greater vascularity. Finally, the supporting structures are not as strong, allowing airway collapse.

Viruses, mainly parainfluenza, respiratory syncytial virus, and influenza account for infectious croup in 85% of the cases. The viruses causing epidemics of croup vary annually, seasonally, and according to geographic area.

No viruses are specific for croup. One child may be susceptible to croup when infected with a virus, whereas another child manifests only mild upper respiratory symptoms with the same virus. Once a child has had croup, however, he is likely to have it again with subsequent infections by a different virus. The relation to allergy is unclear but apparently insignificant. The incidence of croup is higher in males than in females and is highest in cold climates.

Hemophilus influenzae is the major pathogen in the 15% of croup cases due to bacterial infection. Bacterial croups are more acute and severe, leading to more deaths than croups due to viruses; they must be distinguished so that appropriate medical therapy can be given. Most patients with viral croup are from 3 months to 3 years old, whereas those with bacterial croup most often are between 2 and 12 years of age. It is uncommon for a child to have a first bout of viral croup after 2 years of age.

ACUTE EPIGLOTTITIS

Acute epiglottitis is a true pediatric emergency. It must be recognized and treated immediately because it is life-threatening. The fatality rate was from 8% to 12% in hospitalized patients but is improving with better intensive care and airway management. As many as 50% of the cases require an airway during the peak of symptoms, although the type and indications vary among institutions. The infection is usually caused by *Hemophilus influenzae*.

Epiglottitis is characterized by a rapid onset of symptoms of less than 24 hours' duration. The patient is febrile, toxic, and significantly apprehensive. Classically the child between 2 and 12 years of age prefers to sit up with his jaw slung forward, drooling and refusing to swallow. The voice is muffled rather than hoarse. Direct examination would reveal an enlarged, boggy, and bright red epiglottis that looks like a cherry in the back of the throat. There is usually inspiratory stridor as well as suprasternal retraction and tachycardia. The lateral roentgenogram of the neck shows a swollen epiglottis with normal subglottic airway diameter (Fig. 30-6).

Epiglottitis often can be diagnosed "from the doorway" by the classic appearance of the child and the history. Physical examination may aggravate the child sufficiently to provoke spasm and complete airway obstruction. *For this reason, any examination that provokes the child, and, specifically, direct examination of the epiglottis should be made only when there is provision for immediate intubation or tracheostomy.* Complete examination should take place only after therapy has started and an airway has been guaranteed. Roentgenograms of the lateral neck provide perhaps the safest way to diagnose an enlarged epiglottis, if good quality films are immediately available. If, however, symptoms progress rapidly, submitting the patient to the procedure may delay therapy or induce total airway obstruction. Under no conditions should a child be forced to lie down for x-ray films, examination, or blood tests when there is a reasonable suspicion of acute epiglottitis.

ACUTE LARYNGITIS, LARYNGOTRACHEITIS, AND LARYNGOTRACHEOBRONCHITIS (LTB)

In contrast to acute epiglottitis, the above-mentioned syndromes generally are caused by viruses and have different courses and prognoses. Initial bouts of viral croup occur between 6 months and 3 years of age. There is an antecedent upper respiratory infection with cough, rhinorrhea, and fever for 2 to 3 days before the onset of a harsh, barking cough and inspiratory stridor. The onset of the stridor characteristically is at night after the child has been asleep. The patient

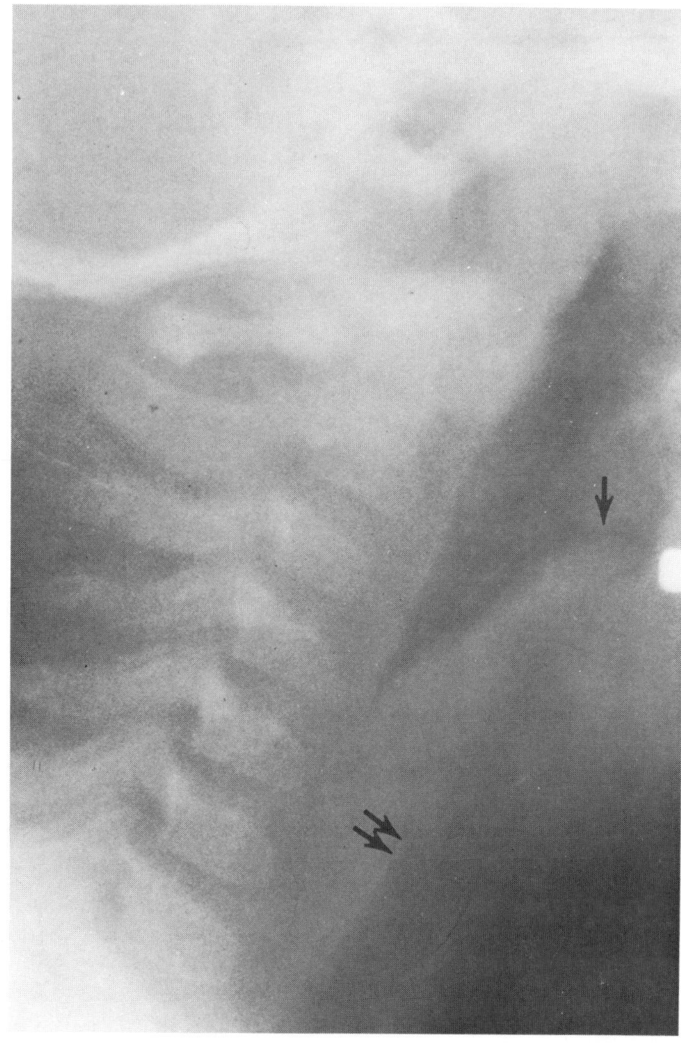

Fig. 30-6. Epiglottitis seen in a lateral view of the airway. The single arrow indicates the markedly swollen epiglottis. The double arrows indicate a normal subglottic airway.

appears apprehensive but not toxic. By the time stridor has developed, defervescence may have already occurred.

The airway obstruction in viral croup owing to inflammatory swelling presents a typical appearance on x-ray film of the lateral neck. The extent of airway involvement determines the prognosis. If infection involves large segments of airway, fever and signs of distal airway obstruction may be present (e.g., intercostal retractions, expiratory wheezes, and rales). Progressive plugging of bronchi may cause severe cyanosis and respiratory insufficiency.

LARYNGEAL DIPHTHERIA

Bacterial croup owing to *Corynebacterium diphtheriae* has been uncommon in the United States for many years. The incidence, however, may increase as the rate of infant immunizations decreases, according to current, unfortunate trends.

The patient presents with several days of rhinorrhea that is typically serosanguineous, with slow onset of the croup syndrome and fever. He appears very toxic. The gray adherent membrane of diphtheria is present on the tonsils and posterior pharynx. If the membrane dislodges, acute airway obstruction may develop.

A similarly located membrane may be seen with infectious mononucleosis and, rarely, with *Staphylococcus aureus* infections. These membranes are not as adherent and do not cause bleeding when removed. They do not carry the same dire prognosis of laryngeal diphtheria unless they cause critical airway obstruction.

DIAGNOSIS OF UPPER AIRWAY OBSTRUCTION

Progressive upper airway obstruction presents with inspiratory stridor and suprasternal and subcostal retractions. The respiratory rate rarely exceeds 45 to 50/min; it slows with increasing obstruction. The heart rate per minute ranges from 120 to 140, and then increases to 160 or above with decompensation. (The baseline heart rate may be higher if the child is febrile.) An indication of serious decompensation in an afebrile infant is an increased heart rate above the baseline with a simultaneous decreased respiratory rate. As air hunger increases, the patient appears more and more anxious and has no moments of rest from his increased work of breathing.

Late in the course, the intensity of stridor and degree of respiratory distress decrease as decompensation occurs. The patient's anxiety gives way to exhaustion and obtundation. Just before death from total obstruction, bradycardia with very shallow respirations occurs. Superficially, the patient appears to be resting comfortably after previously struggling for each breath.

Analysis of arterial blood gases during the course reveals progressive hypoxemia with increasing obstruction. There is no carbon dioxide retention or acidosis until late in the course after the degree of obstruction has become critical.

THERAPY

Early institution of appropriate therapy is life-saving in most cases of proximal airway obstruction. It is essential to recognize the probable cause and degree of airway obstruction as soon as possible with the least amount of trauma to the patient. If acute epiglottitis is present, *immediate* steps must be taken to provide an airway by *tracheostomy* or *intubation*. Waiting for evidence of critical obstruction does not allow enough time to create an airway once that point has been reached. Total obstruction and death may occur immediately at any time during the acute phase of epiglottitis. If complete obstruction does occur before an airway has been established, transtracheal insertion of a 14- to 16-gauge intravenous needle may be temporarily life-saving. Because there is at least a 50% chance for critical airway obstruction requiring an airway, overall mortality is improved dramatically when any patient with acute epiglottitis is given an airway immediately after diagnosis.

The airway may be needed for as little as 12 hours; thus there is more tendency toward using intubation.[12,27] Antibiotics such as chloramphenicol and ampicillin, specific for *Hemophilus influenzae*, are given parenterally.

Some pediatric intensive care units successfully care for children with epiglottitis without routinely intubating patients as soon as the diagnosis is made.[14] If critical airway obstruction develops, ventilation is done by bag and mask until an emergency tracheostomy has been completed. Such a treatment plan means a pediatric surgeon must be at the bedside throughout the acute course; thus this cannot be advocated for most cases, since the consequences of delayed airway establishment and anoxia are too serious.

In other upper airway obstructions owing to infection, any treatment or diagnostic procedure must be done without increasing the patient's anxiety. Treatment is often best administered with a parent's assistance. Frequently, just holding and comforting the patient while providing moist oxygen is more effective in decreasing airway obstruction than is forcing him to undergo a frightening inhalation treatment. If a child is sleeping comfortably (not in agonal obtundation from critical obstruction), he should not be disturbed for therapy or unnecessary laboratory work or vital signs. Good cardiac and respiratory monitors (e.g., an impedance pneumograph) will allow undisturbed rest and still provide adequate parameters for estimating the degree of obstruction.

The classic treatment of croup involves the use of a mist tent, which provides a humidified environment with increased ambient oxygen. Mist tent therapy is most effective if a parent is involved by holding the patient's hand and providing reassurance. It should not be used if it increases apprehensions that the parent cannot allay. When the patient is febrile, cooled mist helps keep body temperature down but may also make him too cold.

Antibiotics are used in bacterial croup and should be given parenterally. In general, if a child appears toxic, is febrile, or has a leukocytosis or a concurrent otitis media, antibiotics are given after blood and throat cultures have been obtained. If laryngeal diphtheria is suspected in an unimmunized child, antitoxin is given in addition to large doses of penicillin.

The use of corticosteroids to reduce mucosal edema in croup is controversial and has been based largely on personal preference and clinical experience rather than on experimental evidence of efficacy in acute croup. Overlap of clinical diagnoses makes comparison of clinical studies difficult, but some controlled studies are available.[31,45] Steroids may be aerosolized or given systemically. Steroids are given for less than 72 hours in most cases, and thus should not interfere with immune defense mechanisms significantly during that time.

Racemic epinephrine has seemed to avert the need for intubation or tracheostomy in many patients. It is delivered by IPPB, nebulization by mask, or by mouthpiece.

Syrup of ipecac traditionally has been used to relieve spasm in some cases of croup, particularly in older children who have repeated episodes of croup. It now seems inappropriate in view of available inhalation techniques; a failure may result in a vomiting child who is likely to aspirate with no improvement of respiratory distress.

Rarely, in some cases of bacterial croup caused by *Staphylococcus* or *C. diphtheriae*, bronchoscopy may be needed to remove membranes that critically narrow the airway. Complete membranous casts of the large airways may be removed.

The patient with croup needs close observation in order to avoid respiratory failure owing to critical airway obstruction. When this occurs or is imminent, the patient should be given an alternate airway, either by tracheostomy or intubation. The selection of either airway should be based on the expertise of the personnel caring for the patient. Excellent results are achieved by either technique when the need is appropriately anticipated. In most cases of croup the airway is needed for 2 days or less. During that time intensive nursing care and pulmonary hygiene are essential.

If tracheobronchitis results in the production of copious secretions, chest physiotherapy and postural drainage may be necessary to maintain airway patency. This is best accomplished when an alternate airway is in place, since vigorous suctioning and physiotherapy may stimulate laryngospasm.

BRONCHIOLITIS

Bronchiolitis is usually caused by a viral infection of the lower respiratory tract that causes obstruction of the most distal airways. The symptoms generally present in infants younger than 18 months of age and primarily younger than 6 months of age.

The decreased airway diameter results from inflammatory edema and cellular infiltrate or proliferation. There may be direct obstruction from mucus plugs, cellular debris, or mucosal sloughing. The remainder of the lung parenchyma is remarkably uninvolved. Air trapping and overinflation develops distal to the involved bronchioles. The principal effect of the diffuse small airway obstruction is interference with gas exchange. Hypoxemia occurs early in the course, whereas carbon dioxide retention occurs only in the most severe cases.

Most cases are attributed to infection with the respiratory syncytial virus, although other viruses, particularly parainfluenza and adenovirus, may be involved.[17] Usually family members or other close contacts have upper respiratory symptoms.

CLINICAL MANIFESTATIONS

The illness begins as an upper respiratory infection with clear rhinorrhea and cough. The cough often is paroxysmal, as in pertussis (whooping cough). After several days, signs of distal airway obstruction develop with intercostal retractions, wheezing and fine rales, severe tachypnea, tachycardia, and, frequently, a hyperexpanded chest. The temperature may be normal or only mildly elevated.

Usually there is an inability to feed or retain feedings; thus dehydration is a frequent problem. The course of the illness may be very short or may persist for up to 2 weeks. The most severe symptoms rarely last more than 2 or 3 days. Bronchiolitis owing to adenovirus infection, however, is often fulminating and prolonged.

The chest roentgenogram appears remarkably normal when compared to the degree of distress. There is hyperinflation with an increase in anteroposterior diameter and general hyperlucency. Expiratory films demonstrate areas of hyperinflation and collapse. Bronchioles seen on end appear thickened or appear as increased linear markings.

The mortality rate is low except in epidemics, when evidence of disseminated viremia is present (especially from adenovirus), or when there are superimposed bacterial infections. Recovery generally is complete, but there may be some correlation between childhood bronchiolitis and the development of chronic obstructive respiratory disease later in life and asthma. A complete review of bronchiolitis is available.[48]

TREATMENT

Treatment is supportive, involving maintenance of adequate hydration and oxygenation. Humidified oxygen therapy is indicated if hypoxemia is present. Antibiotics are needed only if there is evidence of bacterial infection. Steroids may aid in decreasing bronchiolar edema, but supporting evidence for their use is not strong. If respiratory failure occurs, ventilation is indicated to improve oxygenation. Low levels of positive end-expiratory pressure (PEEP) may be useful when the pulmonary compliance is decreased.

PERTUSSIS

Pertussis (whooping cough) is a respiratory disease primarily affecting young children but now occurring with increasing frequency in adults. Infants younger than 1 year of age usually need hospitalization for close observation during the time of maximal mucus production and coughing.

Bordetella pertussis is the etiologic agent in classic whooping cough, but infection caused by *B. parapertussis* or adenovirus is indistinguishable except by laboratory test. The disease is highly communicable.

The course is divided into three stages. The first is the *catarrhal* stage that lasts 2 weeks. It is an upper respiratory infection. This stage progresses into the *paroxysmal* stage, which is the most serious stage for the young infant. Cough paroxysms are characterized by short, repetitive bursts during a prolonged exhalation, followed by a strong inspiratory effort that generates the "whoop." The paroxysms may continue until a mucus plug is dislodged or vomiting and exhaustion develop. Infants younger than 6 months of age rarely demonstrate a classic whoop but frequently have paroxysms prolonged enough to cause severe hypoxia, CNS depression, or seizures. Their inability to clear dislodged mucus plugs or aspirated vomitus makes them susceptible to total airway obstruction. The paroxysmal stage lasts 4 to 6 weeks and resolves into the *convalescent* phase where the paroxysms are less pronounced.

Treatment includes the use of hyperimmune globulin in all patients exposed to the disease, those who have severe disease, or those younger than 2 years of age. Its administration tends to decrease the severity and duration of the symptoms but is effective only when the illness is due to *Bordetella pertussis*. Erythromycin or ampicillin are effective against *B. pertussis in vitro* and are generally used in infants, although there is evidence that the time course of the paroxysmal stage is probably unaffected.

Between paroxysms the patient is relatively asymptomatic. Because paroxysms can be induced by oral feeding and crying, the resting infant should be left undisturbed. A paroxysm often can be aborted by distraction.

Because the disease is communicable, infants must be isolated but must never be left unattended. It is essential to have suctioning available because it may be necessary to clear a mucus plug or emesis at the end of a paroxysm. Seizures or apnea is frequent in infants with pertussis.

ASPIRATION OF FOREIGN BODIES

When a young child presents with sudden onset of wheezing or coughing, the aspiration of a foreign body should be considered. This situation occurs most frequently in young toddlers who habitually taste everything they can get into their mouths. Because of poor cough reflexes and incomplete chewing, they may aspirate virtually anything. Their parents may be able to cite the precise time of onset of symptoms and to identify the aspirated substance. They describe the child, who had been playing or eating earlier, as suddenly beginning to cough and then gradually developing audible wheezing or a "whistle." Often the aspiration is recalled only retrospectively, after anxiety over their child's acute illness has subsided.

Because of poorly developed collateral ventilation and smaller diameter of the major airways in young children, complete obstruction occurs more often than in older children, and thus atelectasis in a major lung segment may develop. If obstruction is incomplete, the foreign particle may act as a ball valve and cause distal hyperinflation. If the foreign body lodges in a distal airway and does not incite generalized bronchospasm, it may remain undetected in an asymptomatic child for an extended period and appear as atelectasis in an x-ray film obtained for other reasons. More often secondary infection develops in the atelectatic segment, and the child is brought to the doctor's attention as having pneumonia with persistent atelectasis.

Two basic classes of foreign bodies cause problems: inert, metallic objects and oily or vegetable particles. Substances that are inert, such as pieces from plastic toys, produce symptoms that relate to the location of the foreign body. If it remains mobile, the particle may be heard clicking against the airway with coughing or breathing. If it lodges in a bronchus, wheezing over that particular lobe may be heard. Once bronchospasm has been established, wheezing throughout the lung fields may develop. If the particle is sharp, direct injury to the airway may result, with bleeding or perforation.

If the foreign body is vegetable, or oily like bacon, a more severe reaction develops. Such particles, particularly peanuts, beans and corn, can swell in size as they absorb fluid. Oily particles are especially irritating since they cause acute, severe swelling of the mucosa and marked bronchospasm in addition to physical obstruction.

Foreign body aspiration is diagnosed on the basis of history and the findings of localized symptoms. Chest roentgenograms are helpful in localizing the affected airway, especially if the material is radiopaque. The right lung, particularly the right middle and right lower lobes, is more often involved than is the left because of the acute angle of the left main bronchus and of the bronchus to the right upper lobe. The chest roentgenogram may reveal either atelectasis or distal air trapping. Occasionally, air trapping may be so severe as to cause atelectasis in the compressed adjacent lobes. Because it is difficult to get cooperation from a young toddler in obtaining deep inspiratory and expiratory films to detect the air trapping, it is helpful to obtain a cross-table decubitus film on the suspected side, using the child's body weight to create the "expiratory" film (Fig. 30-7).

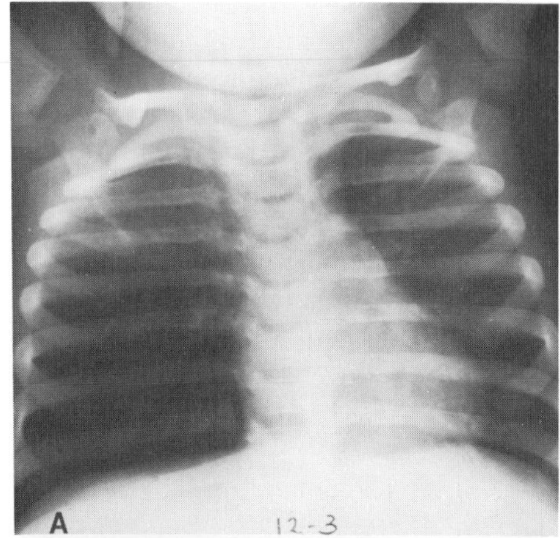

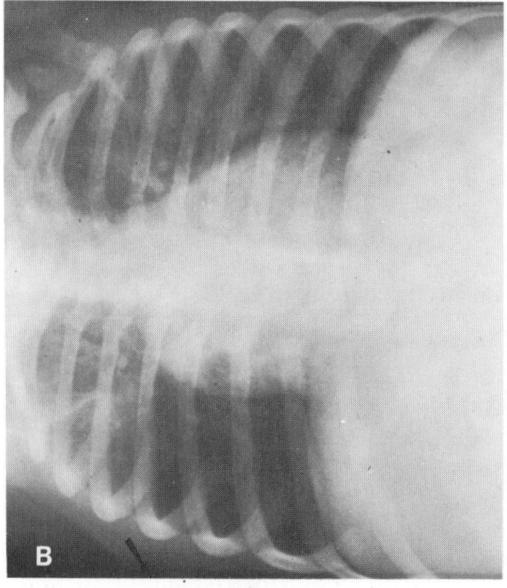

Fig. 30-7. *(A)* Foreign body aspiration in an 18-month-old child who aspirated a piece of crayon. Air is trapped in the middle and lower lobes on the right, as compared to the left and the right upper lobes. There is mild cardiac and mediastinal shift toward the left because of the air-trapping on the right. *(B)* Right lateral decubitus view. In the dependent position the right middle and lower lobes do not empty the air as does the right upper lobe. The arrow indicates a board on which the child is resting.

The treatment of foreign body aspiration depends on early recognition of the cause of the respiratory distress. Removal of the aspirated material at the earliest possible time is essential. Because direct localization of the particle (or particles) in the reactive mucosa is often difficult, an experienced endoscopist is needed. Symptomatic relief may be obtained temporarily by using bronchodilators such as racemic epinephrine by inhalation or parenteral aminophylline, but these should be used only as adjuncts to the definitive treatment of removal. If infection is induced by the foreign body, antibiotic therapy appropriate for the tracheal flora present is indicated. Occasionally, postural drainage and percussion will dislodge a particle.[26] This is particularly helpful if multiple small particles cannot be moved by endoscopy or lavage. Because the dislodged particle may then relocate near the larynx and cause obstructive laryngospasm, an emergency airway should be placed cautiously. The Heimlich maneuver may be useful in older children and is described in Chapter 38.

HYDROCARBON PNEUMONITIS

Ingestion of petroleum products accounts for about 5% of all accidental ingestions in the United States by children younger than 5 years of age. Hydrocarbon ingestions are the second most common reason for admission to the hospital because of accidental poisoning. Fatalities from ingestion of hydrocarbons are decreasing, although the frequency of ingestions is not changing significantly.

Hydrocarbon ingestion may cause pneumonitis, weakness, confusion, irritability, coma, gastrointestinal irritation, myocardiopathy, renal damage, or hepatosplenomegaly. Most fatalities are from pulmonary insufficiency, with 25% to 40% of hydrocarbon ingestions causing respiratory symptoms.

At the time of ingestion there is a burning sensation of the mouth that leads to gagging, choking, and coughing. There may be transient dyspnea and cyanosis. Within 30 minutes after ingestion intercostal retractions and fever may be present, but the onset of symptoms may be delayed for several hours. Often mild retractions, tachypnea, and tachycardia are the only signs of pulmonary involvement. If symptoms are to develop, the onset of tachypnea is usually within the first 6 hours after ingestion. Even in the absence of other symptoms or signs in the first hours after ingestion, tachypnea is an indication for hospital admission for observation of worsening respiratory symptoms.

Symptoms progress during the first 24 hours, plateau for variable periods, and usually subside by the second to fifth days. If pulmonary damage is severe, hemorrhagic pulmonary edema with respiratory failure and circulatory collapse occur within the first 24 hours after ingestion. Symptoms may persist for several weeks but generally resolve more rapidly than they do in adult poisonings.

Roentgenograms may be positive within 30 minutes after ingestion before symptoms appear or may remain normal despite severe clinical symptoms. X-ray abnormalities tend to lag behind the clinical course, reach their peak at 72 hours, and, occasionally, persist for up to several weeks (Fig. 30-8).

Initially the x-ray films have fine perihilar densities that extend peripherally. There may be atelectasis or consolidation of the densities with distal emphysema. Pleural effusion, pneumatoceles, and cysts may develop.

Although up to 75% of patients who ingest hydrocarbons will have abnormalities on chest roentgenogram, only one fourth to one half of these will develop respiratory symptoms.

Most evidence points to aspiration as the cause of pneumonitis, rather than gastrointestinal absorption. In animal experiments where aspiration is prevented, ingestion of very high quantities is needed before pulmonary changes develop. These doses are sublethal and are rarely achieved in children, whereas development of pneumonitis is frequent.

On pathologic examination the lungs appear hyperemic with hemorrhagic pulmonary edema, atelectasis, interstitial inflammation, vascular thromboses, and necrotizing bronchopneumonia. Hyalinized membranes may be present in the bronchi.

Comparisons with animal models suggest that, although the symptoms abate within a few days, the

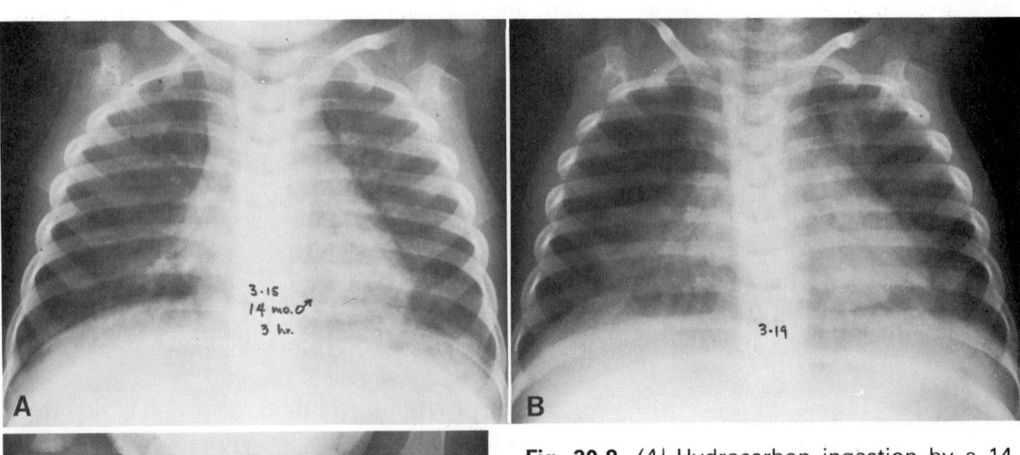

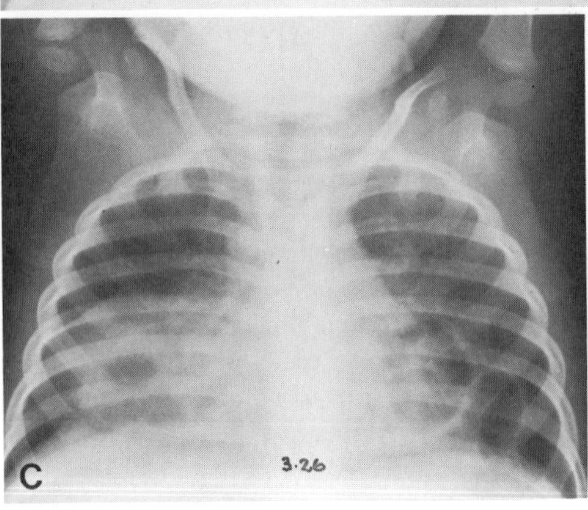

Fig. 30-8. *(A)* Hydrocarbon ingestion by a 14-month-old who drank lamp oil 3 hours before this x-ray film was taken. There are patchy infiltrates at both bases. *(B)* The same patient 4 days after ingestion. The infiltrates have become more solid and coalescent in the middle and left lower lobes. *(C)* The same patient 11 days after ingestion. Multiple pneumatoceles have formed in the areas of previous coalescent pulmonary disease, most prominent on the left. The patient was asymptomatic at this time except for mild tachypnea.

pulmonary parenchymal damage may progress and persist for many weeks.[11] Many of the changes clinically and pathologically suggest abnormalities in surfactant activity. Experimental evidence indicates that hydrocarbons, which are lipid solvents, affect the tension-reducing properties of surfactant. Giammona suggests that the initial pulmonary injury may result from the interaction of the hydrocarbon with surfactant rather than from direct parenchymal destruction.[13]

Hydrocarbons decrease the ability of the lungs to clear bacteria. The mechanism by which this occurs is not clear, but bacterial complications of pneumonia and abscess occur. The effect of ingestion on pulmonary mechanics has not been documented. There appears to be ventilation/perfusion inequality because hypoxemia with normal carbon dioxide tensions has been documented.

Aspiration is the principal hazard from hydrocarbon ingestion. For this reason vomiting should not be induced. The use of lavage to remove any residual toxin is controversial, and, because it may induce gagging and vomiting, its use should be seriously questioned. Steroids have been used to prevent inflammation and fibrosis. Studies in humans and animals indicate that large doses of steroids are not of benefit in preventing the acute inflammation[48] and in decreasing the number of days of symptoms or hospitalization.

Antibiotic therapy has been used routinely because of possible superinfection. Evidence for infection is difficult to ascertain clinically because of the regular occurrence of fever, leukocytosis, and roentgenographic changes. Most mild to moderate ingestions do not appear to be complicated by infection. If the pneumonitis is severe or if the patient is very toxic, has preexisting pulmonary disease, or has strong evidence of infection, antibiotic therapy should be used.

Oxygen therapy is indicated if there is laboratory evidence of hypoxemia. Assisted ventilation is given if respiratory failure develops. Because of predisposition to pneumothorax, the patient should be given low-pressure ventilation. A trial of continuous positive pressure breathing is indicated if acidosis or carbon dioxide retention is not significant. If there is evidence of bronchospasm, bronchodilators given parenterally or by aerosol may be beneficial. Postural drainage with chest physiotherapy is provided if there is obtundation, atelectasis, or production of copious secretions.

DROWNING

Drowning causes about 10% of accidental deaths annually in the United States, and many of the victims are young children. Death from drowning occurs from hypothermia or asphyxia with or without aspiration of water into the lungs. When drowning is in cold water ($\leq 20°C$), the changes of asphyxia are delayed so that survival after longer submersion is possible. If a victim survives submersion after rescue for at least 24 hours, he is a case of "near-drowning." With improved recognition of immediate life-saving techniques at the scene, faster transport to receiving hospitals, and aggressive emergency room resuscitation, more victims survive the initial insult only to suffer the consequences of severe anoxia. Treatment of drowning, then, has to include both cardiorespiratory resuscitation and prevention of the effects of anoxia that occur in the several days afterwards.

In drowning, acute ventilatory insufficiency causes severe hypoxemia, tissue hypoxia, and acidosis. There are also transient changes in electrolyte concentrations and circulating blood volume, but the major problem in the victims that reach emergency rooms is anoxia resulting from marked ventilatory insufficiency. In the lungs, there is increased capillary permeability that allows the development of alveolar edema, which, in turn, decreases lung compliance. There is a loss of the type II alveolar lining cell and also a loss of surfactant. The diffusion defect that develops with edema and atelectasis leads to marked arteriovenous shunting of unoxygenated blood through the pulmonary system, increasing the alveolar–arterial difference with a significant ventilation–perfusion inequality. Anoxic cerebral damage with increased intracranial pressure contributes to pulmonary shunting.

Frequently, with salt-water aspiration, there also is aspiration of other foreign materials (e.g., sand and diatoms). These materials cause chemical irritation or direct obstruction. A significant degree of bronchospasm develops from the foreign bodies or from the water itself. Atelectasis with compensatory emphysema results.

In freshwater immersion some hemodilution and hemolysis may occur owing to the rapid absorption of hypotonic solution into the circulation, whereas saltwater aspiration leads to hemoconcentration. In either case, there is circulatory overload that is poorly handled by the anoxic myocardium, leading to pulmonary edema.

The roentgenographic picture of drowning typically is that of fluffy, nodular, confluent, or homogeneous infiltrations that vary in size and density (Fig. 30-9). The areas of infiltration may increase in the first 24 hours but resolve over the next week. Pneumonia, pulmonary hemorrhage, and atelectasis often are present.

CLINICAL COURSE

The drowning victim may present to the emergency room in any of several cerebral states that can progress. Although the patient may be awake and alert, his pulmonary or cerebral function may deteriorate considerably over the next 24 hours, and thus continued assessment is essential. The level of consciousness may change rapidly with clinical signs lagging behind changes in intracranial pressure. At the other end of the spectrum is the patient who presents in deep coma from more severe brain injury. Therapy to prevent or to reverse increased intracranial pressure has to be applied early and aggressively by continuous monitoring of intracranial pressures, osmotic and diuretic agents, barbiturate coma, mechanical hyperventilation, muscle relaxation or paralysis, maintenance of hypothermia to core temperature of 30°, chlorpromazine, and steroids.

Respiratory support includes application of CPAP or PEEP of 5 to 10 cm H_2O as needed to reverse pulmonary edema; increased FI_{O_2} to maintain the Pa_{O_2} at 150 mm Hg for higher cerebral oxygen; hyperventilation to maintain the Pa_{CO_2} at 30 mm Hg to decrease intracranial blood volume; controlled ventilation of a medically paralyzed patient to minimize muscle rigidity; and decreased intracranial pressure.

During therapy there must be strict attention to bronchial hygiene with a plan of therapy carefully coordinated *not* to increase intracranial pressure. Suctioning of airways or positioning with chest physiotherapy must be done without causing wide swings in Pa_{CO_2} and Pa_{O_2}, increased jugular venous pressure, or increased patient resistance and muscle activity.

The less severely affected victim of partial submersion may not require assisted ventilation to clear pulmonary edema, although intermittent positive pressure ventilation for short periods by mask or mouthpiece may help to relieve bronchospasm and atelectasis if the patient is alert. An elevated oxygen environment should be provided.

The outcome of the drowning primarily depends on the extent of anoxic damage that occurs during the first few minutes. Most patients who reach the emergency room will survive, although those most severely affected may suffer profound and irreversible brain

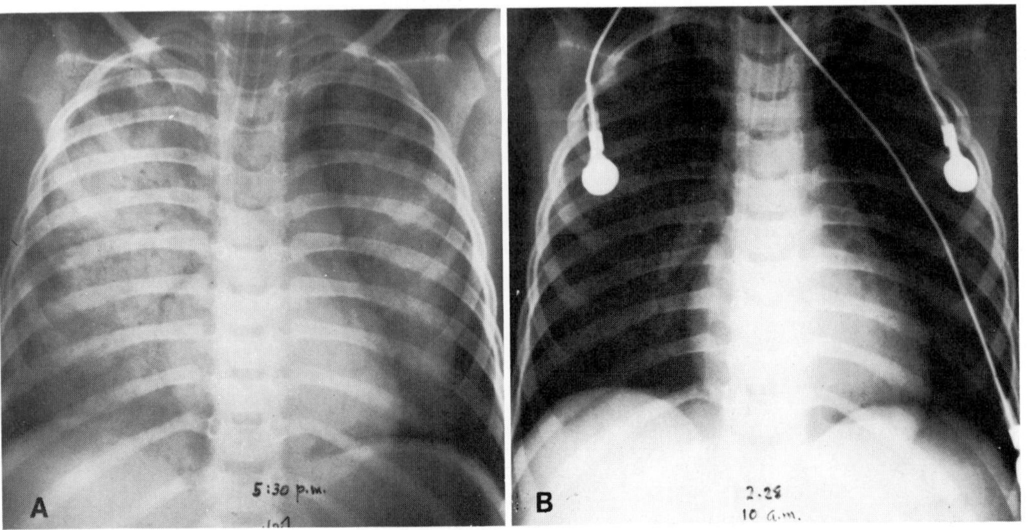

Fig. 30-9. *(A)* A 4-year-old child found in a swimming pool in a state of near drowning. There is diffuse alveolar density throughout both lungs, consistent with pulmonary edema. Note the normal heart size and typical air bronchograms in the partially consolidated lungs. *(B)* The same patient 24 hours after immersion. The pulmonary edema has cleared, and the heart and lungs are normal.

damage and require prolonged, and perhaps permanent, nursing-home care.

More complete attention to preventing further anoxic brain damage after resuscitation has improved the prognosis for most near-drowning victims and makes a coordinated medical and respiratory effort well worth the challenge.[6]

REFERENCES

1. Boushey HA et al: Bronchial hyperreactivity. Am Rev Respir Dis 121:389, 1980
2. Bureau MA et al: Late effect of nocturnal mist tent therapy related to the severity of airway obstruction in children with cystic fibrosis. Pediatrics 61:842, 1978
3. Chai H, Newcomb RW: Pharmacologic management of childhood asthma. Am J Dis Child 125:757, 1973
4. Chase HP, Long MA, Lavin MH: Cystic fibrosis and malnutrition. J Pediatr 95:337, 1979
5. Cohen HI: The role of infection of childhood asthma. Pediatr Ann 6:771, 1977
6. Conn AW, Edmonds JF, Barker GA: Cerebral resuscitation in near-drowning. Pediatr Clin North Am 26:691, 1979
7. Coomey JOO, Levinson H: Physical pain in childhood asthma. Pediatrics 58:537, 1976
8. Cystic Fibrosis Foundation: 1976 report on survival studies of patients with cystic fibrosis. Atlanta, Cystic Fibrosis Foundation, April, 1978
9. Dodge RR, Burrows B: The prevalence and incidence of asthma and asthma-like symptoms in a general population sample. Am Rev Respir Dis 122:567, 1980
10. Downes JJ et al: Intravenous isoproterenol infusion in children with severe hypercapnea due to status asthmaticus. Crit Care Med 1:63, 1973
11. Eggleston PA et al: Radiographic abnormalities in acute asthma in children. Pediatrics 54:442, 1974
12. Faden HS: Treatment of Haemophilus influenzae Type B epiglottitis. Pediatrics 63:402, 1979
13. Giammona ST: Effects of furniture polish on pulmonary surfactant. Am J Dis Child 113:658, 1967
14. Glicklich M, Cohen RD, Jona JZ: Steroids and bag and mask ventilation in the treatment of acute epiglottitis. J Pediatr Surg 14:247, 1979
15. Godfrey S, Balfour–Lynn L, Konig P: The place of cromolyn sodium in the long term management of childhood asthma based on a 3- to 5-year study. J Pediatr 87:465, 1975
16. Gurwitz D et al: Perspectives in cystic fibrosis. Pediatr Clin North Am 26:603, 1979
17. Henderson FW et al: The etiologic and epidemiologic spectrum of bronchiolitis in pediatric practice. J Pediatr 95:183, 1979
18. Hyatt AC et al: A double-blind controlled trial of anti-Pseudomonas chemotherapy of acute respiratory exacerbations in patients with cystic fibrosis. J Pediatr 99:307, 1981
19. Kelly HW, Murphey S: Efficacy of a 12-hour sustained release preparation in maintaining therapeutic serum theophylline levels in asthmatic children. Pediatrics 66:97, 1980
20. Kershnar H et al: Treatment of chronic childhood asthma with beclomethasone dipropionate aerosols. II. Effect on pituitary-adrenal function after substitution for oral corticosteroids. Pediatrics 62:189, 1978
21. Kulczycki LL, Schauf V: Cystic fibrosis in blacks in Washington, D.C. Am J Dis Child 127:64, 1974
22. Kuzemko JA: Natural history of childhood asthma. J Pediatr 97:886, 1980
23. Lake KB, Van Dyke JJ, Rumsfeld JA: Combined topical pulmonary and systemic gentamycin: The question of safety. Chest 68:62, 1975
24. Lamarre A, Reilly BJ, Bryan AC: Early detection of pulmonary function abnormalities in cystic fibrosis. Pediatrics 50:291, 1972
25. Landau LI, Phelan PD: The spectrum of cystic fibrosis: A study of pulmonary mechanics in 46 patients. Am Rev Respir Dis 108:593, 1973
26. Law D, Kosloske AM: Management of tracheobronchial foreign bodies in children: A reevaluation of postural drainage and bronchoscopy. Pediatrics 58:362, 1976
27. Lazoritz S, Saunders BS, Bason WM: Management of acute epiglottitis. Crit Care Med 7:285, 1979
28. Leffert F: Asthma: A modern perspective. Pediatrics 62:1061, 1978
29. Leffert F: The management of acute severe asthma. J Pediatr 96:1, 1980
30. Leffert F: The management of chronic asthma. J Pediatr 97:875, 1980
31. Leipzing B et al: A prospective randomized study to describe the efficacy of steroids in treatment of croup. J Pediatr 94:194, 1979
32. Management of asthma. American Academy of Pediatrics section on Allergy and Immunology. Pediatrics 68:874, 1981
33. Marks MI: the pathogenesis and treatment of pulmonary infections in patients with cystic fibrosis. J Pediatr 98:173,1981
34. McNicol KN, Williams HB: Spectrum of asthma in children. I. Clinical and physiological components. Br Med J 4:7, 1973
35. Mitchell I et al: Bronchial hyperreactivity in cystic fibrosis and asthma. J Pediatr 93:744, 1978
36. Motoyama EK, Gibson LE, Zigas CJ: Evaluation of mist tent therapy in cystic fibrosis using maximum expiratory flow volume curve. Pediatrics 50:299, 1972
37. Pierson WE, Bierman CW, Kelley VC: A double-blind trial of corticosteroid therapy in status asthmaticus. Pediatrics 54:282, 1974
38. Shwachman H, Kulczycki LL: Long-term study of 105 patients with cystic fibrosis. Am J Dis child 96:6, 1958
39. Sly R, Baniei B, Faciane J: Comparison of subcutaneous terbutaline with epinephrine in the treatment of asthma in children. J Allergy Clin Immunol 59:128, 1977
40. Soleymani Y, Weiss NS, Sinnott EC: Management of life-threatening asthma in children. Am J Dis Child 123:533, 1972
41. Stern RC et al: Treatment and prognosis of lobar and segmental atelectasis in cystic fibrosis. Am Rev Respir Dis 118:821, 1978
42. Taussig LM, Belmonte MM, Beaudry PH: Staphylococcus aureus empyema in cystic fibrosis. J Pediatr 84:724, 1974
43. Taussig LM et al: A new prognostic score and clinical evaluation for cystic fibrosis. J Pediatr 82:380, 1973
44. Taussig LM, Smith SM, Blumenfeld R: Chronic bronchitis in childhood: What is it? Pediatrics 67:1, 1981
45. Tunnessen WW Jr, Feinstein AR: The steroid-croup controversy: An analytic review of methodologic problems. J Pediatr 96:751, 1980
46. Weinberger M: Management of asthma—a correction. Pediatrics 69:663, 1982

47. Weinberger MM, Bronsky, EA: Evaluation of oral bronchodilator therapy in asthmatic children. J Pediatr 84:421, 1974
48. Wohl MEB, Chernick V: Bronchiolitis. Am Rev Respir Dis 118:759, 1978
49. Wolfsdorf J, Kundig H: Dexamethasone in the management of kerosene pneumonia. Pediatrics 53:86, 1974

BIBLIOGRAPHY

General Topics

Cloutier MM, Loughlin GM: Chronic cough in children: A manifestation of airway hyperreactivity. Pediatrics 67:6, 1981

Kattan M: Long-term sequelae of respiratory illness in infancy and childhood. Pediatr Clin North Am 26:525, 1979

Keens TG: Exercise training programs for pediatric patients with chronic lung disease. Pediatr Clin North Am 26:517, 1979

Lyrene RK, Truog WE: Adult respiratory distress syndrome in a pediatric intensive care unit: Predisposing conditions, clinical course, and outcome. Pediatrics 67:790, 1981

Newth CJL: Recognition and management of respiratory failure. Pediatr Clin North Am 26:617, 1979

Stone HH: Pulmonary burns in children. J Pediatr Surg 14:48, 1979

Zimmerman SS, Truxal B: Carbon monoxide poisoning. Pediatrics 68:215, 1981

Asthma

Bierman CW, Pierson WE: The pharmacologic management of status asthmaticus in children. Pediatrics 54:245, 1974

Canavan JW, Ellerstein NS, Sullivan TD: Intravenous administration of aminophylline in asthmatic children taking theophylline orally. J Pediatr 97:301, 1980

Fireman P et al: Teaching self-management skills to asthmatic children and their parents in an ambulatory care setting. Pediatrics 68:341, 1981

Harfi H, Hanissian AS, Crawford LV: Treatment of status asthmaticus in children with high doses and conventional doses of methylprednisolone. Pediatrics 61:829, 1978

Kattan M, Gurwitz D, Levison H: Corticosteroids in status asthmaticus. J Pediatr 96:596, 1980

Kattan M et al: The response to exercise in normal and asthmatic children. J Pediatr 92:718, 1978

Katz RM, Rachelefsky GS, Siegel S: The effectiveness of the short- and long-term use of crystallized theophylline in asthmatic children. J Pediatr 92:663, 1978

Kim SP, Ferrara A, Chess S: Temperament of asthmatic children: A preliminary study. J Pediatr 97:483, 1980

Landau LI: Outpatient evaluation and management of asthma. Pediatr Clin North Am 26:581, 1979

Lee HS: Comparison of oral and aerosol adrenergic bronchodilators in asthma. J Pediatr 99:805, 1981

Lulla S, Newcomb RW: Emergency management of asthma in children. J Pediatr 97:346, 1980

Shapiro GG et al: Effectiveness of terbutaline and theophylline alone and in combination in exercise-induced bronchospasm. Pediatrics 67:508, 1981

Weinberger M: Theophylline for treatment of asthma. J Pediatr 92:1, 1978

Welliver RC, Kaul A, Ogra PL: Cell-mediated immune response to respiratory syncytial virus infection: Relationship to the development of reactive airway disease. J Pediatr 94:370, 1979

Cystic Fibrosis

Brasfield D et al: The chest roentgenogram in cystic fibrosis: A new scoring system. Pediatrics 63:24, 1979

Shwachman H, Mahmoodian A, Neff RK: The sweat test: Sodium and chloride values. J Pediatr 98:576, 1981

Stern RC et al: Course of cystic fibrosis in 95 patients. J Pediatr 89:406, 1976

Stern RC et al: Treament and prognosis of massive hemoptysis in cystic fibrosis. Am Rev Respir Dis 117:825, 1978

Epiglottitis and Viral Group

Barker GA: Current management of croup and epiglottitis. Pediatr Clin North Am 26:565, 1979

Battaglia JD, Lockhart CH: Management of acute epiglottitis by nasotracheal intubation. Am J Dis Child 129:334, 1975

Cherry J: The treatment of croup: Continued controversy due to failure of recognition of historic, ecologic, etiologic and clinical perspectives. J Pediatr 94:352, 1979

Corkey CWB et al: Radiographic tracheal diameter measurements in acute infectious croup: An objective scoring system. Crit Care Med 9:587, 1981

Gardner HG et al: The evaluation of racemic epinephrine in the treatment of infectious croup. Pediatrics 52:52, 1973

Gurwitz D, Corey M, Levison H: Pulmonary function and bronchial reactivity in children after croup. Am Rev Respir Dis 122:95, 1980

Milko DA, Marshak G, Striker TW: Nasotracheal intubation in the treatment of acute epiglottitis. Pediatrics 53:674, 1974

Molteni RA: Epiglottitis: Incidence of extraepiglottic infection. Pediatrics 58:526, 1976

Zach MS, Schnall RP, Landau LI: Upper and lower airway hyperreactivity in recurrent croup. Am Rev Respir Dis 121:979, 1980

Bronchiolitis

Dunsky E: Bronchiolitis: Differentiation from infantile asthma. Pediatr Ann 6:459, 1977

Gurwitz D, Mindorff C, Levison H: Increased incidence of bronchial reactivity in children with a history of bronchiolitis. J Pediatr 98:551, 1981

Stokes GM et al: Lung function abnormalities after acute bronchiolitis. J Pediatr 98:871, 1981

Aspiration

Christie DL, O'Grady LR, Mack DV: Incompetent lower esophageal sphincter and gastroesophageal reflux in recurrent acute pulmonary disease of infancy and childhood. J Pediatr 93:23, 1978

Eade NR, Taussig LM, Marks MI: Hydrocarbon pneumonitis. Pediatrics 54:351, 1974

Hight DW, Philippart AI, Herzler JH: The treatment of retained peripheral foreign bodies in the pediatric airway. J Pediatr Surg 16:694, 1981

Drowning

Dean JM, Kaufman ND: Prognostic indicators in pediatric near-drowning: The Glasgow coma scale. Crit Care Med 9:536, 1981

Laughlin JJ, Eigen H: Pulmonary function abnormalities in survivors of near drowning. J Pediatr 100:26, 1982

31

Differential Diagnosis of Various Obstructive Pulmonary Diseases and Implications for Therapy

George G. Burton

The terms chronic obstructive pulmonary disease (COPD) and chronic obstructive airways disease (COAD) are widely and often inappropriately applied to a sizable group of distinct conditions (*see* below). Although there certainly are some common denominators between them, the terms tend to lump together what optimally should be thought of as independent disorders. The term COPD, as such, is not listed in standard hospital medical-record department nomenclatures as a complete discharge diagnosis. As Moser has pointed out, one reason for this somewhat artificial grouping probably was our early dependence on the spirometer as a major tool in pulmonary diagnosis.[16] Any patient who took longer than normal to exhale all his air into a spirometer was said to have "obstructive pulmonary disease." Although physiological testing techniques and therapeutic concepts have progressed considerably in recent years, it still is convenient to use the term *obstructive pulmonary disease* (note the absence of the word "chronic") in interpreting pulmonary function data. On the other hand, the etiology, pathogenesis, and course of each entity differ, as do several aspects of therapy that often make a significant difference in the final outcome.

The obstructive pulmonary disorders discussed in this chapter include upper airways obstruction, chronic bronchitis, extrinsic and intrinsic asthma, emphysema, bronchiectasis, and nonspecific small airways disease. Bronchiolitis and cystic fibrosis, additional obstructive pulmonary diseases seen most often in children and young adults, are discussed in detail in Chapter 30.

Figure 31-1 is a stylized model of a typical intrathoracic airway divided, for purposes of simplicity, into three compartments: the lumen, the wall, and the surrounding or supporting parenchymal structures. The site of airways obstruction may range from the oropharynx to the alveoli. An ability to localize the site of the obstruction correctly has great implications for rational therapy and is now readily done by flow-

THE OBSTRUCTIVE PULMONARY DISEASES

Upper (central) airways obstruction
Chronic bronchitis
Intrinsic asthma (bronchial asthma)
Extrinsic asthma (asthmatic bronchitis)
Other "asthmas"
Pulmonary emphysema
Bronchiectasis
Small airways disease
Bronchiolitis*
Cystic fibrosis (mucoviscidosis)*

*Discussed in Chapter 30.

COMPONENTS OF AIRWAYS OBSTRUCTION*

Lumenal Obstruction: Plugging with mucus; aspirated gastric contents; aspirated foreign bodies; artificial airways and appurtenances (*e.g.,* tracheotomy cuffs); endobronchial tumors; redundancy of the tongue in coma, in obesity, or after a cerebrovascular accident.

Wall Disorders Narrowing Lumen: Smooth muscle constriction (true bronchospasm); mucosal or submucosal edema and inflammation; tumors; tracheal stenosis; laryngospasm; peribronchial fibrosis.

Extramural Wall Occlusion: Tumors and lymph nodes compressing wall; emphysema; small airways occlusive disease; interstitial pulmonary edema; pleural effusion; pneumothorax.

**See* Figure 31-1.

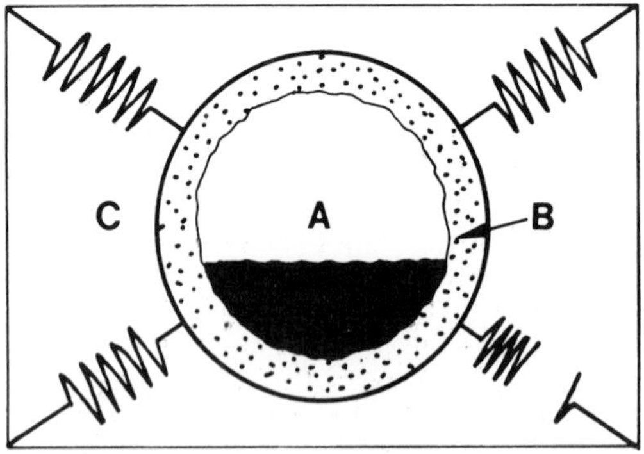

Fig. 31-1. Schematic model of an intrathoracic airway. Three compartments are illustrated. *(A)* The airway lumen and its contents. *(B)* The airway wall. *(C)* The surrounding parenchymal structures.

volume loop analysis and the volume of isoflow test. When one mentions obstructive lung disease or increased airway resistance to most respiratory care workers, the concept of bronchospasm immediately comes to mind, with its attendant therapeutic implications. Some of the various components of airways obstruction as related to the model in Figure 31-1 are listed above. As one can see from a perusal of this list, *much* more than simple smooth muscle constriction might be the cause of airway obstruction, yet it is the *only* one of the causes that can be entirely relieved by usual bronchodilator therapy!

With the exception of *upper* airways obstruction, the various obstructive pulmonary diseases tend to be chronic or recurrent. Recent years have seen increased recognition of each disease entity as being multifactorial in etiology and pathogenesis, and attempts have been made to design rational treatment by selecting several potentially helpful modalities from the options available. A list of such options appears on page 789.[8] These are the component parts of a good respiratory hygiene program and should at least be considered in each case of obstructive airways disease. Especially beneficial modalities are discussed in the paragraphs dealing with *treatment* at the conclusion of the sections discussing each specific obstructive pulmonary disease.

UPPER AIRWAYS OBSTRUCTION

The upper airway may, and often does, become obstructed by various pathologic processes. This portion of the air conducting passages serves as a humidifier, particulate scrubber, and temperature conditioner for inspired air. When the nasal passages are obstructed, as often happens in sinusitis, adenoiditis, nasal polyposis, nasal septal deviation, or trauma, the patient is forced to become an obligate mouth breather, thus depriving himself of these physiological advantages. Drying of the lower (distal) airway is one result, as surely as if the upper airway had been bypassed by an endotracheal tube or tracheotomy.

Table 31-1 lists some of the known relationships between lower obstructive pulmonary disease and

Table 31-1. Common Associations Between Disease Processes in the Upper and Lower Respiratory Tracts

UPPER RESPIRATORY TRACT DISEASE	LOWER (DISTAL) RESPIRATORY TRACT DISEASE
Allergic rhinitis (hay fever) Nasal polyps hypertrophied tonsils and adenoids	Bronchial asthma and cystic fibrosis
Chronic sinusitis	Bronchiectasis
Increased upper airway resistance (mechanism unknown)	Emphysema
Glottal paresis following cerebrovascular accident or intubation	Aspiration pneumonitis

disease processes in the upper airway. Therapeutic attention to disease in the upper airway (e.g., nasal polypectomy in bronchial asthma) will often result in an improved pulmonary condition itself. The *oropharynx* can be obstructed by mucus, saliva, aspirated food, or, after trauma, with blood and other foreign material. Prompt removal of such material by suctioning will often relieve the patient's dyspnea and may be all that is needed to ensure adequate gas exchange.

Obstruction of the upper airway may occur simply because of redundancy of the tongue in a comatose patient. Insertion of an oropharyngeal airway may relieve the obstruction. Intermittent upper airways obstruction at the level of the base of the tongue associated with obesity and hypoventilation particularly during sleep (obstructive sleep apnea) is being reported with increasing frequency. Failing weight loss, tracheostomy relieves all features of the syndrome.

The *larynx* may be the sight of obstruction in cases of infection, tumors, vocal cord paresis or paralysis, or trauma. *Acute laryngotracheobronchitis* is the correct name to apply to childhood "croup." This condition is associated with stridor and, in severe cases, with intercostal retraction, flaring of the alae nasae, circumoral pallor, and cyanosis. Treatment of laryngotracheobronchitis includes humidification and warming of inspired air, appropriate antibiotics, steroids, and, in severe cases, inhalation of an aerosol of a sympathomimetic amine, such as racemic epinephrine.

COMPREHENSIVE RESPIRATORY CARE FACTORS

General
- Patient and family education
- Avoidance of smoking and other inhaled irritants
- Avoidance of infection
- Proper environment
- High fluid intake
- Proper nutrition

Medications
- Bronchodilators
- Expectorants
- Antimicrobials
- Corticosteroids
- Cromolyn sodium
- Digitalis
- Diuretics

Respiratory Therapy
- Aerosol therapy
- Intermittent positive pressure breathing
- Oxygen therapy

Rehabilitation Medicine
- Physical therapy modalities
- Relaxation exercises
- Breathing retraining
- Postural drainage
- Reconditioning exercises
- Psychosocial rehabilitation
- Vocational rehabilitation

(Hodgkin JE et al: Chronic obstructive airway diseases: Current concepts in diagnosis and comprehensive care. JAMA 232:1243, 1975)

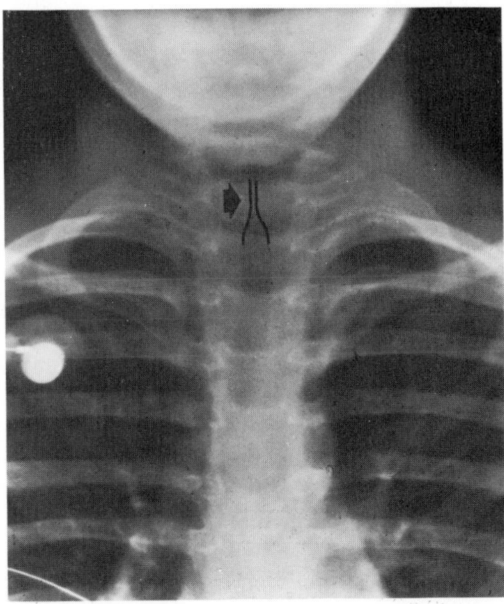

Fig. 31-2. Subglottic edema following postanesthetic extubation. The arrow indicates the area of tracheal narrowing. At the time of this x-ray, the child had intercostal retraction, circumoral cyanosis, tachycardia (heart rate = 170), and the arterial P_{O_2} was 40 mm Hg.

The airway below the larynx may be obstructed in cases of *subglottic edema*, illustrated in Figure 31-2. This relatively rare condition occurs after irritation and inflammation of the subglottic mucosa. It may occur after either short- or long-term intubation once the endotracheal or tracheostomy tube has been removed. Some workers routinely aerosolize a mixture of epinephrine, saline, and a topical steroid such as triamcinolone after extubation to prevent this complication. Otherwise, treatment is essentially the same as in laryngotracheobronchitis.

Probably the most serious central airway obstructive disease is post-tracheotomy *tracheal stenosis* or *tracheomalacia*. Although many etiologic factors are probably involved in stricture formation, the combination of pressure necrosis of the mucosa, suctioning trauma, and infection remain most important. Dunn and coworkers have investigated the etiology of tracheal damage following tracheal intubation.[5] The sidewall pressure of old, nonprestretched tracheostomy cuffs often exceeded the systemic blood pressure, and pressure necrosis was an inevitable result. Even with the newer, high-compliance, low-pressure tracheostomy cuffs, some degree of injury to the mucosal tissue after prolonged intubation is almost invariable, however slight the trauma from suctioning alone.[21]

If enough mucosal trauma and infection occur, the cartilage of the trachea is actually eroded and tracheograms may be diagnostic. The success of surcheal wall is weakened and may actually rupture, with the subsequent development of a tracheoesophageal fistula. Both tracheal stenosis and tracheomalacia often require surgical correction.

The most important "therapeutic" aspect of tracheal stenosis and tracheomalacia is prevention. If a tracheal stricture is suggested by flow-volume loop analysis, bronchoscopy, tomograms of the area, or tracheograms, may be diagnostic. The success of surgery is limited by the relatively short length of trachea that can be successfully sectioned and reanastomosed. The replacement of damaged portions of trachea with prosthetic devices is still in its infancy.

Conditions such as thyroid goiter, enlarging aortic arch aneurysms, or malignancy may compress the major airway from without, also compromising the diameter of the central airway.

PHYSICAL FINDINGS OF UPPER AIRWAYS OBSTRUCTION

Obstruction to nasal breathing may be evident in allergic rhinitis and nasal polyposis. Tenderness over the sinuses may be found in patients with acute or chronic sinusitis. Transillumination of the sinuses may be poor.

Chronic cough is often seen. In one recent series, postnasal drip accounted for this symptom is nearly 50% of patients studied.[10]

A most common finding is that of respiratory *stridor*, as in croup. A loud, brassy cough is said to be highly suggestive of tracheomalacia. Neither the cough nor the stridorous "whooping" is characteristically productive of sputum.

Loud *snoring*, interspersed with periods of apnea, is highly suggestive of the obstructive sleep apnea syndrome.

In some patients with central airways obstruction, the tracheal lumen is reduced to almost one half its normal size before significant symptoms such as exertional dyspnea occur.

LABORATORY DIAGNOSIS

The chest roentgenogram is usually normal, and routine pulmonary function tests findings may be misleading. Endoscopy, dye contrast studies, and sinus roentgenographic studies may be helpful. Analysis of the flow-volume loop has been found to be useful in diagnosing and localizing lesions of the large airways.[6,14]

CHRONIC BRONCHITIS

Chronic bronchitis, as a clinical syndrome, has been arbitrarily defined as cough with sputum production during at least 3 months of the year for at least 2 consecutive years. The term chronic mucus hypersecretion, as suggested by Thurlbeck, may be a more descriptive identifier.[26] Any productive cough that persists for several weeks, in the absence of other problems, is suggestive of bronchitis; whether it is "chronic" is a moot point. Epidemiologic studies indicate that the incidence of chronic bronchitis is between 10% and 25% of all adults in the general population.

The primary pathophysiology involves mucosal swelling and hypertrophy, inflammation, and excess production of thick, tenacious secretions in the airways. Secondary problems include a vicious cycle of recurrent infection and bronchospasm. Accentuated vagal stimulation also leads to increased bronchomotor tone. The lesion most characteristically found in the larger bronchi consists of an increased size and number of the submucous glands. The gland acini, their lumina, and ducts are filled to overflowing with mucus. The ratio of the thickness of the submucous gland layer to that of the bronchial wall is referred to as the "Reid index" and is increased in bronchitis. In the smaller bronchi and bronchioles, excessive numbers of mucus-producing "goblet" cells are frequently found in the epithelial lining layer. The thickness of the basement membrane is increased, and there is a variable cellular infiltrate composed largely of lymphocytes and plasma cells. Along the epithelial surface, denuding of the cilia occurs in often random fashion. Across these so-called skip areas, sputum can be moved only by coughing or suctioning.

Foremost among the causative factors is tobacco smoking, with perhaps 90% of patients being smokers. Particulate air pollutants found in the dusty work environment (e.g., mining, blasting) are also associated with the production of bronchitis, and gaseous pollutants, such as nitrogen oxide and sulfur dioxide, have been shown under experimental conditions to produce hypersecretion and to diminish ciliary activity. Considerable evidence shows that infection may be an additional factor of importance.

Prevention is related to abstinence from cigarette smoking and, to a lesser extent, avoidance or modification of the dusty or fume-laden workplace.

Respiratory mucus, a primitive and ubiquitous substance, is poorly understood (*see* Chap. 16). It has vast importance in the pathogenesis of various obstructive diseases (particularly chronic bronchitis and cystic fibrosis), but a precise or even working understanding of its biochemistry, pharmacology, physiology, and physical properties (rheology) remains one of the unsolved problems in medicine. Although overproduction of mucus is characteristic of bronchitis, occasional cases of "dry" bronchitis may occur. This is particularly true in areas of low ambient humidity.

HISTORY

The characteristic history is one of slowly but progressively worsening cough and sputum production of many years' duration. Cough is the most disabling symptom. Dyspnea on exertion is a common component and may finally bring the patient with "smoker's cough" to medical attention.

Less frequently, productive cough and exertional dyspnea may develop after a severe respiratory infection. The development of peripheral edema occurs late in the disease as a result of associated cor pulmonale.

PHYSICAL FINDINGS

Positive physical findings do not occur until late in the disease. At that time, physical examination shows expiratory prolongation, as in the emphysematous patient. Often, especially in exacerbations of chronic bronchitis, inspiration is also prolonged, since luminal occlusion from bronchial inflammation and secretions does not entirely disappear with inspiration. Percussion of the chest is usually normal; auscultation reveals variously pitched wheezes and rales. These sounds are usually quite loud and are caused by the bronchial narrowing and secretions.

Patients with chronic bronchitis are sometimes called "blue bloaters" or "nonfighters" because they have bouts of hypoxia, hypercapnia, and right heart failure with peripheral edema. They are cyanotic and edematous secondary to the cor pulmonale. These changes relate to the severe amount of ventilation–perfusion mismatching (largely shunt) that occurs in bronchitis.

PULMONARY FUNCTION TESTING

The pulmonary function profile of bronchitis is shown in Table 31-2. A major point of separation from emphysema is that patients with bronchitis have normal pulmonary elastic recoil and relatively normal diffusion capacities, which is understandable because they do not have disruption of alveoli. Flow rates during both expiration and inspiration are reduced, al-

Table 31-2. Pulmonary Function Profiles of Obstructive Pulmonary Diseases

DISEASE	ELASTIC RECOIL	STATIC COMPLIANCE	AIRWAY RESISTANCE	RV/TLC	D_{LCO}	BRONCHO-DILATOR RESPONSE
Bronchitis	Normal	Normal	↑	Normal to ↑	Normal to slightly decreased	2+
Asthma	Normal (↓ in acute attack)	Normal (↑ in acute attack)	↑	Normal to ↑	Slightly decreased normal or ↑	4+
Emphysema	↓	↑	↑ or normal	↑	Markedly ↓	0
Small airways disease	Normal	Normal	Normal	Normal or slightly increased	Normal	0

though the reduction is expiratory flow is usually more pronounced. Air trapping is an inconstant finding in bronchitis, depending on the severity of the airways obstruction.

SPUTUM CHARACTERISTICS

As a rule the sputum is mucoid, thick, and tenacious. The sputum may be purulent, depending on whether the patient is simultaneously infected. Generally, sputum production is more common in the morning.

COURSE

The course of the chronic bronchitic case depends on the number of acute exacerbations. In England, where this condition is very prevalent, total disability from chronic bronchitis may occur by the time the patient is 45 years of age.

TREATMENT

Besides bronchodilator therapy and hydration (which is all-important), there is little specific treatment for chronic bronchitis other than the cessation of cigarette smoking and avoidance of known airway irritants. Water (e.g., 10 to 12 glasses/day) is the safest and most effective expectorant. The use of glyceryl guaiacolate as an expectorant has now been largely abandoned, but use of saturated solution of potassium iodide (SSKI) may be helpful (see Chap. 20).

When specific pathogens can be identified from the sputum, appropriate antibiotic therapy may be necessary. Failing the isolation of a specific pathogen, the empiric use of ampicillin, amoxicillin, or trimethoprim-sulfamethoxazole may be helpful. Very severe, acute exacerbations of bronchitis require intravenous hydration, antibiotics, intravenous aminophylline, inhaled beta-2 adrenergic bronchodilator therapy, bland aerosol inhalation, controlled oxygen therapy, chest physical therapy, and occasionally total ventilator support. Whether the use of continuous antibiotics for prophylaxis is of value is debatable. Steroid and desensitization therapy is of no value. Clapping and postural drainage may be helpful in patients with excessive sputum. Occasionally bronchoscopy is helpful during acute exacerbations in order to aspirate inspissated mucus plugs and to reverse atelectasis.

ASTHMA

Asthma may be defined as a group of disease states in which reversible, widespread airways obstruction oc-

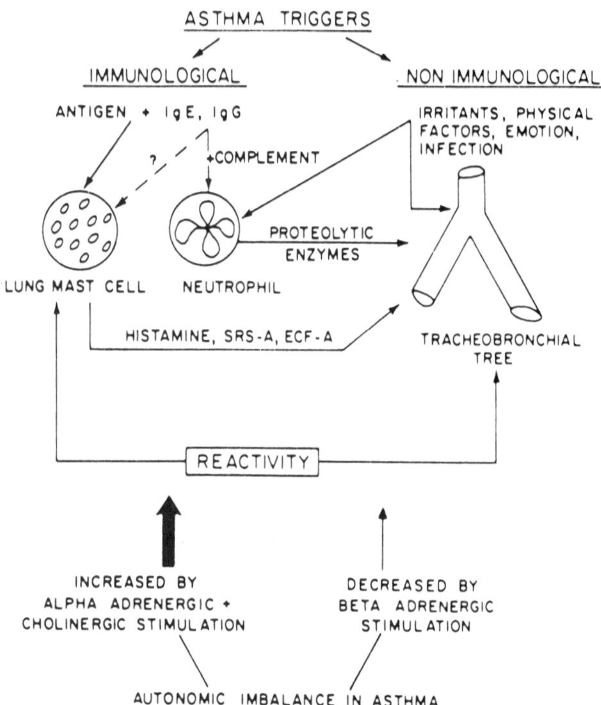

Fig. 31-3. In bronchial asthma, airway obstruction appears to be the result of nonspecific noxious stimuli or immunologic phenomena, or both. One attractive hypothesis is that the basic abnormality is an imbalance between factors responsible for relaxation of bronchial smooth muscle and stability of mast cells. Mediator release may be controlled through maintenance of adequate cAMP levels in these tissues. Agents that lower cAMP or stimulate cholinergic receptors facilitate bronchial smooth muscle contraction and mediator release. (Wilson AF, Galant SP: Recent advances in the pathophysiology of asthma. West J Med 120:463, 1974. Used with permission)

curs. About one half of patients with asthma may be classified as having either clearcut extrinsic asthma (bronchial asthma) or intrinsic asthma (asthmatic bronchitis.) This classification is being recognized more and more as one of significant clinical usefulness.

Asthma has been estimated to afflict between 8 to 10 million people in the United States, and the mortality rate of intractable asthma (status asthmaticus) may be as high as 20% to 50%. Since the publication of the first edition of *Respiratory Care*, much new information relating to cellular and molecular biology, neuropharmacokinetics, smooth muscle physiology, and immunology has accumulated, all of which enhances our ability to diagnose precisely, and to treat more wisely, this common disorder.

The "asthmatic state" is characterized by hyperreactivity of the airways to inhaled, ingested, or otherwise acquired stimuli that would ordinarily produce few, if any, symptoms in the nonasthmatic person. The hyper-reactive state is characterized by smooth muscle spasm, edema, inflammation, and mucus hypersecretion, all of which converge to produce striking resistance to air flow.

The etiology and pathogenesis of asthma is actually much more complex than the above would indicate. In the last 10 years, two separate but distinctively linked theories have been postulated to account for the "asthmatic state:" the theory of beta-adrenergic blockade; and the theory of autonomic imbalance (the so-called neurogenic) theory.

The *theory of beta-adrenergic blockade* postulates that there is congenital or acquired diminished responsiveness of beta-adrenergic receptors in asthmatic patients. These receptors, among other things, are responsible for *normal* bronchomotor tone (relaxation). This theory implies that, in the bronchial smooth muscle, diminished responsiveness to beta-adrenergic stimulation is due to reduced accumulation of intercellular cyclic AMP (cAMP). This situation would favor smooth muscle contraction (Fig. 31-3).

An important counterpart of the beta-adrenergic blockade theory is that cells other than bronchial smooth muscle cells are involved. Mast cells in the lung (Fig. 31-4) and blood basophils, when sensitized

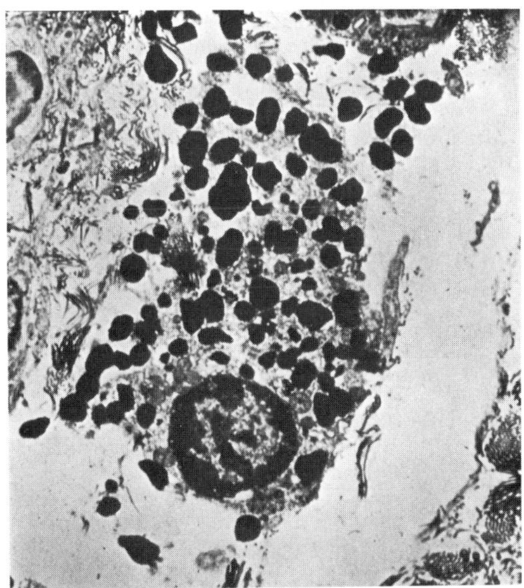

Fig. 31-4. Degranulating sensitized submucosal mast cell following antigenic challenge. Multiple lysozomal packets thought to contain bronchoconstrictor and vasodilator substances are being released from the cell.

Table 31-3. Mast Cell Mediators of Immediate Hypersensitivity

PREFORMED	BIOLOGIC PROPERTIES
Histamine	Contract smooth muscle; increase vascular permeability; stimulate sensory receptors; enhance or inhibit eosinophil migration
Eosinophil chemotactic factor of anaphylaxis (ECF-A)	Eosinophil and neutrophil chemotaxis
Eosinophil chemotactic factor—Oligopeptides	Eosinophil and neutrophil chemotaxis
Neutrophil chemotactic factor	Neutrophil and eosinophil chemotaxis
Heparin	Anticoagulation
Lung kallikrein of anaphylaxis (LK-A)	Kinin generation (contract smooth muscle; increase vascular permeability; stimulate sensory receptors)
NEWLY GENERATED	
Slow-reacting substance of anaphylaxis (SRS-A)—a leukotriene	Contract smooth muscle; increase vascular permeability
Platelet activating factor(s)	Platelet aggregation and degranulation
Lipid chemotactic factors	Neutrophil chemotaxis
Prostaglandins	Control bronchomotor tone

(From Middleton E Jr: Kinds of asthma: Part II. Park Ridge, Illinois, CME publication of the American College of Chest Physicians, 1980)

with IgE antigen-specific antibody, release chemical mediators of anaphylaxis (Table 31-3) following exposure to antigen. The release system again is characterized by a relative decrease in cAMP or an increase in cyclic GMP (cGMP). Release of mediators is inhibited *in vitro* by beta-adrenergic agents (e.g., isoproterenol) and is enhanced by alpha-adrenergic agents such as norepinephrine and phenylephrine. Cholinergic agents (e.g., acetylcholine) tend to increase mediator release by increasing cellular levels of cGMP, an effect that can be blocked by the parasympatholytic agent atropine.

Finally, the locally released chemical mediators of anaphylaxis exert their respective effects on smooth muscle, blood vessels, and mucous glands; these effects are not modulated properly because of the "blocked" beta-adrenergic system previously discussed.

The *neurogenic theory* is based on the presence of a vagally mediated, cholinergic bronchoconstrictor response to irritant challenge. Stimulation of subepithelial receptors in the airways results in a bronchoconstrictor response. Both the afferent and efferent portions of this response are carried in the vagus nerve. The response can be stimulated by cholinergic agents and histamine and blunted or abolished by atropine.

This reflex is more active when the bronchial epithelium is denuded, as after infection, and thus may be very important in the pathogenesis of intrinsic asthma.

EXTRINSIC (BRONCHIAL) ASTHMA

Bronchial asthma is a clinical syndrome that reflects a hyperreactive state of the bronchial airways to multiple factors including extrinsic allergens such as pollens, dusts, and danders. The antigenic fraction of pollens and danders appears to be absorbed directly onto the nasal and hypopharyngeal airways and does not need to be deposited deep in the lung, as was originally thought.

These sensitizing substances, when inhaled (or, in the case of foodstuffs, ingested) call forth, in genetically atopic persons, formation of sensitizing antibody (IgE or *reagin*). With subsequent reintroduction of the antigen, antigen–antibody reaction on the by-then sensitized basophils and mast cells occurs.

By definition, bronchial asthma is a disease that usually begins in childhood, in a patient with a strong personal or family history of allergy. Antedating symptoms may be those of hay fever, eczema, or food allergy. Type I hypersensitivity (immediate reaction), mediated by immune globulin E, plays an important role in the syndrome. This is demonstrated by the "wheal and flare" reaction to antigen-specific skin tests. A secondary bronchoconstrictive response may occur 6 to 8 hours after an irritant challenge. Administration of cromolyn sodium will block both the immediate and the secondary responses; corticosteroids will block only the late reaction. The mechanism of the "late response" has yet to be explained satisfactorily.

"*Not all that wheezes is asthma.*" In his excellent and concise monograph on important pulmonary diseases, Mitchell lists a number of other conditions not mediated by IgE that may produce wheezing (*see* p. 795).[29] These conditions may coexist with each other or with true asthma.

Whatever the inciting factor or mechanisms involved, the effect of airways obstruction at first depends on the site and the degree of the obstruction. With mild airways obstruction, patients will breathe nearer the total lung capacity with resultant increased oxygen consumption and increased cardiac output. Although the symptoms and signs of airway obstruction are most characteristic in asthma, dyspnea is more closely related to the elevated lung volume at which the patient is breathing, presumably because of an increased work of breathing at higher lung volumes, where the compliance of lungs and chest wall is greatly reduced. Pulmonary blood flow and volume will be increased, leading to an increase in the diffusion capacity.

If the airways obstruction is severe enough or other still poorly defined parenchymal changes occur, shunting and hypoxemia will result. Finally, with exhaustion, carbon dioxide retention and respiratory and metabolic acidemia may develop.

PHYSICAL EXAMINATION

There may be no physical findings during a period of total remission. An acute asthmatic attack may be preceded by an apparent upper respiratory infection or "hay fever," with nasal and conjunctival itching, congestion, and discharge.

During an acute attack, dyspnea, expectoration of mucoid sputum, overexpansion of the chest, wheezing, and rhonchi will be found. With more severe attacks, cyanosis, sweating, and dehydration may occur.

In children, the so-called allergic salute (a horizontal wiping of the nose with the finger or hand), "rabbit nose" (constant wiggling and wrinkling of the nose), frequent night sweats, or "allergic shiners" (dark circles under the eyes) all may be early and suspicious signs of allergy. Eczema during infancy is an early sign of allergy as well.

An ominous physical finding in severe asthma is that of pulsus paradoxus, where there may be a greater than 25 mm Hg decrease in both systolic and diastolic blood pressures during inspiration. A high pulse rate (in excess of 130/min) is another ominous sign and may be due to either hypoxemia or medication (e.g., aminophylline) effect. Progression from easily heard to negligible wheezing may *not* be a sign of relief of bronchoconstriction; on the contrary, it may *herald* almost complete airway obstruction ("locked lung") and is of grave prognostic impact unless successfully treated.

PULMONARY FUNCTION TESTING

The pulmonary function profile of asthma is shown in Table 31-2. Narrowing of the airways results in reduced airflow rates and increased airway resistance. A key pulmonary function abnormality in the asthmatic patient is the *reversibility* of the elevated airway resistance with bronchodilator drugs. Unlike bronchitis and emphysema, there is often striking improvement in expiratory flows following inhaled bronchodilator treatment. The carbon monoxide diffusion capacity is normal or increased, using the single-breath method; however, it may be decreased using the steady-state method. The lung usually has a normal elastic recoil.

Static lung volumes are variable, depending on the degree of airways obstruction. As mentioned earlier, during an attack, the functional residual capacity, residual volume, and total lung capacity are increased. During remission, the lung volumes may be normal.

Recent work has indicated that the patient's own estimate of the severity of his asthma is often better than that of the examining physician.[22] These perceptions should certainly not go unheeded in managing the patient's asthmatic condition.

Hypoxemia and preterminal carbon dioxide retention are secondary to profound ventilation–perfusion abnormalities within the lung.

DISEASES ACCOMPANIED BY WHEEZING

- Acute and chronic bronchitis and bronchiolitis due to bacteria, viruses, or fungi
- Inhalation of irritants (*e.g.,* smoke [including tobacco], dusts, fumes, chemicals, and air pollutants)
- Exercise-induced bronchospasm
- Acute left ventricular failure or so-called cardiac asthma
- Bronchial obstruction by an intraluminal foreign body
- Neoplasm (*e.g.,* bronchial adenoma or carcinoma causing partial localized obstruction)
- Carcinoid syndrome
- Drug-induced causes (*e.g.,* cholinergic drug intoxication, beta-adrenergic blockade [propranolol], and overuse of isoproterenol cartridges)
- Acute pulmonary embolism
- Miscellaneous conditions, occasionally associated with wheezing (*e.g.,* polyarteritis nodosa, Löffler's syndrome, tropical eosinophilia, extrinsic allergic alveolitis, and aspirin hypersensitivity [which is generally associated with nasal polyps or sinusitis])

(Ward GW, Mitchell RS: Bronchial asthma. In Mitchell RS (ed): Diagnosis of Clinical Pulmonary Disease. St. Louis, CV Mosby, 1974)

Other Useful Diagnostic Tests in Asthma

Airway challenge (bronchial provocation) tests, various skin tests, and the relatively recently developed radioallergosorbent test (RAST) are sometimes useful diagnostic tests.

In the laboratory, the hyperactive airway responds with bronchoconstriction when challenged by very low concentrations of some of the actual mediators of immune response, including histamine, prostaglandin F_2, and a cogener of acetylcholine, methacholine. Doses $1/1{,}000^{th}$ to $1/10{,}000^{th}$ smaller than would evoke a response in a normal person call forth increased airway resistance in the asthmatic patient within minutes. Similar responses may be obtained by direct inhalation of fumes and suspect dusts and mold extracts, but these tests should only be performed in specialized laboratories with sensitive equipment (e.g., body plethysmography) and experienced personnel.

Skin tests have been used for many years to identify specific antigens responsible for the allergic reaction. If positive, they provide a rough estimate of antigen-specific antibody in the area of skin pricked, scratched, or injected with antigen intradermally. Current consensus is that these tests should probably be performed in adults only occasionally (since there is only a 5–25% correlation between inhaled antigen response and positive skin-test results). Skin test specifically is much higher in childhood bronchial asthma, where, of course, antigen-specific IgE is a vital component of the immune response. Wherever these tests are performed, faculties and personnel should be available to treat any acute, unforeseen anaphylactic response.

The RAST is the first commercially available test that directly measures specific IgE antibodies in the patient's serum.[30] As with skin testing, complete RAST surveys are not inexpensive. As with the skin test, clinical correlation must be made between known, real-life exposure reactions and positive test results. Correlation between positive skin tests and the RAST is 75% to 90% generally and nearly 100% in profound hypersensitivity states. At present, indications for use of the RAST appear to be for corroboration of doubtful skin test results; for standardization of "immune targeted" antigens; in children with skin conditions such as eczema that would preclude skin testing; in patients who cannot stop medications (e.g., corticosteroids, which would invalidate skin test results); in the diagnosis of IgE-mediated food sensitivity; and in the diagnosis of IgE-mediated sensitivity to industrial agents.

Routine Laboratory Studies

Blood eosinophilia is usually present in the patient not on corticosteroids. Slight leukocytosis with an otherwise normal differential is common. Sputum Gram's stain and cultures are usually unrewarding but should be done in case an infectious component is present. Serum electrolytes, glucose, and creatinine studies should be used as indicated.

SPUTUM

The sputum is characteristically clear, thick, and tenacious. It contains larger than normal amounts of mucopolysaccharide and neuraminic acid. Sputum is characteristically laden with eosinophils and may demonstrate small casts of the terminal bronchioles (Curschmann's spirals). Microscopic examination may show precipitated mucopolysaccharide-protein complexes known as Charcot–Leyden crystals and bits of exfoliated ciliated respiratory epithelium (creola bodies).

Because the mediators of anaphylaxis may also depress mucociliary function, patients may actually expectorate little sputum until bronchodilation and rehydration have been effected.

COURSE

The course of bronchial asthma is extremely variable. More than one half of the involved children outgrow their illness by 20 years of age; one third may be bothered on and off through adult life with attacks of bronchospasm. As far as is currently known, the disease does not develop into emphysema.

TREATMENT

Current therapy for asthma includes adequate therapy during the asymptomatic as well as symptomatic interval. Patient education regarding recognition of significant signs and symptoms is vital.

Vigorous bronchial hygiene is indicated. Specific therapy to consider includes strict avoidance of known allergens, desensitization with antigens, use of corticosteroid drugs, and use of the drug cromolyn. Inhalation of cromolyn sodium has been effective in about 50% of patients with extrinsic asthma. This agent apparently blocks the release of chemical mediators of bronchospasm such as histamine and SRS-A from sensitized mast cells. It is not a bronchodilator. Its use has resulted in a reduction of attacks, decreased need for corticosteroids, and a lessened need for hospitalization.

Inhalation of beclomethasone dipropionate or triamcinolone acetonide has been shown to reduce markedly the frequency and severity of bronchospasm. The advantage of these agents over inhaled dexamethasone and oral corticosteroids is that they provide the airway benefit of steroids and yet avoid the systemic side-effects. The use of bronchodilator prostaglandins, particularly prostaglandin E_1 (PGE_1), is still in the experimental stage.

Bronchodilators should be used vigorously but certainly not abused. Rational dosage regimens for these agents are described in Chapter 20. Concomitant use of inhaled as well as systemic bronchodilator agents, especially the beta-2 stimulators, seems to be gaining favor.[25] Combined use of theophylline with beta-2 stimulators is also in current favor. Oxygenation, oral or intravenous hydration, and humidification of inspired air are vital to therapeutic success.

Status asthmaticus is a term used to describe severe attacks of asthma refractory to standard therapy. Long delays before seeking treatment, incomplete assessment of the severity of attacks, overuse of inhaled bronchodilator and sedative drugs and underuse of corticosteroids are predisposing factors. Markedly labile asthmatic patients, and patients with progressive carbon dioxide retention, are at particular risk of sudden death from status asthmaticus. For a severe attack, hospitalization may be necessary for ventilatory support, oxygen therapy, intravenous hydration, and intravenous aminophylline and corticosteroids. Corticosteroids should be given in dosages high enough to induce eosinopenia; the dosage varies greatly from patient to patient.[9] Sedatives and narcotics are contraindicated unless the patient is being ventilated artificially. Tracheobronchial lavage and suctioning by bronchoscopy may be needed if thick, tenacious mucus persists despite the foregoing vigorous therapy. Multiple mucus plugs may be aspirated with this technique. Removal of the carotid body (glomectomy) has been advocated, but no scientific data support the use of this technique at present.

INTRINSIC ASTHMA (ASTHMATIC BRONCHITIS)

Intrinsic asthma is a condition in which a series of events similar to those described for extrinsic (bronchial) asthma is initiated by unknown mechanisms. No definite immunologic precipitants can be detected by currently available techniques. The genetic history of allergy is not nearly as strong as that in extrinsic asthma. Often there is a history of infection. Division into these two types of asthma may be somewhat artificial; indeed, patients often do not fit exactly into either one of these categories. Those who meet my criteria for asthmatic bronchitis meet the American Thoracic Society criteria for both chronic bronchitis and bronchial asthma. The typical history is that of a patient who, in midlife, develops pneumonia or some other respiratory tract infection. After this clears, he is left with a syndrome indistinguishable from episodic bronchial asthma.

Wheezing and cough productive of mucopurulent, thick, viscid sputum and severe episodic respiratory distress constitute the full-blown condition. This disease is much more common than is usually recognized. Many patients are told that they have chronic bronchitis and are disappointed when it does not respond to standard therapy. The key to diagnosis lies in finding eosinophils in expectorated secretions or in the blood. The presence of *sputum eosinophilia* is of immediate prognostic significance; it indicates that the patient has a prominent component of *reversible* airways obstruction. If the clinical situation warrants, oral, parenteral, or inhaled corticosteroids are indicated. As in bronchial asthma, the corticosteroid dosage should induce both blood and sputum eosinopenia.

PULMONARY FUNCTION FINDINGS

As would be expected, pulmonary function findings are a cross between those of chronic bronchitis and bronchial asthma. Bronchodilator reversibility of the reduced expiratory air flows is usual. Depending on the severity of airways obstruction, air trapping may be present.

TREATMENT

Specifics of treatment include the judicious use of oral steroids, often in short courses, starting with 40 to 60 mg of prednisone and tapering to 0 mg over 7 to 10 days. The use of alternate-day steroids and inhaled triamcinolone acetonide or beclomethasone dipropionate provides the steroid benefit and yet avoids undesirable systemic side-effects. Disodium cromoglycate is less efficacious in this syndrome, although there have been scattered case reports of its successful use. Desensitization is generally not helpful, unlike the situation in IgE-mediated extrinsic asthma. Attention to coincident infection is important, and broad-spectrum antibiotic use at the first sign of a chest infection is rewarding. Adequate fluid intake is obviously important.

COURSE

The course of this disease is variable. If treatment is continued for long enough (e.g., as long as 2 years), many such patients will have no further recurrences of the illness. However, some patients will continue to need appropriate therapy indefinitely.

OTHER FORMS OF ASTHMA

Other forms of asthma are now well recognized but will not be discussed here. They include exercise-induced asthma, asthma during or after cold air exposure, aspirin-induced asthma, and many forms of occupational asthma. Allergic bronchopulmonary aspergillosis is another noteworthy inclusion in the list of atypical asthmas. The reader is referred to a recent publication for additional information.[7]

PULMONARY EMPHYSEMA

Pulmonary emphysema may be defined as enlargement of the distal air spaces, with alveolar fragmentation and breakdown of the alveolar septa. Associated with the disruption of alveoli is a loss of lung elasticity. Much of the expiratory obstruction in emphysema appears to be mechanical (see Zone C, Fig. 31-1). Chapter 9 points out the manner in which the terminal bronchioles and alveolar ducts depend on the alveolar parenchyma for support. This support is lost in emphysema, and the terminal airways tend to collapse during expiration. Further, the cartilaginous plates that normally surround the segmental and subsegmental bronchi become atrophic and their distribution less organized.[27] The significance of this latter finding remains unclear. It appears that these lesions are part of a general atrophic process rather than an otherwise significant factor in the pathogenesis of emphysema or airways obstruction.

Terminal airways obstruction secondary to poor airways support is only one part of the admittedly

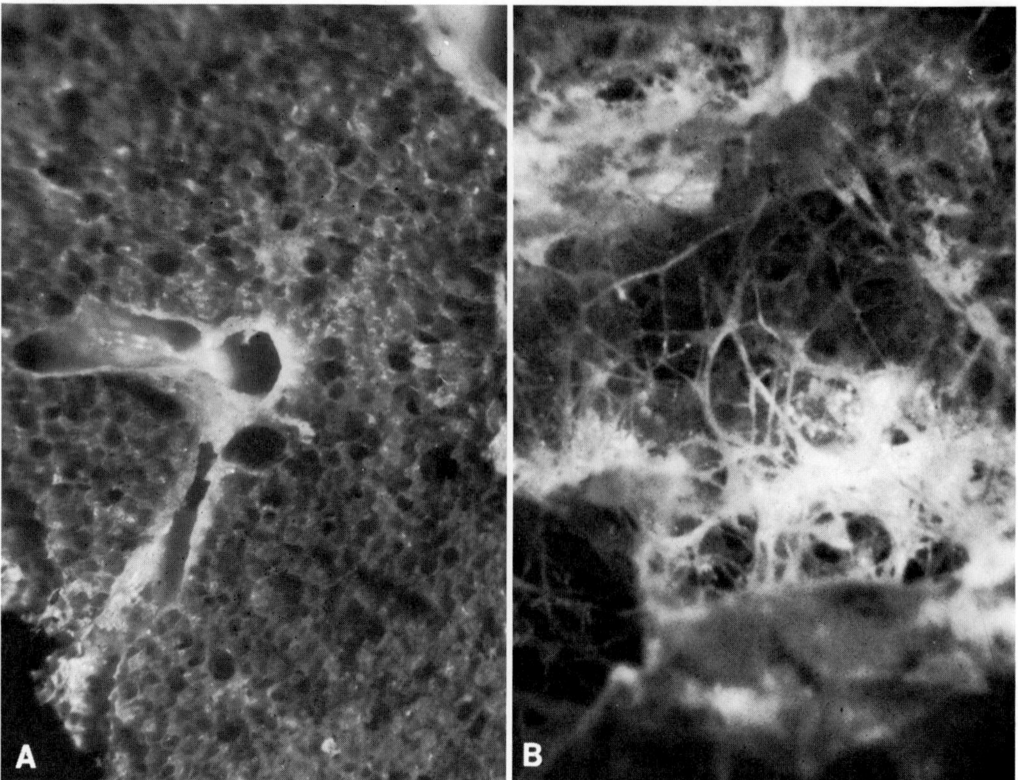

Fig. 31-5. Photomicrographs illustrating alveolar enlargement and disruption in panacinar emphysema *(B)* compared to normal adult lung *(A)*. Magnification is similar (× 15) in both panels.

complicated pathophysiology of pulmonary emphysema. The patient with emphysema tends to retain secretions and to develop repeated infections easily, particularly when the emphysema is of the *centrilobular* variety, associated with chronic bronchitis. About 80% to 90% of patients with chronic obstructive pulmonary disease have combined chronic bronchitis and emphysema.

In *panlobular* (panacinar) emphysema, the primary abnormality appears to be alveolar fragmentation (Fig. 31-5) and air trapping. The entire acinus is involved, whereas in centrilobular emphysema the major problem is with the respiratory bronchioles. The essential feature of this condition is loss of parenchymal substances and alveolar enlargement, as mentioned earlier. In fact, the pathology of emphysema is quite complex and is worth considering by all those who would treat the disease intelligently.[19]

Certain cognate lung conditions resemble emphysema in many ways and must be excluded in the differential diagnosis, including pyogenic lung ascesses, "honeycomb lung" characteristic of end-stage pulmonary fibrosis, many inflammatory conditions of the alveolar wall, sarcoidosis, and bronchiolectasis.

Unilateral translucency of the lung *(MacLeod's syndrome)* is a condition in which one lung is more radiolucent than the other. Resected specimens from these lungs show widespread bronchitis or bronchiolitis obliterans, with air trapping on the affected side. Emphysema is widespread throughout, with enlargement of the alveoli and hypoplasia of the pulmonary arteries. This condition is usually seen in childhood. Patients with this syndrome are usually asymptomatic. Deep expiration films reveal air trapping in the translucent lung. Pulmonary angiography shows filling only of the proximal pulmonary artery, in contrast to normal central and peripheral filling seen on the normal side. Bronchography demonstrates patchy bronchiolitis obliterans on the affected side.

Several other types of emphysema should be mentioned. One is so-called *compensatory emphysema,* a condition in which lung units (lobules or lobes) may enlarge, not in terms of function, but rather in terms of space occupation by filling the thoracic volume previously occupied by now atelectatic, fibrotic, or previously surgically removed segments of lung tissue.

"*Senile emphysema*" occurs in older people whose tendency toward a "barrel chest" deformity is well known. In this condition, kyphotic changes in the spine result in upward and outward displacement of the thoracic ribs in the direction of inspiration. The lung follows chest wall motion normally, and the alveolar spaces tend to become somewhat larger (Fig. 31-6). The enlargement of air spaces with aging is not of the magnitude seen in pulmonary emphysema, and the physiological sequelae are minimal at best.

By far the most common and clinically important types of emphysema are those associated with airways obstruction due to bronchitis and bronchiolitis (centrilobular emphysema) or, in the case of panlobular emphysema, due to poor terminal airways support. The bronchitic elements are partly reversible.

ETIOLOGY AND PATHOGENESIS

Much is known about the etiology and the pathogenesis of emphysema, but all evidence is still not in.[11,24] *Cigarette smoking* seems to be easily the most common cause, although inhalation of certain *atmospheric pollutants,* particularly oxidants, dusts, and cadmium vapors, is also thought to cause breakdown of alveoli. The precise role of *infection* in the etiology of emphysema is at present unclear, but some evidence suggests that focal *mechanical factors,* such as retained intraluminal secretions and air trapping, can indirectly lead to breakdown of alveolar tissue. Chemical factors associated within infection, such as neutrophil-derived proteases, have also been implicated.

That certain genetic factors have an important part to play in the development of emphysema has been known for some time. The discovery of *antitrypsin deficiency* associated with emphysema has opened up an entirely new vista of complex etiologic factors that may eventually lead to emphysema.[12] Alpha-1-antitrypsin is the major component of alpha-1-globulin in normal adult plasma. In patients with a genetic deficiency of this factor, proteases contained in leukocytes and perhaps alveolar macrophages result in destruction of lung parenchyma. Severe (homozygous) deficiency of alpha-1-antitrypsin accounts for only a very small proportion (1–2%) of all cases of emphysema. Intermediate (heterozygous) alpha-1-antitrypsin deficiency states probably predispose to milder forms of emphysema and chronic bronchitis. Identification of these heterozygotes, which compose between 10% and 20% of the total emphysematous population, is important so that genetic

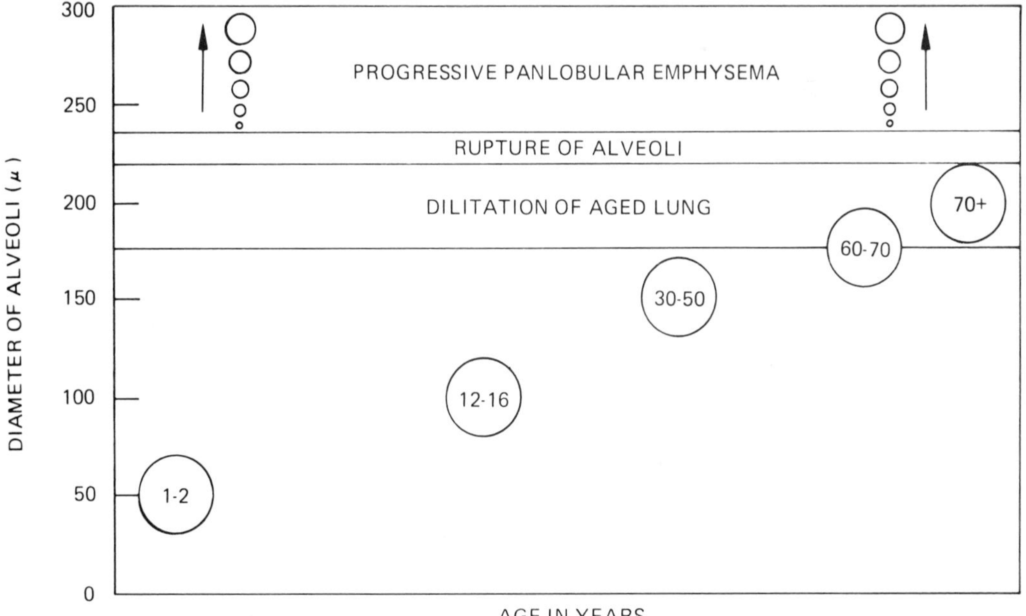

Fig. 31-6. Alveolar size as a function of age. Note that the alveolar diameter in emphysema greatly exceeds the normal for age. The increased alveolar volume results in poor intrapulmonary gas mixing.

counseling can be given and the patients urged not to smoke and to avoid other airway irritants.[15]

Very severe emphysema may accompany other manifestations of Marfan's syndrome, a connective tissue disorder generally thought to be genetically determined, although poorly understood. Similarly, enlargement of the distal air spaces is seen in some forms of cystic fibrosis. Such information has now led to the rather clear belief that there is, at least to some extent, a genetic predisposition to emphysema that is further aggravated by environmental factors, most notably cigarette smoking and air pollution.

PATHOPHYSIOLOGY

In classic panlobular emphysema, ventilation, diffusion, and perfusion are all involved to some extent. Regional alveolar *ventilation* is decreased primarily because of the decreased elastic recoil of the lungs, poor support of the terminal airways, air trapping, and poor intra-alveolar gas mixing in the involved areas. In association with chronic bronchitis (the "blue bloater" syndrome), overall alveolar hypoventilation may occur, associated with a reduced response to hypoxic and hypercapneic respiratory stimuli.

Enlargement of the distal air spaces increases the intraluminal distance for molecular gas *diffusion*. Pulmonary diffusion is further reduced because of loss of alveolar surface membrane and regional and generalized pulmonary vasoconstriction. Hypoxemia and pressure by adjacent distended alveoli may reduce perfusion to otherwise normal alveoli, further resulting in a reduced capillary blood volume and a decreased diffusion capacity.

Finally, emphysema can be thought of as a *perfusion* abnormality in which hypoxemia causes generalized pulmonary arterial vasospasm and shunting of blood away from even relatively normal areas of lung. Further, the distortion of the pulmonary microcirculation results in slowing of the pulmonary capillary blood flow and in vascular thrombosis in some cases. Coincident inflammation and infection of the lung may participate in some of the vascular abnormalities just described. Hypertrophy of the media in the walls of the pulmonary arterioles may reflect pulmonary hypertension.

The argument as to whether pulmonary hypertension and right heart failure cause, or are associated with, concomitant left heart failure continues.[4,13,23]

HISTORY

Exertional dyspnea is the earliest symptom of emphysema. The patient may complain of a productive cough. As has been mentioned elsewhere, the patient may attribute the mild exertional dyspnea to his "being out of shape" and his cough to "that cigarette cough again!" The conscious awareness of these critical symptoms, particularly in a relatively inactive populace, is thus often a very slowly developing affair.

As emphysema worsens, other symptoms, such as loss of appetite, weight loss, position-dependent breathing, inactivity, and depression, develop. Cough and sputum production may worsen although this is not part of the primary symptom complex. In short, the symptoms of emphysema are so nonspecific that they may be overlooked or attributed to something else.

PHYSICAL FINDINGS

In more advanced cases of emphysema, the characteristic "barrel chest" deformity (*see* Fig. 13-1) with low-lying, immobile diaphragms, hyperresonance to percussion, decreased to absent breath sounds, and cor pulmonale with hepatomegaly and peripheral edema may be present. Expiratory prolongation is present and tactile fremitus diminished. Chest expansion will be reduced, and the patient will use the accessory muscles of respiration to breath.

The patient may elect to sit at the side of the bed in the typical arms-braced "emphysematous habitus," wherein the insertions of the accessory respiratory muscles are fixed, making for easier gas exchange. Heart sounds will be distant to absent. Often heart sounds will be heard and right ventricular heaves palpated only in the epigastrium. Movements of the chest and abdominal musculature may be asynchronous.[2]

LABORATORY DATA AND PULMONARY FUNCTION TESTING

The chest roentgenogram will characteristically show overexpansion, low-lying diaphragms, and a vertical heart. The lung parenchyma will be hyperlucent, and the peripheral vascular markings may be diminished. All of these findings are nonspecific and may occur in other obstructive airway conditions, such as severe bronchial asthma. Although the roentgenogram is useful in diagnosing emphysema, it may be overinterpreted in the hands of an unskilled observer. The lateral chest roentgenogram is of more help in this regard (Fig. 31-7). It may show flattening of the diaphragm, an increased retrosternal air space, and perhaps some intercostal bulging of lung parenchyma between the rib margins. Again, all these findings are nonspecific.

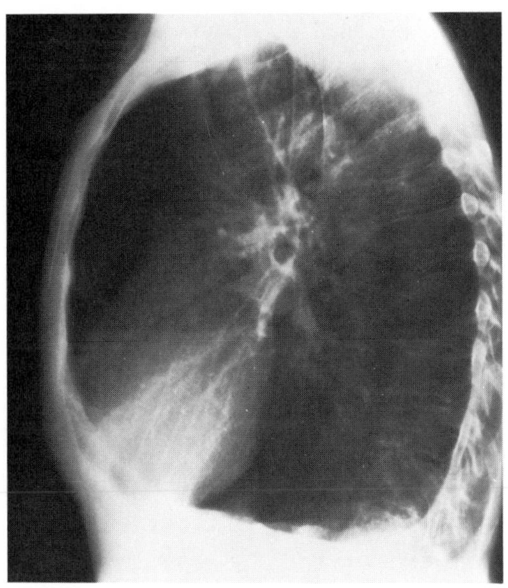

Fig. 31-7. Lateral chest x-ray in pulmonary emphysema. Note the increased anteroposterior diameter, low-lying diaphragms, and increased volume of the retrosternal air space.

Filling of the lower half of the retrosternal space with heart shadow may indicate right ventricular hypertrophy.

Airway resistance may be increased or normal, depending on whether a bronchitic component is present. The flow-volume loop has a characteristic shape, as described in Chapter 11. In straight-forward pulmonary emphysema, there will be no bronchodilator response. The carbon monoxide diffusion capacity will be decreased. In the genetically determined variant, alpha-1-antitrypsin will be decreased to absent.

The elevated residual volume to total lung capacity ratio reflects expiratory airways collapse and air trapping but, again, is a nonspecific finding in many of the obstructive airway diseases. Collapse of small airways during expiration prevents normal lung deflation even during tidal breathing, and washout of helium or nitrogen will show nonuniformity of ventilation (asynchronous emptying of respiratory units with varying time constants) when breath-by-breath analysis is done.

Arterial blood gas analysis will usually show hypoxemia. Carbon dioxide retention may be present. In patients with relatively good matching of ventilation to perfusion (the so-called pink puffers), normal blood gas concentrations are maintained fairly well until late in the disease. In patients with predominant chronic bronchitis (blue bloaters), significant hypoxemia with carbon dioxide retention is more common.

In panlobular emphysema secondary to alpha-1-antitrypsin deficiency, one characteristically loses perfusion at the lung bases, as noted in ventilation-perfusion lung scans. In centrilobular emphysema, on the other hand, most of the problem is at the apices, with the bases being relatively spared. Decreased ventilation with prolonged washout is seen in lung scans in the areas of involvement.

SPUTUM

Sputum production may be lacking, particularly in panlobular emphysema. If bronchitis complicates the disease, then the sputum may be mucopurulent, thick, and tenacious. No specific diagnostic cellular elements or chemical constituents have been identified in the sputum of patients with emphysema *per se*.

COURSE

The prognosis in emphysema, once diagnosed, is poor. The 5-year mortality after diagnosis in some series is higher than 50%. This mortality rate is analogous to that in lymphoma, a malignant disease of the hematopoietic system.

The even higher mortality of cor pulmonale can be reduced, with vigorous bronchial hygiene and supplemental oxygen therapy, from 70% at 2 years to something less than 30% over the same period. The course of pulmonary emphysema is *more* favorable if it is complicated by bronchitis because this latter complication is in itself treatable.[20] However, when the many implicated etiologic agents actually *destroy* lung parenchyma, then the process is irreversible, and the long-term outlook thereafter is grim.

Accelerated deterioration is found in patients with recurrent infection, coincident left ventricular failure, coronary artery disease, obesity, pulmonary embolism, and pneumothorax.[3]

SPECIFIC TREATMENT

The first and most important step in treating emphysema is that of treating frequently coexisting bronchitis. For those patients who have uncomplicated panlobular emphysema, the treatment perforce is supportive. In these patients, pulmonary rehabilitation (see Chap. 27), including exercise training, not only improves morbidity, but also dramatically reduces hospitalization rates after diagnosis.

The use of "pursed-lip breathing" (*i.e.*, inhaling through the nose, followed by a slow exhalation through pursed lips) has been shown to improve gas exchange.[17] This technique is particularly useful to help relieve dyspnea, especially when the ventilatory requirement has increased (*i.e.*, with exercise).

The use of oxygen at home should be considered in any patient with chronic obstructive airway disease who has a resting Pa_{O_2} less than 55 torr on room air. Oxygen use may be advisable, even with a room air Pa_{O_2} above 55 torr, if an intensive exercise program has been outlined, in order to decrease the likelihood of cardiac arrhythmias and lactic acidosis during exercise. If the Pa_{O_2} is less than 50 torr on room air, the patient should be considered a candidate for continuous or at least nocturnal oxygen therapy.[18,28]

Except for the occasional patient in whom resection of a bullous area may be helpful, there is no specific surgical treatment for emphysema *per se*. Lung transplantation is still in its infancy, and replacement of deficient antiproteases such as alpha-1-antitrypsin is not yet practical.

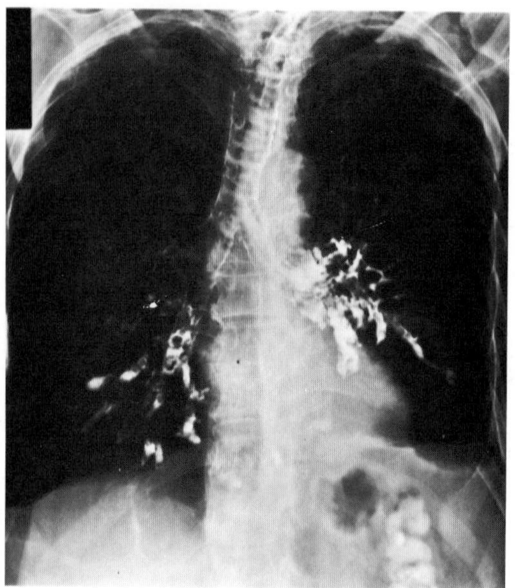

Fig. 31-8. Chest x-ray in saccular bronchiectasis. Note the dilated peripheral airways, which in this bronchogram are filled with contrast material (compare with Figure 14-5).

BRONCHIECTASIS

Bronchiectasis may be defined as a process destructive of the bronchial wall itself, which is diagnosed by bronchography and associated with purulent sputum. Two major types of bronchiectasis are recognized: the saccular type (Fig. 31-8), where enlarged, grapelike dilatations of the airway fill with pooled purulent material and where actual erosion of the airway itself occurs; and that type in which minor fusiform dilations of the airway occur (cylindrical or tubular bronchiectasis). This latter condition is commonly associated with chronic bronchitis and is actually a severe form of chronic bronchitis itself. A mixture of these two basic types of bronchiectasis may also occur.

ETIOLOGY AND PATHOPHYSIOLOGY

The etiology and pathophysiology of both varieties of chronic bronchiectasis are somewhat obscure. Infection clearly plays a major role in this disease process. A history of pertussis ("whooping cough") in childhood is common, but the relation is neither fully understood nor firmly established. Patients with repeated attacks of pneumonia and bronchitis develop areas in which the epithelial surface is denuded of cilia, with peribronchial inflammation, fibrosis, alternate narrowing and dilatation of the airways, and finally necrosis and erosion of portions of the bronchial wall itself. Hypertrophy and hyperplasia of the bronchial (systemic) circulation in the area of the bronchiectatic segment are common and may account for some, if not all, of the hemoptysis. There may be anastomoses between the bronchial and pulmonary vessels, right-to-left shunts, pulmonary hypertension, and cor pulmonale.

Kartagener's syndrome is a recognized genetic variant of saccular bronchiectasis. This syndrome comprises chronic sinusitis, situs inversus, and chronic saccular bronchiectasis. The exact genetic nature of the syndrome has yet to be worked out, but the bronchiectasis is classic and similar to that seen in other forms of generalized saccular bronchiectasis (agammaglobulinemia and cystic fibrosis). The "*immotile-cilia*" *syndrome* may be related to this condition and surely could be involved in the etiology and pathogenesis of secretion retention.[1]

Central airway bronchiectasis is sometimes seen complicating aspergillous mucus plugging.

Saccular bronchiectasis may follow *aspiration* of a foreign body or may follow a severe and *necrotizing pneumonitis* or *tuberculosis*. In these situations, the bronchiectasis is usually localized to the original area of damage.

HISTORY AND PHYSICAL FINDINGS

The common history is that of cough productive of large amounts of purulent, often foul-smelling or bloody sputum. The sputum volume may total several cupfuls daily. Its odor may be that of associated pseudomonas or anaerobic bacterial infection. The sputum, when allowed to stand, has a typical three-layered appearance (*see* Chap. 19), as is also seen in cases of lung abscess. Repeated bouts of pneumonia and hemoptysis are common complaints on history-taking. Sinusitis occurs in a high percentage of patients, even those who do not have associated Kartagener's syndrome. Some patients lose considerable protein in their sputum and become thin and emaciated; others develop classic symptoms of cor pulmonale and resemble the typical "blue bloater" patient in every way. *"Dry bronchiectasis,"* without much sputum production, may occur, particularly in areas of low ambient humidity.

In addition to other findings of expiratory obstruction, coarse rales during inspiration are heard over the involved lobes or segments. Occasional wheezes are heard during expiration as well. Breath sounds are much harsher and more intense than those heard in emphysema; the chest is "noisy," and the diagnosis is often readily made during auscultation by a trained observer. The dependent parts of the lung are those usually involved, most notably the basilar segments of the lower lobes. However, any lobe may be involved, especially in the postpneumonic or post-tubercular variety of the illness.

Nailbed clubbing and cyanosis are seen when the patient develops chronic hypoxia.

LABORATORY FINDINGS

Laboratory findings in chronic bronchiectasis are nonspecific. The plain chest film may show "honeycombing" or be normal. Serum protein electrophoresis may demonstrate elevation of the gamma globulin fraction, indicating chronic infection and inflammation, or hypogammaglobulinemia or agammaglobulinemia in bronchiectasis associated with these latter two conditions. The sputum is filled with much polymorphonuclear debris, and a culture yields a mixed flora, including anaerobic bacteria, fusiform organisms, and spirochetes. The spirogram is that of straightforward obstructive pulmonary disease. There is little, if any, bronchodilator response.

Consideration that bronchiectasis may be present is important in completely evaluating the patient with chronic obstructive pulmonary disease. If persistent findings occur in one segment or lobe, then further studies, including bronchography, are mandatory. Bronchography is the only valid method for demonstrating bronchiectasis accurately.

COURSE

The course of bronchiectasis depends on the severity of the disease. The prognosis is poor if the disease is undiagnosed and untreated. Several studies have shown that long-term survival depends on the number of infectious exacerbations. If exacerbations can be held to a minimum by institution of a comprehensive respiratory care program, the patient may look forward to a long, fairly active, and relatively symptom-free life. Exsanguination from bronchial hemorrhage is decidedly rare.

SPECIFIC TREATMENT

In bronchiectasis, as in cystic fibrosis, especially meticulous bronchial hygiene is necessary. The key therapeutic endeavor here involves vigorous specific chest physical therapy techniques such as percussion, vibration, and postural drainage (discussed in Chap. 26). Specific antibiotic therapy is indicated in acute exacerbations. If the disease process is localized to one segment or lobe, removal of that portion of the lung by surgery may be indicated. Autogenous antibacterial vaccine and gamma globulin therapy have been tried with generally poor results.

SMALL AIRWAYS DISEASE

Not all patients fall clearly into the diagnostic categories listed above. Among such patients are those with what is now being called "small airways obstructive disease." This condition may simply represent early bronchitis or bronchiolitis too mild to be detected by routine simple tests of pulmonary function. The presenting complaints of such patients are usually minimal or absent. If symptoms are present, they are usually those of cough or mild dyspnea on exertion. Many of these patients are cigarette smokers who have been identified as abnormal in various health screening or research programs.

The lungs of such patients have normal elastic recoil, but the small airways (less than 2 mm in diameter) are unstable and tend to close at higher than normal lung volumes. These airways are inflamed;

there is excess mucus and an increased number of goblet cells. At present, we do not know whether this inflammation is reversible, although some encouraging evidence suggests that it is. (Pulmonary function abnormalities in smokers [*see* below] improve upon cessation of smoking.) Small airways disease may be a precursor of chronic bronchitis or emphysema, but these relationships are far from being firmly established. Patients who react to air pollutants with increased closing volumes or frequency-dependency of compliance (*see* Chap. 11) are also thought to have "twitchy airways"—small airways obstructive disease.

PHYSICAL FINDINGS

If any physical findings are present, they consist of minimal expiratory prolongation, a few scattered expiratory wheezes, and, occasionally, atelectatic basilar rales on deep inspiration.

PULMONARY FUNCTION TESTING

The pulmonary function testing pattern of small airways obstructive disease is shown in Table 31-2. Since only 10% to 20% of the resistance to air flow is caused by the small airways, airway resistance is not increased, and thus spirometry and body plethysmographic measurements of airway resistance are normal. However, forced respiration at high frequencies requires that more pressure work be done on the lung, and compliance falls at these frequencies (frequency-dependent compliance). As mentioned above, the closing volume is also increased (*i.e.*, terminal respiratory units are not ventilated at low lung volumes and in areas where alveoli tend to be small anyway, such as in dependent portions of the lung).

Density-dependent flow-volume curves comparing air and helium (volume of isoflow test) show that curves with less dense helium are not as affected by the turbulence created by disease in the small airways as they are when air is breathed. The net result of premature small airways closure is uneven and decreased alveolar ventilation, and mild hypoxemia as a result of the $\dot{V}/\dot{Q}$ mismatch.

SPUTUM CHARACTERISTICS

Sputum production is not usual; when it is expectorated, it has no special identifying features.

TREATMENT

Whether long-term bronchodilation therapy is helpful is not as yet known. Certainly, irritants such as cigarette smoke and air pollutants should be avoided.

SUMMARY

By way of review, I direct the reader's attention to Table 31-2. Separating the obstructive pulmonary diseases into specific groups has been shown to have a number of advantages. Specific management is best related to the specific type of abnormality present, and the opportunity for ultimately unraveling the causes of "COPD" is enhanced to the patient's benefit. The "bread-and-butter" business of respiratory care involves in-depth understanding and comprehensive treatment of the various obstructive pulmonary diseases. Differential diagnosis is a good beginning point.

REFERENCES

1. Afzelius BA: "Immotile-cilia" syndrome and ciliary abnormalities induced by infection and injury. Am Rev Respir Dis 124:107, 1981
2. Ashutosh K et al: Asynchronous breathing movements in patients with chronic obstructive pulmonary disease. Chest 67:553, 1975
3. Burke RN, George RB: Acute respiratory failure in chronic obstructive pulmonary disease: Immediate and long-term prognosis. Arch Intern Med 132:865, 1973
4. Christianson LC, Shah A, Fisher VJ: Quantitative left ventricular cineangiography in patients with chronic obstructive pulmonary disease. Am J Med 66:399, 1979
5. Dunn CR, Dunn DL, Moser KM: Determinants of tracheal injury by cuffed tracheostomy tubes. Chest 65:128, 1974
6. Haponik EF et al: Abnormal inspiratory flow-volume curves in patients with sleep-disordered breathing. Am Rev Respir Dis 124:571, 1981
7. Hodgkin JE (ed): Chronic obstructive pulmonary disease: Current concepts in diagnosis and comprehensive care. Am Coll Chest Physicians, Park Ridge, IL, 1979
8. Hodgkin JE et al: Chronic obstructive airway diseases: Current concepts in diagnosis and comprehensive care. JAMA 232:1243, 1975
9. Horn BR: Total eosinophil counts in the management of bronchial asthma. N Engl J Med 292:1152, 1975
10. Irwin RS, Corrao WM, Pratter MR: Chronic persistent cough in the adult: The spectrum and frequency of causes and successful outcome of specific therapy. Am Rev Respir Dis 123:413, 1981
11. Kilburn KH: New clues for the emphysemas. Am J Med 58:59, 1975
12. Laurell CB, Eriksson S: Electrophoretic alpha$_1$-globulin pattern of serum in alpha$_1$-antitrypsin deficiency. Scand J Clin Lab Invest 15:132, 1968

13. Matthay RA et al: Right and left ventricular exercise performance in chronic obstructive pulmonary disease: Radionuclide assessment. Ann Intern Med 93:234, 1980
14. Miller RD, Hyatt RE: Evaluation of obstructing lesions of the trachea and larynx by flow-volume loops. Am Rev Respir Dis 108:475, 1973
15. Mittman C et al: Smoking and chronic obstructive lung disease in alpha$_1$-antitrypsin deficiency. Chest 60:214, 1971
16. Moser KM: The chronic obstructive pulmonary diseases. Respir Care 20:377, 1975
17. Mueller RE, Petty TL, Filley GF: Ventilation and arterial blood gas changes induced by pursed lip breathing. J Appl Physiol 28:784, 1970
18. Nocturnal Oxygen Therapy Trial Group: Continuous or nocturnal oxygen therapy in hypoxemic chronic obstructive lung disease: A clinical trial. Ann Intern Med 93:391, 1980
19. Reid L: The Pathology of Emphysema. London, Lloyd–Luke, 1967
20. Renzetti AD Jr, McClement JH, Litt BD: The Veterans Administration Cooperative Study of Pulmonary Function. III. Mortality in relation to respiratory function in chronic obstructive pulmonary disease. Am J Med 21:115, 1966
21. Sackner MA et al: Pathogenesis and prevention of tracheobronchial damage with suction procedures. Chest 64:284, 1973
22. Shim CS, Williams MH Jr: Evaluation of the severity of asthma: Patients versus physicians. Am J Med 68:11, 1980
23. Slutsky RA et al: Right and left ventricular dysfunction in patients with chronic obstructive lung disease. Assessment by first-pass radionuclide angiography. Am J Med 68:197, 1980
24. Snider GL: The pathogenesis of emphysema—Twenty years of progress. Am Rev Respir Dis 124:321, 1981
25. Tashkin DP et al: Sites of airway dilatation in asthma following inhaled versus subcutaneous terbutaline. Comparison of physiologic tests with radionuclide lung images. Am J Med 68:14, 1980
26. Thurlbeck WM: Aspects of chronic airflow obstruction. Chest 72:341, 1977
27. Thurlbeck WM et al: Bronchial cartilage and chronic obstructive lung disease. Am Rev Respir Dis 109:73, 1974
28. Timms RM et al: Selection of patients with chronic obstructive pulmonary disease for long-term oxygen therapy. JAMA 245:2514, 1981
29. Ward GW, Mitchell RS: Bronchial asthma. In Mitchell RS (ed): Diagnosis of Clinical Pulmonary Disease. St Louis, CV Mosby, 1974
30. Wide L et al: Diagnosis of allergy by an in vitro test of allergen antibodies. Lancet 25:1105, 1967

32

Respiratory Care in the Coronary Care Unit

Dale J. Wilms • Philip M. Gold
Michael J. Farrell • Suzanne C. Lareau

Intensive care technology, with its beginnings in postsurgical recovery rooms and coronary care units (CCUs), continues to flourish and expand.[56] Increasing technological sophistication, public expectations, and medicolegal concerns contribute to an increasing use of intensive care facilities. While debates continue over admission criteria and intensive care cost-effectiveness, the need for specialized care persists.[66]

Coronary care units in the United States annually admit more than 1.5 million patients with suspected acute ischemic heart disease.[56] Although 50% of these patients are ultimately found not to have acute ischemic events, about 10% require major diagnostic studies or therapeutic procedures such as CPR, cardioversion, intubation, or placement of arterial, central venous, or pulmonary artery and capillary "wedge" catheters.[55,66]

Ventricular arrhythmias continue to cause a significant number of prehospital deaths in cardiac patients, but the increasing availability of lay persons trained in basic life support, as well as skilled paramedical personnel, have improved the survival of the prehospital arrest victim. Successful resuscitation has been performed in 60% to 80% of selected subgroups of such patients.[47]

Although a team approach involving medical, nursing, and other allied health specialists is best for many patient problems, nowhere is this concept more important than in the CCU. While ventricular fibrillation and asystole are final mechanisms of cardiac arrest, respiratory, renal, hepatic, central nervous system, or metabolic dysfunctions are frequent precipitating events. Moreover, even in patients with seemingly isolated cardiac problems, failure of the other major organ-systems often creates formidable management problems.

ACUTE MYOCARDIAL ISCHEMIA

SIGNS AND SYMPTOMS

Chest pain, although not invariably associated with acute myocardial ischemia, is the major presenting symptom of acute myocardial ischemia. There are, however, multiple etiologies of chest pain, and the intensity of pain does not always correlate with the seriousness of the underlying disorder. This fact often is not appreciated by the patient, who tends to equate all chest pain with cardiac disease. The classic angina pain associated with myocardial ischemia consists of a heavy pressure or bandlike constricting sensation in the chest, associated with exercise or emotional stress. Angina usually lasts a few minutes and subsides with rest or nitroglycerin. Characteristically substernal in origin, anginal pain may radiate in any direction, including shoulders, back, arms, or teeth. Radiation of pain to the ulnar aspect of the left arm has been considered a characteristic of ischemic heart disease. Braunwald calls this the "left-arm myth," noting that any thoracic disorder affecting the deep afferent fibers of the upper thoracic nerves can produce this pattern of pain radiation.[11]

The protean manifestations of myocardial ischemic pain make it difficult to delineate from other causes of chest pain. Musculoskeletal pain is generally of a sharper nature, related to movement, and may be identified by finding tenderness over the affected area during physical examination. Pleural pain is also sharp and exacerbated by breathing. Esophageal pain is usually associated with gastrointestinal disorders such as gastroesophageal reflux, indigestion, dysphagia, or weight loss. Other disorders such as dissecting thoracic aortic aneurysm may have characteristics similar to all the above conditions. The differential diagnosis must also include emotional disorders that are expressed as chest pain. The anxious or depressed patient may complain of a substernal aching or tightness. Hyperventilation may lead to tetany of the chest wall as well as the peripheral extremities and accentuate such pain. Hyperventilation and increased adrenergic tone may cause minor ST segment and T-wave changes in the ECG that further confound the diagnosis. Pulmonary embolism may mimic myocardial ischemia with dyspnea, cyanosis, oppressive chest pain, and hypotension. Finally, the diagnostician must remember that two or more diseases may plague the same patient concurrently. Thus discovering a relatively benign disease of the chest does not necessarily rule out a more serious one.

Physical findings in myocardial ischemia without infarction are nonspecific and may include pallor, sweating, transient hypotension, and cardiac arrhythmias.

LABORATORY ABNORMALITIES

Differentiation of myocardial ischemia from an acute myocardial infarction (AMI) requires the discovery of consistent laboratory and electrocardiographic abnormalities in an appropriate clinical setting. The patient with suspected AMI is admitted to the CCU based on his clinical history and ECG. Laboratory confirmation requires hours to days. Increasingly sophisticated enzymatic studies help make interpretation of abnormalities more specific. The MB isoenzyme of creatine phosphokinase (CPK) is found almost exclusively in the myocardium, and the rapidly migrating LDH_1 isoenzyme predominates in the heart.[11] Both are elevated in an AMI. Radionuclide scans, vectorcardiography, echocardiography, and angiography are useful in determining the location and extent of myocardial injury.[57]

ACUTE MYOCARDIAL INFARCTION

PATHOPHYSIOLOGY

In a very complete review of acute myocardial infarction, Oliva convincingly demonstrates that, despite years of investigation, the pathophysiology of AMI is still unclear.[51] Coronary artery thrombosis is associated with most fatal transmural myocardial infarctions, but the sequence of events leading to thrombus formation is not well defined.

Hypercoagulability is present in some patients with myocardial infarction, perhaps due to increased concentrations of clotting factors, increased platelet aggregation, or depressed fibrinolytic activity. The temporal relationship of these factors to AMI and their relative importance still must be elucidated.

Coronary arterial spasm in an otherwise normal coronary artery has been demonstrated to cause severe reversible myocardial ischemia in a condition known as Prinzmetal angina.[27] Maseri and colleagues demonstrated that coronary arterial spasm with or without coronary atherosclerosis could produce myocardial infarction.[48] Some of their patients also had postinfarction thrombus formation demonstrated either angiographically or at postmortem. Oliva and Breckenridge demonstrated coronary arterial spasm superimposed on high-grade atherosclerotic obstruction in 6 of 15 patients with AMI.[52] As investigations continue into the pathophysiology of myocardial infarction, the treatment modalities are being expanded. Surgical revascularization, vasodilator therapy, percutaneous transluminal coronary angioplasty, thrombolytic therapy, and blockade of platelet aggregation are all undergoing extensive clinical trials.[10,39]

SIGNS AND SYMPTOMS

The pain of myocardial infarction is similar in quality and location to that of angina but generally is of longer duration and greater intensity. It, too, is poorly localized substernally and is often accompanied by nausea, dyspnea, diaphoresis, and often the "angor animi" or sense of impending doom or dissolution that causes the patient marked distress.[16]

In a general sense, myocardial infarction is associated with either electrical or mechanical dysfunction, or both. Arrhythmias still cause a significant number of prehospital deaths, although care in the CCU with prophylactic therapy and prompt recognition and treatment of arrhythmias has decreased the associated mortality.[36]

CLINICAL CLASSIFICATIONS

Left ventricular function influences the eventual outcome of the patient with myocardial infarction. Killip and Kimball have classified AMI patients into four groups: class I, no clinical signs of cardiac failure; class II, heart failure with rales, S_3 gallop, and venous hypertension; class III, frank pulmonary edema; and class IV, cardiogenic shock with hypotension and peripheral vasoconstriction.[36] Pulmonary edema was also noted in most class IV patients. Table 32-1 shows the incidence of cardiac arrests and in-hospital deaths in each of these groups. CPK and LDH_1 values (see above) correlate well with infarct size and, in general, increase from class I to class IV. However, congestive failure can occur in the face of a relatively small infarct.[57]

With the advent of pulmonary artery catheterization using Swan–Ganz or other balloon-tipped flotation catheters, hemodynamic data are now readily obtainable, and the functional status of the left ventricle can be more accurately quantified. Using catheterization data, Forrester and colleagues have described a group of hemodynamic subsets based on the cardiac index (CI) and pulmonary capillary wedge pressure (PWP).[25] They are defined as follows: H-I, normal with PWP less than or equal to 18 mm Hg and CI greater than 2.2 liters/min/m^2; H-II, pulmonary congestion without peripheral hypoperfusion, PWP greater than 18 mm Hg, and CI greater than 2.2 liters/min/m^2; H-III, hypoperfusion without pulmonary congestion, PWP less than or equal to 18 mm Hg, and CI less than 2.2 liters/min/m^2; and H-IV, pulmonary congestion and peripheral hypoperfusion, PWP greater than 18 mm Hg, and CI less than 2.2 liters/min/m^2. There is about a 70% correlation between Forrester's hemodynamic subsets and Killip and Kimball's clinical classes.[36] More important than predicting survival rates, hemodynamic information can be used in patient management (*see* below).

Table 32-1. Incidence of Cardiac Arrest and Hospital Mortality*

CLASS	I	II	III	IV
Incidence cardiac arrest, %	5	15	46	77
Hospital mortality, %	6	17	38	81

*Based on data of Killip T, Kimball JT: Treatment of myocardial infarction in a coronary care unit. Am J Cardiol 20:457, 1967. *See* text for description of infarction class.

PULMONARY FUNCTION CHANGES WITH AMI

Arterial hypoxemia occurs commonly in patients with AMI.[23,65,69] The degree of hypoxemia correlates well with the severity of pulmonary vascular congestion. Ventilation–perfusion mismatch, increased pulmonary arteriovenous shunting, and, to a much lesser degree, diffusion abnormalities all contribute to the hypoxemia.[23,28,29,65] In severe left ventricular failure associated with pulmonary edema or cardiogenic shock, alveolar hypoventilation often contributes significantly to the hypoxemia.

Closing volume, a measurement of small airways function, is increased in AMI.[28,29] The precise pathogenesis of this abnormality is not known but may be related to a combination of factors, including mucosal edema of the small airways, changes in transmural pressure of the airways, and changes in regional pulmonary compliance. Gray and colleagues found reduced lung volumes (TLC, VC, FRC, and RV) to be the most consistent pulmonary function abnormality in AMI.[28] Reduction in volumes correlated well with the severity of left ventricular failure and pulmonary vascular congestion. A reversible bronchospastic component has not been demonstrated.[32]

Pulmonary perfusion is also abnormal in AMI. Normally, because of gravitational forces, perfusion is greatest in the pulmonary bases in the upright patient. Studies using ^{133}xenon have demonstrated a relative shift of perfusion toward the apices after AMI. This occurs even with normal cardiac output and normal pulmonary artery wedge pressures.[29] Pulmonary arteriovenous shunting may contribute up to one third of the hypoxemia observed in uncomplicated AMI, and its relative contribution to hypoxemia tends to increase as pulmonary vascular congestion worsens.[23,28,29,65,69]

CHEST RADIOGRAPH IN AMI

The chest radiograph (CXR) in an uncomplicated AMI may be normal. When abnormalities occur, they may be related to the degree of congestive heart failure present (Fig. 32-1). McHugh and associates correlated radiographic findings with hemodynamic data.[46] They

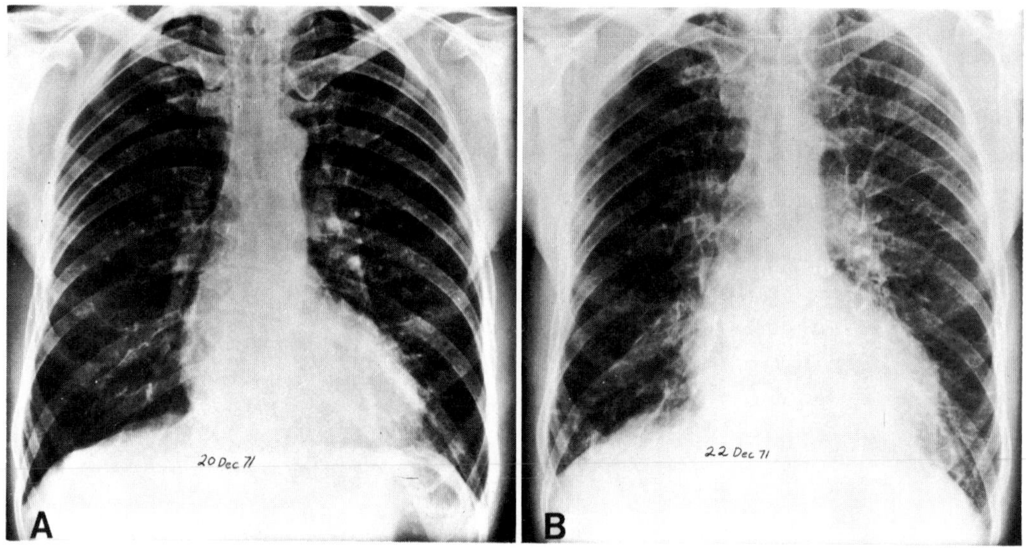

Fig. 32-1. Interstitial pulmonary edema developing 2 days after an acute myocardial infarction. *(B)* Note the Kerley A, B, and C lines, indicative of interstitial edema and lymphatic obstruction. The original roentgenogram *(A)* was taken at admission to hospital. Progressive, but not extremely severe, dyspnea had developed over the 2-day period.

graded the CXR into four categories of severity of left ventricular failure: 0, absent; 1, mild; 2, moderate; and 3, severe. A pulmonary capillary pressure of 18 mm Hg or greater separated grades 0 and 1 left ventricular failure from grades 2 and 3. Generally, as the PWP increased, the CXR findings became more pronounced. At a PWP of 18 mm Hg, the earliest changes observed are those of redistribution of flow to the upper lobes of the lung. With a PWP of 18 to 22 mm Hg, there is a decreased definition of medium-sized pulmonary vessels and the development of a perihilar haze along with increased prominence of the outer zone vessels. Periacinar rosette formation occurs at PWP levels of 22 to 25 mm Hg. There is a 58% agreement between the radiographic classification and Killip and Kimball's clinical severity classification.[36]

McHugh and colleagues found significant discrepancies between PWP and CXR findings in 10% of their cases.[46] In some patients with abnormally elevated PWP, there was a lag before CXR abnormalities occurred. Conversely, other patients had lingering CXR abnormalities, although their PWP has returned to normal following treatment. Patients in cardiogenic shock developed CXR abnormalities despite normal or low PWP. Interestingly, in McHugh's study, increased pulmonary artery size, pleural effusion, cardiomegaly, and Kerley B lines on the CXR were *not* consistent predictors of the severity of left ventricular failure.

TREATMENT

Pharmacologic Therapy

A major goal of coronary care is to achieve an optimal relation between cardiac output and myocardial oxygen consumption. Heart rate, ventricular wall tension, and the rate of myocardial fiber shortening all influence myocardial oxygen consumption. As an example, isoproterenol has been shown to increase cardiac output but also increases myocardial oxygen consumption.[49] Therapy based on hemodynamic subsets is summarized in Figure 32-2.

In subset H-I, the patient likely needs no hemodynamic intervention. The H-II patient with elevated PWP will usually respond to diuretics, peripheral vasodilators, or inotropic agents.[26] As initial therapy, diuretics are the usual option and do not increase myocardial oxygen demand. If hypertension is present or elevated systemic vascular resistance is found on hemodynamic evaluation, a vasodilator such as nitroprusside may be the preferred therapy. If arterial pressure is maintained in a physiologic range, this agent will lower capillary pressure while heart rate and cardiac index remain stable. If cardiomegaly exists, inotropic agents such as dopamine, dobutamine, or digitalis may decrease ventricular dilatation and wall tension and thereby decrease PWP and oxygen demand.[3]

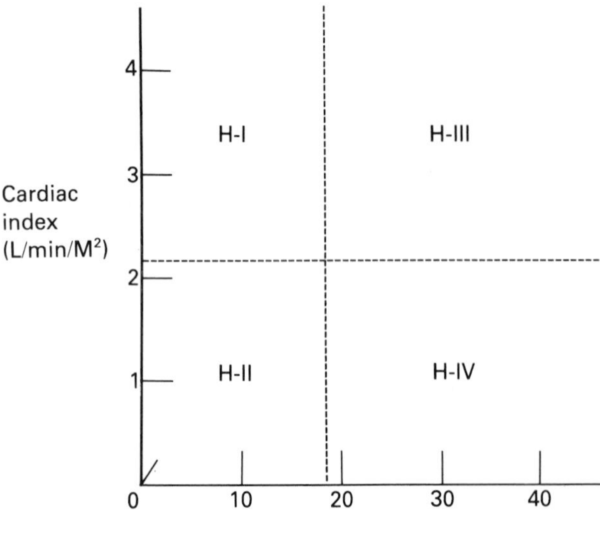

Fig. 32-2. Therapy based on hemodynamic subsets (data of Forrester et al).[25] H-I = no intervention; H-II = diuretics, peripheral vasodilators, inotropic agents; H-III = volume expansion, peripheral vasodilators, increase heart rate; H-IV = manipulation of all modalities, possible aortic balloon assist.

Patients in subset H-III have peripheral hypotension and a low-normal PWP. Starling's law of the heart states that the strength of cardiac contraction is proportional to myocardial fiber length. The PWP is related to left ventricular end-diastolic volume. Therefore, if the PWP—that is, left ventricular end-diastolic volume—is low, it may be beneficial to augment this volume with crystalloid or colloid infusion. Starling curves can be plotted to find the PWP that is associated with the optimal cardiac output. Such manipulation may increase myocardial oxygen consumption. Elevated systemic vascular resistance may be present in the H-III group of patients. When detected, it is the hemodynamic parameter best manipulated, and vasodilator therapy should be used. Cardiac output can be increased in the patient with bradycardia by using medications or by transvenous cardiac pacing.

Patients in subset H-IV have a dismal prognosis if untreated. This group may respond to afterload reduction with vasodilators but often requires manipulation of all the aforementioned modalities.[26,57] If patients are unresponsive to medical management, intrathoracic balloon assist should be considered. This device consists of a balloon positioned in the descending thoracic aorta. The balloon is inflated during diastole and deflated during systole. Thus, afterload is reduced and coronary blood flow augmented.

Use of Oxygen

Although oxygen supplementation for patients with documented or suspected myocardial ischemia is standard practice in most cardiac care units, there is little clinical evidence that oxygen therapy is beneficial if the patient is normoxemic. A significant number of patients with AMI have arterial hypoxemia, usually resulting from ventilation–perfusion abnormalities, and for these patients restoration of normoxemia is of potential benefit for multiple organ systems.[29] In support of the routine use of supplemental oxygen, abnormal breathing patterns and marked oxygen desaturation during sleep have been documented in normal males.[8] These abnormalities are more prevalent in obese subjects or in those with COPD and have been associated with an increased frequency of premature ventricular contractions.[7]

Some deleterious effects of supplemental oxygen have been noted. High inspired oxygen concentrations (FI_{O_2}-about 0.9) administered by means of close-fitting face masks have been shown to increase systemic vascular resistance and to decrease cardiac output.[35] At oxygen flows of 6 liters/min or less administered by mask or nasal cannula, this effect has not been seen.[41]

It has been theorized that increasing arterial oxygen tension in the patient with AMI might improve oxygenation in the area adjacent to the infarct and thus reduce the final size of the infarct. However, administering oxygen to a patient with normal arterial oxygen saturation results in only a 0.3 vol % increase in blood oxygen content for each 100 mm Hg increase in arterial PO_2. Maroko and associates studied the effects of supplemental oxygen on ST-segment elevations and CPK activity in dogs with experimentally induced coronary occlusion.[45] They found that the group of animals given 0.40 FI_{O_2} had less ST-segment changes and less depression of CPK activity when compared to a group breathing room air. Using an FI_{O_2} of 1.0 did not appear to decrease myocardial ischemia further. Controlled clinical studies have failed to demonstrate any benefit of oxygen supplementation in the nonhypoxemic patient. A prospective study of 200 patients given either room air or oxygen at 6 liters/min by mask showed no difference in mortality, incidence of arrhythmias, use of analgesics, or systolic time intervals between the groups.[58] Hyperbaric oxygenation has also been used in treating AMI, but clinical series have not shown improvement in mortality or clinical course.[71]

Accordingly, the use of supplemental oxygen in patients with AMI remains controversial. The theoretical advantages of supplemental oxygen use have not been supported by clinical trials in humans. However, because of evidence of sleep-induced oxygen desaturation in males, encouraging results of animal experimentation, and a strong tradition in use, supplemental oxygen will likely remain an integral part of the therapy for ischemic heart disease.

Mechanical Ventilation in AMI

The indications for initiating mechanical ventilatory support as well as the parameters for maintaining ventilation and weaning are well described elsewhere and apply equally to pulmonary edema as to the adult respiratory distress syndrome. A few aspects of mechanical ventilation are particularly important to consider in patients with cardiac disease. During positive pressure ventilation, intrathoracic pressure increases above atmospheric pressure during inspiration and falls to atmospheric levels at the end of expiration. This results in decreased venous return during inspiration, particularly when an element of volume depletion exists. This, in turn, may cause reduced cardiac output with resultant hypotension.

Cardiovascular compensatory mechanisms subsequently lead to increases in heart rate and arterial and venous resistance that result in increased cardiac work and myocardial oxygen consumption. The use of positive end-expiratory pressure (PEEP) may likewise impede venous return. Increased intrathoracic pressure causes decreased systemic venous pressures that increase transcapillary flow and further decrease venous return. Traditionally, the problem of decreased cardiac output has been treated with volume expansion or the use of sympathomimetic pressor agents to minimize the decrease in venous return.[3] Several groups of investigators have demonstrated that, in many instances, even very high levels of PEEP can be used with intermittent mandatory ventilation (IMV) without significantly altering cardiac output.[21,37] Other investigators have demonstrated a decrease in cardiac output and mean arterial pressure with the use of PEEP despite normal cardiac filling pressures as measured by pulmonary capillary wedge pressures.[13] This suggests primary depression of myocardial contractility and has been noted more consistently at higher levels of PEEP. Culver and colleagues have demonstrated that raising pleural pressure without changing lung volume causes atrial transmural pressure and cardiac output to decrease in the same manner as does reducing preload by partial vena caval occlusion.[17] This same group of investigators showed that raising lung volume to increase juxtacardiac pressures could result in increased right atrial pressure, decreased ventricular filling, and decreased cardiac output. Other investigators have demonstrated similar changes in cardiac function at high levels of PEEP.[44] Jardin and coworkers demonstrated echocardiographically a leftward displacement of the interventricular septum during PEEP.[33] This septal movement restricted left ventricular filling and decreased cardiac output.

Noninvasive methods to assess cardiovascular status in respiratory failure are being developed, including chest radiography, various modes of echocardiography, radionucleotide angiocardiography, and thallium scanning.[2,5] In most clinical settings, however, systemic arterial pressure monitoring and pulmonary artery pressure monitoring are still used. The intrathoracic position of the pulmonary artery catheter is critically important in determining the validity of the data obtained. Pulmonary artery wedge pressure is supposed to reflect left atrial pressure. West demonstrated that the distribution of blood flow within the lung depends on the mechanical pressures exerted in and on the pulmonary blood vessels.[70] If the PWP is to reflect left atrial pressure, the pulmonary venous pressure must exceed alveolar pressure. Flow-directed catheters are expected to locate in a dependent portion of the lung where pulmonary venous pressure exceeds alveolar pressure. However, Shasby and colleagues found that in 43% of 30 patients studied, the pulmonary artery catheter lodged near or above the left atrium.[62] These and other investigators have demonstrated poor correlation between PWP and measured left atrial pressures when the pulmonary artery catheter was above the left atrium.[60,62,67] The more dependent the catheter placement in reference to the left atrium, the less the values obtained will be affected by increasing levels of PEEP.[60] Both anteroposterior and lateral chest roentgenograms are necessary to confirm catheter placement.

The actual measurement and the interpretation of PWP in patients on PEEP are often difficult because it is not known how much of the increased intrapleural pressure is transmitted to the PWP. Pulmonary arterial and wedge pressure measurements should be taken at the end of expiration since, at this point, there is no air movement and intrapleural pressure is at a static baseline.[6] Graphic analysis of pressure data appears to be more reliable than digital readings, particularly in patients who have some spontaneous respirations.[43] DeCampo and Civetta have shown that brief discontinuation of PEEP can be accomplished safely for several seconds in most patients; however, this is discouraged because it is the hemodynamic state of the patient on the ventilator that is of interest.[19] Downs and Douglas found that interruption of positive airway pressure in dogs created profound cardiovascular changes and that the measurements obtained did not reflect the actual cardiovascular status of animals.[20] The degree of transmission of intrathoracic pressure to PWP depends on lung compliance. Estimations of the effect of PEEP on PWP can be made by subtracting 1/5 to 2/5 of the PEEP value from PWP.[15] Intrapleural pressures can be measured directly or approximated with an intraesophageal balloon; however, both of these methods are technically cumbersome.

AMI AND OBSTRUCTIVE LUNG DISEASES

Because cigarette consumption can be an etiologic factor in both AMI and chronic obstructive pulmonary diseae (COPD), the concurrence of these diseases in the CCU is not unusual. At times, distinguishing between an exacerbation of COPD and AMI with left ventricular dysfunction may be difficult. The findings in both disease complexes may be similar. Both types of patients may present with cough, dyspnea, and chest pain. Physical examination in both conditions can reveal crackles, jugular venous distention, peripheral edema, and third heart sounds. Lung hyperinflation may change the voltage and axis of the electrocardiographic complexes and alter the cardiac silhouette on CXR. Large emphysematous bullae may obscure the vascular congestion usually seen in left ventricular failure. When the two diseases coexist, exacerbation of one may precipitate worsening of the other. Left ventricular failure in the patient with COPD leads to interstitial and alveolar congestion and further compromise of gas exchange, which can result in respiratory failure. An exacerbation of COPD with hypoxia, acidosis, and increased work of breathing may lead to arrhythmias and worsening myocardial ischemia.[68]

A wide variety of arrythmias occur in patients with COPD. These appear more commonly at night partly because of abnormal breathing patterns in patients with COPD during sleep.[24,61] Boysen and colleagues demonstrated that the oxygen desaturation during sleep in some patients with COPD is associated with elevated pulmonary artery pressures.[9] Low-flow oxygen can diminish or abolish the nocturnal fall in oxygen saturation, prevent elevation of pulmonary artery pressure, and decrease the frequency of arrhythmias. Oxygen administration should follow the guidelines listed elsewhere in this book as they pertain to the patient with COPD.

At times, medication effective in treating one of the obstructive lung disease processes may be detrimental in the cardiac condition, or *vice versa*. Theophylline preparations and beta agonists, the mainstay of bronchodilator therapy in COPD, can be particularly arrhythmogenic in AMI, and risk–benefit considerations become particularly important. *The risk of arrhythmias and progressive ischemic damage owing to persistent hypoxia in the bronchospastic patient is much greater than the risk of arrhythmias provoked by carefully administered bronchodilators.* Aminophylline should be given as a continuous infusion with close monitoring of blood concentrations. The maintenance dose, based on ideal weight, should be decreased by at least 50% in patients with evidence of cardiac failure.[55]

Aerosolized sympathomimetic agents are very effective bronchodilators and cause less cardiovascular effects than do the same medications administered parenterally.[59,63] This is particularly true of the newer agents that are selective beta-2 agonists. Albuterol, a beta-2 selective agonist, has been shown to produce better bronchodilation and fewer cardiovascular side-effects than isoproterenol, a nonselective beta agonist.[40] The bronchodilator should not be delivered by an intermittent positive pressure breathing (IPPB) device because of potential adverse cardiovascular effects.[31] By altering ventilation–perfusion relationships, bronchodilation may transiently worsen hypoxia, making oxygen supplementation very important in these patients.[38] Propranolol and other beta-2 blocking agents, which may be used in limiting infarct size and controlling arrhythmias in AMI, may cause deterioration in pulmonary function even in the nonbronchospastic patient with COPD.[14,53]

COMPLICATIONS OF CPR

Because of the nature and severity of their illnesses, many patients present to CCUs after having received CPR. The resuscitation procedure itself can result in various complications, from endotracheal tube misplacement to visceral rupture.[50] Some of these complications are listed in Table 32-2. Compromise of airway function or gas exchange related to aspiration is a common complication of CPR.[18] Aspiration is frequently related to an altered state of consciousness and may occur even in healthy people during sleep.[42] Although not always clinically distinguishable, three aspiration syndromes have been identified.[4] All cause direct injury to the respiratory tract, infection, or obstruction of the airway.

During CPR, aspiration of substances (primarily gastric contents) that cause direct chemical injury to the respiratory tract can rapidly provoke respiratory difficulties.[4,12] Although the degree of pulmonary damage depends on the volume and pH of the gastric contents, signs and symptoms of respiratory compromise usually occur within 2 hours of the event.[4,12] These comprise fever, cough, bronchospasm, and tachypnea and may progress to apnea and cardiovascular collapse.[4,12,30] The injury pattern approximates that of a chemical burn or toxic reaction, and treatment is initially supportive.[4] In its severest form, aspiration may progress to the adult respiratory distress syndrome.

Instillation of buffering solution or bronchoalveolar lavage is not indicated since the damage to the respiratory epithelium occurs within minutes.[4,30] Prophylactic antibiotics are also not indicated. They do not prevent development of infections and may select a bacterial flora more resistant to antimicrobials.[12,30] Development of secondary bacterial infections because of impaired clearance and ineffective immune mechanisms is common, and the patient's secretions and clinical course must be monitored closely.

If infection, as characterized by fever, leukocytosis, and pulmonary infiltrates, develops, antibiotic use should be guided by Gram's stain and culture data. Corticosteroids do not improve the outcome of gastric aspiration and should not be used.[12,30]

Aspiration of pathogenic bacteria colonizing the upper airway (usually a less fulminant process than aspiration of gastric contents) presents as a pulmonary infection with fever and purulent sputum. This occurs several hours to days after aspiration of oropharyngeal contents.[4,42] Anaerobic bacteria are common pathogens in this type of infection.

Aspiration of particulate material leads to airway obstruction. Large objects such as food may obstruct the larynx or trachea, whereas smaller particles may lodge more distally in the airways. Such aspiration may result in cough, dyspnea, and bronchospasm and can lead to atelectasis or obstructive emphysema.[4]

Table 32-2. Complications of CPR

Complications of CPR
Vomitus
Upper airway obstruction
Aspiration pneumonia
Foreign body (tooth) aspiration
Endotracheal tube misplacement[64]
Esophageal rupture[34]
Mainstem bronchus intubation
Chest wall trauma
Rib fracture
Sternal fracture
Flail chest
Pneumothorax
Damage to viscera
Esophageal rupture
Gastric hemorrhage or rupture[1]
Liver laceration
Central access complications
Pneumothorax
Hemopericardium[18]
Vascular occlusion[22,54]
Arrhythmias
Infection

Such patients are at particular risk of developing recurrent pneumonitis, lung abscess, and empyema. Once the obstruction has been removed by cough, postural maneuvers, or bronchoscopically, such infection generally respond quickly to antibiotic therapy.

Rib fractures often occur as a result of CPR.[50] If these are extensive enough to cause paradoxical motion of a chest wall segment, a "flail" chest exists. If this segment is large enough to cause significant respiratory compromise, mechanical ventilation should be initiated. Generally the patient should be sedated or paralyzed and maintained on a volume ventilator in a control rather than patient-cycled mode.[30]

During CPR, pneumothorax may develop as a result of rib fractures or lung puncture associated with the placement of central venous lines. A tension pneumothorax may lead to rapid deterioration of the patient and can be relieved temporarily by needle aspiration. An intercostal catheter or tube thoracostomy is needed for definitive therapy of a pneumothorax. Occasionally persistent intrathoracic bleeding requiring surgical repair is associated with rib fractures or central line placement.[30]

SUMMARY

Coronary care units continue to increase in number and degree of sophistication. Establishing the correct diagnosis in the subjects presenting with chest pain or dyspnea can be difficult, particularly for patients with COPD. Patients with AMI may need only monitoring and minor interventions or may demand invasive hemodynamic and respiratory monitoring and pharmacologic manipulation. Patients with AMI often have or develop multiorgan system abnormalities that require treatment. Thus an integrated management plan involving physician, nursing, and paramedical specialists is imperative if optimal care is to be delivered to the CCU patient.

REFERENCES

1. Aquilar J: Fatal gastric hemorrhage: A complication of cardiorespiratory resuscitation. J Trauma 21:573, 1981
2. Askenaige J et al: Echocardiographic estimates of pulmonary artery wedge pressure. N Engl J Med 305:1566, 1981
3. Ayres SM: Ventricular function. In Shoemaker WC, Thompson WL (eds): Critical Care, Vol 1. Fullerton, CA, Society of Critical Care Medicine, 1980
4. Bartlett JG, Gorbach SL: The triple threat of aspiration pneumonia. Chest 68:560, 1975
5. Berger HJ, Matthay RA: Noninvasive radiographic assessment of cardiovascular function in acute and chronic respiratory failure. Am J Cardiol 47:950, 1981
6. Berryhill RE, Benumof JL, Rauscher A: Pulmonary vascular pressure readings at the end of exhalation. Anesthesiology 49: 365, 1978
7. Block AJ, Flick MR: Cardiac arrhythmias in chronic obstructive lung disease: Effects of low flow oxygen administration. Am Rev Respir Dis (Suppl) 113:126, 1976
8. Block AJ et al: Sleep apnea, hypoxemia and oxygen desaturation in normal subjects. N Engl J Med 300:513, 1979
9. Boysen PG et al: Nocturnal pulmonary hypertension in patients with chronic obstructive pulmonary disease. Chest 76:536, 1979
10. Braunwald E: Coronary spasm and acute myocardial infarction—new possibility for treatment and prevention. N Engl J Med 299:1301, 1978
11. Braunwald E: Chest pain and palpitation. In Isselbacher KJ et al (eds): Principles of Internal Medicine, 9th ed. New York, McGraw–Hill, 1980
12. Bynum LJ, Pierce AK: Pulmonary aspiration of gastric contents. Am Rev Respir Dis 114:1129, 1976
13. Cassidy SS et al: Cardiovascular effects of positive end-expiratory pressure in dogs. J Appl Physiol 44:743, 1978
14. Chester EH, Schwartz HJ, Fleming GM: Adverse effect of propranolol on airway function in non-asthmatic chronic obstructive lung disease. Chest 79:540, 1981
15. Civetta JM: Invasive catheterization. In Shoemaker WC, Thompson WL (eds): Critical Care, Vol 1. Fullerton, CA, Society of Critical Care Medicine, 1980
16. Conn HL: Congestive heart failure. In Conn HL, Horwitz O (eds): Cardiac and Vascular Disease. Philadelphia, Lea & Febiger, 1971
17. Culver BH, Marini JJ, Butler J: Lung volume and pleural pressure effects on ventricular function. J Appl Physiol 50:630, 1981
18. Davison R et al: Intracardiac injections during cardiopulmonary resuscitation. JAMA 244:1110, 1980
19. De Campo T, Civetta JM: The effect of short-term discontinuation of high-level PEEP in patients with acute respiratory failure. Crit Care Med 7:47, 1979
20. Downs JB, Douglas ME: Assessment of cardiac filling pressure during continuous positive-pressure ventilation. Crit Care Med 8:285, 1980
21. Downs JB, Douglas ME, Sanfelippo PM: Ventilatory pattern, intrapleural pressure and cardiac output. Anesth Analg 56:88, 1977
22. Elliott CG, Zimmerman GA, Clemmer TP: Complications of pulmonary artery catheterization in the care of critically ill patients. Chest 76:647, 1979
23. Fillmore SJ et al: Blood-gas changes and pulmonary hemodynamics following acute myocardial infarction. Circulation 45:583, 1972
24. Flick MR, Block AJ: Nocturnal vs. diurnal cardiac arrythmias in patients with chronic obstructive pulmonary disease. Chest 75:8, 1979
25. Forrester JS et al: Medical therapy of acute myocardial infarction by application of hemodynamic subsets, Part 1. N Engl J Med 295:1356, 1976
26. Forrester JS et al: Medical therapy of acute myocardial infarction by application of hemodynamic subsets, Part 2. N Engl J Med 295:1404, 1976
27. Gensini GC: Coronary artery spasm and angina pectoris. Chest 50:709, 1975
28. Gray BA et al: Alterations in lung volume and pulmonary function in relation to hemodynamic changes in acute myocardial infarction. Circulation 59:551, 1979
29. Hales CA, Kazemi H: Pulmonary function after uncomplicated myocardial infarction. Chest 72:350, 1977
30. Hinshaw HC, Murray JF: Diseases of the Chest, 4th ed. Philadelphia, WB Saunders, 1980
31. Hodgkin JE, Webster JS: IPPB: Worthwhile for which patient? J Respir Dis 3:97, 1982
32. Interiano B et al: Interrelation between alterations in pulmonary mechanics and hemodynamics in acute myocardial infarction. J Clin Invest 52:1994, 1973
33. Jardin F et al: Influence of positive end-expiratory pressure on left ventricular performance. N Engl J Med 304:387, 1981
34. Kassels SJ, Robinson WA, O'Bara KJ: Esophageal perforation associated with esophageal obturator airway. Crit Care Med 8:386, 1980
35. Kenmore ACF et al: Circulatory and metabolic effects of oxygen on myocardial infarction. Br Med J 4:360, 1968
36. Killip T, Kimball JT: Treatment of myocardial infarction in a coronary care unit. Am J Cardiol 20:457, 1967
37. Kirby RR et al: High level positive end expiratory pressure in acute respiratory insufficiency. Chest 67:156, 1975
38. Kvale PA et al: Continuous or nocturnal oxygen therapy in hypoxemic chronic obstructive lung disease. Ann Intern Med 93:391, 1980
39. Levy RI et al: Percutaneous transluminal coronary angioplasty—a status report. N Engl J Med 305:399, 1981
40. Light RW, Taylor RW, George RB: Albuterol and isoproterenol in bronchial asthma. Arch Intern Med 139:639, 1979
41. Loeb HS et al: Effects of low-flow oxygen on the hemodynamics and left ventricular function in patients with uncomplicated acute myocardial infarction. Chest 60:352, 1971
42. Lorber B, Swenson RM: Bacteriology of aspiration pneumonia. Ann Intern Med 81:329, 1974

43. Maran A: Variables in pulmonary capillary wedge pressure: Variation with intrathoracic pressure, graphic and digital recorders. Crit Care Med 8:102, 1980
44. Marini JJ, Culver BH, Butler J: Mechanical effect of lung distention with positive pressure on cardiac function. Am Rev Respir Dis 124:382, 1981
45. Maroko PR et al: Reduction of infarct size by oxygen inhalation following acute coronary occlusion. Circulation 52:360, 1975
46. McHugh TJ et al: Pulmonary vascular congestion in acute myocardial infarction: Hemodynamic and radiologic correlations. Ann Intern Med 76:29, 1972
47. McIntyre KM et al: Standards and guidelines for cardiopulmonary resuscitation (CPR) and emergency cardiac care (ECC). JAMA 244:453, 1980
48. Miseri A et al: Coronary vasospasm as a possible cause of myocardial infarction. N Engl J Med 299:1721, 1978
49. Mueller HS et al: Hemodynamics, coronary blood flow and myocardial metabolism in coronary shock: Response to l-norepinephrine and isoproterenol. J Clin Invest 49:1855, 1970
50. Nagel EL et al: Complications of CPR. Crit Care Med 9:424, 1981
51. Oliva PB: Pathophysiology of acute myocardial infarction, 1981. Ann Intern Med 94:236, 1981
52. Oliva PB, Breckenridge JC: Arteriographic evidence of coronary arterial spasm in acute myocardial infarction. Circulation 56:366, 1977
53. Opie LH: Myocardial infarct size. Am Heart J 100:531, 1980
54. Parish JM et al: Etiologic considerations in superior vena cava syndrome. Mayo Clin Proc 56:407, 1981
55. Paterson JW, Woolcock AJ, Shenfield GM: Bronchodilator drugs. Am Rev Respir Dis 120:1149, 1979
56. Pozen MW et al: The usefulness of a productive instrument to reduce inappropriate admissions to the coronary care unit. Ann Intern Med 92:238, 1980
57. Rackley CE et al: Modern approach to myocardial infarction: Determination of prognosis and therapy. Am Heart J 101:75, 1981
58. Rawles JM, Kenmore ACF: Controlled trial of oxygen in uncomplicated myocardial infarction. Br Med J 1:1121, 1976
59. Rossing TH et al: Emergency therapy of asthma: Comparison of the acute effects of parenteral and inhaled sympathomimetics and infused aminophylline. Am Rev Respir Dis 365, 1980
60. Roy R et al: Pulmonary wedge catheterization during positive end-expiratory pressure ventilation in the dog. Anesthesiology 46:385, 1977
61. Rude RE, Miller JE, Braunwald E: Efforts to limit the size of myocardial infarcts. Ann Intern Med 95:736, 1981
62. Shasby DM et al: Swan-Ganz catheter location and left atrial pressure determine the accuracy of the wedge pressure when positive end-expiratory pressure is used. Chest 80:666, 1981
63. Simonsson BG, Svedenblad H, Strom B: Bronchodilatory and circulatory effects of two doses of a B_2-agonist (terbutaline) inhaled with IPPB in patients with reversible airway obstruction. Scand J Respir Dis 57:252, 1976
64. Stauffer JL et al: Complications and consequences of endotracheal intubation and tracheostomy. Am J Med 70:65, 1981
65. Storstein O, Rasmussen K: The cause of arterial hypoxemia in acute myocardial infarction. Acta Med Scand 183:193, 1968
66. Thibault GE et al: Medical intensive care. Indications, interventions and outcomes. N Engl J Med 302:938, 1980
67. Tooker J, Huseby J, Butler J: The effect of Swan-Ganz catheter height on the wedge pressure-left atrial pressure relationship in edema during positive-pressure ventilation. Am Rev Respir Dis 117:721, 1978
68. Unger M et al: Potentiation of pulmonary vasoconstrictor response with repeated intermittent hypoxia. J Appl Physiol 43:662, 1977
69. Valencia A, Burgess JH: Arterial hypoxemia following acute myocardial infarction. Circulation 40:641, 1969
70. West JB: Regional differences in the lung. Chest 74:426, 1978
71. Wynne JW et al: Disordered breathing and oxygen desaturation during sleep in patients with chronic obstructive pulmonary disease. Chest 73:301, 1978

BIBLIOGRAPHY

Bone RC (ed): Adult respiratory distress syndrome. Clin Chest Med 3, No. 1, 1982

Oliva PB: Pathophysiology of acute myocardial infarction. Ann Intern Med 94:236, 1981

Rude RE, Miller JE, Braunwald E: Efforts to limit the size of myocardial infarcts. Ann Intern Med 95:736, 1981

Shoemaker WC, Thompson WL (eds): Critical Care, Vols 1 and 2. Fullerton, CA, Society of Critical Care Medicine, 1980, 1981

33

Pulmonary Embolism and Infarction

Steven E. Levy • Myron Stein

INCIDENCE AND IMPORTANCE

Venous thrombosis with subsequent embolization of the lungs is probably the most common pulmonary disease encountered in the hospitalized patient. The importance of this disease is emphasized by recent estimates that there are about 200,000 deaths per year in the United States caused by pulmonary embolism. In 100,000 of these deaths, it is the sole cause, and in the remaining 100,000 it is the major contributing cause. The incidence of symptomatic episodes of pulmonary embolism is estimated to be 630,000 per year, which would make this disease half as common as acute myocardial infarction.

The diagnosis is not established in about two thirds of the patients suffering an embolic episode, and it is in this group of 400,000 patients that most fatalities occur (about 120,000). With appropriate therapy less than 10% of patients suffering from pulmonary embolism will die if they survive the initial hour after the embolic event. Thus the major problem in managing this disease is recognition and diagnosis. This becomes particularly difficult in the patient with underlying nonembolic pulmonary disease in whom respiratory therapy may be indicated (e.g., the patient with chronic obstructive airway disease, the postoperative patient with atelectasis, or the patient who has aspirated for any of several reasons).

In regard to therapy, the primary goal of treatment is prevention of further venous thrombosis with anticoagulation, allowing natural thrombolytic mechanisms to lyse the thromboemboli in the pulmonary arteries. The primary role of respiratory therapy in treating the patient with pulmonary thromboembolism is supportive, using the administration of oxygen to correct the arterial hypoxemia that may be typically a consequence of acute pulmonary embolism. Other respiratory therapy modalities, including periodic hyperinflation of the lungs, administration of aerosols, and chest physiotherapy, have no proven therapeutic effect in pulmonary embolism.

ETIOLOGY AND PATHOLOGY

Pulmonary thromboembolism denotes the passage of a thrombus into a pulmonary artery, with subsequent obstruction of blood supply to lung tissue. In most patients who suffer a symptomatic embolic event, the thrombi initially form in the deep veins of the calves and then propagate proximally into the deep veins of the thighs and pelvis. From these sites the thrombi break off and travel through the venous circulation through the right heart into the lungs. Symptomatic embolic events from thrombi forming in the upper extremities or the right cardiac chambers do occur but are uncommon.

Pulmonary infarction is an infrequent consequence of thromboembolic obstruction of the pulmonary arteries, occurring in no more than 10% of embolic events. Infarction is characterized by hemorrhagic consolidation of the lung and is often associated with pleuritis and a pleural effusion, which frequently is hemorrhagic. When actual necrosis of lung tissue occurs, the infarction is said to be "complete" and will heal by organization and fibrosis over several weeks. If necrosis does not occur, the infarction is said to be "incomplete" and may resolve in a few days with restoration of normal lung architecture. The thromboemboli themselves typically are lysed over a period of weeks to months, with restoration of normal pulmonary arterial perfusion to the lung parenchyma. Rarely the thromboemboli organize, resulting in permanent obstruction of the pulmonary arteries with serious clinical and hemodynamic consequences.

The mechanisms of thrombus formation in the venous system involve stasis, alterations in the coagulability of the blood, and damage to the veins. Clinical evidence of venous damage manifested by signs of thrombophlebitis is not detected in most patients with pulmonary embolism and, even when present, does not usually manifest itself until after the embolic event. Venous stasis is very likely to be important in the genesis of venous thrombosis in the setting of bed rest, prolonged immobility, cardiac failure, pregnancy, obesity, chronic obstructive airway disease, and the postoperative state. Hypercoagulability, although difficult to measure by coagulation studies, is probably important in the setting of hip fractures, the administration of oral contraceptives, malignancy, hematologic disorders, pregnancy, the postoperative state, and antithrombin III deficiency. Patients in respiratory failure may be particularly likely to develop venous thrombosis and pulmonary embolism.

PATHOPHYSIOLOGY

The diagnosis and subsequent treatment of pulmonary thromboembolism must be based on a firm understanding of the pathophysiologic changes that occur as a consequence of thromboembolic obstruction of the pulmonary arteries. These changes are complex, involving alterations in pulmonary and cardiac hemodynamics, pulmonary gas exchange, pulmonary mechanics, and ventilatory control.

The magnitude of disordered cardiopulmonary function after an embolic event is a function of two factors: the extent of pulmonary arterial obstruction, which will vary depending on the size and number of the thrombi that impact into the pulmonary arteries; and the functional state of the lungs and the heart before the embolic event. Thus the patient with preexisting obstructive lung disease or cardiac failure is more likely to manifest serious symptoms and signs after embolization. Moreover, the patient with preexisting cardiac or pulmonary disease is more likely to die of an embolic event. People with normal heart and lung function can tolerate massive embolization of the pulmonary arteries and still survive with appropriate specific and supporting therapy.

Much of the current knowledge on the pathophysiology of this disease has been obtained from studies performed on experimental animals subjected to pulmonary embolism. This has been necessary because of the difficulty and risk of performing extensive physiological studies in acutely ill patients. However, if an appropriate model is used (e.g., embolization of the lungs by venous thrombi formed *in vivo*), the changes that occur are similar to those seen in humans. In the following discussion, the extrapolation of these experimental observations will be so noted. A presentation of the pathophysiology of pulmonary thromboembolism must provide a mechanism to explain the development of [1] pulmonary hypertension with right ventricular failure and shock; [2] breathlessness with rapid, shallow respirations (tachypnea) and hyperventilation (low arterial Pa_{CO_2} with an elevated arterial pH); [3] arterial hypoxemia; and [4] pulmonary infarction.

Pulmonary hypertension is the most important and dangerous physiological alteration after pulmonary embolization. It occurs primarily as a consequence of the decreased functional cross-sectional area of the pulmonary arterial tree, with an increase in pulmonary vascular resistance. To maintain cardiac output, the right ventricle must generate higher pressures (*i.e.*, pulmonary hypertension). The normal pulmonary artery pressure is 25/10 mm Hg, with a mean pulmonary artery pressure no greater than 15 mm Hg. Thus *pulmonary hypertension can be defined as an increase in mean pulmonary artery pressure above 15 mm Hg.*

Most patients with symptomatic acute pulmonary embolism manifested by breathlessness have an elevated mean pulmonary artery pressure, usually in excess of 20 mm Hg. With increasing pulmonary arterial occlusion, the severity of pulmonary hypertension increases but is ultimately limited by the maximal function of the right ventricle. The normal, nonhypertrophied right ventricle can generate a mean pulmonary arterial pressure of about 35 to 40 mm Hg or systolic pressure of 50 to 55 mm Hg. When pulmonary vascular obstruction increases beyond the limits of right ventricular function, the right ventricle fails, with a fall in forward cardiac output and the development of shock (*i.e.*, peripheral vasoconstriction; diaphoresis; a weak, thready pulse; decreased urine output or oliguria; and changes in sensorium). An important characteristic of this form of shock is the association with an increased central venous or right atrial pressure, in contrast to other shock states where the cardiac filling pressures tend to be low, *e.g.*, septic shock and shock due to blood loss.

Clinical observations demonstrate a rough correlation between the extent of pulmonary arterial obstruction as determined by pulmonary angiography and the degree of pulmonary hypertension. Existing evidence suggests that active pulmonary vasoconstriction contributes to the development of pulmonary hypertension both in experimental animals and humans. A dog subjected to pulmonary embolization with autologous *in vivo* thrombi develops active constriction of the pulmonary arteries. The vasoconstriction in the dog is mediated partly by the release of serotonin from platelets that have aggregated on the thromboembolus as it passes through the venous circulation into the pulmonary arteries. Additional humoral substances may be involved in humans, including other vasoactive amines, various prostaglandins, and leukotrienes. No convincing evidence suggests that reflex pulmonary vasoconstriction occurs. The development of arterial hypoxemia may be of great importance in producing additional pulmonary arterial constriction. Current evidence suggests that active pulmonary vasoconstriction plays a less important role in the development of pulmonary hypertension than does mechanical obstruction of the pulmonary arteries. The development of right ventricular failure with shock is usually seen only in the event of massive embolization of pulmonary arteries, wherein 60% to 70% of the pulmonary arterial beds have been occluded.

Breathlessness (dyspnea) with rapid shallow respirations (tachypnea) occurs in almost all patients after a symptomatic episode of pulmonary thromboembolism. This symptom is difficult to explain on the basis of the mechanisms thought to be operative in other patients with breathlessness and airway or parenchymal lung disease. With airway or parenchymal lung disease, there are usually significant alterations in lung mechanics, either increased airway resistance or decreased lung compliance. To maintain a normal volume of ventilation, one must increase the work of breathing to overcome the mechanical alterations, and the increased work of breathing is in some manner sensed as breathlessness, possibly by receptors in the muscles of the chest wall that can relate the movement of the respiratory system to the excess effort expended.

Although there are changes in lung mechanics after pulmonary embolism, they are usually mild and probably not sufficient by themselves to cause breathlessness. In this regard, recent experimental studies in animals on the humoral and reflex events that occur immediately after an embolic event may provide an explanation. Located in the alveolar wall are receptors known as juxtapulmonary capillary receptors or *J receptors*, which are stimulated by increased interstitial fluid pressure, humoral agents (*e.g.*, serotonin), and microemboli. When these receptors are stimulated, the response is rapid, shallow breathing, which is the typical pattern seen after pulmonary embolism in humans. This pattern of breathing is usually associated with alveolar hyperventilation and a respiratory alkalemia.

Another type of receptor, the irritant receptor, may also be involved. This receptor is located in the airway epithelium and can be stimulated by humoral substances, changes in lung compliance, bronchoconstriction, and irritants such as cigarette smoke. Stimulation of these receptors may cause tachypnea and cough. When these intrapulmonary receptors are stimulated in the experimental animal, there is an increased afferent nerve impulse activity in the vagus nerve supplying the lung, with subsequent stimulation of respiratory neurons in the medulla of the brain. This afferent input to the respiratory center presumably mediates the development of the rapid, shallow breathing pattern. It has been suggested, but not proved, that this increased level of vagal discharge to the respiratory center may be sensed as breathlessness. Currently, it is not known how or where the dyspneic sensation develops in the cerebrum. Most patients with pulmonary embolism and breathlessness have pulmonary hypertension when subjected to right heart catheterization and pulmonary angiography. This increase in pressure may effect an increase in interstitial fluid pressure in the lung, stimulating the J receptors, with additional stimulation by the humoral substances that are thought to be released. However, these reflex changes are not likely to be the only mechanism in the causation of breathlessness and the abnormal breathing pattern after pulmonary embolism (see below).

The physiological hallmark of pulmonary vascular occlusion is the development of an increase in dead-space or "wasted" ventilation. Following occlusion of the pulmonary arteries, the nonperfused lung units cease to accomplish gas exchange, but, in the absence of infarction, ventilation continues. Ventilation to these units is "wasted" in a functional sense because there is little or no carbon dioxide or oxygen exchange. The ventilation–perfusion ratio ($\dot{V}A/Q$) in these units is near infinity, and, as will be described, this alteration in lung function can sometimes be detected by radioisotope lung scanning. A more direct approach is to measure the physiological dead-space/tidal volume ratio (VD/VT). With the increase in dead-space ventilation, total ventilation of the lungs must increase to maintain normal carbon dioxide and oxygen exchange. The increase in total ventilation may be an additional factor in the development of breathlessness. If ventilation does not increase (e.g., in the patient on a ventilator with a fixed rate and tidal volume), hypercapnia with hypoxemia will ensue.

Although the nonspecific development of high $\dot{V}A/Q$ lung units is characteristic of acute pulmonary embolism, some changes that occur serve to decrease ventilation to the embolized lung units, including bronchoconstriction and pneumoconstriction in the embolized lung units, possible changes in pulmonary surfactant in the embolized lung units, and infarction. With cessation of perfusion, the carbon dioxide tension in the embolized lung units falls to low levels, resulting in smooth muscle constriction in the terminal lung units, which causes a shrinkage and stiffening of the embolized lung unit (pneumoconstriction) and smooth muscle constriction in the bronchi (bronchoconstriction). These alterations in alveolar and airway mechanics effect a shift in ventilation away from the embolized lung units but never to the extent that the $\dot{V}A/\dot{Q}$ ratio is restored to normal.

Within 12 to 24 hours, the embolized, nonperfused lung units may become deficient in producing surfactant, the lipoprotein secretion that serves to maintain the stability of the peripheral lung units. Without adequate amounts of surfactant, the embolized lung units may become stiff and collapse, thereby shifting ventilation away from the units. Infarction of the embolized lung unit shifts the ventilation to more normally perfused lung units.

These changes in lung mechanics and structure are the result of pulmonary ischemia. In addition humorally mediated changes are a consequence of changes involving the thromboembolus. In experimental thromboembolism in the dog, pulmonary resistance increases (bronchoconstriction) and pulmonary compliance falls (pneumoconstriction) immediately after embolization, and similar changes probably occur in humans. The observed acute decrease in maximal expiratory flow rate in persons with angiographically documented pulmonary thromboembolism is probably a consequence of bronchoconstriction, and the decrease in lung volume seen radiographically after acute pulmonary embolism, manifested by elevation of the diaphragms, may well be the result of the pneumoconstriction. In an experimental animal, these changes are due to the release of serotonin from platelets that have aggregated on the thromboembolus as it traverses the venous circulation. The transient nature of the radiographic changes that occur in humans, as well as the changes in maximal expiratory flow rates, is consistent with the possibility that they are humorally mediated. The changes can be prevented in animals by administration of heparin before embolization. In humans, heparin appears to lessen the degree of bronchoconstriction. Even if these changes in lung mechanics occur in humans, it is unlikely that they are the major factor in the development of persistent dyspnea because they are transient and of mild severity.

These mechanical changes are of more importance in the development of *arterial hypoxemia*, which is a common occurrence after pulmonary thromboembolism. However, the presence of a normal Pa_{O_2} does not exclude the diagnosis. Various mechanisms have been proposed as the cause of arterial hypoxemia, including a decrease in diffusing capacity owing to a reduced surface area of the alveolar–capillary membrane, abnormally rapid passage of blood through a pulmonary capillary bed decreased in volume, ventilation–perfusion abnormalities, atelectasis, and right-to-left shunting. Alveolar hypoventilation cannot be invoked since these patients usually hyperventilate.

Obstruction of the pulmonary vascular bed does result in a decreased diffusing capacity of the lung, but it is variable in degree and not usually sufficient to account for arterial hypoxemia at rest. A shortened transit time may be an important factor in hypoxemia during exercise but not at rest. Although there is evidence in humans that arterial hypoxemia after embolism may be partly due to right-to-left shunting secondary to atelectasis (which can be partially reversed by deep breathing), most evidence favors ventilation–perfusion imbalance as the primary cause of arterial hypoxemia at rest.

Following thromboembolism in a dog, a $\dot{V}A/\dot{Q}$ imbalance does develop. The following explanation has been proposed to explain the VA/Q imbalance and may also account for the development of atelectasis with right-to-left shunting: After embolism, release of

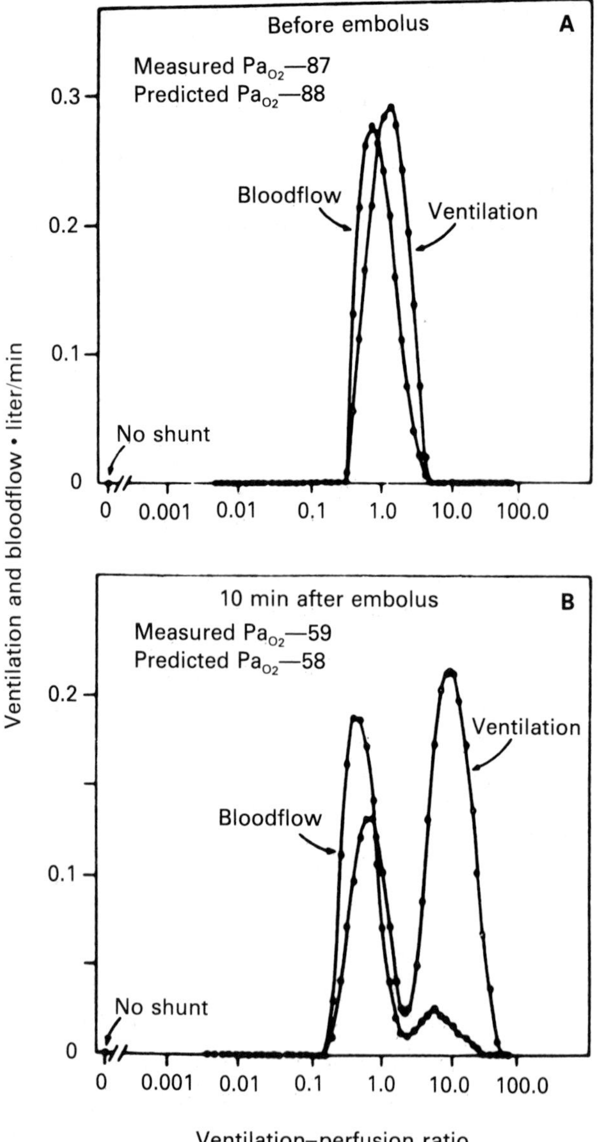

Fig. 33-1. Distributions of ventilation–perfusion ratios *(A)* before and *(B)* after experimental pulmonary thromboembolism in a dog. Note that embolization caused a region of high ventilation–perfusion ratios and that the main body of the distribution had its ventilation–perfusion ratio somewhat reduced. These changes were sufficient to account for the fall in arterial Pa_{O_2} to 59 mm Hg. (Reprinted with permission from West JB: Pulmonary Pathophysiology—The Essentials, p 129. Baltimore, Williams & Wilkins, 1977).

serotonin or other humoral agents into the pulmonary circulation induces nonuniform constriction of distal airways and terminal lung units, with a decrease in ventilation of these units with respect to their perfusion (*i.e.*, low $\dot{V}A/\dot{Q}$ ratios and a fall in Pa_{O_2}). When these changes are severe, atelectasis can occur with right-to-left shunting. This explanation is supported by the observation that heparin, when given *before* the release of thromboemboli in a dog, prevents, to a significant degree, changes in lung mechanics and a fall in Pa_{O_2}. Thus the disturbance in ventilation–perfusion relationships after embolization is characterized by the development of high $\dot{V}A/\dot{Q}$ lung units, as manifested by an increased VD/VT, and as manifested by a decreased arterial Pa_{O_2} and widened A-a Pa_{O_2} difference (Fig. 33-1).

In a recent interesting series of experiments on dogs, Fisher and colleagues postulated that postembolic decreases in Pa_{O_2} are due to shifting of perfusion to poorly ventilated areas of lung (low VA/Q). However, their experimental model included complex perturbations, and therefore may not resemble clinical pulmonary embolism in humans.

There is as yet insufficient understanding of the metabolic effects of pulmonary arterial obstruction to explain the development of *pulmonary infarction.* The lung parenchyma is protected by three sources of oxygen supply: the bronchial arteries, the pulmonary arteries, and the airways. In most clinical situations where infarction develops, there is either impairment of the bronchial circulation as a consequence of previous lung disease or pulmonary vascular congestion secondary to cardiac failure. Dalen and colleagues have observed that thromboembolism of a large pulmonary artery alone is not associated with pulmonary infarction. When a peripheral pulmonary artery suffers vascular occlusion, influx of bronchial artery blood may produce alveolar hemorrhage. In the presence of congestive heart failure and pulmonary venous hypertension, the hemorrhage does not resolve, and tissue necrosis (infarction) results. Pulmonary hemorrhage may resemble infarction on the chest radiograph but may be transient, lasting 4 to 5 days. Pulmonary hemorrhage or infarct may contribute to dyspnea and tachypnea by producing painful, shallow respirations owing to pleuritis. The role of endorphins, if any, in mitigating the effects of painful respirations or dyspnea is not known at present.

The natural history of these pathophysiological changes is determined primarily by the rapidity with which the thromboemboli lyse. In humans this is a dynamic process. The thrombi begin to lyse immediately after the embolic event, and within a matter of hours to days sufficient lysis will occur to allow reperfusion of embolized lung units, with a lessening of the physiological alterations and thereby the symptoms and signs of the embolic event. The rare emboli that fail to lyse result in permanent obstruction of the pulmonary vascular bed. If the residual obstruction is massive, chronic pulmonary hypertension will occur (see below).

CLINICAL MANIFESTATIONS

Symptoms and signs of pulmonary thromboembolism are nonspecific, and thus the diagnosis is often difficult to establish without resorting to more precise and definitive diagnostic procedures. Clinical findings that do occur are variable both in frequency and in intensity. They depend on the extent of pulmonary vascular occlusion, the functional state of the heart and the lungs before embolization, and the development of pulmonary infarction. It is particularly important to distinguish between the clinical findings in the patient with embolization alone and those in the patient having embolization with infarction. Because most embolic events do not result in infarction, the classic clinical picture occurs infrequently and is one of the major reasons why the disease is not diagnosed in many patients.

In the absence of infarction, embolization is almost invariably manifested by the abrupt onset of breathlessness. Unless the extent of embolic obstruction is severe, this may be the only subjective manifestation of the embolic event. When massive pulmonary embolization occurs with obstruction of more than 50% to 60% of the pulmonary vascular bed, severe pulmonary hypertension results and may be manifested by the development of substernal chest pain similar to the sensation experienced by patients with myocardial ischemia. The mechanism of the pain is unclear but may be secondary to subendocardial ischemia.

When, as a consequence of severe pulmonary outflow obstruction, the right ventricle fails with a decrease in cardiac output and perfusion to vital organs such as the brain, lightheadedness or syncope may occur. These latter symptoms are, however, *infrequent* because massive embolization is uncommon. In most patients breathlessness will be the only symptom of the embolic event. It may be fleeting in nature or persistent, and is usually exacerbated by physical exertion. The embolic event will usually occur in a patient with one or more of the previously described predisposing conditions.

On physical examination, the patient with acute pulmonary embolism will usually manifest an increase in respiratory rate (tachypnea) greater than 20/min and an increase in heart rate (tachycardia) greater than 90/min. Evidence of pulmonary hypertension as manifested by increased intensity of the pulmonary second sound or an abnormal splitting of the second sound with a widened and fixed split occurs less frequently and is usually only clearly manifested when the mean pulmonary artery pressure is greater than 25 to 30 mm Hg. With massive embolism and a marked increase in pulmonary vascular resistance, there will be evidence of right ventricular overwork and failure as manifested by a right ventricular lift, a right ventricular gallop, and distension of the jugular veins with an elevation of jugular venous pressure. Arterial hypotension with evidence of peripheral vasoconstriction may be seen, as well as central cyanosis.

One of the most striking findings in the patient with acute pulmonary embolism without infarction is the absence of any abnormal physical findings on examination of the lungs. It is this combination of acute breathlessness with no apparent pulmonary abnormality that should strongly suggest the diagnosis. Although wheezing has been described in some patients with acute pulmonary embolism, it occurs infrequently and is more likely to be seen in patients who have underlying bronchial disease such as asthma. Evidence of peripheral venous thrombosis on physical examination is seen in less than 50% of patients.

When embolic obstruction of the pulmonary arteries results in the development of pulmonary infarction, the clinical picture will be more typical. Cough, hemoptysis, pleuritic pain, and physical findings comprising signs of pulmonary consolidation with dullness and bronchial breathing, signs of pleuritis with a friction rub, or signs of pleural fluid will be present. Fever is also a common finding. Most patients who sustain a pulmonary infarct will usually manifest the symptoms and signs of embolization in addition to those of infarction. It is possible, but difficult to prove, that some patients develop infarction as a consequence of a small peripheral embolus but do not obstruct enough of the pulmonary vascular bed to cause pulmonary hypertension with breathlessness.

Leukocytosis, with an increase in sedimentation rate, occurs frequently in the patient with pulmonary infarction, as does an elevated LDH, normal SGOT, and elevated bilirubin, the so-called diagnostic triad. Unfortunately, these findings are nonspecific and of minimal diagnostic value. Arterial hypoxemia occurs frequently in association with alveolar hyperventilation. This again is a nonspecific finding, since most of the diseases with which pulmonary embolism is confused are usually associated with arterial hypoxemia. The measurement of "wasted ventilation" by determination of the physiological dead-space to tidal volume ratio (VD/VT) has been advocated as a useful diagnostic procedure but again is limited in applicability to those patients who have no other underlying cardiac or pulmonary disease. As is true of many pulmonary function tests, an abnormality may not be specific for a disease but is a consequence of many conditions that alter lung structure.

In the absence of massive embolism, the electrocardiogram is not very helpful, aside from showing tachycardia or nonspecific ST changes. The development of a rightward shift in axis, right ventricular strain, the classic S_1-Q_3-T_3 pattern, or P pulmonale is seen only with massive pulmonary embolism, and then not consistently.

Before the development of lung scanning and pulmonary angiography, the chest roentgenogram was the most useful laboratory diagnostic aid (*see* Chap. 14). In many patients with embolization without infarction, the chest roentgenogram is completely normal. When there are abnormalities, they include diaphragmatic elevation (a manifestation of pneumoconstriction) and avascular lung zones (Westermark's sign). With the development of infarction, pulmonary infiltrates are seen. They are not invariably the typically described triangular-shaped densities abutting on the pleural surface but may appear as consolidated or atelectatic densities, often with pleural effusions. In contrast to most pneumonias, the radiographic lesions are usually bilateral.

DIFFERENTIAL DIAGNOSIS

The diagnosis of pulmonary thromboembolism with or without infarction necessitates differentiating this disease from other diseases that can cause similar clinical and laboratory findings. Ultimately this requires lung scanning, and in some patients pulmonary angiography, to be specific or definitive. These techniques, which can visualize the pattern of distribution of pulmonary blood flow (radioisotope lung scans) and the anatomy of the pulmonary arteries (pulmonary angiography), have made it possible to approach the diagnosis of suspect pulmonary embolism systematically.

The first step in the diagnosis of pulmonary embolism and infarction is a high degree of suspicion based on suggestive clinical symptoms and signs. The second step includes the performance of routine laboratory tests, including chest roentgenogram, electrocardiogram, complete blood count, and arterial blood gas analysis with the measurement of pH, Pa_{CO_2}, and Pa_{O_2}. If all of these tests are consistent with the diagnosis and the clinical picture is very typical, further studies may not be needed before instituting anticoagulant therapy. This is an infrequent occurrence.

Most patients who present with breathlessness and *nonembolic* cardiac or pulmonary disease will have abnormal test results. The differential diagnosis of pulmonary embolism without infarction includes acute myocardial infarction, dissecting aneurysm, bacteremic shock, and anxiety states. In the differential diagnosis of pulmonary infarction, pneumonia, atelectasis, heart failure, and neoplasm must also be considered. In most patients additional studies are needed to establish the diagnosis.

The third step in evaluating a patient with suspected pulmonary embolism is the performance of a perfusion lung scan. This test is performed by the intravenous infusion of radiolabeled macroaggregates of human serum albumin, which are of sufficient size that they do not pass through the pulmonary capillaries but rather lodge there. As the macroaggregates pass through the right heart, they are mixed uniformly with the blood in the right ventricle and then distributed throughout the lungs in a pattern that corresponds to regional pulmonary blood flow. When the lungs are scanned with an appropriate imaging device (rectilinear scanner, scintillation camera), the distribution of pulmonary blood flow can be assessed. In contrast to the chest roentgenogram, where only one or two views of the lungs are needed, perfusion lung scanning requires viewing the lungs in the anterior, posterior, and both lateral projections to evaluate overall perfusion of the lungs. *An abnormality in the distribution of pulmonary blood flow detected by perfusion lung scanning is a nonspecific finding.* Abnormalities in the distribution of pulmonary blood flow are the usual consequence of any pulmonary or cardiac disease that affects lung structure or function.

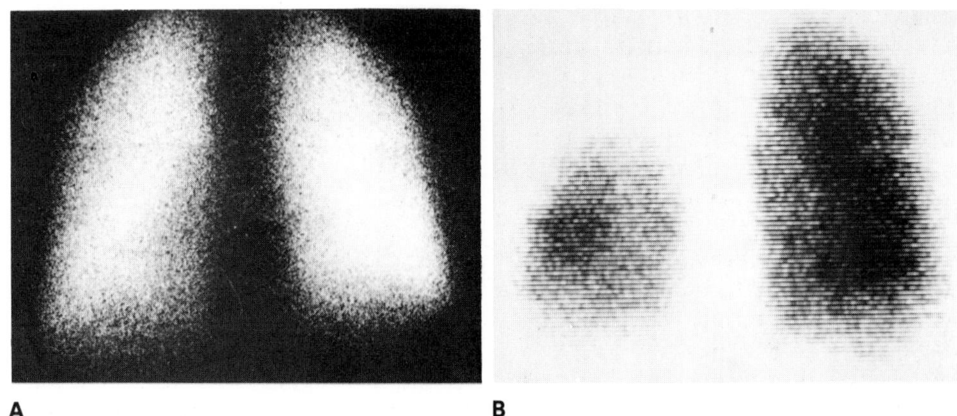

Fig. 33-2. Pulmonary scintiscans (posterior view). *(A)* Normal perfusion scan. *(B)* Perfusion scan showing a lobar defect involving the right upper lobe, consistent with pulmonary embolism but caused by a bronchogenic carcinoma.

Thus perfusion lung scan abnormalities, being nonspecific, never establish an etiologic diagnosis. This has led to many errors in diagnosis (Fig. 33-2).

The typical defect seen on the perfusion lung scan is an area of absent to markedly reduced radioactivity that conforms to a lung subsegment, lobe, or entire lung. Nonsegmental defects, which cross the boundary between adjacent lung segments, are more typical of nonembolic pulmonary diseases. One of the most important considerations in the interpretation of the perfusion lung scan is to correlate radiographic abnormalities, if present, with perfusion lung scan abnormalities. If the perfusion lung scan demonstrates abnormalities that correspond with radiographic abnormalities, the scan is considered to be "indeterminate" (Fig. 33-3), with the likelihood of pulmonary embolism ranging from 25% to 50%. Thus the "indeterminate" perfusion lung scan is of limited diagnostic value. Moreover this is the most frequent scan pattern found in patients with suspect pulmonary embolism who undergo lung scanning. The demonstration of a perfusion defect is more helpful when the chest roentgenogram is *normal*. However, even when a typical perfusion defect with a normal chest roentgenogram is observed, the probability of pulmonary embolism may be as low as 50%.

The usefulness of perfusion lung scanning can be increased when combined with ventilation lung scanning. The distribution of ventilation can be evaluated by the inhalation of a breath of xenon-133, with a subsequent imaging of the lungs with a scintillation camera to determine the distribution of ventilation. If an abnormality in the distribution of perfusion is a consequence of parenchymal lung disease involving airways or alveoli, a defect in ventilation similar to the perfusion defect will be found. Such a defect in the presence of a normal chest roentgenogram is said to be a "matched ventilation–perfusion defect." A "matched" defect does not usually occur after pulmonary embolization but does not conclusively rule out pulmonary embolism.

Emboli in the absence of infarction do not usually cause a persistent decrease in ventilation of the embolized lung unit, and the ventilation scan will typically show normal ventilation in the area of diminished perfusion (Fig. 33-4). This type of defect—that is, areas of diminished perfusion with normal ventilation in the presence of a normal chest roentgenogram—is called a "mismatch." The specificity of this combined defect is much greater than that of a perfusion defect alone and has been shown to be a manifestation of angiographically proven emboli in 80% to 100% of instances when the perfusion defects are of moderate size or greater (more than 25% of segmental volume) and are multiple. The scans, however, *never* provide specific anatomical information. If the diagnosis of pulmonary embolism is still in doubt after ventilation–perfusion scanning and it is necessary to establish a definitive diagnosis, pulmonary angiography is indicated. It is the only test that can provide specific and definitive evidence on the presence of pulmonary emboli.

Pulmonary angiography is a procedure that has minimal risks to the patient unless severe pulmonary

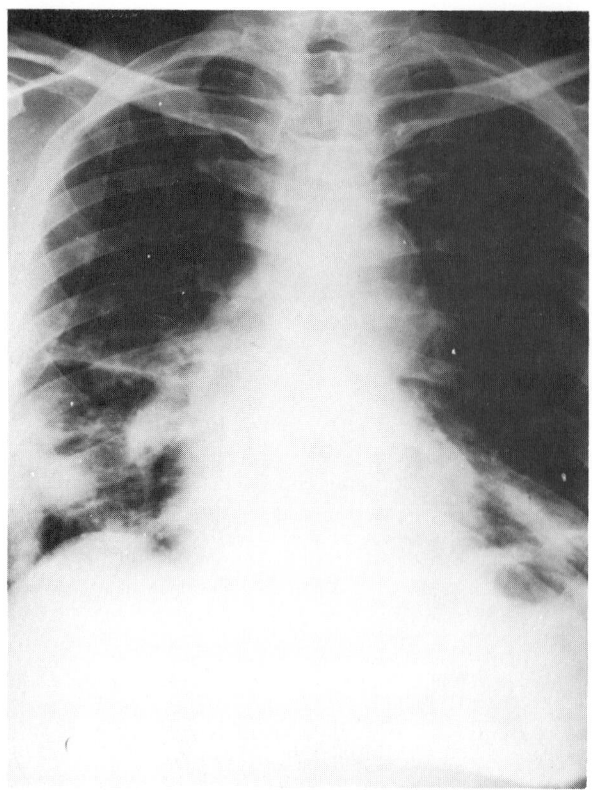

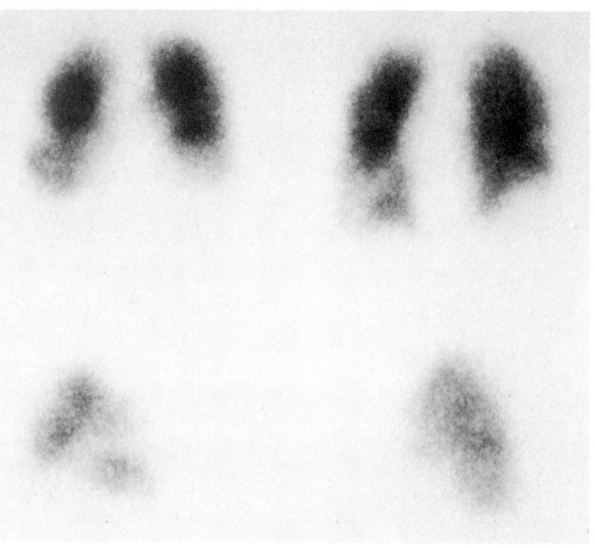

Fig. 33-3. Findings in a patient with dyspnea, pleurisy, and hemoptysis. *(A)* Chest roentgenogram demonstrating bibasilar atelectatic and infiltrative changes consistent with pulmonary embolism and infarction or pneumonitis. *(B)* Pulmonary perfusion scintiscans: Upper left, anterior view; upper right, posterior view; lower left, right lateral view; lower right, left lateral view. Perfusion defects correspond to the roentgenographic defects. This scan is "indeterminate." Pulmonary angiogram (not shown) demonstrated thromboemboli.

hypertension (mean pulmonary artery pressure greater than 45 mm Hg) or shock is present.

Pulmonary angiography requires the positioning of a suitable catheter in the pulmonary artery (*i.e.*, right heart catheterization). A radiopaque dye is rapidly injected into the pulmonary artery, and rapid serial roentgenograms are taken. The findings that are diagnostic of embolism are the presence of a filling defect within the artery and a "cutoff" of the artery (Fig. 33-5). The filling defect results from incomplete filling of the lumen of the thrombus-occluded artery with contrast material. The "cutoff" is seen as an abrupt termination of the contrast material within the artery as a consequence of total obstruction by an embolus. Another advantage of performing pulmonary angiography is that the pulmonary artery pressure can be measured to assess the severity of the embolic event. It is also possible at this time to measure cardiac output and quantitate the pulmonary vascular resistance.

When the lung scan is completely normal in a patient with suspect pulmonary embolism and has been performed within 48 to 72 hours of the acute episode, the likelihood of pulmonary embolism as a cause of symptoms suggesting embolization (e.g., breathlessness) is very remote. A normal perfusion scan, however, does not exclude possible small peripheral pulmonary emboli, which might cause infarction with pleurisy but not breathlessness. This type of embolic event cannot be diagnosed by conventional angiography either, and there is no reliable method of making a definitive diagnosis of this type of pulmonary embolism. Fortunately, life-threatening embolic disease is rarely, if ever, a consequence of small, peripheral emboli. In the Urokinase Pulmonary Embolism Trial, 150 patients with angiographically

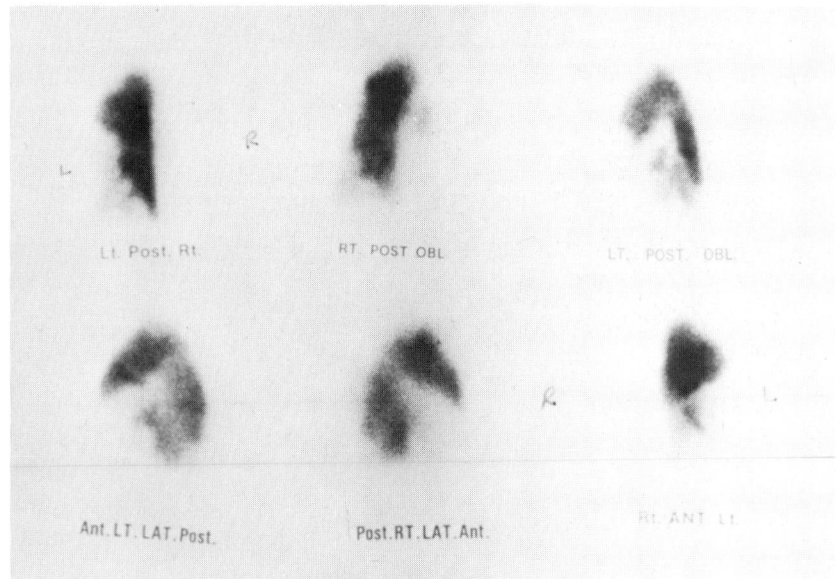

A

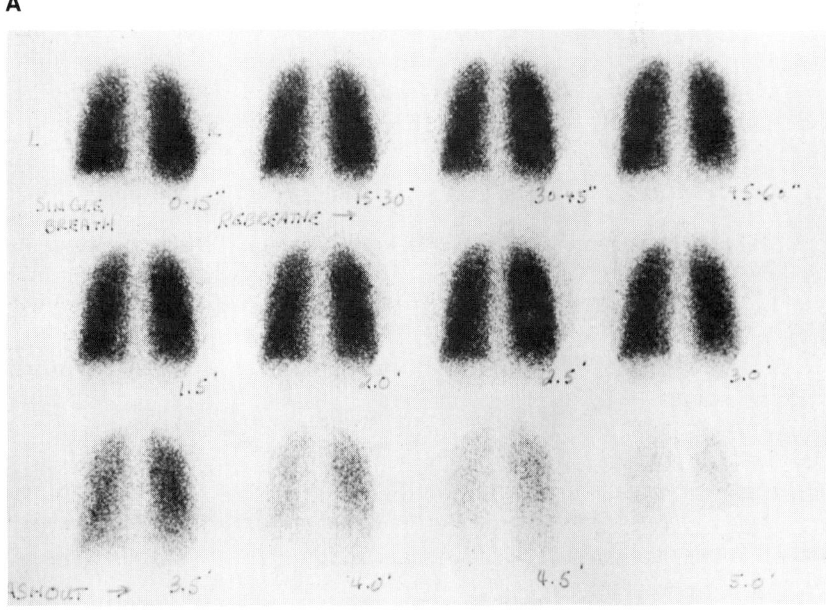

B

Fig. 33-4. Pulmonary scintiscans in a patient with chronic dyspnea and recurrent pleurisy with hemoptysis. Chest roentgenogram was normal. *(A)* Perfusion scan. There is absent perfusion to the entire right lung. *(B)* Ventilation scan. Ventilation to both lungs is normal. This $\dot{V}/\dot{Q}$ scan is a "mismatch" because of pulmonary thromboembolism (*see* Fig. 33-5).

proven emboli had lung scans, and in none was the scan completely normal. Currently, it is thought that a completely normal, well-performed perfusion lung scan rules out the possibility of arteriographically detectable emboli.

Other procedures that may be helpful in evaluating the patient with suspected pulmonary embolism are those tests designed to detect venous thrombosis, including venography, ^{125}I-fibrinogen scanning, impedance plethysmography, and tests that reflect coagulation disturbances, including measurement of fibrin-split products and fibrin monomer complexes. However, failure to demonstrate venous thrombosis or coagulation abnormalities does not exclude the diagnosis.

The diagnosis of pulmonary thromboembolism is particularly difficult to establish in the patient with underlying, previously diagnosed pulmonary disease, whether obstructive or restrictive. In such patients, both a ventilation and perfusion scan must be done.

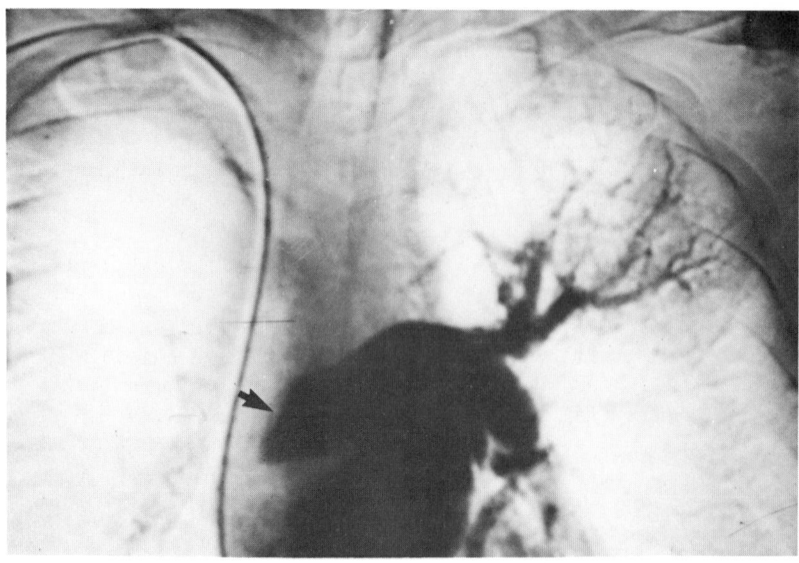

Fig. 33-5. Pulmonary angiogram in a patient with $\dot{V}/\dot{Q}$ "mismatch" (*see* Fig. 33-4). Posteroanterior chest film shows the catheter that has been passed through the superior vena cava, through the right atrium and ventricle, and into the pulmonary trunk. The pulmonary trunk, both main pulmonary arteries, and several lobar and segmental arteries in the left lung are opacified by the injected contrast. A large filling defect, "cut off," in the right main pulmonary artery diagnostic of embolism is seen *(arrow)*. Additional filling defects can be seen in the left lower lobe arteries.

In the patient with a normal chest roentgenogram, a "matched" defect suggests strongly that the symptoms and signs are not a consequence of pulmonary embolism. However, in the presence of pulmonary infiltrates (e.g., the patient with pneumonia, atelectasis, or heart failure), a "matched" defect might well be due to an embolic event with infarction. If the diagnosis is to be established or excluded with certainty, pulmonary angiography is mandatory.

In summary, the diagnosis of pulmonary embolism in most patients can be established with reasonable certainty from the clinical evaluation, chest roentgenogram, electrocardiogram, and perfusion lung scan. In some patients, a ventilation scan will be needed to determine whether or not the perfusion defect is a consequence of parenchymal lung disease or primary vascular disease, and, in a smaller number of patients, pulmonary angiography will be necessary.

PROGNOSIS AND NATURAL HISTORY

To appreciate the impact and the effect of anticoagulant therapy of pulmonary thromboembolism, one should review the natural history of untreated embolic disease. The mortality following the initial thromboembolic event has been estimated to be about 25%. This figure may be misleading, being both an overestimate and an underestimate. In the patient with compromised cardiopulmonary function, who is at greater risk to develop thromboemboli, there is a greater likelihood that he will die after the initial embolic event. Those patients who have normal cardiopulmonary function most likely have a lower incidence of mortality after the initial embolic event.

Once the embolic event has occurred and the patient has survived, the chances of recurrence without therapy and subsequent fatality are great, with approximately 50% of patients experiencing a recurrent episode. In about half of these embolic episodes a fatality occurs. With anticoagulant therapy the recurrence rate is reduced to about 5%, and fewer of the recurrences will be fatal. Thus the initial outcome of a thromboembolic episode is largely predetermined by the patient's cardiopulmonary status and the extent of embolization. The subsequent response will depend primarily on the adequacy of anticoagulant therapy. With adequate therapy, resolution by lysis of the thrombi begins immediately and may be reasonably complete within 14 days after the embolic event, with similar resolution of the cardiopulmonary functional alterations, symptoms, and signs. Recurrent embolism is unlikely unless a predisposing factor persists (e.g., persistent cardiac failure or long-term immobility).

THERAPY

Any discussion of the treatment of pulmonary thromboembolism must include consideration of [1] prophylactic therapy in the patient who is predisposed to venous thrombosis and embolism; [2] therapy of the acute embolic event; and [3] the prevention of further embolism in the patient who has experienced an acute embolic event.

PROPHYLACTIC THERAPY

The optimal therapy of pulmonary thromboembolism would be a reliable, consistent method to prevent venous thrombosis. Toward this end the correction of any predisposing factor is of great importance (e.g., early ambulation after surgery). In many patients, however, this is not easily accomplished, for example, after a myocardial infarction or hip fracture. Recently there has been great interest in developing therapeutic modalities that will prevent venous thrombosis and thereby prevent thromboembolism.

The most promising approaches have been directed at the prevention of coagulation with drugs that either prevent the generation of thrombin or inhibit platelet aggregation. In the latter instance, aspirin and dipyridamole, drugs that can inhibit platelet aggregation, have been used, among others. Controlled studies of each drug used independently have not demonstrated any convincing decrease in the incidence of ^{125}I-fibrinogen-detectable venous thrombi in the legs postoperatively.

The most promising results to date have been achieved with heparin in low doses, which prevents the generation of thrombin. When given before and after surgery in a dose of 5000 units subcutaneously every 12 hours, there is a significant decrease in the incidence of ^{125}I-fibrinogen-detectable calf vein thromboses in treated patients. When given in this way, there is little or no effect on coagulation, specifically on the thrombin clotting time. Similar results have been obtained in patients with postmyocardial infarction when the heparin was given every 8 hours, although there was a slight prolongation of the activated partial thromboplastin time (APTT). Low-dose heparin, however, has not been effective in the prophylaxis of deep venous thrombosis and pulmonary embolism in patients with hip fractures or after hip surgery. Clinically significant bleeding has not been a problem with the use of low-dose heparin.

Although low-dose heparin appears to be effective in certain situations in preventing venous thrombosis, it is of no value in treating established acute thromboembolic disease. One might anticipate that this type of prophylactic therapy in the patient with chronic obstructive pulmonary disease, particularly when in respiratory failure, might be beneficial in decreasing the incidence of venous thrombosis and pulmonary embolism. In a single reported study, low-dose heparin, 5000 units subcutaneously every 8 hours, produced a significant decrease of pulmonary emboli in respiratory intensive care unit patients. Although the increased incidence of gastrointestinal bleeding encountered in patients in respiratory failure may argue against the routine use of low-dose heparin in such patients, the reported study failed to demonstrate significant increases in frequency or severity of gastrointestinal hemorrhage. However, low-dose heparin was believed to be contraindicated in a large number of intensive care patients. Also, the duration of therapy and the effectiveness of prophylactic heparin in preventing deaths owing to pulmonary embolism in such patients have not been established.

TREATMENT OF THE EMBOLIC EVENT AND PREVENTION OF FURTHER EMBOLISM

After an embolic episode, therapy is directed at two goals: First, supportive therapy is used to maintain cardiopulmonary function and relieve breathlessness, pain, and hypoxemia until the thrombi begin to lyse; and second, and more important, is the prevention by anticoagulation of further venous thromboses and embolization. It is only in those infrequent instances where these goals cannot be achieved that surgical therapy may be indicated. Supportive therapy includes the administration of oxygen in concentrations sufficient to raise the Pa_{O_2} to greater than 60 to 70 torr, analgesics for relief of severe pleuritic pain if present, and vasoactive drugs if cardiac failure with a depression of cardiac output occurs. Isoproterenol given by intravenous drip (2–4 mg/500 ml of 5% dextrose in water) may be effective in this event because of its pulmonary vasodilator effect and its inotropic effect on the heart. Metaraminol may also be effective.

Although digitalization may not be very effective therapy, it may be used if there is cardiac failure. There probably is no contraindication to its use as long as the patient is adequately oxygenated. In regard to oxygen therapy, [1] the arterial hypoxemia responds well to modest increases in inspired oxygen concentrations (e.g., 6–8 liters/min via a nasal cannula) because the mechanism of hypoxemia is primarily a $\dot{V}A/\dot{Q}$ abnormality; [2] these patients rarely hypoventilate and there is no need to fear respiratory depression as a consequence of raising the arterial oxygen tension; and [3] one should not expect significant relief of breathlessness with oxygen therapy since the cause of the breathlessness presumably has other origins.

The mainstay of therapy for pulmonary thromboembolism is directed at preventing further venous thrombosis. Most patients, if they survive the immediate hemodynamic effects of the embolic event, will recover as the thrombi spontaneously lyse. The prevention of further venous thrombosis is accomplished by anticoagulation, which is initiated with heparin rather than an oral anticoagulant because of the rapid action of heparin. The oral anticoagulants do not become effective for at least 4 to 6 days, and during this period the patient is most likely to suffer recurring embolic episodes as a consequence of continuing venous thrombosis. Heparin can be administered by either of two intravenous methods: as a bolus of 5000 to 7500 units every 4 to 6 hours, or by continuous pump infusion with the goal of prolonging the clotting time to two to two and one-half times normal. The precise methods of heparin administration, dose, monitoring, and duration of therapy have not been established.

When given by continuous pump infusion, a loading dose of 2000 to 3000 units is given, followed by 1000 units per hour. Regardless of the method, the adequacy of anticoagulation should be assessed by periodic determinations of APTT. When given by the bolus method, the APTT should be determined ½ hour to 1 hour before the next dose of heparin.

With adequate anticoagulation, the likelihood that the patient will experience further venous thrombosis with recurrent embolization is low (*i.e.*, less than 5–10%), unless there is a significant predisposing factor, such as intractable cardiac failure or a defect in antithrombin III. Once supportive therapy and anticoagulant therapy have been instituted and the patient is improving, the major decision that remains is the question of how long to continue the anticoagulant therapy. In the patient who can be identified as having definable causes of venous thrombosis that can be reversed (e.g., the postoperative state in an otherwise healthy person), anticoagulation need be continued only until the patient is *fully* ambulatory—usually a minimum of 8 to 10 days. In this regard, as soon as the patient's hemodynamic and respiratory status has stabilized and begun to return to normal, ambulation is very important in preventing further venous thrombosis and embolization. In the patient with no definable cause for thromboembolism, anticoagulation should be continued empirically for 6 months, changing from heparin to an oral anticoagulant during the first week of therapy. In the patient in whom an irreversible predisposing factor persists (e.g., chronic congestive heart failure, pulmonary hypertension owing to pulmonary embolism, recurrent episodes of pulmonary embolism after cessation of therapy), anticoagulant therapy probably should be continued indefinitely.

The only absolute contraindication to the use of heparin is a hemorrhagic disorder or active bleeding. The incidence of morbidity and mortality related to hemorrhagic complications associated with heparin therapy must be considered in treating the patient who has presumed pulmonary thromboembolism. In the patient in whom the diagnosis is firm, the risk of not treating is far greater than the risk of treating. However, the complications of heparin therapy are significant, with bleeding occurring in 10% to 20% of patients treated by the bolus method. However, this increased incidence of bleeding may be related to the administration of larger doses of heparin when given by the intermittent bolus method. Women older than 65 years of age are even more likely to experience hemorrhagic complications, for reasons that are not clear. Other patients may also have an increased risk of complicating hemorrhage: elderly men and those with recent gastrointestinal bleeding, liver disease, and abnormal coagulation. For this reason, if there is any question about the diagnosis, pulmonary angiography should be considered seriously before anticoagulant therapy is instituted or continued.

Therapy directed at lysis of the thromboemboli (thrombolytic therapy) has been the subject of a number of recent studies. The drugs that have been evaluated are urokinase and streptokinase, both of which activate and accelerate the rate of clot lysis during the first 24 to 48 hours after the initial thromboembolic event. During this time, patients receiving thrombolytic therapy may have greater resolution of hemodynamic abnormalities and more rapid restoration of perfusion. However, a comparison of patients treated with anticoagulation only versus anticoagulation plus thrombolytic therapy did not demonstrate any significant difference in the resolution of symptoms, mortality, or cardiopulmonary abnormalities 2 weeks after the embolic event. Moreover, the incidence of bleeding in the patient treated with thrombolytic drugs was significantly greater. The situations wherein thrombolytic therapy may prove most useful is in the patient with massive pulmonary embolism and shock, thus effecting a "medical pulmonary embolectomy." Thrombolytic therapy is also recommended for the patient with onset of deep venous thrombosis of recent origin. Recently, a National Institutes of Health Consensus Conference recommended increasing use of these thrombolytic drugs. The reader is referred to recent reviews about indications, contraindications, monitoring, and continuing controversies regarding these agents (*see* Bibliography under Therapy).

SURGICAL THERAPY

A surgical approach to the treatment of acute pulmonary thromboembolism is indicated only when anticoagulation fails to prevent recurrent thromboembolism or in the patient in whom anticoagulation is contraindicated. In these instances vena caval interruption or embolectomy may be used. Several methods have been developed to interrupt the passage of the venous thrombi through the inferior vena cava, including ligation of the inferior vena cava, plication of the vena cava with sutures or a clip, placement of a "harpstring grid" of sutures across the vena cava, and more recently, placement of an "umbrella" in the vena cava.

In most instances, regardless of the method used to interrupt the vena cava, subsequent thrombosis at the site of interruption occurs, thus converting the nonocclusive modalities into a total occlusion. Inasmuch as the patient who fails to respond to anticoagulation therapy usually has underlying cardiac, pulmonary, or other predisposing disease, it is not surprising that when vena caval interruption is indicated, there is significant morbidity and mortality related to the procedure itself. Although recurrent embolization is unlikely to occur during the immediate period after the ligation, recurrent embolization does subsequently occur in a significant percentage of patients (10–20%). This suggests that when medical therapy fails, the ultimate prognosis is poor, with the likelihood of further embolization and mortality being great. Whenever the vena cava is interrupted, continued anticoagulation therapy should be considered, unless contraindicated, to minimize the chances of complications related to venous disease developing in the lower extremities.

Rarely, patients with massive pulmonary embolism will not die immediately but will survive for a period ranging from several hours to several days, experiencing progressive deterioration of cardiac and pulmonary function. In such patients, if thrombolytic therapy and anticoagulation therapy have failed, pulmonary embolectomy may be indicated. Few patients will fall into this category, inasmuch as the natural history of the disease is spontaneous lysis of the thrombi with improvement in cardiac and pulmonary

Table 33-1. Observations Before and After Pulmonary Thromboendarterectomy (PTE)

	BEFORE PTE	AFTER PTE
Dyspnea	Present with mild exertion	None with moderate exertion
Vital capacity, *liters*	5.2	4.1
Total lung capacity, *liters*	6.9	5.2
Airway mechanics	Normal	Normal
Diffusing capacity (single breath), *ml/min/mm Hg*	31	36
Pa_{O_2}, *mm Hg*		
Rest	59	104
Exercise*	40	88
Minute volume, *liters/min*		
Rest	20.0	5.1
Exercise*	117.0	42.5
Physiologic dead space/tidal volume, %		
Rest	51	32
Exercise*	61	28

*At similar power output before and after PTE.

function with the institution of appropriate therapy. Thus if the patient can be kept alive for 24 hours, he will usually recover. If pulmonary embolectomy is necessary, it should be undertaken only if adequate facilities for open-heart surgery with cardiopulmonary bypass are available. Pulmonary angiography should always be performed to verify the diagnosis before surgical therapy.

A small number of patients have not had resolution of their pulmonary emboli. These patients have chronic pulmonary thromboembolism, and, if the pulmonary vascular obstruction is great, they may have disabling, chronic pulmonary hypertension. They may experience progressive dyspnea on exercise, hypoxemia increased by exercise, large dead space ventilation, and increases in pulmonary artery pressure (Table 33-1). The normal diffusing capacity observed in the patient described in Table 33-1 may be due to filling of the pulmonary capillary bed via bronchial arteries or retrograde filling from pulmonary veins. Perfusion lung scans and pulmonary arteriograms in this subject demonstrated no perfusion of the right lung and partial vascular obstruction of the left, findings that did not change over an 8-month period despite a course of adequate anticoagulation (Fig. 33-4). After pulmonary thromboendarterectomy, perfusion lung scans (Fig. 33-6), and exercise, tolerance (Table 33-1) improved dramatically. Four months after the surgical procedure, the patient was jogging 4 miles daily. Although chronic pulmonary embolism is a rare complication, it is likely that increasing follow-up of pulmonary embolism will lead to discovery of increasing numbers of such patients. Hopefully, the mechanisms involved in failure of thrombus lysis will be uncovered in the near future.

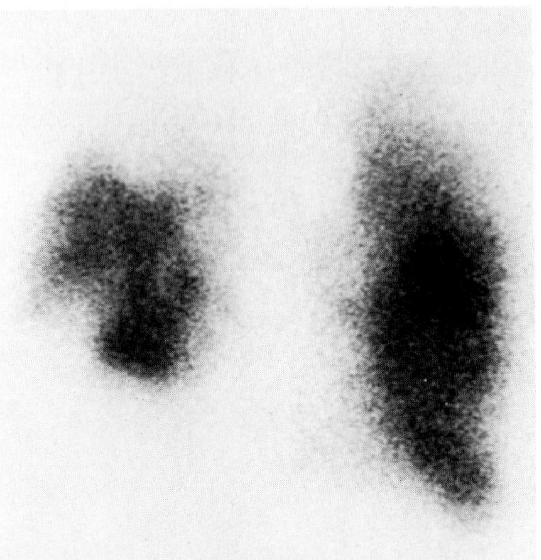

Fig. 33-6. Pulmonary perfusion scintiscan in patient with $\dot{V}/\dot{Q}$ "mismatch" (*see* Figs. 33-4, 33-5) following pulmonary thromboendarterectomy. There has been significant reperfusion of the right lung and improved perfusion to the left lower lobe.

SPECIAL CONSIDERATIONS IN THE PATIENT ON A VENTILATOR WHO DEVELOPS A PULMONARY EMBOLUS

As discussed previously, patients with chronic obstructive airway disease are likely to develop pulmonary thromboembolism, and the diagnosis can be very difficult, particularly in the patient in respiratory failure and on a ventilator. The clinical findings that should suggest pulmonary embolism include the abrupt worsening of breathlessness, for which no apparent explanation can be found (*i.e.*, secretions, bronchospasm, pneumothorax, or acute cardiac failure). Usually there will be no specific clinical findings that will allow one to make the diagnosis, and reliance must be placed on physiological studies, lung scanning, and pulmonary angiography. Although not specific, the measurement of "wasted ventilation" may be very useful in this situation, particularly if previous baseline measurements have been done. With embolization, there will be an abrupt increase in the physiological dead space to tidal volume ratio. In the patient who has limited ventilatory capacity or in the patient who is on a ventilator and cannot increase minute ventilation, the consequence of the increase in "wasted ventilation" will be a decrease in "effective" alveolar ventilation with a sudden rise in Pa_{CO_2}. The Pa_{O_2} will also fall abruptly, and the fall will be out of proportion to the rise in Pa_{CO_2}. Thus the abrupt development of increased breathlessness with tachycardia and tachypnea in a patient on a respirator, with an abrupt increase in Pa_{CO_2} in the absence of any change in total minute ventilation, strongly suggests the development of pulmonary embolization. Recognizing the limitations of lung scanning in such a patient, pulmonary angiography is probably the diagnostic procedure of choice. The use of low-dose heparin prophylactically in such patients may prevent this unwanted complication.

BIBLIOGRAPHY

Incidence and Importance

Dalen JE, Alpert JS: Natural history of pulmonary embolism. Prog Cardiovasc Dis 27:259, 1975

Etiology and Pathology

Castleman B: Pathologic observations on pulmonary infarction in man. In Sasahara AA, Stein M (eds): Pulmonary Embolic Disease. New York, Grune & Stratton, 1965

Freiman DG: Pathologic observations on experimental and human pulmonary thromboembolism. In Sasahara AA, Stein M (eds): Pulmonary Embolic Disease. New York, Grune & Stratton, 1965

Kakkar VV, Flanc C, Howe CT et al: Natural history of postoperative deep vein thrombosis. Lancet 2:230, 1969

Pathophysiology

McIntyre KM, Sasahara AA: Hemodynamic and ventricular responses to pulmonary embolism. Prog Cardiovasc Dis 27:175, 1974

Stein M, Levy SE: Reflex and humoral responses to pulmonary embolism. Prog Cardiovasc Dis 27:164, 1974

Thomas DP, Gurewich V, Ashford TP: Platelet adherence to thromboemboli in relation to pathogenesis and treatment of pulmonary embolism. N Engl J Med 274:953, 1966

Thomas DP et al: Mechanism of bronchoconstriction produced by thromboemboli in dogs. Am J Physiol 206:1207, 1964

Clinical Manifestations

Goodwin JF: Clinical diagnosis of pulmonary thromboembolism. In Sasahara AA, Stein M (eds): Pulmonary Embolic Disease. New York, Grune & Stratton, 1965

Sasahara AA: Clinical studies in pulmonary thromboembolism. In Sasahara AA, Stein M (eds): Pulmonary Embolic Disease. New York, Grune & Stratton, 1965

Simon M: Plain film and angiographic aspects of pulmonary embolism. In Moser KM, Stein M (eds): Pulmonary Thromboembolism. Chicago, Yearbook, 1973

Diagnosis and Differential Diagnosis

Ashburn WL, Moser KM: Pulmonary ventilation and perfusion scanning in pulmonary thromboembolism. In Moser KM, Stein M (eds): Pulmonary Thromboembolism. Chicago, Yearbook, 1973

Biello DR et al: Ventilation-perfusion studies in suspected pulmonary embolism. Am J Roentgenol 133:1033, 1979

Moser KM: Diagnostic measures in pulmonary embolism. Basics of RD 3, No. 5, 1975

Tow DE, Simon AL: Comparison of lung scanning and pulmonary arteriography in the detection and follow-up of pulmonary embolism. The Urokinase Pulmonary Embolism Trial Experience. Prog Cardiovasc Dis 27:239, 1975

Tow DE et al: Validity of measuring regional pulmonary blood flow with macroaggregates of human serum albumin. Am J Roentgenol Radium Ther Nucl Med 96:664, 1966

Wagner HN, Strauss HW: Radioactive tracers in the differential diagnosis of pulmonary embolism. Prog Cardiovasc Dis 27:271, 1975

Therapy

Sasahara AA: Therapy for pulmonary embolism. JAMA 229:1795, 1974

Silverglade AJ: Thromboembolism: Diagnosis and treatment. West J Med 120:219, 1974

Thrombolytic Therapy in Thrombosis: A National Institutes of Health Consensus Development Conference. Ann Intern Med 93:141, 1980

Urokinase pulmonary embolism trial: Phase 1 results. Urokinase Pulmonary Embolism Trial Study Group. JAMA 214:2163, 1970

Urokinase-streptokinase embolism trial: Phase 2 results. JAMA 229:1606, 1974

34

Respiratory Care of the Neurologic/ Neurosurgical Patient

Edward J. O'Connor

The purpose of this chapter is to provide an introductory understanding of respiratory control and the neurologic illnesses that cause respiratory dysfunction. Several neuromedical abnormalities exhibit subtle respiratory changes, but others can produce, or be complicated by, life-threatening pulmonary disorders.

Nearly 50% of deaths in most neuromedicine or neurosurgery units are secondary to respiratory causes. When respiratory abnormalities are life-threatening, the very survival of the neuromedical or neurosurgical patient often depends on the quality of respiratory care. The many advances in respiratory therapy help to ensure that the improving neurologic patient will not perish from pulmonary complications. As will be pointed out, application of some of these techniques is not without hazard because of certain physiological considerations. The many different neurologic problems that cause respiratory dysfunction can be studied further in those sources listed in the Bibliography.

CONTROL OF RESPIRATION

The respiratory control system can be conceptualized as an integrated mechanism comprising three parts: afferent mechanisms, central controller, and efferent mechanisms. Although respiration will continue in an isolated brain-stem preparation, normal respiration depends on intact afferent pathways to adjust ventilation to changing metabolic demands.

SENSORS

The afferent mechanisms, or sensors, include the peripheral arterial chemoreceptors, central chemoreceptors, and lung receptors. The *peripheral* arterial chemoreceptors mediate the immediate ventilatory increase produced by hypoxemia and increased hydrogen ion. These receptors are located in the carotid bodies near the bifurcation of the common carotid artery and in the aortic bodies near the aortic arch. Their central projections are carried in the carotid sinus and vagus nerves, primarily toward the nucleus tractus solitarius in the medulla.

Chemoreceptor discharge of the carotid bodies is increased by decreased Pa_{O_2}, increased Pa_{CO_2}, and decreased pH, whereas aortic body chemoreceptor discharge is increased only by decreased Pa_{O_2} and, to a lesser extent, by an increased Pa_{CO_2}. The precise mechanism for transduction of chemical stimuli to nerve action potential is not clear.

Central receptors are located near the ventral surface of the medulla and project toward the respiratory integrating site in the medulla.[21] These chemoreceptors, located in the medulla, provide a delayed (about 60 sec) response of increased ventilation to increases in alveolar carbon dioxide. This response occurs even after denervation of the peripheral chemoreceptors and suggests that the central chemoreceptors are not in immediate equilibrium with arterial blood. The central chemoreceptors are sensitive to changes in body levels of carbon dioxide, as perceived by changes in the brain extracellular fluid or cerebrospinal fluid pH.

The three major types of *lung receptors* are the pulmonary stretch receptors, the irritant receptors, and the type J receptors. The phasic pulmonary stretch receptors are located in the smooth muscle of the airways and are activated by lung inflation. The afferent discharge is carried by the vagus nerves to the brain stem and tends to limit the respiratory excursions. This is the classic Hering–Breuer reflex. Recent studies indicate that, in humans, this reflex occurs only at tidal volumes of one and one-half to two times resting levels.[5,35]

The irritant receptors lie in the epithelial cells of airways and are excited by chemical and mechanical irritants. When stimulated, the reflex effects include hyperpnea and bronchoconstriction.

The type J receptors probably are located near the walls of the pulmonary capillaries and are activated by pulmonary congestion, but the reflex effect during normal respiration is not clear.

CENTRAL CONTROLLER

The sensors provide ongoing information for the central integration of respiratory control. Since the respiratory muscles are mainly skeletal and have no inherent rhythm, they cannot function without nervous system control. The central nervous system control of respiration is divided into two components: voluntary respiration and automatic respiration. The voluntary system, which originates in the forebrain, has its expression in our speech, nonverbal communication, and emotions. The automatic system regulates breathing to maintain normal oxygenation and acid–base balance.

Lumsden's classic experiments on the cat brainstem respiratory system led him to conclude that brain-stem transection at the quadrigeminal plate had no effect on automatic respiration, whereas transection at the cervical medullary junction caused cessation of all respiratory movements. He also proposed that three brain-stem centers were associated with respiration: a pneumotaxic center in the rostral pons; an apneustic center near the pontomedullary junction; and a medullary center.[17,18] Recent information suggests that the pneumotaxic center tunes the respiratory pattern, primarily by setting lung inspiratory cutoff and modulating respiratory response to afferent stimuli. No specific apneustic center has been identified, and apneusis is considered a general phenomenon of sustained inspiration due to prolonged discharge of medullary inspiratory neurons resulting from an impaired inspiratory cutoff mechanism.

The medulla alone can spontaneously generate respiration. When parts of the medulla are destroyed, respiration ceases. The respiratory medulla comprises two bilateral neuronal columns: One, the dorsal respiratory group (DRG), is located in the ventrolateral aspect of the nucleus tractus solitarius and contains inspiratory cells; the other, the ventral respiratory group (VRG), is located in the nucleus ambiguous/nucleus retroambigualis and has inspiratory and expiratory neurons.

The DRG neurons project to the VRG, not *vice versa*, and also to the contralateral spinal cord. Since the DRG is part of the nucleus tractus solitarius, it receives afferent projections from the carotid sinus and vagus nerves that may then be incorporated into a respiratory motor response. It has been suggested that the DRG is the origin of the rhythmic drive to the VRG and that a primary site of respiratory rhythmic generation lies near the DRG. The VRG projects primarily to the spinal cord and innervates spinal respiratory motoneurons as well as phrenic motoneurons.

The axons of the cortical (voluntary) and medullary (automatic) respiratory neurons descend in spinal cord white matter. The descending cortical tracts travel in the posterolateral columns, whereas the axons of the VRG and DRG cross midline in the region of the obex and descend in the ventrolateral columns of the cord. This anatomical separation of the two pathways occasionally results in striking clinical abnormalities characterized by normal or near-normal breathing while awake but by severe hypoventilation, or apnea, during sleep or inattention. This syndrome, which has been seen in bilateral cervical chordotomy,[27] medullary infarcts,[8] poliomyelitis,[32] syringomyelia, encephalitis,[6] and other medullary lesions, is due to disruptions of the automatic respiratory system. It has been called *Ondine's curse*, after the water nymph of German legend who mortally cursed her suitor with loss of involuntary function.[27] Cases with intact involuntary respiration but paralyzed voluntary breathing have been described (respiratory apraxia).

ABNORMAL BREATHING PATTERNS IN DISEASE-STATES

Respiratory abnormalities are commonly seen in patients with stupor and coma. These respiratory changes, when recognized, can be helpful in diagnosis and are of localizing value (Fig. 34-1).[25]

Posthyperventilation Apnea

Normally, if the arterial P_{CO_2} is lowered by a period of hyperventilation, most subjects will continue to breathe regularly but with a reduced tidal volume until the Pa_{CO_2} returns to normal. However, in subjects with metabolic disease or bilateral forebrain disease, there may be an abnormally long period of apnea after hyperventilation.

Cheyne–Stokes Respiration

Cheyne–Stokes is a pattern of breathing in which phases of hyperpnea regularly alternate with phases of apnea. The variation in breathing is usually that of volume and not frequency (*see* Fig. 34-1A). It is seen occasionally in normal persons during sleep. However, sustained Cheyne–Stokes respirations usually imply a neurologic, cardiac (e.g., congestive heart failure), or metabolic abnormality. In patients with neurologic disease, its presence usually implies bilateral dysfunction in the hemispheres or diencephalon, and sometimes as far caudally as the pons.[23] If the apneic periods result in net alveolar hypoventilation, intravenous aminophylline may be used. Oxygen administration should be guided by periodic arterial blood gas measurements.

Specific causes of Cheyne–Stokes respiration are listed below (lower left-hand column).

CLINICAL CONDITIONS ASSOCIATED WITH CHEYNE–STOKES RESPIRATION

Central Nervous System Abnormalities
- Normal people given morphine or sedatives
- Older people in sleep
- Elevation of intracranial pressure (especially at the brain-stem level)

Cardiovascular System Disease
- Cardiac failure, hypertension, uremia, and coronary artery disease (the latter associated with cerebrovascular disease)

Respiratory System Disease
- Alveolar hypoventilation, especially with terminal interstitial lung disease

Hyperventilation

Sustained rapid and deep ventilation is commonly seen in patients with upper brain-stem injury. Although it was formerly believed that such lesions can cause central neurogenic hyperventilation (*see* Fig. 34-1B), it now appears that such cases are uncommon if one applies strict criteria for this state and excludes pulmonary congestion as a cause. Although hyperventilation is known to be associated with metabolic encephalopathies, it may occasionally be due to primary central nervous system abnormalities, usually infiltrating tumors of the brainstem.[24,26]

Apneusis

Apneusis (*see* Fig. 34-1C) refers to a prolonged pause at full inspiration. It is seen in humans but not commonly. A more frequent abnormality is end-inspiratory pauses alternating with end-expiratory pauses. Apneusis implies an extensive lesion (e.g., infarct) in the lower pontine tegmentum.

Ataxic Breathing

Ataxic breathing (*see* Fig. 34-1E) has an unpredictable irregular pattern with both deep and shallow breaths. It represents a disruption of medullary groups that produce respiratory rhythmicity and is due to lesions in the dorsomedial part of the medulla. Cluster breathing (*see* Fig. 34-1D) with irregular pauses and gasps may be seen in medullary lesions. *Biot's breathing*, associated with meningitis or basal encephalitis, is one type of ataxic breathing.

In addition to the abnormalities of respiration mentioned above, several states of altered respiratory control are not due to *known* central nervous system diseases.

Primary Alveolar Hypoventilation

Primary alveolar hypoventilation has been ascribed to defective respiratory control when it occurs without primary cardiorespiratory disease. This syndrome is characterized by chronic hypoventilation, which is more severe during sleep and which can be improved by voluntary hyperventilation.

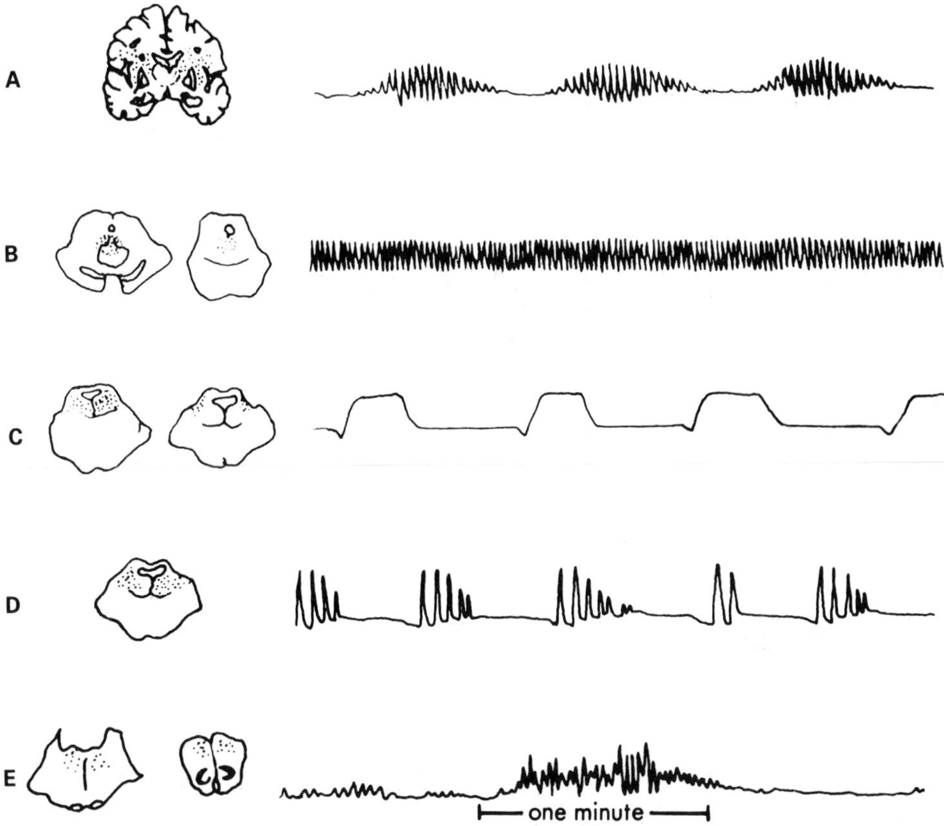

Fig. 34-1. Abnormal respiratory patterns associated with pathologic lesions *(shaded areas)* at various levels of the brain. The dotted areas in the brain and brain stem represent the postulated sites of lesions producing the various rhythm abnormalities. Tracings are by chest–abdomen pneumograph; inspiration reads up. *(A)* Cheyne–Stokes respiration. *(B)* Central neurogenic hypervention *(C)* Apneusis. *(D)* Cluster breathing. *(E)* Ataxic breathing (*see* text). (Plum F, Posner JB: The Diagnosis of Stupor and Coma, 2nd ed. Philadelphia, FA Davis, 1972)

Sleep Apnea

There are several reports of patients with primary (central) alveolar hypoventilation who have had episodes of apnea during sleep.[11] Nocturnal phrenic nerve pacing has been useful in treating this disorder,[15] as well as in central alveolar hypoventilation with known neurologic disease (Ondine's curse).[27]

The sleep apnea syndromes have received considerable attention recently.[14] Patients with this abnormality have periods of apnea during sleep that last longer than 10 seconds and that occur more than 30 times in 7 hours of sleep. The apnea may be obstructive, nonobstructive (central), or of mixed type. The obstructive type, caused by upper airway obstruction, is most common. The apneic episodes are associated with hypoxia, hypercapnea, and acidosis, but chronic hypoventilation is usually absent. Diagnosis is discussed in Appendix C.

Sudden Infant Death Syndrome

There are similarities between the sleep apnea syndromes and the sudden infant death syndrome (SIDS). Some infants in whom SIDS occurs have demonstrated episodes of prolonged apnea and excessive periodic apnea.[28] In addition, some patients with each syndrome have demonstrated elevated sleeping Pa_{CO_2} levels and insensitivity to carbon dioxide inhalation.[13,29] Although primary alveolar hypoventilation, SIDS, and sleep apnea syndromes share some features, their fundamental interrelationship is not clear.

RESPIRATORY DISORDERS IN NEUROMUSCULAR DISEASE

The motor unit is the anatomical entity that generates power and movement. This unit comprises the anterior horn cell, peripheral nerve, myoneural junction, and muscle fiber. In a large limb muscle, each anterior horn cell innervates from 400 to 1000 muscle fibers that interdigitate with muscle fibers of other motor units. Diseases that affect any part of the motor unit most commonly present as weakness or fatigability. Table 34-1 lists the common neuromuscular diseases.

The respiratory symptoms of neuromuscular disease are similar to those of intrinsic lung disease, although the pathophysiology is quite different. Exertional or resting dyspnea associated with hypoxemia is the hallmark. In neuromuscular disease, the main respiratory abnormality is respiratory muscle weakness. During quiet breathing, the diaphragm is the principal muscle, whereas the intercostal muscles stabilize the chest wall. Expiration is usually a passive phenomenon without muscle contraction. Thus, in respiratory insufficiency associated with neuromuscular disease, the primary respiratory disorder is inspiratory weakness. Intercostal muscle weakness may result in a decreased resting lung volume with lung underinflation, airway closure, atelectasis, and decreased alveolar ventilation. If the abdominal muscles are also weak, the cough reflex may be inadequate to prevent aspiration, particularly when dysphagia is present.

In neuromuscular disease, respiratory muscle strength must be assessed regularly, particularly in acute disease when strength may change abruptly.

There are several nonspecific tests of respiratory muscle strength (e.g., forced vital capacity and maximum voluntary ventilation). The *most specific* measurements are maximal static inspiratory and expiratory pressures (PI max and PE max) (see Chap. 25). These measurements are not affected by intrinsic lung disease and can be easily performed at the bedside.[2,3] A more complicated, invasive technique is that of measuring transdiaphragmatic pressure gradients.

Acute muscle weakness may be accompanied by life-threatening respiratory muscle paralysis. It is extremely important to observe the *trend* of muscle strength to anticipate respiratory insufficiency. The medical team should follow the patient's symptoms, signs, blood gases, and tests of respiratory muscle strength for any suggestion of ventilatory failure. If there is uncertainty, the patient should be followed closely in a unit where there is specialized medical, nursing, and respiratory care.

Table 34-1. Classification of Common Neuromuscular Diseases

I. *Anterior Horn Cell* (neuronal)

- Spinal muscular atrophies (Werdnig-Hoffmann; Kugelberg-Welander)
- Motor neuron disease (ALS)
- Poliomyelitis

II. *Peripheral Nerve* (neuropathy)

- Metabolic (uremia, hepatic failure)
- Endocrine (diabetes, thyroid)
- Toxic (*e.g.,* lead, arsenic, vincristine, Dilantin)
- Hereditary (Charcot–Marie–Tooth)
- Immunologic (Guillain Barré, lupus erythematosus, rheumatoid arthritis)
- Vitamin deficiency

III. *Neuromuscular Junction*

- Myasthenia gravis
- Botulism

IV. *Muscle* (myopathy)

- Dystrophies (Duchenne, FSH, limb girdle, CPEO)
- Myotonic disorders
- Congenital myopathies (central core, rod, myotubular)
- Periodic paralysis
- Inflammatory myopathies (polymyositis, dermatomyositis)
- Metabolic myopathies (glycogen and lipid storage diseases)
- Endocrine myopathies (thyroid, adrenal)
- Toxic myopathies (*e.g.,* alcohol, chloroquine)

MOTOR NEURON DISEASE

Motor neuron disease is a progressive disorder of deterioration in the motor neuron cell. It is clinically manifested according to the location of the cells most affected, from the anterior horn cell of the spinal cord to the motor cells of the cerebral cortex. *Amyotrophic lateral sclerosis* (ALS), *progressive bulbar palsy*, and *adult spinal muscular atrophy* all present with symptoms and signs of weakness, atrophy, fasciculations, and, in ALS, with upper motor neuron signs. The disease usually has a progressive course, and death commonly is due to respiratory complications, either aspiration and pneumonia or respiratory failure, or both. There is no specific treatment for the disease except for maintaining the optimal medical, physical, and psychological condition of the patient. There are reports of patients with motor neuron disease presenting with respiratory insufficiency,[31] but this generally occurs late in the disease.

Despite the usually dismal prognosis, long-term mechanical ventilation in the home or skilled nursing facility is being offered more frequently.[4,30]

PERIPHERAL NERVE DISEASE

The most common acute disorder of peripheral nerve function is the *Guillain-Barré syndrome*. This is a descriptive entity with progressive motor weakness and areflexia that is commonly preceded by a viral infection, surgery, or inoculation. Sensory symptoms and signs, cranial nerve signs, and sphincter disturbances may also be present. The diagnosis is supported by the finding of abnormal cerebrospinal fluid (elevated protein, few cells) and slowed nerve conduction.[22] The progression of the weakness is rarely longer than 4 weeks, after which recovery gradually ensues.

Life-threatening respiratory involvement has been reported in up to 20% of cases, and, before mechanical ventilation, it was the major cause of mortality. Ventilatory failure, which can occur abruptly, must be monitored carefully. Ventilatory assistance should be provided as soon as respiratory compromise has been detected. Meticulous suctioning of the oropharynx and the airways is mandatory.

Most patients have good potential for functional recovery within 6 months, which emphasizes the need for meticulous respiratory care. When respiratory failure occurs, it is usually protracted, and the complications are mainly those of prolonged intubation with a tracheostomy tube.[12]

DISEASE AT THE MYONEURAL JUNCTION

Myasthenia gravis is an immune-mediated disorder characterized by weakness and fatigability of voluntary muscle. The etiology appears to be a specific functional abnormality at the myoneural junction, but the exact process remains unexplained. A refractory type of this syndrome, associated with malignant tumors (in particular oat-cell carcinoma of the lung), is recognized—the so-called Eaton-Lambert syndrome.

The diagnosis of myasthenia gravis is based on clinical features (electrophysiological properties and pharmacologic testing).[9] Respiratory muscle weakness and ventilatory failure are common in myasthenia gravis, occurring in about 20% of patients. Several factors may precipitate deterioration, such as adjustment of anticholinergic medication, initiation of steroid therapy (usually in the first 3–10 days), surgery, and infections. In patients with marginal ventilatory reserve, it is imperative that respiratory strength be monitored frequently, since ventilatory failure can occur rapidly and insidiously. Assisted ventilation should be provided when ventilatory failure is imminent.

It is very important to recognize when dysphagia and aspiration are occurring, because the potential for developing bronchopneumonia is great. Careful attention to feeding, postural positioning and drainage, and general pulmonary hygiene is mandatory.

A useful assessment in determining residual pulmonary reserve in these patients is the comparison between tidal volume (V_T) and vital capacity (VC). When the VC is less than three times the V_T, severe impairment is present, and aggressive bronchial hygiene is mandatory. When VC approaches V_T or is less than 1 liter, ventilatory support is indicated or its need is imminent.

MUSCULAR DISORDERS

A host of primary muscle disorders (Table 34-1) have associated pulmonary involvement at one time or another in their course. The interested reader is referred to the Bibliography for more extensive information in this area.

TOXIC AND METABOLIC ENCEPHALOPATHIES

Toxic or metabolic abnormalities involving the brain commonly result in respiration abnormalities.[25] Usually these abnormalities are nonspecific expressions of diffuse brain-stem dysfunction, but sometimes the respiratory alterations stand out from other neurologic changes. Posthyperventilation apnea, Cheyne–Stokes respirations, and hyperventilation are often exhibited by patients with metabolic brain disease.

Respiratory changes (e.g., hypoventilation or hyperventilation) can reflect adjustments to metabolic acid–base disturbances or can result from specific metabolic diseases that affect respiration *per se* (e.g., hypothyroidism or hyperthyroidism). Careful clinical observation combined with arterial blood gas analysis usually leads to accurate diagnosis (see Chap. 12).

The main causes of metabolic acidosis in encephalopathic patients are uremia, diabetes, lactic acidosis, and acid poisons. These can usually be differentiated by clinical means and simple laboratory tests.

Respiratory alkalosis that occurs in encephalopathic patients has several main causes: hepatic coma, salicylism, gram-negative sepsis, and pulmonary diseases. These can usually be differentiated by the clinical setting and appropriate laboratory tests.

Hypoventilation in encephalopathic patients is due to either metabolic alkalosis or respiratory depression with acidosis. Respiratory depression with acidosis is a dangerous problem and can be due to central respiratory depression from sedatives, narcotics, or brain-stem injury, as well as from primary lung disease. When respiratory depression is severe, ventilatory support is necessary.

Salicylate poisoning is unusual in that it sometimes causes an early respiratory alkalosis, followed by a respiratory acidosis, and then mixed metabolic and respiratory acidosis. This sequence is believed to be due to an early increase in tissue carbon dioxide production as well as to direct brain-stem stimulation, which causes hyperventilation and respiratory alkalosis. This is followed by central respiratory depression and an accumulation of metabolic acid groups, hence respiratory and metabolic acidosis. The complete sequence is seen most often in infants, whereas adults more commonly exhibit respiratory alkalosis.

STATUS EPILEPTICUS

Status epilepticus is currently classified as [1] convulsive status epilepticus in which the epileptic patient with seizures does not recover to a normal alert state between repeated tonic–clonic attacks; [2] nonconvulsive status epilepticus such as absence status and complex partial status in which there is a prolonged "twilight" state; or [3] continuous partial seizures or "epilepsia partialis continua" in which consciousness is preserved.[7]

Convulsive status epilepticus is a neurologic emergency and should be terminated as soon as possible to reduce morbidity and mortality. During seizures, ventilation can be reduced by overzealous use of sedating drugs, by aspiration of food, or by "aspiration" of the tongue, resulting in an obstructed central airway.

An oral airway should be inserted and oxygen always administered initially. An endotracheal tube may need to be inserted if continuous infusion of diazepam (Valium) or intravenous loading with phenobarbital is to be used after unsuccessful early attempts to control convulsive status.

Unexpected, unexplained death has been noted in epileptic patients and may be related to neurogenic pulmonary edema.[33]

THE CRANIUM: PHYSIOLOGICAL CONSIDERATIONS

The cranium has a volume of 1200 to 1400/cm^3. The brain takes up to 80% of the space, whereas the rest is occupied by cerebrospinal fluid and blood in the arteries and veins. Because the brain is about 75% water, the intracranial contents are largely fluid and incompressible. Since the adult skull is rigid, the intracranial volume remains fixed, and any process that tends to add volume must do so by reducing the volume of other intracranial constituents. Under normal conditions, intracranial pressure (ICP) remains relatively constant, despite alterations in brain size, cerebrospinal fluid volume, and cerebral blood volume.

Initially, a space-occupying lesion adds volume, and cerebrospinal fluid is reduced by expression of the fluid into the spinal dural sac. Further compensation occurs by a decrease in cerebral blood volume. When a mass continues to expand, the elasticity of the system diminishes, and eventually ICP rises. The rapidity of the rise in intracranial pressure depends on the rate of expansion of the mass; slow-growing masses are tolerated much longer. However, if the lesion is acute, as in cerebral hemorrhage, the elasticity of the system is soon exceeded, and even small changes in volume produce large changes in ICP.

The brain under normal conditions receives about 800 ml/min of blood. Average blood flow in the brain is 50 ml/100 g/min, but there is a difference between gray matter (80–100 ml/100 g/min) and white matter (10–20 ml/100 g/min). Cerebral blood flow (CBF) varies according to resistance of the cerebral vasculature and the cerebral perfusion pressure. Changes in Pa_{CO_2} can cause profound changes in CBF. Because carbon dioxide is a potent stimulus to cerebral vasodilation, CBF doubles when PCO_2 is increased from 40 mm Hg to 80 mm Hg and is halved when PCO_2 falls to 20 mm Hg. Changes in Pa_{O_2} have little effect on the cerebral vessels until the Pa_{O_2} falls below 50 mm Hg, when a distinct increase in CBF occurs; at a Pa_{O_2} of 30 mm Hg, CBF more than doubles.

Cerebral perfusion pressure (CPP) is the difference between systemic arterial pressure (SAP) and the intracranial pressure (CPP = SAP − ICP), since the pressure inside cerebral veins is practically the same as the intracranial pressure. Any significant, uncompensated rise in ICP will reduce CPP and cause a decrease in CBF. If the reduction in CBF is sufficient, ischemic injury to the brain may occur.

The cerebral blood flow does not passively depend on arterial pressure. The normal brain has a capacity to maintain CBF despite wide changes in systemic blood pressure. CBF is relatively constant when arterial pressure is reduced to 60 mm Hg or raised to 160 mm Hg. This phenomenon has been termed *autoregulation*.

These interrelationships of cerebral blood flow, arterial pressure, and intracranial pressure may not hold true in pathologic states of the brain itself, and associated intracranial hypertension may develop.

NEUROSURGERY AND NEUROTRAUMA

SPINAL INJURY

Most acute cervical spinal cord lesions are due to trauma with associated fracture/dislocation, pure fracture, or dislocation with ligamentous instability. When the upper cervical cord is affected above C3, phrenic outflow is lost, as is intercostal and abdominal muscular function. Complete respiratory failure occurs, and death follows unless emergency care is immediately available. More commonly, the traumatic cervical lesion is lower and phrenic outflow is preserved, although quadriplegia occurs with loss of intercostal and abdominal muscle function. The patient must then be carefully observed for any early cephalad extension of the lesion that would compromise diaphragmatic function. Since the diaphragm is the primary muscle of quiet breathing, the quadriplegic patient can usually maintain adequate tidal volumes but has a reduced vital capacity.

Meticulous bronchial hygiene must be provided to avoid any pulmonary complications (*i.e.*, infection, atelectasis, pulmonary embolism) that would further compromise respiration. Initial management should include assessment of arterial blood gases and vital capacity, as well as any history of pulmonary disease. Physiotherapy should be directed toward increasing the contribution of accessory muscles of respiration in breathing and coughing.

HEAD INJURY

Head injury (Fig. 34-2) is a frequent cause of altered sensorium, and seriously injured patients may be comatose. Patients with head trauma who are unconscious run a great risk of airway obstruction. Initial evaluation of such patients should be directed toward the establishment of an effective airway. This may necessitate proper positioning, an oropharyngeal airway, endotracheal intubation, or even tracheostomy.[34]

Inexpert attempted intubation should be avoided because the associated coughing and choking will cause a rise in ICP. The stomach should be kept empty by intermittent aspiration through a nasogastric tube. Standard sterile suctioning techniques should be used (see Chap. 21). During the suctioning period, the patient is at risk from hypoventilation. This, along with the induced coughing, may result in an increase in ICP; accordingly, the suctioning period should be as brief and atraumatic as possible. Preoxygenation with 100% oxygen for 5 minutes is also indicated.

Head and chest trauma frequently occur together, particularly in vehicular traffic injuries. This worsens

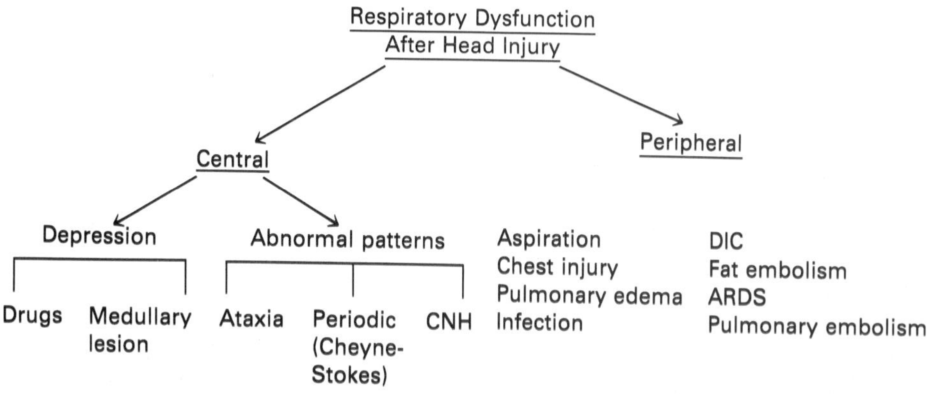

Fig. 34-2. Respiratory sequela of head injury. CNH = central neurogenic hyperventilation; DIC = disseminated intravascular coagulation; ARDS = adult respiratory distress syndrome. (Jennett B, Teasdale G: Management of Head Injuries. Philadelphia, FA Davis, 1981)

the eventual outcome, and care should be directed simultaneously to both injuries (see Chap. 37).

Neurogenic pulmonary edema is characterized by the rapid development of pulmonary edema after an acute central nervous system lesion. The clinical disorders include head trauma, intracranial hemorrhage, and seizures. The mechanism is probably related to a centrally mediated massive sympathetic discharge that produces intense vasoconstriction and shifting of blood from the high-resistance systemic circulation to the low-resistance pulmonary circulation. This results in an increased pulmonary blood volume, which, because of the hydrostatic effect of increased pulmonary capillary pressure, produces pulmonary edema.[34]

The aim in managing respiratory dysfunction in patients with head injury is to maintain adequate oxygenation, prevent carbon dioxide retention, and sometimes to control intracranial pressure. Controlled ventilation should be considered if adequate ventilation and arterial oxygenation cannot be maintained despite a clear airway or if controlled hyperventilation is necessary to reduce intracranial hypertension. With the use of intracranial pressure monitoring, the effect of controlled hyperventilation on intracranial pressure can be readily assessed and used in the overall management of cerebral edema. Although controlled hyperventilation *does* cause an initial reduction in ICP, a recent study indicates that maximal reduction occurs within 10 minutes, with a gradual return to previous levels within 80 minutes.[16]

When PEEP is used to maintain oxygenation, a rise in intracranial pressure can occur[1] that may be prevented by keeping the head up at 30°.[10]

Barbiturates have been shown to reduce acutely raised ICP and are sometimes used at special centers in the aggressive management of head injury.[19,20] However, the levels of barbiturates used produce coma, and, because of respiratory depression, ventilatory support is inevitable and meticulous pulmonary toilet must be provided.

REFERENCES

1. Apuzzo MLJ et al: Effect of positive end expiratory pressure ventilation on intracranial pressure in man. J Neurosurg 46:227, 1977
2. Black LF, Hyatt RE: Maximal respiratory pressures: Normal values and relationship to age and sex. Am Rev Respir Dis 99:696, 1969
3. ———: Maximal static respiratory pressures in generalized neuromuscular disease. Am Rev Respir Dis 103:641, 1971
4. Bradley WG: Respirator support in amyotrophic lateral sclerosis. Ann Neurol 13:466, 1983
5. Clark FJ, von Euler C: On the regulation of depth and rate of breathing. J Physiol 222:267, 1972
6. Cohn JE, Kuida H: Primary alveolar hypoventilation associated with western equine encephalitis. Ann Intern Med 56:633, 1962
7. Delgado–Escueta AV, Wasterlain C, Treiman DM, Porter RJ: Current concepts in neurology: Management of status epilepticus. N Engl J Med 306:1337, 1982
8. Devereaux MV, Keane JR, Davis RL: Automatic respiratory failure associated with infarction of the medulla. Arch Neurol 29:46, 1973
9. Drachman DB: Myasthenia gravis. N Engl J Med 298:136, 186, 1978
10. Frost EAM, Gildenberg PL: Effects of positive end expiratory pressure in intracranial pressure and compliance in brain injured patients. J Neurosurg 47:195, 1977
11. Glenn WWL et al: Combined central alveolar hypoventilation and upper airway obstruction. Am J Med 64:50, 1978
12. Gracey DR, McMichan JC, Divertie MB, Howard FM Jr: Respiratory failure in Guillain-Barré syndrome. Mayo Clin Proc 57:742, 1982
13. Guilleminault C, Peraita R, Soquet M, Dement WC: Apneas during sleep in infants: Possible relationship with sudden infant death syndrome. Science 190:677, 1975
14. Guilleminault C, Tiikian A, Dement WC: The sleep apnea syndromes. Ann Rev Med 27:465, 1976
15. Hyland RH et al: Primary alveolar hypoventilation treated with nocturnal electrophrenic respiration. Am Rev Respir Dis 117:165, 1978
16. James HE et al: Treatment of intracranial hypertension. Analysis of 105 consecutive continuous recordings of intracranial pressure. Acta Neurochir 36:189, 1977
17. Lumsden T: Observations on the respiratory centers in the cat. J Physiol 57:153, 1923
18. Lumsden T: Observations on the respiratory centers. J Physiol 57:354, 1923
19. Marshall LF, Smith RW, Shapiro HM: The outcome with aggressive treatment in severe head injuries: II. Acute and chronic barbiturate administration in the management of head injury. J Neurosurg 50:26, 1979
20. Miller JD: Barbiturates and raised intracranial pressure. Ann Neurol 6:189, 1979
21. Mitchell RA et al: Respiratory responses mediated through superficial chemosensitive areas on the medulla. J Appl Physiol 18:523, 1963
22. National Institute of Neurological and Communicative Disorders and Stroke, Ad Hoc Committee: Criteria for diagnosis of Guillain-Barré syndrome. Ann Neurol 3:565, 1978
23. North JB, Jennett S: Abnormal breathing patterns associated with acute brain damage. Arch Neurol 31:338, 1974
24. Plum F: Mechanisms of 'central' hyperventilation. Ann Neurol 11:636, 1982
25. Plum F, Posner JB: The Diagnosis of Stupor and Coma, 3rd ed. Philadelphia, FA Davis, 1980
26. Rodriguez M, Baele PL, Marsh HM, Okazaki H: Central neurogenic hyperventilation in an awake patient with brainstem astrocytoma. Ann Neurol 11:625, 1982
27. Severinghaus JW, Mitchell RA: Ondine's curse—failure of respiratory center automaticity while asleep. Clin Res 10:122, 1962
28. Shannon DC, Kelly DH: SIDS and near-SIDS. N Engl J Med 306:959, 1022, 1982
29. Shannon DC, Kelly DH, O'Connell K: Abnormal regulation of ventilation in infants at risk for sudden-infant-death syndrome. N Engl J Med 297:747, 1977

30. Sivak ED, Gipson WT, Hanson MR: Long-term management of respiratory failure in amyotrophic lateral sclerosis. Ann Neurol 12:18, 1982
31. Sivak ED, Streib EW: Management of hypoventilation in motor neuron disease presenting with respiratory insufficiency. Ann Neurol 7:188, 1980
32. Solliday NH et al: Impaired central chemoreceptor function and chronic hypoventilation many years following poliomyelitis. Respiration 31:177, 1974
33. Terrence CF, Rao GR, Perper JA: Neurogenic pulmonary edema in unexpected, unexplained death of epileptic patients. Ann Neurol 9:458, 1981
34. Theodore J, Robin ED: Speculations on neurogenic pulmonary edema. Am Rev Respir Dis 113:405, 1976
35. Von Euler C, Herrero F, Wexler I: Control mechanisms determining rate and depth of respiratory movements. Respir Physiol 10:93, 1970

BIBLIOGRAPHY

Berger AJ, Mitchell RA, Severinghaus JW: Regulation of respiration. N Engl J Med 297:92, 138, 194, 1977

Weiner WJ (ed): Respiratory Dysfunction in Neurologic Disease. Mt. Kisco, New York, Futura, 1980

Williams MH: Disturbances of respiratory control. Clin Chest Med 1:1, 1980

35

Acute Respiratory Failure: Classification, Differential Diagnosis, and Introduction to Management

Roger C. Bone

Most clinicians caring for acutely ill patients in critical care units today agree that acute respiratory failure is one of the most common life-threatening processes encountered in children and adults. Whether superimposed as an acute exacerbation of advanced chronic obstructive lung disease or developing in patients with previously healthy lungs (e.g., adult respiratory distress syndrome, myasthenia gravis, botulism, or sepsis), management of the patient with respiratory failure requires an organized approach.[11,14,16] The purpose of this chapter is to outline such an approach, implementation of which is one of the continuing, and constantly changing, challenges of critical care medicine.

HISTORY

In the 1940s, two major causes of respiratory failure were bulbar and anterior horn cell poliomyelitis and barbiturate overdose. Poliomyelitis was essentially eradicated by the development of specific, effective vaccines. Barbiturate overdose was initially treated with central nervous system stimulants and gastric lavage. With the importance of an effective airway and of continuous mechanical ventilation in comatose patients appreciated, the prognosis rapidly improved for patients suffering from barbiturate overdose. In the 1960s, readily available blood gas analysis provided a realistic appreciation of the true incidence of respiratory failure. Clinicians became aware of significant hypoxemia resulting from shock, myocardial infarction, and burns, as well as from acute pulmonary problems *per se*. The modern era of treatment of respiratory failure began about this same time, when practitioners from diverse backgrounds such as internal medicine, anesthesiology, surgery, respiratory therapy, pediatrics, and neurology developed a coordinated approach to the care of patients with respiratory failure. Now, critical care units are an integral part of all moderately large to large hospitals. About one half to one third of patients in any medical or surgical intensive care unit receive mechanical ventilation at some point during their disease process.

In the 1970s, respiratory failure was frequently diagnosed. Patients treated during that period had less mortality attributed to progressive hypoxemia and more deaths attributed to multiorgan failure. Presumably, in earlier times, severely ill patients did not live long enough for multiorgan failure to develop. Gastric stress ulcers, disseminated intravascular coagulation, sepsis, hypotension, opportunistic infections, cardiac arrhythmias, occult or overt left ventricular failure, acute renal failure, and iatrogenic starvation were recognized earlier and in increasingly large numbers of cases.

The extremely high cost of caring for critically ill patients became appreciated, as did the equally high incidence of iatrogenic complications occurring in such patients.[1,18]

DEFINITION

Acute respiratory failure (ARF) cannot be generically defined, but a useful definition that applies to most causes of respiratory failure can be offered. Acute respiratory failure may be said to be present when

1. the patient is acutely dyspneic;
2. the Pa_{O_2} is less than 50 mm Hg breathing room air;
3. the Pa_{CO_2} is greater than 50 mm Hg; or
4. the arterial *p*H shows significant respiratory acidemia.

Many patients with ARF do not fulfill all four components of this definition, but most will have at least two of the four components.

DIAGNOSIS AND TREATMENT

ARF may occur as a result of malfunction in one or more of the seven systems shown in Figure 35-1. Table 35-1 outlines an abbreviated approach to diagnosis (by blood gas abnormalities only) and treatment.

Respiratory failure from alveolar and airway disease in adults can be subdivided into that characterized by hypoxemia and hypercapnea (predominantly patients with chronic obstructive lung disease) and that characterized by hypoxemia alone (predominantly patients with acute lung injury, the adult respiratory distress syndrome).

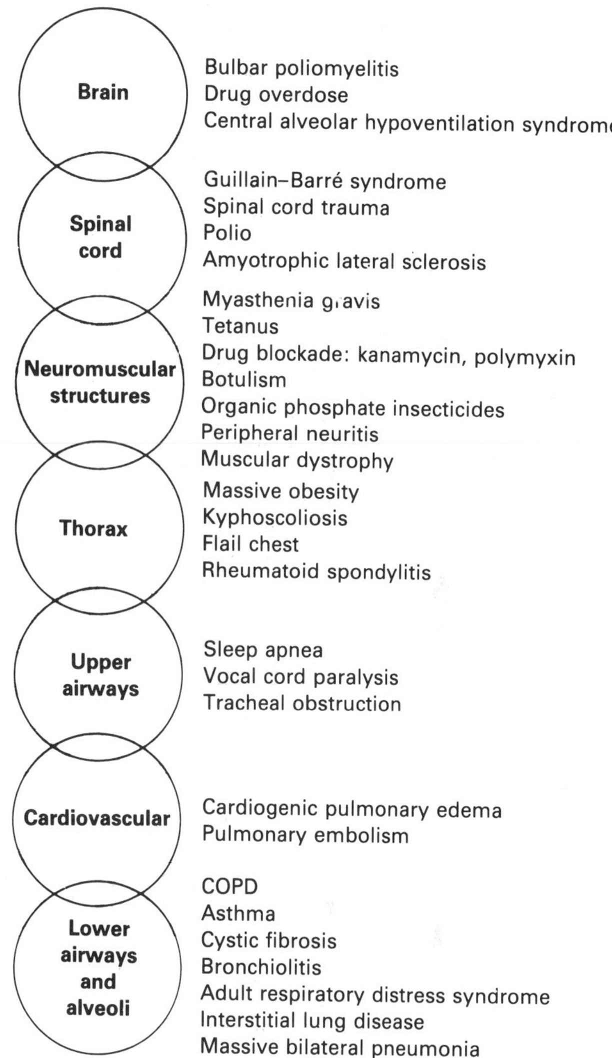

Fig. 35-1. Causes of acute respiratory failure.

TREATMENT OF HYPOXEMIC, HYPERCAPNEIC RESPIRATORY FAILURE

The major risk of the use of high concentrations of oxygen in the patient with hypercapnic respiratory failure is the iatrogenic precipitation of progressive hypercapnea from relief of the hypoxic drive to breathing.[7] The correct dose of oxygen to use in respiratory failure is that which satisfies tissue needs for oxygen but does not produce carbon dioxide narcosis or oxygen toxicity. Thus the proper concentration of oxygen is that which produces an adequate but not excessive arterial oxygen tension (generally thought to be between 50–60 mm Hg).

Since the introduction of the concept of controlled oxygen therapy by Barach[3] and its practical implementation by Campbell,[9,10] the administration of progressive increments of inspired oxygen has become the usual therapy for patients with ARF secondary to chronic obstructive lung disease and its exacerbations. Most such patients respond to an increased fraction of inspired oxygen (FI_{O_2}) by an improvement in arterial hypoxemia and, in conjunction with other therapy, an improvement in clinical status. However, some patients experience progressive hypercapnia and acidosis with resultant confusion, stupor, or coma even when the FI_{O_2} is only moderately increased. These latter patients may require an artificial airway and mechanical ventilation.

Table 35-1. Acute Respiratory Failure

CAUSES	DIAGNOSIS AND TREATMENT
BRAIN	
Clinical examples Bulbar poliomyelitis Drug overdose Central alveolar hypoventilation syndrome	**A.** Arterial blood gases show a decreased Pa_{O_2} and increased Pa_{CO_2}. **B.** Adequate oxygenation is no problem if patient is given assisted ventilation. **C.** Special situations **1.** For bulbar poliomyelitis, assisted ventilation is usually necessary. **2.** For narcotics, Darvon, and Talwin, Narcan (Naloxone HCl) in a dose of 0.4 mg (1 ml) may be given to reverse respiratory depression. This dose can be repeated in 2 to 3 minutes. **3.** For central alveolar ventilation, phrenic nerve pacing has been used, but upper airway obstruction has been noted after phrenic pacing.
SPINAL CORD	
Clinical examples Guillain–Barré Spinal cord trauma Poliomyelitis	**A.** Arterial blood gases show a decreased Pa_{O_2} and increased Pa_{CO_2}. **B.** Adequate oxygenation is no problem if patient is given assisted ventilation. **C.** Special situations **1.** For spinal cord disease, intubation and mechanical ventilation should be instituted when patient's vital capacity <1000 ml or <10 ml/kg body weight, or both. **2.** Rocking beds, pneumatic belts, cuirass ventilation, and "iron lung" may be attractive alternatives to long-term, if not permanent, intubation and mechanical ventilation.
NEUROMUSCULAR STRUCTURES	
Clinical examples Myasthenia gravis Tetanus Drug-induced neuromuscular blockage (*e.g.*, curare, neomycin, kanamycin, streptomycin, polymyxin) Botulism Organic phosphate insecticide poisoning	**A.** Arterial blood gases show a decreased Pa_{O_2} and increased Pa_{CO_2}. **B.** Adequate oxygenation is no problem if patient is given assisted ventilation. **C.** Special situations **1.** Intubation and mechanical ventilation should be instituted when patient's vital capacity <1000 ml or <10 ml/kg body weight. **2.** In myasthenia gravis, intubation and assisted ventilation should also be instituted when patient is unable to clear secretions from airway and saliva from mouth. **3.** In tetanus, good debridement of wound, penicillin, and human tetanus antitoxin are used. Valium is often used for sedation and Pavulon (pancuronium bromide) for paralysis.

Table 35-1. ***(Continued)***

CAUSES	DIAGNOSIS AND TREATMENT
NEUROMUSCULAR STRUCTURES *(continued)*	
	4. Neomycin, kanamycin, and streptomycin produce a competitive blockage at the myoneural end plate, which may be reversed by neostigmine. Polymyxin B, colistin, and possibly kanamycin produce a noncompetitive blockage, which may be helped by intravenous calcium gluconate. **5.** In botulism, treatment includes antitoxin. **6.** In organic phosphate insecticide poisoning, atropine, 1 to 2 mg i.m. and 2-PAM (pyridine aldoxime methiodide) may combat the cholinesterase inhibition.
THE THORAX AND ABDOMEN	
Clinical examples Kyphoscoliosis Massive obesity Muscular dystrophy Flail chest Rheumatoid spondylitis	**A.** Arterial blood gases show decreased Pa_{O2} and increased Pa_{CO2}. **B.** Adequate oxygenation is no problem if patient is given assisted ventilation. **C.** Special situations **1.** Patients with kyphoscoliosis usually have severe spinal deformity before hypoventilation occurs. **2.** Massive obesity is a major risk factor for accentuating other causes of respiratory failure. **3.** In flail chest associated with chest contusion or adult respiratory distress syndrome, intubation with mechanical ventilation and positive end-expiratory pressure is often indicated.
UPPER AIRWAYS	
Clinical examples Obstructive sleep apnea Vocal cord paralysis Tracheal obstruction Epiglottitis/laryngotracheitis Large tonsils and adenoids Postextubation laryngeal edema	**A.** Arterial blood gases show decreased Pa_{O2} and increased Pa_{CO2}. **B.** Adequate oxygenation is no problem if patient is given assisted ventilation. **C.** Special situations **1.** Obstructive sleep apnea is usually improved by tracheostomy. **2.** Epiglottitis/laryngotracheitis and postextubation laryngeal edema may be helped by antibiotics (*e.g.,* ampicillin) for infection. Corticosteroids are used for laryngeal edema and aerosolized microNEFRIN (racemic epinephrine) as a decongestant to reduce edema. **3.** Tracheal obstruction by tumor or stricture may be corrected surgically.
CARDIOVASCULAR AND THROMBOEMBOLIC	
Clinical examples Cardiogenic pulmonary edema Pulmonary embolism	**A.** Arterial blood gases show a decreased Pa_{O2} and a decreased Pa_{CO2} (respiratory alkalosis).

(continued)

Table 35-1. Acute Respiratory Failure

CAUSES	DIAGNOSIS AND TREATMENT
CARDIOVASCULAR AND THROMBOEMBOLIC *(continued)*	
	B. Oxygen mask or high-flow oxygen by nasal cannula often needed to treat hypoxemia. C. Intubation and mechanical ventilation usually not needed unless acidotic or impending cardiovascular collapse. D. Special situations 1. Pulmonary edema secondary to left ventricular failure is treated with diuretics, digoxin, unloading agents, fluid, and salt restriction. 2. Pulmonary embolism is treated with heparin or fibrinolytic agents, or both.
ALVEOLI AND LOWER AIRWAYS	
Clinical examples Chronic obstructive pulmonary disease Asthma Cystic fibrosis Bronchiolitis Adult respiratory distress syndrome Interstitial lung disease	A. Arterial blood gases in chronic obstructive lung disease usually show a decreased Pa_{O_2} and increased Pa_{CO_2}. In asthma, usually a decreased Pa_{O_2} and Pa_{CO_2} are seen except in late stages, when a decreased Pa_{O_2} and increased Pa_{CO_2} are seen. In ARDS, a decreased Pa_{O_2} and Pa_{CO_2} are seen except in late stages, when an elevated Pa_{CO_2} can be seen. B. Special situations 1. For COPD and ARDS, *see* text and Chapters 31 and 36. 2. For asthma, cystic fibrosis, bronchiolitis, and interstitial lung disease, *see* text and chapters on these topics.

The rationale for controlled oxygen therapy is that most patients with chronic obstructive lung disease who develop acute respiratory failure have reversible problems such as airways infection, bronchospasm, retained secretions, congestive heart failure, or other conditions that have resulted in decreased alveolar ventilation. Low concentrations of oxygen are used to produce an acceptable Pa_{O_2}, whereas other therapy is directed toward reversing the factors that precipitated the respiratory failure. The goal is to maintain adequate oxygenation without significantly worsening respiratory acidosis. Thus adequate oxygenation may result from improvement of the Pa_{O_2} from 40 to 60 mm Hg, rather than to absolute "normal" Pa_{O_2} values. This leads to a substantial increase in oxygen delivery to the tissue, since such Pa_{O_2} values are on the steep portion of the oxyhemoglobin dissociation curve.

Air-entrainment oxygen masks, such as Venturi masks, can deliver a precise dose of oxygen. These devices use the Bernoulli principle by passing oxygen through a restriction and entraining room air to provide precise concentrations of oxygen ranging from 24% to 50%, depending on the mask. If the original Pa_{O_2} on room air is known, a reasonable estimate of the Pa_{O_2} that will be achieved in patients with hypercapnic respiratory failure resulting from a specific Venturi mask is shown in Figure 35-2.[8,12] If the Venturi mask is not available or feasible, then a nasal cannula at flow rates of 0.25 to 2 liters/min can be used to treat hypoxemia (low-flow oxygen therapy). Arterial blood gases should be measured at frequent intervals, usually every 30 minutes for the first 1 to 2 hours, or until it is certain that an acceptable Pa_{O_2} has been achieved without the precipitation of hypercapnia and respiratory acidosis. Simultaneously, bronchodilators, antibiotics, and other measures are used as indicated to treat the primary cause of acute respiratory failure.

The patient should be managed in an intensive care unit, since life-threatening changes in oxygenation and acid–base balance may occur on a minute-to-minute basis. Most patients with chronic obstructive lung disease respond favorably to this regimen, and adequate oxygenation is usually achieved without the precipitation of severe hypercapnia. Despite these precautions, if the patient does hypoventilate and significant hypercapnia does occur, care should be taken to avoid complete removal of oxygen. At this time, mechanical ventilation should probably be considered.

The likelihood of carbon dioxide narcosis developing despite controlled oxygen therapy can be predicted with some certainty (Fig. 35-3) and is a function of admission Pa_{O_2} and *p*H. Experience has shown that not all patients need to be intubated simply because they have a slightly increased Pa_{CO_2} after being given oxygen. Slight carbon dioxide retention should be considered a tolerable, adaptive response to oxygen administration (Fig. 35-4).[15] At least initially, a major therapeutic goal in hypoxemic, hypercapnic respiratory failure is to avoid endotracheal intubation and mechanical ventilation, if possible. The reasons for this are [1] the complications of intubation are more frequent with hypoxemic hypercapnic respiratory failure; [2] the need for ventilatory support, once applied, is usually more prolonged, and weaning is difficult; and [3] the physiological profile of these patients make it more likely that they can be managed without artificial support.

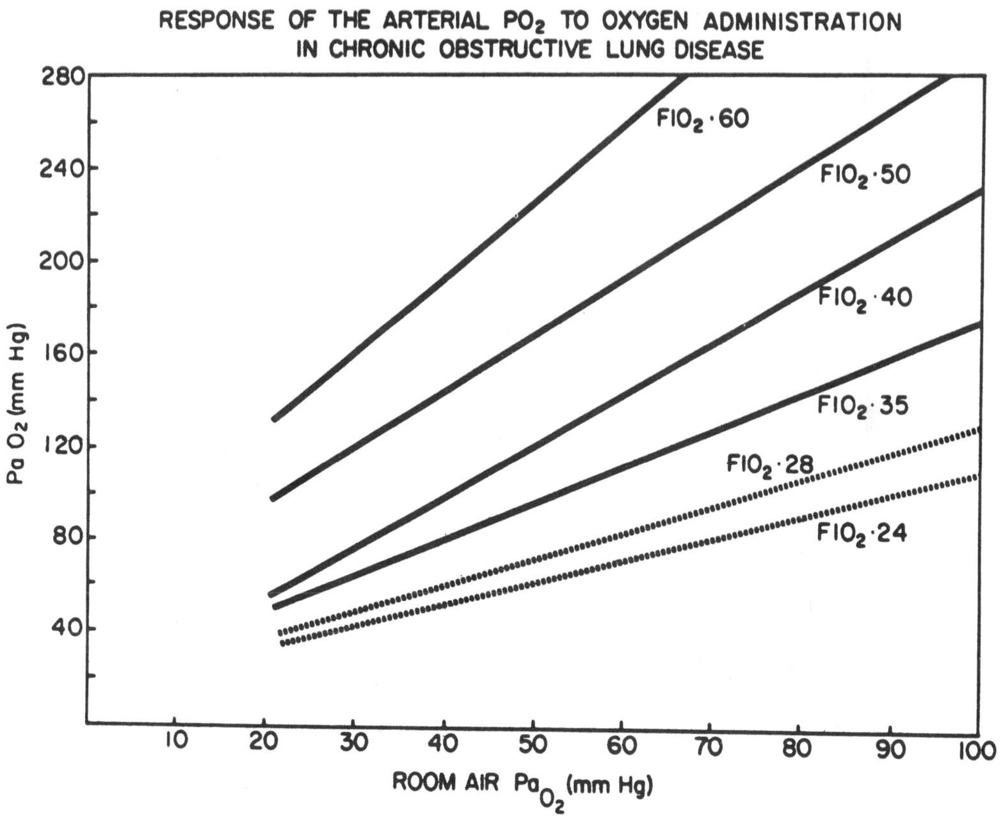

Fig. 35-2. Regression lines for different inspired percentages of oxygen (FI_{O_2}). Each line gives the expected arterial oxygen tension (Pa_{O_2}) for oxygen therapy based on the patient's room air Pa_{O_2} and applied FI_{O_2}. The relationships were determined with patients in acute respiratory failure *(dashed lines)* and stable patients *(solid lines)*.

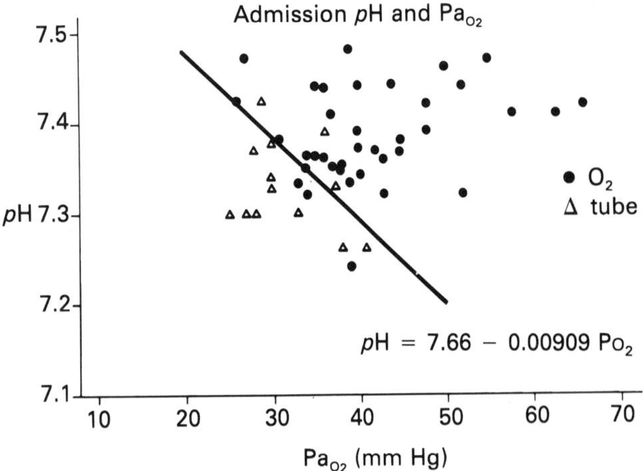

Fig. 35-3. Arterial oxygen tension (Pa_{O_2}) and *p*H at admission. Patients developing somnolence on controlled oxygen therapy were generally severely hypoxemic or had a combination of moderate hypoxemia and acidemia. This figure demonstrates the importance of hypoxemia and acidemia as risk factors for the development of carbon dioxide narcosis on controlled oxygen therapy. The line separating high- from low-risk patients was found by discriminant analysis ($pH = 7.66 - 0.00919\ P_{O_2}$). Δ = intubated patients; ● = nonintubated patients. (Bone RC, Pierce AK, Johnson RL Jr: Controlled oxygen administration in acute respiratory failure in chronic obstructive pulmonary disease: A reappraisal. Am J Med 65:896, 1978)

If intubation is performed, however, it should be done with a high-compliance, low-pressure cuffed endotracheal tube. Usually, ventilator tidal volumes of 8 to 12 ml/kg are sufficient. The inspiratory flow rate should be regulated carefully to allow adequate time for full expiration to avoid air trapping. In most cases, an inspiratory to expiratory (I:E) ratio of 1:3 is satisfactory. The respiratory rate may have to be decreased to achieve this. Again, the goal of ventilator therapy is not normalization of blood gases. If chronic carbon dioxide retention has been present before illness, decreasing arterial Pa_{CO_2} to normal levels causes alkalosis and may make it more difficult to wean the patient from the respirator. Thus an arterial Pa_{CO_2} level that results in a normal pH is an acceptable goal for initial treatment. All changes from admission baseline in arterial Pa_{CO_2} and pH should be made gradually, since rapid changes may cause significant alkalosis with resultant cardiac arrhythmias, convulsions, or both.

Monitoring of vital signs, tidal volume, respiratory rate, compliance, arterial blood gases, electrocardiogram, and fluid and electrolyte balance is routine for all patients. Careful monitoring of such patients is particularly important during sleep because there is often greater bronchosecretion, poorer secretion clearance, worse oxygen desaturation, worse pulmonary hypertension, and cardiac arrhythmias. In selected patients, particularly those in whom left ventricular failure is suspected, a flow directed pulmonary artery catheter may be used, but the data must be interpreted with caution, particularly in patients with chronic obstructive lung disease on ventilators. Rapid swings in the intrapleural pressure in such patients will cause reliance on the mean pulmonary artery pressure to be in error. The pulmonary wedge pressure should be read at end-expiration, and even then its values should be compared closely with the patient's clinical condition before alterations are made.

Treatment with antibiotics, bronchodilators, and other therapeutic maneuvers are described in detail in other chapters of *Respiratory Care*.

TREATMENT OF HYPOXEMIC, NORMOCAPNEIC RESPIRATORY FAILURE

The prototype of hypoxemic, normocapneic respiratory failure is the adult respiratory distress syndrome (ARDS),[2,13] discussed in detail in Chapter 36. The reader is referred to this chapter for pertinent details of the pathophysiology and treatment of this condition, in which mortality may be greater than 75% in patients needing long-term oxygen therapy with an FI_{O_2} of 0.50 or greater.

ARDS may be largely preventable if it is anticipated and appropriate measures are instituted in the immediate postinjury period. Respiratory failure in ARDS is self-perpetuating, since hypoventilation and alveolar closure, as may occur postinjury, lead to further atelectasis and hypoxemia. Simple measures in the postoperative or postinjury period that may abort respiratory failure at an early phase are listed below.

PROPHYLACTIC MEASURES TO PREVENT ARDS

1. Restore circulatory blood volume promptly after shock.
2. Leave endotracheal tube in place until postoperative patient is fully awake and ventilation adequate.

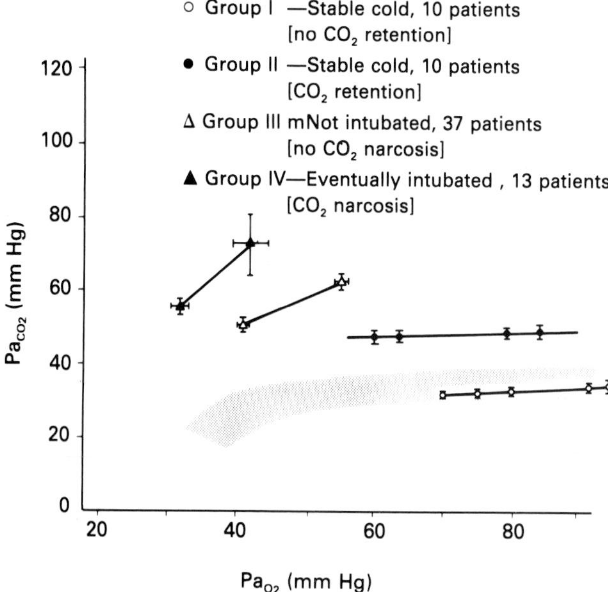

Fig. 35-4. Mean values for admission Pa_{O_2}–Pa_{CO_2}–plotted with Pa_{O_2} and Pa_{CO_2} at point of greatest hypercapnia after oxygen administration in four separate groups of patients with chronic obstructive pulmonary disease. The hatched area represents a normal human response to various inspired oxygen tensions during *(lower portion)* and after *(upper portion)* acclimatization to high altitudes. Horizontal and vertical bars indicate standard error of the mean for the Pa_{O_2} and Pa_{CO_2}, respectively. (Bone RC, Pierce AK, Johnson RL Jr: Controlled oxygen administration in acute respiratory failure in chronic obstructive pulmonary disease: A reappraisal. Am J Med 65:896, 1978)

3. Encourage sighing (deep breathing) in postinjury period.
4. Change patient position frequently.
5. Use blood filters for blood transfusion exceeding 4 units.
6. Use antibiotics and adrenocorticosteroids early for suspected sepsis.
7. Use hyperalimentation early for major injury with inadequate nutrition.

The treatment of all causes of ARDS includes providing adequate tissue oxygenation by respiratory and circulatory support.[6] Regardless of the inciting agent in ARDS, once the alveolar–capillary membrane has been damaged, the clinical problems are similar. The therapeutic goal in all causes of ARDS is to support the patient until the integrity of the alveolar–capillary membrane has been reestablished. The critical factors in treatment of ARDS are [1] optimal distention of alveoli to increase functional residual capacity; [2] maintenance of tissue perfusion; and [3] control of the primary problem. Because the basic physiological event in this syndrome is alveolar collapse, major efforts are made to obtain optimal distention of alveoli.

A major problem in ARDS is the potential development of oxygen toxicity. The toxic effects of increased oxygen concentrations were described by Smith in 1899.[17] Continuous exposure of animals to 100% oxygen leads to death within a few days. Pulmonary oxygen toxicity in humans was demonstrated by Barber and colleagues in a prospective study of ten patients with irreversible brain damage.[4] One group of patients received air and the other, 100% oxygen. Greater impairment of pulmonary physiology was detected in the oxygen-treated patients. The pathologic changes of oxygen toxicity include endothelial proliferation and perivascular edema. Later, pulmonary fibrosis occurs.

Because of the danger of oxygen toxicity, patients with ARDS should be treated with the lowest concentration of oxygen that provides adequate oxygenation. Clinical manifestations of oxygen toxicity have not been shown to develop if the inspired oxygen concentration is less than 50%.

DIAGNOSIS OF DETERIORATION OF RESPIRATORY STATUS IN VENTILATOR PATIENTS

In patients who develop worsening respiratory failure while on ventilator support, the cause for such deterioration may not always be apparent. The use of static and dynamic pressure-volume curves has been advocated to separate airways obstructive problems such as retained secretions and bronchoconstriction from parenchymal disorders such as atelectasis, pulmonary edema, and other causes of increased lung water, and pneumonia (Fig. 35-5).[5] The technology involved is simple and noninvasive and will identify the presence of complicating factors in the already ill patient.

TERMINOLOGY OF MECHANICAL VENTILATION

In this chapter, only three terms will be used from the multiple synonyms available. *Intermittent positive pressure ventilation* (IPPV) usually implies that a me-

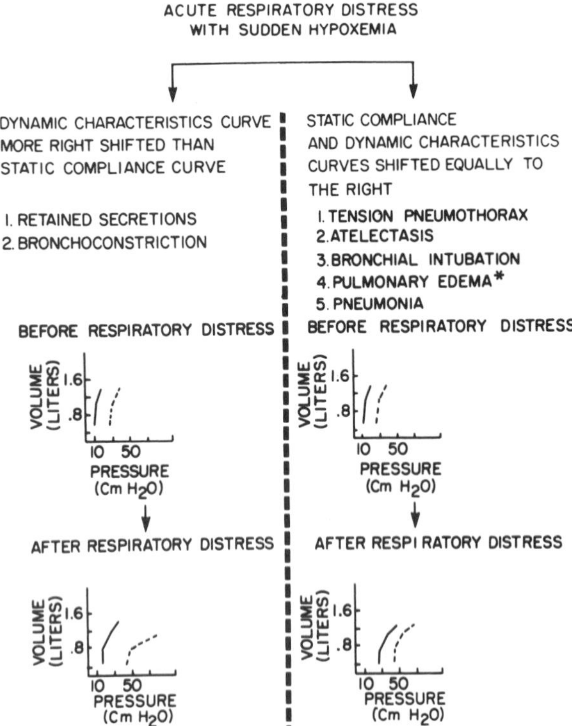

Fig. 35-5. Causes of acute respiratory distress in patients receiving assisted ventilation. After acute respiratory distress in patients treated with mechanical ventilation, static compliance curves and curves for dynamic characteristics compared to the same curves plotted before respiratory distress will assist in differential diagnosis of causes for acute respiratory distress. Idealized curves obtained before and after respiratory distress categorized by their pattern of abnormality are shown. *Solid curves* represent static compliance curves, and *dashed curves* represent curves for dynamic characteristics. *Asterisk* indicates cardiogenic and noncardiogenic pulmonary edema (adult respiratory distress syndrome). (Bone RC: Diagnosis of causes for acute respiratory distress by pressure-volume curves. Chest 70:740, 1976)

chanical respirator forces a ventilating gas mixture into the lungs. Exhalation is passive and results from the recoil of the lung and chest wall. Flow ceases at end-expiration when alveolar pressure equals atmospheric pressure.

Positive end-expiratory pressure (PEEP) refers to positive pressure of selected magnitude at end-expiration that is maintained throughout expiration (Fig. 35-6, Fig. 35-7). With *continuous positive airway pressure* (CPAP), above-ambient pressure is maintained throughout the respiratory cycle in the spontaneously breathing patient.

PEEP of significant magnitude used in a normal lung will markedly decrease cardiac output because of a decrease in preload to the heart. When alveolar pressure exceeds pulmonary arterial pressure, no blood flow occurs, as shown in Figure 35-8, and a zone 1 alveolus is produced. As long as ARDS results in uniform disease, less alveolar pressure is transmitted to the blood vessels. However, if the disease is patchy or excessive levels of PEEP are used, either maldistribution of pressure or excessive alveolar pressure can decrease cardiac output or cause regional lung damage such as alveolar rupture and pneumothorax.

Recruitment of collapsed alveoli by PEEP may take 30 minutes or longer. Discontinuance of PEEP prematurely results in rapid collapse. Thus PEEP should be maintained until alveoli are sufficiently stable to remain open without PEEP. General principles for the use of ventilator therapy in ARDS are outlined below.

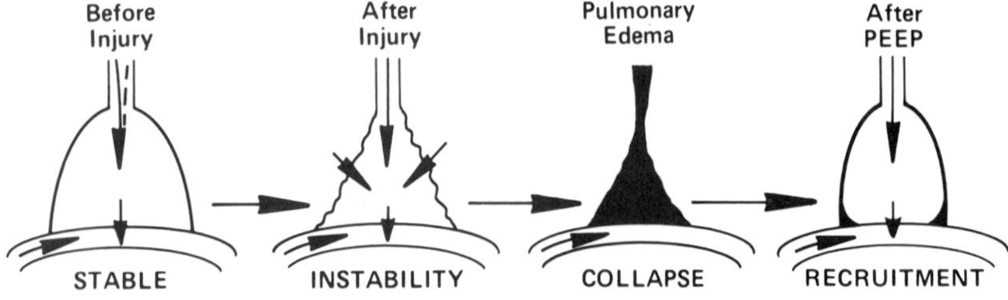

Fig. 35-6. The adult respiratory distress syndrome is characterized by an unstable alveolus, resulting in alveolar collapse and perfusion of unventilated alveoli (intrapulmonary shunt). With positive end-expiratory pressure (PEEP), the increase in alveolar pressure at end-expiration prevents partial or complete collapse of unstable alveoli. PEEP may also recruit unstable alveoli. The net beneficial result is a reduction in intrapulmonary shunt owing to an improvement in ventilation–perfusion relationship in diseased lung units. (Bone RC: Treatment of severe hypoxemia due to the adult respiratory distress syndrome. Arch Intern Med 140:85, 1980. Copyright 1980, American Medical Association)

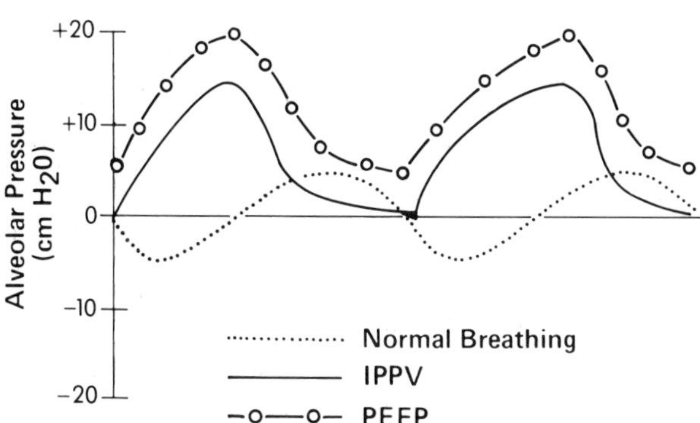

Fig. 35-7. With spontaneous breathing, alveolar pressure is negative in inhalation and positive in exhalation. With IPPV, when alveolar pressure returns to atmospheric and a slight negative alveolar pressure is generated by the patient (not shown in figure), the ventilator forces a certain predetermined volume into the lung. With positive end-expiratory pressure (PEEP), if the patient is controlled, inspiration begins when the alveolar pressure reaches a preset level of PEEP (5 cm H_2O in this example). (Bone RC: Treatment of severe hypoxemia due to the adult respiratory distress syndrome. Arch Intern Med 140:85, 1980. Copyright 1980, American Medical Association)

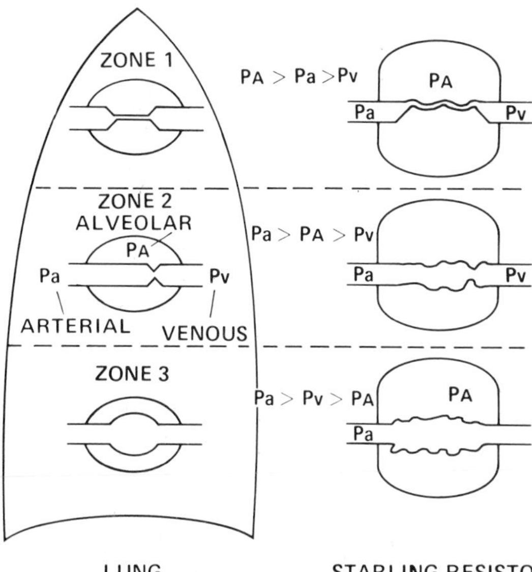

Fig. 35-8. The pulmonary capillary bed has flow characteristics of a Starling resistor. In the Starling resistor, when chamber pressure exceeds downstream pressure, flow is independent of downstream pressure. However, when downstream pressure exceeds chamber pressure, flow is determined by the upstream–downstream difference. Alveolar pressure is the same throughout the lung. Pulmonary arterial pressure increases down the lung. There may be a region at the top of the lung (zone 1) where pulmonary arterial pressure falls below alveolar pressure. Thus zone 1 will occur whenever alveolar pressure exceeds pulmonary arterial pressure. This may occur when the pulmonary arterial pressure is decreased, as in hypovolemia, or when alveolar pressure is increased, as with the application of positive end-expiratory pressure. Zone 1 produces an alveolar dead space. In zone 2, pulmonary arterial pressure increases and exceeds alveolar pressure. In zone 2, blood flow is determined by the difference between arterial and alveolar pressure. In zone 3, blood flow is determined by the arteriovenous pressure difference. (Bone RC: Treatment of severe hypoxemia due to the adult respiratory distress syndrome. Arch Intern Med 140:85, 1980. Copyright 1980, American Medical Association)

VENTILATOR THERAPY FOR ARDS

1. Use volume-cycle ventilators.
2. Use tidal volumes and PEEP that maintain "optimal compliance."
3. Keep inspired oxygen concentration as low as possible, consistent with adequate arterial ($Pa_{O_2} > 60$ mm Hg) and mixed venous oxygenation ($P\bar{v}_{O_2} > 30$ mm Hg).
4. Keep inflation pressure as low as possible.
5. Provide adequate humidification.
6. Provide positive end-expiratory pressure if an inspired oxygen concentration of >50% is required for greater than 24 hours.

OPTIMAL COMPLIANCE AND MONITORING

Frequent determination of static compliance of the lungs and chest wall may allow one to pick tidal volumes and PEEP that put the lung in the range of optimal compliance (Fig. 35-9). In the range of optimal compliance, the incidence of pulmonary barotrauma (pneumothorax, pneumomediastinum, and subcutaneous emphysema) is least, and tissue oxygen delivery may be maximal.

Several studies have shown that despite an increased Pa_{O_2}, significant reduction in cardiac output and mixed venous oxygen tension may occur from PEEP (Fig. 35-10). In the patient with severe ARDS, improvement in tissue oxygenation is the goal. Since oxygen delivery is the product of cardiac output and arterial oxygen content, cardiac output or some index of change in cardiac output should be made as PEEP is altered. If cardiac output or mixed venous oxygen tension ($P\bar{v}_{O_2}$) decreases as PEEP is increased, a reduction in oxygen delivery to the tissue may have occurred. If PEEP results in decreased cardiac output,

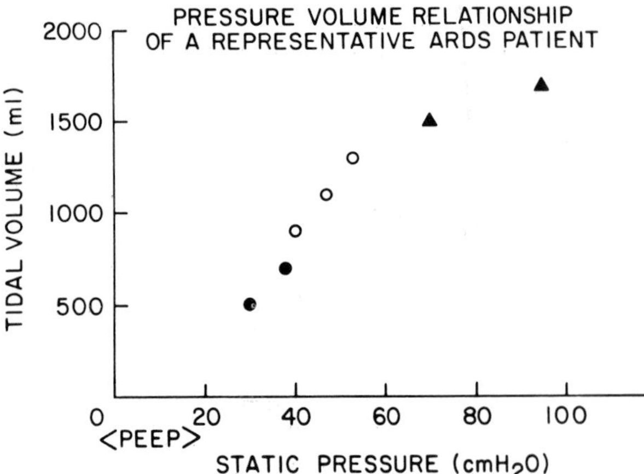

Fig. 35-9. Static pressure volume relationship of the lungs and thorax in ARDS. Each observation represents the inflation hold manometer pressure on the ventilator *(horizontal axis)* obtained for the tidal volume indicated on the vertical axis. Static compliance = tidal volume/inflation hold pressure − PEEP pressure. In this example, PEEP pressure is 10 cm H_2O. Compliance for tidal volumes is indicated by ● = 25 m/cm H_2O; ○ = 30 ml/cm H_2O; Δ = 25 and 20 ml/cm H_2O. (Bone RC: Treatment of severe hypoxemia due to the adult respiratory distress syndrome. Arch Intern Med 140:85, 1980. Copyright 1980, American Medical Association)

the patient may be hypovolemic and cardiac filling pressure too low to be maintained in the presence of PEEP. In this case, fluid loading is indicated. Alternatively, the patient may have primary cardiac dysfunction and require inotropic agents. A properly positioned pulmonary artery catheter allows measurement of the pulmonary capillary wedge pressure (PCWP), which reflects the filling pressure of the left ventricle. When PEEP is used, the positive alveolar pressure can influence the reliability of the PCWP. This results from transmission of PEEP to the microvasculature. If the transmitted alveolar pressure exceeds left atrial pressure, the vessels may be collapsed, as demonstrated in zone 1 of the Starling resistor model (see Fig. 35-8). In this case, the PCWP may be artificially high because it reflects alveolar pressure.

INDICATIONS FOR EXTUBATION

Guidelines for discontinuing mechanical ventilation are discussed in detail in Chapter 25. The large number of criteria underscores the fact that none is foolproof. Each roughly assesses baseline ventilation and oxygen transfer capability and reserve. Regardless of the criteria for extubation, maintenance of satisfactory arterial blood gases during a trial of spontaneous ventilation must be achieved by means of a T-tube attached to the airway or from the reservoir of an intermittent mandatory ventilation (IMV) apparatus. With IMV, the patient breathes spontaneously while still being administered a diminishing number of assisted breaths per minute. Although IMV is popular, whether it is a superior method of weaning awaits controlled trials of weaning methods. By decreasing mean intrathoracic pressure, IMV might decrease the incidence of pneumothorax or depression of cardiac output resulting from a high ventilating pressure or high levels of PEEP. Since cessation of mechanical ventilation may result in increased airway closure, CPAP of 2 to 10 cm H_2O may be used to decrease microatelectasis on transition from mechanical to spontaneous ventilation.

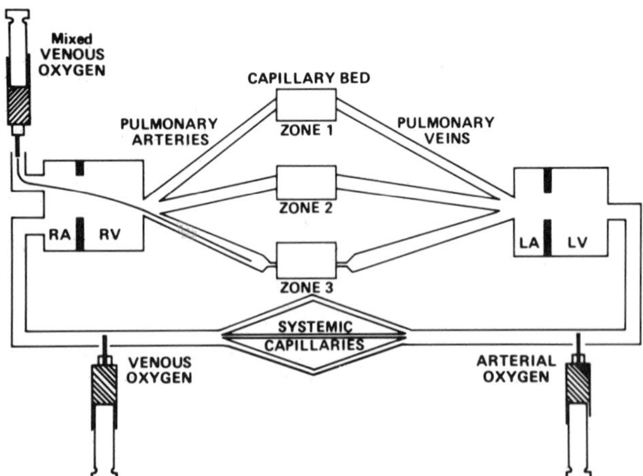

Fig. 35-10. Oxygen can be obtained from the arterial, peripheral venous, or mixed venous blood. Arterial blood provides essential information about lung function. In certain circumstances, the Pa_{O2} may increase despite a deterioration in oxygen delivery to tissue. For example, the application of PEEP in a relatively hypovolemic patient with ARDS might increase Pa_{O2} but depress cardiac output. In this situation, the arterial–mixed venous oxygen content difference may increase, reflecting the decreased cardiac output. A decreased $P\bar{v}_{O2}$ (taken from a pulmonary artery catheter) gives important information about decreased tissue oxygenation despite improvement of arterial oxygenation. (Bone RC: Treatment of severe hypoxemia due to the adult respiratory distress syndrome. Arch Intern Med 140:85, 1980. Copyright 1980, American Medical Association)

REFERENCES

1. Abramson NS et al: Adverse occurrences in intensive care units. JAMA 244:1582, 1980
2. Ashbaugh DG et al: Acute respiratory distress in adults. Lancet 2:319, 1967
3. Barach AL: Physiological methods in diagnosis and treatment of asthma and emphysema. Ann Intern Med 12:454, 1938
4. Barber RE, Lee J, Hamilton WK: Oxygen toxicity in man—a prospective study in patients with irreversible brain damage. N Engl J Med 283:1478, 1970
5. Bone RC: Diagnosis of causes for acute respiratory distress by pressure-volume curves. Chest 70:740, 1976
6. Bone RC: Treatment of severe hypoxemia due to the adult respiratory distress syndrome. Arch Intern Med 140:85, 1980
7. Bone RC: Treatment of respiratory failure due to advanced chronic obstructive lung disease. Arch Intern Med 140: 1018, 1980
8. Bone RC, Pierce AK, Johnson RL: Controlled oxygen administration in acute respiratory failure in chronic obstructive pulmonary disease: A reappraisal. Am J Med 65:896, 1978
9. Campbell EJM: Management of respiratory failure. Br Med J 2:1328, 1964
10. Campbell EJM, Gabbis T: Mask and tent for providing controlled oxygen concentration. Lancet 1:468, 1966
11. Martin L: Respiratory failure. Med Clin North Am 61:1369, 1977
12. Mithoefer JC, Keighley MB, Karetzky MS: Response of the arterial P_{O_2} to oxygen administration in chronic pulmonary disease. Ann Intern Med 74:328, 1971
13. Murray JF: Mechanism of acute respiratory failure. ARRD 115:1071, 1977
14. Pontoppidan H, Geffin B, Lowenstein E: Acute respiratory failure in the adult. N Engl J Med 287:690, 1972
15. Rahn H, Otis AB: Man's response during and after acclimatization to high altitude. Am J Physiol 157:445, 1949
16. Seriff NS, Khan F, Lazo BJ: Acute respiratory failure: Current concepts of pathophysiology and management. Med Clin North Am 57:1539, 1973
17. Smith JL: Pathological effects due to increased oxygen in air breathed. J Physiol 24:19, 1899
18. Zwillich CW et al: Complications of assisted ventilation. Am J Med 57:161, 1974

36

Adult Respiratory Distress Syndrome (High Permeability Pulmonary Edema)

Kevin B. Lake

From the battlefields of this century has emerged a form of respiratory failure not previously described. The adult respiratory distress syndrome ("shock lung") was not recognized during the War Between the States despite the large number of soldiers who died of respiratory ailments during that conflict. Even during World War I most of those who died from respiratory causes did so because of atelectasis or pneumonia, although by that time posttraumatic pulmonary insufficiency had been described.[2] Military surgeons in World War II coined the term "wet lung" to apply to those casualities without direct chest trauma, but usually with significant blood loss, who presented with dyspnea, crackles, and wheezes on chest examination and whose chest radiographs demonstrated abnormalities ranging from minimal atelectasis to what appeared to be severe pulmonary edema. These "wet lung" patients frequently developed progressive respiratory insufficiency, were found to be at high risk for emergency surgery, and were more difficult to resuscitate than were similarly traumatized patients without these findings.

During the Vietnam War, "wet lung" became known as "Da Nang lung," and it was the special circumstances of this period that allowed the observations made during World War II to be confirmed and extended.[2] These special circumstances and observations included [1] survival after massive trauma and blood loss in those who would have died at the front in previous wars; [2] evacuation by helicopter within 15 to 20 minutes after injury to sophisticated treatment centers; [3] rapid treatment and recovery from initial shock and trauma; and [4] development of respiratory failure after a latent period of 12 to 48 hours.

During the next decade, parallels to this wartime experience were recognized in civilian hospitals, and terms such as "stiff lung," "postperfusion lung," "wet lung," "shock lung," "white lung," and "respirator lung" were added to our vocabulary. All the terms listed in Table 36-1 describe what is essentially one entity: high permeability pulmonary edema (HPPE).

Today all physicians who care for critically ill patients should understand how to recognize and manage this syndrome. The discerning reader will note substantial changes in the current discussion from the first edition of *Respiratory Care*[31] because of the rapid and remarkable advances in our understanding of both the pathophysiology and the management of this syndrome.

DEFINITION

HPPE can be defined most succinctly as those forms of pulmonary edema with normal cardiac function associated with the accumulation of protein-rich fluid

Table 36-1. Synonyms for HPPE

White lung
Shock lung
Da Nang lung
Liver lung
Respirator lung
Wet lung
Pump lung
ARDS
Congestive atelectasis
Progressive pulmonary consolidation
Posttraumatic pulmonary insufficiency
Adult hyaline membrane disease

in the interstitial or intraalveolar spaces. In terms of clinical recognition, the following should be sought.

- Clinical: dyspnea, tachypnea
- Radiologic: diffuse interstitial and alveolar infiltrates
- Physiological: refractory hypoxemia, reduced pulmonary compliance
- Pathologic: edema, hemorrhage, microemboli, hyaline membrane formation

Even though there is a wide variation in etiology, the similar clinical, radiologic, and pathologic pictures have allowed the gathering together of, under the single heading HPPE, a variety of illnesses that have a phase in common which meets the definition of the syndrome as given above. Although the neonatal respiratory distress syndrome certainly meets the criteria, it is a separate entity discussed in detail elsewhere.

Because the pathologic picture is so consistent from patient to patient regardless of the etiology, it has been suggested that all previous synonyms be abandoned in favor of the term that is most descriptive of this syndrome: HPPE.[45] The changing terminology for this syndrome recalls a passage from "The Waltz of the Toreadors."*

GENERAL: And how is medical science progressing?
DOCTOR: No further. We have found other terms far less vague than the old ones to designate the same complaints. It's a great advance linguistically.

*Anouilh J: The Waltz of the Toreadors, translated by Hill L, p 17. New York, Coward–McCann, 1953

Table 36-2. Conditions Superficially Resembling HPPE

Cardiac pulmonary edema
Acute hypersensitivity lung disease
Chronic interstitial fibrosis
Respiratory failure secondary to obstructive airway disease, with pneumonitis

A partial list of conditions that superficially resemble HPPE appears in Table 36-2. However, major differences in pathophysiology, pathology, and therapy justify their exclusion. Only when other factors such as shock, sepsis, oxygen toxicity, or aspiration are involved can these conditions be considered for inclusion, provided that they fulfill the other criteria.

ETIOLOGY

Some medical and surgical settings in which HPPE has been described are listed in Table 36-3. Reports

Table 36-3. Causal Factors Related to HPPE

Aspiration of gastric contents
Hydrocarbon ingestion
Drug ingestion and overdose
Trauma and hemorrhagic shock
Chest
Abdominal
Other
Near-drowning
Smoke and gas inhalation
Disseminated intravascular coagulation
Septic and nonseptic shock
Fat and air embolism
Severe pneumonitis
Viral
Bacterial
Fungal
Mycoplasma
Oxygen toxicity
Homologous blood transfusion
Radiation pneumonitis
Postperfusion (cardiopulmonary bypass)
Fluid overload
Anaphylaxis
Narcotic overdose
Uremia
Hemorrhagic pancreatitis
Neurogenic pulmonary edema
High-altitude pulmonary edema

that describe new clinical settings for HPPE are continuously being published.[17,42] Although management of all patients with HPPE is similar in terms of such basics as oxygenation and fluid balance, therapy may be quite different in terms of treating the underlying disorder—for example, infection, neurogenic pulmonary edema, and aspiration. In a critically ill patient with HPPE after major trauma, for instance, the physician might face the concurrent problems of sepsis, fat embolism, and oxygen toxicity. Although difficult, it is important to assess the contribution of each of these factors so that proper management can be provided.

HPPE may be thought of as the pulmonary counterpart of acute tubular necrosis of the kidney (ATN). Just as ATN may occur in previously normal or abnormal kidneys, so too may HPPE occur in normal or abnormal lungs. However, unrecognized underlying disease in these organs may more easily predispose to development of the acute injury state.

PATHOPHYSIOLOGY

Despite the diverse etiologies that lead to the lung injury seen in HPPE, no common pathway has been found. The multiple factors discussed below are of varying importance depending on the cause of the initial injury. Clearly, however, the pathologic injury to the lung is remarkably similar from case to case. In some forms of HPPE such as sepsis, aspiration, and neurogenic pulmonary edema, the pathophysiology is reasonably well understood, in many others, it is not. Because not everyone who is ill with one of the disorders listed in Table 36-3 develops HPPE, it should be appreciated that incompletely understood protective mechanisms exist. Whether genetic, immunologic, or other factors confer this protection is unknown.

The major site of injury in the lung is the alveolar–capillary membrane (ACM). Normally this membrane is permeable only to small molecules (water-electrolytes). The balance between the Starling forces of osmotic and hydrostatic pressures plus the effectiveness of lymph flow serve to keep the interstitium of the lung relatively dry. The protein content of edema fluid is less than 50% of serum in hydrostatic pulmonary edema but rises with HPPE.[16] This fact serves as the basis for a test to recognize the presence of HPPE (*see* p. 861).

Severe central nervous system injury such as trauma, cerebrovascular accidents, tumors, and sudden increases in cerebrospinal fluid pressure may produce HPPE. Massive hypothalamic sympathetic neural discharge leads to systemic vasoconstriction with redistribution of large volumes of blood into the pulmonary circuit, producing severe elevation of the hydrostatic pressure.[45,65] Increased interstitial protein has also been found, suggesting the injury is due to not only the increased pressure but also the increased capillary permeability.[45] These changes may be extraordinarily rapid.[65] Massive pulmonary edema was found in autopsied Vietnam War casualties who died within minutes after head trauma. Other processes that produce cerebral hypoxia such as shock and ascent to high altitude may operate by a similar mechanism.[45] Figure 36-1 summarizes a similar condition, *i.e.*, the proposed mechanisms of neurogenic pulmonary edema.

Factors that can produce HPPE by direct injury to the lung include aspiration of gastric contents, which can either lead to mechanical obstruction or, more important, produce an acid burn to the airway when the *p*H is equal to, or less than, 2.5.[19] Although the major event is the rapid necrosis of the alveolar type I pneumocyte, the capillary endothelium is also injured, allowing protein and cellular elements to escape from the intravascular space. Oxygen in high concentration (approximately 50% or higher) causes damage to cellular DNA and membrane lipids presumably by the action of superoxide radicals (O_2^-) and hydrogen peroxide (H_2O_2). Radiation injures the alveolar epithelium and capillary endothelium usually 1 to 3 months after the initial exposure.[47] Other causes of direct injury to the alveolar membrane include near-drowning (osmotic effect?) and inhalation of toxic gases.

Studies of patients with combat injuries have revealed intravascular microaggregates in the lung of fibrin and blood cells (platelets and leukocytes). Trauma and perhaps other processes such as sepsis, drowning, and burns cause the release of thromboplastins that form fibrin clots in the peripheral blood, and these, along with platelets and leukocytes, are filtered out in the lung. If this were a massive and widespread process, physiologic dead space should increase, but this has not been uniformly demonstrated. The thrombotic state would normally be expected to be short because of the action of plasminogen on the fibrin clot. In many cases of HPPE, however, especially after trauma, production of plasminogen activation inhibitors by the liver is enhanced.[61] Thus fibrinolysis is prevented and microemboli remain. Disseminated intravascular coagulation (DIC) may also play a role in some patients. Whether

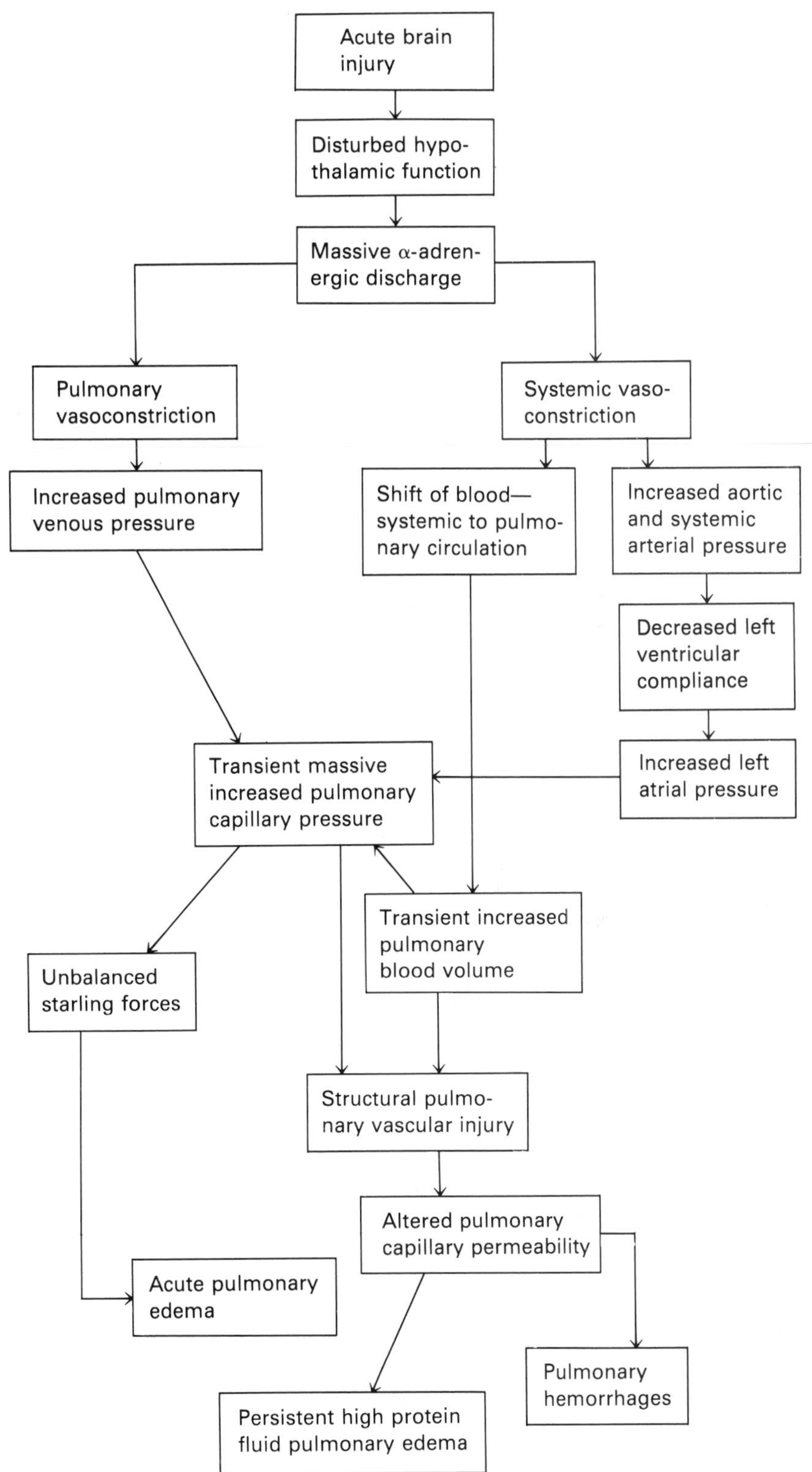

Fig. 36-1. Mechanism of neurogenic pulmonary edema. (Robin ED: Neurogenic pulmonary edema. Am Rev Respir Dis 113:405, 1979)

Table 36-4. Mechanisms by Which Humoral Substances May Participate in Alveolar–Capillary Membrane Injury

Increased permeability of capillary endothelium
Histamine
Endotoxin
Fibrinogen degradation products
Increased capillary hydrostatic pressure
Histamine
Serotonin
Prostaglandin endoperoxides
Prostaglandin F_2
Thromboxane

(Connors AF Jr, McCaffree DR, Rogers RM: The adult respiratory distress syndrome. In Cotsonas NJ Jr et al (ed): Disease-A-Month. Copyright 1981 by Year Book Medical Publishers, Inc., Chicago)

this is primary or a result of capillary endothelial damage is not known.

A number of hormones and vasoactive substances are found in the blood of patients with HPPE. The role that each plays in the genesis of the syndrome has not been well described, but as a group they are clearly important.

Histamine increases vascular permeability and produces vasoconstriction of the pulmonary veins.[6] Serotonin, which is present in mast cells and platelets, raises hydrostatic pressure and may be a major cause of HPPE and pulmonary hypertension.[50] The role of bradykinin is uncertain but is thought to be important because of its ability to stimulate leukocyte migration, which in turn may cause damage by release of chemical mediators.[43] Prostaglandin production leads to platelet aggregation and thrombosis and also to the release of chemical mediators. This has been best shown with thromboxane (T_XA_2), which is metabolized from endoperoxide PGG_2. Bacterial endotoxin increases capillary membrane permeability, a reaction that may be indirectly mediated by complement. Fibrinogen is split into D and E fragments by plasmin, but it is the D fragment that (in a rabbit model) increases capillary permeability.[36] The polymorphonuclear leukocyte (PMN) may participate in the inflammatory process by releasing lysosomal proteases and by releasing H_2O_2 and O_2^- directly. Additional evidence for the role of this cell in the ACM injury was presented in a recent study showing increased elastolytic activity from the PMNs of patients with HPPE.[34] A summary of humoral events is shown in Table 36-4.

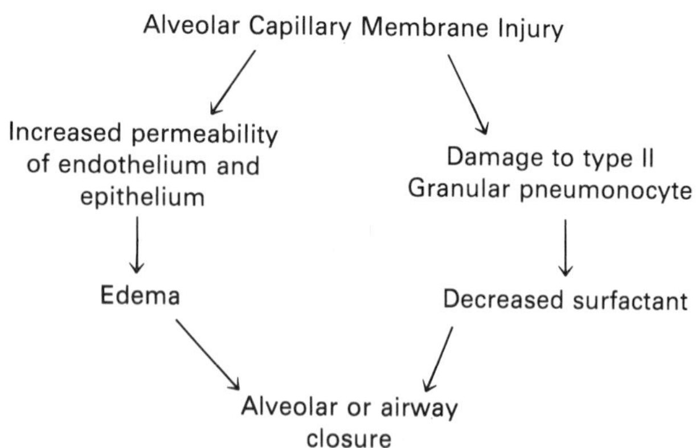

Fig. 36-2. Consequences of alveolar capillary membrane injury.

Other significant changes occur in the alveoli and respiratory bronchioles. The granular type II pneumocyte is responsible for producing surfactant. This phospholipoprotein lowers the surface tension in the alveolus and contributes significantly to its stability. Surfactant activity is reduced in HPPE either because of destruction of the type II pneumocyte or because of inactivation of surfactant. In either case the surfactant concentration falls, and the alveolus becomes unstable and tends to collapse unless filled with fluid from the interstitial space. Such alveoli can no longer participate in gas exchange. Previously normal gas exchange sites thus become a tangled mass of interstitial and alveolar edema, along with hemorrhage and focal atelectasis (Fig. 36-2).

Interstitial edema collects around terminal airways, compressing and obliterating them. This further reduces lung volume and leads to even less compliance. As the leak grows larger, fluid, protein, and blood cells collect in the interstitium and alveoli. Lymph channels that normally would evacuate these elements are compressed. Since many poorly ventilated units continue to receive blood, the shunt fraction ($\dot{Q}s/\dot{Q}t$) goes up. In other areas where vasoconstriction and microemboli occur, wasted ventilation (V_D/V_T) increases. The net result is $\dot{V}/\dot{Q}$ mismatching and hypoxemia.

Although cardiac function is usually normal in patients with HPPE, a myocardial depressant factor has been described in some patients with gram-negative sepsis, in some with nonsurviving hemorrhagic shock, and in some who have been on a myocardial depressant drug.[35] What this "factor" is and how it works is unknown.

The basic pathophysiology of HPPE and its interrelationships is shown in Figure 36-3.

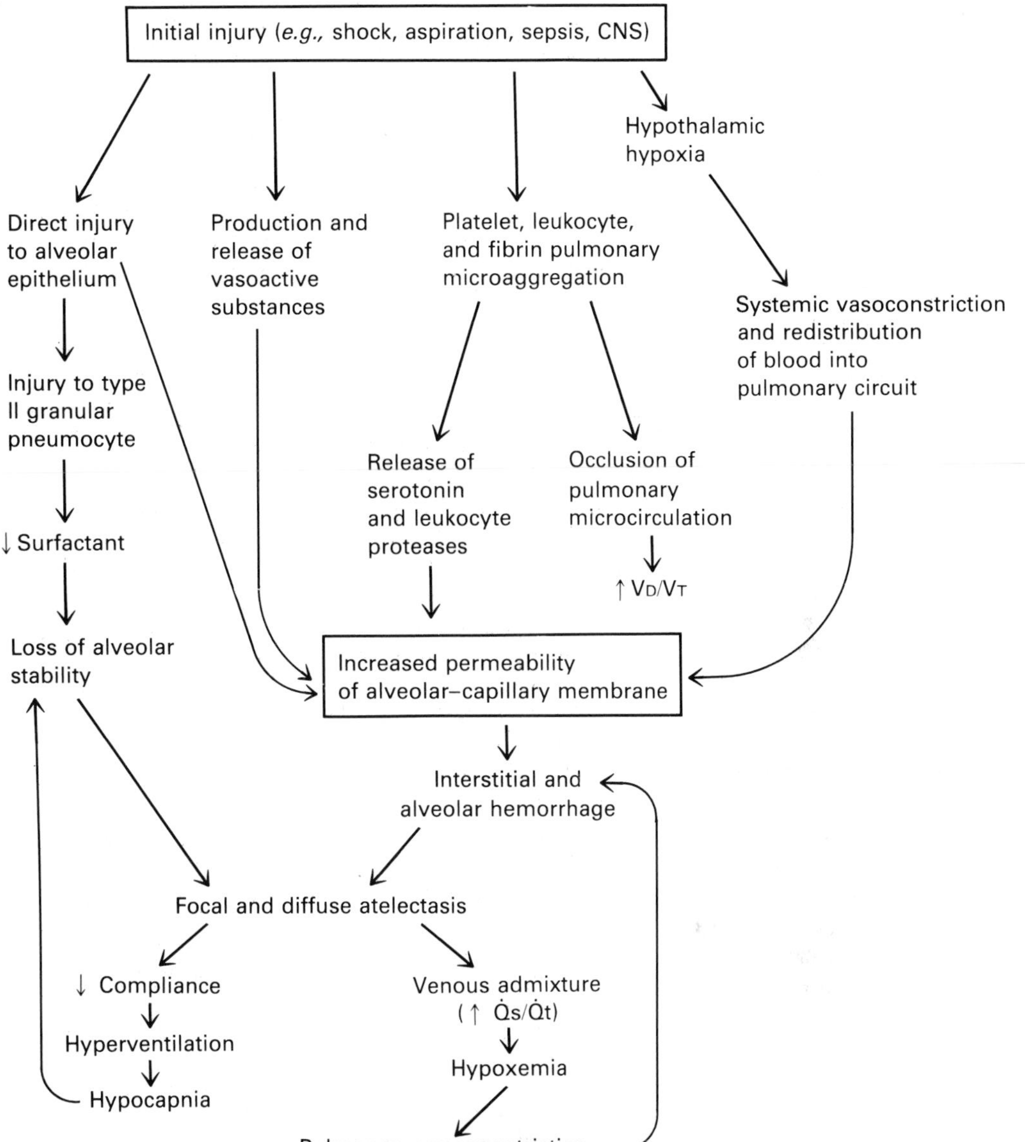

Fig. 36-3. Proposed pathophysiology of HPPE.

Table 36-5. Summary of Physiological Abnormalities in HPPE

Hypoxemia
Normal or low Pa_{CO_2} in early stages; high Pa_{CO_2} in late stages
Normal or high *p*H in early stages; low *p*H in late stages
Increased minute ventilation
Increased work of breathing
Increased wasted ventilation
Increased venous admixture
Decreased vital capacity
Decreased functional residual capacity
Decreased lung compliance

Once the pathophysiology of HPPE is understood, the various physiological abnormalities as outlined in Table 36-5 are easily understood. Some, such as the increased minute ventilation and decreased vital capacity, can be measured conveniently at the bedside, whereas others, such as increased shunt or work of breathing, require special equipment or invasive procedures.

CLINICAL FINDINGS

Although HPPE is easy to recognize in its advanced stages, the early, sometimes subtle, findings may be missed unless actively sought. The physician must be alert for development of the syndrome in those clinical states identified as substrates for the development of HPPE. By recognizing the syndrome early and confirming it with clinical and laboratory measurements, appropriate action can be taken at a time when the prognosis is still favorable. Also, by making an early diagnosis, the clinician may avoid compounding the problems by mishandling oxygen, respirators, fluids, and drugs.

Onset may be almost immediate, as in neurogenic pulmonary edema, or may be delayed 6 to 48 hours after the injury. The early symptoms are dyspnea, restlessness, and cough, alone or in combination. Dyspnea, however, may not appear early in the young, healthy person who can easily double or triple his minute ventilation at rest. In the patient on a respirator, the first finding may be that of an increase in the pressure required to deliver a given tidal volume (indicating a decreasing pulmonary compliance).

On physical examination, increased work of breathing with hyperpnea, grunting respirations, cyanosis or pallor, and intercostal and suprasternal retraction are usually evident. Tachypnea, diaphoresis, and mental obtundation also occur frequently. Early on, chest auscultation may be normal, and only as the syndrome becomes more advanced will various kinds of wheezes and crackles be heard. Increased breath sounds are a late finding. Physical findings that might give a clue to the underlying etiology should be sought, such as skin, conjunctival, and retinal findings in fat embolism and singed nasal hairs and palatal erythema in pulmonary burns.

The differential diagnosis may, at times, be difficult. Hemodynamic monitoring is useful in separating cardiogenic from noncardiogenic pulmonary edema. Pulmonary thromboembolism (PTE) is an unusual cause of HPPE and may be a difficult diagnosis to establish. In a patient on a respirator with "white lungs" by radiograph, a low compliance, and severe refractory hypoxemia, only a pulmonary angiogram will exclude a diagnosis of PTE. This procedure, however, carries a high risk in a critically ill patient with HPPE. The decision to treat for PTE may be a difficult one. Fibrinolytic therapy is contraindicated, heparin is relatively contraindicated, and interruption of the inferior vena cava is a major therapeutic intervention requiring angiographic confirmation.

Diagnosis of HPPE by those who first see the patient before hospitalization should not be difficult in the proper clinical setting. The presence of dyspnea, tachypnea, shallow respirations, and cyanosis, the lack of wheezes or crackles, and no evidence of heart failure should alert the observer to the possibility of this diagnosis.

LABORATORY DATA

Tests of gas exchange, oxygen delivery and consumption, and mechanical function of the lung are useful in evaluating and managing HPPE. All other tests, such as the various chemistries and measurements of blood cells, are important only as they help the physician to understand the patient more completely or yield clues to an underlying etiology.

The *sine qua non* for establishing the diagnosis remains a lowered Pa_{O_2}, which is poorly responsive to increased concentrations of oxygen in the inspired air. A more precise way in which to express this is by the alveolar–arterial oxygen gradient ($(A\text{-}a)D_{O_2}$). Normally the $(A\text{-}a)D_{O_2}$ should be less than 15 torr on room air, but, in severe HPPE, values of 200 to 500 torr and greater are recorded. This information conveys more about the efficiency of oxygen transfer than the Pa_{O_2}

determination alone, especially when followed serially. It may also be useful to measure the shunt fraction ($\dot{Q}s/\dot{Q}t$), the oxygen content (Ca_{O_2}), and oxygen consumption ($\dot{V}O_2$). It is most convenient to calculate the $\dot{V}O_2$ with a pulmonary artery catheter in place, at which time the cardiac output (CO) and arterial and mixed venous oxygen contents can be calculated. $\dot{V}O_2$ is then determined by the Fick principle; $\dot{V}O_2 = CO \times (a\text{-}v)D_{O_2}$. Alveolar ventilation remains high until late in the course of HPPE. A "normal" Pa_{CO_2} in a very dyspneic, hypoxemic patient is not "normal" and when present, suggests seriously diseased lungs that no longer can increase alveolar ventilation in response to hypoxemia and other stimuli.

The pH normally rises as the Pa_{CO_2} falls (uncompensated respiratory alkalemia). Failure to do so signifies the presence of metabolic acidemia, which, in the face of shock and hypoxemia, is most commonly a result of lactic acidosis. This can be confirmed by direct measurement of blood lactate.

Pulmonary artery pressure (PAP), pulmonary capillary wedge pressure (PCWP), and CO are usually normal but, if abnormal, give useful information to guide therapy.

Tests of pulmonary mechanics reveal decreasing static and dynamic compliance and reduction in lung volumes, particularly the functional residual capacity (FRC). Significant obstruction to air flow is usually not a problem unless there is preexisting airway disease or there are large volumes of secretions.

A sensitive test is needed that can detect HPPE at an early phase when fluid is starting to collect in the lung interstitium. Current approaches to this problem have included the use of radioactive tracers, thermodilution techniques, and transthoracic electrical impedance measurements. A recent international conference on this subject was not able to recommend any of these techniques. The chest roentgenogram remains the standard for assessing lung water.[55]

A recently described test that may prove useful compares total protein in the tracheal aspirate to total protein in the plasma (tracheal protein/plasma protein). In cardiogenic pulmonary edema the ratio is usually less than 0.5, whereas in HPPE the tracheal protein value is close to the plasma level.[54]

RADIOGRAPHIC FINDINGS

The chest roentgenogram may be normal early during HPPE, but as the syndrome progresses it always becomes abnormal (Figures 36-4, 36-5). The radiologic picture is the result of movement of fluid out of the injured alveolar capillary into the interstitium and, in later phases, into the alveolus itself. There must, however, be a large increase in lung water before the chest roentgenogram becomes abnormal. This is why roentgenograms frequently are normal during the early stages of HPPE. During this time when the chest film is normal, a considerable degree of microatelectasis may be present.

Although it is easy to recognize HPPE when it reaches the appearance seen in Figure 36-5A, one needs a sensitive eye to detect early changes. Subtle findings such as thickened or blurred margins of bronchi or vessels should be sought. An elevated diaphragm consistent with a reduced FRC should be looked for. Except for the increased heart size typical of left ventricular failure, the roentgenogram of HPPE may be difficult to discriminate from that of cardiogenic pulmonary edema.

The first roentgenographic changes are those of fine and coarse reticulation (Fig. 36-4A), which then progress to give the lung a ground-glass appearance. When fluid spills into the alveoli, a typical airspace alveolar filling pattern is seen (Fig. 36-5A,B,C). Pleural effusion is not part of the typical HPPE chest roentgenographic presentation. Terminally, when consolidation and coalescing infiltrates are seen, there may be few recognizable air spaces, and at this point the term "white lung" is applicable (Fig. 36-5A).

The rapidity with which radiographic resolution takes place depends on not only the amount of fluid, but also its composition and associated pathologic changes. Fluid with a low protein content and a minimum of cells and other formed elements may resolve within hours to several days (Fig. 36-4A,B,C). Large amounts of blood usually resolve in a few days, whereas fluid with a distinct inflammatory component requires weeks for maximum resolution.

PATHOLOGY

The pathologic lesion in HPPE is similar no matter how the lesion arrives at the ACM—by inhalation or by the blood. Autopsies of those dying from shock or after trauma reveal the lungs to be involved more frequently than any other organ.[38]

On gross examination the lungs are heavy, hemorrhagic, and congested, with only a minimal amount of air. When placed in water or fixative solution, they sink. On sectioning, only a small amount of fluid can be expressed; such lungs have the appearance of liver.

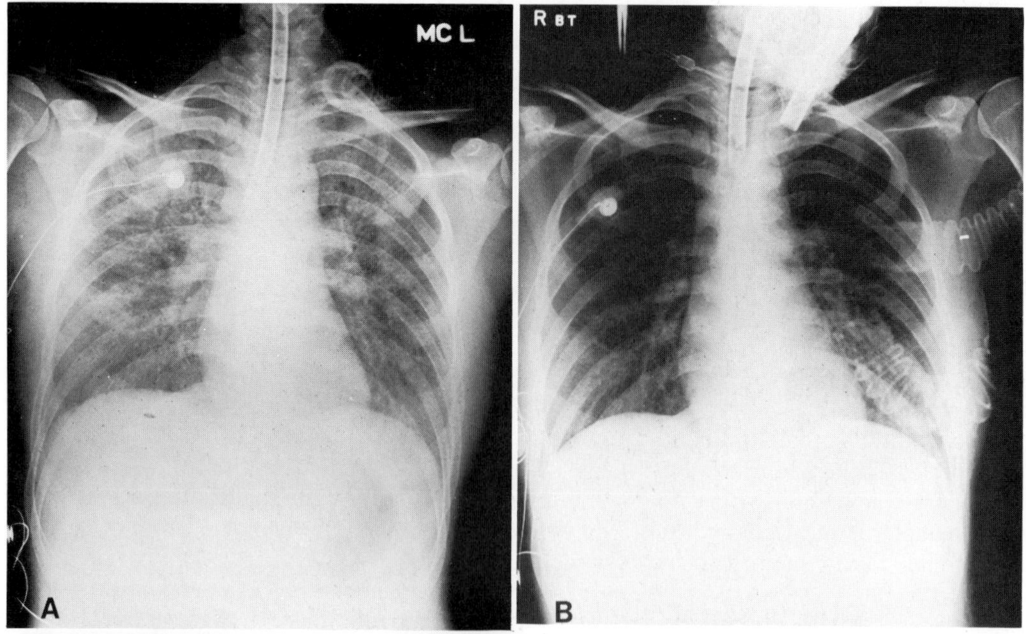

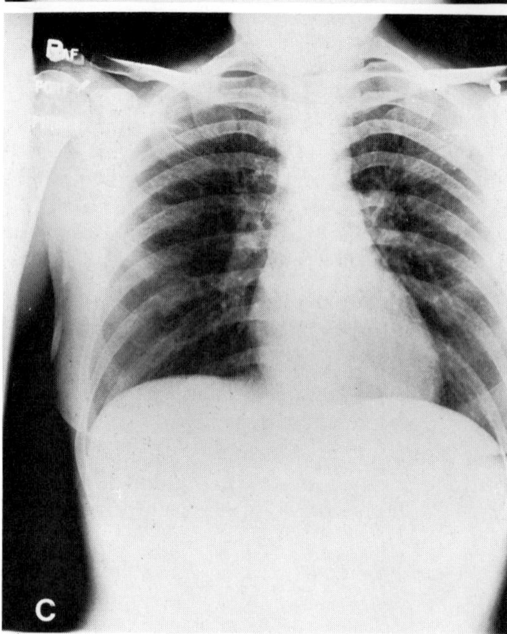

Fig. 36-4. *(A)* Diffuse alveolar and interstitial involvement in a 23-year-old woman with viral pneumonia and generalized urticaria who had been given a cephalosporin antibiotic. Note the accidental passage of the nasotracheal tube into the right mainstem bronchus. Compliance was low, and high levels of inspired oxygen were needed. *(B)* Seventeen hours after admission, the patient's roentgenogram has cleared markedly. *(C)* Forty-eight hours after admission, the roentgenogram has almost returned to normal. This probably represents HPPE on the basis of drug-induced urticaria.

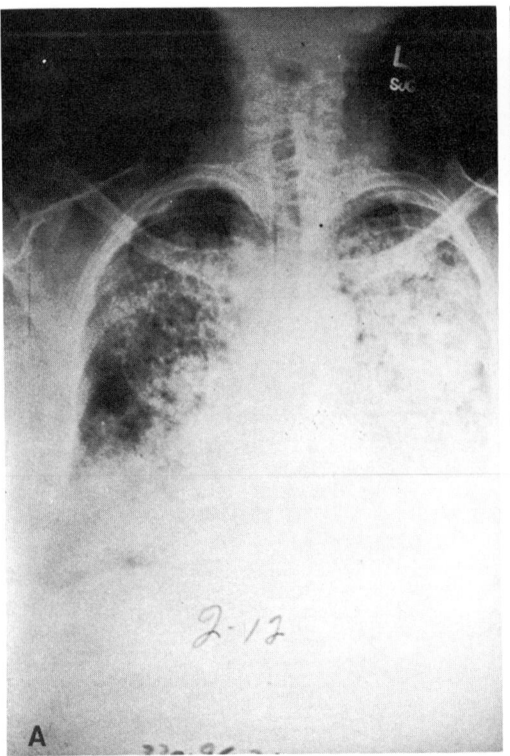

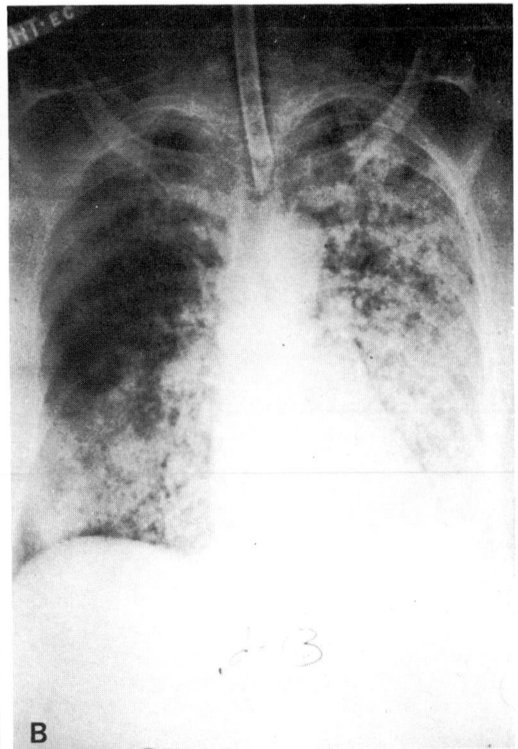

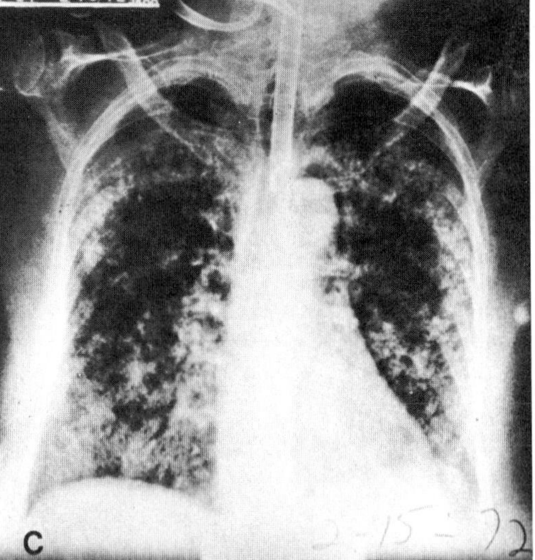

Figure 36-5. *(A)* Severe influenza A pneumonia and HPPE in a 42-year-old black woman. *(B)* Twenty-four hours later there is marked improvement. *(C)* Seventy-two hours after admission, the patient continues to improve clinically and roentgenographically.

Table 36-6. Pathology: The Lung's Response to Injury

Exudative phase (24–96 hrs)
Alveolar and interstitial edema
Capillary congestion
Destruction of type I alveolar cells
Early hyaline membrane formation
Proliferative phase, cellular (3–10 days)
Increased type II alveolar cells
Cellular infiltrate of the alveolar septum
Organization of hyaline membranes
Proliferative phase, fibrotic (>7–10 days)
Fibrosis of hyaline membranes and alveolar septum
Alveolar duct fibrosis, typical lesion

(Connors AF Jr, McCaffree DR, Rogers RM: The adult respiratory distress syndrome. In Cotsonas NJ Jr et al (ed): Disease-A-Month. Copyright 1981 by Year Book Medical Publishers, Inc., Chicago)

In late deaths, especially after prolonged therapy, the lungs are small and fibrotic with emphysematous blebs. Generally, secretions in the large airways are not significant, nor is there grossly visible obstruction of the major pulmonary vessels.

The HPPE injury can be divided into three phases (Table 36-6).[8,26] During the early exudative phase (24–96 hrs), there is edema of the interstitial and alveolar spaces, and thickening of the ACM due to blood and inflammatory products occurs (Fig. 36-6A,B). Hyaline membranes that are seen early are formed from necrotic type I pneumocytes, fibrin, and plasma proteins. The type I pneumocyte is more susceptible to injury than is the capillary endothelium.

During the proliferative phase (3–10 days), the type II pneumocytes increase in number and may form a complete covering of the alveolar surface, as compared to the 5% of the surface area they normally cover. Alveolar lining cell hyperplasia, increased intraalveolar exudate, and capillary congestion are also seen (Fig. 36-6C,D).

During the fibrotic phase (>7–10 days), marked interstitial and intraalveolar fibrosis is present (Fig. 36-6E). Hyaline membranes that were so prominent earlier have been transformed into fibrous tissue.

Oxygen is a frequent cause or contributor to HPPE. High concentrations of oxygen may lead to interstitial edema within 48 hours, and by 3 to 7 days necrosis and sloughing of the capillary endothelium and alveolar epithelium are present.

Electron microscopy has significantly advanced our understanding of HPPE.[1] Figure 36-7A shows the normal intraalveolar septum with the delicate alveolar epithelium and capillary endothelium, even where they are fused. It is over the thin nonfused portion of the ACM (approximately one half of the surface) where most of the gas exchange takes place. The granular pneumocyte with its large number of organelles is the site of surfactant production and other metabolic activities.

The acute phase is seen electron microscopically within 24 hours. The essential finding is pulmonary edema due to capillary leakage. Various numbers of erythrocytes, leukocytes and macrophages, and fibrin are found in the alveolar fluid (Fig. 36-7B). The cytoplasmic extensions of the type I pneumonocyte are destroyed early, but the type II pneumonocyte appears to resist injury. Hyaline membranes are also seen at this stage. One surprising finding has been the lack of any conspicuous visible capillary leak despite the large amount of fluid, protein, and blood cells that obviously is crossing the capillary endothelium. Overall, however, pulmonary architecture is preserved.

The electron microscopic picture in the subacute and chronic phase (days to weeks) is that of tissue fibrosis and loss of pulmonary architecture (Fig. 36-7C). Edema is much less obvious, and capillaries are few in number. One of the striking findings is that of marked proliferation of the type II pneumocyte.

THERAPY

GENERAL CARE

Lives that would have been lost from HPPE a few years ago now frequently can be saved. Current standards of care require the ability to make certain measurements that can be used as guides to therapeutic intervention. Listed in Table 36-7 are a number of such measurements needed to follow these extremely ill patients. Although different clinical settings will require different measurements, the more critically ill the patient, the more parameters will be needed to assess the situation adequately.

Central to the management of HPPE is prevention or correction of the underlying disorder and a vigorous attempt to correct reversible components of the clinical picture. Electrolyte and acid–base disturbances should be treated as judiciously as is feasible. Serious metabolic acidemia (pH equal to or less than 7.10) may be cautiously corrected up to a pH of no more than 7.25 to 7.30 with sodium bicarbonate. A given level of acidemia is better tolerated by the body

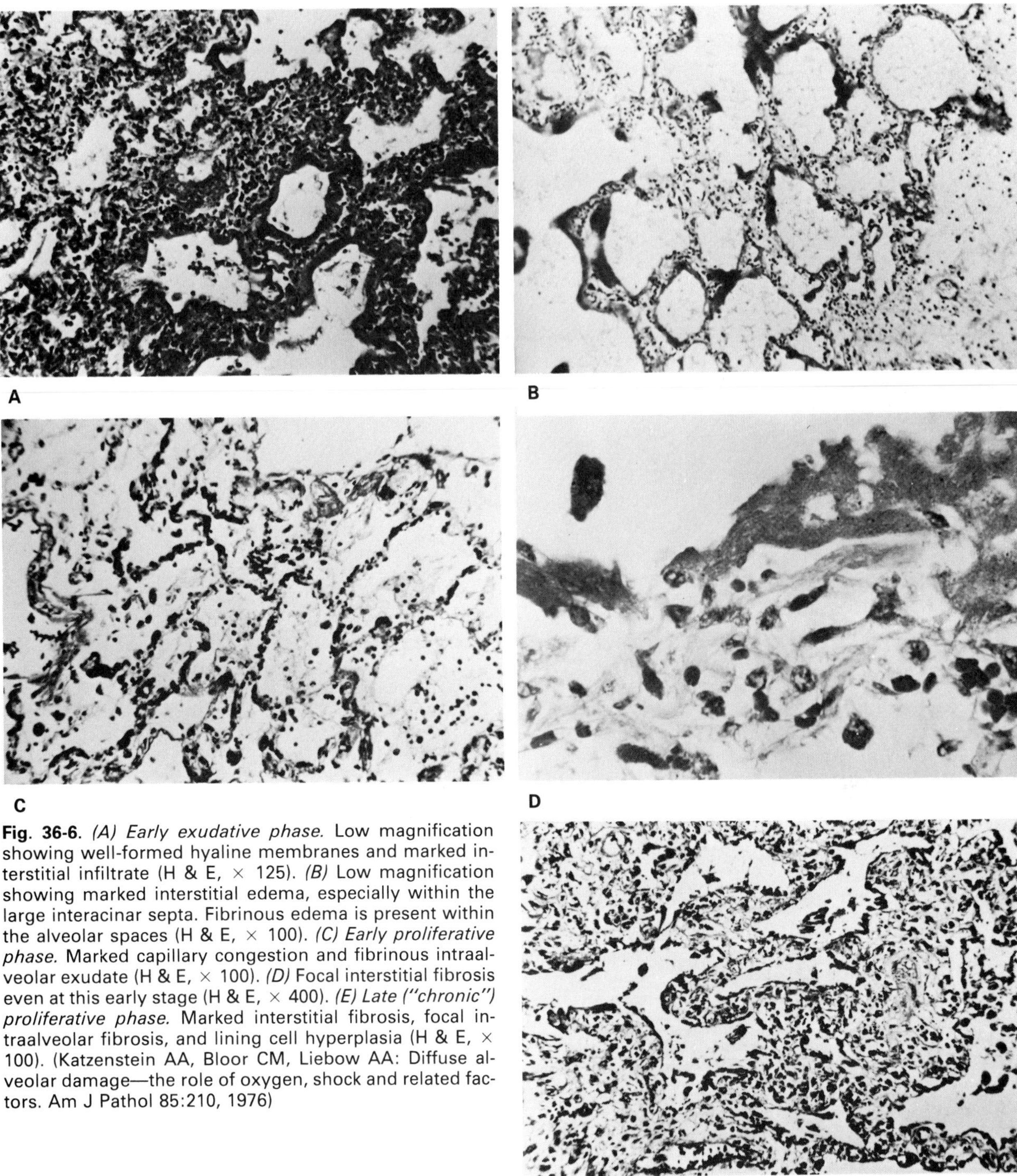

Fig. 36-6. *(A) Early exudative phase.* Low magnification showing well-formed hyaline membranes and marked interstitial infiltrate (H & E, × 125). *(B)* Low magnification showing marked interstitial edema, especially within the large interacinar septa. Fibrinous edema is present within the alveolar spaces (H & E, × 100). *(C) Early proliferative phase.* Marked capillary congestion and fibrinous intraalveolar exudate (H & E, × 100). *(D)* Focal interstitial fibrosis even at this early stage (H & E, × 400). *(E) Late ("chronic") proliferative phase.* Marked interstitial fibrosis, focal intraalveolar fibrosis, and lining cell hyperplasia (H & E, × 100). (Katzenstein AA, Bloor CM, Liebow AA: Diffuse alveolar damage—the role of oxygen, shock and related factors. Am J Pathol 85:210, 1976)

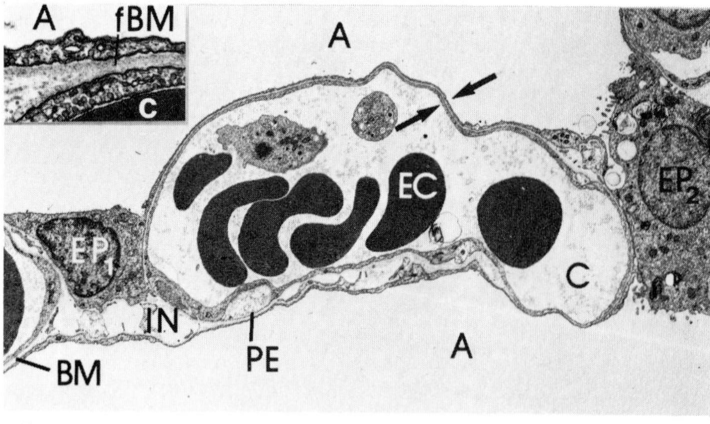

A

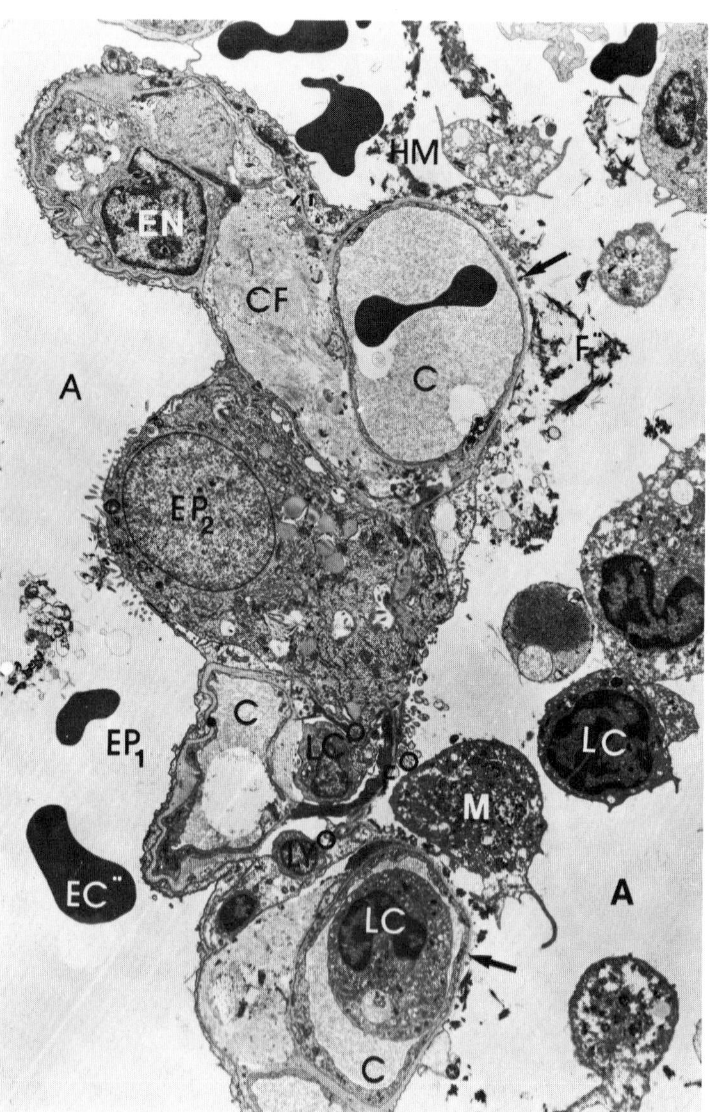

B

Fig. 36-7. *(A)* Normal interalveolar septum of the human lung. Note that the gas exchange barrier is extremely thin on one side of the septum *(arrows)* (original magnification, × 1500). *Inset:* Transition from thick to thin blood–gas barrier, where epithelial and endothelial basement membrane become fused *(fBM)*. A = alveolar space; C = capillary; EC = erythrocyte; EP_1 = type I squamous epithelial cell; IN = interstitium; BM = basement membrane; PE = pericyte; EP_2 = type II granular epithelial cell. *(B)* Alveolar and interstitial edema in a patient who died 24 hours after the onset of acute respiratory failure due to septicemia. Interstitial blood constitutents are marked with °, blood cells and fibrin in the alveolar space with ″. Arrows indicate areas of destroyed type I squamous epithelial cell (original magnification, × 3600). HM = hyaline membrane; EN = endothelium; CF = collagen fibers; C = capillary; A = alveolar space; EP_2 = type II granular epithelial cell; EP_1 = type I squamous epithelial cell; LC = leukocyte; F = fibrin; LY = lymphocyte; EC = erythrocyte. *(C)* Alveolar septa showing the interstitium broadened by edema, fibers, and free cells. Capillaries *(C)* are scarce. Slitlike alveolar spaces (indicated by x's) are lined by type II epithelial cells (EP_2) (original magnification, × 1920). LC = leukocyte; (° = interstitial); Mx = alveolar macrophage in mitosis; FC = fibrocyte. (Bachofen M, Weibel ER: Alterations of the gas exchange apparatus in adult respiratory insufficiency associated with septicemia. Am Rev Respir Dis 116:589, 1977)

Table 36-7. Measurements to Guide Therapy in HPPE

Frequent examination of patient
Temperature, pulse, and respiratory rate
Intake–output and body weight
Heart monitor and complete electrocardiogram
Tracheobronchial secretions: amount, appearance, Gram's stain, culture
Clinical: CBC, serum proteins, serum and urine electrolytes, renal function, coagulation profile, liver function, appropriate cultures
Ventilator: volume, pressure required, dead space, O_2 concentration, assist or control, IMV, PEEP, CPAP
Pulmonary function: vital capacity, tidal volume, minute ventilation, peak negative pressure, peak positive pressure, ventilator inspiratory plateau pressure
Hemodynamic and blood gas: systemic, arterial, and pulmonary artery pressure, PCWP, arterial *p*H, P_{CO_2}, P_{O_2}, hemoglobin, P_{50}, central venous oxygen tension ($P\bar{v}_{O_2}$) and oxygen consumption ($\dot{V}O_2$)
Mass spectroscopy: FRC, $\dot{V}O_2$, $\dot{V}CO_2$

than the same level of alkalemia. Prevention of fever, chills, and restlessness are important in reducing oxygen consumption and may be critical to survival when tissue oxygenation is marginal.

Just as in asthma and other forms of obstructive airway disease, bronchial hygiene is important when secretions, mucosal edema, and bronchospasm are present. Elevation of the head and chest will increase the vital capacity by reducing the pressure of the abdominal viscera on the diaphragm. Chest wall pain is best managed with analgesics and regional nerve blocks rather than strapping of the chest, which interferes with normal ventilatory mechanics. Collections of air, fluid, or blood in the pleural space inhibit normal ventilation and should be removed.

FLUID BALANCE

Fluid management is difficult in those who are seriously ill with HPPE. On the one hand, an excess of

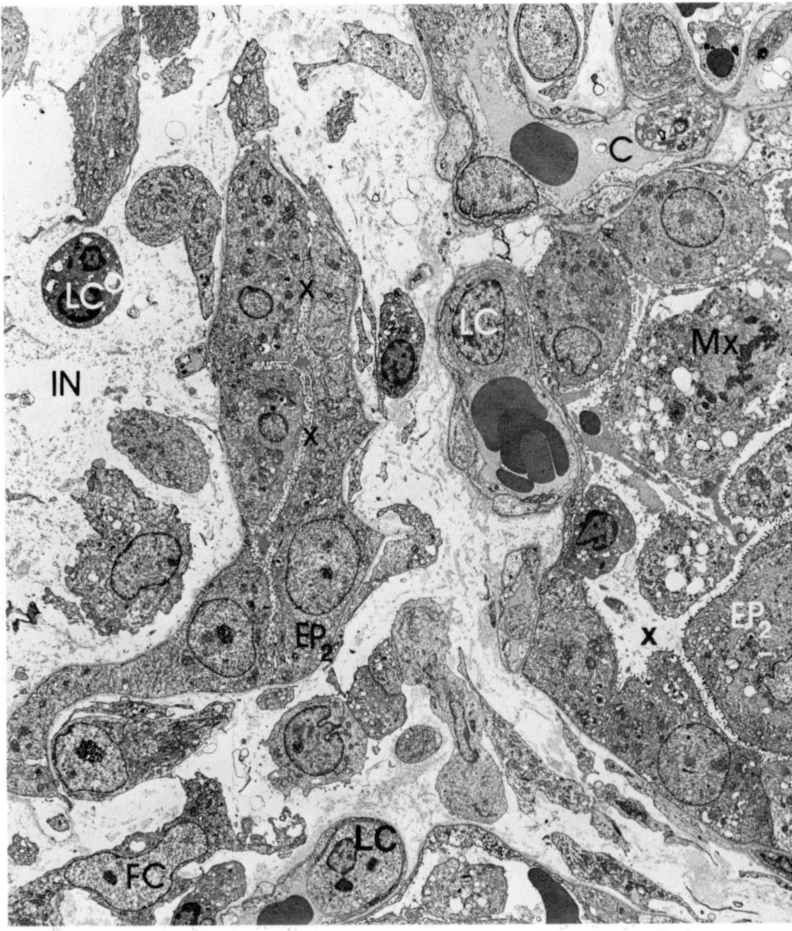

Fig. 36-7 *(continued)* **C**

fluid simply pours out through a leaky capillary membrane into the lung parenchyma; on the other hand, the volume-depleted patient is prone to develop hypotension with mechanical ventilation and positive end-expiratory pressure.

Serum oncotic pressure frequently is reduced either because of failure of protein synthesis (overwhelming illness) or through losses of protein. Because of the reduced osmotic pressure, fluid tends to move out of the vascular space (Starling forces). With leakage of protein into the interstitial and intraalveolar spaces, even more fluid is drawn out of the intravascular space. The leakage of protein also contributes to the formation of hyaline membranes.

Patients on respirators generally require less fluid than do patients not on respirators for the following reasons.[8]

1. Decreased insensible loss from the respiratory tract
2. Renal
   a. Increased antidiuretic hormone
   b. Decreased renal blood flow
   c. Alteration of intrarenal distribution

The patient's volume status must be monitored rigorously. This includes strict intake and output measurements, daily body weights, arterial blood pressure, and in many cases measurement of CO, PAP, and PCWP. Failure to lose 300 to 500 g/day in a catabolic state while only on intravenous fluids indicates increased free water retention.[44]

The goal of fluid therapy is to give just enough fluid to maintain a minimum PCWP that provides an adequate cardiac output and acceptable tissue oxygenation (see below). Although serious controversy continues over whether to use crystalloids or colloids, the current practice of many is to use crystalloids,[22,52] especially when the capillary leak is presumed to be large.

OXYGEN THERAPY

The most pressing problem in the use of oxygen is to provide acceptable tissue oxygenation with an FI_{O_2} equal to or less than 0.5. (Many options are open; see Fig. 36-8.)

Under circumstances where oxygen delivery is reduced, such as in anemia, hypoxemia, or decreased cardiac output, compensatory mechanisms come into play in order to maintain adequate oxygen consumption.[11,64]

The most important such mechanism is increased extraction of the oxygen delivered ($(a\text{-}v)D_{O_2}$). Other compensatory mechanisms include [1] local vasodilation and increased tissue perfusion and [2] shifts in the oxyhemoglobin dissociation curve. Again, under normal physiologic circumstances regional perfusion is determined by oxygen needs, and, when decreases in oxygen delivery occur, blood flow may be shifted from organs of low use to organs of high use to utilize maximally the available oxygen. Because of these regulatory forces it has been shown that oxygen consumption is related to tissue needs and is independent of oxygen delivery, except at very low levels where a direct relation exists between consumption and delivery.[7]

Recent work has suggested, however, that unlike the normal state described above, patients with HPPE have a direct relation between oxygen delivery and oxygen consumption. Again, unlike the normal state, $(a\text{-}v)D_{O_2}$ did not vary (in one study) with changes in oxygen delivery.[10] Patients on PEEP with HPPE have failure of peripheral perfusion distribution so that much of the blood goes to organs with low extraction ratios.[37] This may be related to increased amounts of circulating vasoactive substances.

Although a mixed venous oxygen tension may be a reliable indicator of tissue oxygenation in normal persons, it can be very misleading in patients with critical illnesses, including HPPE. A large part of the cardiac output may be going to organs with low extraction ratios (as described in HPPE), or there may be arteriovenous shunting at the tissue level. In either case, the central venous oxygen tension ($P\bar{v}_{O_2}$) will be falsely elevated and tissue hypoxia may go unrecognized.[21] Likewise serum lactate or lactate/pyruvate ratios have been found to be insensitive and inadequate measurements of tissue hypoxia until severe hypoxia is present.[25] Unfortunately there are no good independent measurements of tissue oxygenation. The most practical means of measuring tissue hypoxia is to calculate oxygen consumption by the Fick principle (see Laboratory section). *If some maneuver that increases oxygen delivery (e.g., blood transfusion, digitalis) results in increased oxygen consumption, one may conclude that an unmet oxygen need existed before that maneuver.*

Without controlled studies it is difficult to provide guidelines for the adequacy of oxygenation, but the following are suggested.[3,9]

1. Oxygen delivery $>$ 600 ml/min/m^2
2. Cardiac index $\geq$ 4.5 liters/min/m^2

3. Oxygen consumption (V_{O2}) $\geq$ 156 ml/min/m^2

These must be considered baseline. Certainly those who are seriously ill or who have complications such as fever or sepsis will require more blood and oxygen.

From a practical viewpoint, numbers should act only as guides and not as substitutes for clinical judgment. Bedside assessment of tissue oxygenation (e.g., brain, kidney, heart) can be just as valuable, if not more so, than a number representing whole body oxygenation. Not all patients with HPPE need sophisticated monitoring and determination of all of the above parameters of oxygenation. These measurements ought to be reserved for those who are not improving, for those who are deteriorating, or for cases where the adequacy of tissue oxygenation is questionable.

The risk of oxygen toxicity increases exponentially at high FI_{O_2}. Generally concentrations of less than 0.5 do not produce toxicity. Other factors to consider in the oxygen toxicity equation are the length of time on a high FI_{O_2}, the condition of the underlying lung, and perhaps other aggravating factors (e.g., shock, fluid overload, aspiration, sepsis). The sicker the patient and the longer the need for high concentrations of oxygen, the greater the likelihood of toxicity. Another problem with 100% oxygen is resorption atelectasis, which occurs when all of the nitrogen is washed out of lung units with low $\dot{V}/\dot{Q}$'s, which then leads to collapse of such lung units.

The extracorporeal membrane oxygenator occasionally has been responsible for temporarily sustaining life in patients with severe HPPE who could not be oxygenated at acceptable FI_{O_2}'s by any other means. This technique may provide an acceptable level of oxygenation and allow the concentration of inspired oxygen to be reduced. Unfortunately, this requires a team approach, has many technical problems, is very expensive, has not been shown to reduce mortality and therefore should be considered, at this time, investigational.[66]

VENTILATOR CARE

The major indication for the use of a ventilator in HPPE is a failure to oxygenate the patient at an acceptable FI_{O_2}. Alveolar hypoventilation is an infrequent reason. Currently only volume ventilation can be recommended. An endotracheal tube is placed either orally or nasally. The nasal route is preferred because of better tube stability and greater patient comfort, including easier swallowing and allowing the mouth to be closed. Although an endotracheal tube may be left in place for at least 7 to 10 days[32] (and some believe much longer) before tracheostomy needs to be done, tracheostomy should be considered at the outset if the clinical status of the patient suggests a need for prolonged assisted ventilation.

Continuous positive pressure ventilation (CPPV) is a means of providing a supraambient pressure to the airway throughout the respiratory cycle. It may be administered as continuous positive airway pressure (CPAP), which is the nonventilator mode, or by positive end-expiratory pressure (PEEP), the ventilator mode.

After intubation one of several approaches may be taken. In patients with milder forms of HPPE, 5- to 15-cm CPAP may be used. Alternatively, the patient can be placed on the ventilator with tidal volumes of 12 to 15 cc/kg (twice normal), with PEEP added only if adequate oxygenation has not been obtained. In more severely ill patients, high tidal volumes with PEEP will be required at the outset. Ventilation with large tidal volumes has been shown to prevent further atelectasis and to retard progressive hypoxemia.[20,59,62] In early studies with patients on normal tidal volumes (6–8 cc/kg), atelectasis developed unless periodic hyperinflations (sighs) were given.[39] Not only is there no evidence that patients on large tidal volumes have no therapeutic benefit from adding sighs, but such sighing of patients on large tidal volumes increases the risk of pneumothorax and pneumomediastinum.

When a patient is placed on the ventilator, a decision must be made as to the mode of ventilation. The control mode is used in patients who cannot supply any of their ventilatory needs, such as those who are paralyzed, heavily sedated, or deeply comatose. A more alert patient may be placed on assist-control, which allows him to breathe at his own rate but delivers a predetermined volume with each breath. Intermittent mandatory ventilation (IMV) is a form of controlled breathing that allows breathing at the patient's own rate and volume, with a preset number of breaths/minute at a given volume interspersed by the respirator. IMV is the preferred method and offers the following advantages: [1] It allows the patient to do some of the work of breathing; [2] because of the lower mean pleural pressure (versus assist-control or control), higher levels of PEEP can be used; [3] it decreases the likelihood of asynchronous ventilation; [4] the Pa_{CO_2} can be more easily controlled; and [5] weaning can take place gradually.

If frequent ventilator breaths at high tidal volumes do not achieve acceptable oxygenation, then increasing amounts of PEEP are added. At this point it

Nasal prongs (Max $F_{IO_2} \leq 0.35$)
↓
Face masks ≤ (Max FI_{O_2} 0.5)
↓
Face mask with
one-way valve,
reservoir, and
tight fit (Max FI_{O_2} 0.9–1.0)
↓
Intubate
↓
CPAP (5 cm H_2O–15 cm H_2O)
↓
IMV with VT = 12–15 cc/kg and PEEP
↓
Increasing BUR to point of control—
↑ PEEP as tolerated
↓
Paralyze patient and keep on
VT = 12–15 cc/kg and
adjust rate and PEEP to
maximize oxygenation without
adversely affecting CO

Fig. 36-8. Sequential steps to improve oxygenation in HPPE.

is a matter of adjusting inspiratory flow (starting at 40–50 liters/m), the back-up rate (BUR), FI_{O_2}, tidal volume, and the level of PEEP to achieve the therapeutic endpoint. All this is to be done with close attention to making certain that hemodynamic function is not compromised. The Pa_{CO_2} should be kept between 35 and 45 torr to avoid bronchoconstriction, cardiac arrhythmias, cerebral hypoxia, and hypokalemia. There is no way to predictably foresee the outcome of a change made on the ventilator, and therefore each change must be accompanied by a set of arterial blood gases. Of course, blood gases must also be obtained after any significant change in the patient's clinical condition. The sequential steps in improving oxygenation in patients with HPPE are outlined in Figure 36-8.

Frequently, patients on respirators become uncomfortable and restless. It may be necessary only to attend to some minor need or to suction out the hypopharynx. Sedatives and narcotics can be used if the blood pressure is maintained. Narcotics have the advantage of being quickly reversible with naloxone if blood pressure drops to unacceptable levels. Occasionally, in a difficult or combative patient, paralysis with curare or one of its analogues, such as pancuronium bromide, may be used. Because it does not release histamine as does curare, pancuronium bromide is preferred.[46] When a patient on a respirator suddenly requires more pressure to deliver the same tidal volume, the following should be considered.

1. Worsening of the primary disorder
2. Pneumothorax
3. Atelectasis
4. Increasing airway resistance (e.g., secretions, bronchospasm)
5. Mechanical dysfunction of the respirator or tubing

A useful way of separating which of the above might be responsible is to measure both the static and the dynamic compliance. The static compliance measures the elastic properties of the lungs and is given by the formula

$$C_{static} = \frac{\text{tidal volume}}{P_{plateau} - \text{PEEP}}.$$

The dynamic compliance on the other hand measures both the elastic and the resistive forces in the lungs and is given by the formula

$$C_{dynamic} = \frac{\text{tidal volume}}{P_{peak} - \text{PEEP}}.$$

A decrease in the dynamic compliance without a decrease in the static compliance suggests an increase in airway resistance caused by excessive secretions or bronchospasm, among other causes. However, a decrease in both the dynamic and the static compliances points toward some change in the lungs' elastic properties—for example, pneumothorax, atelectasis, or worsening of the underlying disorder.

If the clinical situation permits, CPAP is preferred over PEEP for the following reasons.[49,52]

1. PEEP increases pleural pressure more than does CPAP, thereby decreasing venous return and ultimately cardiac output
2. CPAP is more effective than PEEP in maintaining oxygen delivery and tissue oxygenation by mechanism 1 above
3. Higher levels of end-expiratory pressure can be used with CPAP than with PEEP

Although the impairment of venous return by PEEP seems certain, a recent report suggests that the decrease in cardiac output may be mediated by a leftward displacement of the interventricular septum, which then restricts left ventricular filling.[24] Clearly, however, whatever the benefits or drawbacks of PEEP, it does not decrease lung water.[5,41]

The terms "optimal PEEP" and "best PEEP" are defined by different groups in different ways. One group defines it on the basis of compliance and delivery of oxygen,[58] another on the reduction of intrapulmonary shunt,[14] and yet another by the amount of PEEP that reduces intrapulmonary shunt to a preselected goal of 15%.[18] Suter and associates have suggested that maximum oxygen delivery takes place at the point of maximum pulmonary compliance.[58] It seems, however, that the wrong question is being addressed; instead of asking "At what point is oxygen transport at a maximum?" the question should be "What evidence is there of tissue hypoxia?" PEEP (or anything else) should be "optimal" when tissue oxygen needs have been met, at an FI_{O_2} equal to or less than 0.5. Certainly a minimum oxygen delivery is required, but no published data show that achieving the maximum oxygen delivery possible has any effect on the clinical course. Patients in Suter's study were on the assist-control mode, and there were no attempts to volume load the patients to increase oxygen delivery. Suter's study has been criticized because of erroneous measurements of compliance in those with very high PEEP or with a very low compliance.[8] Also, several other investigators were unable to confirm his data.[23,60] Kirby, on the other hand, has shown that with the IMV mode and volume loading, very high levels of PEEP ("super PEEP") can be tolerated.[27] Indirect measurements such as compliance should never serve as a substitute for more direct determinants of oxygenation in the critically ill patient.

A pulmonary-artery balloon flotation catheter (e.g. Swan–Ganz) is useful in critically ill patients for monitoring CO, $P\bar{v}_{O_2}$, PAP, and PCWP. Generally PEEP up to 15 mm Hg has a minimal effect on the PCWP.[56] Several situations occur, however, in which PCWP does not reflect left atrial pressure (LAP),[48,51] including [1] misplacement of the catheter; [2] vessels collapsing because the PEEP transmitted to the microvasculature exceeds the LAP ("Starling resistor effect"), resulting in a dissociation between PCWP and the LAP; [3] inadequate intravascular volume; and [4] placement of the catheter with an eccentric balloon at a bifurcation that may not occlude the lumen.

The values for PCWP should be measured while on the respirator.[13] Removal of the patient from the respirator decreases mean pleural pressure and increases venous return, distorting the hemodynamics that existed while the patient was on the respirator. A normal PCWP is about 8 to 12 mm Hg. Fluid loading in an attempt to increase cardiac output, and therefore oxygen delivery, can be done, but generally the PCWP should not be pushed beyond 18 mm Hg.

High oxygen tensions lead to oxygen toxicity, and increased pressures and volumes to the lung produce barotrauma, thereby increasing the risk of pneumothorax or pneumomediastinum. Sophisticated clinical judgment is needed to balance the requirements for tissue oxygenation against possible lung injury with the ventilator and high concentrations of oxygen.

STEROIDS

There are little objective data that deal with the benefits of corticosteroids in HPPE. A number of mechanisms have been suggested as reasons why corticosteroids should be useful in the syndrome, including [1] maintenance of capillary and cell membranous structure; [2] stabilization of lysosomal membranes; [3] modification or prevention of platelet aggregation; [4] enhancement of surfactant production; [5] opposition to the effects of fatty acids on lung tissue; [6] inhibition of leukocyte adherence to pulmonary vascular walls; [7] increased capillary flow; and [8] inhibition of complement-mediated damage.

Prolonged corticosteroid use may predispose to an increased incidence of infection. This has been shown clearly only with regard to tuberculosis. No significant complications seem to result from a short course of corticosteroids (less than 3 days) at any dose.

Although controversy continues, recent work has shown corticosteroids to be beneficial in sepsis.[8] Corticosteroids may also be useful in aspiration pneumonia,[57] fat embolism,[53] and chemical injuries to the airway.[63] In the absence of any significant complications from short-term high-dose corticosteroids, it seems reasonable to use doses as high as 30 mg/kg methylprednisolone sodium succinate or its equivalent every 8 hours for 1 or 2 days in selected critically ill patients.

Despite the zeal with which certain preparations are promoted as the "corticosteroid of choice," most authorities believe that it does not make any difference which product is used as long as it is used in equivalent doses.

ANTIBIOTICS

Because bacterial infection is rarely the cause of HPPE, it is unusual for antibiotics to be indicated in the initial management. Recently described cases of mycoplasma pneumonia[17] and miliary tuberculosis[42] as causes of HPPE would, of course, be exceptions. The use of prophylactic antibiotics is futile and may simply lead to a superinfection with highly resistant organisms (e.g., *Pseudomonas* sp.).

Bacterial infection that complicates HPPE, however, is not rare. Purulent sputum, increasing pulmonary infiltrates, fever, or leukocytosis alone or in combination should alert the clinician to the possibility of bacterial infection in order that appropriate smears and cultures can be made. Without those findings, what may look like infection (e.g., a tracheal aspirate that grows pathogenic bacteria) may represent only colonization.

It is difficult for the clinician to resist "covering" with antibiotics a critically ill patient, especially when he feels that bacterial infection has not been excluded. He should resist such therapy, however, until reasonably certain clinical and laboratory grounds exist for such treatment.

One possible use of prophylactic antimicrobial therapy is in the patient with aspiration and poor dentition. In this case, where infection with anaerobes is likely, it is reasonable to administer 5 to 6 million units of penicillin G per day for the first few days of HPPE.

The use of aerosolized pulmonary antibiotics in the face of bacterial infection seems reasonable. However, no controlled studies in the literature support their use. Limited experience by Klastersky suggests that certain pulmonary infections may be prevented[29] and also treated more effectively by aminoglycoside tracheal lavage.[28,30] Generally the systemic route should be used for established bacterial infections. Combining tracheal lavage with full systemic doses of aminoglycosides can produce dangerously high serum levels.[33]

VASOACTIVE AGENTS

If a vasoactive drug is required, then an agent with primary beta activity should be used. When oxygen delivery is insufficient despite ventilator support and maximum volume loading, then low-dose dopamine can be used to augment cardiac output and renal blood flow, thereby increasing oxygen delivery.

OTHER PHARMACOLOGIC APPROACHES

When the PCWP is elevated, digitalis and diuretics may be needed to treat heart failure. At times digitalis will also be needed to manage cardiac rhythm disturbances, although such arrhythmias are frequently related to abnormal blood gas values or electrolyte disturbances.

Just as the role of DIC and microemboli in HPPE is unclear,[4] so, too, is the therapeutic use of heparin. Regardless of theoretical advantages, the major concern with the use of heparin is serious bleeding in tissues that are already injured. Except for preventing tissue damage directly related to ongoing DIC, the use of heparin in HPPE cannot be recommended.

NUTRITION

There are heavy energy costs with respiratory failure. Adequate nutrition must be provided to patients who have lost 10% of their usual body weight or who cannot eat or absorb nutrients.[40] This can be done enterally or systemically with a peripheral vein (partial peripheral) or central vein (total hyperalimentation). The enteral route is, of course, preferred. The usual nasogastric tube does not necessarily protect against aspiration, and therefore a small feeding tube (Dubhoff or Keofeed) should be used.

The basic caloric requirement is given in Table 36-8. In a critically ill patient who may be febrile or septic, this basal figure must be multiplied by 1.5 to 2.0.[40] If total energy needs cannot be met with 5 to 6 mg/kg of dextrose, then the remainder of the calories should be given as fat. Excessive amounts of carbohydrate produce hyperglycemia, fatty infiltration of the liver, and increased production of carbon dioxide. This increased carbon dioxide production may complicate and prolong ventilator weaning. Giving large amounts of carbohydrate does not increase protein

Table 36-8. Harris–Benedict Equations* for Calculating Basal Energy Expenditure (BEE) in Calories

Women

$$BEE = 655 + (9.6 \times W) + (1.8 \times H) - (4.7 \times A)$$

Men

$$BEE = 66 + (13.7 \times W) + (5 \times H) - (6.8 \times A)$$

*W = usual weight in kilograms; H = height in centimeters; A = age in years.

sparing. Amino acid requirements vary between 1.5 and 2.0 g/kg/day depending on the seriousness of the illness and the degree of catabolism present at the start of alimentation.

COMPLICATIONS

Complications occur both as part of HPPE and as a result of therapy (see Table 36-9). Although these complications are indeed very real, their classification is somewhat artificial. Examples of such complications are listed below.

1. Atelectasis may be either part of the syndrome or due to faulty placement of an endotracheal tube (*see* Fig. 36-4A).
2. Disturbances of heart rhythm may be due to hypoxia, electrolyte disturbances, or excessive use of digitalis.
3. Sepsis may be unavoidable or due to poor technique or contaminated equipment.

Regardless of how one might choose to classify them, the point to remember is that continuing close observation is needed by the clinician to maximize the patient's chances of recovery without intercurrent complications.

The use and the misuse of ventilators deserve special comment. Mechanical failure of the respirator, such as alarms not working (or having been turned off during suctioning and not having been turned on again afterward), invites disaster. Respirators such as the Bear I have buttons that can be potentially dangerous—for instance, "alarm silence" and "stand by." Gram-negative pneumonias with organisms such as *Pseudomonas* and *Serratia* are seen less frequently now that more standardized methods of equipment maintenance have been established.

The patient who has a very low compliance and who is receiving high-volume ventilation with PEEP at rapid respiratory rates is at an increased risk of developing a rapidly fatal pneumothorax. In these high-risk patients, physicians knowledgeable in chest tube insertion must be immediately available.

Table 36-9. Complications of HPPE

Medical complications
Aspiration
Disseminated intravascular coagulation
Sepsis
Fat embolism
Heart failure
Malnutrition
Cardiac conduction disturbances
Pulmonary fibrosis
Stress ulcers (gastric)
Gastrointestinal hemorrhage
Atelectasis
Complications resulting from therapy
Fluid overload
Volume depletion and shock
Anaphylaxis
Overmedication
Acidosis or alkalosis
Gastric distention
Complications from an endotracheal tube or tracheostomy (*e.g.*, laryngeal stridor, tracheal stenosis, tracheomalacia)
Airway obstruction secondary to untreated secretions, bronchospasm, and so forth
Complications resulting from ventilator use
Hypoxemia and hypoxia
Hypocarbia and hypercarbia
Oxygen toxicity
Barotrauma
Resorption atelectasis (100% oxygen)
Technical: *e.g.*, alarm silence, standby, etc.
Bacterial pneumonia
Pneumothorax
Pneumomediastinum
Subcutaneous emphysema
Reduced cardiac output

PROGNOSIS

The survival of the patient and his residual pulmonary function depends on the etiology and severity of the illness, the sophistication of the medical, respiratory therapy, and nursing staffs, complications arising during the course of the illness, and the patient's previous pulmonary and medical health. Patients treated with modern modalities of therapy in sophisticated institutions should have a survival rate in excess of 50%. One large study reported 80% survival.[12]

In seriously ill patients with HPPE who are not improving or who are deteriorating, consideration must be given to transferring such patients to institutions that have the technical sophistication to manage such critically ill patients.

Some degree of prognostic value has been attached to the magnitude of the shunt fraction seen during the illness. This is reasonable since it gives an expression of both cardiac output and amount of collapsed alveolar tissue. Shunts of more than 30% are usually associated with some degree of pulmonary insufficiency, and, although shunts of 50% have been seen in HPPE survivors, those who exceed 60% die.

Pulmonary mechanics have reportedly returned to normal in 4 to 6 months, but abnormalities of gas exchange (e.g., DL_{CO} and exercise $(A\text{-}a)D_{O_2}$) may persist.[15]

REFERENCES

1. Bachofen M, Weibel ER: Alterations of the gas exchange apparatus in adult respiratory insufficiency associated with septicemia. Am Rev Resp Dis, 116:589, 1977
2. Bergofsky EH: Pulmonary insufficiency—shock lung. Am J Med Sci 264:93, 1972
3. Bland R, Shoemaker WC, Shabot MM: Physiologic monitoring goals for the critically ill patient. Surg Gynecol Obstet 147:833, 1978
4. Bone RC, Francis PB, Pierce AK: Intravascular coagulation associated with the adult respiratory distress syndrome. Am J Med 61:585, 1976
5. Bredenberg CE, Webb WR: Experimental pulmonary edema—the effect of unilateral PEEP on the accumulation of lung water. Ann Surg 189:433, 1979
6. Brigham KL, Owen PJ: Increased sheep lung vascular permeability caused by histamine. Circ Res 37:647, 1975
7. Cain SM: Oxygen delivery and uptake in dogs during anemic and hypoxic hypoxia. J Appl Physiol 42:228, 1977
8. Connors AF, McCaffree DR, Rogers RM: The adult respiratory distress syndrome. DM (Disease-a-Month) 27(4), 1981
9. Czer LS, Appel P, Shoemaker WC: Pathogenesis of respiratory failure (ARDS) after hemorrhage and trauma. Crit Care Med 8:513, 1980
10. Danek SJ et al: The dependence of oxygen uptake on oxygen delivery in the adult respiratory distress syndrome. Am Rev Respir Dis 122:387, 1980
11. Daniel A et al: The relationships among arterial oxygen flow rate, oxygen binding by hemoglobin and oxygen utilization in chronic cardiac decompensation. J Lab Clin Med 91:635, 1978
12. Douglas ME, Downs JB: Pulmonary function following severe acute respiratory failure and high levels of positive end-expiratory pressure. Chest 71:18, 1977
13. Downs JB, Douglas ME: Assessment of cardiac filling pressure during continuous positive-pressure ventilation. Crit Care Med 8:285, 1980
14. Downs JB, Klein EF, Modell JH: The effect of incremental PEEP on PaO_2 in patients with respiratory failure. Anesth Analg 52:210, 1973
15. Elliott CG, Morris AH, Cengiz M: Pulmonary function and exercise gas exchange in survivors of adult respiratory distress syndrome. Am Rev Respir Dis 123:492, 1981
16. Fein A et al: The value of edema fluid protein measurement in patients with pulmonary edema. Am J Med 67:32, 1979
17. Fischman RA et al: Adult respiratory distress syndrome caused by mycoplasma pneumoniae. Chest 74:471, 1978
18. Gallagher TJ, Civetta JM, Kirby RR: Terminology update: Optimal PEEP. Crit Care Med 6:323, 1978
19. Glauser FL, Millen JE, and Falls R: Effects of acid aspiration on pulmonary alveolar epithelial membrane permeability. Chest 76:201, 1979
20. Hedley–Whyte J, Pontoppidan H, Morris MJ: The relation of alveolar to tidal ventilation during respiratory failure in man. Anesthesiology 27:218, 1966
21. Hiller C, Bone R, Wilson F: Comparison of tissue and mixed venous oxygen tension in endotoxin shock. Am Rev Respir Dis 119:127, 1979
22. Hopewell PC: Adult respiratory distress syndrome. Basics of RD 7:No. 4, 1979
23. Hudson L et al: Does compliance reflect optimal oxygen transfer with positive end-expiratory pressure (PEEP)? (abstr). 43rd Annual Scientific Assembly, American College of Chest Physicians, 1977
24. Jardin F et al: Influence of positive end-expiratory pressure on left ventricular performance. N Engl J Med 304:387, 1981
25. Jobsis F, LaManna J: Kinetic aspects of intracellular redox reactions. In Robin E (ed): Extrapulmonary Manifestations of Respiratory Disease. New York, Marcel Dekker, 1978
26. Katzenstein AA, Bloor CM, Leibow AA: Diffuse alveolar damage—the role of oxygen, shock, and related factors. Am J Pathol 85:210, 1976
27. Kirby RR et al: High level positive end-expiratory pressure (PEEP) in acute respiratory insufficiency. Chest 67:156, 1975
28. Klastersky J et al: Endotracheal gentamicin in bronchial infections in patients with tracheostomy. Chest 61:117, 1972
29. Klastersky J et al: Endotracheally administered gentamicin for the prevention of infections of the respiratory tract in patients with tracheostomy: A double blind study. Chest 65:650, 1974
30. Klastersky J et al: Endotracheally administered antibiotics for gram-negative bronchopneumonia. Chest 75:586, 1979
31. Lake KB, Rumsfeld JA: Adult respiratory distress syndrome ("shock lung"). In Burton GG, Gee GN, Hodgkin JE (eds): Respiratory Care, A Guide to Clinical Practice. Philadelphia, JB Lippincott, 1977
32. Lake KB, Van Dyke JJ: Prolonged nasotracheal intubation. Heart Lung 9:93, 1980
33. Lake KB, Van Dyke JJ, Rumsfeld JA: Combined topical pulmonary and systemic gentamicin: The question of safety. Chest 68:62, 1975
34. Lee CT et al: Elastolytic activity in pulmonary lavage fluid from patients with adult respiratory-distress syndrome. N Engl J Med 304:192, 1981
35. Lefer AM: Role of a myocardial depressant factor in shock states. Mod Concepts Cardiovasc Dis 42:59, 1973
36. Luterman A, Manwaring D, Curreri PW: The role of fibrinogen degradation products in the pathogenesis of the respiratory distress syndrome. Surgery 82:703, 1977
37. Manny J, Justice R, Hechtman HB: Abnormalities in organ blood flow and its distribution during positive end-expiratory pressure. Surgery 85:425, 1979
38. Martin AM, Soloway HB, Simmons RL: Pathologic anatomy of the lungs following shock and trauma. J Trauma 8:687, 1968
39. Mead J, Collier C: Relation of volume history of lungs to respiratory mechanics in anesthetized dogs. J Appl Physiol 14:669, 1959
40. Michel L, Serrano A, Malt RA: Nutritional support of hospitalized patients. N Engl J Med 304:1147, 1981
41. Miller WC et al: Effect of PEEP on lung water content in experimental noncardiogenic pulmonary edema. Crit Care Med 9:7, 1981
42. Murray HW et al: The adult respiratory distress syndrome associated with miliary tuberculosis. Chest 73:37, 1978
43. Murray JF: Mechanisms of acute respiratory failure. Am Rev Respir Dis 115:1071, 1977
44. Pontoppidan H, Geffin B, Lowenstein E: Acute respiratory failure in the adult. N Engl J Med 287:690, 1972
45. Robin ED: Permeability pulmonary edema. In Fishman AP, Renkin EM (eds): Pulmonary Edema. Bethesda, American Physiologic Society, 1979

46. Roizen MF, Feeley TW: Pancuronium bromide. Ann Intern Med 88:64, 1978
47. Roswit B, White DC: Severe radiation injuries of the lung. Am J Roentgenol 129:127, 1977
48. Roy R et al: Pulmonary wedge catheterization during positive end-expiratory pressure ventilation in the dog. Anesthesiology 46:385, 1977
49. Shah DM et al: Continuous positive airway pressure versus positive end-expiratory pressure in respiratory distress syndrome. J Thorac Cardiovasc Surg 74:557, 1977
50. Sibbald W, Peters S, Lindsay RM: Serotonin and pulmonary hypertension in human septic ARDS. Crit Care Med 8:490, 1980
51. Shin B, Ayella RJ, McAslan TC: Pitfalls of Swan-Ganz catheterization. Crit Care Med 5:125, 1977
52. Simmons DH et al: Adult respiratory distress syndrome—Interdepartmental Clinical Case Conference, University of California, Los Angeles (specialty conference). West J Med 130:218, 1979
53. Solliday NH, Shapiro BA, Gracey DR: Adult respiratory distress syndrome. Clinical conference in pulmonary disease for Northwestern University—McGaw Medical Center, Chicago. Chest 69:207, 1976
54. Staub NC: "State of the art" review. Pathogenesis of pulmonary edema. Am Rev Respir Dis 109:358, 1974
55. Staub NC, Hogg JC: Conference report of a workshop on the measurement of lung water. Crit Care Med 8:752, 1980
56. Stevens PM: Positive end-expiratory pressure breathing. Basics of RD 5:No. 3, 1977
57. Sukumaran M et al: Evaluation of corticosteroid treatment in aspiration of gastric contents: A controlled clinical trial. Mount Sinai J Med 47:335, 1980
58. Suter PM, Fairley HB, Isenberg MD: Optimum end-expiratory airway pressure in patients with acute pulmonary failure. N Engl J Med 292:284, 1975
59. Sykes MK, Young WE, Robinson BE: Oxygenation during anaesthesia with controlled ventilation. Br J Anaesth 37:314, 1965
60. Tenaillon A et al: Optimal positive end-expiratory pressure and static lung compliance. N Engl J Med 299:774, 1978
61. Vaage J: Intravascular platelet aggregation and acute respiratory insufficiency. Circ Shock 4:279, 1977
62. Visick WD, Fairley HB, Hickey RF: The effects of tidal volume and end-expiratory pressure on pulmonary gas exchange during anesthesia. Anesthesiology 39:285, 1973
63. Welch GW et al: The use of steroids in inhalational injury. Surg Gynecol Obstet 145:539, 1977
64. Woodson RD, Wills RE, Lenfant C: Effect of acute and established anemia on O_2 transport at rest, submaximal and maximal work. J Appl Physiol 44:36, 1978
65. Wray NP, Nicotra MB: Pathogenesis of neurogenic pulmonary edema. Am Rev Resp Dis 118:783, 1978
66. Zapol WM et al: Extracorporeal membrane oxygenation in severe acute respiratory failure. JAMA 242:2193, 1979

BIBLIOGRAPHY

General

Connors AF, McCaffree DR, Rogers RM: The adult respiratory distress syndrome. DM (Disease-a-Month) 27(4), 1981

Simmons DH et al: Adult respiratory distress syndrome—Interdepartmental Clinical Case Conference, University of California, Los Angeles, (specialty conference). West J Med 130:218, 1979

Pathogenesis

Anderson RR et al: Documentation of pulmonary capillary permeability in the adult respiratory distress syndrome accompanying human sepsis. Am Rev Respir Dis 119:869, 1979

Murray JF: Mechanisms of acute respiratory failure. Am Rev Respir Dis 115:1070, 1977

Robin ED: Permeability pulmonary edema. In Fishman AP, Rankin EM (eds): Pulmonary Edema. Bethesda, American Physiology Society, 1979

Staub NC: "State of the art" review. Pathogenesis of pulmonary edema. Am Rev Respir Dis 109:358, 1974

Pathology

Bachofen M, Weibel ER: Alterations of the gas exchange apparatus in adult respiratory insufficiency associated with septicemia. Am Rev Respir Dis 116:589, 1977

Katzenstein AA, Bloor CM, Leibow AA: Diffuse alveolar damage—the role of oxygen, shock and related factors. Am J Pathol 85:210, 1976

Therapy

Oxygen

Bland R, Shoemaker WC, Shabot MM: Physiologic monitoring goals for the critically ill patient. Surg Gynecol Obstet 147:833, 1978

Cain SM: Oxygen delivery and uptake in dogs during anemic and hypoxic hypoxia. J Appl Physiol 42:228, 1977

Danek SJ et al: The dependence of oxygen uptake on oxygen delivery in the adult respiratory distress syndrome. Am Rev Respir Dis 122:387, 1980

Ventilators

Shah DM et al: Continuous positive airway pressure versus positive end-expiratory pressure in respiratory distress syndrome. J Thorac Cardiovasc Surg 74:557, 1977

Stevens PM: Positive end-expiratory pressure breathing. Basics of RD 5(3), 1977

Venus B, Jacobs HK, Lim L: Treatment of the adult respiratory distress syndrome with continuous positive airway pressure. Chest 76:257, 1979

Walkinshaw M, Shoemaker WC: Use of volume loading to obtain preferred levels or PEEP. Crit Care Med 8:81, 1980

Steroids

Sibbald WJ et al: Alveolo-capillary permeability in human septic ARDS. Effect of high dose corticosteroid therapy. Chest 79:133, 1981

Nutrition

Michel L, Serrano A, Malt RA: Nutritional support of hospitalized patients. N Engl J Med 304:1147, 1981

Prognosis

Rotman HH et al: Long-term physiologic consequences of the adult respiratory distress syndrome. Chest 72:190, 1977

Yahav J, Lieberman P, Molho M: Pulmonary function following the adult respiratory distress syndrome. Chest 74:247, 1978

37

Respiratory Care of the Surgical Patient

Robert H. Bartlett

Respiratory complications are the single largest cause of morbidity and mortality in surgical patients. Much of the surgeon's time is spent preventing or treating such conditions. Respiratory complications may occur in any patient subjected to anesthesia and operation, but the patient who needs an operation on the chest or the lung itself is at particularly high risk. In this chapter I shall review the definitions of postoperative pulmonary complications, the pathophysiology of pulmonary insufficiency as seen in surgical patients, and the current guidelines for prevention and treatment.

As a corollary, a segment of this chapter is entitled Surgical Care of the Respiratory Patient. This serves to introduce common surgical procedures such as bronchoscopy, tracheostomy, and thoracotomy. Conditions of the chest wall, pleural space, lung parenchyma, and airways that commonly require operative management are also discussed. More detailed information on any of these topics can be found in a recent monograph.[3]

Major changes in pulmonary function occur after anesthesia and major operative procedures. These changes occur in all patients and progress to clinically obvious pulmonary insufficiency in a small percentage. If patients with preexisting chronic or acute lung disease must undergo operation, the effects of the operation will be appreciated earlier and more readily because the patient has less pulmonary reserve.

Abnormal lung function owing to the basic disease (e.g., pancreatitis, massive transfusion, fat embolism from fracture) or postoperatively owing to the normal response to operation may be present in varying degrees and goes under many names. The clinical picture may range from minor atelectasis, hypoventilation, or positional ventilation–perfusion abnormalities to the syndromes of adult respiratory distress, or so-called wet lung.

The terms atelectasis and ARDS are merely part of a continuum of physiological changes. It is not helpful to isolate segments of this continuum with specific names. In the following discussion, I shall focus on the alterations in pulmonary structure and function that accompany anesthesia and major operations, and then discuss how these changes might add to, or be affected by, other factors that affect lung function.

POSTOPERATIVE CHANGES IN LUNG FUNCTION

USUAL AND CUSTOMARY POSTOPERATIVE CHANGES

After any major operation, changes occur in function as a result of alveolar atelectasis. These changes occur in all patients but are generally not routinely detected.[19] Aside from shallow tidal ventilation and some decreased breath sounds at the lung bases, the patient shows no signs of respiratory abnormality. On direct measurement lung volumes are decreased (particularly residual volume, expiratory reserve volume, functional residual capacity, and vital capacity). Compliance is decreased because of the decrease in FRC. The work of breathing is increased for the same reason (*i.e.*, more pressure is required to inhale a given volume into the decreased lung air space). Further evidence that alveoli are not being ventilated is absolute or relative arterial hypoxemia, which occurs with the patient breathing room air or 100% oxygen, indicating that nonventilated alveoli are being perfused (transpulmonary shunting).

These changes in lung function are present immediately after operation, then progress slowly over 1 to 2 days, and return to normal in most patients. The extent and duration of abnormality are related to the site of operation, the duration of operation and anesthesia, quality of postoperative care, and preexisting pulmonary status. These changes in pulmonary function for a typical laparotomy patient are shown in Figure 37-1.

The extent and the duration of these abnormalities are greatest for operations on the thorax and upper abdomen and progressively decrease as the site of operation moves more distally and more superficially on the body structures. These changes may occur after only 1 to 2 hours of general anesthesia if careful attention is not paid to maximal lung inflation during anesthesia.[12] They are superimposed on the patient's preexisting lung status. If, for example, the patient requires operation for pancreatitis 2 weeks after the onset of disease, he may already have pleural effusions, increased pulmonary capillary permeability, and existing transpulmonary shunting and will not tolerate any further deterioration of lung function. Likewise, the patient with preexisting chronic obstructive lung disease with high airway resistance, maximal work of breathing, and minimal functional lung tissue preoperatively may proceed to carbon dioxide retention if the work of breathing is only slightly increased after an operation.

Several factors contribute to these changes in pulmonary function, but shallow breathing with incomplete alveolar inflation is the common denominator.

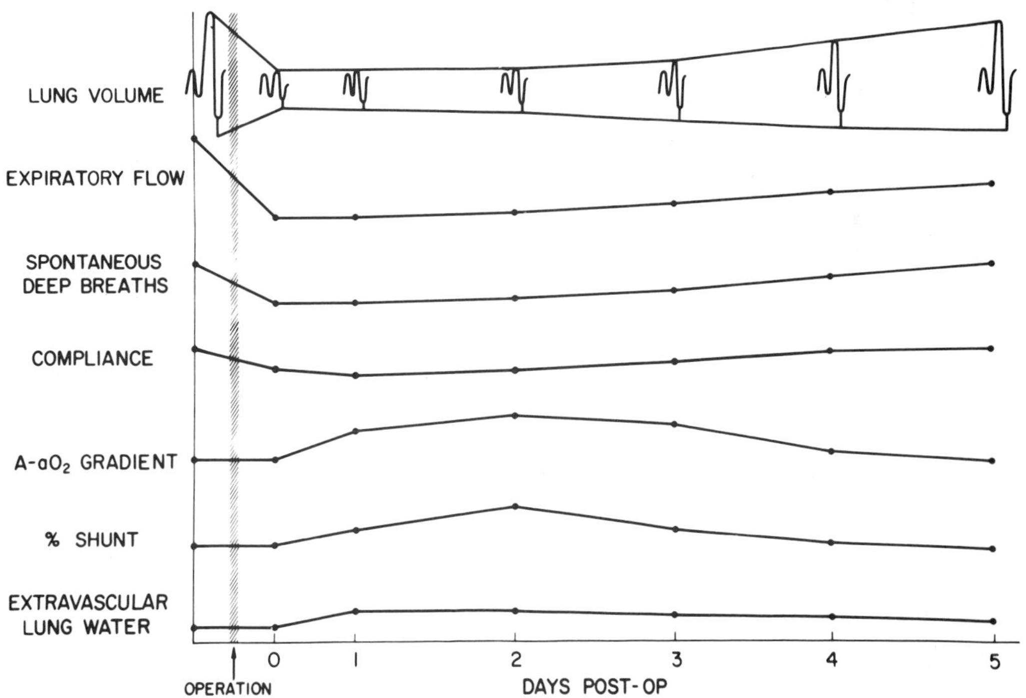

Fig. 37-1. Usual and expected changes in pulmonary function after an abdominal operation. Note the transient nature of the abnormalities, all of which have returned to normal by the fifth postoperative day (*see* text). (Bartlett RH: Post-traumatic pulmonary insufficiency. In Cooper P, Nyhus L (eds): Surgery Annual. New York, Appleton–Century–Crofts, 1971)

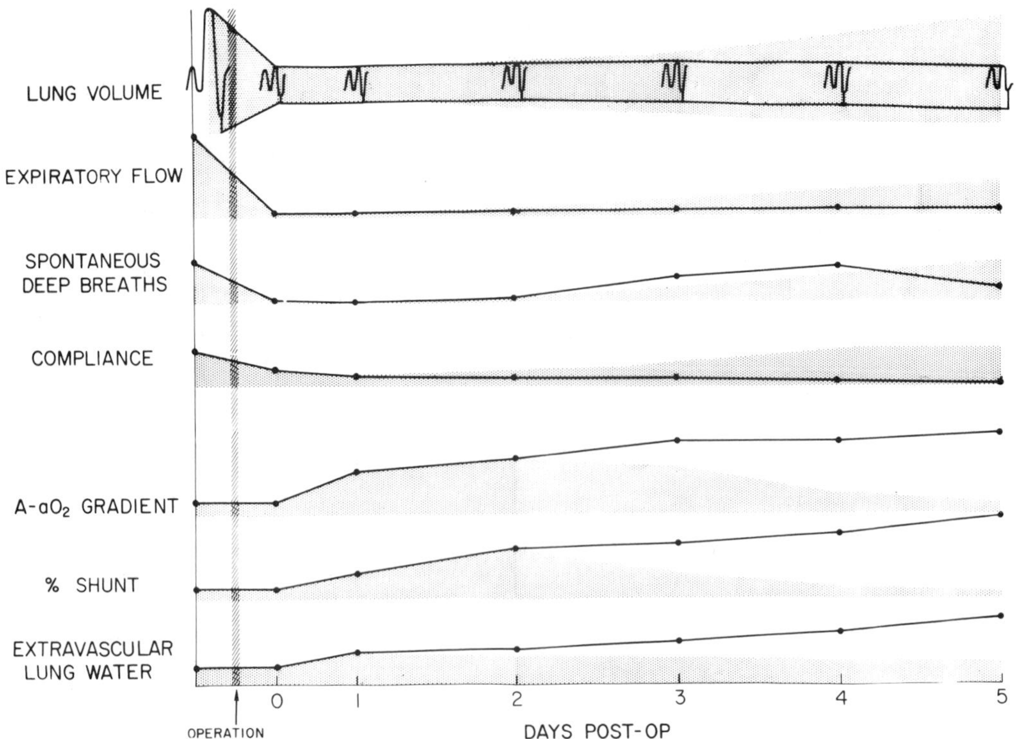

Fig. 37-2. Progression from the normal response (*see* Fig. 37-1) to pulmonary failure after an abdominal operation. The shaded areas outline the expected *normal* postoperative course. (Bartlett RH: Post-traumatic pulmonary insufficiency. In Cooper P, Nyhus L (eds): Surgery Annual. New York, Appleton–Century–Crofts, 1971)

If spontaneous deep breaths to maximal lung inflation are eliminated from the pattern of breathing, alveolar collapse begins within 1 hour and progresses rather rapidly to produce significant transpulmonary shunting. Several studies have shown that patients postoperatively lack the normal pattern of spontaneous deep breaths[20,34] because of severe pain, anesthetics, or narcotic drugs. Further evidence supporting this observation is the fact that the postoperative changes in lung function can be returned toward normal by instituting maximal inflation, deep breathing exercises at regular intervals.[6] Excessive tracheobronchial secretions, aspiration of oral or gastric contents, and intraoperative fluid overload or blood transfusion may be additional contributing factors to the postoperative changes described above.

POSTOPERATIVE PULMONARY COMPLICATIONS

If the pattern of decreased lung volume and shunting progresses rather than returns to normal, it becomes clinically evident within 2 to 4 days after operation. Decreased lung volume is detectable as decreased breath sounds on physical examination, and atelectatic areas may be visible on chest x-ray film. Shunt-produced hypoxemia leads to an increased ventilatory rate and the sensation of dyspnea.

Severe hypoxemia may cause cyanosis. Atelectasis causes fever and pooling of mucus secretions in nonventilated areas, leading to an apparent increase in sputum production. This sequence of events is diagrammed in Figure 37-2, where physiological changes that become clinically obvious as pulmonary "complications" are compared to the normal pattern of lung changes and recovery after operation. Against this background of changes that normally accompany major operations, a more complete picture of pulmonary pathophysiology in the surgical patient can be drawn.

PATHOGENESIS AND PATHOPHYSIOLOGY

Abnormal patterns of breathing postoperatively are a major factor in the development of postoperative re-

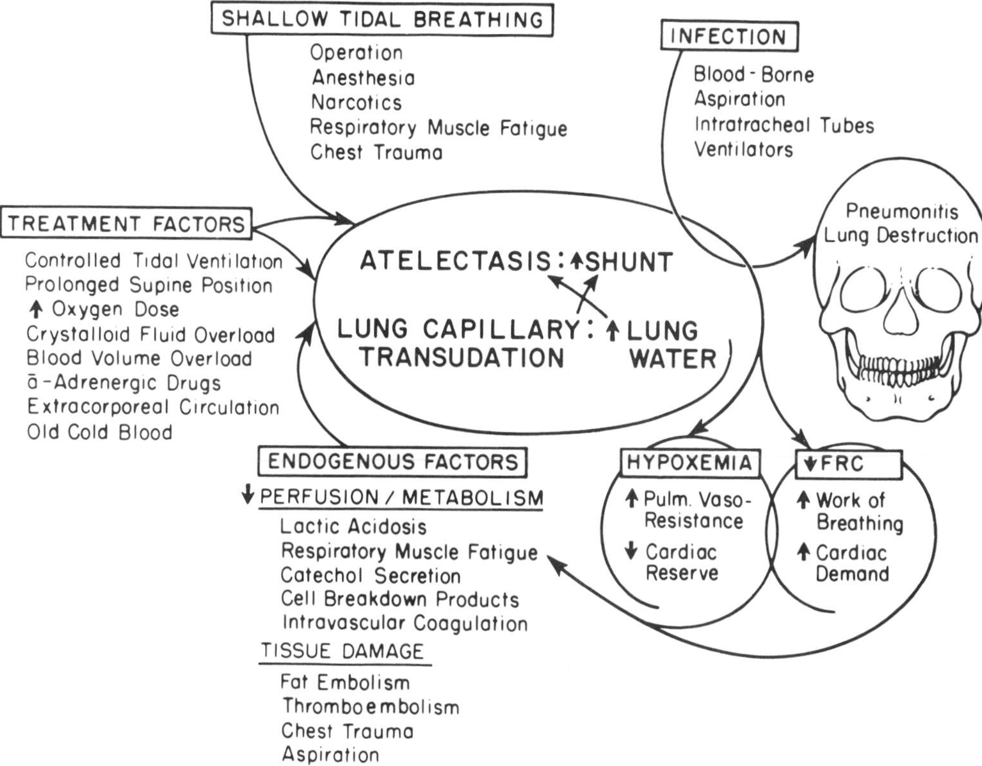

Fig. 37-3. Interaction of factors involved in the development of post-traumatic pulmonary insufficiency. (From Bartlett RH: Post-traumatic pulmonary insufficiency. In Cooper P, Nyhus L (eds): Surgery Annual. New York, Appleton–Century–Crofts, 1971)

spiratory complications. In any specific patient, however, other factors that actually cause lung damage may be more important causes of pulmonary insufficiency (*see* Fig. 37-3). These factors can be divided into [1] ventilatory or airway mechanisms; [2] humoral or hydrostatic mechanisms acting at the *capillary* level; and [3] direct lung trauma. Bacterial infection or progressive fibrosis are the final common pathways of severe pulmonary insufficiency resulting from any of these mechanisms.

VENTILATORY FACTORS

Abnormal ventilation (Table 37-1) will cause altered pulmonary function as outlined above. The abnormal pattern of tidal breathing without spontaneous deep breaths after operation is a good example of this phenomenon. A patient lying on his back in bed will preferentially ventilate the superior lobes while the blood flow will preferentially go to dependent lobes. This ventilation–perfusion imbalance itself will result in hypoxemia. If it progresses over time, lower lobe alveoli begin to collapse in the pathogenetic pathway,

Table 37-1. Ventilatory Factors Resulting in Pulmonary Insufficiency

CAUSES

- Shallow/incomplete inflation
  - Spontaneous breathing
  - Mechanical ventilation
  - Obstructed airways
- Absorptive atelectasis
  - ↑ FI_{O_2}
- Alveolar damage (↓ surfactant)
  - Infection
  - Drowning
  - Circulating lipase
- ↑ Lung water

EFFECTS

- Transpulmonary shunting
- Hypoxemia
- Hyperventilation
- ↓ Compliance
- ↑ Work of breathing
- ↑ Risk of infection
- ↑ Lung water (?)

as outlined above. Alveolar collapse will occur in any patient who remains in one position for a prolonged period and in whom the pattern of breathing is that of shallow tidal ventilation. It should be emphasized that 600-cc breaths delivered with a mechanical ventilator will lead to alveolar collapse, in the same fashion as shallow spontaneous breathing, if regular maximal inflations are not carried out.

Foreign materials inhaled by means of the airway may contribute to pulmonary insufficiency in surgical patients. Aspiration of blood, gastric juice, or other gastric contents damages the respiratory mucosa and may reach the alveolar level, causing direct damage to alveoli and capillaries. Vomiting with aspiration is a constant concern in patients who have suffered acute trauma, head injury patients, patients requiring gastric feedings, and patients undergoing general anesthesia.

When vomiting occurs and aspiration is even suspected, vigorous treatment measures should be undertaken immediately. (This will be discussed in a later section.) Tissue may also be damaged by inhalation of toxic vapors; in surgical patients this is most commonly smoke inhalation, often associated with surface burn injury. The pathogenesis of pulmonary lesions from smoke inhalation with or without burn is also discussed below.

CAPILLARY FACTORS

The second category of conditions that may lead to lung damage is that which occurs at the capillary level (Table 37-2). Increased pulmonary hydrostatic pressure, decreased plasma oncotic pressure, or increased capillary permeability may all occur in the surgical patient. All will cause increased pulmonary extravascular water and deterioration of lung function.

Hydrostatic and Humoral Factors

In Figure 37-4, the factors regulating fluid flux in the lung are shown, although the actual mechanisms are not as simple as illustrated.[28] For example, interstitial pressure itself, the oncotic effects of interstitial protein, and the effects of lymph flow are not illustrated. However, fluid flux is a net function of the hydrostatic pressure that tends to force fluid out of the vascular space, on the one hand, and the oncotic pressure that tends to pull fluid in, on the other hand.

High hydrostatic pressure or low oncotic pressure will result in accumulation of fluid in the extravascular space. If the pulmonary endothelium is damaged, fluid may leak into the extracellular space at normal hydrostatic or oncotic pressures. The mechanisms and the effects of increased extravascular water are shown in Table 37-2. Pulmonary vascular resistance increases owing to periarteriolar cuffing. Ventilation–perfusion imbalance is created by peribronchiolar and alveolar compression. Shunting occurs if the alveoli become completely collapsed or filled with fluid. Finally, boggy atelectatic areas of lung are ideal breeding grounds for bacterial pulmonary infection.

Table 37-2. Capillary Factors Resulting in Increased Lung Water and Pulmonary Insufficiency

CAUSES
↑ Capillary filtration pressure
↑ Hydrostatic pressure
LV failure
↑ Pulmonary vascular resistance
↑ Pulmonary artery pressure (?)
↓ Oncotic pressure
Hypoproteinemia
Crystalloid overload
Pulmonary capillary damage
Airway
Bloodborne
Direct trauma
Atelectasis (?)
EFFECTS
↑ Pulmonary vascular resistance
↑ Small airway resistance
↓ FRC, compliance
↑ Risk of infection
V/Q imbalance, hypoxemia

Well-intentioned therapy done in the normal course of treatment or resuscitation may cause increased lung water. Examples are replacement of blood or plasma loss with *crystalloid solution* that must equilibrate into the entire extracellular space, including that in the lung. Exogenous inappropriate fluid replacement or overload of this type along with endogenous production of the water of metabolism during hypermetabolic states combines to make increased total body extracellular fluid the major cause of pulmonary extravascular water collection. This fact is compounded by the decreased oncotic pressure that results when protein is lost or replaced with noncolloid-containing fluids. When plasma proteins are diluted in this way, lung interstitial proteins are diluted also; thus the oncotic gradients stay unchanged, whereas the entire extracellular space expands.[15]

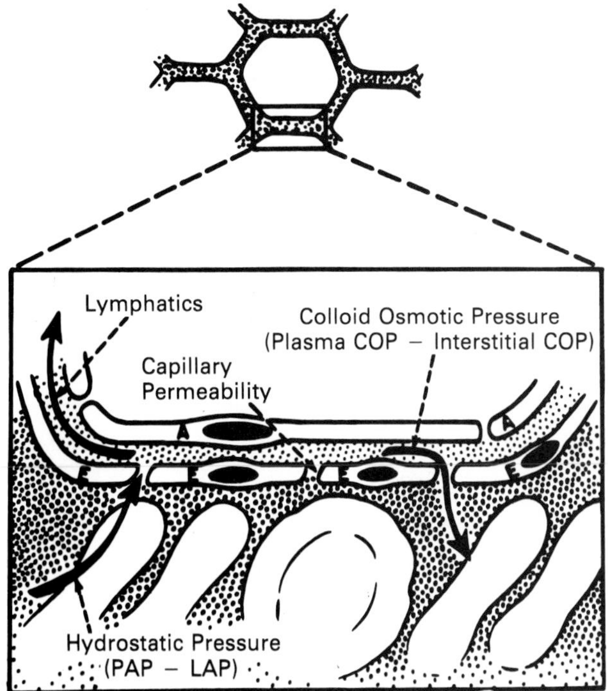

Fig. 37-4. Forces that control fluid flux at the alveolar–capillary membrane. COP = colloid osmotic pressure; LAP = left atrial pressure; PAP = pulmonary artery pressure. A = alveolar epithelium; E = capillary endothelium.

The pulmonary capillary endothelium is the first major vascular bed to "see" any toxic substance arising from peripheral organ metabolism or perfusion of ischemic or infected tissue. The venous effluent from an underperfused tissue (whether localized to a single organ, as in arterial embolism, or the entire body, as in any type of shock) arrives directly at the lung where pulmonary capillary damage occurs. *Humoral substances* such as lysosomal enzymes and bacterial endotoxin or particulate materials such as microemboli, major thromboemboli, platelet aggregates, and fat particles may lodge in the pulmonary capillary bed.

As these materials are cleared, leaky pulmonary capillaries are left behind, resulting in the accumulation of extravascular water. If the material trapped in pulmonary capillaries includes large amounts of platelets, secondary effects caused by platelet breakdown products, notably serotonin, are also seen. In major thromboembolism, for example, hypoxemia occurs because of ventilation–perfusion imbalance owing to bronchial spasm, presumably secondary to serotonin released from platelets.

The pulmonary effects of materials released into the venous blood in shock entrain a particularly vicious circle. Increased pulmonary vascular resistance and hypoxia resulting from the capillary damage lead to decreased cardiac output and peripheral oxygen delivery, adding to the shock state and perpetuating the pulmonary lesion.

Left ventricular failure with increased left atrial pressure will result in pulmonary transcapillary transudation, which may be subtle or grossly obvious, as in conventional heart failure with overt pulmonary edema. Left ventricular pressures may waiver at the point of high left atrial pressure for short periods of time, even minutes, resulting in a transient increase in lung water, and then return to a balanced state. This situation may not lead to severe pulmonary edema in itself but probably places the lung in a more vulnerable position in the presence of coexisting minor capillary damage.

PREVENTION OF PULMONARY COMPLICATIONS

PREOPERATIVE MEASURES

With an understanding of the pathogenesis and mechanisms of potential lung damage in surgical patients as outlined above, one can draw up guidelines to prevent pulmonary complications (Tables 37-3, 37-4).

If a patient is scheduled for an elective operative procedure, as much time as is necessary should be spent measuring lung function, correcting abnormalities where present, and changing conditions that may predispose to pulmonary complications. This is particularly true in patients with preexisting cardiopulmonary disease. Preoperative patients are advised to train for a major operation as one would train for an

Table 37-3. Treatment Modalities Used to Prevent Alveolar Collapse

- Maximum inflation
  - Yawn maneuver
  - Continuous positive pressure breathing (CPPB)
  - Incentive spirometry
  - Mechanical ventilator (IPPV)
    - Large tidal volume
    - "Sigh" and IMV
    - Positive end-expiratory pressure (PEEP)
- Airway cleaning
  - Chest physiotherapy
- ↓ FI_{O_2}
- ↓ Lung water

Table 37-4. Treatment Modalities Used to Prevent Accumulation of Lung Water

Capillary filtration pressure
- Avoid left ventricular failure
- Maintain oncotic pressure

Pulmonary capillary damage
- Prevent
  - Endotoxemia
  - Shock
  - Ischemia
  - Disseminated intravascular coagulation
- Avoid
  - ↑ Airway pressure (?)
  - ↑ FI_{O_2}

Maintain alveolar inflation

athletic event. The respiratory muscles should be exercised and specific breathing maneuvers learned.

Factors that may decrease the efficiency of ventilation should be corrected, including cessation of smoking, elective weight loss in grossly obese patients, and treatment of existing bacterial infection (chronic bronchitis) with culture-specific antibiotics, where indicated. Patients with a known tendency to bronchospasm should become accustomed to bronchodilator treatment preoperatively, and the effect of bronchodilators on pulmonary mechanics should be directly measured, particularly in patients with known bronchospastic disorders such as asthma.

An excellent test of preoperative lung function is to measure arterial blood gas levels while the patient breathes room air. These are useful as a measure of overall lung function and as a baseline for postoperative comparisons.

If the patient is hypoxemic breathing air, if he has a history of asthma, intermittent bronchospasm, wheezing, or any other significant lung disorder, or if the proposed operation is to be on the lung itself, pulmonary mechanics should be measured (lung volumes and flows). These measurements should be made with and without bronchodilators, if indicated. If the values are abnormally low (less than 80% of predicted), training and exercise in specific breathing maneuvers should be carried out and function testing repeated until the ventilation is normal or has reached a stable plateau. Conversely, if the patient has no history of respiratory problems and has a normal examination of the chest (including x-ray), no further pulmonary function testing is indicated.

Although much has been written about specific flow or volume tests and their correlation with postoperative pulmonary complications, abnormal pulmonary function is rarely a contraindication to operation except where the operation involves resection of lung tissue itself.

The flow and volume tests that correlate best with poor postoperative lung function are vital capacity, timed vital capacity, and maximal breathing capacity.[17] These tests are completely effort-dependent, so that the surgical patient with abdominal or chest pain, poor abdominal muscle function from disease, or general debility from cancer or infection may perform poorly on these tests for reasons completely unrelated to lung function. Routine preoperative flow and volume testing on all patients is costly and unnecessary.

Included in preoperative preparation should be efforts to minimize pulmonary extravascular water leakage intraoperatively and postoperatively. This includes adequate nutrition (and parenteral supplementation, if necessary) to assure a normal total serum protein concentration, and therefore a normal plasma oncotic pressure. Left ventricular function should be assisted pharmacologically if signs of left ventricular failure exist. Prophylactic digitalis should be used in elderly patients, primarily to avoid rapid atrial fibrillation postoperatively rather than for general toning of the left ventricle.

The patient with preexisting lung disease requires special consideration. Preparation related to bronchospasm or chronic bronchitis has been discussed. The patient with acute pulmonary insufficiency, increased lung water, and atelectasis secondary to an acute disorder such as pancreatitis or systemic sepsis will often improve during the operation and postoperative mechanical ventilation.

The patient with severe, chronic obstructive lung disease should be improved as much as possible with bronchodilators, treatment of chronic bronchitis, if present, nutrition, and breathing and coughing training. If the pulmonary disorder is very severe (Pa_{O_2} [air] < 50 torr, or carbon dioxide retention), prolonged postoperative intubation and mechanical ventilation should be anticipated and the patient advised accordingly.

INTRAOPERATIVE MEASURES

Intraoperatively, several things may minimize the risk of postoperative pulmonary complications. The operation may directly *improve* pulmonary function (e.g., by repairing a mitral valve or a large abdominal wall hernia) or may improve factors that, of themselves, are causing pulmonary insufficiency (such as draining of an empyema, removing a foreign body, or resecting dead tissue).

The surgeon plans his operative procedure to simultaneously treat the patient and to avoid factors that may cause postoperative complications of any sort. With regard to the pulmonary system, this includes the following: Abdominal incisions should be planned to minimize postoperative pain and to maintain the strength of the abdominal wall for forced inspiration; and transverse incisions should be used whenever possible, particularly in patients with chronic heavy sputum production who will have to cough excessively after operation.

Gastrostomy should be considered to avoid prolonged nasogastric intubation. Bone fragments should be manipulated as gently as possible to avoid possible marrow embolism. Veins under negative pressure (e.g., in the brain) must be managed carefully to avoid air embolism. Prolonged periods of vascular stasis should be avoided as much as possible and systemic heparinization used whenever vascular occlusion is unavoidable.

When gastrointestinal function is impaired by operation, a few minutes spent in assuring good postoperative nutrition (hence, good postoperative oncotic pressure and muscular function) will always be well spent, such as inserting a centrally placed venous catheter for hypertonic glucose administration. If the patient has a history of pulmonary embolism or existing deep venous thrombosis in the legs, prophylactic inferior vena cava plication should be considered when abdominal procedures are done.[9]

A large portion of the intraoperative prevention of pulmonary complications is carried out by the anesthesiologist. Maintaining large tidal volume ventilation (10–15 cc/kg) during operation has been emphasized repeatedly. Particularly during long procedures, alveoli will begin to collapse unless regularly hyperinflated at least every hour. The anesthesiologist contributes greatly toward preventing pulmonary complications by avoiding crystalloid fluid overload during operation. Blood and protein losses can be replaced with Ringer's lactate solution during operation. Overzealous pursuit of such therapy contributed to the epidemic of pulmonary insufficiency known as the adult respiratory distress syndrome (ARDS) in the late 1960s (*see* Chap. 36). Generally, blood or plasma lost during operation should be replaced with blood or plasma. Moderate amounts of saline-type solutions are permissible, but caution should be observed.

Mechanical ventilation should be continued postoperatively until the adequacy of spontaneous ventilation has been clearly established. The action of paralytic drugs should be reversed completely and a vital capacity at least twice the tidal volume documented before extubation.

ROUTINE POSTOPERATIVE MEASURES

Postoperatively, both the surgeon and the patient must participate in preventing pulmonary complications. In the recovery room, the endotracheal tube should be maintained in place as long as is necessary, as noted above. Patients with preexisting pulmonary dysfunction or those at high risk of pulmonary complications may need to be left intubated and maintained on mechanical ventilation for hours or days after operation.

Abundant evidence suggests that the well-ventilated alveolus is less susceptible to humoral capillary damage than is the atelectatic alveolus.[2] In my institution, elderly, debilitated patients, patients with major cardiac procedures, and patients with extensive trauma, multiple fractures, pancreatitis, dead tissue, or severe peritonitis are commonly left intubated and maintained on mechanical ventilation 12 hours or more postoperatively. When the patient is fully alert and awake, when his perfusion and cardiac status are stable, and when the blood and extracellular fluid volumes are demonstrated to be normal, *then* the patient is ready for spontaneous ventilation and extubation.

Deep breathing exercises, clearing of sputum and mucus, and avoidance of prolonged periods in the supine position must begin in the recovery room. Profound hypoventilation, ventilation–perfusion imbalance, and resultant hypoxemia are the rule in the patient awakening from anesthesia. For this reason, it is common practice to administer moderate amounts (5–10 liters/min) of supplemental oxygen to all patients in the recovery room. This is a wise precaution for the first hour or two after anesthesia, but this practice is really prophylactic only against hypoxic arrhythmias and may actually be slightly detrimental to lung function by suppressing whatever deep breathing may result from moderate degrees of hypoxemia. Consequently, supplemental oxygen should not be administered for more than a few hours unless serial blood gas analyses so dictate.

Airway cleaning, suctioning, expectorant drugs, mist inhalation, and mucolytic agents are all useful in patients with preexisting chronic bronchitis or thick, tenacious tracheobronchial secretions. However, these maneuvers and agents may not be necessary in patients who maintain the lung adequately inflated by *emphasis on inspiratory maneuvers*. A compulsion to force patients to cough dominates much of the thinking on postoperative pulmonary care. Coughing maneuvers are painful in thoracotomy or laparotomy patients and should not be necessary if the lung remains well ventilated.

Breathing maneuvers, and devices designed to encourage those maneuvers, are important adjuncts to postoperative care. Since shallow breathing, the lack of spontaneous deep breaths, and alveolar collapse are the steps that lead to postoperative pulmonary complications, respiratory maneuvers must be those that emphasize maximal lung inflation.[7,31] Emphasis on breathing out (coughing, tracheal stimulation, "blow bottles") will do nothing to accomplish alveolar inflation, save the preparatory inspiration the patient may take before that maneuver. The more emphasis that is placed on the inhaled volume and inspiratory pressure, the more effective the maneuver will be.

Postoperative breathing maneuvers are compared in Figure 37-5. As can be seen, spontaneous deep breathing exercise fulfills these criteria best. Inflation with a mechanical ventilator (IPPB) is useful theoretically but in controlled studies has not been shown to decrease the incidence of pulmonary complications.[7] The reasons for the failure of IPPB lie not in the theory but in the usual method of practice. Regular alveolar inflation must be carried out at frequent intervals, preferably every hour, to be effective. IPPB is usually done for periods of minutes with long hours between "treatments."

Maximal inhaled volumes must be assured; however, the volumes delivered by IPPB are regulated by pressure. The more the atelectasis, the lower the compliance, and the less volume is delivered by the ventilator to reach the cycling pressure of the IPPB device. Hence, the desired inhaled volume is not assured. Finally, many patients involuntarily swallow with each blast of the ventilator in the mouth, resulting in gastric distention, compression of the dia-

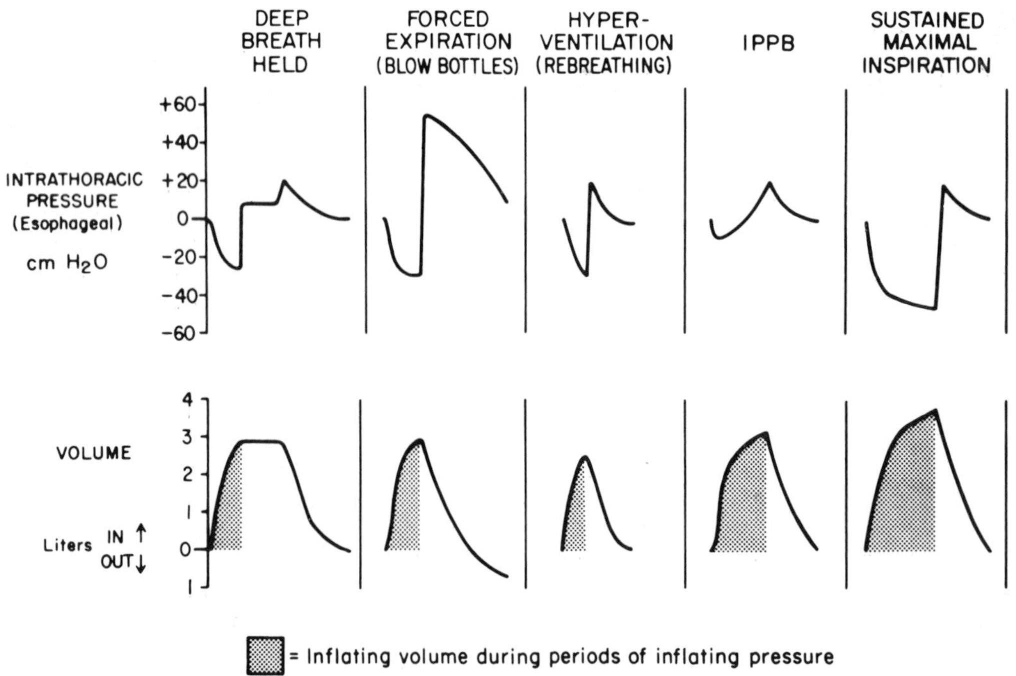

Fig. 37-5. A comparison of respiratory maneuvers used to inflate the lung. The best maneuver has the largest volume inhaled during periods of inflating (negative) pressure (shown as shaded area). (Bartlett RH, Brennan MD, Gazzaniga AB et al: Studies on the pathogenesis and prevention of postoperative pulmonary complications. Surg Gynecol Obstet 137:925, 1973)

phragm, and further compromise of pulmonary function.

Several authors have emphasized the ineffectiveness of routine IPPB in preventing pulmonary complications.[10,11] This does not mean that IPPB is not a useful method of treatment. On the contrary, in patients who are too obtunded, in those too weak to carry out spontaneous breathing maneuvers, or in those with already established atelectasis, IPPB is very useful. In those circumstances, however, the device should be used frequently, preferably each hour, and monitored by direct measurement of exhaled volumes, with maximum volume inflation attempted with each breath.

Deep inspiratory maneuvers can be done spontaneously but are better done with the use of a device that will record the volume inhaled and "reward" the patient for his efforts. Such a device is the *incentive spirometer*. When using this device, the patient can see his inspired volume with each breath, and the total breathing excursions in a period of time are recorded on a counter. Consequently, the physician, respiratory therapist, and patient can all be assured that the proper maneuver is being done, and frequently enough to maintain alveolar inflation. The regular use of deep breathing exercises using an incentive spirometer has been shown to decrease the incidence of pulmonary complications from about 30% to about 10%.[6]

Another method of preventing postoperative atelectasis is the application of continuous positive airway pressure (CPAP) with a tight-fitting face mask. Initial reports of this technique show improved alveolar inflation.[16] The potential complications of mask CPAP (gastric distension, vomiting and aspiration, patient discomfort) did not occur in the initial series but remain a cause for concern. This technique, perhaps combined with "mask" IPPB, may prove useful in patients who are extubated but who cannot or will not breathe deeply.

Whatever method is used to accomplish maximal inflation must be carefully taught to the patient *preoperatively*. Most patients cannot learn breathing exercises in a painful, narcotized, postoperative state. Recent reviews and discussion of postoperative pulmonary prophylaxis are available.[5,22,26]

Frequent change of position and early ambulation will minimize fluid collection in the dependent portions of the lung. Postoperative nutrition should be maintained. If the patient must go without oral intake for more than 4 or 5 days, total parenteral nutrition is advisable for several reasons, not the least of which is to maintain the strength of the respiratory effort. Fluids must be managed carefully to avoid overloading the extracellular space and diluting the serum proteins.

Pulmonary thromboembolism from deep veins of the leg or pelvis is a constant threat in the postoperative patient. Patients older than 40 years of age and patients with cancer constitute a particularly high-risk group. Several methods have been proposed to prevent deep venous thrombosis, including anticoagulation, drugs that inhibit platelet function, applying pressure to the legs with plastic wraps or stockings, and frequent active or passive lower leg exercises (*see* Chaps. 26, 33).

Regularly exercising the muscles is the easiest of these maneuvers, has the least complications, and is advised for all postoperative patients. Again, early ambulation will also promote venous flow in the deep veins of the leg.

Even if all the above steps are followed, postoperative pulmonary complications will still occur in about 15% of thoracotomy patients, less than 10% of laparotomy patients, and in progressively smaller numbers of patients with extremity, head and neck, or pelvic surgery. Pulmonary complications usually occur because the patient cannot pursue maximum inflation exercises or because some combination of fluid infusion and pulmonary capillary damage has led to interstitial pulmonary edema. Early vigorous treatment of such complications will almost always reverse the situation. Rarely, a postoperative patient progresses to severe pulmonary insufficiency, requiring further intensive care.

TREATMENT OF POSTOPERATIVE PULMONARY INSUFFICIENCY

Treatment of pulmonary insufficiency in the surgical patient, as in any patient, has two major goals: to expand collapsed alveoli and maintain or return lung volumes to normal; and to decrease extravascular water in the lung and return pulmonary capillary permeability to normal.

TREATMENT AIMED AT ALVEOLAR INFLATION

Treatment aimed at alveolar inflation is outlined in Table 37-5. The cornerstone is to establish large vol-

Table 37-5. Treatment Modalities Used to Reverse Alveolar Collapse

Maximum inflation
Yawn
CPPB
Mechanical ventilator
IPPV, TV, IMV
CPPB (+PEEP)
Airway cleaning
Suctioning
Chest physical therapy
Use least possible FI_{O_2}
Decrease lung water
Treat lung infection
Optimize nutrition

ume inflation by merely instituting breathing exercises, perhaps with the assistance of an incentive spirometer. In most patients, atelectasis can be treated successfully by merely intensifying breathing exercise efforts. If adequate volumes cannot be generated by the patient in this manner, then mechanical assistance is necessary, initially with intermittent positive pressure breathing with a mechanical ventilator, without intubation. As mentioned earlier, this must be done with direct volume measurements and often requires high pressures with the IPPB device (40 to 50 cm of water). Efforts at alveolar inflation must be combined with cleaning and dilating the airway, where necessary.

When an area of lung is not ventilated, mucus secreted in the bronchi draining from that lung segment becomes thickened and impacted, which hinders efforts at reexpansion. This mucus should be cleared by chest physical therapy (percussion) and postural drainage.

Hydration and nebulized bronchodilator and mucolytic drugs via the airway may be used. Coughing will help to expel mucus from airways that have been inflated distally. Coughing will not dislodge mucus from airways leading to nonventilated areas of lung. In this situation mucus must be removed directly with tracheal suction or bronchoscopy. I prefer bronchoscopy as the initial step in managing any postoperative patient with major atelectasis.

Tracheal suctioning (see Chap. 21) will exacerbate hypoxia if not done properly. The catheter is passed through the nose, verified as passing through the larynx by a change in voice, and connected to oxygen at 5 liters/min. Then, 5 cc of saline is injected and the oxygen reconnected for several coughing breaths. Suction is applied for no longer than 15 seconds, then oxygen is resumed. This process is continued until the suction return is clear (1–5 min). ECG monitoring should be done during and after suctioning. Atropine is given for bradycardia.

Routine endotracheal suctioning is practiced on many surgical services. In adults the value of this technique lies primarily in stimulation of deep breathing associated with the vigorous coughing that it induces. If that is the intent, then deep breathing can be easily accomplished by other means without the potential vagal complications associated with tracheal suctioning. In other words, *routine* tracheal suctioning has no rational place in the care of postoperative adult patients.

In infants the size of the airway is such that a very small amount of mucus (which would be insignificant in a larger patient) may cause major tracheal or bronchial occlusion. Infants breathe rapidly with a large ventilation of the dead space, leading to drying of the tracheal secretions, and may have difficulty coughing material from the lower trachea or from the bronchi. Consequently, routine endotracheal suctioning can be valuable in the postoperative management of infants following operations on the thorax or upper abdomen.

In both infants and adults, if adequate ventilation cannot be established with the methods mentioned above, endotracheal intubation and continuous mechanical ventilation are instituted. As with bronchoscopy, I favor this type of management. I consider mechanical ventilation to be indicated when the inspiratory force during a Müller maneuver is less than 20 cm of water, when the vital capacity is less than twice the tidal volume, or if the patient is severely hypoxemic (Pa_{O_2} less than 50 torr breathing room air). If any one of these indications exist and cannot be reversed by the measures mentioned above, intubation and mechanical ventilation are carried out. The same criteria apply for extubating the patient. Intubation with spontaneous breathing and continuous positive airway pressure (5–10 cm of water) without mechanical ventilation are standard therapy in the respiratory distress syndrome of the newborn and are commonly used when that condition is complicated by a surgical procedure. CPAP is reportedly useful in some adults with respiratory insufficiency associated with absence of surfactant. Generally, if the patient requires intubation, the use of the mechanical ventilator is also indicated (see Chap. 36).

The principles outlined above for spontaneous respiration apply equally well to mechanical ventilation. Emphasis is placed on maximum alveolar inflation with every breath. The goal is to return the FRC to normal and to maintain it there. The use of large tidal volumes will assure that alveoli distal to narrowed airways are well inflated with each breath. The use of positive end-expiratory pressure will offset the effects of decreased surfactant and minimize absorption atelectasis when high concentrations of oxygen are needed. Mechanical ventilation must be regulated by volume, either by using a volume ventilator or by continuously measuring exhaled volume when using a pressure-cycled ventilator. The inspired oxygen should be regulated to the lowest level needed to give a Pa_{O_2} between 60 and 90 torr. Inspiratory pressure is determined by the inspired volume. In patients with severely decreased FRC, inspiratory pressures of 60 to 80 cm of water may be necessary to deliver volumes of 10 cc/kg. As alveoli become reinflated (FRC increases), the pressure needed to deliver this volume decreases. If high airway pressures are required, the staff must be constantly alert to possible pneumothorax.

Positive end-expiratory pressure (PEEP) helps to maintain alveolar inflation and should be used whenever FRC is decreased. When PEEP is used, tidal volume is decreased to avoid high peak inspiratory pressure. The increase in mean intrathoracic pressure impedes venous return and decreases cardiac output. Therefore, a level of PEEP and tidal volume is selected that gives optimal alveolar inflation and oxygen delivery. Usually this is the PEEP level associated with the best pulmonary compliance.[29]

The respiratory rate should be regulated by the patient's respiratory center, if possible. The ventilator is set at a very low rate (5–8 breaths/min) and the patient allowed to breathe at a more rapid rate, triggering the ventilator to regulate the Pa_{CO_2} at 40 torr (assist technique; *see* Chap. 24). In a comatose patient or a patient in whom the assist mode cannot be used, the rate should be set to maintain the Pa_{CO_2} at 40 torr. With large tidal volumes and minimal lung dysfunction, this may require the addition of a rebreathing volume between the ventilator and the patient to avoid hypocapnea. Direct access to the airway allows adequate humidification, delivery of nebulized drugs, and easy access for tracheal cleaning and suctioning where appropriate.

Airway access is gained by direct endotracheal intubation in all patients except those with laryngeal trauma or possible cervical spine injury. With the exception of these latter conditions, emergency tracheostomy for airway access is never indicated. Tracheostomy is always safer when done over an endotracheal tube in a previously intubated patient. Tracheal intubation should always be carried out before tracheostomy. The endotracheal tube is uncomfortable and precludes the patient from moving about easily and from eating. Tracheostomy provides easier access to the airway and allows the patient to move about and eat and drink without difficulty; it may, however, have a higher incidence of direct tracheal complications. These various factors balance out after 48 to 72 hours of ventilator management via endotracheal tube, and a tracheostomy is usually advised if mechanical ventilation is needed beyond that time.

Whether airway access is maintained by means of direct endotracheal intubation or tracheostomy, several principles are important in avoiding tracheal damage (discussed extensively in Chap. 21), including avoiding high-pressure, low-volume occlusive cuffs that may damage the tracheal mucosa; inserting a shock-absorbing piece of tubing between the ventilator and the patient; and putting a swivel connector in the circuitry to avoid torsion of the tube when the patient moves. Care in suctioning, management of the ventilator patient, and weaning from mechanical ventilation are discussed in Chapter 25 and Appendix H.

Monitoring the patient on mechanical ventilation requires frequent blood gas analysis (*see* Chaps. 12 and 39). If the patient requires ventilator support for longer than 24 hours, the best practice is to place an indwelling arterial cannula, preferably in a radial or ulnar artery, to avoid repeated arterial punctures.

TREATMENT OF INCREASED LUNG WATER

Lung water can be decreased by decreasing the entire extracellular fluid space; decreasing the hydrostatic pressure in the pulmonary capillary bed; and increasing the plasma oncotic pressure without increasing the oncotic pressure in the interstitial fluid of the lung (Table 37-6). Mechanical positive pressure ventilation is *not* listed as a means to decrease lung water. In fact, positive pressure ventilation with PEEP actually increases lung water slightly, probably by stretching the pulmonary tissue. Mechanical ventilation will improve gas exchange in patients with pulmonary edema by overcoming $\dot{V}/\dot{Q}$ imbalance associated with bronchodilator or alveolar thickening but will not decrease lung water itself.

Patients with simple atelectasis do not need treatment for increased lung water except by avoiding fluid overload and cardiac failure. Increased lung water requires treatment when diffuse interstitial

Table 37-6. Treatment Modalities Used to Reverse Established Increases in Lung Water

↓ Capillary filtration pressure
Inotropic drugs
↓ Pulmonary artery pressure
Diuresis or dialysis
↑ Oncotic pressure
Concentrated albumin
Dehydration
Treat pulmonary capillaries
↓ FI_{O_2}
↓ Airway pressure (?)
Steroids (?)
Platelets (?)
Lung inflation

fluid collection is evident by x-ray film and by the hospital course. For example, the patient who has had an episode of septicemia, one who has had an episode of disseminated intravascular coagulation or fat embolism, one with peritonitis or revascularization of ischemic tissue, or one who received 4 liters of Ringer's lactate solution during a 3-hour operation would be likely to have increased lung water in association with other pulmonary problems.

Decreasing pulmonary hydrostatic pressure by improving left ventricular function is done pharmacologically and can, and should, be done in all patients with major pulmonary insufficiency. If the patient has received large infusions of citrate in the form of banked blood or plasma substitutes, a transient myocardial depression may occur, which can be reversed with calcium infusion. A long-acting inotropic drug such as digoxin should be instituted and may be supplemented with a short-acting inotrope such as dopamine.

The effectiveness of this treatment can be determined only by measuring cardiac output and left atrial (or pulmonary capillary wedge) pressure directly. This requires insertion of a pulmonary artery catheter. Pulmonary artery and wedge pressure monitoring and mixed venous blood sampling are nearly as important as direct arterial blood gas sampling in managing the patient with pulmonary insufficiency who has a major increase in lung water. The exact position of the pulmonary artery catheter must be carefully determined and the pressure tracings properly interpreted, which requires continuous display on an oscilloscope and careful selection of the end-expiratory point for pressure readings.

Total extracellular fluid volume is reduced by forced diuresis or dialysis if the patient is in renal failure. Diuresis is induced with a potent diuretic such as furosemide or mannitol. The course of diuresis is followed with careful measurement of body weight daily and measurement of fluid intake and output hourly. Usually the postoperative patient with pulmonary insufficiency will be found to be 4 to 5 kg overloaded, primarily with extracellular fluid.

Adequate treatment of increased lung water must include removing the excess extravascular fluid (returning the patient to his baseline weight) and establishing continued diuresis until the patient is in 1 to 3 liters of negative water balance and is maintained in this condition.[23,27] This major decrease in total extracellular fluid volume will be accompanied by a minor decrease in pulmonary extracellular fluid volume, but this change may be enough to improve pulmonary function greatly. Use of diuretic drugs will remove water, sodium, and potassium at differing rates so that all must be monitored carefully and frequently. Usually water is removed in excess of electrolyte so that with extreme forced diuresis a hypernatremic, hyperosmotic state will result. Serum sodium concentrations should be monitored closely. Diuresis has reached its limit when the serum sodium is between 140 and 150 mEq/liter.

Diuresis is combined with colloid loading to increase plasma oncotic pressure transiently, which forces the movement of fluid from the extravascular to the intravascular space. This should be done concomitantly with diuresis because most agents used for colloid loading, such as albumin, have a molecular weight between 50,000 and 100,000 and will gradually find their way into the extracellular space within 4 to 12 hours after infusion. The advantages of colloid loading come during the first hour or two after infusion and before the colloid load joins the lymphatic system and is subsequently metabolized.

Although some animal studies suggest a deleterious effect of albumin loading in pulmonary insufficiency,[18] treatment of human subjects with colloid loading (and diuresis) is usually highly successful. The technique should be used when capillary integrity has been restored, as determined by response to small initial doses.[4,24]

SPECIFIC CONSIDERATIONS

GASTRIC ASPIRATION

Vomiting with subsequent aspiration is a dreaded complication for the surgeon and the anesthesiologist.

Elective operations are always done after 12 hours of fasting so that the stomach will be empty. However, emergency procedures or elective procedures in patients with intestinal obstruction may be associated with vomiting at any time during the procedure. The patient is most likely to vomit during the induction of anesthesia. Whenever an emergent procedure is planned, a nasogastric tube should be placed first and the stomach emptied as much as possible. Anesthesia should be induced abruptly and followed immediately by endotracheal intubation, or intubation should be achieved before induction of anesthesia. Even with these precautions, aspiration of gastric contents will occur occasionally. If aspiration is suspected before or during the operation, an endotracheal tube should be passed, the balloon inflated, and the trachea irrigated and aspirated vigorously. If aspiration is documented by return of gastric contents from the trachea, a short course of steroids and large-volume ventilation may avoid subsequent aspiration pneumonitis.[14]

Postoperatively, the patient who has aspirated should always be suctioned vigorously with saline lavage until clear. Any patient who may have aspirated food particles (some would say any patient who aspirates) should undergo bronchoscopy with a conventional rigid bronchoscope, careful examination of all bronchi, vigorous lavage, and aspiration. Most patients who have aspirated should be maintained on large-volume mechanical ventilation until physiological and x-ray film studies indicate that any lung damage is resolving.

FAT EMBOLISM

A small percentage of patients with extensive fractures develop the clinical syndrome of fat embolism, which is due to pulmonary embolization of neutral fat globules from the marrow cavity and is often associated with embolization of megakaryocytes and other marrow cells. Hypoxemia and bilateral patchy pulmonary infiltrates beginning 12 to 36 hours after trauma are typical of this lesion. Associated findings include a falling hematocrit, hemolysis, high fever, cerebral symptoms, petechiae (particularly in the anterior axillary folds, sclerae, and eyelids), and possibly fat globules in the urine, blood, or sputum. Pulmonary capillary damage occurs in this condition, apparently due to sterile inflammation from fatty acids released as the triglyceride particles break down in the lung parenchyma.

Steroids have been shown to decrease the inflammation and hence the mortality from this lesion, although they must be given early and in large doses. Intubation and mechanical ventilation are indicated as soon as the syndrome has been diagnosed. Care must be taken to maintain the patient's fluid balance as "dry" as possible since the pulmonary capillaries leak, even at normal hydrostatic pressures. This is often difficult in patients who have multiple system trauma and may have active bleeding or oliguria at the same time that the pulmonary lesion develops. Intravenous heparin and alcohol, suggested by some, have not proved to be useful drugs in the clinical treatment of this disorder.

SMOKE INHALATION

Several investigators have demonstrated a generalized increase in capillary permeability (including that of the pulmonary capillaries) after a small body surface burn. The more extensive the burn, the greater the capillary leakage. For reasons outlined earlier in this chapter, the pulmonary capillary bed shows signs of increased capillary permeability first, in the form of increased lung water. This phenomenon has confused clinicians caring for patients with smoke inhalation syndrome for many years. The problem has recently been clarified by Zawacki,[33] who found smoke inhalation injury to be a relatively mild pulmonary insult but a major insult when combined with body surface burn, as is often the case in humans.

The toxic materials in smoke are carbon monoxide, heat, various aldehydes and other organic materials, and other organic compounds in the vapor state. Materials that are totally combustible (such as natural gas or gasoline) burn to carbon dioxide and water, producing certain toxic organic compounds and causing minimal lung damage when inhaled in smoke.[1] On the other hand, wood, paint, upholstery, and the like burn incompletely, yielding various toxic vapors in addition to the usual products of combustion. These vapors are damaging to the respiratory epithelium and alveoli. Heat in smoke is a minimal factor that causes lung damage because air is such a poor heat conductor. Deep lung damage from heat is unusual unless the thermal injury is conveyed by hot steam.

Carbon monoxide is the major toxic material in smoke. It does not damage the lungs but renders the brain hypoxic by association with hemoglobin, creating potentially lethal brain damage. Patients with smoke inhalation injury without a surface burn usually pass through a period of mild pulmonary insufficiency and recover completely unless irreversible brain damage or metabolic acidosis has occurred because of carboxyhemoglobinemia. Patients with the same degree of smoke inhalation and a moderate surface burn are subject to serious pulmonary insufficiency with combined atelectasis and increased lung water, usually requiring intubation, mechanical ventilation, and efforts to reduce lung water as outlined above.

BACTERIAL PNEUMONITIS AND PULMONARY THROMBOEMBOLISM

Because these problems so often complicate otherwise uneventful surgery, the reader is urged to review the topics of bacterial pneumonitis (*see* Chap. 19) and pulmonary thromboembolism (*see* Chap. 33).

CHEST TRAUMA

Direct injury to the chest may cause damage to the chest wall, lung parenchyma, diaphragm, airway, and other intrathoracic structures such as the heart and great vessels. These injuries are usually associated with hemothorax or pneumothorax. Life-threatening hypoventilation may result from injuries to the chest wall or from alveolar collapse caused by fluid or blood in the pleural space. Emergency treatment includes placement of a large chest tube to empty the pleural space and reexpand the lung and mechanical ventilation if spontaneous breathing is inadequate.

Blunt trauma to the chest may be caused by any direct blow but is most commonly associated with motor vehicle accidents. Most rib fractures do not require specific treatment other than intercostal nerve block to relieve pain. Fractured ribs should, however, always suggest more serious injuries to internal organs. Fracture of the ribs or sternum may create a segment of the chest wall that moves inward in response to the negative pressure created during spontaneous inspiration. This is referred to as paradoxical motion, and the floating segment of the chest wall is referred as a *"flail"* segment or *flail chest*. A small amount of paradoxical motion with no physiological side-effects does not require specific treatment. Hypoxemia or carbon dioxide retention associated with the flail chest injury indicates lung contusion and requires intubation and ventilation.

If air or fluid is detected in the pleural space, a large test tube should be placed (Figure 37-6). If a patient with minor chest injuries requires immediate operation for other problems (such as a ruptured spleen or head injury), prophylactic chest tubes should be placed on both sides to eliminate the possibility of a tension pneumothorax or hemothorax developing during anesthesia. Mechanical ventilation is required for patients with major flail segments and lung contusion or chest injury complicating other serious multiple system injuries. The use of corticosteroids for 1 or 2 days in severe lung contusion decreases mortality and morbidity in both experimental animals and patients.[30] The risk of infection should be balanced against possible benefits of this treatment

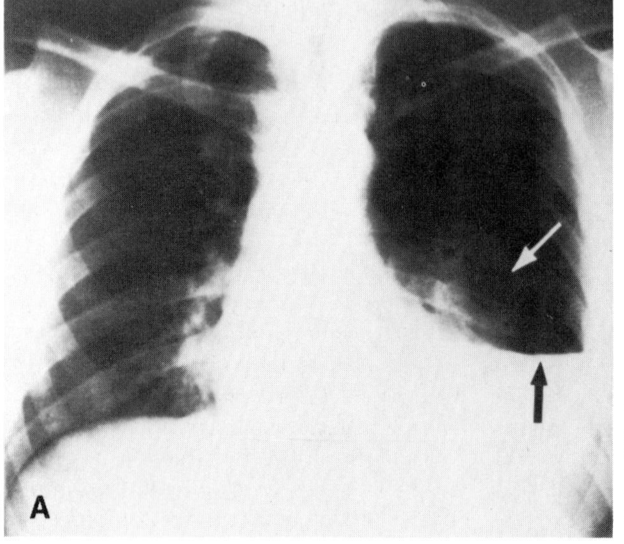

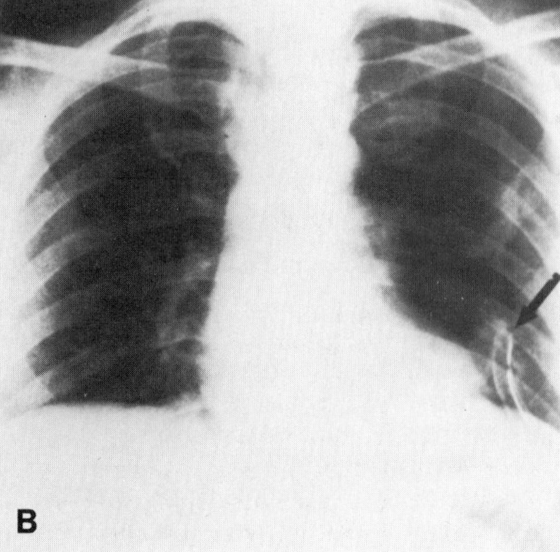

Fig. 37-6. Chest x-rays showing *(A)* hemopneumothorax with collapse of the lung and *(B)* same patient after treatment with chest tube.

in patients with multiple injuries. Operation is rarely necessary for blunt injury to the chest but may be needed for injury to the heart, aorta, bronchus, esophagus, or diaphragm. Operation for stabilization of rib and sternal fractures should be considered in any patient with multiple fractures or a large flail segment.

Penetrating trauma occurs from gunshot wounds, stab wounds, and some crushing injuries. Any hole between the pleural space and skin will result in a "sucking chest injury." In this circumstance air is inhaled into the pleural space during inspiration, filling the pleural space and eliminating the pressure gradient that would normally cause the lung to inflate, resulting in atelectasis of that lung. If the chest wall injury allows air to be inhaled into the pleural space but prevents the egress of air (a "flap valve" effect), a tension pneumothorax results, with hypoventilation and blockage of venous return. Bleeding into the pleural space from the chest wall or lung complicates this problem.

Penetrating chest injury is treated by placing a chest tube to drain accumulated air and blood. This maneuver, along with appropriate replacement of blood lost, will usually return cardiac output and respiration to normal quite promptly. Bleeding from the lung itself will usually subside because the lung vasculature is a low-pressure system. Air leaks from the lung usually seal within a day or two. Prolonged major air leaks should suggest injury to a large bronchus, trachea, or esophagus that requires operative repair. Massive bleeding (more than half of the blood volume in 12 hours or less) suggests injury to the heart, a major vessel, or an intercostal artery and should be treated by thoracotomy and direct repair. The possibility of penetrating injury through the diaphragm involving abdominal viscera should always be considered.

RESPIRATORY CARE AFTER THORACOTOMY AND PULMONARY RESECTION

The principles of pathogenesis , prevention, and management of pulmonary problems after thoracic operations are those described in the early part of this chapter. Some patients require resection of part or all of the lung for infection, cancer, congenital abnormalities, or (rarely) trauma. If the remaining lung is normal, removal of lung tissue does not cause a major physiological deficit. However, pulmonary resection creates unique problems because the "empty" space that was formerly occupied by the lung tissue must be managed very carefully or poor healing and infection may result. If pleural space infection, leak from the closed bronchus, or pulmonary failure occur after pulmonary resection, challenging ventilatory problems result.

SURGICAL CARE OF THE RESPIRATORY PATIENT

The *pleural "space"* is the space between the parietal and visceral pleural surfaces. Normally it is filled with a few cubic centimeters of clear fluid that serves to lubricate the services as they slide past each other during normal breathing. In abnormal conditions the pleural space can fill with air (pneumothorax), blood (hemothorax), plasma, serum or lymph (hydrothorax or pleural effusion), or pus (pyothorax, empyema). Anything in the pleural space compresses the underlying lung and causes atelectasis. Any fluid (with or without air) in the pleural space is subject to infection by direct contamination or blood-borne bacteria. Fluid detected by examination and x-ray film should be removed to establish a diagnosis and to prevent subsequent infection.

Aspiration of fluid or air from the chest is called *thoracentesis* and is usually done to remove fluid. Placement of a tube to establish more permanent drainage of the pleural space is called *thoracostomy, closed thoracostomy, or tube thoracostomy.*

Pleural effusion may be associated with systemic edema or with pulmonary edema caused by congestive heart failure or lung capillary leakage. In addition, infection, infarction, or cancer in the lung itself may result in accumulation of fluid in the pleural space. If a pleural effusion becomes infected with bacteria, an inflammatory reaction results that creates an abscess in the pleural space (an empyema). An empyema will usually form in the most dependent area of the pleural space and will become walled off from the remaining space by acute inflammation at the walls of the abscess, which seals the visceral and parietal pleura together around the abscess (pleural symphysis). An empyema, like any other abscess, is treated by establishing external drainage, usually with a chest tube or (if the empyema is chronic and walled off) by removing segments of ribs overlying the empyema to allow free external drainage.

Pneumothorax may occur after trauma or operation on the lung or after rupture of lung tissue (spontaneous pneumothorax). Pneumothorax is treated by placement of a chest tube to remove the air from the pleural space. When air is removed, the leaking area of lung is brought into a position with the parietal pleura that usually results in spontaneous healing or sealing of the air leak. If the air leak from the lung is major (more than half the tidal volume with each breath) or prolonged (more than 5 days), the condition is referred to as a bronchopleural fistula and may require operation for repair.

SPECIFIC PROCEDURES

Thoracentesis for removal of fluid is done with the patient in a sitting position, inserting the needle where fluid has been detected, usually in the posterior axillary line. The skin, rib periosteum, and pleura are the only pain-sensitive structures in the chest wall. These areas are liberally anesthetized with local anesthetic, and a needle (mounted on a syringe with a stopcock) is advanced into the pleural space and fluid removed. Thoracentesis should be a painless procedure. Meticulous sterile conditions must be maintained (Fig. 37-7).

Tube thoracostomy is also done under local anesthesia (Fig. 37-8). A tube placed for pneumothorax is placed in the third or fourth interspace in the midaxillary line and directed to the apex of the pleural space. A tube placed to remove blood, with or without air, is placed in the sixth or seventh interspace in the midaxillary or posterior axillary line and then directed posteriorly. Local anesthesia is used for chest tube placement. Regional anesthesia by intercostal block should be done for placement of large chest tubes. In adults, an incision large enough to insert one finger is made two interspaces below the point where the chest tube will enter the pleural space. Subcutaneous tissue and muscle are bluntly dissected with a large clamp and with the finger. The clamp is forced into the pleural space, followed by an exploring finger to be sure that the lung is not adherent. The tube is advanced to the desired position, the clamp on the tube removed, and the air or fluid in the pleural space drained into a valved system. In small children a finger-sized hole is too large, and a smaller dissection should be done. *Trocars* are large pointed rods or tubes that have been used for introducing chest tubes. These instruments commonly result in injury to the lung and should never be used for tube thoracostomy.

Once the chest tube has been properly positioned, it should be attached to a system that allows free egress of fluid or air but prevents aspiration of external air into the chest. This is commonly accomplished with a water seal valve. In addition, suction may be applied to the chest tube to facilitate air or fluid removal.

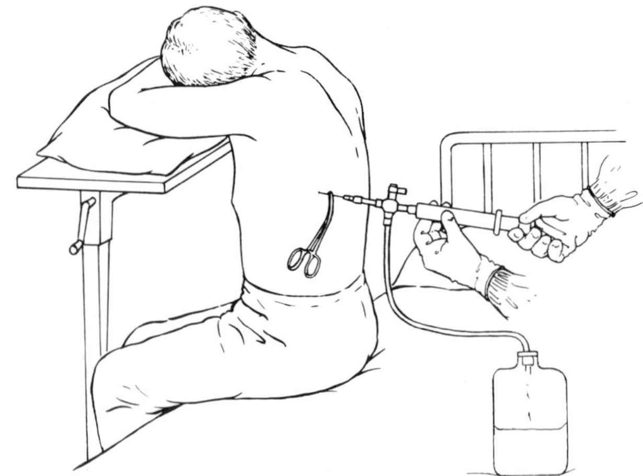

Fig. 37-7. Technique for thoracentesis.

Bronchoscopy is a procedure that involves placement of a viewing instrument into the trachea and bronchi to diagnose or treat lung and airway problems. The respiratory therapist may be called on to assist with bronchoscopy and thus should be familiar with this technique.[25] The *flexible bronchoscope* is made up primarily of fiberoptic bundles that carry illuminating light into the bronchus and reflected light back to the lens, which allows direct visualization of the airways. The tip of the bronchoscope can be manipulated with a series of levers. Parallel channels of the bronchoscope can carry irrigating fluid and flexible biopsy forceps and can be used for suctioning at the end of the instrument. The flexible bronchoscope is small and maneuverable and can be used through an endotracheal tube in ventilator patients; it can reach far into the segmental and subsegmental bronchi. The *rigid bronchoscope* is a long, straight metal tube with a light at the tip. The rigid bronchoscope can be used to manipulate the wall of the trachea and bronchi; the large lumen allows aspiration of large particles, but vision is limited to the lobar and some segmental bronchi. Hence, the rigid bronchoscope is used if large particles must be cleared from the airways or if fixation or mobility of the tracheal wall is in question.

During bronchoscopy the mouth, pharynx, larynx, and airways are anesthetized with topical anesthetic. The bronchoscope is passed into the lower airways, and appropriate studies and lavage are carried out. The assistant to the bronchoscopist must be sure that all equipment is in proper working order, adjust the light or power source, and supply local anesthesia, irrigating solution, and suction as needed.

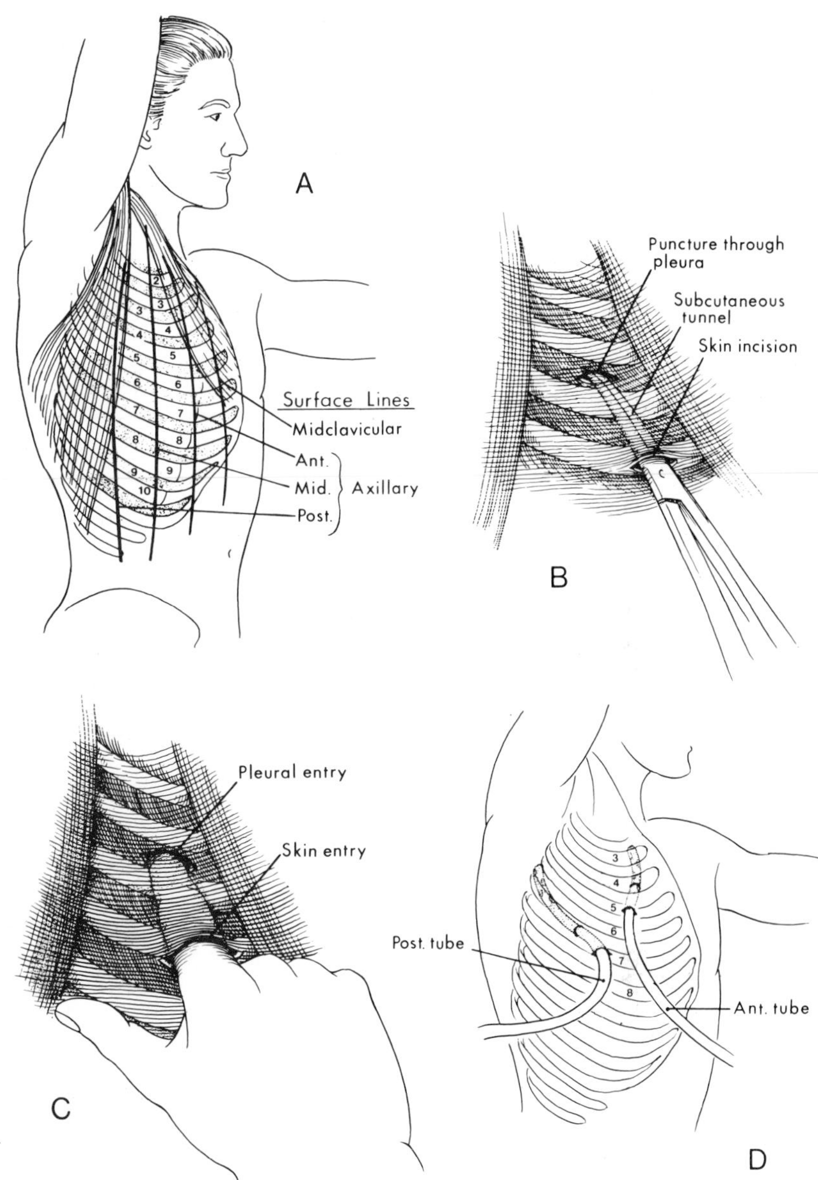

Fig. 37-8. Technique of chest tube placement. A = landmarks; B = dissecting with hemostat; C = exploring with finger; D = proper tube placement.

Tracheostomy is an operation in which a tube is placed through the skin of the neck into the trachea.[21] This is needed if the upper airway is occluded or if the patient requires prolonged ventilatory support. Although endotracheal intubation can be maintained for weeks at a time, there are many advantages to direct tracheostomy for prolonged ventilator support (less resistance, easier tracheal suctioning, less damage to the larynx, and the ability of the patient to eat by mouth). The major advantage of tracheostomy over endotracheal intubation is that it is much more comfortable for the patient and does not require prolonged sedation. If the operation is properly done, the advantages of tracheostomy far outweigh any advantages of prolonged endotracheal intubation. Formerly a proponent of prolonged intubation, I now favor tracheostomy for airway access in any patient who needs mechanical ventilation for more than a few days (Fig. 37-9).

With the rare exceptions of cervical spine injury or laryngeal occlusion, tracheostomy is always an elective operation done with an endotracheal tube in

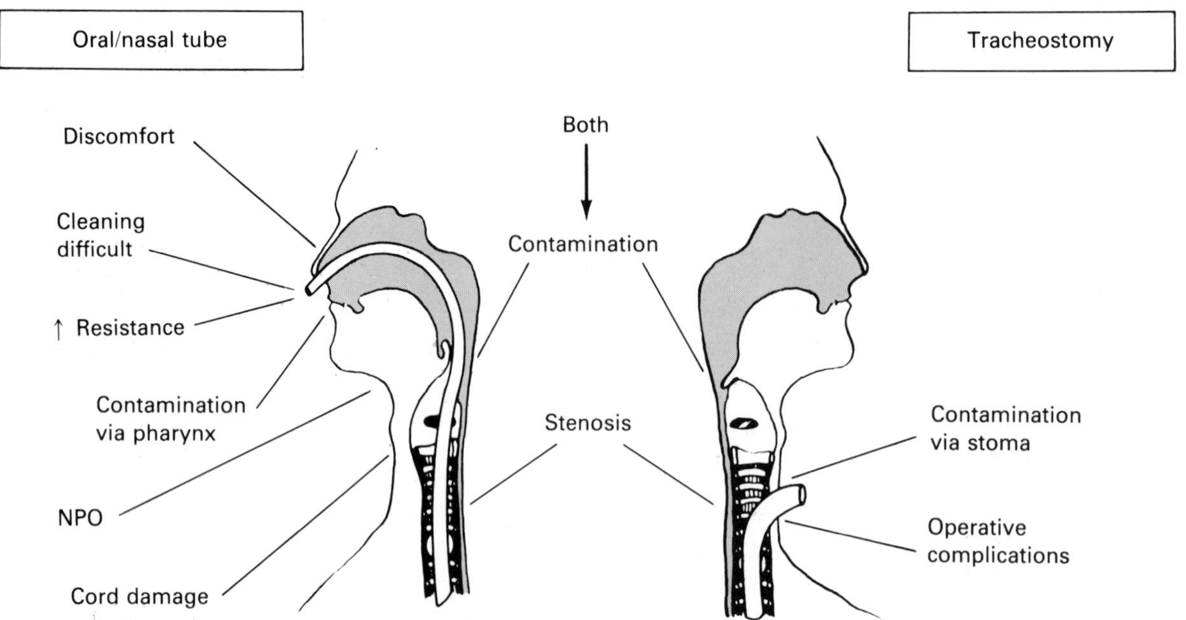

Fig. 37-9. Potential complications of endotracheal intubation and tracheostomy. Balloon cuff complications are common to both.

place. Tracheostomies are conventionally done through the second tracheal cartilage. This operation can be easily done in a well-equipped intensive care unit under local anesthesia and requires excellent lighting, suction, exposure, and hemostasis. Tracheostomy done through the cricothyroid membrane was formerly an emergency procedure only. This operation is quicker and easier to do but may damage the cricoid cartilage or vocal cords. It has recently been shown that this type of tracheostomy is acceptable for chronic and elective airway access as long as damage to the cricoid cartilage is avoided.[13] Usually tracheostomy is done because the patient has pulmonary failure and needs ventilator support. This requires coordination between the surgeon and the nurse or respiratory therapist. Often the endotracheal tube balloon is punctured as the trachea is entered, so that the tracheostomy tube must be prepared and available as soon as the trachea has been opened. Under direct vision and with the patient on the ventilator, the endotracheal tube is pulled back until the tracheal lumen has been exposed. The tracheostomy tube is placed, the endotracheal tube completely removed, and the ventilator attached to the tracheostomy tube. When the ventilator is attached to the tracheostomy tube, the operative field is contaminated. It is not necessary to use separate sterile ventilator tubing for this transition.

EXTRACORPOREAL MEMBRANE OXYGENATION

When acute pulmonary insufficiency becomes severe and prolonged enough to carry a high mortality risk with continued therapy, extracorporeal membrane oxygenation (ECMO) may provide total life support for all organs while new and innovative treatment is pursued. This technique is an extension of cardiopulmonary bypass, in which an artificial lung and pumping system are substituted for the lungs and heart during cardiac surgery. Large catheters are placed into the heart or great vessels under local anesthesia. A diagram of a typical ECMO system is shown in Figure 37-10. The patient is anticoagulated with heparin and venous blood is drained from the patient, oxygen added, and carbon dioxide removed; the arterialized blood is then pumped back into the patient. In this way the artificial lung takes over the function of the normal lung, allowing removal of the patient from a ventilator, even though severe lung disease exists.

ECMO has been evaluated extensively in adults with severe acute respiratory failure. The results of a

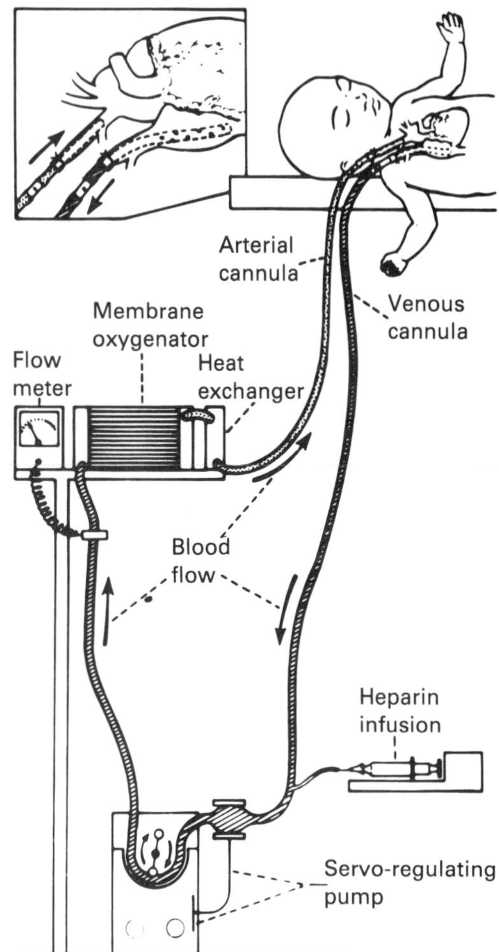

Fig. 37-10. Extracorporeal membrane oxygenation system.

comparative study between ECMO and conventional ventilator treatment showed 90% mortality in both groups.[32] The cause of death in these patients was fibrosis or infection in the lung. The results of ECMO in adult respiratory failure may improve as new perfusion techniques are employed or ways of preventing pulmonary fibrosis developed.

The use of ECMO in newborn respiratory failure, on the other hand, has shown very promising results.[8] Recovery and survival occurred in 25 of the 45 moribund infants we have treated with ECMO. Other investigators have shown similar results.

SUMMARY

Respiratory care in the surgical patient includes prevention and treatment of the single largest cause of complication and death—respiratory insufficiency and failure. Ventilation–perfusion imbalance leading to total alveolar collapse is found to some extent in almost every surgical patient. An increase in pulmonary extravascular water volume frequently complicates this situation. Prevention and treatment of pulmonary insufficiency, therefore, are aimed at achieving and maintaining normal FRC, normal hemodynamics, and normal pulmonary capillary permeability.

REFERENCES

1. Achauer BM, Allyn PA, Furnas DW et al: Pulmonary complications of burns: The major threat to the burned patient. Ann Surg 177:311, 1974
2. Bartlett RH: Post-traumatic pulmonary insufficiency. In Cooper P, Nyhus L (eds): Surgery Annual. New York, Appleton-Century-Crofts, 1971
3. Bartlett RH: Respiratory Care in Surgery. Surg Clin North Am 16, No. 6. Philadelphia, WB Saunders, 1980
4. Bartlett RH: Cardiopulmonary complications of pancreatitis. In Dent TL (ed): Pancreatic Disease. New York, Grune & Stratton, 1981
5. Bartlett RH: Editorial: Postoperative pulmonary prophylaxis: Breathe deeply and read carefully. Chest 81:1, 1982
6. Bartlett RH, Brennan MD, Gazzaniga AB et al: Studies on the pathogenesis and prevention of postoperative pulmonary complications. Surg Gynecol Obstet 137:925, 1973
7. Bartlett RH, Gazzaniga AB, Geraghty TR: Respiratory maneuvers to prevent postoperative pulmonary complications. A critical review. JAMA 224:1017, 1973
8. Bartlett RH, Gazzaniga AB, Huxtable RF et al: Extracorporeal circulation (ECMO) in neonatal respiratory failure. J Thorac Cardiovasc Surg 74:826, 1977
9. Bartlett RH, Yahia C: Management of septic chemical abortion with acute renal failure. N Engl J Med 281:747, 1969
10. Baxter WD, Levine RS: An evaluation of intermittent positive pressure breathing in the prevention of postoperative pulmonary complications. Arch Surg 98:795, 1969
11. Becker A et al: The treatment of postoperative pulmonary atelectasis with intermittent positive pressure breathing. Surg Gynecol Obstet 111:517, 1960
12. Bendixen HH, Hedley–Whyte J, Laver MR: Oxygenation in surgical patients during general anesthesia with controlled ventilation. N Engl J Med 269:991, 1963
13. Brantigan CO, Growe B: Cricothyroidotomy: Elective use in respiratory problems requiring tracheostomy. J Thorac Cardiovasc Surg 71:72, 1976
14. Broe PJ, Toung TJK, Cameron JL: Aspiration pneumonia. Surg Clin North Am 60:1551, 1980
15. Demling RH, Manohar M, Will JA et al: The effect of plasma oncotic pressure on the pulmonary micro-circulation after hemorrhagic shock. Surgery 86:323, 1979
16. Greenbaum DM, Millen JE, Eross B et al: Continuous positive airway pressure without tracheal intubation in spontaneously breathing patients. Chest 69:615, 1976
17. Hodgkin JE, Dines DE, Didier EP: Preoperative evaluation of the patient with pulmonary disease. Mayo Clin Proc 48:114, 1973
18. Holcroft JW, Trunkey DD, Lim RC: Further analysis of lung water in baboons resuscitated from hemorrhage shock. J Surg Res 20:291, 1976

19. Lee AB, Kinney JM, Turino G et al: Effects of abdominal operations on ventilation and gas exchange. J Natl Med Assoc 61:164, 1969
20. Okinaka AJ: The pattern of breathing after operation. Surg Gynecol Obstet 125:785, 1967
21. Orringer M: Endotracheal intubation and tracheostomy. Surg Clin North Am 60:1447, 1980
22. Pontoppidan H: Mechanical aids to lung expansion in non-intubated surgical patients. Am Rev Respir Dis 122:109, 1981
23. Powers SR, Shah D, Ryon D et al: Hypertonic mannitol in the therapy of acute respiratory distress syndrome. Ann Surg 185:619, 1977
24. Puri V, Weil MH, Michaels S et al: Pulmonary edema associated with reduction in plasma oncotic pressure. Surg Gynecol Obstet 151:344, 1980
25. Ratliff JL: Bronchoscopy in respiratory care. Surg Clin North Am 60:1497, 1980
26. Shapiro BA: IPPB therapy is indicated preoperatively and postoperatively in some patients with pulmonary disease. In Eckenhoff JG (ed): Controversy in Anesthesiology. Philadelphia, WB Saunders, 1979
27. Skillman JJ, Parikh BM, Tanenbaum BJ: Pulmonary arteriovenous admixture: Improvement with albumin and diuresis. Am J Surg 119:440, 1970
28. Staub NC: State of the art review: Pathogenesis of pulmonary edema. Am Rev Respir Dis 109:358, 1974
29. Suter PM, Fairley HB, Isenberg MD: Optimum end expiratory pressure in patients with acute pulmonary failure. N Engl J Med 292:284, 1975
30. Trinkle JK, Richardson JD, Franz FL et al: Management of flail chest without mechanical ventilation. Ann Thorac Surg 19:355, 1975
31. Vandewater JM: Preoperative and postoperative techniques in the prevention of pulmonary complications. Surg Clin North Am 60:1339, 1980
32. Zapol WM, Snider MT, Hill SD et al: Extracorporeal membrane oxygenation in severe acute respiratory failure: A randomized prospective study. JAMA 242:2193, 1979
33. Zawacki BE, Jung RC, Joyce J et al: Smoke, burns, and the natural history of inhalation injury in fire victims. Ann Surg 185:100, 1977
34. Zikria BA, Spencer JL, Kinney JM et al: Alterations in ventilatory function in breathing patterns following surgical trauma. Ann Surg 179:1, 1974

38

Cardiopulmonary Resuscitation

Hugh E. Stephenson, Jr.

Sudden cessation of cardiac output (usually called "cardiac arrest") is an emergency encountered by almost every practicing member of a health care team. In the adult population, it is the most common mode of death. The actual incidence of sudden cardiac arrest may be as high as 30% of all natural deaths; ineffectual resuscitation is still alarmingly frequent. This situation can be improved only by the dissemination of knowledge about the various aspects of cardiac arrest and resuscitation to every person who may have the opportunity to apply the principles presented here.

Sudden cessation of cardiac output in a hospital setting continues to have a marked lethality despite widespread advances over the last quarter century, which include the introduction of closed-chest cardiac compression, mouth-to-mouth artificial ventilation, and defibrillation through the unopened chest. The overall success rate of cardiac resuscitative efforts unfortunately remains at a rather constant rate. In 1968, a 16% success rate was achieved among 5076 arrests collected from the literature. (By a successful cardiac resuscitation, one infers that the patient left the hospital as a viable individual.) Five years later, a 13% success rate was reported among 5718 cases of cardiac arrests.

I have collected an additional 4188 cases from the literature and note that 641, or 15.3%, were successfully resuscitated. To a minor extent, these studies may be misleading in that they include a mixture of resuscitative attempts. Some occurred before hospitalization. In addition, they represent results of a broad cross-section of community and university hospital experiences; they also include a number of coronary care units where success rates are considerably higher. The overall success rate is about 13% to 16% for those arrests occurring within hospitals.

With the organization of a "stat team" comprising a cardiology fellow, surgery resident, anesthesiology resident, internal medicine resident, nurse, and respiratory therapist, long-term survival increased from 17.6% of pre-stat team resuscitations to 23.8% of resuscitations in which the stat team participated.[18]

Most persons closely involved in cardiopulmonary resuscitative efforts are optimistic that the many years spent in the teaching of basic life support, as well as an intensification and further sophistication of definitive life-support measures, are now beginning to yield significant dividends. At present, *all* categories of personnel within the hospital setting must be competent to deal with the cardiopulmonary arrest victim. High on the list is that group involved in respiratory care. These persons are highly trained in the pathophysiology of the cardiopulmonary system and are heavily committed to the care of this group of high-risk patients.

This chapter attempts to provide the respiratory care worker with the basic information needed for cardiopulmonary resuscitation. The field of cardiopulmonary resuscitation is a broad one, however, and encompasses many varied circumstances and situations that are difficult to include in a relatively brief presentation. Additional references for selected reading have been provided in the Bibliography.

A large proportion of the unsuccessful attempts at cardiac resuscitation result from a delay in diagnosis and the subsequent delay in instituting effective resuscitative efforts. A cardiac arrest is basically a 3- to 4-minute emergency. This *time factor* must be continually before us in any consideration of cardiac arrest and resuscitation. There is a time period during which reversibility and resuscitation are possible in almost every case of cardiac arrest. No time must be wasted in attempts to locate a consultant, use various ineffective stimulants, question the accuracy of monitoring devices, or otherwise allow the short period of time to pass in pursuing useless diagnostic procedures. Fortunately, with knowledge of cardiac arrest and resuscitation becoming more widespread today, there seems to be earlier recognition of the problem. Cardiac arrest has become less often a completely unexpected event. We are alerted by much information accumulated from intensive care and coronary care units to conditions likely to produce cardiac standstill or ventricular fibrillation. Nevertheless, even in these carefully controlled areas, cardiac arrest may frequently surprisingly appear.

Within recent years the training of paramedics, firemen, policemen, lifeguards, and other rescue workers in the application of on-site cardiopulmonary resuscitation techniques has accelerated. Likewise, training in basic resuscitation techniques has been extended into the high schools of the nation and among the lay public. It seems logical that medical and allied health personnel should be exposed as early as possible to well-designed training in all of the ramifications of effective cardiopulmonary resuscitation. Unfortunately, some medical workers are completely lacking in the knowledge of even basic resuscitation techniques.

Each successful cardiac resuscitation attempt may require a slightly different approach as far as definitive care is concerned. In fact, some cases require a most sophisticated therapeutic approach and one that is beyond the scope of this chapter. The basic life-support efforts will generally, however, require a uniform technique.

A wide variety of etiologic factors may be involved in cardiac arrest. Usually these factors are ones that produce sudden severe cardiac arrhythmias (e.g., myocardial infarction), decreased coronary artery perfusion, decreased myocardial function, or decreased cardiac output. Electrolyte imbalance, vagal stimulation, acid–base disturbances, and other factors may also be responsible for cardiac arrhythmias. Biochemical, toxic, and anatomical changes may be responsible for any of the above factors. Although cardiac arrest owing to myocardial circulatory insufficiency is the most commonly encountered cause of cardiac arrest, a multitude of other causes may be encountered, including factors that result in sudden decrease in cardiac output, such as exsanguinating hemorrhage, pericardial tamponade, pulmonary embolism, or valvular heart disease.

HISTORY

Our understanding and appreciation of progress in cardiopulmonary resuscitation may well be augmented by a brief review of man's historic efforts to restart the stilled heart.

Interestingly, closed-chest massage considerably antedates direct or open-chest massage. The former method fell into disuse for many years in favor of direct or open-chest massage. Indeed, when the first edition of the textbook *Cardiac Arrest and Resuscitation* appeared in 1958, closed-chest cardiac massage was not directly mentioned as such. It was, however, stated:

> . . for some time it has been noted occasionally that a suspected case of cardiac arrest will respond successfully following a strong blow to the chest in the precordial area. Unfortunately, it is seldom a documented case. . . . An apparent case of cardiac arrest with multiple episodes responded twice in a period of several days to a strong blow on the precordium and [it was] urged that such a procedure be carried out in all cases before any incision [is] made. Mention should be made that on more than one occasion a heart in cardiac arrest has resumed normal nodal rhythm following a rather severe precordial concussion. As a general rule, precordial concussion refers to a sharp or abrupt blow with a folded fist upon the lower portion of the sternum or precordium.

Today the method of closed-chest cardiac massage is obviously considered to be a major part of the armamentarium of the physician in cases of cardiac arrest.

A HISTORIC REVIEW OF PROGRESS IN CARDIOPULMONARY RESUSCITATION

1543 Resuscitation in animals was described by Andreas Vesalius.

1628 William Harvey published his pioneer description of the circulation of blood and described resuscitation of a pigeon.

1679 Johann Wepfer described resuscitative efforts on a pharmacologic basis in *Circutae aquaticae historia et noxae.*

1755 John Hunter did classic experiments in resuscitating animals in Scotland.

1842 In his London surgery, E. Erichsen found that ligature of the coronary arteries caused death in dogs.

1850 Cardiac defibrillation was described for the first time by M. Hoffa and Carl Ludwig.

1858 Fifty cases of death from chloroform anesthesia were described by the London physician John Snow.

1871 Electropuncture of the heart for purposes of resuscitation was recommended by F. Steiner, an assistant of Billroth in Vienna.

1874 The method of Moritz Schiff for open-chest massage was first published by T. G. Hake in England. This year also brought the first description of a method of closed-chest resuscitation in animals by Louis Mickwitz in Dorpat, Estonia.

1878 Evidence that blood actually circulated during external heart massage was published by R. Boehm of Dorpat: *Concerning Resuscitation after Poisoning and Asphyxiation.*

1880 Ringer's solution was developed in London by Sidney Ringer, who also studied the action of blood salts on the activity of the heart.

1891 Using a modification of König's method, Maas, in Germany, was able to resuscitate two patients with cardiac arrest in incidents involving anesthesia, using closed-chest massage.

1898 A signal year in cardiac resuscitation: T. Tuffier achieved for the first time temporary return of the heartbeat and respiration by direct heart massage. Direct heart massage was also attempted by Gallet, de Liege, and Michaux in France. Moritz Schiff's resuscitative experiments were repeated by Tuffier, also in France.

1900 Direct heart massage was performed by Prus and repeated in Geneva by F. Batelli, who discovered a method of defibrillation with alternating current.

1901 The first complete resuscitation of a patient by direct heart massage was performed by Kristian Igelsrud in Norway. The French surgeon Mauclaire recommended the transdiaphragmatic approach for direct heart massage, and at the Fifth International Congress of Physiologists in Turin, J. Locke maintained cardiac action in the isolated heart of a rabbit for about 7 hours. Kuliabko of St. Petersburg stimulated isolated bird and mammalian hearts to beat and finally succeeded in postmortem restoration of cardiac activity in a human child.

1902 Sir W. A. Lane used the subdiaphragmatic approach to resuscitate successfully a patient's heart with direct massage, assisted by Gray.

1904 Probably the most thorough discussion of cardiac resuscitation, up to that time, was presented by Maurice d'Halluin in his book *Résurrection du coeur,* published in France.

1914 Indirect cardiac massage was described by Crile in his book *Anemia and Resuscitation,* published in the United States.

1915 By injecting a dye into the right ventricle and tracing its path, J. A. Gunn and P. A. Martin established additional proof of the auxiliary circulation during heart massage. This was done in Britain.

1947 Beck performed the first successful electrical defibrillation of the human heart. This milestone was reached after more than 10 years of research and technique and apparatus development.

(continued)

1952 Thoracic electrical stimulation was used in Boston by P. M. Zoll to induce heart beats in patients with Stokes–Adams syndrome.

1954 J. O. Elam and his group revived the concept of effective mouth-to-mouth insufflation as an ideal artificial ventilatory technique.

1955 The first successful resuscitation of a myocardial infarction victim with subsequent ventricular fibrillation occurring *outside the hospital* took place on June 22, 1955, in Cleveland. A physician suffered an apparently fatal heart attack and was carried into the nearby emergency room where his chest was opened and ventilation begun. The heart was successfully defibrillated, and the physician returned to his practice, where he continued until retirement at age 70.

1958 The present method of closed-chest cardiac massage was developed at Johns Hopkins Hospital in Baltimore by Kouvenhoven, Jude, and Knickerbocker.

By the time the fourth edition of *Cardiac Arrest and Resuscitation* was published in 1974, the method of closed-chest resuscitation was presented in detail.

Actually, attempts at closed-chest compression of the thorax antedate even those of Maas. The first application of such compression was probably performed by John Hovard in the mid-18th century. He himself abandoned the method, however, after he had the misfortune to break several ribs of a patient during a demonstration in front of a police inspector. Although several workers reported success thereafter with the technique of closed-chest compression, nearly 200 years were to elapse before it became popular and entrenched.

Efforts to train physicians and others in the techniques of cardiac resuscitation go back at least 26 years. In September 1950, at Bellevue Hospital, a course on cardiac resuscitation was offered periodically by the New York University Postgraduate Medical School. In that same year a course was presented by Beck and Leighninger in Cleveland.

Many interesting historical vignettes could be related on this subject. One such vignette concerns Charles C. Guthrie (Fig. 38-1). As one of the pioneers in vascular surgery, Guthrie, along with his associates, did a great deal of original investigative work on cardiopulmonary resuscitation during the early part of this century. Along with Alexis Carrel, Guthrie first showed that vascular anastomoses could be done with consistently successful results in animals. They pioneered in organ transplantation and replantation of limbs. In 1908, Pike, Guthrie, and Stewart published their work on resuscitation which had been started in 1903 in the physiological laboratories of Western Reserve University, before their work in the Hull Physiological Laboratories of the University of Chicago. They made numerous attempts to start the heart without recourse to opening the thoracic cavity. In commenting on extrathoracic massage, they state

> Rhythmical compression of the thorax over the heart by means of the hands has given fairly good results in certain stages of the heart stoppage; the time when such massage is effective is, however, much too limited to

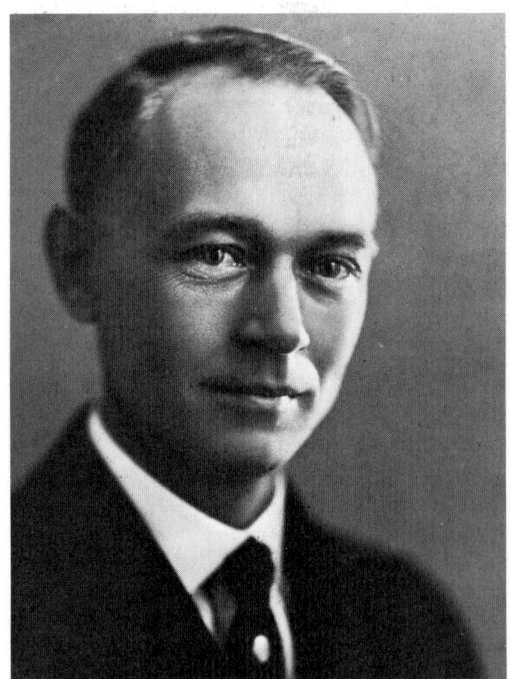

Fig. 38-1. Charles Claude Guthrie, pioneer in vascular surgery, who worked with Alexis Carrel at the Hull Physiological Laboratory at the University of Chicago in 1905 and 1906. They were active in many aspects of organ transplantation and vascular surgery. In addition, Guthrie investigated the comparative advantages of closed- and open-chest resuscitation almost 70 years ago.

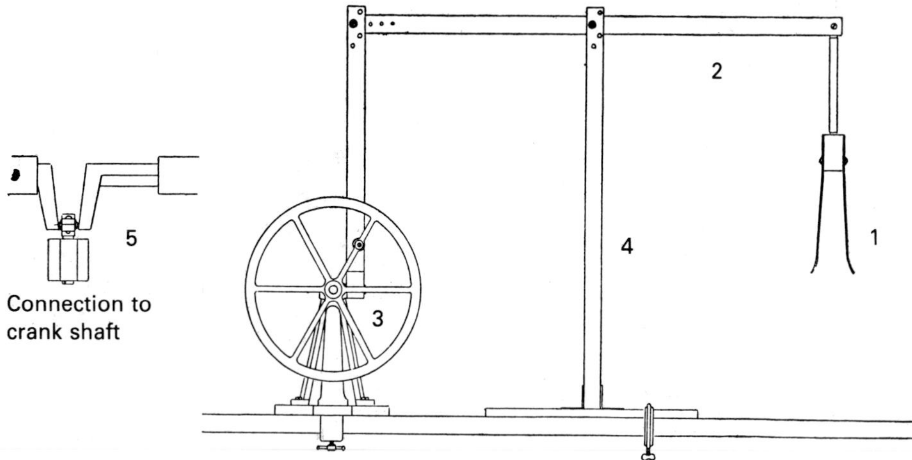

Fig. 38-2. In an effort to develop an effective means of closed-chest cardiac compression, J. L. Kessler, working with Guthrie, developed the apparatus pictured here, which was a predecessor of closed-chest compression units developed almost 7 decades later. A hand-operated crank (3) operated a chest compression bellows (1).

> make the method a sure one. Rhythmical compression of the thorax is efficient up to three to five minutes after the cessation of the external pulse, but it is probable that in every case of successful resuscitation by this method, the heart has not entirely ceased beating.[12]

They cite one case of successful resuscitation of a cat by closed-chest massage, done on May 21, 1905. They further comment that rhythmical compression of the thorax of a large dog at a necessary rate for resuscitation was exceedingly laborious and that it was difficult for them to maintain massage for a sufficiently long time. This prompted them to devise a machine for closed-chest compression. Figure 38-2 may well represent the first closed-chest compression machine. Pike, Guthrie, and Stewart credit one of their associates, J. L. Kessler, as the designer.

Interestingly, these workers also tied a cannula in the pericardial sac and connected the pericardium with a syringe filled with water. Rhythmic pressure on the syringe was applied to increase the intrapericardial pressure. Years later in Milan, Bencini reported a "pneumomassage" technique very similar to this.[2]

In 1954, J. O. Elam and his group revived the concept of effective mouth-to-mouth insufflation as an ideal method for artificial ventilation. Elam has continued to pioneer in various aspects of cardiopulmonary resuscitation, particularly artificial ventilation.[10]

Establishing an entirely accurate historical perspective of the various aspects of artificial ventilation in cardiac resuscitation is extremely difficult because many of our present efforts stem from activities going back at least to Biblical days. Mouth-to-mouth resuscitation is such an example.

WHO IS RESPONSIBLE FOR ADMINISTERING CPR?

Obviously cardiac arrest can no longer be regarded as an emergency confined to the hospital. Since either sudden cardiac standstill or ventricular fibrillation may occur in or outside the hospital, there must be a total commitment by the entire medical community to the idea that most cases of cardiac arrest are salvageable if adequate measures are applied within a sufficient time limit. In the hospital this commitment implies the presence of a *cardiac resuscitation committee.* Operating under the direction of this committee will be a day and night resuscitation or "stat" team, an ongoing hospital training program, and proper maintenance of all resuscitation equipment. A meaningful record system is essential.

Responsibility for successful cardiac resuscitation by the hospital includes at least the following definitive steps.

1. All hospital personnel should have proper instruction in at least basic methods of cardiopulmonary resuscitation regardless of their staff positions.

2. Mandatory attendance should be required for regularly scheduled conferences relating to cardiac resuscitation.
3. Repetitive practice sessions in procedures such as cardiac compression, electrical defibrillation of the heart, artificial ventilation, and related techniques should be provided for all members of the staff.
4. Proper resuscitative equipment should be in working condition and easily accessible in all parts of the hospital at all times.

A day-to-day review of resuscitative efforts within the hospital will inevitably improve the techniques and results of resuscitation and will demonstrate areas of weakness in communication and equipment needs. Coordination of such a review is an important function of the resuscitation committee.

The resuscitation committee should be set up as a permanent hospital committee. There should be regular meetings and active supervision of the resuscitation team. The composition of this team will vary with the type of hospital being served. In some hospitals, a medical resident or fellow in cardiology, a surgical resident, a respiratory therapist, and an anesthesiologist may constitute the team. The composition of the team will, however, vary from hospital to hospital. The committee is responsible for providing a continuing program of resuscitation instruction to all hospital personnel because of the rapid turnover of personnel in most institutions.

The committee should have an especially designated office or area devoted to its function. If resources permit, the employment of a secretary by this committee will aid in maintaining all records of resuscitation and in collecting data for the committee, as well as maintaining an effective library on the subject. The secretary should be responsible for scheduling retraining sessions at periodic intervals and for maintaining and supervising the use of cardiac resuscitation teaching slides, audiovisual aids, and training manikins.

A monthly schedule delineating the daily assignment of each member of the resuscitation team is needed so that each team member will remain in the hospital at all times when he is on call. Periodic drills should be conducted to determine the efficiency and promptness of the team's response to resuscitation calls. Frequently the junior members of the team will have night duty. It is essential that the cardiac resuscitation team feel confident that each member, regardless of the hour, is well versed in all aspects of resuscitation. The team must have the full support of the administrative structure with enough delegated responsibility to carry out its task. The team's budgetary needs should receive high priority.

Soon after every instance of cardiac arrest, a critique session must be held. The sooner the session is held, the more significance it will have. Technical errors will be more likely to be visible, suggestions will be more pertinent, and the overall benefit to all personnel will be greatly increased.

Record keeping in connection with a hospital's plan of action is important. Thus far there has not been a generally accepted cardiac arrest report form; obviously each record should have sufficient identifying data and information on the events leading to the arrest and the underlying pathology of a possibly contributory nature. Notes should be made of how the arrest was diagnosed and under what conditions, what the initial resuscitative efforts were and how soon after the arrest they were employed, what kind of ventilation and cardiac massage were given, and what drugs were given, as well as the time and dosage.

A sample flow-chart of the type in use at the University of Missouri–Columbia Health Sciences Center appears in Figure 38-3. It is completed by the personnel present at the time of the cardiac arrest.

Data sheets on cardiac arrests should be reviewed each month by the cardiopulmonary resuscitation committee, and any obvious shortcomings or deficiencies in the program should be noted carefully so that steps can be taken toward their correction. Only then may one obtain a comprehensive picture of the sequence of events with a satisfactory degree of accuracy. Only an accurate analysis of what has been done can lead the committee toward the always elusive goal of 100% successful resuscitation.

The matter of *communication* is vitally important in initiating cardiopulmonary resuscitative efforts. The telephone loudspeaker paging system, pocket page systems, or vital paging systems may all be involved, but a definite plan must be worked out whereby the most rapid and expeditious assembling of the team occurs. In areas of the hospital covered by a single nurse, this nurse may be diverted from her role of making initial resuscitative efforts while she notifies the switchboard, or a single telephone operator frequently must notify individual house staff members in numerous on-call rooms, and during this period the switchboard is diverted from other functions. These approaches clearly are unacceptable.

A recorded alert message may well be designed into the telephone system of an institution that be-

UNIVERSITY OF MISSOURI-COLUMBIA
MEDICAL CENTER
TRAUMA & CARDIO-PULMONARY
RESUSCITATION RECORD

VITAL SIGNS

Time	B/P	Pulse	Resp.	Pupils

Date: ________ Location: ________

Resuscitation Started: ________ Stopped: ________

Intubated by: ________ Time: ________

Ventilator: ________ $\%O_2$ ________

Airway: ________

Medication Nurses Signatures: ________

Ordering Physicians Signature: ________

Pt's. Post-Code Status: ________

PROCEDURES/ LAB WORK

TIMES/DOSAGES/INITIALS

$NaHCO_3$										
Lidocaine										
Epinephrine										
Atropine										
Defibrillation										

IV SOLUTIONS

Started	Amount, Solution, Medication	Stopped	Amount Rec'd	Initials

Recording Nurse:

MR-076B-Z-79

Sheet # ________

Fig. 38-3. Sample of a flow chart used to record the events that occur during a cardiopulmonary arrest.

comes operative whenever a certain low-digit number is dialed or even when certain handsets are lifted. These techniques might well be in the anesthesia department, the anesthesia on-call room, the emergency room, the physicians' on-call room, the heart station, the intensive care unit, the interns' quarters, and certain other on-call rooms or physicians' offices, as well as respiratory therapy offices, certain conference rooms where physicians are likely to be, and certain outpatient facilities. The hospital administration must, of course, be responsible for a workable system of emergency alert. With increasing sophistication of electronic equipment, many possibilities suggest themselves. Since time continues to be the key factor in all successful resuscitative efforts, the best hospital plan of action will revolve around the most efficient means of assembling the staff to allow rapid institution of resuscitative procedures.

In many situations, the elevator system may provide the stumbling block in speedy institution of resuscitative efforts. The use of automated control equipment, activated by the same telephone or paging system described above, may be used to activate a locking relay that interrupts the normal elevator traffic and diverts the car to the floor where an emergency equipment cart is located. A second car bypasses other floors and automatically transports personnel to the floor where the emergency exists.

Hospital preparations for the emergency of cardiac arrest will include provision of one or more readily accessible portable resuscitation carts that will contain such essential equipment as a resuscitation board, airways, direct current defibrillator, suction apparatus, positive pressure ventilator, venous cutdown set, laryngoscope and endotracheal tubes, drugs for emergency use (such as epinephrine, sodium bicarbonate, calcium chloride, lidocaine, procainamide, and atropine), and a portable electrocardiogram recorder. To avoid the obvious problem with nonfunctioning equipment, outdated or missing drugs, and inadequacy of vital pieces of equipment, a *designated* person or department should have responsibility for cleaning, replacing, and checking equipment. This department may vary from hospital to hospital (for example, nursing service, respiratory therapy, or central service department). Defibrillator paddles and patient electrodes must be cleaned conscientiously and the monitor–defibrillator checked at least twice a week by a technician who goes to each area in which a unit is located. Each machine is plugged into a standard electrical outlet and turned on, and the leads are connected to a heart stimulator to test its particular operation.

"CARDIAC ARREST": DIAGNOSIS

Cardiac arrest seldom occurs without warning signs of some sort, but these signs may be most subtle and extremely varied. All too frequently the blood pressure and pulse suddenly disappear, and, on inspection, the heart is found to be in complete standstill or, more often, in fibrillation. Even in a hospital setting, cardiac arrest may well represent a "sudden and unexplained" occurrence, and, on very sophisticated intensive care wards, life-threatening arrhythmias may occur without warning.

There is a period of time during which reversibility (and resuscitation) is possible in *almost every case* of cardiac arrest. More patients lose their chance for total recovery during the very critical period between an arrest and diagnosis than at any other time in the resuscitative period. While the absence of heart sounds on auscultation usually will indicate inadequate cardiac output, complete cardiac standstill is not necessarily implied. Prolonged stethoscopic auscultation should be avoided. The time factor obviously precludes spending much time in reviewing what may be unreliable evidence of heart action, once the blood pressure has fallen to zero and the pulse has ceased. Generally, however, heart sounds resume about the same point that circulation does.

Abrupt cardiopulmonary failure may not always have a cardiac basis but may simply involve respiratory failure with subsequent cardiac arrhythmia or arrest. Hyperventilation and convulsive action may characterize sudden hypoxia or complete anoxia, or there may eventually be agonal, gasping respiratory activity. The blood pressure usually rises temporarily only to fall precipitously. These abrupt failures may occur after various instances of airway obstruction, near-drowning, drug overdose, electrical shock, and other causes. Ventilatory disturbances *per se* are not infrequent causes of cardiac arrhythmias. Hypoxia and hypercarbia may not be as easy to identify as one might assume because few patients show classic signs of these conditions.

Unfortunately, on occasion, the first thing noted is cessation of respiration, when actual circulatory arrest may have been present initially. Sudden cessation of heart action frequently may be followed by a few agonal respiratory efforts. In any case, if effectiveness of respiration is difficult to ascertain quickly, one should conclude that ventilation is inadequate regardless of the cause.

Ophthalmologic evidence of cardiac arrest has received attention, but, as with most of the so-called classic signs, there is room for considerable dispute.

Pupillary diameter does increase markedly when circulatory arrest occurs, but, because there is an appreciable lag (30–40 sec) between cessation of cardiac output and full pupillary dilatation, it is desirable that resuscitation be started before such dilatation occurs. The pupils may, indeed, be very small, even after death in certain cases, specifically if the patient has received morphine sulphate or other opiates. Patients who are receiving atropine, quinidine, or epinephrine, as well as those under hypothermia, may continually exhibit varying degrees of pupillary dilatation. Funduscopic examination may show segmentation of the retinal venous columns and disappearance of the retinal arterial pattern within a minute or so of cessation of cardiac output. Although these findings are of considerable diagnostic value, they are rather academic, since other physical findings are more easily discernible, and at an earlier stage.

"Cardiac arrest" continues to be a wastebasket diagnosis, but no better term is available in discussing problems related to the acutely arrested circulation. Many different terms have been substituted to denote more precisely the actual situation, but without any success. The term cardiac arrest serves a useful purpose despite some of the obvious disadvantages implied by the designation. Most instances that require cardiopulmonary resuscitation present no initial clear-cut delineation of the etiology involved, thus obviating use of a more appropriate term for the state of an acutely arrested heart, whether it be in ventricular fibrillation or in asystole.

Definitions of cardiac arrest range from a description of the clinical picture of cessation of circulation (unconsciousness, pulselessness of large arteries, cyanosis, and apnea in a person who had not been expected to die at the time) to failure of the heart action to maintain an adequate cerebral circulation in the absence of a causative or irreversible disease.

EMERGENCY AIRWAY MANAGEMENT*

The importance of providing and maintaining an adequate patent airway in emergency situations which arise in the general medical–surgical institution has been established. There are numerous mechanical methods for providing a patent airway, including those techniques of hyperextension of the neck, nasal and oral airways, and endotracheal devices. The superior expertise of the anesthesiologist and nurse anesthetist is recognized in providing this care; but, in many hospitals anesthesiologists and nurse anesthetists may not be available to provide immediate emergency airway management in situations where time is a critical factor. Therefore, it is reasonable and correct to assume that under these circumstances, respiratory therapy personnel, after being qualified by medical direction, are suitable individuals to provide such airway management.

*Position statement on emergency airway management adopted by the American Association for Respiratory Therapy and its Board of Medical Advisors in 1973.

AIRWAY MANAGEMENT AND VENTILATION

Many aspects of airway management and ventilation have been discussed elsewhere in *Respiratory Care*. Although some duplication is desirable for emphasis, most of the material on this subject pertains particularly to the patient who needs artificial ventilation because of a cardiopulmonary arrest.

The well-trained respiratory therapist is an especially valuable member of any hospital resuscitation team because of his intimate knowledge and proven competency in the acquisition and maintenance of an adequate airway and proper ventilation. Unquestionably, the failure of many resuscitative attempts rests with inadequate management of the airway and ventilation. In fact, one of the most difficult aspects of training personnel in cardiopulmonary resuscitation is centered in this area.

Currently, trained respiratory therapists are experienced in emergency airway management; some states have statutes specifically allowing them to intubate patients when no person with more advanced skills is present (*see* below).

The background of the respiratory therapist includes a thorough education in airway anatomy and physiology and the hazards and complications of airway maintenance. In addition, the work requires them to possess good psychomotor skills. Table 38-1 illustrates that when this foundation is supplemented by an adequate training program, with regular opportunities given to attempt emergency intubation, the respiratory therapist can perform this life-saving procedure safely and effectively.

The basic life-support measures relating to artificial ventilation as adopted by the National Conference on Standards for Cardiopulmonary Resuscitation and Emergency Cardiac Care at the Washington Conference in May 1973, and the changes made in 1980, need to be continually stressed in all teaching efforts of hospital personnel.[17] Except in certain circum-

Table 38-1. Complications of Emergency Endotracheal Intubation Attempts, Classified by Intubator Status

	STATUS OF INTUBATOR				
COMPLICATION	*Respiratory Care Personnel*	*Emergency Department Physician*	*Anesthesiologist*	*Nurse Anesthetist*	*Staff Physician*
Prolonged intubation (>3 min)	0	3	1	0	2
Aspiration	0	0	1	0	0
Esophageal intubation	7	13	2	0	5
Right mainstem bronchial intubation	3	0	3	0	2
Oral trauma	0	1	0	0	0
Unsuccessful attempt	3	4	0	0	0
Arrhythmias	0	0	1	0	1
Total complications	13	21	8	0	10
Number of attempts	74	29	30	5	5
Percentage of complications/attempt	18	72	27	0	200

(Cokley JM, Smith DJ: Emergency endotracheal intubation by respiratory care personnel in a community hospital. Respir Care 26:336, 1981)

stances with a witnessed cardiac arrest or in a person who is being monitored, first attention should be directed toward establishing an adequate airway followed by ventilation. To ensure that the victim's airway is opened, his head is first tilted backward as far as possible by the operator, who places his hand beneath the patient's neck and lifts, while, with his other hand, he tilts the patient's head by pressure on the forehead (Fig. 38-4). The neck is extended, and the tongue is thus lifted away from the back of the throat. In teaching airway management to others, the respiratory therapist must continually emphasize the frequency with which the tongue can occlude the airway by dropping against the back of the throat. The hypopharynx is opened in 70% to 80% of unconscious patients simply by tilting the head backward.

Frequently one observes spontaneous respiration immediately after an adequate airway has been established, but of course with a full cardiopulmonary arrest both artificial ventilation and circulation are required. *Rescue breathing* must be started promptly either by mouth-to-nose or mouth-to-mouth breathing. If the latter technique is used, one pinches the patient's nostrils together with the thumb and index finger of the hand, which is also exerting continuous pressure on the forehead to maintain the tilted head. One then blows into the patient's mouth after taking each of four, deep, quick breaths while making a tight seal with one's mouth around the patient's mouth. By turning one's head toward the patient's chest, one can observe chest expansion. By seeing the chest rise and fall, by noting the resistance and compliance characteristics of the patient's lungs as they expand, and by hearing and feeling the air escape during exhalation, one is assured of air exchange.

One of the most common errors in resuscitation of the unconscious patient lies in failing to maintain an open airway! In the flurry of attention to the diverse matters involved in meeting the crisis of cardiopulmonary arrest, one may temporarily lose sight of the obviously simple physiological fact that there must be a clear, open pathway for oxygen to reach the lungs of the patient before any other resuscitative activities, no matter how sophisticated, will help him.

In our experience, one of the most difficult aspects of training personnel for cardiopulmonary resuscitation has been in establishing the patent airway and adequate ventilation. We have been impressed with the difficulty many physicians have had in establishing "ventilation," even on the Resusci–Anne manikin. In cases of cardiac arrest where resuscitation of the heart cannot be achieved, it will frequently be noticed that *adequate exchange of air in the lungs is not occurring.* Diverse problems may arise in the establishment of the airway, but basically two simple situations present themselves over and over again: The base of the tongue may have shifted posteriorly to occlude the airway by pressure against the posterior

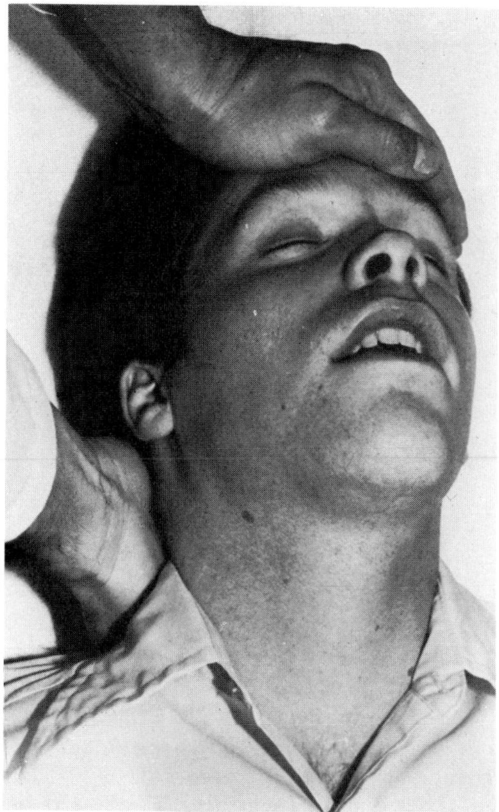

Fig. 38-4. The head tilt method of opening the upper airway (*see* text).

pharyngeal wall; or the neck may be flexed on the anterior chest wall (Fig. 38-5B).

COPING WITH AIRWAY OBSTRUCTION

Complete obstruction of the airway for longer than 5 minutes will cause death. Infants may tolerate slightly longer periods of asphyxia, but the time-honored 4- to 5-minute period is a good average to remember and is an accurate indicator of how rapidly the airway obstruction must be relieved. Of course, the oxygenation status of the patient at the start of the period of asphyxia is directly related to his ability to withstand the insult. The resulting hypoxia and the accumulation of carbon dioxide obviously represent an emergency of almost the same proportions as sudden cessation of cardiac output. The heart may continue to beat, in fact, for several minutes under conditions of asphyxia, but all available oxygen stores are rapidly depleted, cardiac output becomes ineffective, and ventricular fibrillation may be initiated.

It is estimated that foreign body obstruction of the airway ranks sixth as a cause of accidental death in the United States. The National Safety Council estimates that there were 3100 deaths in 1975 from foreign body obstruction of the airway. Most airway obstructions occur during eating, with pieces of meat being the usual obstructing agent. Associated elevated blood alcohol levels, loose dentures, or poorly chewed food may be contributing factors.

Airway obstruction should be easily recognized, but this is not always the case. Merely positioning the patient improperly, with neck muscles and head relaxed and the neck in a partially flexed position, may be sufficient to obstruct the airway, even if the tongue does not become so relaxed as to press against the posterior pharyngeal wall. Not all victims of airway obstruction become cyanotic. An actual vasodilatation may be set off by the hypoxemia that is present. Even the color of the nail beds, mucous membranes, or conjunctiva may be misleading, particularly if the patient is dark-skinned. One cannot rely on the presence or absence of noticeable respiratory movements. Patients somnolent from hypercarbia or those suffering from massive drug overdoses may present in such a profound state of hypoventilation that one may need to hold a wisp of cleansing tissue in front of the patient's mouth or nose to detect any air movement. Obstruction of the airway need not, of course, be complete. If the degree of obstruction is severe enough, intrathoracic pressure fluctuations are increased along with the efforts of breathing. Gradually, however, the respiratory centers become less sensitive to the usual stimuli caused by increasing carbon dioxide tension.

Severe or even complete airway obstruction is indicated by marked activity of the accessory muscles of respiration in the neck, supraclavicular, and intercostal areas. If the airway obstruction is complete, one will hear no sounds of air flow; if it is incomplete, various degrees of noise intensity may be provoked, depending on the degree of obstruction. Crowing, gurgling, wheezing, or snoring may be indications of partial airway obstruction. The experienced respiratory therapist can frequently suspect an obstruction at either the bronchial, laryngeal, or hypopharyngeal level, depending on the character of the noise.

Breathing efforts are stimulated first by partial airway obstruction, and then normal or low Pa_{CO_2} and normal or low Pa_{O_2} determinations may be seen. Shortly before coma, apnea, or cardiac arrest, the Pa_{O_2} rapidly decreases and the Pa_{CO_2} increases.

Safar, who has effectively addressed himself to the management of emergency airway control, rec-

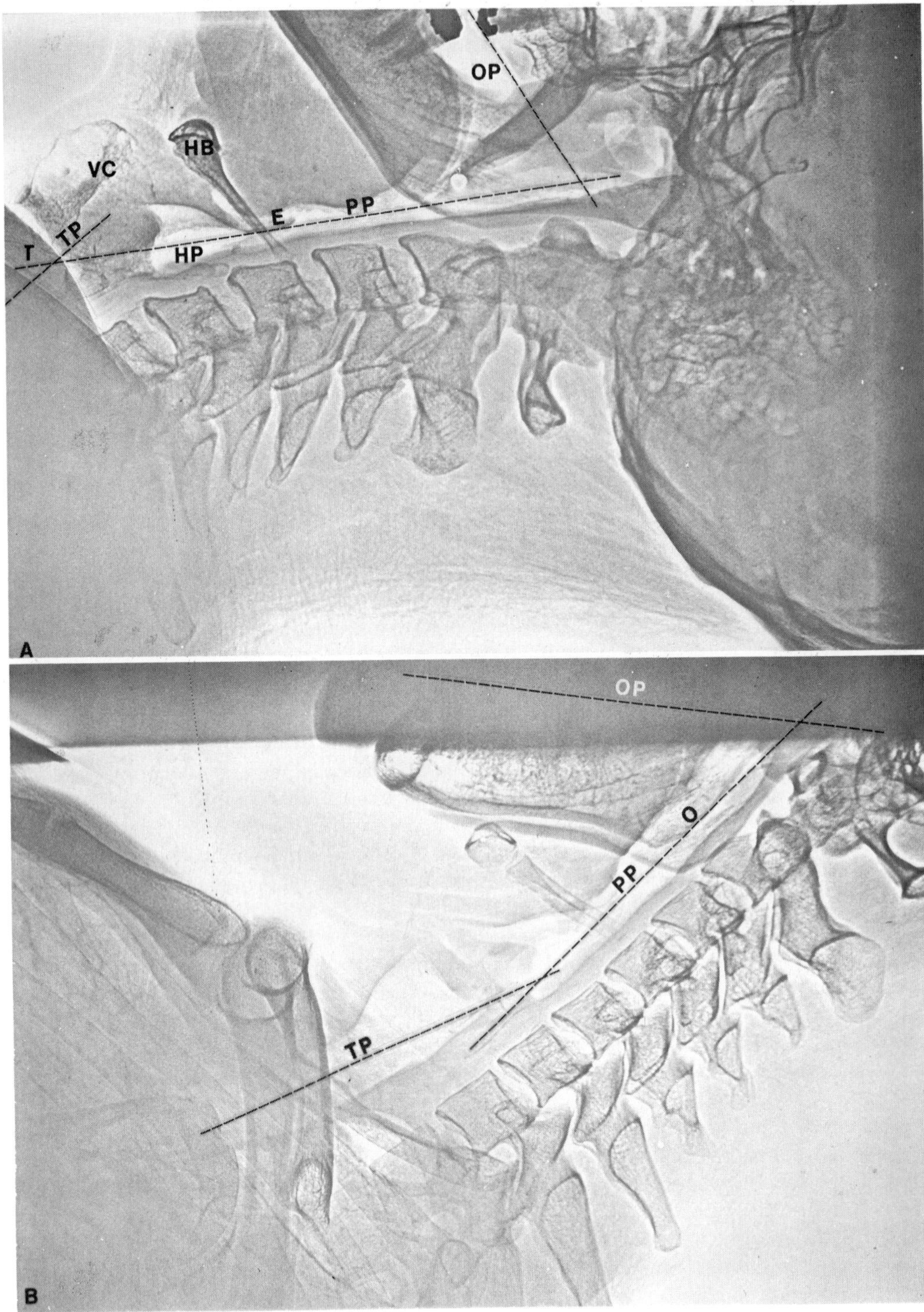

Fig. 38-5. Xeroradiographs of the head and neck in various positions in which intubation might be attempted. *(A)* The pure supine or "neutral" position. *(B)* Head and neck flexed, demonstrating marked angulation between the oral and pharyngeal planes and constriction of the pharyngeal air column. *(C)* Head and neck hyperextended. Note the angulation between the pharyngeal and tracheal planes. *(D)* The "sniffing" or modified Jackson position, the optimal choice because of the minimal angulation between the pharyngeal and

(continued)

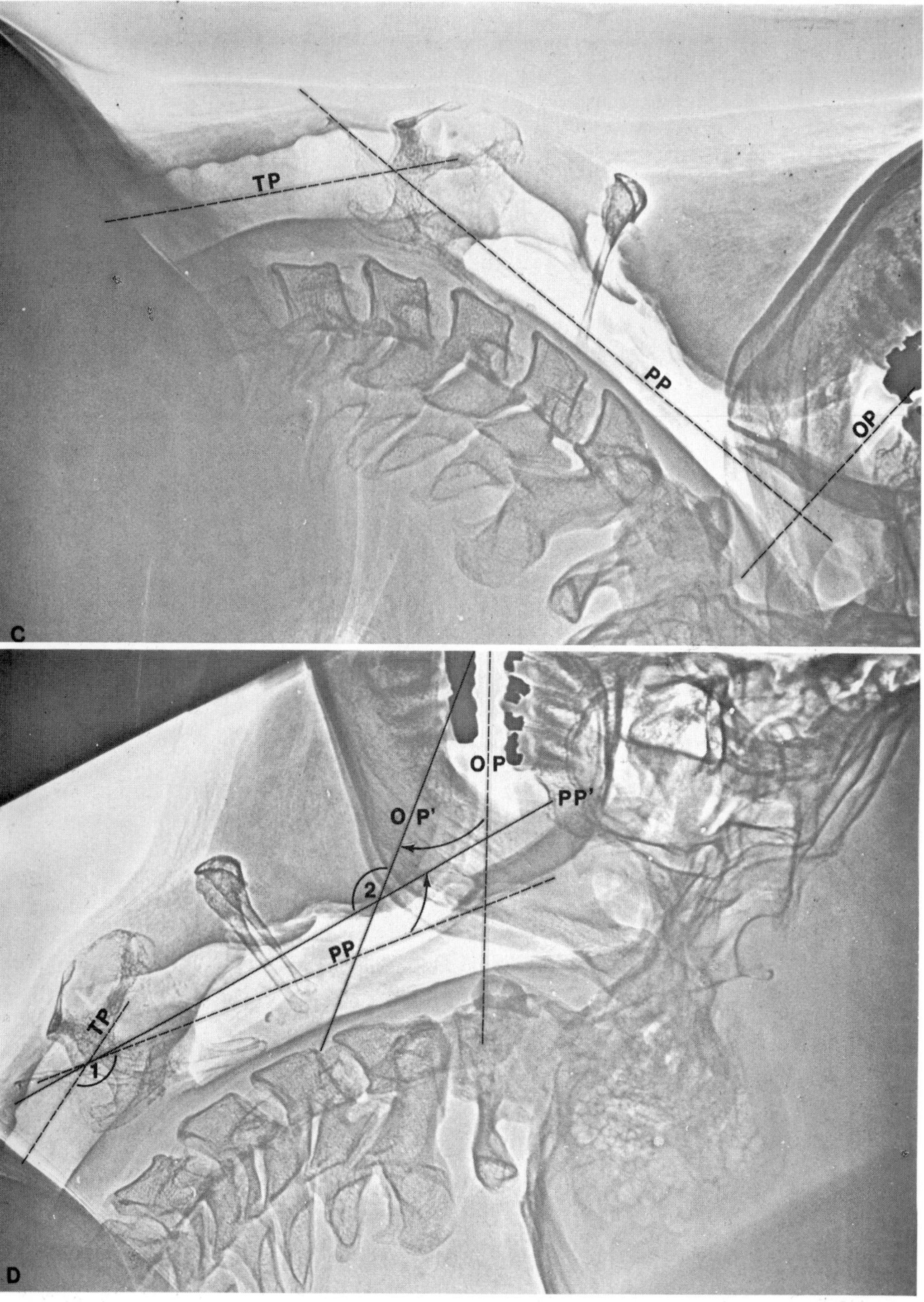

tracheal planes. Arrows in *D* indicate the effects of finger pressure on the thyroid cartilage and lifting upward and forward of the head, which optimize angles 1 and 2 for easiest intubation. T = trachea; TP = tracheal plane; VC = vocal cords; HP = hypopharynx; HB = hyoid bone; E = epiglottis; PP = pharyngeal plane; PP′ = pharyngeal plane with forward head tilt; OP = oral plane; OP′ = oral plane in sniffing position.

ommends that with each step taken for control of upper airway obstruction, one must make efforts at positive pressure inflation with either exhaled air (16–19% oxygen), compressed air, or 100% oxygen.[24] He stresses that airway obstruction may be overcome, at least partly, by positive pressure inflation, which may also help overcome laryngospasm, if present.

Safar places emphasis on seven specific points in the management of the airway.

1. *Positioning.* The unconscious patient should be placed in a supine position with the head tilted back. The patient should not be placed in the prone position because the face becomes inaccessible for mouth-to-mouth respiration and such a position may further promote mechanical obstruction.
2. *Tilting the head backward* (*see* Fig. 38-5C). This is, perhaps, the most effective step in promoting an open airway in the unconscious patient. By placing one hand under the patient's neck and the other hand on the patient's forehead (see Fig. 38-4), the tissues within the larynx and the mandible are stretched and the base of the tongue is lifted away from the posterior pharyngeal wall. In some instances, elevation of the patient's shoulders may further facilitate the tilting of his head. The patient's mouth will usually open when the head is tilted back, and this may indeed be helpful when there is a partial or complete nasal obstruction.
3. *Positive airway pressure.* One may apply mouth-to-mouth or mouth-to-nose respiration by exhaling into the patient's air passages. This may well help to overcome any obstruction by increasing the pressure gradient for airflow and by dilating the air passages.
4. *Forward displacement of the mandible.* In approximately one fifth of the patients, the preceding three steps will not result in an open airway, and an additional maneuver should be performed—namely, the forward displacement of the mandible, which can be done simply by lifting with hand at the ascending rami or by placing the thumb in the mouth and pulling the mandible forward. If the mouth does open with the backward tilting of the head, then the patient's lips and teeth should be separated in the event that an expiratory nasal obstruction is present. This procedure is called the "triple airway maneuver" (Fig. 38-6).

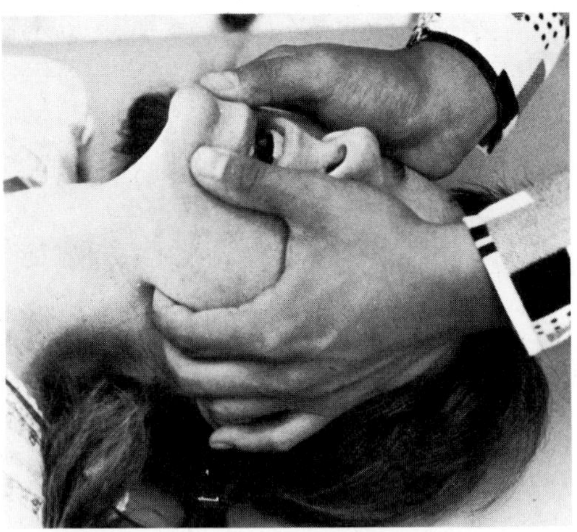

Fig. 38-6. The "triple airway" maneuver. Forward displacement of the mandible results in further opening of the upper airway (*see* also Fig. 38-5D).

5. *Foreign body in the back of the pharynx.* By turning the patient's head to the side, pushing the mouth open, and wiping the pharynx and mouth clean, the fingers may quickly remove a foreign body that may be in the back of the pharynx; on the other hand, suction may be necessary. Obviously one must not risk further spinal cord damage by twisting the cervical spine in cases of possible neck fracture.
6. *Artificial oral airways* (*see* Chap. 21). To hold the base of the tongue forward and to maintain the lips and teeth in an open position, one may need to use oral airways. A nasopharyngeal tube may be particularly valuable in the patient with trismus (spasm of the jaw muscles). The familiar S-shaped oral pharyngeal airway may be used as may the simple, comma-shaped Guedel airway. If a nasopharyngeal tube is not available, the mouth may be forced open by sliding the index finger backward between the cheek and the teeth and then wedging the tip of the index finger behind the last molars. If the jaws are not clenched, the tube may be inserted by forcing the mouth open with the thumb and index finger crossed while inserting the tube over the tongue and twisting it into position. With the Brook airway, hyperextension of the victim's head prevents any throat obstruction by the tongue. Unlike the oral pharyngeal airway, it is unlikely to stimulate vomiting and thereby cause aspiration of the gastric contents in the partially comatose patient. (A word of caution: an oral airway

may occasionally reach beyond the pharynx and obstruct the air passage by impacting the epiglottis. This obviously must be avoided.)

7. *Tracheal intubation.* When the tracheobronchial tree must be suctioned rapidly, when gastric contents have been aspirated, and when the above steps have been ineffective in maintaining adequate oxygenation, rapid insertion of an endotracheal tube is indicated. Obviously, in many emergency situations, an endotracheal tube and the proper insertion material may not be available but should be part of the equipment on every ambulance and emergency cart. The endotracheal tube will not be tolerated easily by the conscious or even the partially conscious patient. The respiratory therapist, of course, will have become well versed in using the endotracheal tube and will be able to intubate the trachea rapidly. In difficult cases, intubation over a fiberoptic stylet laryngoscope may be necessary (Fig. 38-7).

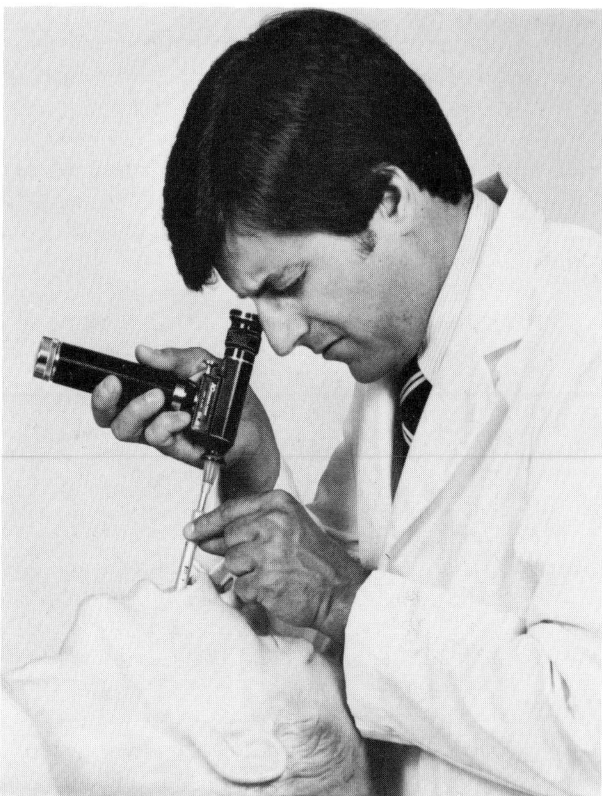

Fig. 38-7. The fiberoptic stylet laryngoscope is a new development that aids in intubation during airway obstruction. It uses the principle of fiberoptics, combined with a malleable stylet. The endotracheal tube is advanced while visualization is maintained. It is of particular aid when movement of the mouth, jaw, head, and neck is limited.

An additional consideration in the all-important matter of maintaining an open airway is the condition frequently termed the "café coronary." This refers to the clinical observation that suggests an apparent sudden heart attack when actually there has been inadvertent aspiration of a bolus of food with airway obstruction and often death. Aspirated foreign bodies are responsible for an inordinately large percentage of accidental deaths in the young child as well.

Few emergency care measures have received such widespread interest among laymen as has the so-called *Heimlich maneuver* for removing the foreign body obstruction of the airway by manual upper abdominal compression.[13] The victim whose airway is suddenly obstructed by a large object or food cannot cough, speak, or breathe if the obstruction is complete. After clutching at his throat, the victim becomes cyanotic and collapses. If the strangling victim can cough, speak, or breathe, no actions are necessary because his own spontaneous coughs will likely be more effective than any artificial cough maneuver. One must act immediately, however, if the patient cannot cough, speak, or breathe. Two to four back blows should be delivered quickly, and, if ineffective, one should encircle the person's upper abdomen with one's arms and deliver a series of four to six compressions (Fig. 38-8). The foreign body will often be coughed up and out. If there is still no improvement, repeat the back blows and the abdominal compression efforts.

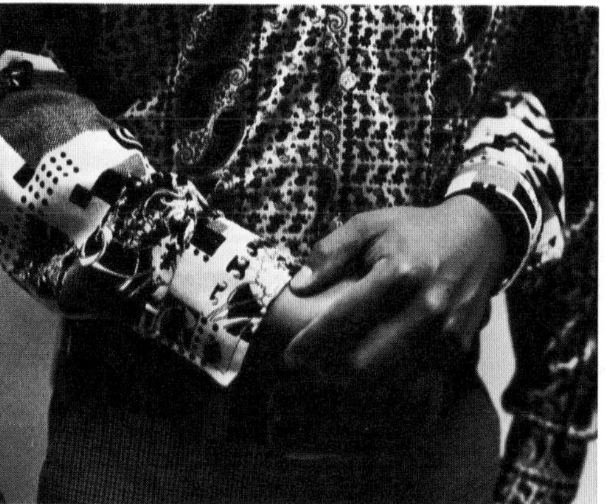

Fig. 38-8. The Heimlich maneuver, used to expel aspirated food or other objects from the trachea and oropharynx. The technique is discussed in detail in the text.

MANAGEMENT OF THE UNWITNESSED CARDIAC ARREST

1. Kneel at the patient's side.
2. Determine unconsciousness.
3. If the patient is unconscious, tilt the head and check for breathing.
4. If the patient is not breathing, give four quick breaths.
5. If unable to ventilate, use the tongue–jaw lift maneuver and attempt one-finger extrication.
6. Palpate for carotid pulse. If the patient is pulseless, begin external cardiac massage.†
7. If this ventilation is still unsuccessful, roll the patient toward you onto his side and deliver a series of two to four back blows.
8. Next, roll the patient onto his back and deliver a series of four to six supine inward compressions beneath the axillae.
9. Repeat tongue–jaw lift and one-finger extrication because the foreign body may now have been forced into a position where one may be able to retrieve it.
10. If still unsuccessful, attempt mouth-to-nose ventilation.
11. If still unable to ventilate the patient, repeat the series of back blows, chest compressions, tongue–jaw lift, and finger extrication maneuvers between attempts to ventilate, since the muscles of the throat become increasingly relaxed as the patient becomes more hypoxic, and thus one's efforts may become increasingly effective.

*The procedures should be done in the order listed and performed as rapidly as possible.
†Cardiac massage may then be continued by a second rescuer, using the single rescuer technique, or cardiac compression may be delivered intermittently.

If a previously unwitnessed victim of strangulation is encountered in the unconscious state, one obviously will not be aware of the presence or absence of a foreign body and should proceed as one would for an unwitnessed cardiac arrest, as outlined below.

In an infant, back blows are aided by gravity. With the patient in a head-down position, the foreign body will occasionally drop out of the mouth. External cardiac compression is obviously of little value for a foreign object obstruction unless cardiac arrest and aspiration coexist.

Investigative work by Guildner shows that airflow and pressures resulting from a low chest squeeze are markedly greater than those resulting from an abdominal squeeze.[11] The low chest squeeze can easily and quickly be applied in the horizontal position. Guildner recommends that if one witnesses a "café coronary" and the victim cannot talk, cough, groan, or breathe, total obstruction is likely present, and one should quickly position oneself behind the victim (often still standing or sitting), lean him forward, and apply the low chest squeeze promptly and vigorously. He emphasizes that the technique can be used in children by placing only one arm around the chest, or in infants by picking them up and inverting the infant over the arm of the rescuer, where a quick compression is delivered between the child's shoulder blades.

Guildner has compared the three techniques for opening an airway obstructed by the tongue: neck lift, chin lift, or jaw thrust. Consistently, the chin-lift technique provides the most consistent adequate airway. In a surprisingly large number of unconscious patients, he found that the head-tilt method does not relieve the airway obstruction produced by the backward movement of the tongue when the jaw is relaxed. He believes that the lower jaw often needs support to lift the tongue sufficiently away from the throat to provide an open airway. When the chin is lifted, the lower jaw moves forward, and with it the tongue. Another advantage of the chin-lift maneuver is that it will facilitate holding the patient's dentures, if present, securely in position.

For a more detailed discussion of management of the obstructed airway, the reader is referred to recent specific instructions offered for situations where the patient is sitting, standing, conscious, or unconscious. Comparisons are made of the effectiveness of chest thrusts, abdominal thrusts, and back blows in each of these situations.[26]

MOUTH-TO-MOUTH ARTIFICIAL RESPIRATION

An effective pulmonary resuscitation unit lies within each person. The air around us contains more than 20% oxygen and about 0.04% carbon dioxide. Exhaled air contains 16% to 19% oxygen and approximately 4% carbon dioxide. By instinct, one will ordinarily breathe more deeply when applying mouth-to-mouth resuscitation, thereby enhancing the quality (higher FE_{O_2}, lower FE_{CO_2}) and quantity of his expired air. The apneic patient, therefore, will consequently receive twice his normal tidal volume of air, which will contain as much as 18% oxygen and as little as 2% carbon dioxide. After about 15 seconds or perhaps 5 inflations, the victim's lungs will contain nearly the normal alveolar concentrations of oxygen and carbon dioxide.

The method of mouth-to-mouth artificial respiration, or "expired air resuscitation," was first described in the late 18th century. At that time it was recommended that the larynx be pressed against the spine to prevent entry of air into the stomach. The method was not then widely used because expired air was not considered to be of great value and was even thought by some to be harmful. Bellows were constructed for the use of fresh air and were sometimes used for artificial respiration.

The techniques of rescue ventilation have already been discussed briefly. During mouth-to-mouth respiration, the patient's nose should be compressed with one hand, while the other hand should be used to make pressure over the upper abdomen and epigastrium in order to prevent distention of the stomach by air. Before expiration, the operator should take a deep inspiration and immediately apply his widely opened mouth to the mouth of the patient and make a forcible exhalation. Upon seeing this technique demonstrated, the novice is inevitably surprised at the degree of inflation produced by this method. The patient's chest will expand quite noticeably as the air is blown into his mouth, and when the operator raises his mouth from that of the patient, a rush of air will distinctly be heard coming from the patient's lungs. Forcible pressure on the patient's chest may augment expiration. As in all methods of artificial respiration, one must be quite sure to bring the tongue forward, since it may occlude the oral pharynx. One should exhale twice his normal resting tidal volume (about 1000 ml).

While delivering such a breath, the rescuer should turn his head toward the victim's chest to observe chest expansion. He then quickly takes a series of 4 inhalations, exhaling about 1000 cc each time into the patient's airway. This should be done as rapidly as possible.

During single-rescuer CPR, two quick breaths, without allowing time for full lung deflation between breaths, are delivered to the patient after each cycle of 15 chest compressions.

During two-rescuer CPR, a breath is interposed during the upstroke of every fifth chest compression (*i.e.*, every 5 seconds).

One should be aware of several precautions and possible pitfalls inherent in the procedure of mouth-to-mouth resuscitation. Because of the limited endurance of the person performing the resuscitation, the probability of physical fatigue must be considered. Although the operator may experience a degree of hypocapnia from his prolonged efforts and may therefore experience some vertigo, the decrease in the carbon dioxide concentration of the blood will not be sufficient to cause any real discomfort, particularly if additional personnel are available to take over the procedure at the appropriate time.

According to some workers, the mouth-to-mask or mouth-to-tube method is advantageous over the simple mouth-to-mouth procedure in that both hands of the operator are available to maintain patency of the upper airway. The operator can also sense any increase in pulmonary resistance by the amount of exertion it takes for deflation of his own lungs. In addition, the mouth-to-tube method of respiration has several points in its favor besides that of preventing hypocapnia in the operator. Cross-contamination between the operator and the patient is prevented if a disposable filter is placed in the breathing tube. The method can be continued for long periods, and no special position of the patient is required by the operator. The equipment is minimal in expense, and adequate ventilation is ensured despite abnormalities in either airway resistance or lung compliance. Of course, if a breathing tube is available, a resuscitation bag will usually be also, thus obviating the general need for mouth-to-tube respiration.

Another drawback in the mouth-to-mouth procedure is that, in some instances, the operator may be exposed to the danger of pulmonary tuberculosis or other infectious diseases. Anaerobic suppurative disease of the lungs, with its associated foul odor, makes the problem increasingly difficult. Additionally, there may be reluctance on the part of the rescuer to contact the lips of a dying patient. Prevention of cross-contamination can be implemented by the use of a handkerchief, and of course the mouth-to-tube method will also obviate this objection.

Esophageal insufflation and gastric dilatation present potential problems. The operator may press his hand on the epigastrium of the subject periodically to prevent dilatation from occurring. Moreover, pressure on the sternum may provoke regurgitation of stomach contents into the upper airway. Both active and passive regurgitation and air venting into the esophagus can be prevented by compressing the esophagus against the cricoid cartilage displaced posteriorly. This may be done by applying posterior pressure to the skin over the anterior surface of the cricoid and by compressing the esophagus between the cricoid and the anterior surface of the cervical vertebrae. Moderate pressure will prevent air from entering the esophagus, and gastric contents can also be kept from regurgitating through it. Two fingers of the hand supporting the chin and tongue are free to displace the cricoid backward with sufficient pressure to occlude the esophagus. Care must be used that pressure is applied to the cricoid cartilage and not to the thyroid cartilage.

Lung rupture is also possible, particularly in the event that too much expiratory effort is applied by the operator, especially in infants. With the very young infant, a mere puffing motion with the cheeks may suffice and will obviate any danger from too much pressure.

The patient who has had a laryngectomy will have a permanent stoma connecting his trachea directly to the skin, recognized as an opening at the front of the base of the neck. Direct mouth-to-stoma artificial ventilation will be needed should these individuals need rescue breathing; neither head tilt nor jaw thrust maneuvers will be needed. When a rescuer blows into a patient's temporary tracheostomy tube, the rescuer must, with his hand or with a tightly fitting face mask, seal the patient's nose and mouth to prevent leakage of air. This problem can, of course, be prevented if the tracheostomy tube is provided with an inflatable cuff.

MOUTH-TO-NOSE RESPIRATION

As an alternative to mouth-to-mouth respiration, mouth-to-nose respiration may be useful in some instances. The use of nasopharyngeal airways has already been mentioned. The person applying artificial respiration may be unable to seal his mouth completely around the patient's mouth, if transient rigidity, trismus, or convulsions are present. In such cases, mouth-to-nose respiration will be a viable alternative. The patient with a broken jaw may have his teeth wired together, but blowing between the teeth has been successful in these cases. It may become necessary to open the patient's mouth or to separate his lips to allow the air to escape during exhalation, since the soft palate may cause obstruction of the nasopharynx.

In infants and small children, the rescuer may cover both the mouth and the nose of the child with his mouth. He will, of course, use less volume than is used in adults to inflate the lung *once every 3 seconds*. Forceful backward tilting of the neck of the infant may obstruct breathing passages because of the marked pliability of the neck. Therefore, the tilted position should not be exaggerated.

The nasal insufflation route has a number of advantages, not the least of which is the lowering of the chances of gastric regurgitation and subsequent aspiration. It is generally accepted that the occurrence of gastric inflation depends on the pressure in the upper airways. When this exceeds 25 cm H_2O, gastric inflation is uniformly produced. This almost never occurs with pressures below 15 cm H_2O. With the increased resistance to airflow via the nasal route as compared to the oral route, there is a reduction of the air pressure in the pharynx and at the gastric cardia. Rubin has demonstrated that regurgitation is less likely to occur in instances of expired air resuscitation when the nasal inflation route is used.[22] The use of the mouth-to-nose technique eliminates such maneuvers as pinching the nostrils or resting the cheek against the nostrils to prevent an air leak. Not only is the incidence of nasal blockage extremely low (probably less than 2%), but the tilt angle is less critical with use of the mouth-to-nose technique.

FACE MASKS

Certainly needing at least as much emphasis in instruction as endotracheal intubation is the appropriate use of face masks. It has been urged that the endotracheal tube be reserved for later stages of cardiac resuscitation when prolonged maintenance is needed and when the tube can be inserted in a relatively leisurely manner into an already oxygenated patient. It cannot be stressed often enough that valuable time should not be expended in passing an endotracheal tube during the early stages of resuscitation, when simple mouth-to-mouth or face mask and bag techniques can more quickly ventilate the patient. The face masks include the simple oronasal mask, the oronasal mask with mouthpiece, and the oronasal mask with bag or bellows. Such masks are successfully used by most physicians, but in the hands of the inexperienced air leakage may occur. Inspiration may occur through the nose, and expiration may be blocked by a valving action of the soft palate.

RESPIRATORY BAGS

Since the AMBU bag was developed by Rubin and reported in the literature in 1955,[21] various types of mask-bag systems have evolved that now deliver high concentrations of enriched oxygen (Fig. 38-9). The AMBU (air-mask bag unit) bag provides a satisfactory method of artificial respiration using manual compression of the bag, or it may be attached to an endotracheal tube. Self-inflating resuscitator bags do achieve adequate ventilation when they are used with tight-fitting face masks or when connected to an en-

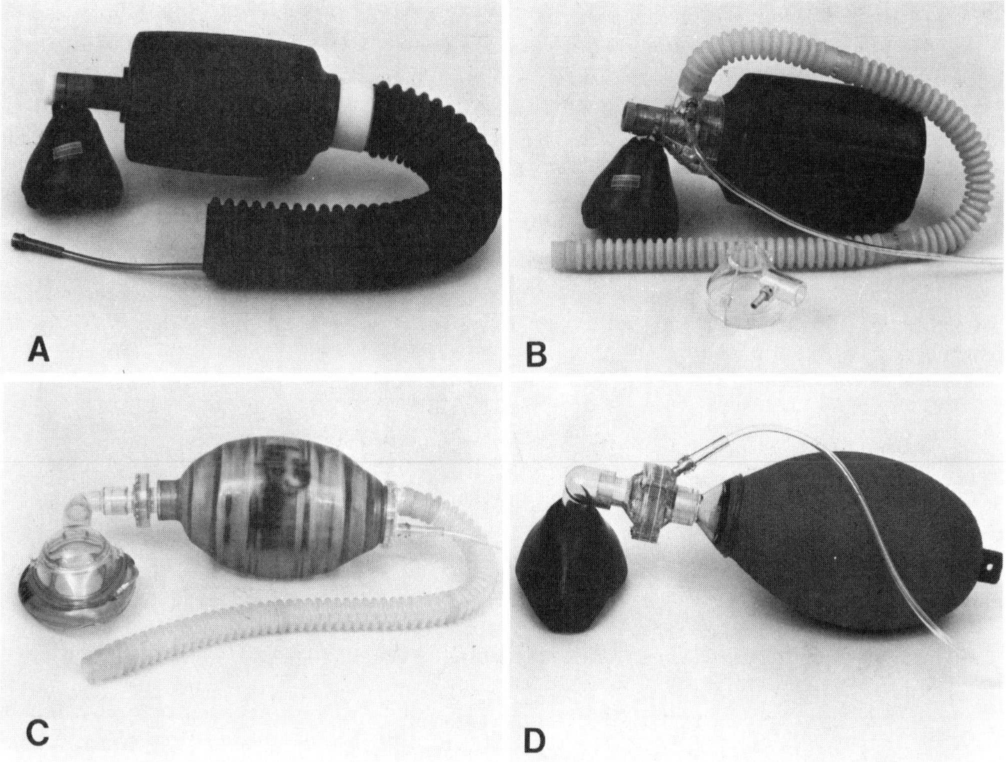

Fig. 38-9. Various types of hand resuscitator units. *(A)* Hope II bag (new style) provides an $F_{I_{O_2}}$ of 90% to 95%. *(B)* Hope bag (old style) provides $F_{I_{O_2}}$ of 35% to 40%. With the Blount adaptor (clear plastic shield) and the 80 cm O_2 reservoir tubing, as shown in this picture, an $F_{I_{O_2}}$ of 90% to 95% can be achieved. *(C)* Laerdal bag provides $F_{I_{O_2}}$ of 50% to 60%. With the 40 cm O_2 reservoir tubing, as shown in this picture, an $F_{I_{O_2}}$ of 75% to 80% can be obtained. With 80-cm reservoir tubing, an $F_{I_{O_2}}$ of 90% to 95% can be achieved. *(D)* Puritan Bennett resuscitator bag provides $F_{I_{O_2}}$ of 35% to 40%. At 10 to 15 liters/min O_2 flow, tidal volumes of approximately 800 cc, and 12 to 20 inflations/min can be achieved by all devices pictured. (Hodgkin JE, Foster GL, Nicolay LI: Cardiopulmonary resuscitation: Development of an organized protocol. Crit Care Med 5:93, 1977)

dotracheal tube or a tracheostomy tube. There are at least ten commonly used resuscitative bags, and testing of various bags has resulted in the conclusion that all do give an increased concentration of oxygen with an increase in oxygen flow.

Criteria for selection of an adequate bag-valve-mask unit should include the following.

1. Self-refilling capability.
2. A valve system that will not permit rebreathing and will not jam with an oxygen flow of 15 liters/min.
3. Capability to perform satisfactorily at extremes of temperature and under common environmental conditions.
4. Availability in both adult and pediatric sizes.
5. No pressure pop-off valve except in pediatric sizes.
6. An adequate system to ensure the delivery of 95% oxygen, with standard 15/22 mm connecting fittings.
7. A face mask made of transparent material soft enough to ensure a tight facial seal.
8. Performance characteristics that make it suitable for manikin practice.
9. PEEP capability of 0 to 12 cm H_2O pressure.
10. Ability to monitor airway pressure.

An esophageal airway and a compact carrying unit should accompany all such devices. The performance of various resuscitation units has recently been critically reviewed (see Bibliography).

Table 38-2. Weights, Dimensions, and Numbers of Parts of Eight Adult Manual Resuscitators

RESUSCITATOR	WEIGHT		DIMENSIONS		NUMBER OF PARTS
	Resuscitator *g*	*Reservoir* *g*	*Resuscitator (Length × Diameter)* *cm*	*Reservoir (Length)* *cm*	
Ambu Mark II	340	NA*	33 × 13	NA	5
Hope I	240	NA	28 × 13	NA	7
Hope II	280	210	32 × 12	107	11
Hudson Lifesaver	330	90	28 × 11	53	10
Laerdal II	350	50	36 × 14	88	10
Penlon	245	140	28 × 11	114	6
Puritan PMR	430	NA	34 × 14	NA	13
Robertshaw	340	NA	28 × 11	NA	8

(LeBouef LL: 1980 assessment of eight adult manual resuscitators. Respir Care 25:1136, 1980)
*NA = reservoir not available.

Table 38-3. Percentage of Oxygen Concentration and Percentage of Demand Ventilation in Eight Adult Manual Resuscitators

RESUSCITATOR	PERCENTAGE OF OXYGEN CONCENTRATION				PERCENTAGE OF DEMAND VENTILATION	
	Normal Bag Reinflation		*Slow Bag Reinflation**			
	Without Reservoir	*With Reservoir*	*Without Reservoir*	*With Reservoir*	*Through Bag*	*Through Valve*
Ambu Mark II	76	—	85	—	48	52
Hope I	44	—	50	—	50	50
Hope II	34	74	40	85	51	49
Hudson Lifesaver	—	73	—	84	63	37
Laerdal II	36	65	69	96	58	42
Penlon	—	73	—	97	97	3
Puritan PMR	38	—	59	—	0	100
Robertshaw	50	—	58	—	76	24

(LeBouef LL: 1980 assessment of eight adult manual resuscitators. Respir Care 25:1136, 1980)
*Slow reinflation time of 3 to 4 seconds.

Table 38-4. Self-Reinflation Times, Average Stroke Volumes, and Maximum Cycling Rates in Eight Adult Manual Resuscitators

		AVERAGE STROKE VOLUME				MAXIMUM CYCLING RATE	
		One Hand		*Two Hand*			
RESUSCITATOR	SELF-REINFLATION TIME *sec*	*Male ml*	*Female ml*	*Male ml*	*Female ml*	*At 25°C min*	*At −7°C min*
Ambu Mark II	0.56	952	702	999	987	76	39
Hope I	0.63	852	835	1,163	1,103	77	51
Hope II	0.76	1,211	806	1,452	1,073	64	40
Hudson Lifesaver	2.84	952	858	1,132	1,080	22	17
Hudson Livesafer without O_2 adapter	0.90	—	—	—	—	63	—
Laerdal II	0.68	1,146	1,038	1,302	1,272	70	48
Penlon	0.39	696	680	775	748	106	70
Puritan PMR	0.98	944	954	1,389	1,170	52	16
Robertshaw	2.93	927	849	1,039	977	20	15
Robertshaw without O_2 adapter	0.93	—	—	—	—	64	—

(LeBouef LL: 1980 assessment of eight adult manual resuscitators. Respir Care 80:1136, 1980)

Hand resuscitators should be evaluated on weight, dimensions, percentage of oxygen delivery capability, volume, self-reinflation time, maximum cycling rate, and number of parts. Tables 38-2, 38-3, and 38-4 detail these variables. No hand resuscitator seems "perfect" for all situations and institutions. The PMR-2 in child and adult models would appear to be the nearest to a "perfect" hand resuscitator. It features two accessory items that seem to be clinically very useful: an in-line airway manometer to reflect peak airway pressure; and a combination exhalation PEEP valve (Fig. 38–10).

ESOPHAGEAL OBTURATOR AIRWAY

A relatively new concept in emergency ventilation is the esophageal obturator airway (Fig. 38-11), which can be passed with ease after rather minimal training and provides excellent ventilation.[8] It also prevents aspiration of gastric contents. This airway consists of

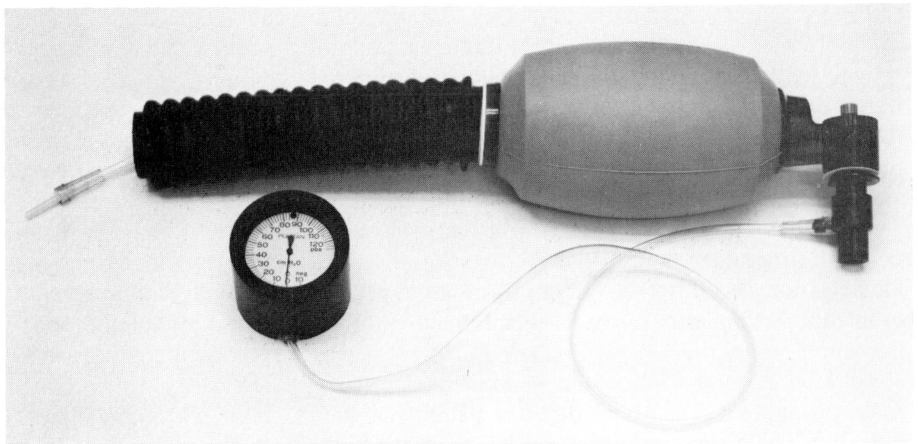

Fig. 38-10. Puritan Bennett Adult PMR-2 shown with optional airway manometer. Both adult and child models can be equipped with PEEP valve, adjustable from 4 to 14 cm H_2O pressure.

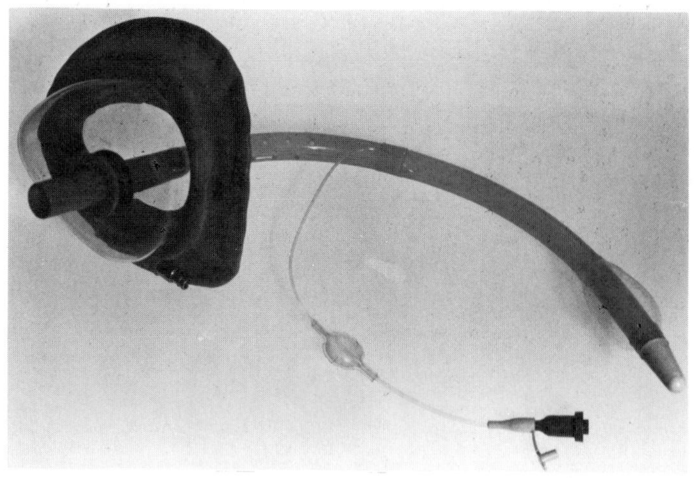

Fig. 38-11. An esophageal airway (*see* text for description).

an endotracheal tube so modified that it is inserted into the esophagus instead of into the trachea. It is mounted on a transparent mask with an inflatable cuff seal. Another inflatable cuff just proximal to the soft rubber obturator blocks the distal end of the tube. Air is injected into this silastic cuff, distending it symmetrically when the attached plastic syringe and check valve are put into operation. The syringe can then be removed without escape of air. Sixteen serial openings are located in the upper third of the tube, and the sum of the diameter of these openings exceeds the diameter of the tube itself.

Insertion of the tube requires little or no visualization of the anatomical structures, since the rescuer merely grasps the mandible between the thumb and index finger and lifts with one hand while he inserts the tube into the mouth and pharynx and advances it into the esophagus with the other hand. The distal cuff is then inflated.

The mask is fitted over the face, and the rescuer proceeds to perform mouth-to-airway resuscitation. The obturator blocks the distal end of the esophageal airway while the air escapes from the openings in the upper portion of the tube and inflates the lungs. Since the openings are located in the posterior portion of the mouth and the upper portion of the pharynx, oral secretions do not generally interfere with ventilation. These tubes are reusable, provide at least as much ventilation as does mouth-to-mask ventilation (since air does not pass into the stomach), and are far easier to introduce than are the standard endotracheal tubes. Personnel who plan to use the esophageal airway should be trained first on an anatomically suitable manikin and on actual anesthetized patients, where possible. The airway should never be introduced into a conscious patient.

Inadvertent tracheal introduction of the tube may occasionally occur but has not proved to be a problem in over 1000 insertions made in actual CPR cases by highly trained personnel. If the chest rises, the obturator is in the esophagus; if the chest does not rise, the obturator is in the trachea. In the latter case the tube is immediately removed and some other form of artificial ventilation used until it can be placed properly.

The tube should not be removed until appropriate steps have been taken. Adequate suction should be available to clear the airway, if necessary, because vomiting frequently occurs upon removal of the tube. Obviously, the cuff on the esophageal airway should always be deflated before its removal. The mask may be removed at the time the patient resumes spontaneous respiration, but the tube should be left in place until the patient is reacting or is sufficiently conscious to permit extubation under the above-mentioned conditions.

The stomach may be decompressed before the removal of the esophageal airway in either of two ways.* After passing a nasogastric tube to the area of the cuff in the esophagus, it can be temporarily deflated while the nasogastric tube is passed into the stomach, and then reinflated while the stomach is being decompressed. Alternatively, the unconscious patient may have an endotracheal tube introduced while the esophageal obturator airway remains in place. The esophageal airway can be removed after the cuff on the endotracheal tube has been inflated without any hazard of aspiration of stomach contents. Recently, several instances of a ruptured esophagus

*Newer modifications of the esophageal airway are now available that allow gastric suctioning with the tube in place.

have been reported with the use of the esophageal airway. Overinflation of the cuff must be avoided. Only 30 ml of air should be used in inflating the distal cuff so as not to overdistend the esophagus.

The size of the tube (which comes in one adult size only) does not overdistend any normal adult, flaccid esophagus. The tube is so designed that the inflatable cuff always lies proximal to the carina of the trachea, even in tall people. It may lie deeper in the esophagus in small or short people but will not extend into the stomach. Rapid and careless introduction of this tube, as with any similar procedure, could naturally cause some damage to the mucosa and wall of the esophagus, but proper training and care should obviate this problem.

The appeal of the esophageal airway rests largely on the ease with which physicians and paramedical personnel can be trained in its use, in contrast to the training of persons in tracheal intubation. In general, critical reports of its use in the recent literature have been enthusiastic.[25] Critics of the esophageal airway point out that the inflated cuff is too small to prevent gastric distention and regurgitation uniformly, except in small people. Face and head injuries may preclude use of the obturator airway. In addition, blind insertions of the esophageal airway device into the trachea, producing total airway obstruction and massive gastric distention, have been encountered. If the inflated esophageal cuff is inadvertently withdrawn before deflating, esophageal lacerations may be provoked.

CRICOTHYROID MEMBRANE PUNCTURE

If all the emergency measures listed above fail, cricothyroid puncture and insertion of a 6-mm tube have been recommended for adults. Cardiac arrest may be associated with a number of respiratory difficulties that do indeed respond poorly to the usual methods of artificial respiration, such as acute obstructive laryngeal edema in anaphylactic reactions of various etiology, hemorrhage into neck tissue fascial planes, and epiglottitis or blockage of the larynx by particulate matter such as food. If there is noticeable inability to inflate or deflate the lungs on mouth-to-mouth or mouth-to-nose respiration, high airway obstruction of this nature may be suspected. High insufflation pressure may partially relieve these obstructions, and further extension of the neck may also be helpful, as well as pushing the mandible forward to prevent obstruction of the pharynx by the tongue. If ventilation is still inadequate, a puncture of the cricothyroid membrane is the quickest, simplest, and safest means of establishing a temporary airway.

There are several advantages to this approach through a relatively avascular membrane. It is easily reached, owing to its superficial position and adjacent landmarks of cartilage. The cricothyroid space is large and can accept fairly large tubes. Because of the heavy posterior projection of the cricoid cartilage, posterior perforation is unlikely. An elective tracheotomy can be done at a later date, if necessary. The cricothyroid membrane approach should not be used much beyond 24 hours.

In this technique the larynx is stabilized between the left thumb and middle finger. The skin is incised with scalpel or scissors over the cricothyroid space, and the instrument is then guided down the index finger to puncture the membrane.

A mini-tracheotomy may be elected in which a standard intravenous transfusion needle is inserted into the trachea through the cricothyroid membrane. This technique is used in instances of airway obstruction where anesthetic apparatus is unavailable. At pressures reached during obstructed inspiration, the volume of air that can be drawn into the needle is believed to be sufficient to prevent asphyxia and to enable the patient to make forced expiratory efforts. Such insertion of a size 13 needle may temporarily restore an adequate airway to the infant but probably will not do so in the child or adult with acute obstruction of the upper airway. Even the percutaneous insertion of a size 13 needle into the trachea of an infant is not always an easy procedure to accomplish technically.

Cricothyroid membrane puncture, to be effective, should generally be done with a large-bore cannula of at least 6 mm size to allow for breathing, suctioning, or ventilation.

TRACHEOTOMY

Emergency tracheotomy is rarely indicated in the initial phase of cardiopulmonary resuscitation and is now rarely, if ever, done by any but experienced surgeons. Other, more effective means are available for supplying oxygen to the lungs, and the time required to perform a tracheotomy is usually excessive. If a cricothyroid membrane puncture is not elected, however, one may perform a tracheotomy using essentially the same indications. In instances of multiple fractures and injuries around the nose and mouth with considerable bleeding, a tracheotomy may prove to be necessary. In any event, the procedure must be carried out under well-controlled conditions, preferably in the operating room with the patient well oxygenated. A change of the airway from an endotracheal tube to a tracheostomy tube should be considered between 72 hours and 7 days (see Chap. 21), although the time lag need not be as long if it is obvious that the patient will need an artificial tracheal airway for a prolonged period because of severe crushing injury of the chest or a head injury.

Tracheotomy is not a procedure to be undertaken lightly. An occasional death does occur from massive tracheal hemorrhage. Patients with tracheostomies require continuous observation by experienced personnel, and complications of the procedure include severe endotracheitis, pneumothorax, improper tube positions, aspiration, delayed arterial bleeding, atelectasis, diminution of the tracheal lumen, mediastinitis, and wound infections.

MECHANICAL BREATHING DEVICES

Mechanical resuscitator-respirators have obvious advantages (*see* Chap. 24). An obvious disadvantage, however, is their general inability to alert one to increased airway resistance. Therefore, either airway-to-mouth or bag breathing should probably be recommended until there is reasonable certainty that an adequate airway actually exists. Safar and associates point out several disadvantages inherent in the use of pulmonary resuscitators.[24] Airway obstruction is difficult to detect and difficult to treat because of a lack of pressure reserve. Mask leakage, which is common during emergency artificial ventilation, leads to failure in cycling of pressure-cycled apparatus. The rate, pressure, volume, and flow for each inhalation cannot be changed instantly, according to the changing resistances encountered in the patient. Lung–thorax compliance and airway resistance vary greatly from patient to patient, and within each patient during the course of resuscitation. The use of hand-operated equipment such as bags or bellows probably offers the best method of positive pressure ventilation during resuscitation. Additionally, closed-chest cardiac compression does not lend itself effectively to a combination with positive pressure-cycled ventilators, since airway pressure increases with each compression of the chest, causing premature termination of the inflation cycle, followed by insufficient ventilation. Moreover, these are "demand valves" and may be used to deliver 40%, 70%, 85%, or 100% oxygen to spontaneously breathing patients. Flow rate is adjustable to 5, 10, or 15 liters/min. An adult/child selector modifies a safety vent to 60 cm H_2O pressure in adults and 40 cm H_2O in the child mode.

Manually triggered, oxygen-powered devices are generally easier to use effectively (Fig. 38-12). They

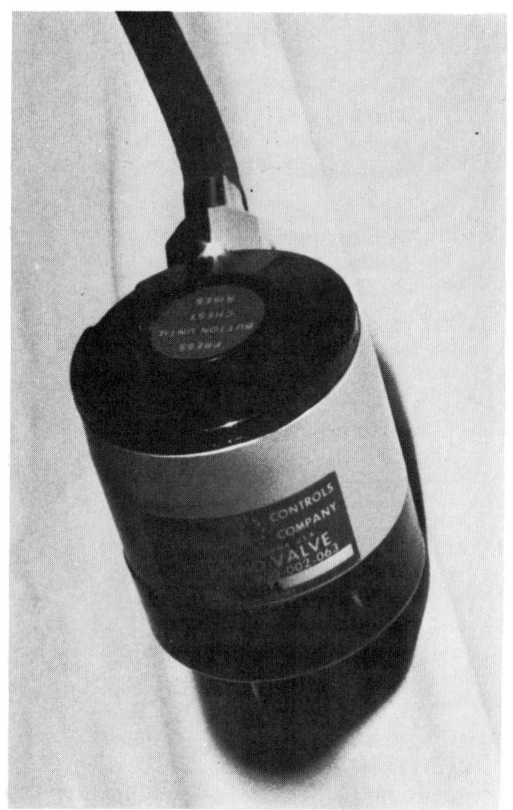

Fig. 38-12. A manually triggered hand resuscitator (Elder valve), powered by source gas, usually 100% oxygen. The operator can easily cycle respirations with closed-chest compression using such a device.

are particularly effective in situations where a tight airway seal cannot be achieved, owing to their capability to deliver exceedingly high airflow rates. These devices also have the advantage of interposing additional breaths between chest compressions. Moreover, these units are "demand valves" and may be used to deliver 100% oxygen to the spontaneously breathing patient.

If a manually triggered, oxygen-powered resuscitator is used, it should be able to provide certain capabilities. Flow rates of 10 liters/min or more are needed, and the safety pressure release valve should open at 60 cm H_2O, although this high instantaneous flow rate will usually result in gastric distension unless a cuffed endotracheal tube or cuffed esophageal obturator/airway is used. These units should provide 100% oxygen and should operate satisfactorily under varying environmental conditions, including all temperature extremes. Such units should have a standard 15-mm to 22-mm coupling for mask, esophageal airway, endotracheal tube, and tracheal tubes. They should have a rugged, breakage-resistant design that is compact and easy to hold, and the trigger should be positioned so that both hands of the rescuer can remain on the mask to hold it in position while supporting and tilting the jaw and keeping it elevated.

SUCTION DEVICES

Both portable and installed suction equipment should be available for resuscitative emergencies. The portable unit should be adequate for pharyngeal suction and the installed suction unit sufficiently powerful to provide an airflow of over 30 liters/min at the end of the delivery tube, and a vacuum of at least 300 mm Hg when the tube is clamped. The amount of suction should, of course, be controllable for use on children and intubated patients. Either a Y or T connection, or a lateral opening, should be provided between the suction tube and the suction source for an off–on control. The tube should reach the airway of any patient, regardless of his position, and the suction apparatus must be designed for easy cleaning and decontamination.

If a nasogastric tube is to be used for gastric decompression, preferably it should be inserted after the airway has been isolated by an endotracheal intubation. If gastric distension interferes with adequate ventilation, however, a nasogastric tube may be inserted by well-trained personnel.

USE OF 100% OXYGEN

The patient may be receiving only expired air during the immediate rescue phase of cardiopulmonary resuscitation. If the bag-mask unit is used, he will receive room air, and one should strive to administer 100% oxygen, if possible.

BELLOWS

As a device for respiratory support, the bellows is almost always avoided. Such use was flatly condemned by the National Conference on Standards for Cardiopulmonary Resuscitation and Emergency Cardiac Care.[17] All of these devices suffer common design flaws, and even professional rescuers cannot provide adequate lung ventilation when applying compression with bellows devices.

ELECTROPHRENIC RESPIRATION

Interest in electrophrenic stimulation as an emergency respiratory measure has been rather dormant during the last 30 years. An electrophrenic stimulator for providing artificial respiration either by direct application to the phrenic nerve in the neck or by application of current over the appropriate cutaneous area was part of the original mobile cardiac resuscitation cart developed at Bellevue Hospital in 1951. My own clinical experience with electrophrenic stimulation has not been extensive, but it does appear that it would be helpful to the patient experiencing prolonged inadequate spontaneous respiration or to the patient in whom a delayed return to spontaneous respirations occurs.

Interest in electrophrenic stimulation is attributed to Daggett and associates, who compared electrical stimulation with positive–negative pressure breathing under different conditions.[6] They found that under barbiturate intoxication, intracaval electrophrenic stimulation is a more effective method of ventilatory support than is positive–negative pressure. Cardiac output consistently appears to be higher and ventilation more physiologic, as measured by the carbon dioxide tension and pH. Cardiac arrhythmias were not noted. In shock, positive pressure breathing may depress cardiac output and arterial pressure. Electrophrenic stimulation does not carry this complication. Active contraction of the diaphragm by phrenic nerve stimulation prevents disuse atrophy of respiratory musculature, which is thought to occur during prolonged periods of ventilatory support by a positive pressure respirator. During stimulation of the phrenic nerve, apnea occurs, as mediated through the vagus nerve, and therefore no effort of spontaneous respiratory activity counters artificial efforts. Further, negative pressure breathing that takes place during electrophrenic stimulation promotes increased venous return to the heart. Adequate ventilation of the contralateral lung has been demonstrated during stimulation of the right phrenic nerve. Thus the procedure shows some promise but, at present, is not widely used clinically.

CHEST COMPRESSION (CARDIAC MASSAGE)

INDICATIONS

When I refer to the term "*cardiac arrest*," I am speaking of the sudden, superficially unexplained, and unexpected cessation of an effective cardiac output. Such cessation may be characterized either by the absence of all cardiac activity, which is cardiac asystole, or by the sudden onset of ventricular fibrillation, a wild, uncoordinated, and disorganized myocardial contraction resulting in the complete absence of any effective cardiac output. Occasionally, a third condition may be involved: The heart may be beating feebly but at such a depressed rate or with such an ineffective stroke volume that the net result is very much the same as with cardiac asystole or ventricular fibrillation. In any event, all three conditions require *immediate* efforts to establish circulation artificially in order that irreversible brain damage may not occur. Statistically, most cardiac resuscitative efforts will be applied to the patient with myocardial infarction or sudden ventricular fibrillation. Cardiac arrests do occur, however, in victims of near-drowning and accidental electrocution as well as in victims of lightning shock, anaphylactic shock, chest injuries, certain poisonings, and hemorrhagic shock.

Most deaths from acute myocardial infarction occur within 24 hours after the onset of the symptoms, and at least 50% of these deaths occur within the first 2 hours. The incidence of ventricular fibrillation after an acute myocardial infarction is not necessarily related to the size of the infarct, since the electric stability of the heart is a fragile affair, and various hypoxic changes in the myocardium may trigger electric discharges sufficient to throw the heart into fibrillation.

Patients with Stokes–Adams disease may suddenly experience cardiac arrest without any warning. Stokes–Adams disease is a term applied to many of the conditions characterized by sudden failure of the ventricles to contract, and it may be associated with markedly slowed idioventricular beats, ventricular tachycardia, or ventricular fibrillation. Currently, a large percentage of diagnosed Stokes–Adams cases are successfully managed with long-term implantation of electric or nuclear cardiac pacemakers.

Cardiac arrest may occasionally follow carotid sinus pressure, pressure on the globe of the eye with resultant vagus stimulation, or any surgical manipulation of a viscus that causes traction on a branch of the vagus nerve. Hypercapnic or hyperpotassemic patients are particularly susceptible to the vagal influence in the etiology of cardiac arrest. The severely burned patient, in particular, may have an increased serum potassium level as a result of tissue breakdown. Patients with obstructive jaundice (caused by a stone in the common duct or a tumor of the papilla of Vater or head of the pancreas) may also be markedly sensitive to vagal influences.

Pericardial tamponade may result in ineffective cardiac output and may produce very much the same results as a sudden cardiac arrest. This condition may be caused by a penetrating wound to the chest or by cardiac contusion in automobile accidents, such as "steering wheel injuries." The relief of the cardiac tamponade is, indeed, urgent.

Which should one start first: closed chest resuscitative efforts or artificial ventilation? One may debate the eminence of each of these priorities. Unless the cardiac arrest is witnessed from its onset, one should first establish an open airway and start pulmonary ventilation at the onset of the resuscitative effort. The most crucial consideration is, of course, that of adequate cerebral circulation. Therefore, first priority involves artificial augmentation of the circulation with oxygenated blood. Obviously the circulating blood, if unoxygenated, will have a limited value. Likewise, a well-ventilated lung will have no value to the patient unless the circulation is moving. It bears reemphasis that one effort without the other is virtually worthless. It is unfortunate that often, in the excitement of an emergency, this fact is overlooked. In rare situations of marked cardiopulmonary collapse, while the heart is still beating, the patient will be revived by artificial ventilation alone, but one cannot rely on such an eventuality.

TECHNIQUE OF CLOSED-CHEST COMPRESSION

The patient should be placed in the supine or flat position, preferably on a hard, nonyielding surface, while efforts are made to compress the heart between the sternum and the thoracic vertebrae. When this maneuver is properly instituted, sufficient cardiac output is achieved to maintain adequate cerebral circulation as well as adequate blood flow to the myocardium and to other vital tissues (up to 35% of the normal blood flow). Intermittent pressure is applied to the lower third of the sternum with the minimum possible pressure to the adjacent rib cage. This can be accomplished by using the base of the palm. Ideally, one should be positioned directly over the patient with the elbows rigidly extended and with the pressure exerted from the shoulders downward. If the pressure is directed at an angle to the chest wall, it is more likely to produce complications such as rib fractures and soft tissue injuries. Too vigorous application of the initial compression is a tendency of the uninitiated. One usually begins with an intermittent depression of the sternum, which gradually increases in depth as the sternum and the rib cage become slightly more mobile and elastic.

The operator positions himself at either side of the patient and places the heel of one hand over the lower half of the patient's sternum, and the heel of the other hand on top of the first hand. (The lower hand must not be placed over the lower tip of the sternum.) The sternum is then displaced downwardly toward the spine for about 1½ to 2 inches. It should be held down for a fraction of a second and then released rapidly. Contact with the chest is maintained during relaxation; a rate of 60 to 80 compressions per minute is probably best in most cases. In children, however, the rate should be increased to between 80 and 100 compressions per minute. Undue fatigue in the operator can be avoided if he uses the entire weight of his body, rather than just the strength of his arms, in applying the compressions. The fingers should be carefully maintained in a raised position to avoid undue pressure on the rib cage.

In children the principles are the same, but much less pressure is used. In small children the force of the heel of one hand is ordinarily sufficient, and with infants moderate pressure should be applied, with the tips of the fingers only, to the center of the sternum. Care must be used in applying this pressure because the infant's myocardium is easily bruised. The depression of the infant's sternum will be for a distance of one half to three fourths of an inch. Young children require three fourths to 1½ inches. Small infants may also have the chest encircled with the hands while the midsternum is compressed with both thumbs.

Two immediately applicable measures may be helpful at the very start of closed-chest resuscitative efforts. Placing the patient in a supine position with the head slightly downward produces an actual, significant, rapid, and demonstrable increase in blood flow to the brain. To stretch that delicate time period between reversibility and irreversibility of cerebral cortical activity, the head-down position appears to have merit. Additionally, the Trendelenburg position tends to prevent aspiration of vomitus and gastric contents after pressure on the sternum and epigastrium, and it also has the advantage of decreasing the likelihood of air embolization to the brain in the relatively rare cases where such emboli form. Second, elevation of the patient's lower extremities provides sudden augmentation of venous filling of the heart and may even produce a desired effect simply by stretching the cardiac fibers. With elevation of the legs, venous return may be increased by making as much as 1000 ml of additional blood available. In some instances, wrapping the extremities with elastic bandages may provide additional venous blood return in amounts that are significantly beneficial.

Evaluating the effectiveness of closed-chest compression is desirable. If a blood pressure cuff is available, maintenance of a systolic blood pressure above 60 to 70 mm Hg indicates that the cardiac output is adequate to sustain life. Otherwise, a palpable pulse and maintenance of the pupils in the constricted state generally indicate satisfactory augmentation of the circulation.

The use of transcutaneous oxygen and carbon dioxide sensors during CPR is an interesting new development. These sensors are basically the same electrodes used in conventional blood gas machines. $Ptco_2$ and $PtcCO_2$ values are linearly related to arterial gas tensions if patients are not in shock. It has also been demonstrated in experimental animals that, during hypovolemic shock, $PtcPO_2$ falls with the decreased cardiac index (CI) and oxygen delivery, whereas the $PtcCO_2$ values rise and correlate inversely with flow. The schematic shown in Figure 38-13 demonstrates this situation.

SIMULTANEOUS CLOSED-CHEST AND MOUTH-TO-MOUTH RESUSCITATION (SINGLE RESCUER TECHNIQUE)

If one is alone with the patient, how does one combine external cardiac compression with intermittent positive pressure artificial ventilation? The best combination lies in alternating two mouth-to-mouth lung inflations with 15 chest compressions at about 1-second intervals (Fig. 38-14). With only one operator, chest compression should be given at a more rapid rate: approximately 80 compressions/min. Two full lung inflations are delivered in rapid succession, within 5 or 6 seconds, without allowing full exhalation between breaths. In the event that a second person is available to apply artificial respiration, he should *interpose* one deep lung inflation after every fifth sternal compression. Interposed breathing must occur without any pause in compressions, since cerebral perfusion drops to zero when there is a cessation of compression.

The person administering closed-chest resuscitation will count aloud as follows: "one one-thousand, two one-thousand, three one-thousand, four one-thousand." At each count of "five one-thousand," the person responsible for the mouth-to-mouth effort will administer one good exhalation to the mouth of the patient. In effect, one can imagine one is blowing the compression hands off the chest wall as one exhales just at the end point of the fifth compression. The reversal of roles between the two rescuers should be so coordinated that *no* interruption of perfusion

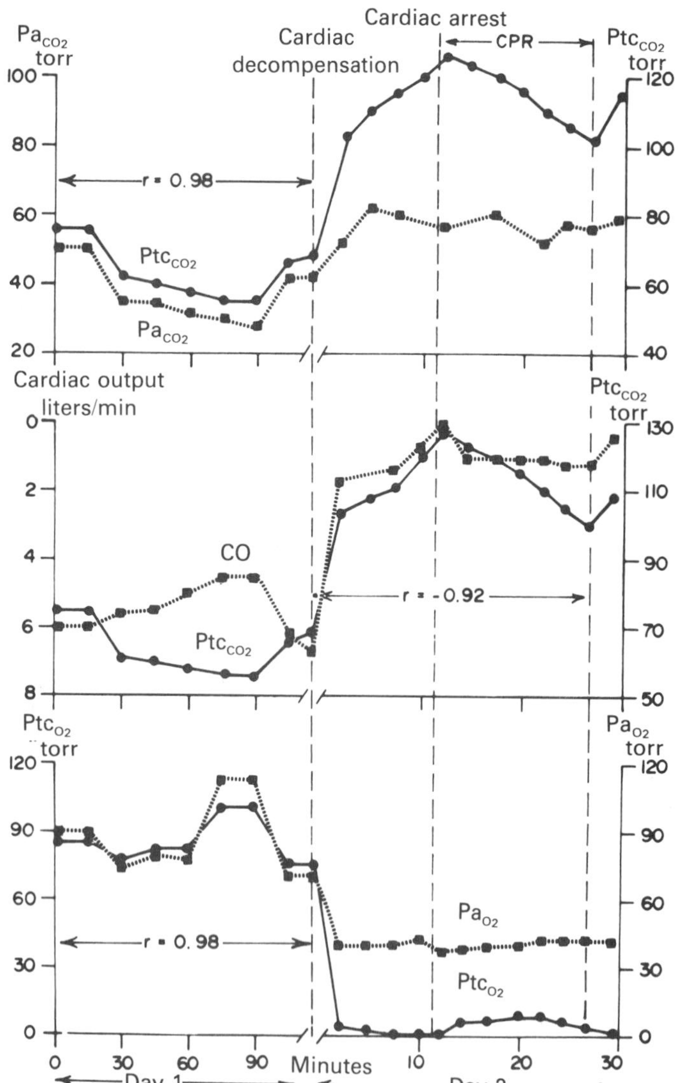

Fig. 38-13. Ptc_{CO_2}, Pa_{CO_2}, cardiac output *(CO)*, Ptc_{O_2}, and Pa_{O_2} during cardiac decompensation, cardiac arrest, and CPR in an adult ICU patient. Two-day time course of Ptc_{CO_2} and Pa_{CO_2} *(upper section)*; Ptc_{CO_2} and cardiac output (CO plotted inversely, *i.e.*, with zero at the top to 8 liters/min at the bottom of the scale) *(middle section)*; and Ptc_{O_2} and Pa_{O_2} *(lower section)*. Note during the first day the close trend of Ptc_{CO_2} with Pa_{CO_2} and Ptc_{O_2} with Pa_{O_2}, while the patient has adequate blood flow (CO 4 liters/min). During day 2, the CO drops to below 2 liters/min, and Ptc_{CO_2} rises while the Ptc_{O_2} falls. Note how Ptc_{CO_2} correlates with the reciprocal of CO *(middle section*, r = −0.92). Also note how Ptc_{CO_2} responds to CPR by a decrease of more than 20 torr *(upper section)*. (Tremper KK, Shoemaker WC: Continuous CPR monitoring with transcutaneous oxygen and carbon dioxide sensors. Crit Care Med 9:417, 1981. Copyright © 1981 by The Williams & Wilkins Co., Baltimore)

occurs. Even with the most effective technique of closed-chest resuscitation, the perfusion rate remains only one third that of normal. *Obviously, any departure from the proper technique will drop perfusion to an ineffective level.*

If, after prolonged efforts, the person administering the chest compression tires, it may be desirable to change operators. In this case, the count by the person compressing the chest may be as follows (adhering to the previously counted rhythm): "next time change on *three*." After administering a breath to the patient on the word "three," the person administering the mouth-to-mouth technique will move immediately to the chest area and place his hands alongside those of the compressor of the chest so that he is entirely ready to shove these hands aside and continue with the count "four one-thousand" at the proper time in the next cycle. The other person will immediately move to the head of the patient and be ready to administer the next breath to the patient on the following count of five.

We have observed that even personnel who are experienced and quite effective at either of these techniques alone may prove to be quite awkward at the two-person changeover. Practice with manikins is essential.

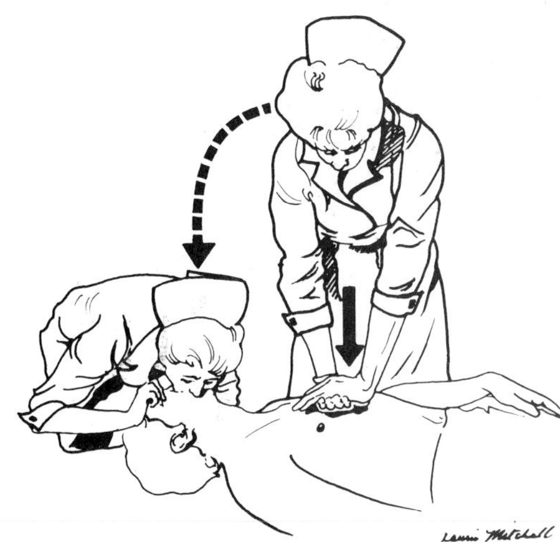

Fig. 38-14. The single-rescuer technique of cardiopulmonary resuscitation. Two mouth-to-mouth lung inflations are followed by 15 chest compressions at about 1-second intervals.

There is a real necessity for practice on manikins by all health care personnel likely to be in the position to apply cardiopulmonary resuscitation. If the recording Resusci–Anne manikin can be used for a demonstration and various hospital personnel are allowed to demonstrate their techniques, amazing inadequacies of the procedure will almost invariably be seen, even by persons considered to be quite experienced in resuscitation.

The recording manikin has two distinct aids to teaching closed-chest massage and mouth-to-mouth breathing. First, a series of lights on a panel beside the manikin indicates the effectiveness of the efforts applied. A single green light glows at the instant of sufficient pulmonary ventilation, and, independently, a red light and an amber light demonstrate the effectiveness of the chest compression, the red light indicating either misapplied chest compression or an effort of too great a magnitude, and the amber light indicating correctly applied compression of the proper magnitude. It is not at all uncommon that the supposedly experienced resuscitator will, at first, fail to illuminate the proper lights.

The second feature of this manikin involves an internal recorder that delivers, through a slit in the side of the manikin, an ECG-type printout on a paper strip, showing the "cardiovascular" effectiveness of the efforts applied.

It is important that the respiratory therapist be tested on adequate psychomotor skills for the ability to deliver a near-perfect "Recording Annie" strip. For example, the initial four ventilations must be properly stair-stepped with ventilations of proper strength. The period from termination of ventilation to the beginning of chest compression without pulse should not be longer than 5 seconds. Compression should be of proper duration without bouncing or jerking efforts. With the two-man rescue technique, there should be no pause for ventilation while compressing.

A training session with a recording manikin quickly separates the "bone crushers," the too gentle chest "caressers," and the ineffectual "puffers" from the truly life-saving administrators of correctly applied cardiopulmonary resuscitative measures!

Rhythmic sternal compression may have some value in artificial *respiration*. It is generally believed, however, to be of rather minimal value. Safar and associates attempted to evaluate this feature under several different conditions.[24] In 30 curarized patients with natural airways, no respiratory tidal exchange was produced by using closed-chest compression. The head was unsupported, and there was probable upper airway obstruction. If the airway was improved with elevation of the shoulder and backward tilting of the head, some improvement in the respiratory tidal exchange occurred, but this was still minimal. If an artificial airway was introduced, tidal volumes as high as 390 ml were recorded, with tidal volume being inversely proportional to *rate* of chest compression. They also studied tidal exchange in 12 patients in whom resuscitative attempts had been started with closed-chest massage while an endotracheal tube was in place. No basic tidal exchange was detectable, and it was therefore assumed that closed-chest compression should not be relied on to produce much tidal exchange. It does seem, however, that an occasional patient has benefited in this fashion. Adult patients with more rigid chests probably receive less benefit than does the younger person.

As described in recent CPR guidelines,

> two full lung inflations must be delivered in rapid succession, within a period of four to five seconds, without allowing full exhalation between the breaths. If time for full exhalation were allowed, the additional time required would reduce the number of compressions and ventilation that could be achieved in a one-minute period.
>
> The carotid pulse should be palpated periodically during CPR to check the effectiveness of external chest compression or the return of a spontaneous effective heartbeat. This should be done after the first minute of CPR and every few minutes thereafter. It should be checked particularly when a second rescuer arrives to determine the effectiveness of external chest compressions and to confirm pulselessness.

> The compression rate for two rescuers is 60 per minute. When performed without interruptions, this rate can maintain adequate blood flow and pressure and will allow cardiac refilling. This rate is practical because it avoids fatigue, facilitates timing at a rate of one compression per second, and allows optimal ventilation and circulation by permitting the swift interposition of an inflation at the upstroke of each fifth compression without any pause in compressions (5:1 ratio). The rate of 60 compressions per minute allows breaths to be interposed without any pauses.[26]

As previously mentioned, if the cardiac arrest occurs in a hospital bed, a firm support should be provided beneath the patient's back when CPR is performed. A simple serving tray or support of similar size is useful but not best. Optimally, a bed board should extend from the shoulders to the waist and across the full width of the bed. A special cardiac arrest board is available that has a shape conducive to positioning the patient's neck in the properly extended position. Spineboards should be used for ambulance services and mobile support units. They are also useful for extricating and immobilizing patients. They may be used directly on the floor of the emergency vehicle or on a wheeled litter. Actually, the floor may be the best place for applying closed-chest massage. When the patient is on a bed or a high-wheeled litter, the rescuer must stand on a step or chair or kneel on the bed or litter. With a low-wheeled litter, the rescuer can stand at the patient's side.

PRECORDIAL PERCUSSION OR THUMP

The precordial thump is no longer recommended for use as a basic life-support maneuver, although it has been shown to be effective in evoking ventricular depolarization with associated myocardial contraction in asystole. It has also been demonstrated to restore a sinus rhythm when delivered early after the onset of ventricular tachycardia and ventricular fibrillation. It may, however, cause ventricular fibrillation or asystole on occasion when used to treat ventricular tachycardia.

Accordingly, the precordial thump is recommended for use exclusively in the setting of the ECG-monitored patient. As demonstrated in Figure 38-15, it is delivered as a sharp, quick, single blow over the midportion of the sternum, hitting with the bottom, fleshy portion of the fist from about 8 to 12 inches over the chest. The precordial thump is not recommended in pediatric patients.

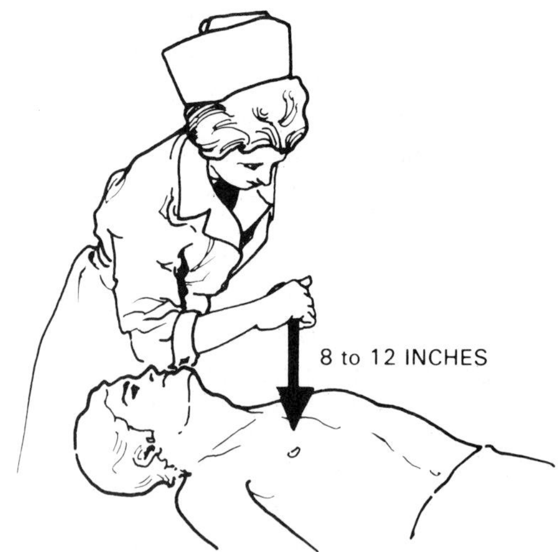

Fig. 38-15. The precordial thump.

MECHANICAL EXTERNAL CARDIAC COMPRESSION

Units are now available commercially that permit adequate variation of chest compression, duration of systole, heart rate, independent use of a ventilator or compressor, ventilation as described, and intermittent prolonged cycling. The performance of these mechanical devices should be similar to that recommended for the manual methods. Although they do afford more regular and uninterrupted CPR than can be administered manually, such devices have limitations: [1] They are relatively heavy and difficult to move because of their associated oxygen tanks and components; [2] they are seldom available at the actual site where the emergency occurs; and [3] they may be difficult to use without accidentally displacing the plunger while moving the patient. Moreover, with long-continued use, the body of the patient may shift sufficiently so that the plunger is applied to an ineffective or even dangerous location. When such devices are used, external cardiac compression must always be started with the manual method first. Personnel who will be using the automatic equipment must have careful and extensive training and manikin practice in the manual method, the mechanical method, and, most important, the proper technique for changing from one to the other without interrupting CPR for more than 5 or 10 seconds at any one time. Use of most commercially available models is limited to adult patients.

Simple, hinged, manually operated mechanical chest compressors can be used for effective external cardiac compression. The stroke should be adjustable from 1½ to 2 inches and should be able to be applied with a very minimal interruption in cardiopulmonary resuscitative efforts. Prolonged effective external cardiac compression may be facilitated with manual chest compressors.

THE "NEW" CPR

The so-called new CPR was proposed by Chandra and colleagues in 1980.[4] Briefly, the technique brings three modifications to the standard resuscitation procedure: high intermediate pressure ventilation (IPPV) simultaneous with external cardiac compression; an external cardiac compressive rate of 40/min, with a compression-relaxation time ratio of 60:40; and abdominal restraint applied by use of military antishock trousers (MAST).

Bircher and associates and Alifimoff and coworkers have reported that common carotid artery blood flow is doubled by use of the abdominal restraint (and tripled by use of open-chest compression of the heart) but that such restraint also causes rupture of the liver, acidemia, and hypoxemia.[1,3] MAST-induced increases in intracranial pressure may also be deleterious to cerebral oxygenation, and prolonged open-chest resuscitation by conventional means has caused lower venous pressure, lower intracranial pressure, higher perfusion pressures, and improved cardiac and cerebral recovery.[1,3]

In a study presented at the Second Wolf Creek Conference, Bircher and associates cited the above findings and supported them with their results from a laboratory study in dogs of open- and closed-chest CPR and the "new" CPR.[3] They concluded that the new CPR could transiently increase common carotid artery blood flow but could lead also to decreased cerebral oxygenation. They pointed out the possible complications mentioned above and concluded that the new technique required tracheal intubation and mechanical equipment that made it an advanced life-support measure, and in this setting defibrillation, drug use, and intravenous fluids should have priority.

Redding's conclusion, in comparing the two methods, was similar.

> Regarding "new" versus "old" CPR, it is clear that there are two valid mechanisms for producing artificial circulation: the classical cardiac pump mechanism and the thoracic pump mechanism. During open-chest cardiac compression, there are no global intrathoracic pressure fluctuations yet the method works very well if performed properly. On the other hand, cough CPR represents a pure form of thoracic pumping in which there is no direct cardiac compression. Both mechanisms operate in varying proportions depending on a number of variables, some yet to be described. In some of these studies, one mechanism was dominant and in others, the other mechanism dominated.
>
> In some forms of new CPR, flow may not be improved because the effectiveness of cardiac compression is compromised at the same time the effectiveness of the thoracic pump is increased. There is a shift from one mechanism to another with no net improvement. It is time to stop arguing about which is the true mechanism and start thinking of ways to recruit both mechanisms simultaneously.[19]

In yet another study presented at the second Wolf Creek Conference, Redding and colleagues concluded that the new CPR not only requires intubation, but also is far more fatiguing to the operator and no more effective than the usual technique in terms of successful resuscitation.[20]

Thus the effect of the new CPR on basic life-support techniques and technology awaits further study and confirmation.

MANAGEMENT OF THE NEAR-DROWNING EPISODE

In cases of near-drowning, immediate resuscitative efforts will already have been made, including mouth-to-mouth ventilation with closed-chest cardiac massage, if indicated. Supplemental oxygen is indicated as early as possible, and mechanical ventilation may need to be applied to ensure maximum ventilatory support while the victim is being transported to the hospital.

As Modell points out, fewer than 15% of near-drowning victims aspirate quantities of water sufficient to produce life-threatening changes in serum electrolyte and hemoglobin concentrations.[16] Therefore the emphasis on fluid and electrolyte changes has switched within recent years to the alterations in pulmonary function and gas exchange.

Arterial hypoxemia is seen with aspiration of minimal quantities of fluid. Obviously, if the arterial hypoxemia is severe, metabolic acidosis will result from the resultant shift to anaerobic metabolism. Modell emphasizes that regardless of whether the hypoxia is caused by aspiration of sea water or fresh water, the end result is the same—mismatch of ventilation and perfusion, or interpulmonary shunt resulting in arterial hypoxemia. To minimize mismatched ventilation/perfusion ratios, one can use positive end-expiratory pressure (PEEP). Carbon dioxide can be removed adequately by providing sufficient mechanical ventilation. Although intermittent mandatory ventilation or continuous positive pressure ventilation is not needed for every patient, intensive pulmonary care is the key to survival in most cases. Certainly, maximal pulmonary therapy should be continued until the patient is able to stabilize his own alveoli (which may have been denuded of surfactant) to match his ventilation/perfusion ratios more closely, thereby producing adequate arterial oxygenation with spontaneous ventilation. Pulmonary support should not be withdrawn prematurely, since these patients may quickly develop pulmonary edema.

Modell emphasizes that considerable variability exists in the clinical status of the patient who has suffered a near-drowning episode. Accordingly, each patient must be treated individually, and therapy must emphasize intensive pulmonary and cardiovascular support. Although steroids and antibiotic therapy have often been recommended in the hospital care of these patients, the clinical experience of Modell and many other workers does not indicate that prophylactic use of corticosteroids or antibiotic therapy improves the patient's chance of survival.

PRECAUTIONS IN CARDIOPULMONARY RESUSCITATION

Although complications and inadequacies of cardiopulmonary resuscitative efforts will inevitably occur, these complications will be minimized by an effective training program that also embodies periodic retraining efforts. The respiratory therapist should be aware of the potential pitfalls and precautions necessary for preventing complications. Some of these complications will be discussed below.

Multiple rib fractures are likely to occur during closed-chest resuscitation, especially in elderly patients, since the rib cage is relatively inflexible. The broken ends of the rib present sharp edges that may lacerate the lung. Various studies report a 24% to 40% incidence of fractured ribs in large series of applications of the technique. It appears that the frequency of rib fracture due to external cardiac massage probably depends on the skill and experience of the person performing the resuscitation. Additionally, 2% of these studies have reported fracture of the sternum during closed-chest massage, as well as at least one case of a fractured scapula. The rescuer's fingers should not rest on the patient's ribs during compression. Interlocking the fingers of the two hands may help to avoid this. Pressure with fingers on the ribs or lateral pressure increases the possibility of rib fracture and costochondral separation.

The incidence of fat embolization after closed-chest massage may be as high as 30% to 50% (Fig. 38-16). The actual mechanism producing the pulmonary fat emboli has been a source of some speculation. There is now some consensus that the compression of bones or the act of bending and compressing bones such as the rib cage may lead to microfractures within the medulla of ribs and sternum, with an increase in marrow pressure. Fat is thus allowed to enter the venous circulation from the marrow. Significantly, marrow embolization may occur without demonstrable fractures. In fact, when one recalls the semiliquid na-

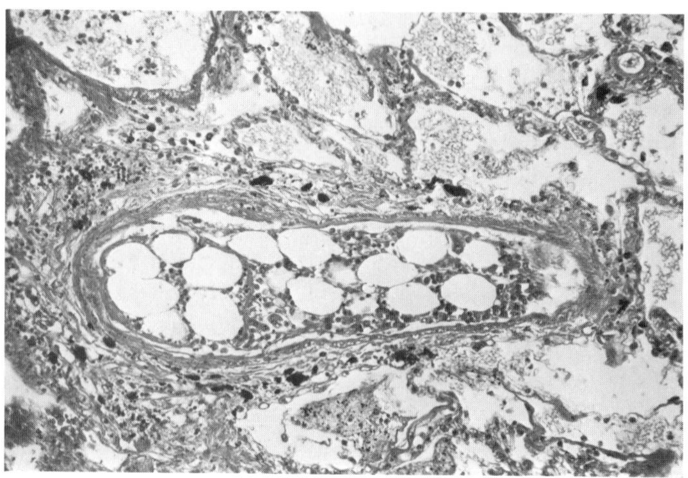

Fig. 38-16. Bone marrow embolism to a pulmonary arteriole from fracture of the sternum, incurred during an unsuccessful CPR attempt. Note the high fat content of the marrow embolus.

ture of the sternal marrow and the communication of the marrow cavities with the venous system, one might wonder if such embolism might not occur even more frequently than is suggested by the reported incidence of successful closed-chest cardiac massage.

Although it has been generally assumed that mental deterioration after cardiac resuscitation is due to the effect of prolonged cerebral anoxia, the question is now as to whether cerebral fat emboli may be considered as another etiologic factor.

Pneumoperitoneum is a recognized hazard of closed-chest cardiac massage in that free abdominal air under sufficient pressures severely compromises ventilation. The mechanism of air entry into the peritoneal cavity may involve a rupture of the wall of a viscus (e.g., esophagus or stomach), and closed-chest resuscitation could, and would, of course, be the precipitating factor. Air extravasated from the pulmonary parenchyma to the mediastinum after external massage may dissect within the esophageal wall to the stomach or intestine (or enter the peritoneal cavity through the serosal surface of the intestine or stomach). Obviously this complication must be recognized and its immediate effects managed simply by aspiration of the air from the abdomen or, in the case of a pneumothorax, from the chest.

Gastroesophageal laceration is a not infrequent complication of closed-chest cardiac massage. The laceration is most commonly a linear one along the lesser curvature of the stomach and extends upward through the fundus and the cardia into the esophagus. The combination of mouth-to-mouth artificial respiration with closed-chest massage is particularly prone to producing such tearing. Pressures as low as 120 to 150 mm Hg will produce mucosal slits in the adult stomach. Varying degrees of hemorrhage have been associated with this complication, and any bleeding from the nose or mouth after resuscitative efforts should alert one to this Mallory–Weiss-type syndrome. Delayed perforation of the transverse colon has appeared as a sequel to mouth-to-mouth resuscitation and external cardiac massage. Edema and interstitial hemorrhage of the bowel wall as well as hematomata of the mesentery and transverse colon doubtless follow the trauma sustained during resuscitation. Ultimately this situation progresses to necrosis and perforation of the bowel wall.

Numerous reports have appeared in the literature of hepatic lacerations after closed-chest cardiac compression. This may well be the most common serious complication of external cardiac compression in infants and children.

Continuous pressure should not be maintained on the abdomen to decompress the stomach while performing closed-chest compression. Such action may "trap" the liver and could cause it to rupture. The patient with pectus excavatum or funnel chest is particularly susceptible to this hazard of sternal depression. In these patients, the funnel chest serves in effect as a "battering ram" to compress the liver forcibly against the vertebral bodies.

Gastric dilatation is a fairly common complication of closed-chest cardiac massage. It can easily occur with pharyngeal pressures of 20 to 25 cm, such as may be commonly used during mouth-to-mouth or bag-and-mask resuscitation. In addition to regurgitation and aspiration pneumonia, several ill effects of overdistension of the stomach occur. Gastric distension may further impair pulmonary function in patients already in difficulty with hypoventilation and hypotension. Moreover, increased vagal tone and decreased venous return to the heart may occur, even to the point of being the actual cause of bradycardia, sinus arrest, or cardiac standstill. Gastric pressure can easily force air out of the stomach, allowing gastric secretions to enter the upper airway and even block the airway. The patient should be in a head-down position if epigastric pressure is being used, and the stomach should be reasonably empty (preferably by passing a gastric tube).

Doubtless there are instances in which direct trauma to the lungs is a hazard of closed-chest resuscitation. Increased right atrial and vena caval pressures during application of the closed-chest technique have been reported by numerous studies, and it seems likely that pulmonary contusion and edema may be more common than has been clinically recognized.

Sudden or jerking motions should be avoided when compressing the chest. The compression should be smooth, regular, and uninterrupted. Quick jabs increase the possibility of injury and produce quick jets of flow; they do not enhance stroke volume or mean flow and pressure.

Certain psychiatric complications of closed-chest cardiac resuscitation have been reported and may be of considerable concern. Severe personality decompensation is occasionally seen in patients subjected to highly mechanized and anxiety-provoking emotional distresses during treatment in areas such as coronary care units, intensive care units, recovery rooms, or burn and trauma units. The postcardiac resuscitation victim is no exception, since he may require prolonged artificial assistance of one type or another. An endotracheal tube may prevent him from communicating easily, and he may be totally unfamiliar with the purpose of the monitoring apparatus and the strange sounds, tubes, and equipment. Usually it is impossible for a patient to remember clearly the events surrounding cardiac arrest followed by successful resuscitation. The emotional adaptation of the patient after a cardiac resuscitation tends to be quite varied. The impersonal nature of his confinement, often in a windowless room, may compound the difficulties. In addition, his psychlogical problems may aggravate an acute brain syndrome provoked by anoxia or hypercapnia. The situation can be helped considerably by giving all possible personal attention and as much direct communication as possible.

The psychiatric study by Druss and Kornfeld on a group of 10 survivors of cardiac arrest is significant.[9] These two physicians wondered how patients might react to the unique and remarkable experience of having been clinically "dead." Their group of 10 patients was taken from 16 patients successfully resuscitated and discharged from Columbia–Presbyterian Hospital and represented a group of 85 patients who had experienced cardiac arrest outside the operating room. Prolonged psychiatric interviews were carried out with patients and relatives and with a control group comprising 10 additional males who had been in the intensive care unit but who had not had a cardiac arrest. Nine of the 10 patients with cardiac arrest had a mild to severe organic brain syndrome that included symptoms of confusion, delusional thinking, and uncontrollable agitation. At least four defense mechanisms were elicited.

1. Denial and isolation
2. Displacement
3. Rejection
4. Hallucinatory or delusional behavior

Eight of the patients reacted by an isolation of affect and by denying that they had been afraid. Eight of the 10 patients experienced dreams of violence and violent death after the cardiac arrest episode. When questioned about their attitude toward death, patients replied that they had been in no pain, and therefore death was believed to be painless. No overt alterations in patients' religious attitudes were uncovered as a result of having experienced clinical "death." Persistent long-term symptoms were often present, the most common being insomnia. Tenseness, anxiety, restlessness, and irritability were common. Difficulty in concentration and a lack of memory for recent events were noted by most of these patients.

Several suggestions have been made by psychiatrists for improving the care of cardiac patients. Much can be done to make the intensive care/coronary care unit a less frightening place. Increasing the degree of privacy would be helpful so that patients would be less aware of the life and death struggle of other patients. Monitoring equipment might be placed outside the unit to reduce some of the frightening aspects to the patient. Each patient experiencing a cardiac arrest should be talked to in detail and given as much reassurance as possible. The psychic trauma to the physician and allied health personnel themselves might well be mentioned. One particular surgeon, for example, was so severely depressed by an occurrence of cardiac arrest during a tonsillectomy that he ceased performing any type of surgery.

The foregoing discussion has dealt with a rather formidable group of possible pitfalls in, and possible complications of, closed-chest cardiac massage. Each of these complications can be minimized by careful attention to details of performance. During cardiac arrest, effective cardiopulmonary resuscitation is required, even if it results in complications, since the alternative to effective cardiopulmonary resuscitation is death.

THE OPEN-CHEST APPROACH IN MODERN MANAGEMENT OF CARDIAC ARREST

Although the respiratory care worker will not be opening the chest for direct cardiac massage, it is important that he be aware of those situations not likely to yield successfully to closed-chest compressive efforts. There are pathophysiological considerations that contribute to ineffective closed-chest compression techniques and that can be managed more effectively by means of the direct or open-chest route.

The effectiveness of closed-chest resuscitation, if properly performed, in establishing an effective tissue perfusion is clearly established. In those situations where closed-chest compression techniques are ineffective, the open-chest approach for direct cardiac compression is a viable alternative that should be part of the physician's armamentarium.

Unfortunately, physicians who have graduated within the past 15 years have had virtually no experience with the open-chest approach for resuscitation. For example, at a recent national conference on ventricular fibrillation, a young physician referred to the days of the "bloody bedside thoracotomy" approach for resuscitation of the fibrillating ventricles. Although conceding that a few of these patients survived, he emphasized that more commonly the heart was considerably damaged by the "scorching" epicardial current and that the patient rapidly died because of the "gaping thoracotomy initially done under the worst possible conditions." This is, of course, at variance with many reported series on open-chest resuscitative efforts. In fact, our initially reported large series of open-chest resuscitative efforts included 1200 cases with a long-term survival of 28%.

Previously discussed factors that lead to failure—undue delay in instituting resuscitation, complications of the procedure itself, and ineffective use of proven ventilatory and cardiac resuscitative efforts—are the most usual contributors to failure. However, new data on monitoring show, as many of us have long suspected, that sternal compression, even under ideal conditions, may result in only borderline perfusion of the brain and vital organs.

Recent data give considerable evidence that the heart serves as a passive conduit during conventional cardiac massage (e.g., as demonstrated by two-dimensional echocardiography that showed no change in ventricular-chamber size during closed-chest compression). Rudikoff and colleagues pointed to the role of generalized increases in intrathoracic pressure rather than to heart compression itself in generating intrathoracic vascular pressure.[23] Additionally, only marginal arterial blood pressure levels (seldom over 40 mm Hg) are achieved by standard, closed-chest CPR.

At present, unfortunately, no highly usable clinical features indicate the time for switching quickly from closed- to open-chest cardiac compression, although poor perfusion, widely dilated pupils, continued anoxic appearance, and poor capillary refilling are helpful.

When adequate perfusion is not quickly apparent in closed-chest attempts, we move decisively to open the left chest, especially in the hypovolemic patient. Inserting the gloved left hand through a fifth or sixth intercostal space, spreading the ribs manually, we carry out manual compression at about 80 times/min. Under these circumstances, it is easy to determine the tone of the myocardium and visually or manually observe the vigor of myocardial contraction as a response to pharmacologic agents. If necessary, the thoracic aorta may be occluded distal to the left subclavian artery, thus allowing the cardiac output to be diverted to augment the coronary and cerebral circulations.

Although no one expects open-chest massage to become one of the *first* lines of CPR effort, it behooves us to be mindful of the technique as a backup in cases where response to closed-chest effort is less than adequate. In the following discussion, emphasis is directed toward those cases that would not otherwise be likely to survive without an open-chest resuscitative effort. At least six general categories of cardiac arrest cases would seem best managed by directly compressing the heart through the open-chest approach. Obviously there are gray areas included where some disagreement may occur.

GROUP 1: ANATOMICAL AND DEVELOPMENTAL ABNORMALITIES THAT WOULD HINDER OR PRECLUDE ADEQUATE CLOSED-CHEST COMPRESSION

In this group of patients one would include those with a pectus excavatum or pectus carinatum deformity of sufficient magnitude as to make external cardiac compression impractical. When the heart's anatomical location is shifted from its more-or-less midline locus and is not positioned between the sternum and the vertebrae, closed-chest compression will be virtually worthless. Vertebral abnormalities such as marked scoliosis, lordosis, and kyphosis may preclude external compression simply because the heart cannot be compressed between the sternum and the vertebrae. Further, any pathologic state shifting the mediastinum produces the same anatomical difficulty (e.g., significant atelectasis may require open-chest resuscitation); in the postpneumonectomy or postlobectomy patient there may be enough shift of the mediastinum, including the heart, to produce a similar difficulty.

GROUP 2: CARDIAC ABNORMALITIES REQUIRING A DIRECT, OPEN-CHEST APPROACH

Several cases may be cited in which a direct, open-chest approach is clearly dictated.

1. When cardiac arrest is associated with a myocardial laceration or puncture requiring direct suture application, open-chest resuscitation is essential. We experienced such a case in a teenage girl who had been stabbed in the left side of the chest. The emergency room chest film was not remarkable, and it was thought that a laceration of the spleen may have oc-

curred. Cardiac arrest ensued, and closed-chest compression was attempted but did not seem adequate. The chest was subsequently opened to reveal a myocardial laceration with exsanguinating hemorrhage. Resuscitation was prompt after the laceration had been sutured between intervals of cardiac compression. The patient made an uneventful recovery.

2. If a known ventricular aneurysm is present, one may be reluctant to use closed-chest compression and may prefer to compress the noninvolved portion of the ventricle selectively by means of the visual approach.
3. Intracardiac obstruction owing to a tumor (e.g., left atrial myxoma) will need to be approached directly.
4. Ventricular herniation after cardiac surgery will require manual relocation of the heart to its position within the pericardial sac and appropriate closure of the pericardium.
5. Cases have been reported of mitral stenosis so severe that cardiac resuscitation could not be successful until an emergency valvotomy had been performed rapidly.
6. Cardiac tamponade is a not infrequent cause of cardiac arrest but is often unsuspected. Venting of the pericardial sac for removal of the offending agent, usually blood, is mandatory before successful cardiac compression can be applied.
7. In a case of right ventricular output obstruction or pulmonary artery obstruction owing to a pulmonary embolism, failure to recognize or suspect the presence of a pulmonary embolus results in failure to resuscitate many cardiac arrest victims. Admittedly, this is often a difficult diagnosis, but one should suspect it if cardiac output is virtually absent despite what appears to be technically correct closed-chest compression. Postoperative patients are, of course, particularly suspect. Pulmonary embolism is a difficult, challenging association with cardiac arrest, but techniques are available to remove the embolism effectively in such instances.

GROUP 3: SITUATIONS IN WHICH EXTERNAL DEFIBRILLATION MAY NOT BE POSSIBLE

Because of the work of Tacker and Geddes, it is becoming increasingly apparent that many commercially available defibrillators cannot deliver a peak current high enough to defibrillate patients weighing more than 80 kg.[27] They emphasize that patients who have had an acute myocardial infarction probably require current levels higher than do noninfarcted patients. Thus patients who weigh more than 100 kg may require open-chest resuscitation if a satisfactory defibrillator is unavailable.

GROUP 4: CARDIAC ARREST PROBLEMS COMPOUNDED BY ADDITIONAL THORACIC PATHOLOGY

The presence of thoracic complications in a case of cardiac arrest suggests the adoption of the open-chest approach.

1. A crushed chest injury or a flail chest may so neutralize the benefit of external compression that the heart should be directly approached. In addition, if exsanguinating hemorrhage is suspected within the chest, its control will require a thoracotomy.
2. A bilateral pneumothorax with grossly inadequate ventilation may be unrecognized until the chest has been opened. Similarly, a tension pneumothorax may so shift the mediastinum that closed-chest compression is inadequate.
3. Right-sided venous air embolism or left-sided arterial embolism to the coronary arteries often is best approached by a direct visualization of the pathology. For example, if a large bolus of air is lodged in the right side of the heart, it can usually be effectively and directly aspirated. Arterial embolization to the heart, although infrequent, can more effectively be dispersed by a direct approach.

GROUP 5: CARDIAC ARREST CASES REFRACTORY TO CLOSED-CHEST RESUSCITATION

Since tissue perfusion is only about 30% of normal under the most ideal closed-chest cardiopulmonary resuscitative efforts, it is not unexpected that closed-chest massage may need to be abandoned for direct massage where signs of inadequate tissue perfusion exist. Cohn and Del Guerico report 11 such patients successfully resuscitated and able to leave the hospital after closed-chest massage had been abandoned in favor of direct cardiac massage with its increased cardiac output.[5] The precise reason for failure of the closed-chest approach may not always be apparent.

GROUP 6: MISCELLANEOUS CASES THAT MAY BENEFIT FROM OPEN-CHEST RESUSCITATION

The final category is a heterogeneous one, composed of patients whose conditions favor an open-chest approach.

1. The elderly emphysematous patient with a large, inelastic anterior–posterior thoracic diameter chest may not be a good candidate for external cardiac resuscitation.
2. Although some patients in the third trimester of pregnancy have been resuscitated with closed-chest techniques, others would probably do best with the open-chest technique. Theoretically, a ruptured liver should be more likely if the closed-chest approach were used.
3. If cardiac arrest occurs while the chest is open during an intrathoracic procedure, the open-chest approach obviously is desirable.
4. If cardiac arrest is due to exsanguinating hemorrhage of an extrathoracic origin, it may be lifesaving if one opens the chest and pinches off the descending thoracic aorta so that the remaining available blood will be circulated to the highly anoxia-sensitive cerebral tissues.
5. In rare situations, such as cardiac arrest that occurs on the operating table in a patient in an upright position, indications for the open-chest approach may arise.
6. Rapid rewarming of the heart may be required for defibrillation, and the direct application of warm saline to the heart and intrathoracic structures is an effective approach.
7. Although many patients with prosthetic heart valves have had successful closed-chest cardiopulmonary resuscitation, there are pitfalls in this approach. The metallic ring of the mitral valve prosthesis may produce damaging pressure in the region of the posterior arteriovenous groove because of the position of the unyielding ring. Myocardial hematomas have been caused by pressure on the myocardium as well as disruption of the ventricle, rupture of a coronary artery, or intractable cardiac conduction disturbances.

Again, the hemodynamic superiority of direct cardiac massage is significant as measured in terms of the cardiac index, mean circulation time, and carotid and systemic arterial blood flow. A more rapid diastolic filling allows a faster stroke rate to achieve greater forward flow of circulation as well as more complete ventricular emptying. Less blood is propelled retrograde into the vena cava with direct cardiac massage. Del Guerico has shown that the cardiac index is more than doubled when the chest is opened during cardiac massage; the mean circulation time in his studies is reduced by more than half.[7]

Closed-chest resuscitation is nevertheless the method of choice in most instances. Because of its immediate availability to, and applicability by, medical and nonmedical personnel, because of the rapidity with which the cerebral circulation can be perfused, and because of the legions of successful closed-chest resuscitations, this technique represents a most significant advance in medicine. Some flexibility of the physician is needed, however, if additional selected cardiac arrest victims are to be resuscitated. Although the general and thoracic surgeon may be required in some of these efforts, the open-chest approach still should remain a part of the well-trained physician's in-hospital capabilities.

PHARMACOLOGIC CONSIDERATIONS

The proper use of drugs, including timing, proper dosage, and intended pharmacologic effect, has a vital role in CPR. A chapter far longer than this one would be needed to present adequately all the details of the very sophisticated pharmacologic routines available to the present-day resuscitator. Therefore, I shall necessarily restrict the present consideration of drugs to those currently in accepted use (Table 38-5). Any discussion of the pharmacology of resuscitation inevitably turns our attention to the four basic properties inherent in a normal beating heart: excitability, contractility, rhythmicity, and conductivity. These properties of the beating heart are the ones we seek to control, inhibit, or enhance. The pharmacologic agents presented will be divided into two categories: essential drugs and useful drugs.

ESSENTIAL DRUGS

Essential drugs recommended by the National Conference to be available for any CPR effort include sodium bicarbonate, atropine sulfate, epinephrine, morphine sulfate, lidocaine, and calcium chloride. Oxygen is also considered since it is obviously essential.[17]

Table 38-5. Drugs Commonly Used in Cardiopulmonary Resuscitation

DRUG	USUAL DOSAGE	INDICATIONS AND REMARKS
Sodium bicarbonate	Adult: 1 mEq/kg. May repeat in 10 min, then 0.5 mEq/kg during CPR Child: 1.2 mEq/kg dose or 0.3 × kg × base deficit	Correction of lactic acidosis due to tissue hypoxia. Use arterial blood gas data to follow effectiveness.
Atropine sulfate	Adult: 0.2–0.6 mg i.v. (up to 2.0 mg) Child: 0.01 mg/kg/dose or 0.3 mg/m^2 (up to 0.4 mg)	1. Sinus bradycardia 2. A-V block 3. Accelerate slow nodal rhythm
Epinephrine	Adult: 5–10 ml (0.5–1.0 mg) of 1:10,000 dilution i.v., 0.3–2.0 ml intracardiac Child: 0.1 ml/kg of 1:10,000 dilution	1. Stimulate the myocardium to contract 2. May repeat every 5 minutes in cases of asystole
Metaraminol bitartrate	Adult: 100 mg/250 ml of 5% D/W; start slowly Child: 25 mg/100 ml in 5% D/W and titrate blood pressure	Correct hypotension
Levarterenol bitartrate	Adult: 2 mg in 250 ml 5% D/W and titrate Child: 2 mg in 250 ml 5% D/W and titrate (0.1 μg/kg/min)	Correct hypotension
Lidocaine	Adult: 50–100 mg bolus i.v., then 1–4 mg/min Child 0.5–1.0 mg/kg q 20–60 min. Titrate at 0.05–0.15 mg/kg/min	Reduce ventricular irritability (*e.g.,* premature ventricular contractions and tachycardia)
Isoproterenol hydrochloride	Adult: 1 mg/250 ml 5% D/W. Start at 1–5 μg/min and titrate Child: 0.1–0.5 μg/kg/min and titrate to desired effect	1. Correct bradycardia 2. Correct hypotension
Calcium chloride (10%)	Adult: 2.5–5 ml i.v. May repeat q 5–10 min Child: 1–4 ml of 10% solution i.v. (Maximum dose of 1 ml/5 kg)	1. Increase force of myocardial contraction 2. Use with caution in digitalized patients
Propranolol	Adult: Give 1 mg/min i.v. up to 4.0 mg total Child: 0.01–0.15 mg/kg given slowly	Inhibit supraventricular and ventricular arrhythmias, particularly those related to digitalis toxicity
Terbutaline sulfate*	Adult: 0.25 mg subcutaneously (not more than 0.5 mg/4 hr) Child: Not recommended	Relieve bronchospasm

(Hodgkin JE, Foster GL, Nicolay LI: Cardiopulmonary resuscitation: Development of an organized protocol. Crit Care Med 5:93, 1977, and the National Conference Steering Committee—standards for cardiopulmonary resuscitation (CPR) and emergency cardiac care (ECC). JAMA 227[Suppl]:837, 1974)

**See* Chapter 20.

Sodium Bicarbonate

Sodium bicarbonate is used to combat the metabolic acidosis that accompanies cardiac arrest and tissue hypoxia. It is administered intravenously in an initial dose of 1 mEq/kg by either bolus injection or by continuous infusion over a 10-minute period. Further administration of sodium bicarbonate after effective circulation has been restored is not usually indicated unless severe hypotension is present. Excessive administration may even be harmful because of sodium loading, hyperosmolarity, and "overshoot" alkalemia. Prefilled syringes and ampules of sodium bicarbonate contain either 44.6 or 50.0 mEq of sodium bicarbonate. If ventricular fibrillation is present, defibrillation should be attempted immediately, before sodium bicarbonate is administered. If effective circulation is not restored after defibrillation and the initial dose of bicarbonate, a repeat dose of 1 mEq/kg should be given. In hospitalized patients, further administration of sodium bicarbonate should be governed by arterial blood gas and *p*H measurements.

Sodium bicarbonate administration must always be accompanied by effective ventilation to remove carbon dioxide from the arterial blood. When blood gas *p*H determinations are not available, one half of the initial dose may be administered subsequently every 10 minutes. Catecholamine drugs such as epinephrine may be given either simultaneously or in rapid succession with sodium bicarbonate. Mixing the two agents before injection is not advisable.

Patients with cardiac standstill or persistent ventricular fibrillation should not receive sodium bicarbonate alone. Repeated doses of epinephrine and sodium bicarbonate should be administered while external cardiac massage and artificial ventilation are continued. This combination of agents may convert a cardiac standstill into ventricular fibrillation, which can then be defibrillated. In ventricular fibrillation, the use of both drugs improves the status of the myocardium and enhances the effectiveness of the defibrillation.

Atropine Sulfate

Atropine sulfate accelerates heartbeat in cases of sinus bradycardia, reduces vagal activity, and enhances atrioventricular conduction. Particularly in cases of hypotension, it is useful in preventing cardiac arrest in severe sinus bradycardia secondary to toxic myocardial infarction. It is indicated for the treatment of sinus bradycardia when the cardiac rate is less than 60 beats/min, accompanied by premature ventricular contractions, or when the systolic blood pressure is less than 90 mm Hg. Its use is indicated for high-degree atrioventricular block when accompanied by bradycardia, but it is of no value in ventricular ectopic bradycardia in the absence of atrial activity. A dose of 0.5 mg is administered intravenously as a bolus and repeated every 5 minutes until a ventricular rate greater than 60 has been achieved. The total dose should not exceed 2 mg except in cases of third-degree atrioventricular block, where larger doses may be needed. Smaller doses of atropine may slow the heart rate by either a peripheral parasympathomimetic or a central vagal-stimulating action.

Epinephrine

Epinephrine, a sympathomimetic catecholamine drug, increases myocardial contractility and perfusion pressures, lowers the defibrillatory threshold, and occasionally restores myocardial contractility itself. With respect to epinephrine, recent guidelines state

> There is convincing evidence that epinephrine is absorbed promptly after instillation into the tracheobronchial tree via an endotracheal tube. If an IV route cannot be established quickly, this route of injection should be used if an endotracheal tube is in place or can be inserted promptly. Until more is known about dose-response relationships after tracheobronchial injection, it is recommended that 1 mg. (10 mL of the 1:10,000 solution) be used for this site of administration. The IV or tracheobronchial routes of injection are strongly recommended, and the intracardiac route of injection should be used only if the other sites of injection are inaccessible. The hazards of intracardiac injection include coronary artery laceration, cardiac tamponade, pneumothorax, and the need to interrupt external chest compressions and ventilation during the period of injection.
>
> Epinephrine can also be administered as a continuous infusion to sustain arterial pressure, heart rate, and cardiac output, although there are preferable approaches to sustaining arterial pressure, particularly in the setting of myocardial infarction. An infusion can be prepared by adding 1 mg. of epinephrine to 250 mL of 5 per cent dextrose in water. Infusion can be started in the adult at 1 μg/min. This dose should increase cardiac output and arterial pressure in most instances.
>
> The recommended dose of epinephrine hydrochloride is 0.5 to 1.0 mg. (5 to 10 mL of a 1:10,000 solution) given IV during the resuscitation effort. It is necessary to repeat this dose at approximately five-minute intervals when given IV because of the short duration of action of epinephrine.[26]

Morphine Sulfate

Morphine is not usually indicated in CPR emergencies. It is used in cases of myocardial infarction to relieve pain and to treat pulmonary edema. Dosage varies from person to person: 2 to 5 mg may be given intravenously every 5 to 30 minutes, as needed.

Small doses of morphine given in increments will usually allow early recognition of respiratory depression or hypotension. Hypotension is most likely to occur in volume-depleted patients or in those with elevation of systemic vascular resistance.

Lidocaine

Lidocaine reduces cardiac irritability and increases the electrical stimulation threshold of the ventricle during diastole, therefore exerting an antidysrhythmic effect. There is no significant change in myocardial contractility, systemic arterial pressure, or absolute refractory period when lidocaine is given in the usual therapeutic doses. It is particularly effective in depressing irritability (ventricular premature contractions or ventricular tachycardia) when successive defibrillation attempts revert to fibrillation. According to recent guidelines,

> There are a number of ways to administer lidocaine to achieve and maintain therapeutic blood levels rapidly. A commonly used technique consists of a bolus injection of about 1 mg/kg of body weight, followed immediately by an infusion of 1 to 4 mg/min., preferably by

means of an infusion pump. Another approach consists of administration of a 75 mg. bolus injection and the simultaneous initiation of an infusion at 2 mg/min. If ventricular ectopy occurs after the initial 75 mg. bolus, an additional 50 mg. bolus can be given every five minutes if necessary, to a total of 225 mg. The concomitant infusion begun at 2 mg/min. is increased by 1 mg/min. after each additional bolus injection to a maximum of 4 mg/min. A somewhat similar dosage program can be used for primary prophylaxis against ventricular fibrillation. Prophylactic administration of lidocaine in the presence of acute myocardial infarction may reduce the incidence of ventricular dysrhythmias and primary ventricular fibrillation.

The dose of lidocaine should be reduced in the presence of a reduction in cardiac output such as may be associated with acute myocardial infarction, congestive cardiac failure, or shock from whatever cause. In such clinical situations, one might begin with half the normal bolus dose and observe the patient closely for signs of both toxic reactions and therapeutic effect. Other investigators have recommended that the usual loading dose be given to such patients and that only the maintenance dosage should be reduced. Most instances of toxic reactions are related to the CNS (e.g., slurred speech, altered consciousness, muscle twitching, and seizures), and once identified, the dosage should be reduced.[26]

Naturally, lidocaine is of no value in cardiac asystole.

Calcium Chloride

Calcium chloride increases myocardial contractility, prolongs systole, and *enhances* ventricular excitability. After rapid intravenous injection, it suppresses sinus impulse formation and can produce sudden death, especially in fully digitalized patients. Calcium chloride is useful in treating profound cardiovascular collapse (electromechanical dissociation); it may restore an electrical rhythm in instances of asystole and may enhance electrical defibrillation.

The dosage varies widely. The usual recommended dosage of calcium chloride is 2.5 to 5 ml of a 10% solution (3.4–6.8 mEq Ca^{++}) injected intravenously as a bolus at 10-minute intervals. Calcium gluconate provides fewer calcium ions per unit volume, and, if it is used, the dosage should be 10 ml of a 10% solution (4.8 mEq). Alternatively, calcium gluceptate may be administered in a dosage of 5 ml (4.5 mEq). Hypercalcemia is a definite hazard of large doses. No form of calcium must be administered at the same time as sodium bicarbonate, since the mixture results in formation of a precipitate.

Alternate Drug Routes

In the event of failure to establish an intravenous lifeline, epinephrine can be effectively instilled directly in the tracheobronchial tree by means of an endotracheal tube, using 1 to 2 mg/10 ml of sterile distilled water. Lidocaine may be similarly used in the amount of 50 to 100 mg/10 ml of sterile, distilled water. Endotracheal use of other drugs for cardiopulmonary resuscitation has not yet been established.

Atropine sulfate (2 mg) or lidocaine (300 mg) may be given intramuscularly to establish therapeutic and prophylactic blood levels for control of dysrhythmia; this route, however, requires the presence of adequate spontaneous circulation.

USEFUL DRUGS

Along with the vasoactive drugs, levarterenol (Levophed) and metaraminol (Aramine), isoproterenol (Isuprel), propranolol (Inderal), and corticosteroids may be included in this category.

Some physicians challenge the use of potent peripheral vasoconstrictors because of the possibility of reducing cerebral, cardiac, and renal blood flow. The choice of a vasoconstrictor or a positive inotropic agent remains controversial in the treatment of cardiac arrest and in the immediate postresuscitative period. Blood pressure must, however, be supported when inadequate cerebral and renal perfusion give evidence of shock, both during cardiac compression and in the postresuscitative period.

In cases of peripheral vascular collapse, identified clinically by hypotension and the absence of significant peripheral vasoconstriction, higher than usual intravenous dosages of levarterenol bitartrate (concentrations of 16 μg/ml) or metaraminol bitartrate (concentrations of 0.4 mg/ml of dextrose in water) should be given intravenously. Metaraminol may be given intravenously as a bolus of 2 to 5 mg every 5 to 10 seconds. Continuous administration is required to maintain a satisfactory blood pressure and adequate urinary output. Both of these drugs are potent vasoconstrictors, and both have a positive inotropic effect on the myocardium. They are especially useful where systemic peripheral resistance is low.

Isoproterenol

If a bradycardia is demonstrated to result, in fact, from complete heart block, isoproterenol hydrochloride should be infused in amounts of 2 to 20 μg/min (1–10 ml of a solution consisting of 1 mg in 500 ml of 5% glucose in water). The flow should be adjusted to increase heart rate to approximately 60 beats/min. This regimen is useful in cases of profound sinus bradycardia that have proved refractory to atropine. An isoproterenol infusion is prepared for use by adding 1 mg of isoproterenol hydrochloride to 500 ml of 5%

dextrose in sterile water; this produces a concentration of 2 μg/ml. One milligram in 250 ml of 5% dextrose produces a concentration of 4 μg/ml.

Propranolol

Propranolol is a β-adrenergic blocking agent with useful antiarrhythmic properties. It is useful in instances of repetitive ventricular tachycardia or repetitive ventricular fibrillation where maintenance of a restored beat cannot be achieved with lidocaine. The usual dose of propranolol is 1 mg intravenously, repeated to a total of 3 mg with careful monitoring. Caution is needed in using this drug in patients with chronic obstructive pulmonary disease, since it may cause bronchoconstriction, or in patients with cardiac failure, in whom it may further reduce cardiac output. Extreme caution must be exercised when propranolol therapy is considered for use in patients who may be critically dependent on β-adrenergic receptor support, including those patients in whom asthma and cardiac failure are suspected. Treatment with propranolol may be particularly hazardous when cardiac function is depressed, as it usually is after cardiac arrest. Propranolol hydrochloride may be administered in boluses up to 1.0 mg i.v. every 5 minutes, usually not exceeding a total dose of 5.0 mg.

Corticosteroids

Prompt treatment of cardiogenic shock or shock lung that occurs as a complication of cardiac arrest may be treated with pharmacologic doses of synthetic corticosteroids (5 mg/kg of methylprednisolone sodium succinate, or 1 mg/kg of dexamethasone phosphate). If cerebral edema is suspected as a complicating factor in cardiac arrest, methylprednisolone sodium succinate in doses of 60 to 100 mg every 6 hours may be beneficial. Postaspiration pneumonitis or other pulmonary complications may indicate use of dexamethasone phosphate in doses of 4 to 8 mg every 6 hours.

Other Drugs

Other drugs such as bretylium tosylate (Darenthin), dopamine hydrochloride (Intropin), dobutamine hydrochloride (Dobutrex), digitalis preparations, sodium nitroprusside (Nipride), nitroglycerin, and certain diuretics have an occasional role. The reader is referred to a discussion of them under advanced life support in recent standards and guidelines.[26]

CPR TRAINING

The respiratory care worker is a prime target for CPR training at a sophisticated level; it is logical to look to him for considerable leadership and assistance in the training of special groups such as policemen, firemen, high-risk industry workers, families with cardiac patients, medical students, and nursing students. Although the American Heart Association and, more recently, the American Red Cross have embarked on massive efforts to train laymen in cardiopulmonary resuscitative techniques, it would appear that we are still at the beginning of our efforts if one views the picture of total need in adequate perspective.

Interestingly, in Norway, mouth-to-mouth resuscitation was made a compulsory school subject in 1960, as part of a first aid course designed to prepare the pupils to treat life-threatening emergencies. Laerdal comments that about 800,000 lay people (one fifth of the population of Norway) have received practical instruction in mouth-to-mouth resuscitation; 400,000 others have been trained or retrained during military service and civil defense and in courses given by volunteer organizations such as the Red Cross.[15] He estimates that almost 1000 lives have been saved by mouth-to-mouth resuscitation during the 15-year period. It is now a law in Norway that all driver's license applicants must be trained and tested in essential first aid. This will mean that 100,000 people per year will be trained or retrained in driving schools.

Obviously, we are not salvaging the potentially overwhelming number of cardiac arrest patients that we may, hopefully, some day be able to reach. Time, of course, continues to be the crux of successful resuscitation. If the percentage of permanent survival is to be enhanced and neurologic deficits are to be reduced, we must eliminate every possible source of delay in beginning basic life-support measures.

The survival rate of patients who suffer cardiopulmonary arrest outside the hospital is, naturally, considerably less than that of those patients who encounter this difficulty in the more favorable environment of the hospital. But with the increasing availability of more widespread training of lay personnel, this situation is one of the more encouraging ones in the total picture at this time.

SUMMARY

Gradual gains here and minimal gains there have provoked a feeling of optimism that we may be embarking on a higher plateau of success in combating the problem of sudden death. Since the largest group of patients requiring CPR involves those patients with acute myocardial infarction, it is in this direction that a preponderance of effort has logically been made. Obviously, mobile coronary care units will continue to increase in effectiveness, and undoubtedly their numbers will increase. Preventive efforts seem likely with further identification of important risk factors. Instruction of the family and associates of the high-risk patient seems a logical extension of this effort. There are encouraging signs that inroads are being made toward salvaging a portion of the 365,000 "coronary deaths" that occur outside the hospitals of the United States each year. These patients are being more effectively reached by community programs of increasingly greater sophistication. Experimental ventricular defibrillation by automated and completely implanted systems appears promising, and the increasing use of electromagnetic tape recorders for continuous monitoring of ECGs to detect previously uninvestigated arrhythmias seems to be a development of the immediate future. The physician may, for example, monitor the patient for varying periods of time and under varying circumstances to select the drug that will give maximal protection to the patient prone to worrisome dysrhythmias.

Any program to effectively diminish the incidence of sudden cardiac arrest must include education of the patient so that he will call for help at the very onset of any sign of trouble. We believe that in the years ahead both the patient and the physician will insist that every hospital develop an adequate program for in-depth training, and that the quality control of resuscitative efforts be maintained at a higher level. We would hope that hospital accreditation agencies will insist on effective and functioning cardiac resuscitation committees responsible for disseminating all new advances in the area of resuscitation, maintaining equipment for resuscitation, and providing current data on all resuscitative efforts, as well as providing continued evaluation of the quality of the program.

Risk factors associated with coronary artery disease and sudden death (e.g., hypercholesterolemia, hypertension, hyperglycemia, excessive cigarette smoking, lack of exercise, and stress factors) are receiving attention. More than three-fourths of the men who suffered instantaneous death in recent studies could be categorized as having two or more of these risk factors. It would obviously be productive to identify these risk factors further and to direct efforts toward alleviating them. Certainly, if the incidence of sudden death is to be reduced, we must get the victim of myocardial infarction to the hospital sooner. Currently, an average of 7 hours elapses between the first onset of symptoms and the arrival of these patients at the hospital. This is presumably because of lack of information on the significance of the symptoms, misinterpretation of the symptoms, or denial of their importance. A relatively minor source of the delay is the unavailability of medical attention. The development of an effective prophylactic antiarrhythmic drug, free of toxicity and side reactions, would be a truly significant advance.

Even though cardiopulmonary resuscitative efforts are promptly instituted, and even though they appear to be technically correct, one continues to see some patients who experience severe neurologic deficits after episodes of cardiac arrest. The explanation has often been obscure and indicates that factors other than the factor of time may be involved. During periods of transient cardiac arrest, serious deficiency of the microcirculation develops and appears to persist even after resuscitative measures have been instituted. After external cardiac massage, patients have been shown to develop an aggregation of formed elements of the blood in the small vessels of the kidneys and lungs. Anaerobic glycolysis in the brain produces lactic acid locally and has a devastating effect on the microcirculation, through aggregation and sludging of formed elements and formation of microemboli and thrombi. Efforts toward recovery of the patency of this microcirculation may well prove fruitful in future cardiopulmonary resuscitative efforts. Administration of steroids and low molecular weight dextran seems to be promising because of their specific antisludging and lysosome membrane stabilization properties. Both drugs not only decrease the cerebral edema, thereby improving perfusion, but also reduce platelet adhesiveness.

One may be called on, at any time, to attempt resuscitation of the heart. Knowledge about cardiac resuscitation has become extensive, and the literature is vast. Because many attempts are in progress to familiarize an ever-growing number of health care personnel with techniques of resuscitation, it is hoped that greater success will be achieved in the future.

The author wishes to thank Morris Hiatt, R.R.T., Manager, Respiratory Therapy Department, University of Missouri Hospital and Clinics, Columbia, MO, for his review of, and contributions to, the sections on intubation, laryngoscopes, resuscitators, bags, and airways.

REFERENCES

1. Alifimoff J et al: Cardiac resuscitability after closed-chest, MAST-augmented and open-chest CPR. Anesthesiology 53[Suppl]:151, 1980
2. Bencini A et al: The pneumomassage of the heart. Surgery 39:375, 1956
3. Bircher N, Safar P, Stewart R: A comparison of standard,

MAST-augmented and open-chest CPR in dogs. A preliminary investigation. Crit Care Med 8:147, 1980
4. Chandra N, Rudikoff MT, Weisfeldt ML: Simultaneous chest compression and ventilation at high airway pressure during cardiopulmonary resuscitation. Lancet 361:175, 1980
5. Cohn JD, Del Guerico LRM: Cardiorespiratory determinants of clinical resuscitation. Sug Forum 16:182, 1965
6. Daggett WM et al; Intracaval electrophrenic stimulation. J Thorac Cardiovasc Surg 51:676, 1966
7. Del Guerico LRM et al: Comparison of blood flow during external and internal cardiac massage in man. Circulation 31:171, 1965
8. Don Michael TA, Lambert EH, Mebran A: Mouth to lung airway for cardiac resuscitation. Lancet 2:1329, 1968
9. Druss RG, Kornfeld DS: The survivors of cardiac arrest. A psychiatric study. JAMA 201:291, 1967
10. Elam JO et al: Artificial respiration by mouth-to-mask method. N Engl J Med 250:749, 1954
11. Guildner CW: A comparison of airway maintenance techniques. *In* Safar P (ed): Advances in Cardiopulmonary Resuscitation. New York, Springer–Verlag, 1975
12. Guthrie CC, Pike FH, Stewart GN: I. The general condition affecting resuscitation, and the resuscitation of the blood and of the heart. J. Exp Med 10:371, 1908
13. Heimlich HJ: A life-saving maneuver to prevent food choking. JAMA 234:398, 1975
14. Kouwenhoven WB, Jude JR, Knickerbocker GG: Closed-chest cardiac massage. JAMA 173:1064, 1960
15. Laerdal A: Quantitative goals in the teaching of cardiopulmonary resuscitation. *In* Safar P (ed): Advances in Cardiopulmonary Resuscitation. New York, Springer–Verlag, 1975
16. Modell JH: Resuscitation after aspiration of chlorinated fresh water. JAMA 185:651, 1963
17. National Conference on Standards for Cardiopulmonary Resuscitation (CPR) and Emergency Cardiac Care (ECC). JAMA 227[Suppl], February 18, 1974
18. Nicolay LI, Hodgkin JE: Positive impact of a CPR team on successful resuscitations. Am Rev Respir Dis 115[Suppl]:146, 1977
19. Redding JS: Commentary on the proceedings: Second Wolf Creek conference on CPR. Crit Care Med 9:432, 1981
20. Redding JS, Haynes RR, Thomas JD: "Old" and "new" CPR manually performed in dogs. Crit Care Med 9:386, 1981
21. Rubin H: A new non-rebreathing valve. Anesthesiology 16:643, 1955
22. Rubin IL et al: Five years of cardiac resuscitation. GP 30(3):96, 1963
23. Rudikoff MT et al: Mechanisms of blood flow during cardiopulmonary resuscitation. Circulation 61:345, 1980
24. Safar P: Recognition and management of airway obstruction. JAMA 208:1009, 1969
25. Schofferman J, Oill P, Lewis AJ: The esophageal obturator airway: A clinical evaluation. Chest 69:67, 1976
26. Standards and guidelines for cardiopulmonary resuscitation (CPR) and emergency cardiac care (ECC). JAMA 244:453, 1980
27. Tacker WA, Geddes LA, Hoff HE: Defibrillation without A-V block using capacitor discharge with added inductance. Circ Res 22:633, 1968

BIBLIOGRAPHY

Introduction

Stephenson HE Jr: Cardiac Arrest and Resuscitation, 4th ed. St. Louis, CV Mosby, 1974

History

Beck CS, Pritchard WH, Feil H: Ventricular fibrillation of long duration abolished by electric shock. JAMA 135:985, 1947

phyxie. Arch Klin Exp Path Pharmacol 8:68, 1878

Crile GW: Anemia and Resuscitation. New York, Appleton Century, 1914

d'Halluin M: Résurrection du coeur, la vie du coeurisole, le massage du coeur. Lille, 1904

Gray HMW: Subdiaphragmatic transperitoneal massage of the heart as a means of resuscitation. Lancet 2:506, 1905

Gunn JA, Martin PA: Intrapericardial medicine and massage in treatment of arrest of the heart. J Pharmacol Exp Ther 7:31, 1915

Harvey W: Lectures on the Whole of Anatomy. Berkeley, University of California Press, 1961

Hoffa M et al: Einige neue Versuchen über Herzbewegung. Z Rationelle Med 9:107, 1850

Kouwenhoven WB, Jude JR, Knickerbocker GG: Closed-chest cardiac massage. JAMA 173:1064, 1960

Kuliabko A: Weitere Studien über die Wiederbelebung des Herzens. Arch Physiol 97:539, 1903

Locke J: The action of Ringer's fluid and of dextrose on the isolated rabbit heart. Zentralbl Physiol 15:490, 1901

Maas A: Die Methode der Wiederbelebung der Herztod nach Chloroform-einatmung. Berl Klin Wochenschr 12:265, 1892

Mauclaire M: La chloroformisation, l'éthérisation et la cocainisation lombaire. Gaz Hop 140:1345, 1901

Mickwitz L: Vergleichende Untersuchungen über die physiologische Wirkung der Salze der alcalien und alcalischen Erden. Doctoral dissertation, Dorpat, 1874

Prus J: Uber die Wiederbelebung in Todesfallen in Folge von Erstickung. Wien Klin Wochenschr 21:486, 1900; Zentralbl Chir (Leipzig) 27:1002, 1900

Safar P: Cardiopulmonary Cerebral Resuscitation. Philadelphia, WB Saunders, 1981

Schif M: Gesammelte Beiträge zur Physiologie. Lausanne, TG Hake, 1874

Snow J: Chloroform and Other Anaesthetics. London, John & Churchill, 1858

Steiner F: Über die Elektro-punktur. Arch Klin Chir 12:741, 1871

Stephenson HE Jr: Charles Claude Guthrie's contribution to cardiac resuscitation. Crit Care Med 9:429, 1981

Vesalius A: De humani corporis fabrica libri septem. Basel 1555

Zoll PM: Resuscitation of the heart in ventricular standstill by external cardiac stimulation. N Engl J Med 247:768, 1942

Airway Management

Applebaum EL, Bruce DL: Tracheal Intubation. Philadelphia, WB Saunders, 1976

Committee on Emergency Services: Report on Emergency Airway Management. Washington DC, National Research Council, National Academy of Sciences, 1976

Conley JM: Emergency endotracheal intubation. Respir Care 26:336, 1981

Emergency Care Research Institute: Evaluation of manually operated resuscitators. Health Devices, 3:164, 1974

LaBouef LL: Assessment of eight resuscitators. Respir Care 80:1136, 1980

Tremper KK, Shoemaker WC: Continuous CPR monitoring. Crit Care Med 9:417, 1981

39

Patient Monitoring Techniques

Robert J. Fallat • John J. Osborn

As respiratory management becomes increasingly complex, so too must the monitoring of the patient. Patient monitoring should not be considered as solely technological; a nurse feeling a pulse or a respiratory therapist watching the chest rise on inspiration is "monitoring" in a most useful and fundamental way. At the present stage of medicine, however, where a cardiac arrest or disconnection of a continuously ventilated patient may result in a disaster within moments, the need for more automated methods has become increasingly apparent.

The development of techniques for cardiopulmonary resuscitation, particularly the advent of electrical defibrillation in 1956, and the readily available ECG technology resulted in the rapid development and application of cardiac monitoring. Subsequent advances in resuscitation and cardiac and renal management have resulted in the survival of many patients, only to have them later demonstrate severe morbidity and mortality from pulmonary failure. More recently, as respiratory monitoring has developed, it has become increasingly apparent that many cardiac arrests were, in fact, precipitated by pulmonary malfunction, indicating the need for more and better respiratory monitoring.

The development of respiratory devices dates back several centuries, but not until the advent of the positive pressure breathing devices in the past three decades has continuous and complete control of ventilation become a reality. The increased prevalence of chronic obstructive pulmonary disease (COPD), with attendant respiratory failure requiring ventilator support, and the increased use of continuous mechanical ventilation following many surgical procedures, as well as a variety of medical conditions (e.g., overdose, neuromuscular disease, trauma, pulmonary edema), have all contributed to the need for more reliable, continuous, automatic ventilator monitoring systems.

Patient monitors are not simply alarm systems. They should provide features that assist in diagnosis; for example, rising ventilator pressure requirements may indicate a new pulmonary process; differentiation of the pressure requirements into resistance and compliance elements may be used to diagnose the source of the problem, as will be described later.

Monitoring can and should be an essential part of optimizing therapy. The "best" tidal volume, pressure, and flow settings on a ventilator or the time to wean a patient from a ventilator currently are largely determined by the experience of the therapist, nurse, or physician. Objective measurements, however, should be used to supplement, and in some cases substitute for clinical "hunches."[10,15] As therapists use such repetitive, reliable, objective measurements, clinical judgment cannot help but improve. Monitors have the potential of providing important physiological information, which the clinician can apply at the bedside.

Yet another function of automated monitors is to free personnel from routine tasks and to provide more accurate records with less expenditure of time by the staff. Finally, automated computer monitors may "close the loop" and provide automated treatment such as control of intravenous infusions.

In the monitoring of the critically ill patient, two general questions must be considered: What measurements should be made, and how often does one make them? The technological availability of a measurement does not, in itself, dictate its need or usefulness. The problem of excess information can be, and frequently is, a bigger problem than too little information. A continuous record of an ECG or of ventilator flows has limited usefulness, but a *change* in the frequency of arrhythmias or respiratory rate, or a *change* in the tidal volume, inspired oxygen concentration, or airway pressure detected before they can significantly alter the patient's condition is essential to optimal management.

In general, one must consider the specific problem expected, its severity, frequency, and critical time lapse permissible before detection, and then monitor accordingly. For example, if a drop in inspired oxygen concentration results in critical hypoxia and cardiac arrhythmias, then the inspired oxygen concentration should be carefully and continuously monitored. In most cases, however, oxygen therapy is supportive and supplemental, and intermittent monitoring of the inspired oxygen concentration (FI_{O_2}) and arterial blood gases is sufficient.

The full scope of monitoring the critically ill patient, of course, cannot be covered in a brief chapter. An outline of a wide range of patient monitoring is shown in Table 39-1. We shall discuss the monitoring of some of the cardiac and respiratory variables in detail. The importance of the integrity of each organ system and the overall clinical and metabolic state of the patient is obvious. Fortunately, renal, hematologic, and metabolic changes usually occur at such a rate that intermittent monitoring of these systems is fairly satisfactory, and automated systems such as metabolic beds and urine drip monitors are used only occasionally. The central nervous system, particularly the brain, is unquestionably the most fragile of organ-systems; it is critically dependent on the integrity of the other organs. Continuous monitoring of CNS function, however, is still in its infancy and largely depends on the clinical art of frequent physical examination.

Practical monitors for intracranial pressure are now available. The application of automatic frequency analysis to simple electroencephalographic signals has resulted in useful monitoring instruments generally called "cerebral function monitors." Both these methods may have real importance in future management of critically ill patients.

CARDIOVASCULAR MONITORING

The ECG is the mainstay of cardiac monitoring. Visual systems with nurse and physician monitoring are routine in any intensive care unit; however, the unreliability of visual monitoring for detecting arrhythmias has been documented.[13] Computer programs are now available that detect arrhythmias with more consistency.[14] More important, clinical personnel are relieved of this tedious and time-consuming task. Within a few years most ECGs in intensive care units will probably be processed automatically, with rhythm strip recordings made only when programmed abnormalities are detected. Abnormalities in the ECG may be *late manifestations* of respiratory, electrolyte, or acid–base disturbances, which should be detected directly.

Arterial pressure determination is a second, well-established part of cardiopulmonary monitoring. Simple percutaneous catheters are available in various diameters and lengths. The short catheter over a needle is readily inserted and is sufficient for short-term monitoring. For more prolonged use, we prefer using longer catheters threaded in over a guide wire by the Seldinger modification of the Cournand technique.

Arterial catheters provide a number of uses, some of which are not yet fully realized. They provide an accurate measure of blood pressure, particularly in the critically ill patient who frequently has such low pressure that accurate measurement is not possible by conventional techniques, and they can save an enormous amount of nursing time. The ready availability of arterial blood for analysis is invaluable in allowing frequent assessment of the pulmonary and metabolic function of the patient. Direct continuous pulse and pressure traces are available and, like continuous ECGs, provide a flood of information that must be properly edited and analyzed to give maximum usefulness. Trend analysis of blood pressure currently must be done by the observer, but a few centers have developed computer capabilities to provide such edited feedback.

Table 39-1. Methods of Monitoring Critical Care Patients

PROBLEM	INTERMITTENT	CONTINUOUS
Routine vital signs	Temperature Pulse Blood pressure	Rectal thermistor ECG Arterial line
	Respiratory rate	Nasal cannula CO_2 change Nasal cannula pressure Chest belt Impedance pneumography
Potential respiratory failure, not on ventilator	Tidal volume Vital capacity Maximum inspiratory force Compliance during IPPB	Chest inductance Spirometry Pressure gauges
	Arterial blood gases	Ear oximetry Nasal cannula CO_2 Arterial catheter Skin monitors
Patient continuously ventilated	All of the above Ventilator pressures, (maximum, plateau, PEEP)	Pneumotachograph O_2 and CO_2 analysis of inspired and expired gas Pressure strain gauges
Shock or hemodynamic instability	All of the above plus cardiac filling pressure, peripheral vasoconstriction, urine output, lactate, venous oxygen	Central venous or pulmonary artery lines Plethysmography Urine drip monitor Skin or tissue *p*H monitors Fiberoptic catheters
Metabolic or renal	Daily weight Intake and output Electrolytes Blood chemistries	Bed balance Controlled infusion Urine drip monitor
Hematologic, particularly disseminated intravascular coagulopathy (DIC)	Blood smear Coagulation panel	Not available
Central nervous system	State of consciousness Reflexes Electroencephalogram (EEG)	Rapid eye movements Continuous EEG Intracranial pressure monitor

Simple observation of "respiratory swings" in the arterial pressure trace can be a very useful guide to blood volume replacement needs or excessive ventilator pressures, as shown in Figure 39-1. The arterial pressure in itself is a measure of tissue perfusion, which is usually as accurate as the many measures of cardiac output that have been derived from analysis of the pulse contours; nevertheless, the development of such contour analysis and its use in the clinical setting have yet to be fully realized.

The first derivative of the arterial pressure has been used as a measure of cardiac contractility, since it numerically expresses the rate of rise of the onset of the pulse, and therefore has a relation to the vigor of left ventricular contraction. We have not found it very useful in practical care because it is subject to large errors owing to damping, or to changes in the peripheral arterial compliance or resistance.

On the other hand, we have found that a pulse-rate derived from the arterial pulse contour is useful in monitoring, partly because it may be easily readable when there is ECG artifact. A normal, steady arterial pulse is extremely reassuring when a loose ECG electrode is projecting a wave that looks just like ventricular fibrillation. It is even more useful if pulse rate is recorded on the same scale, superimposed on the heart-rate derived from the ECG. In the normal patient in sinus rhythm, the two traces coincide. Separation of the two, indicating a pulse deficit, is strong, suggestive evidence of ectopic beats or other arrhythmias. Very premature beats or rapid tachycardia will be counted by the ECG counter but will not show up as pulse-beats, as seen in Figure 39-2.

Complications of arterial catheters include hemorrhage, compromised perfusion distal to the catheter site, infection, and embolization. If care is taken to avoid multiple punctures in a single site, to change lines after 5 to 7 days, and to provide a system for continuous heparinization, the complication rate is minimized.

Cardiac filling pressure is a third common mode of surveillance of the cardiovascular system. Central venous pressure (CVP) catheters inserted percutaneously in antecubital, external jugular, or superficial femoral veins and threaded into the vena cava or right atrium have been in use for many years as a measure of adequacy of right ventricular filling pressure or increase in intravascular volume. Following myocardial infarction, however, or in the presence of significant pulmonary pathology with a rise in pulmonary vascular resistance, the CVP may not be a reliable indicator of *left* ventricular filling pressure and cannot be

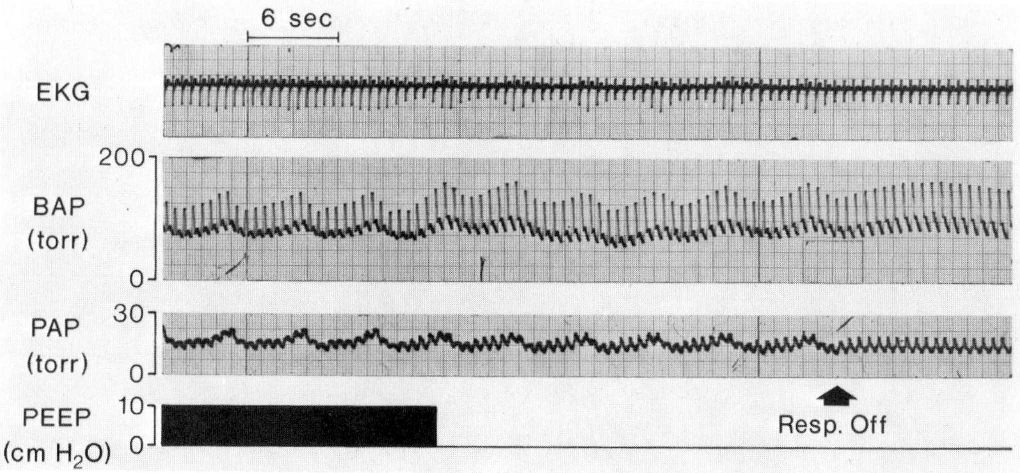

Fig. 39-1. Effect of ventilation and airway pressure on hemodynamics. Variation in pulmonary artery pressure *(PAP)* and brachial artery pressures *(BAP)* with ventilation and positive end-expiratory pressure *(PEEP)* is shown in a patient with severely stiff lungs that required high ventilatory pressures. When PEEP is stopped, there is a rise in the pulse pressure and less of a sinusoidal variation or "swing" with each inspiration in both the PAP and BAP. When the ventilator is turned off, there is a further rise in the pulse pressure and complete loss of the "swing." Note that even the ECG shows a "swing" due to position change of the heart with each inspiration, thus changing the electrical axis; this is not an indication of conduction abnormalities in the heart.

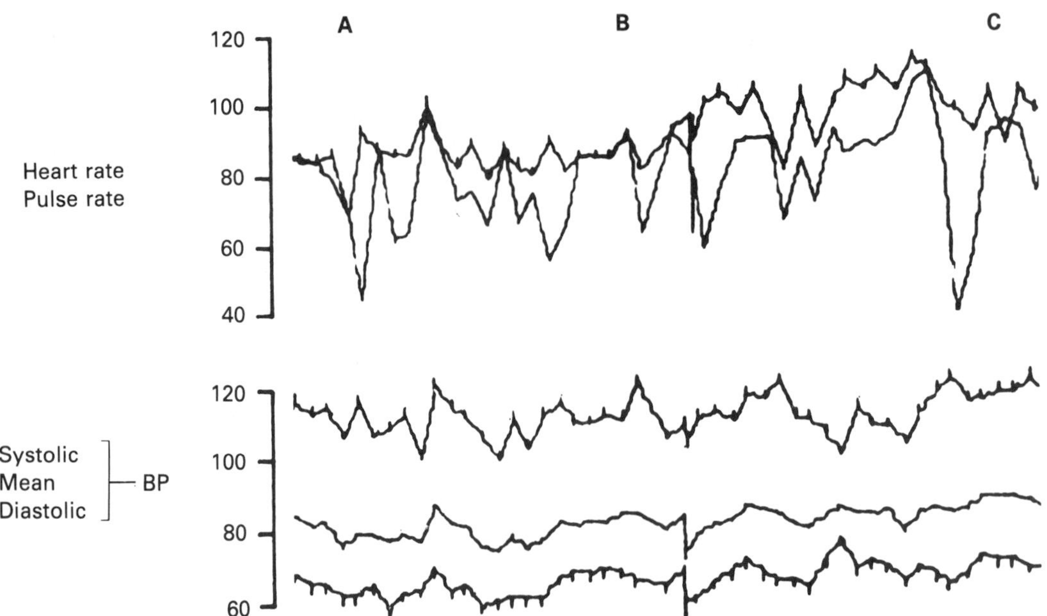

Fig. 39-2. Heart rate/pulse rate differences. An 8-hour computer record of both the heart rate, obtained from the ECG signal, and the pulse rate, obtained from the arterial line. During most of the record there is a marked discrepancy between the two because of atrial fibrillation, when many of the beats are mechanically ineffective and do not produce a measurable rise in pulse pressure. At points *A* and *C*, and particularly at point *B*, there is no "pulse deficit" (*i.e.*, the two rates are the same), each ECG activation produces an effectual pulse, tissue perfusion improves, and there is a measurable narrowing of the pulse pressure because each beat is now effective.

used to guide infusion rates or to avoid or detect the development of pulmonary edema.

The recent development of the Swan–Ganz balloon flotation catheter, which can be inserted readily at the bedside, has provided a much more reliable means of monitoring patients with severe cardiopulmonary decompensation.[23] This catheter allows measurement of both the pulmonary arterial and pulmonary capillary wedge pressure (PCWP). The PCWP more accurately reflects left heart pressures than does either the CVP or pulmonary arterial pressure. The greater reliability of the PCWP as a guide to fluid administration has been well documented.[5]

The pulmonary artery catheter also provides ready accessibility to mixed venous blood, which is perhaps a better indicator than arterial blood of adequate tissue oxygenation. The difference between the arterial and venous oxygen content $C(a - v)O_2$ is inversely related to cardiac output and directly related to oxygen consumption by the well-known *Fick equation:*

$$\frac{O_2 \text{ consumption}}{\text{cardiac output}} = C(a - v)O_2.$$

Thus, when the patient is in a basal state with oxygen consumption constant, changes in $C(a - v)O_2$ are a measure of cardiac output. In addition, a direct measure of cardiac output by thermal dilution can be done readily with the Swan–Ganz catheter.

The problem of differentiating cardiac versus primary pulmonary causes of acute pulmonary edema, as seen in the adult respiratory distress syndrome, is a prime example of the usefulness of pulmonary artery catheters.[22] Arterial and venous catheters are now an essential part of diagnosing acute cardiorespiratory failure and of serving as a useful guide to optimize not only fluid balance and drug therapy, but also respirator settings. For a more complete description of the details of the physiological measurements obtainable with arterial and venous catheters and their use in clinical situations, the reader is referred to the Bibliography.

The complication rates of central venous and Swan–Ganz catheters are not inconsequential. Because they are placed in low-flow vessels, clotting and infection may occur. Perforation of the pulmonary artery by the flow-directed catheter with subsequent hemoptysis has been reported. Cardiac arrhythmias, particularly during insertion, must be monitored carefully. Pneumothorax and hemopneumothorax are other complications. Despite these hazards, these catheters have been invaluable in managing critically ill patients.

RESPIRATORY MONITORING

As outlined in Table 39-1, respiratory monitoring can be divided into two major categories. The first describes monitoring of those patients not on continuous ventilation but who have either significant respiratory disease that warrants intermittent treatment and monitoring or the potential to develop respiratory complications. These patients will be followed primarily by intermittent assessments, although some modes of continuous monitoring are available or are under development. The second category pertains to patients on continuous ventilation. Continuous monitoring of respiratory variables is available in such patients but is not yet widespread.

THE SPONTANEOUSLY BREATHING PATIENT

In the patient not on mechanical ventilation, manual monitoring methods must be used with a frequency and intensity determined by the clinical situation. Patients in shock or in acute pulmonary edema, or recovering from anesthesia or a drug overdose, are all candidates for developing respiratory failure, and therefore should have careful respiratory monitoring. Frequent measures of respiratory rate, tidal volume, and vital capacity may be done easily, and noninvasively, in a cooperative patient, using very simple equipment such as a hand-held spirometer or any of a number of small portable spirometers currently available. In conjunction with arterial blood gas measurements, a relatively complete respiratory assessment can be made. In the less alert or noncooperative patient, vital capacity measurements may not be obtained, but an assessment of approximate lung compliance, by dividing the maximum airway pressure into the tidal volume attained during an IPPB treatment, can be a useful guide to deterioration of lung mechanics.

An additional, intermittent, manual measurement frequently used is the maximal inspiratory and expiratory force or pressure (MIP, MEP). Like the vital capacity or peak flow meter, these are small, hand-held pressure gauges that may be used readily at the bedside (see Fig. 11-12). The information obtained is physiologically similar to the FVC but may be a more sensitive indicator of neuromuscular failure than FVC. It is most commonly used in assessing patients for weaning from ventilators.

In some spontaneously breathing patients, it would be desirable to monitor the respiratory system more continuously. In spontaneously breathing patients, only respiratory rate and perhaps tidal volume can be monitored continuously. There are several modes for following respiratory rates. Perhaps the most convenient is by chest impedance using two of the ECG leads.[8] A thermal dilution catheter placed in the nose can be used to monitor respiratory rate by detecting the change in temperature that occurs with respiration.[3] Recently, respiratory rate and, more particularly, apnea during sleep have been monitored, using a microphone to listen for breath sound over the neck.[12] A number of methods have been used for monitoring respiratory rate and apnea, particularly in infants and neonatal populations, including magnometers, electromyograms, head or body plethysomographs, and esophageal balloons.[12,19]

An informative, noninvasive monitoring technique that we have used to monitor respiratory rate is one of sampling gas for carbon dioxide analysis from a standard two-pronged nasal oxygen cannula. This provides a means of following respiratory rate and also gives some indication of changing arterial P_{CO_2}. Because of dilution in the deadspace of the nasopharynx, the end-tidal P_{CO_2} determined by this method does not as closely approximate arterial P_{CO_2} as does that obtained from a closed system, but is adequate for detecting gross changes in expired carbon dioxide tension (Fig. 39-3).

The monitoring of tidal volume in the nonintubated patient is more difficult. Chest impedance and magnometer methods have been tried but are not reliable owing to the complex configuration of the chest and changing contribution of the chest wall and diaphragmatic contractions to tidal breathing with changes in position.[1] Measuring the changing inductance of the chest and abdomen using two separate insulated wire coils held in place by a mesh suit is reportedly a reliably method for monitoring tidal volume in spontaneously breathing patients.[4] This method measures thoracic gas volume, and therefore differs from exhaled volume measurements because of intrathoracic gas compressibility and blood volume fluctuations. More common clinical use of this device in the intensive care setting awaits further clinical experience.

Too often, the patients likely to develop respiratory failure are not alert or cooperative enough to perform a reliable vital capacity maneuver, and even the

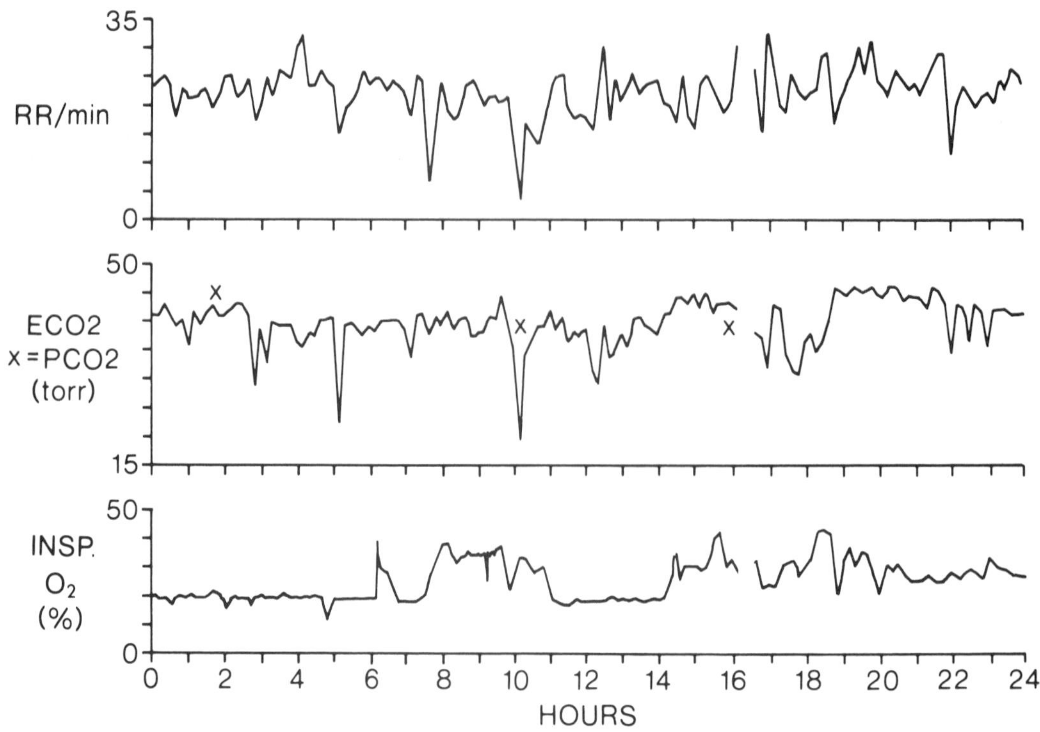

Fig. 39-3. Monitoring using a nasal cannula. A two-pronged nasal cannula routinely used for administering O_2 can be used to sample inspired and exhaled gas. The respiratory rate *(RR)* is easily detected by the change in CO_2. The end-tidal CO_2 is relatively stable and in good agreement with arterial P_{CO_2} measurements shown by *X*. The patient was on room air (FI_{O_2} = 20%) during the first 6 hours, then given O_2 by mask with considerable variation in the FI_{O_2}.

cooperative patient must be left to sleep. Arterial blood gases are an obvious means for defining the gas exchange abnormalities but are invasive, expensive, and intermittent. Several cutaneous oxygen monitors are available that utilize a polarographic oxygen sensor similar to that used in the blood measurement. The skin is heated to 43° to 45°C to "arterialize" the dermal blood flow. These sensors have been used successfully in neonatal and pediatric monitoring and are now routinely used for monitoring the neonatal respiratory distress syndrome. In adults, however, the thickened epidermis results in much higher gradients between the cutaneous oxygen (tc_{O_2}) and arterial blood oxygen (Pa_{O_2}). On average, the Pa_{O_2} is 10 torr lower than the tc_{O_2}, but a wide range from −40 to +20 torr has been reported.[11] Whether this gradient remains constant enough in adult patients to make it a useful trend monitor of oxygenation remains to be investigated.

Cutaneous carbon dioxide monitors are also becoming available. These are of two types: One uses a miniaturized infrared system,[6] shown in Figures 39-4A and 39-4B, the other a modified Severinghaus carbon dioxide electrode system.[2] Both require lower skin temperatures and reportedly give reliable results in monitoring arterial carbon dioxide in adults.[7]

Ear oximetry is another noninvasive means of continuously monitoring gas exchange. This unit sets loosely over the ear, heated to only 39° to 40°C and is comfortable enough for long-term use. Maintaining a good position on the ear is one of the most difficult problems and requires some care (see Fig. 39-4A, C). The instrument has a unique feature of monitoring for blood pulsation; if cardiac output is too low or the unit falls off the ear, pulses are not detected and are indicated by an alarm light. These units have become particularly useful in monitoring sleep apnea and as a noninvasive means of following exercise-induced desaturation. We now use this technique for determination of oxygen needs for patients with COPD or other patients with cardiopulmonary disease; this has obviated the use of multiple arterial blood gas deter-

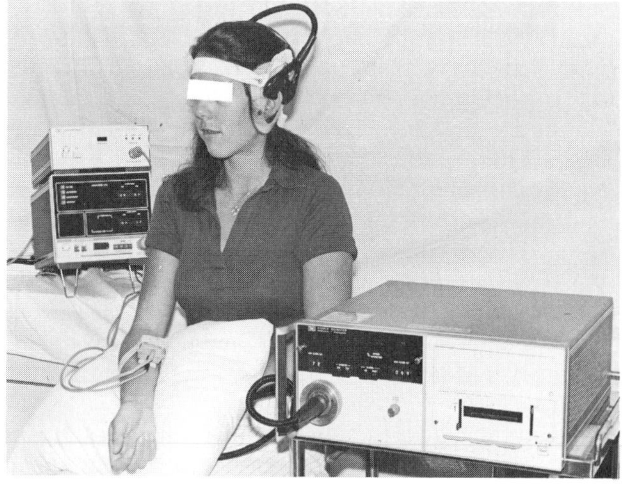

A

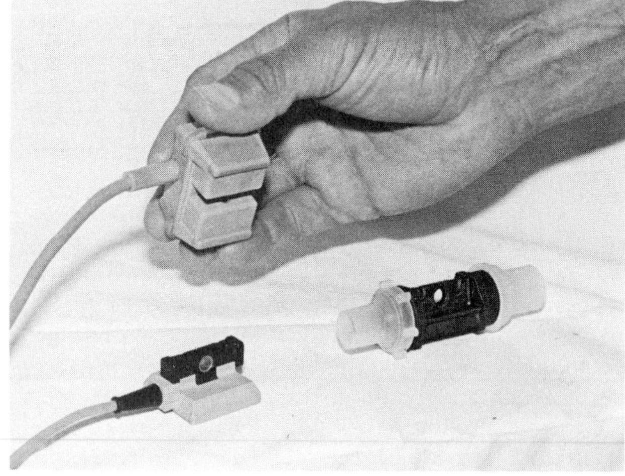

B

Fig. 39-4. *(A)* Noninvasive monitoring of CO_2 by cutaneous infrared analyzer is shown on the model's right forearm. Two wires lead from the monitoring unit on her right. There is no gas sampling. On her ear is the oximeter that is shown in the close-up in Figure 39-4C. *(B)* Close-up of the infrared CO_2 monitor. In the hand is the miniaturized infrared source and detector. The infrared beam is directed through a chamber that may be attached either to the skin for cutaneous measurements (that unit is shown in the lower left) or to an airway insert, as shown on the right. Since the infrared source is at the sight of measurement, no gas sampling is required. *(C)* Close-up of the ear oximeter shows the gap at the index finger which fits loosely over the ear. The ear is heated to 39°, but this is well tolerated for many hours. There are eight infrared wave lengths transmitted through the ear 20 times per second. The box contains a minicomputer that analyzes data continuously and approximates the oxygen saturation from a polynomial equation with eight coefficients.

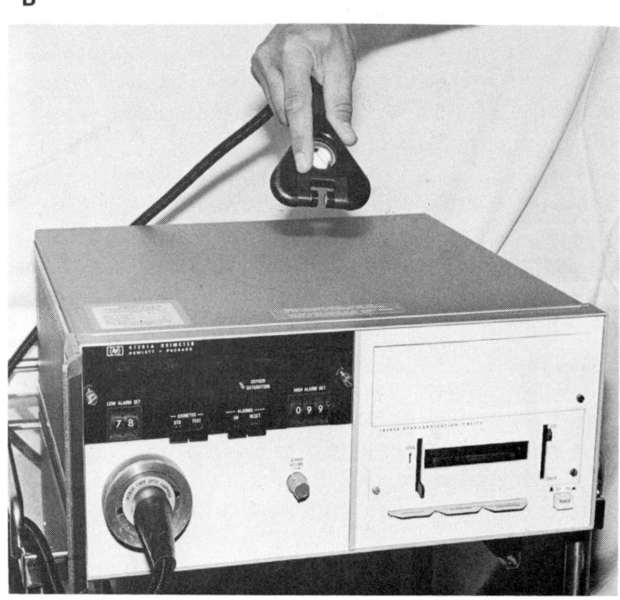

C

mination during exercise or to determine supplemental oxygen requirements.

All of these cutaneous methods for monitoring blood gases have marked limitations in the hemodynamically unstable patient. When perfusion to the tissue being monitored is changing, there will be a change in the gradient from the blood through the skin. Therefore, changes in the measurement may not be true changes in the blood gases but a reflection of the changing perfusion. The ear oximeter detects pulsations and warns the observer that perfusion may be inadequate. Other devices must be checked by obtaining an arterial blood sample. Future experience and technical improvements will undoubtedly see a much wider use of these noninvasive methods.

THE CONTINUOUSLY VENTILATED PATIENT

When the patient is mechanically ventilated, the number of parameters to be monitored increases considerably. Because of the extremely rapid and critical changes that can be induced by ventilators, such monitoring is essential. The slow development of appropriate monitoring devices is somewhat surprising in view of the ease with which measurement devices can be placed in the artificial airway or directly into the ventilators. In monitoring systems that are not computer-based, three basic measurements are readily available: expired tidal volumes, airway pressures, and gas concentrations.

Expired tidal volume from the patient is commonly measured by a volume displacement spirometer that can be equipped with alarms; however, these devices are not fail-safe. For example, failure of the expiratory valve of a ventilator to close fully during inspiration may result in the inspiratory volume's bypassing the patient, going directly into the spirometer, resulting in severe patient hypoventilation. This usually will be detected by a low airway pressure alarm. Alternatively, the incorporation of a pneumotachograph into the patient's airway, or the use of both inspiratory and expiratory pneumotachographs as in the Siemens–Elema ventilator, obviates at least this difficulty. If the airway pressures are quite high, the expired volume measured includes the expansion volume of the tubing; since this can be as high as 5 ml/cm H_2O, a significant portion of the measured expired volume may not reflect effective alveolar ventilation. Here again an in-line pneumotachograph obviates this problem. Pneumotachographs, however, have problems of their own, primarily those of calibration changes resulting from changing gas concentrations and interference from secretions and humidity. Pneumotachographs are now available that are specially designed for intensive care service. They will operate in the presence of tracheal secretions. They do not require warming and weigh only about one tenth as must as the older metal units (Fig. 39-5A).

Airway pressure measurements have always been available on ventilators, and most volume ventilators have built-in alarms to detect high and low limits. Some of the ingenious devices for allowing suctioning, such as the "flip-off" valves on tracheostomy tubes, if open by mistake, allow much of the inspired volume to leak out into the room, but enough pressure still remains not to trip the low pressure alarm. The concurrent use of an expired volume monitor, however, should detect this. The increasing use of positive end-expiratory pressure (PEEP) has resulted in the incorporation of PEEP devices into the newer ventilators. The application of excessive PEEP may have serious hemodynamic and pulmonary consequences. To alleviate this, some ventilators contain a PEEP alarm that detects end-expiratory pressures of 5 cm H_2O greater than the pre-set value (see Chap. 24). In general, monitoring of airway pressures has been done most successfully directly in the ventilators themselves.

Monitoring of gas concentrations, on the other hand, has not been as widespread as we believe is indicated. Oxygen delivery is, of course, frequently critical in the patient on the respirator, and built-in alarms are generally available only on volume ventilators. These alarms, however, generally sense the adequate filling of an oxygen-mixing chamber rather than the concentration directly. Accidental changes in the oxygen control knob or mistaken connection of the oxygen line to an air source is not detected by these monitors. A variety of in-line oxygen measuring devices are available, however, and are relatively inexpensive. Many have both high-limit and low-limit alarms.

Oxygen sensors are basically of four types.

1. A polarographic electrode similar to that used to measure blood oxygen tensions. These have a slow response time so that changes in inspired and expired concentration cannot be detected. A rapidly responding instrument, however, that is based on a miniature polarographic electrode and that allows continuous breath-by-breath measurements is available.
2. A paramagnetic detector has long been available for oxygen monitoring, but this also has a slow response time of several seconds.
3. A third type of oxygen sensor is the fuel cell type. Those operating at high temperatures have a rapid response, allowing continuous monitoring. Less expensive, slow-responding, low temperature portable units are available as pocket monitors or simple in-line detectors.
4. The mass spectrometer can rapidly analyze several gas concentrations simultaneously. In recent years, these instruments have been improved to the point where they are stable enough for use in a clinical setting for prolonged continuous monitoring of several patients at one time. They are relatively expensive and require some engineering and technical competence to maintain reliability.

Carbon dioxide monitoring may seem to be less critical than that of oxygen. To the contrary, because of the relationships of P_{CO_2} to acid–base balance and because of the ease with which small adjustments in ventilator settings can markedly and quickly affect the patient's Pa_{CO_2}, carbon dioxide monitoring becomes even more critical than that of oxygen tension. We believe that carbon dioxide monitoring is most essential to manage effectively the critically ill patient on

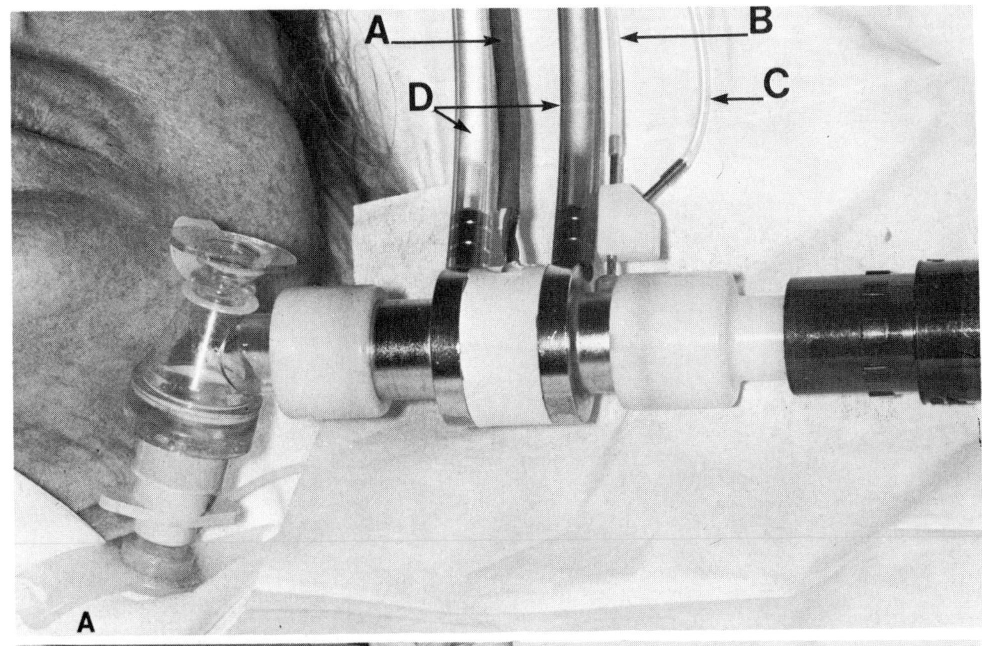

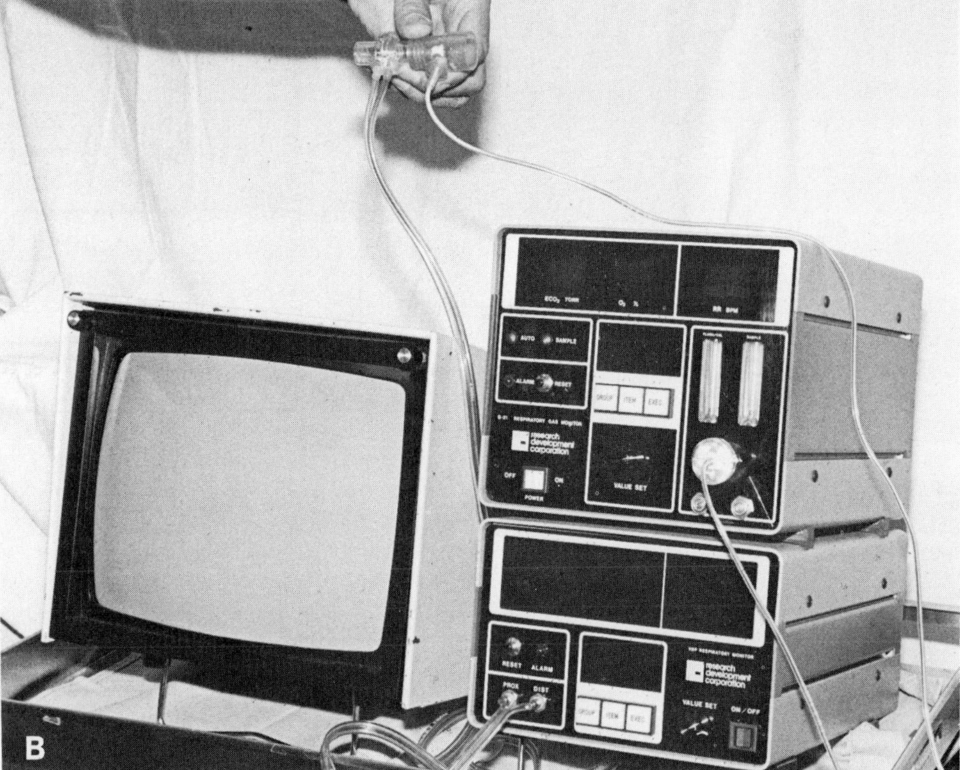

Fig. 39-5. *(A)* Modified pneumotachography. The Fleisch pneumotachograph is in place in a tracheotomized patient. It is heated to 39°C by a coil *(A)*. A gas sampling line *(B)* is flushed with dry gas through line *(C)* when not monitoring to avoid condensation and contamination. Pressure lines *(D)* and gas sampling lines (*B* and *C*) may extend for 6 to 8 feet to the transducers and analyzers housed in a cart. *(B)* The lightweight plastic pneumotachograph is held in the hand. Pressure and flow characteristics obtained from the pneumotachograph are analyzed by the bottom unit on the right, whereas the top unit samples gas for CO_2 and O_2 analyses. The output can then be displayed on a television monitor or a printer. One of these units can monitor alternately two beds continuously.

a ventilator, and that the availability of at least end-tidal carbon dioxide measurements can reduce the guesswork in ventilator adjustment, reduce the need for arterial blood gas determinations, and, most important, reduce morbidity and mortality. Some of the uses of carbon dioxide monitoring of the critically ill patient are listed below, and some examples of these uses will be presented.

As with oxygen monitoring several methods are available for monitoring carbon dioxide. Most common are the instruments based on the infrared absorption of carbon dioxide. These instruments have a rapid response time and are stable if kept free of condensation and secretions by providing either a heated sample line or frequent flushing with a dry gas. The mass spectrometer, of course, is equally effective but considerably more expensive than an infrared carbon dioxide analyzer. Slow-response chromatographic units are available in conjunction with an end-tidal sampler for monitoring only the end-tidal carbon dioxide.

USES OF CARBON DIOXIDE MONITOR

1. Follows arterial P_{CO_2}
2. Follows wasted ventilation (physiological dead space)
3. Defines pattern of ventilation ("fighting the respirator"?)
4. Effects pulmonary blood flow (during cardiac arrest)
5. Analyzes lung function (inequality of ventilation)

COMPUTER-BASED SYSTEMS

If a patient is on continuous ventilation, there are so many "critical variables" (arterial and venous pressures, maximum airway pressures, positive end-expiratory pressures, volume in, volume out, flow rates, respiratory rates, oxygen and carbon dioxide tensions, and so forth) that one wonders how it is possible to monitor such a patient effectively. Clearly, with so many variables to monitor, some computerized system for filtering this mass of information may be not only desirable, but also necessary for optimum management.

Over the past 10 years computerized systems for monitoring cardiac function have been developed by Warner and his colleagues in Salt Lake City, and by Weil and his coworkers in Los Angeles (see Bibliography). They have demonstrated the power of the computer to store and to display multiple physiological variables to provide trend analysis for better management and prognosis of the critically ill patient.

Computerized monitoring of respiratory variables has been more limited but is undoubtedly going to increase considerably in the future. A small mobile digital computer system has been described by Peters and Hilberman.[18]

Powers and coworkers have described a small pulmonary function analyzer that has been used pri-

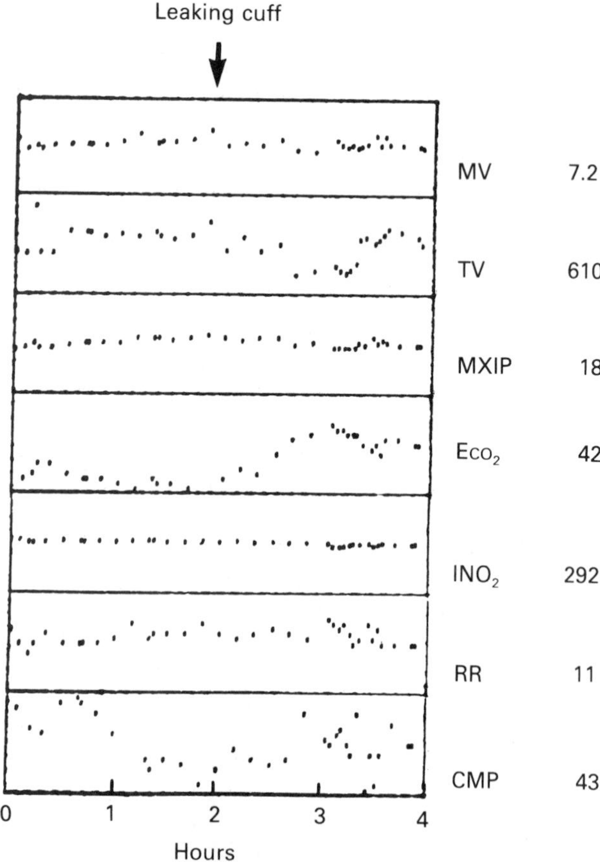

Fig. 39-6. Detection of a leaking cuff. This is a 4-hour record as seen on a bedside television monitor at Pacific Medical Center. Measurements are automatically made every 10 minutes. Shown from the top: minute volume (MV = 7.2 liters); tidal volume (TV = 610 ml); maximum inspiratory pressure (MXIP = 18 cm H_2O); end-tidal CO_2 (E_{CO_2} = 42 torr); inspired O_2 (INO_2 = 292 torr); respiratory rate (RR = 11); compliance (CMP = 43 ml/cm H_2O). As the cuff began to leak *(arrow)*, the TV falls and E_{CO_2} rises. The RR rises to maintain the MV. The nurse then called for more frequent measurements, found the problem, and the TV was raised and E_{CO_2} brought back to a new stable value.

marily for clinical research.[20] They have stressed the usefulness of rather sophisticated bedside measurements of functional residual capacity and oxygen washout curves to optimize ventilator settings, particularly positive end-expiratory pressure. Small portable minicomputer units are now being marketed for bedside pulmonary function analysis, including spirometry, lung volumes, ventilatory volumes, oxygen consumption, and carbon dioxide production. Experience is needed to see how well these adapt to long-term continuous monitoring.

At our institution a rather elaborate respiratory monitoring system has been developed by Osborn and his associates using a large digital computer to monitor nine beds in our hospital as well as beds in remote hospitals linked to the computer by telephone lines.[17] The system has been designed primarily to provide clinically useful variables to physicians, nurses, and therapists at the bedside in order to optimize management and to minimize the time spent collecting and recording such data. A modified Fleisch pneumotachograph (*see* Fig. 39-5A) is placed in the airway and is the only apparatus added to the ventilator system. Currently, a lighter plastic "flap valve" pneumotachograph (Fig. 39-5B) has been developed that provides a stable flow reading, with fewer problems of plugging by mucus and humidity, which changes the calibration. Pressure and gas sampling lines lead to rapid oxygen and carbon dioxide sensors that can be housed in a small portable cart. The system is illustrated in Figure 39-5B. More than 30 cardiopulmonary variables are measured automatically at 10-minute intervals, or more often if desired. Results are available within seconds on a bedside television monitor. Hard-copy printouts and 24-hour plots of the data are routinely provided.

An example of how such a system has proved useful is shown by the 4-hour plots in Figures 39-6 and 39-7. The patient in Figure 39-6 developed a small leak from a deflated cuff on the endotracheal tube. This resulted in a decrease in tidal volume (VT) and a gradual rise in the end-tidal carbon dioxide (ECO_2). The patient responded with an increased respiratory rate (RR) that maintained the minute volume (MV) and prevented a further rise in ECO_2. At this point the nurse noted the changes, requested more frequent analyses, analyzed the problem to be in the leaking cuff, and corrected the leak. Thereafter, the tidal volume rose and the ECO_2 stabilized.

Figures 39-7 and 39-8 demonstrate the usefulness of volume-pressure and compliance measurements, particularly in patients with acute pulmonary edema or adult respiratory distress syndrome, as this patient had. When PEEP was raised from 0 to 5 cm H_2O, one could see a fall in the VT and rise in the ECO_2 that resulted from an air leak around the patient's tracheostomy as well as from the chest tubes secondary to a bronchopleural fistula. The reason for this marked rise in pressure is seen from the volume-pressure plots shown in Figure 39-8. The use of 5 or 10 cm H_2O

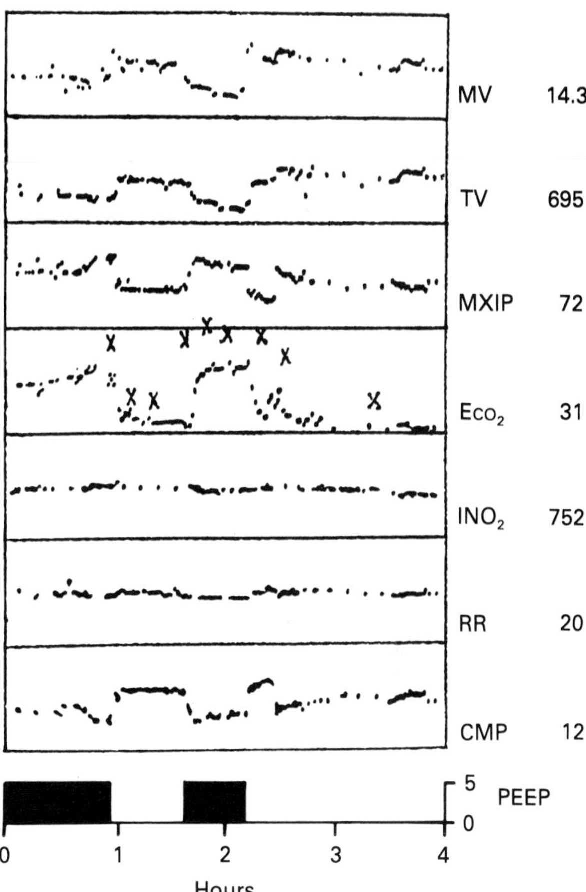

Fig. 39-7. Effect of PEEP on ventilation. A 4-hour record with symbols similar to those in Figure 39-6. The monitor is in continuous mode, so that measurements are made every 40 seconds. When positive end-expiratory pressure (PEEP) is removed, the maximum inspiratory pressure falls and the tidal volume rises, resulting in higher minute volume and a fall in ECO_2. The reverse occurs with the reapplication of PEEP. This adverse effect of PEEP occurs because the lungs are already fully distended, as demonstrated by the fall in compliance with PEEP. As a result, the patient was managed without PEEP and conditions stabilized. Note the good agreement between ECO_2 and Pa_{CO_2} *(X)*, with some increase in the difference during application of PEEP because of increased wasted ventilation.

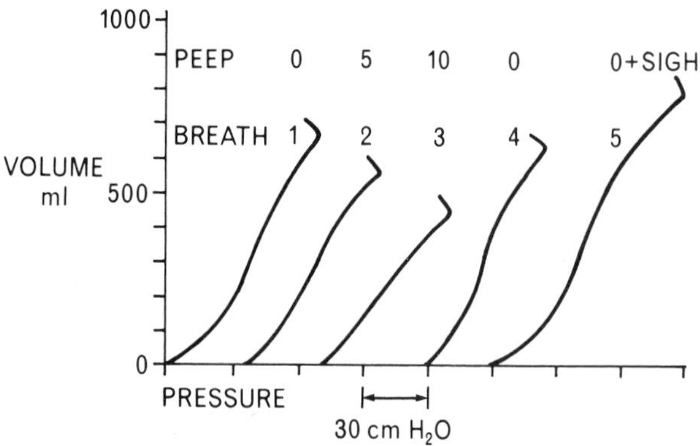

Fig. 39-8. Effect of PEEP on volume–pressure curves. Another display available at Pacific Medical Center is the volume–pressure curves of each inspiration during a 30-second period of monitoring. The small reduction in pressure at the end of inspired volume is due to the inflationary hold that allows the pressure to fall to a "static" or plateau pressure. Note the decline in volume from more than 700 ml to less than 500 ml as 5 and then 10 cm H_2O PEEP is added on the second and third breaths, respectively. The pressure starts at the PEEP pressure and rises to more than 60 cm H_2O in each breath. When a small sigh of only 200 ml is given in the last breath, the peak pressure reaches almost 90 cm H_2O. This is the same severely ill patient shown in Figure 39-7.

PEEP results in lower tidal volume and considerable increase in airway pressure (*i.e.*, a marked fall in compliance as shown). Further, it is seen in Figure 39-8 that with the addition of only a 200-ml increment in tidal volume (a small "sigh"), there is a marked change in the slope of the volume–pressure curve with a marked rise in pressure. These measurements indicate that the patient's lungs are fully distended, and any attempt to inflate the lungs further, either by PEEP or increased VT, results in inordinate pressure increases. One would not expect such manipulation to be helpful in improving oxygenation, which was true in this patient, who actually developed a reduced mixed venous oxygen tension and increased arteriovenous oxygen difference when PEEP was used. These curves are also useful to detect subtle degrees of "fighting" or sucking on the ventilator, and can be used to differentiate between resistance and compliance factors as a cause of increased ventilator pressures.

Respiratory monitoring is particularly useful at certain critical points when a patient's condition is changing or when certain clinical decisions need to be made. One of these is when a patient is first placed on a ventilator or is being shifted from control to assist mode, or from a volume to pressure ventilator, or finally being "weaned" from the ventilator entirely. After it has been determined that the patient's vital capacity is high enough and the alveolar–arterial oxygen gradient low enough to consider the patient for weaning (to a T-piece or to intermittent mandatory ventilation), it is very convenient to monitor his response on a minute-to-minute basis, rather than to rely on multiple blood gas determinations, whose results may not be immediately available. The most useful parameters are tidal volume and ECO_2. If the patient tires and cannot meet adequately the demands of providing his own ventilation, tidal volume falls and the ECO_2 rises sharply. The ability to observe these changes as they are happening can be lifesaving, and, at the least, they decrease the frequency of blood gas analyses during this sometimes very tedious and difficult transition period. Figure 39-9 is an example of use of the monitor system as demonstrated by a 24-hour record during ventilator weaning.

Several examples have been shown of using the ECO_2 to monitor arterial carbon dioxide. It is well known, however, that the ECO_2 differs from the Pa_{CO_2} in a number of pathologic conditions, and therefore use of the ECO_2 might be questioned. This difference in itself, however, has proved useful as a guide to monitoring and diagnosing critically ill patients. Although a difference does exist, it should remain constant so that changes in ECO_2 either reflect changes in Pa_{CO_2} or in the gradient between the ECO_2 and Pa_{CO_2}. In either case, the change may be clinically important and therefore worthy of the effort to monitor carbon dioxide.

The $ECO_2 - Pa_{CO_2}$ gradient is an indicator of wasted ventilation or physiological dead space, which is particularly increased in patients with pulmonary vascular disease such as emboli, a very common and frequently insidious killer of the obtunded, continuously ventilated patient. The use of the $ECO_2 - Pa_{CO_2}$ gradient as an indicator of pulmonary emboli is one potential use of monitoring carbon dioxide. Many other conditions, however, may cause an increase in wasted ventilation or the $ECO_2 - Pa_{CO_2}$ gradient; some are artifactual, such as very low tidal volumes or relatively high external dead space, so that a true end-tidal carbon dioxide cannot be obtained. More important, though, is the fact that virtually any pulmonary pathology may cause an increase in wasted ventilation and arterial $CO_2 - ECO_2$ gradient. The simple maneuver of measuring the gradient after a sighing maneuver has been suggested as a means to differentiate pulmonary emboli from other causes.[9]

There are many other potential uses of expired oxygen and carbon dioxide analysis, since they are indicators of both cardiac output and the distribution

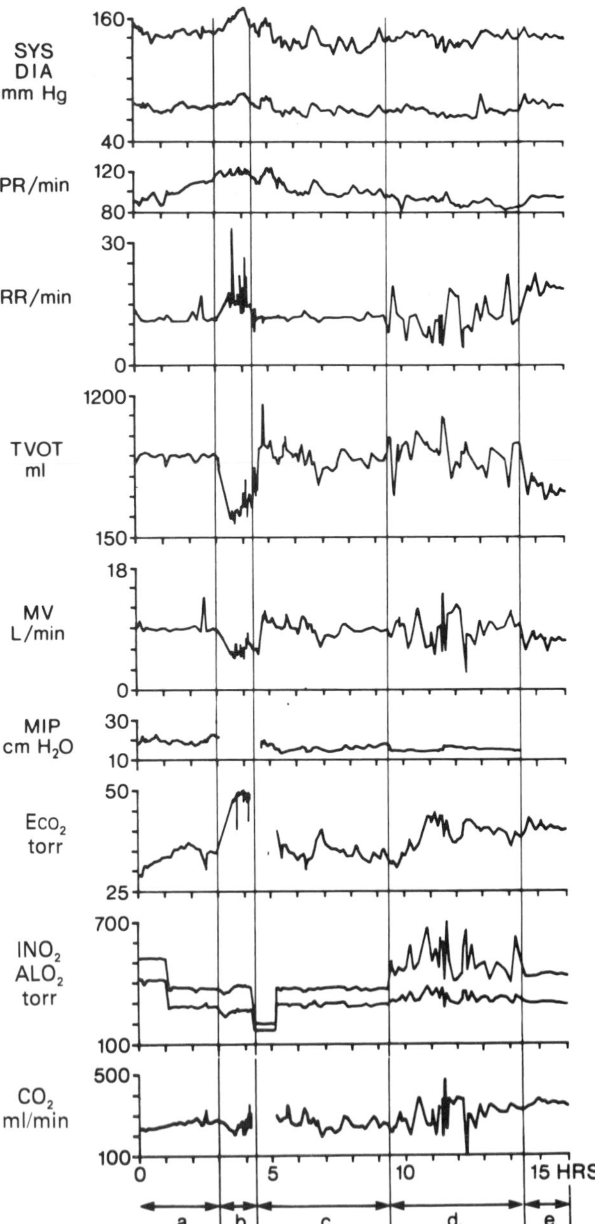

Fig. 39-9. A 24-hour physiologic record of a patient being weaned. This patient was quite stable on a volume ventilator following cardiac surgery (period *a*). He was placed on a T-piece during period *b*, but his TV and MV fell markedly, resulting in a rise in Eco_2 as well as in pulse and BP. He was replaced on the volume ventilator (period *c*), then switched to assist mode on a pressure ventilator *(d)*, which resulted in a much more variable RR and TV and some slight increase in the Eco_2. During period *e*, he was again placed on a T-piece, and although the TV fell slightly and the RR increased, he remained with a stable pulse, BP, and Eco_2 and was successfully weaned. The symbols are similar to those used in Figures 39-6 and 39-7. CO_2 refers here to CO_2 production. INO_2 = inspired O_2 tension; ALO_2 = arterial O_2 tension.

of ventilation and perfusion.[16,21] Whether more detailed analyses of these curves will have future clinical usefulness remains to be seen.

These are only a few examples of how continuous monitoring may be useful in patient management. In general, we would view monitoring not as a collation of simple alarm systems, but as a data-gathering (and reducing) and educational system. By providing accurate clinical and physiological data at the bedside on an ongoing basis, more precise diagnoses and better management of the criticaly ill patient will undoubtedly follow.

REFERENCES

1. Ashutosh K, Gilbert R, Auchincloss H: Impedance pneumograph and magnetometer methods for monitoring tidal volume. J Appl Physiol 37:964, 1974
2. Beran AV et al: An improved sensor and a method for transcutaneous CO_2 monitoring. Acta Anesth Scand (Suppl):68:111, 1978
3. Brown BH: Some new instruments for the continuous monitoring of body temperature, respiration-rate and pulse-rate. Phys Med Biol 11:135, 1966
4. Cohn MA et al: A transducer for non-invasive monitoring of respiration. In Stott FD, Raftery EB, Sleight P et al: (eds): ISAM Proceedings of the Second International Symposium on Ambulatory Monitoring. London, Academic Press, 1975
5. DeLaurentis DA, Hayes M, Matsumoto T et al: Does central venous pressure accurately reflect hemodynamic and fluid volume patterns in the critical surgical patient? Am J Surg 126:415, 1973
6. Eletr S et al: Cutaneous monitoring of systemic pCO_2 on patients being weaned from ventilator. Acta Anesth Scand (Suppl) 68:123, 1978
7. Fallat RJ et al: Lung function in long-term survivors from severe respiratory distress syndrome. Am Rev Respir Dis 113:181, 1976
8. Grenvik A et al: Impedance pneumography: Comparison between chest impedance changes and respiratory volumes in 11 healthy volunteers. Chest 62:439, 1972
9. Hatle L, Rokseth R: The arterial to end-expiratory carbon dioxide tension gradient in acute pulmonary embolism and other cardiopulmonary diseases. Chest 66:4, 1974
10. Hilberman M et al: An analysis of potential physiological predictors of respiratory adequacy following cardiac surgery. J Thorac Cardiovasc Surg 71:711, 1976
11. Huch A, Huch R: Transcutaneous, non-invasive monitoring of pO_2. Hosp Pract 11:43, 1976
12. Krumpke PE, Cummiskey JM: Use of laryngeal sound recordings to monitor apnea. Am Rev Respir Dis 122:797, 1980
13. Lindsay J, Bruckner NV: Conventional coronary care unit monitoring (nondetection of transient rhythm disturbances). JAMA 221:667, 1972
14. Lown B, Motta RV, Besser HW: Programmed "trendescription": A new approach to EKG monitoring. JAMA 232, No. 1:39, 1975
15. Menn SJ, Rarnett GO, Schmechel D: A computer program to assist in the care of acute respiratory failure. JAMA 223:308, 1973
16. Osborn JJ: Monitoring respiratory function. Crit Care Med 2:217, 1974

17. Osborn JJ, Beaumont JO, Raison JCA: Computation for quantitative on-line measurements in an intensive care ward. In Stacy RW, Waxman B (eds): Computers in Biomedical Research. New York, Academic Press, 1969
18. Peters RM, Hilberman M: Respiratory insufficiency: Diagnosis and control of therapy. Surgery 70:280, 1971
19. Polgar G: Comparison of methods for recording respiration in newborn infants. Pediatrics 36:861, 1965
20. Powers SR et al: Studies of pulmonary insufficiency in non-thoracic trauma. J Trauma 12:1, 1972
21. Sobol BJ, Emirgil C, Goyal P et al: The single breath carbon dioxide washout test. Am J Med Sci 257:140, 1969
22. Stevens PM: Editorial: Assessment of acute respiratory failure: Cardiac versus pulmonary causes. Chest 67:1, 1975
23. Swan HJC et al: Catheterization of the heart in man with use of a flow-directed balloon-tipped catheter. N Engl J Med 283:447, 1970

BIBLIOGRAPHY

General Sources

Morgan A et al: Effects of computer controlled transfusion on recovery from cardiac surgery. Ann Surg 179:391, 1973

Osborn JJ et al: Respiratory causes of "sudden unexplained arrhythmia" in post-thoracotomy patients. Surgery, 69:24, 1971. (This article points out the now well-recognized fact that hypoxemia and acid-base disturbances are frequent *precursors* of cardiac arrhythmias)

Powers SR et al: Studies of pulmonary insufficiency in non-thoracic trauma. J Trauma 12:1, 1972. (A discussion of the pulmonary complications of otherwise successful cardiopulmonary resuscitation)

Sheppard LC, Kirklin JW, Kouchoukos NT: Computer-controlled interventions for the acutely ill patient. Comput Biomed Res 4:135, 1974. (This paper, and the one following, explain how computer technology can be used to "close the loop" between diagnosis and therapy. The problem of such computer applications still awaits more extensive clinical trials)

Wiess M: Head trauma and spinal cord injuries: Diagnostic and therapeutic criteria. Crit Care Med 2:311, 1974. (A paper discussing means currently under study whereby central nervous system function can be monitored)

Zoll PM et al: Arrest by external electric stimulation of the heart. N Engl J Med 254:541, 1956. (The first description of successful defibrillation of the heart)

Cardiovascular Monitoring

Jurado R, Matucha D, Osborn JJ: Cardiac output estimation by pulse contour methods: Validity of their use for monitoring the critically ill patient. Surgery 74:358, 1973

Osborn JJ, Beaumont JO, Raison JCA: Measurement and monitoring of acutely ill patients by digital computer. Surgery 64:1057, 1968

Shubin J, Weil MH, Palley N, Affifi AA: Monitoring the critically ill patient with the aid of a digital computer. Comput Biomed Res 4:460, 1971

Stevens PM, Friedman GK, Nicotra MB: The value of flow-directed catheters in cardiorespiratory failure. Am Rev Respir Dis 107:111, 1973

Warner HR, Gardner RM, Toronto AF: Computer-based monitoring of cardiovascular functions in post-operative patients. Circulation 17:68, 1968

Weisel RD, Berger RL, Hechtman HB: Measurement of cardiac output by thermodilution. N Engl J Med 292:13, 1975

Respiratory Monitoring

Rooth G, Hedstrand U, Tyden J: The validity of the transcutaneous oxygen tension method in adults. Crit Care Med 4:162, 1976. (The potential usefulness of this noninvasive technique is discussed)

APPENDICES

A

Pulmonary Function Testing Methodology

Donald W. Herrmann • David Hoover

SPIROMETRY

Spirometry is the most frequently performed test of pulmonary function. It comprises slow, forced vital capacity maneuvers and may also include inspiratory and maximum voluntary ventilation maneuvers.

Originally, most spirometry was performed in the volume time mode because the mechanical characteristics of most spirometers were frequently of the water seal type with a sealed cylinder or bell immersed in water over a support column. A connection to the air space within the bell was provided through the support column for the air entering the spirometer. As air moved into the bell, the cylinder was forced upward. The weight of the bell was balanced through the use of a chain connected to the top of the cylinder, which was run upward over a pulley and then down to a recording pen. The recording pen was filled with ink and could be adjusted to touch the surface of the recording paper, which was wrapped around a rotating cylinder. This recording device was called a kymograph, and its speed of rotation could be adjusted with a switch on the unit. Originally the water seal spirometer bell and the chain connected to it were made of metal. This construction feature resulted in some reduction of spirometer performance during forced maneuvers owing to expansion and contraction of the chain, oscillations in the water level, and the inertial, resistance, and frequency response characteristics. To help with these problems spirometer bells were made of plastic, which significantly enhanced performance.

Water seal spirometers can be classified as "volume displacement devices" because they capture and hold all gas that they measure. Other examples of this type of spirometer are the dry rolling seal and wedge spirometers (Fig. A-1). These are sometimes also referred to as electronic spirometers because many of them do not have a direct mechanical link from a cylinder or bellows movement to a recording device. Instead, an electronic circuit is connected to the moving part of the spirometer and an analogue voltage is provided as an output signal. These electric connections may be accomplished with variable potentiometers that are turned by the mechanical movement of the spirometer, ferrite loops that are moved within a coil of wire, or other types of linkages. Because of the lack of a direct mechanical link to a recording pen, these devices had different performance characteristics than do water seal spirometers. In addition, they could provide a flow output as well as a volume output. Today, some water seal spirometers have been modified to generate a flow signal. The simultaneous availability of both signals allows for production of a flow-volume loop. With this type of curve, the volume movement of the spirometer is generally played on the horizontal axis of the recorder while the instantaneous flow is displayed on the vertical axis.

A second type of spirometer design uses a pneumotachometer. These devices work on a variety of design principles. A common design uses a differential pressure transducer to measure the pressure drop across a fixed resistance within a rigid tube. In this

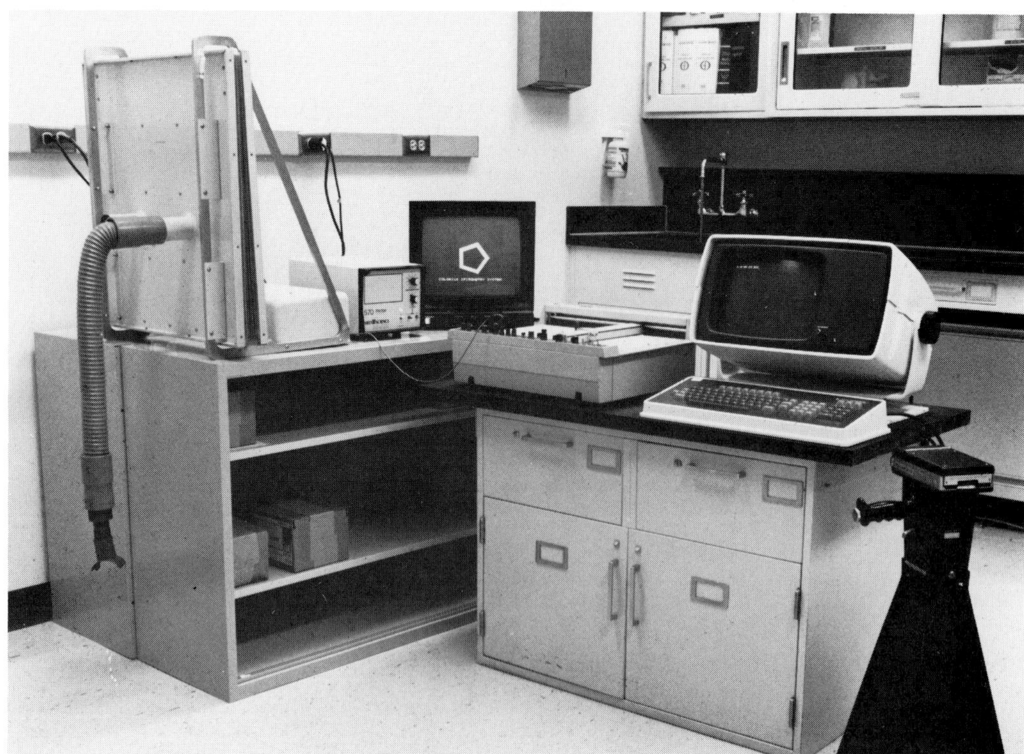

Fig. A-1. A complete spirometry system with wedge spirometer, x–y recorder, graphics terminal, and computer terminal.

type of system, the pressure drop will increase proportionately to the flow moving through the tube. Therefore, the output from this device is a flow rate signal rather than a volume signal. A flow signal is usually electronically integrated to provide a volume output for the production of a flow-volume loop. Pneumotachometer performance may be affected by gas density, gas viscosity, air turbulence, water vapor, and condensation as well as other factors. Therefore the environment in which these devices are expected to work should be carefully monitored. Pneumotachometer-based spirometers are frequently smaller and more easily transported than are volume displacement devices. This makes them convenient for use in screening devices that need to be used in a variety of locations. In addition, the lack of a volume limitation makes them useful in other testing applications besides spirometry, such as exercise testing.

By convention, all spirometry results are reported at body temperature and pressure under saturated conditions (BTPS). This conversion may or may not be necessary depending on the particular components of a given system. For a further evaluation of spirometer systems, the reader is referred to the work by Gardner and Hankinson.[11]

The technologist has a vital role to play in spirometry testing. Subjects need an explanation of the maneuver they are expected to perform and usually a few trial runs before they perform the maneuver acceptably. The technologist must properly instruct and coach the test subject throughout the maneuver and provide the primary checks on the quality and acceptability of the data.

Several variables are computed from the subjects' raw waveforms. The expiratory vital capacity is measured as the largest volume of gas that can be exhaled after the lungs are completely full. If the resting ventilation was recorded with this maneuver, then the expiratory reserve volume, tidal volume, inspiratory reserve volume, and frequency of breathing can be determined. The tidal volume plus the inspiratory reserve volume equals the inspiratory capacity.

If the expiratory vital capacity maneuver was performed as forcefully as possible, additional variables can be determined (Fig. A-2). The FEV_1 is the volume of gas exhaled during the first second. It should be

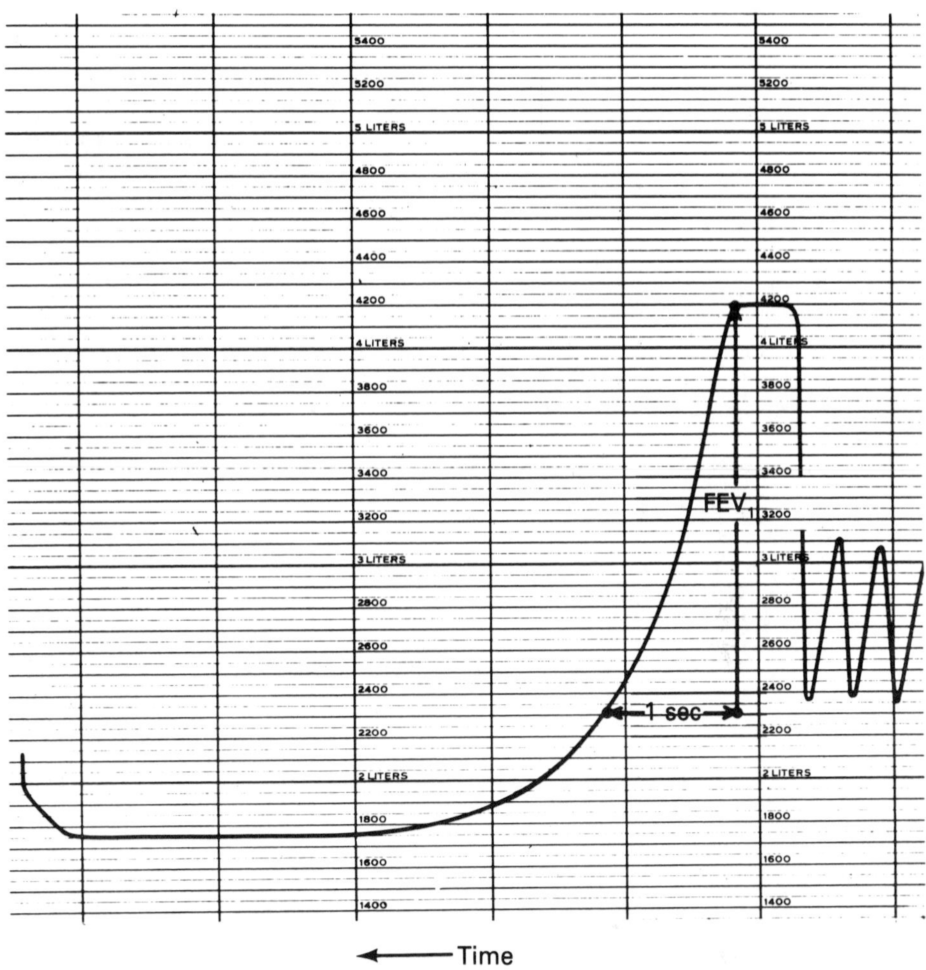

Fig. A-2. Spirogram tracing showing the measurement of FEV_1.

computed through the use of the beginning of breath determination known as backward extrapolation (Fig. A-3). This method corrects for the volume of gas at total lung capacity that is exhaled by the test subject before reaching his best forced effort. This lost volume should be less than 100 ml or 10% of the FVC, whichever is greater. The American Thoracic Society (ATS) published a statement on the standardization of spirometry that contains the following requirements for the forced vital capacity and FEV_1 determination.[1] The spirometer should be able to measure a volume change of at least 7 liters (BTPS) independent of flows between zero and 12 liters/sec. The instrument must be able to accumulate volume for a minimum of 10 seconds and must be accurate to within 50 ml or 3% of the reading, whichever is greater. The resistance to airflow at 12 liters/sec should be less than 1.5 cm H_2O/liter/sec.

The device used to record the raw waveform must provide either a volume-time or a flow-volume trace for the entire duration of the maneuver. If a time base is used, it must be constant throughout the maneuver, and the recording should show a pen displacement of at least 2 cm for each second. Volume sensitivity should be at least 1 cm of displacement per liter and flow sensitivity should be at least 4 mm/liter/sec. A minimum of three acceptable maneuvers should be obtained. Acceptable curves are those which the technologist verifies as being performed with a smooth continuous exhalation, at maximal effort, with a proper start, and without evidence of coughing, glottis closure, premature termination, leaks, or mouthpiece obstruction. In addition, the three acceptable curves should not vary from one another by more than 5% or 100 ml, whichever is greater. The reported FVC and FEV_1 should be the largest observed values for each

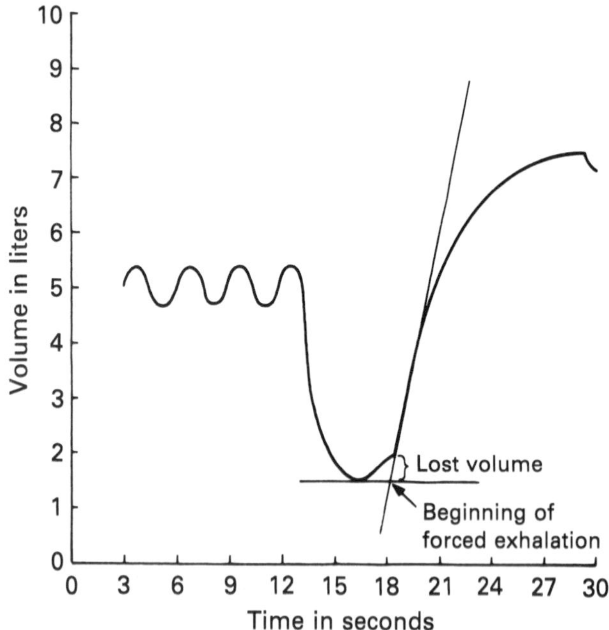

Fig. A-3. The backward extrapolation technique for determining the beginning of forced exhalation (*see* text).

variable even if they are from different curves. The FEF 25%–75% (Fig. A-4) and the instantaneous flows should be obtained from the one curve with the largest sum of FVC and FEV_1. For additional information the reader is referred to the section on quality control and the ATS statement on the standardization of spirometry.

BTPS correction can be made by the following

$$V_2 = \frac{(V_1)(P_1 - P_{H_2O} @ T)(310)}{(P_2 - 47)(T)},$$

where V_2 is the volume corrected to BTPS; V_1 is the volume measured under ambient conditions; 310 is body temperature in degrees Kelvin (37 + 273 = 310); T is the room temperature in degrees Kelvin; (P_2 − 47) is the barometric pressure minus the partial pressure of water vapor at 37°C (47 mm Hg); and (P_1 − PH_2O) is the barometric pressure minus the partial pressure of water vapor at ambient conditions.

HELIUM EQUILIBRATION

Helium equilibration is one of the most commonly used methods of lung volume determination. During this maneuver, the test subject is connected at functional residual capacity (FRC) to a closed system containing a known quantity of helium. As the subject breathes within the system, the helium concentration will gradually fall as gas from the lungs mixes with gas in the closed system (Fig. A-5). This process is enhanced through the use of a blower contained within the circuit that serves to circulate gas throughout all parts of the system. During this procedure, the carbon dioxide from the subject is absorbed within the system and oxygen is consumed from the system. In some laboratories, oxygen is added to the system at a rate equal to the subject's use. This means that the starting and ending volumes of the system are the same. An alternate approach is to start out with more oxygen in the system than the patient requires and to let the volume in the closed system decrease according to the patient's oxygen uptake. In either case, the assumption that the quantity of helium remains constant within the closed system leads to one of the following equations:

$$(VS) \cdot (F_{iHe}) = (VS + FRC) \cdot (F_{fHe}),$$

where VS is the volume of the closed system (including the amount of gas within the spirometer); F_{iHe} is the initial helium concentration within the system; FRC is the functional residual capacity; and F_{fHe} is the final helium concentration in the system after the test subject had equilibrated. In this case the system volume is assumed to be constant. By expanding the right side of the equation and solving for FRC, the following results.

$$\frac{(VS)(F_{iHe} - F_{fHE})}{F_{fHE}} = FRC.$$

If the volume of the closed system is allowed to fall throughout the test, then the following equation applies.

$$(VS_i)(F_{iHe}) = (VS_f + FRC)(F_{fHe}),$$

where VS_i is the initial system volume and VS_f is the final system volume. The following relationship exists between VS_i and VS_f.

$$VS_f = VS_i + \Delta VS,$$

where ΔVS is the change in system volume during subject equilibration. Therefore the equation can be modified to the following.

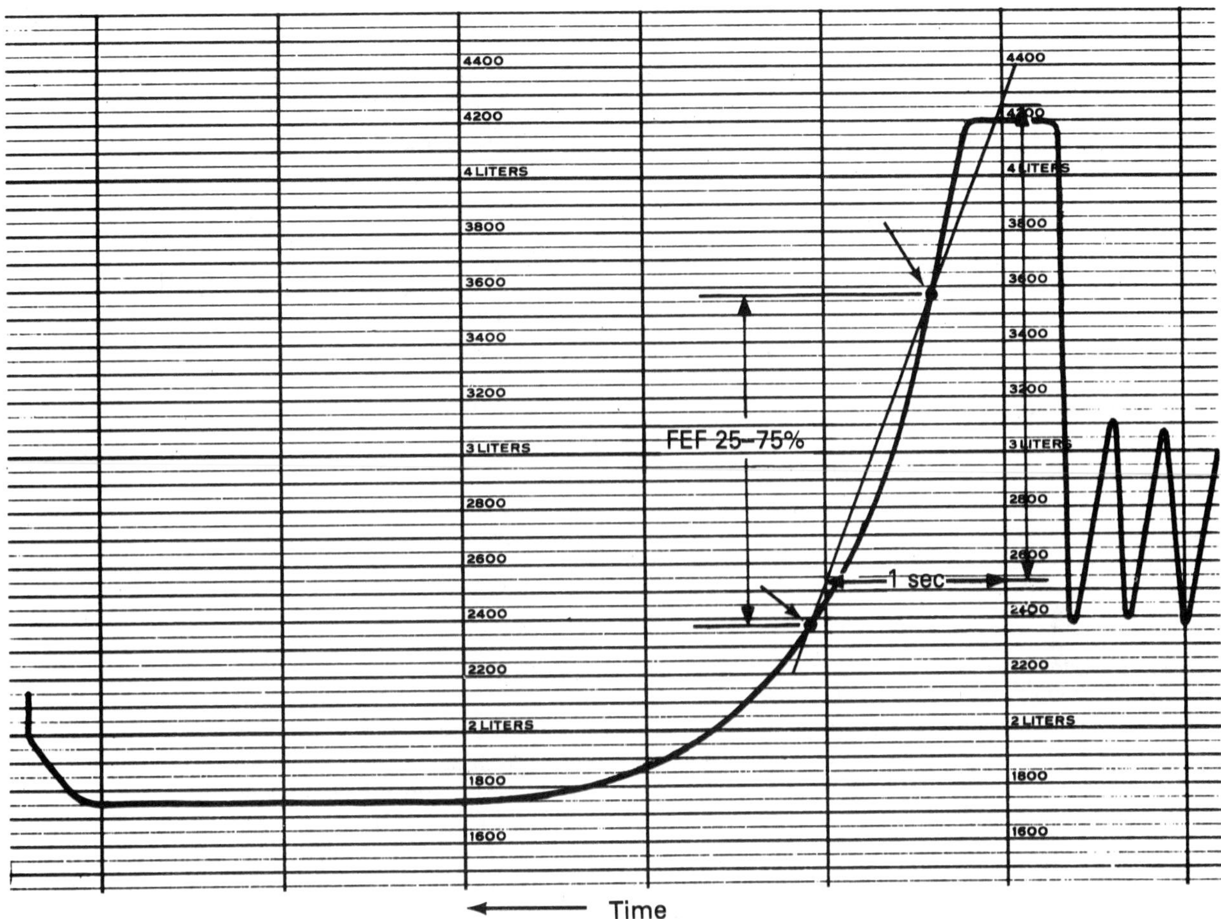

Fig. A-4. Spirogram tracing showing the measurement of $FEF_{25-75\%}$. Arrows indicate the 25% and 75% volume markers.

$$(VS_i)(F_{iHe}) = (VS_i + \Delta VS + FRC)(F_{fHe}).$$

When simplified this equation becomes

$$\frac{(VS_i)(F_{iHe})}{F_{fHe}} - VS_f = FRC.$$

Another form of this equation is

$$\frac{(VS_i)(F_{iHe} - F_{fHe})}{F_{FHe}} - \Delta VS = FRC.$$

Immediately after equilibration, the test subject should perform a vital capacity maneuver so that the expiratory reserve volume, inspiratory capacity, and vital capacity can be used to calculate the residual volume and total lung capacity. Regardless of the method used, all gas removed from the system for the helium analyzer must be returned to the system or a correction applied for the lost gas.

Other factors must be considered when performing this maneuver. First the system must be leak free. This can be tested by generating a helium concentration within the closed system, sealing the system from the atmosphere, and turning on the blower. The helium concentration should remain constant during this process, and the system volume should not change. During patient tests, the blower speed should be adjusted for adequate mixing without producing a pressure against which the subject must breathe.

An accurate value for the system volume must be obtained by, first, washing out the entire system with air so that there is no helium. Then, with a completely empty spirometer, a known quantity of helium should

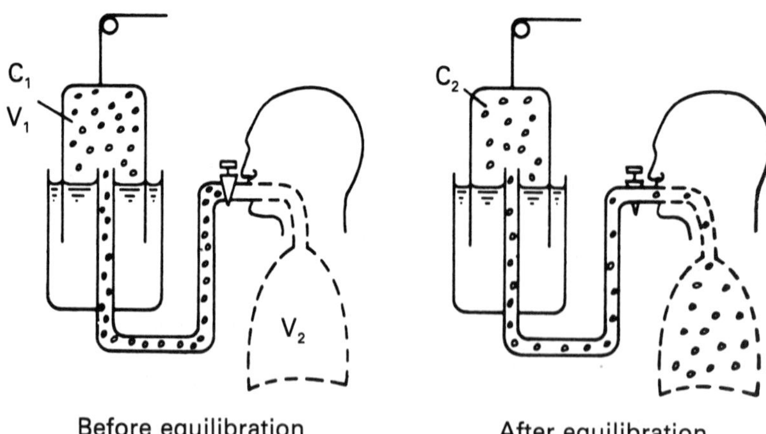

Fig. A-5. The helium equilibration technique. (West JB: Respiratory Physiology: The Essentials, 2nd ed. Baltimore, The Williams & Wilkins Co., 1979)

be injected into the system. Since there was no helium in the system initially, the quantity that was injected must be the total amount within the system. This leads to the following equation.

$$(V_i)(F_{iHe}) + (V\text{A})(F_{tHe}) = (V_i + V\text{A})(F_{fHe}),$$

where V_i is the initial volume of the system with the spirometer empty; F_{iHe} is the starting helium concentration in the system or zero; VA is the amount of added volume as recorded by the system spirometer; F_{tHe} is the helium concentration in the gas that was added; and F_{fHe} is the final helium concentration in the system after the helium injection has been well mixed with the other system gas. This equation simplifies to

$$V_i = \frac{(V\text{A})(F_{tHe} - F_{fHe})}{F_{fHe}}.$$

This process should be repeated until one can reproduce the value for V_i. Any change in the component make-up of the system will necessitate recomputing the value for V_i.

After computing the FRC, one must correct the value obtained for all mechanical deadspace used in the system. Additional corrections can be made to the resulting FRC value for helium absorption, the subject's respiratory exchange ratio, and conversion to BTPS conditions. However, these are somewhat controversial at this time, since there are no commonly accepted methods for handling these corrections. But after all corrections, duplicate measurements should agree within 90 to 160 ml.

Quality control for this maneuver should include on-going testing of a normal subject as well as procedures based on component level checks.

BODY PLETHYSMOGRAPHY

Plethysmography means the measurement of a change in the volume of some object. Body plethysmography is the measurement of a change in lung volume performed while a person is sitting within an enclosed chamber (Fig. A-6). This measurement process is based on Boyle's law, which says that the product of pressure and volume is constant in a closed system if the temperature remains constant ($P \cdot V = K$). If one attempts to apply this equation directly to the measurement of lung volume, it becomes obvious that two of the three elements are not obtainable directly. One can measure the pressure on the lung but not its volume. However, one can measure the change in the lung volume and the change in the pressure on the lung. The basic principle, then, of lung volume measurement in the body plethysmograph is that the volume of a gas-containing closed space can be determined by how its volume changes when certain pressure changes are applied to it. If P_1 is barometric pressure, V_1 is the lung volume we wish to measure, and P_2 and V_2 represent the same system after a pressure and volume change (Δ), then the following results.

$$P_1 \cdot V_1 = K \text{ and } P_2 \cdot V_2 = K$$

implies that

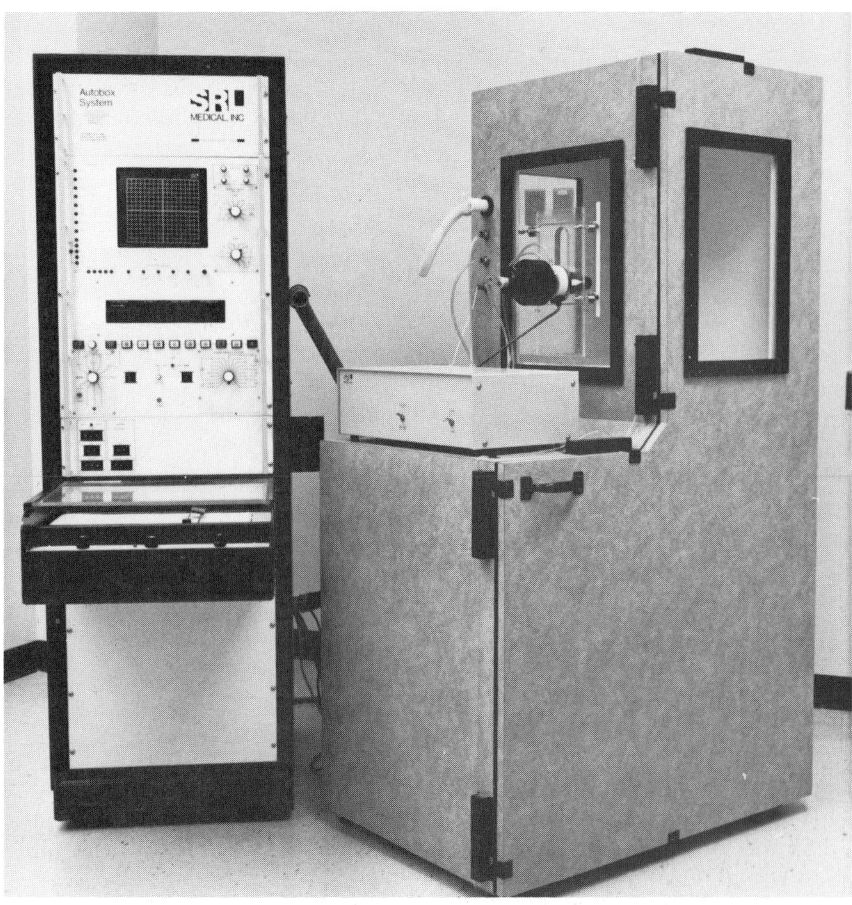

Fig. A-6. One of the newer, fully automated "flow"-type body plethysmographs.

$$P_1 \cdot V_1 = P_2 \cdot V_2.$$
$$P_1 \cdot V_1 = (P_1 + \Delta P) \cdot (V_1 + \Delta V),$$

where ΔP represents the change in pressure and ΔV represents the change in volume.

$$P_1 \cdot V_1 = P_1 \cdot V_1 + P_1 \cdot \Delta V + \Delta P \cdot V_1 + \Delta P \cdot \Delta V.$$

Subtracting the quantity $P_1 \cdot V_1$ from each side yields

$$0 = P_1 \cdot \Delta V + \Delta P \cdot V_1 + \Delta P \cdot \Delta V.$$

The desired variable is isolated by subtracting $\Delta P \cdot V_1$ from each side with the following result.

$$-\Delta P \cdot V_1 = P_1 \cdot \Delta V + \Delta P \cdot \Delta V.$$
$$-\Delta P \cdot V_1 = \Delta V \cdot (P_1 + \Delta P).$$
$$V_1 = \frac{\Delta V \cdot (P_1 + \Delta P)}{-\Delta P}$$

$$V_1 = \frac{\Delta V \cdot (P_1 + \Delta P)}{-\Delta P}$$

The limit of

$$(P_1 + \Delta P) = \Delta P$$

as ΔP approaches 0.

$$V_1 = -\frac{\Delta V}{\Delta P} \cdot P_1.$$

This may be derived in a much simpler way by means of implicit differentiation with respect to either variable. For example,

$$P \cdot V = K$$

implies that

$$P \cdot \frac{\Delta V}{\Delta P} + V = 0$$

and

$$V = -\frac{\Delta V}{\Delta P} \cdot P.$$

Therefore, to measure lung volume one must determine the rate of change of lung volume with respect to lung pressure. This value (assumed to be constant) is frequently determined as the slope of a line on an oscilloscope screen when one is observing mouth pressure and box pressure. For one to assume that the mouth pressure accurately represents the pressure on the lung, there must be no gas flow. For this reason and the fact that Boyle's law requires a closed system, a shutter that can occlude the patient's mouthpiece is used in the breathing circuit. For a change in box pressure to reflect a change in lung volume, we must have a second application of Boyle's law. This time the application is much easier because both pressure and volume can be measured directly. This can, however, be complicated by the fact that the patient, once in the plethysmograph, will displace some of the gas volume and will cause temperature fluctuations.

The type of plethysmograph discussed thus far is known as a "pressure box" because it measures the change in lung volume by measuring pressure changes. These boxes must have a constant volume and be air tight. Other plethysmographs use a spirometer to measure this variable, and hence are called "volume boxes." In these boxes the pressure remains relatively constant while the volume varies. The third type of plethysmograph incorporates a pneumotachograph instead of a spirometer to measure the change in lung volume and is known as a "flow box."

Airway resistance may also be measured in the body plethysmograph by adding a pneumotachograph into the patient breathing circuit. *Resistance* is defined as a pressure drop at a given flow rate. Therefore one must be able to measure the flow rate of the gas entering and leaving the lung while also measuring the pressure difference between the alveoli and the mouth. Alveolar pressure can by measured only when the mouth shutter is closed, necessitating indexing flow and pressure to a third variable. In the pressure box this variable is the box pressure or the indicator of the change in lung volume. During this maneuver the patient is expected to perform a panting maneuver through the mouthpiece first with the shutter open, then when it is closed. The panting maneuver is necessary to this measurement to provide a linear or closed loop relationship between flow and change in lung volume. After obtaining the slopes or tangents of both closed and open shutter breathing, one should calculate the resistance of the airways by dividing one slope or tangent by the other.

$$\frac{\Delta\text{flow}}{\Delta\text{volume}} \div \frac{\Delta\text{P}}{\Delta\text{volume}} = \frac{\Delta\text{flow}}{\Delta\text{P}},$$

where Δ represents the change observed.

The tangent obtained during closed shutter panting may be used to compute lung volume, as explained in the first part of this section. However, the panting maneuver usually elevates the function residual capacity (FRC) above the resting level. Hence this volume is known as *thoracic gas volume* (TGV). Since the airway resistance depends on lung volume, it is frequently indexed against the TGV at which it was measured. This value is known as the *specific airway resistance*. Some laboratories prefer to show the reciprocal of resistance, *airway conductance*, on their reports. It is also indexed against lung volume and is known as *specific conductance*.

Spirometry can also be performed in some body plethysmographs. One advantage of being able to perform these spirometric measurements, specifically the slow vital capacity maneuver, is that it can be performed immediately after a lung volume measurement. This avoids the problem associated with assuming that the patient's FRC was the same during both the plethysmographic measurement in the box and the vital capacity measurement outside the box. Many details are specific to each manufacturer's plethysmograph. The reader is referred to equipment manuals or the findings of DuBois and colleagues for further information.[8,9]

Quality control of the body plethysmograph should be performed on both a component and system level. Pressure transducers, pneumotachs, and system electronics should all be compared at multiple levels to a standard and checked for accuracy and linearity. One method of checking system performance is with the use of an isothermal bottle (Fig. A-7). This consists of a rigid walled container filled with copper sponges or other conductive metal fibers to provide a stable temperature. The amount of gas-containing space within the bottle must be computed and corrected for the volume of gas displaced by the metal fibers. This can be done by filling the bottle with water and accurately measuring its volume with a graduated cylinder. The bottle volume that is displaced by the metal fibers can be computed by multiplying the density of the metal times the weight of the fiber that was added. The bottle is then attached to the patient mouthpiece in the plethysmograph and tested using the standard procedure. The change in lung volume that would be seen in a patient is simulated by pumping about 50 ml of gas into and out of the bottle with a glass syringe-connected to the bottle. Because this maneuver is performed by someone sitting in the box care must be taken to ensure that the person does not breathe during the testing maneuver. This type of test-

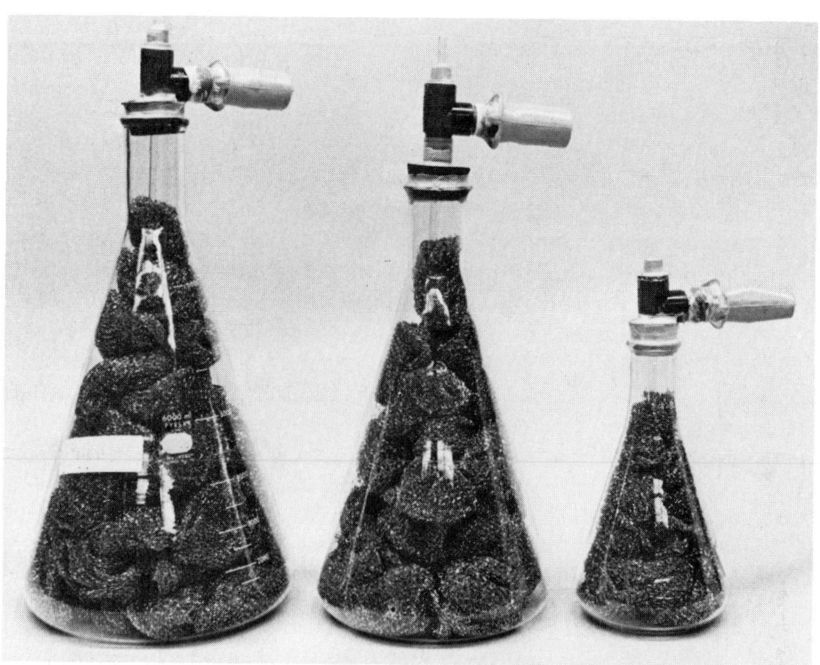

A-7. Example of a series of isomal bottles used to control quality ie body plethysmograph over a se- of volumes.

ing should be carried out with several bottles, each with a different volume. In this way, the linearity and the accuracy of the plethysmograph may be determined.

The airway resistance calibration can be checked through the use of fixed resistors connected to the patient mouthpiece. The resistance must be determined with some other external standard such as a precision flow meter and differential pressure transducer. In addition, these resistors must be within the physiologic range seen in patients and should be constructed to work within laminar flow conditions. When connected between the patient mouthpiece and an isothermal bottle as previously described, the resistor will generate a curve similar to a patient curve that can be used to calculate resistance in the usual way. These types of checks should also be performed at evenly distributed points throughout the working range of the instrument and should include accuracy and linearity determinations. In addition, a member of the laboratory staff should be tested at regular intervals for a complete quality-control program.

NITROGEN WASHOUT

The nitrogen washout procedure assumes that by breathing pure oxygen all nitrogen can be removed from gas-containing spaces of the lung. This is the case in the normal lung but is not true in disease states that prevent air in the lung from communicating with a patent airway. In addition, some patients with poor distribution of ventilation may take much longer to washout than will normal patients. Therefore, the alveolar nitrogen concentration at the end of the test (the nitrogen index) can be used as a rough index of distribution of ventilation. The nitrogen washout test is used to determine the FRC, residual volume (RV), and TLC. The procedure should be performed by connecting the patient to a system that provides pure oxygen for inhalation and a reservoir to collect all exhaled gas. The patient must be at FRC when connected to the system. The oxygen concentration of the inspired gas should be measured and the initial volume and nitrogen concentration of the reservoir determined. This will allow the computation of the initial quantity of nitrogen in the system, which must be subtracted from the total quantity of nitrogen in the system after washout in order to obtain the quantity removed from the patient.

Because oxygen breathing lowers the alveolar nitrogen concentration dramatically, some nitrogen in the blood and other areas of the body enters the lung and is removed along with the nitrogen from the alveoli. This is known as nitrogen excretion and must be subtracted from the final nitrogen quantity within the reservoir in order to determine lung volume accurately. At present, most investigators believe this nitrogen excretion to be about 200 ml/7-min interval.

Because many laboratories constantly sample the exhaled nitrogen concentration during the washout process to look at the distribution of ventilation, a certain quantity of nitrogen will be removed from the system that should have remained for analysis. This should be corrected by either returning the gas to the reservoir after analysis or adding to the computed reservoir value an amount equal to that removed for analysis. This can be computed by multiplying the average nitrogen concentration times the quantity of gas removed. Next, one must correct for the amount of mechanical dead space used during the test and convert to BTPS conditions, since the quantity of nitrogen in the reservoir was measured at room temperature. Last, since the resulting volume of nitrogen represents only a portion of the total gas that makes up the FRC, it must be divided by the original alveolar nitrogen concentration to determine the total FRC. This leads to the following equation.

$$FRC = \frac{(F_{N2}SYSf)\cdot(VSYSf) - (F_{N2}SYSi)\cdot(VSYSi) - N_2E}{FA_{N2}},$$

where FA_{N2} is the test subject's initial alveolar nitrogen concentration; $F_{N2}SYSf$ is the fractional concentration of nitrogen in the reservoir after washout; VSYSf is the ending reservoir volume; $F_{N2}SYSi$ is the initial nitrogen concentration within the reservoir; VSYSi is the initial reservoir volume; and N_2E represents nitrogen excretion.

With this procedure, the operator must have a leak-free system, including the patient interface and all tubing and valves in the system. Methods of quality control could include placing an anesthesia bag with a known quantity of air at the patient connection and checking for the expected result. If this is done, one would ignore the correction for nitrogen excretion. Another method of quality control could be to test a member of the laboratory staff to check for reproducibility. Duplicate measurements in normal subjects should agree to within 200 to 400 ml in adults and 100 to 200 ml in children. Quality control on the individual component level rather than on the system level should include tests of linearity, accuracy, and precision for the gas analyzer and the spirometer used to collect exhaled volume.

SINGLE BREATH DIFFUSING CAPACITY (DL_{CO})

Diffusion is defined as an uptake of gas at a given partial pressure of the gas. The three most commonly used techniques to measure diffusion are the single breath, steady state, and rebreathing methods. This discussion will concentrate on the *single breath technique*, the one used most commonly. Carbon monoxide is used to measure diffusion because of its extremely high affinity for hemoglobin and because one can assume that the pressure gradient across the alveolar capillary membrane is proportional to the alveolar carbon monoxide concentration. The equation used to compute the DL_{CO} is based on the assumption that the rate at which the alveolar carbon monoxide concentration is changing depends on the amount of carbon monoxide left in the alveolar space. This assumption can be expressed by the following differential equation.

$$\frac{\Delta[CO]}{\Delta t} = k \cdot [CO],$$

where k is a constant; Δ[co] is the change in carbon monoxide concentration; and Δt is the change in time.

By separating variables one arrives at the following.

$$\frac{\Delta[CO]}{[CO]} = k \cdot \Delta t.$$

In this form, the equation can be readily integrated on both sides with the following results.

$$\int \frac{\Delta[CO]}{[CO]} = k \int \Delta t$$

implies that

$$Ln[CO] = kt + c,$$

where c is the constant of integration.

Then by taking the antilog of each side of the equation one arrives at

$$[CO]_t = e^{kt} + c.$$

However, at this point c can be evaluated by the following process.

$$e^{kt} + c = e^c \cdot e^{kt}.$$

At t = 0, e^{kt} equals one. Therefore e^c must equal the initial alveolar carbon monoxide concentration (FA_{COi}). Our equation then becomes

$$[CO]_t = FA_{COi} \cdot e^{kt}.$$

If one then substitutes the following value for k into the equation, the result is

$$k = -\frac{(DL_{CO}) \cdot (P_B - 47)}{(TLC) \cdot (60)}.$$

implies that

$$[CO]_t = FA_{COi} \cdot e^{\frac{-(DL_{CO}) \cdot (P_B - 47) \cdot t}{(TLC) \cdot (60)}}.$$

The k is assumed to be negative since the alveolar carbon monoxide concentration must be decreasing constantly. In this equation, $P_B - 47$ is the barometric pressure minus the partial pressure of water vapor at 37°C (47 mm Hg); TLC is the total lung capacity; and 60 converts from seconds to minutes. Then by dividing by the final alveolar carbon monoxide concentration and taking the natural logarithm of both sides of the equation, the following results.

$$\text{Ln}\left(\frac{FA_{CO_i}}{FA_{CO_f}}\right) = \frac{(DL_{CO}) \cdot (P_B - 47) \cdot (t)}{(TLC) \cdot (60)}.$$

FA_{CO_f} is the final alveolar carbon monoxide concentration.

The classic equation for diffusing capacity is

$$DL_{CO} = \frac{(TLC) \cdot (60)}{(P_B - 47) \cdot (t)} \cdot \text{Ln}\,\frac{FA_{CO_i}}{FA_{CO_f}}.$$

Most frequently the patient breathes gas that contains another component (usually helium) used to calculate the TLC. This computation is based on the concentration dilution formula and can be derived in the following way. One starts by assuming that the concentration of inspired helium is known and that the vital capacity is measured during the maneuver. It follows, then, that the amount of helium in the lungs resulted from what was originally there and what was inhaled during the test. This is shown by the following equation.

$$(TLC) \cdot (FA_{He_f}) = (RV) \cdot (FA_{He_i}) + (VC) \cdot (FI_{He}).$$

In this equation TLC represents total lung capacity; RV is residual volume; VC is vital capacity; FA_{He_f} is the final alveolar helium concentration; FA_{He_i} is the initial alveolar helium concentration; and FI_{He} is the inspired helium concentration. However, if one assumes that there was no helium initially in the lung, then the equation simplifies to the following.

$$(TLC) \cdot (FA_{He_f}) = (VC) \cdot (FI_{He}),$$

and total lung capacity is calculated by

$$TLC = \frac{(VC) \cdot (FI_{He})}{(FA_{He_f})}.$$

The initial alveolar carbon monoxide concentration must be corrected because of the dilution due to the residual volume that one assumes to contain no carbon monoxide. Then, by again using the concentration dilution formula, the following results after dropping the term for residual volume.

$$(TLC) \cdot (FA_{CO_i}) = (VC) \cdot (FI_{CO}).$$

In this equation the TLC and VC are the same as previously defined; the FA_{CO_i} is the initial alveolar carbon monoxide concentration; and the FI_{CO} is the fractional concentration of inspired carbon monoxide. By solving for the FI_{CO}, one obtains the following.

$$FA_{CO_i} = \frac{(VC) \cdot (FI_{CO})}{TLC}.$$

However, we are able to show the following from the TLC calculation by helium dilution.

$$\frac{VC}{TLC} = \frac{FA_{He_f}}{FI_{He}}.$$

Therefore by substitution the computed initial alveolar carbon monoxide concentration is given by

$$FA_{CO_i} = \frac{(FA_{He_f}) \cdot (FI_{CO})}{(FI_{He})}.$$

A properly performed maneuver should show constant rapid inhalation to TLC at the start of the test, a breath hold at TLC for about 10 seconds, an appropriate volume of gas allowed to pass before collection starts, and then collection of the sample for analysis. Exhalation should be relatively rapid and constant.

To compute the DL_{CO} properly, one must sample a portion of the patient's exhaled gas. The first part of the exhaled gas contains primarily gas that was sitting in anatomical dead space, and thus should not be sampled. Once gas capture has begun, the gas should be collected until a suitable volume for analysis has been exhaled. One should not include gas from the terminal phase of exhalation, since midexhalation samples more accurately reflect the average alveolar gas concentration. The breath-holding time is computed from the tracing of both volume and time made during the maneuver. Several techniques are available for computing this time. Generally time zero cannot occur before the point at which the patient has inhaled a volume of gas equal to his anatomical dead space, and the final time cannot be later than the time at which the gas collection has ended or earlier than the time at which gas collection had started. Some laboratories like to report the diffusing capacity indexed against the lung volume at which it was measured (DL/VA). An alternative approach to this is to use the TLC measured by the test to help predict the normal DL_{CO}. In either case, diffusion defects can be distinguished from a DL_{CO} that is low simply because of lung volume.

Oxygen and carbon monoxide both compete for the same receptor site on the hemoglobin molecule. Therefore the oxygen concentration in the gas mixture used to measure DL_{CO} should be held constant from test to test. Some laboratories use oxygen concentrations slightly above 21% if the usual barometric pressure in their geographic area is significantly below 760 mm Hg. This is used to maintain an alveolar P_{O_2} equal to the sea level value.

The membrane diffusing capacity and the pulmonary capillary blood volume can be computed in a patient who has had the DL_{CO} measured at several different oxygen concentrations. This computation is based on the following relationship.

$$\frac{1}{DL_{CO}} = \frac{1}{DM} + \frac{1}{\phi Vc},$$

where DM represents the membrane diffusing capacity; Vc is the average volume of blood in the capillary bed in milliliters; and ϕ is the reaction rate of carbon monoxide with hemoglobin in uptake per unit of volume per minute per torr. After computing the DL_{CO}, one must consider the effect of hemoglobin on the result. An anemic patient may have a low DL_{CO} because of low hemoglobin as opposed to any actual diffusion defect. The DL_{CO} will drop about 7% per gram decrease in hemoglobin.[6]

Quality control for the diffusing capacity test must include checks of the spirometer used to measure volume, the gas analyzers, and any instrumentation used to compute breath-holding time. Special attention should be paid to the linearity of the gas analyzers and the development of a correction if alinearity exists.

EXERCISE TESTING

The equipment needed to establish an exercise laboratory will vary according to available personnel, space, test measurements to be made, and the number and type of patients undergoing exercise testing (Fig. A-8). Cost for equipment is considerable.

The cycle ergometer is preferred by many for evaluating the pulmonary patient because workload can be quantified precisely and changed rapidly without difficulty. A predictable metabolic response can be obtained providing that adequate calibration is maintained. The patient can cease work immediately if distress occurs simply by stopping pedaling. The maximum oxygen uptake is usually about 7% lower with a cycle ergometer than with a treadmill; however, ventilation and lactate production are higher. Treadmill exercise uses a greater number of muscle groups to account for the higher oxygen uptake. Testing on the cycle ergometer more commonly produces discomfort in the leg muscles than does treadmill testing.

The treadmill is preferred by some because walking is a much more familiar activity than bicycling. However, it is more difficult to establish a desired workload because of a large number of variables. There is a potential danger to the patient in that the treadmill cannot be stopped quickly should the patient experience distress. Additional treadmill testing problems include size, noise, expense, and patient discomfort.

Basic measurements taken during exercise testing include heart rate, ECG, minute ventilation ($\dot{V}_E$), frequency of breathing (f), and an estimate of the patient's work rate. Cardiac frequency can be determined best by using a cardiac monitor with chest electrodes attached to the patient. Analysis of expired gas volume requires a Tissot spirometer. (A dry gas meter can be used although it is less accurate in that it has a tendency to leak and tends to be alinear.) A mass spectrometer (or CO_2 and O_2 analyzers) and a mixing chamber (or Douglas bag) are required to analyze mixed expired gas concentrations. In addition, tubing, valves, and a stopwatch are needed. A multichannel recorder is highly desirable to record multiple physiological parameters simultaneously.

The capability to sample arterial blood and blood pressure during exercise using an indwelling arterial line and a pressure transducer is very helpful. An ear oximeter or transcutaneous PO_2 monitor can be used as noninvasive substitutes to arterial cannulation for evaluating oxygen levels.

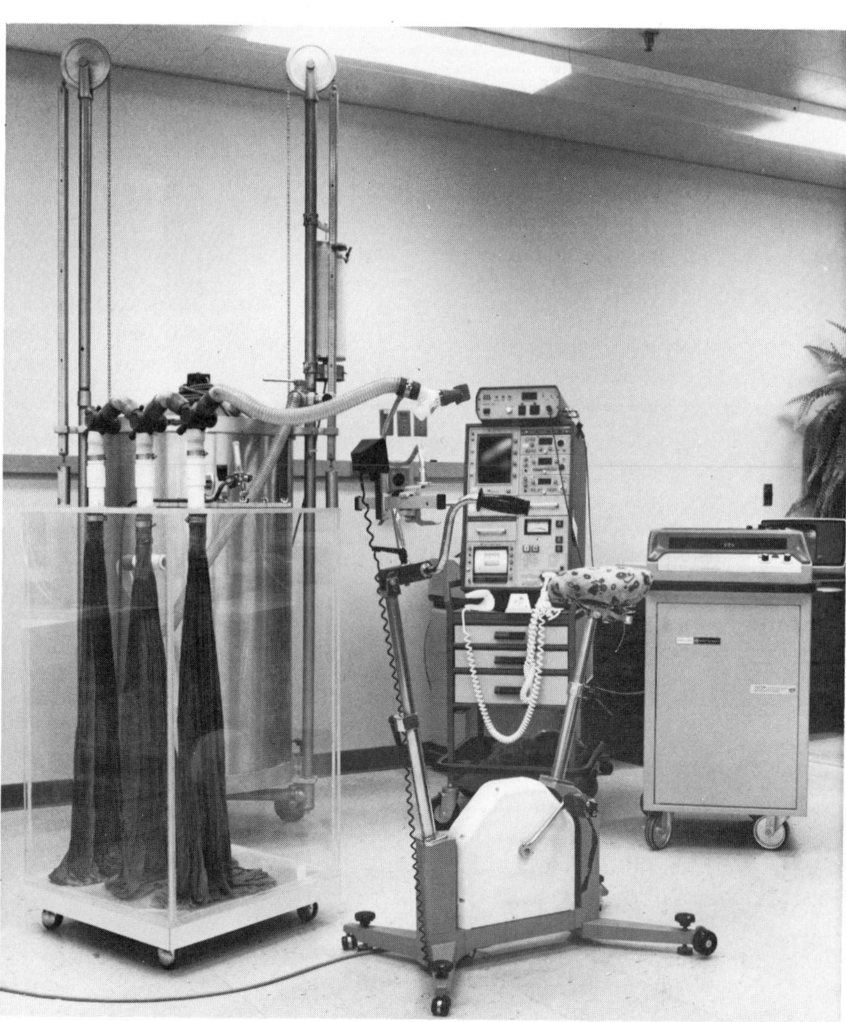

Fig. A-8. Exercise testing laboratory showing gas collection system (Bag in Box), Tissot spirometer, electromechanical bicycle ergometer, hemodynamic monitors, ear oximeter, emergency equipment, and mass spectrometer.

For additional details, the reader is referred to the source references on exercise testing.[3,15,24]

The initial evaluation of a patient before testing should include a complete history and physical examination, ECG to detect unsuspected cardiac disease, pulmonary function testing, and resting arterial blood gas determination. The type of test performed will depend on the training of the personnel, the facilities in the laboratory performing the test, and the type of information being sought.

The procedure should be explained thoroughly to the patient ahead of time. He should be properly positioned on the bicycle and have an opportunity to practice pedaling or walking on the treadmill. Appropriate footwear and clothing are advisable. In most cases collection of ventilation through a mouthpiece with a noseclip in place will be needed. Owing to the patient's general condition (assessed in the initial evaluation), some patients are not suitable candidates for exercise testing—for instance, those with disabling musculoskeletal problems or those with severely disabling cardiopulmonary disorders.

Incremental increases in work intensity can be made after collecting baseline data until the patient reaches the maximum work level tolerated. At each level of exercise the expired gas can be collected and analyzed and the heart rate recorded.

After allowing time for the patient to rest and return to a normal heart rate, the patient's steady-state response can be tested during 4 to 5 minutes of constant exercise. During this time, appropriate collections such as arterial blood gas sample can be obtained. The same procedure can be carried out with patients who need oxygen administration, although this may preclude calculation of expired gas results unless an exact concentration of inspired oxygen is known.

Gas Volumes (*also see* section on Spirometry)

$\dot{V}CO_2$ (ml/min STPD) = FE_{CO_2} × $\dot{V}E$ (liters/min STPD) × 1000.
$\dot{V}O_2$ (STPD) = $\dot{V}E$ (liters/min STPD) × [0.265 (1 − FE_{O_2} − FE_{CO_2}) − FE_{O_2}].

$$R = \text{respiratory exchange ratio} = \frac{\dot{V}CO_2}{\dot{V}O_2},$$

where $\dot{V}CO_2$ = CO_2 production; FE_{CO_2} = expired CO_2 concentration; VO_2 = O_2 uptake; FE_{O_2} = expired O_2 concentration.

In view of the many measurements made in exercise testing and the difficulty at times in establishing accuracy, the development of a valid quality control program is especially important. An error in measurement can compound larger errors in the derived variables.

Work Levels

Mechanical calibration should be checked initially and at regular intervals (at least once a year). Pedaling frequency of some ergometers does not affect the workload with the electromechanical bicycle as long as it is maintained between 40 and 80 cycles/min. Biologic calibration should be performed more frequently (i.e., weekly or monthly) and is achieved by measuring oxygen uptake and heart rate at several work levels by a physically fit member of the laboratory staff. This should be reproducible within ± 5% for a given power output. For the treadmill, the grade and speed should be verified at regular intervals.

Volume and Flow Rates

Dry gas meters, pneumotachographs, transducers, and Tissot spirometers need to be calibrated regularly in order to maintain a high level of dependability. The details for carrying this out are available to the interested reader in several sources.[3,15,24]

Gas Analyzers and Blood Gas Machines

Carbon dioxide and oxygen analyzers should be calibrated with certified gases in the range of 0 to 7% carbon dioxide (±0.02%) and 16% oxygen (±0.03%) as well as with room air (±0.03%). Cylinder calibrating gases do vary sufficiently enough to require verification by the Haldane or Scholander techniques. The mass spectrometer requires calibration against room air. A regular quality control program is now carried out by most blood gas laboratories to ensure reliability of arterial blood gas results.

Integrity of Overall Circuit

By assessing values at rest and at several exercise levels, leaks in the system can be detected along with errors in calculation or gas analyzer response. An R value of 0.7 to 0.85 should normally be seen at rest in a healthy person tested under optimal conditions with an increase to 1.0 with near peak levels of exercise.

TESTING CONTROL OF VENTILATION

Ventilatory response testing is a rather new field. Since its clinical importance is still in an evolving state, testing has not yet been standardized. To conduct ventilatory response testing, the following pieces of equipment are needed.

- **A.** A means of measuring mouth pressure—for example, a transducer attached to a mouthpiece.
- **B.** A means of measuring flow and volume—for example, a pneumotachograph and transducer or a volume displacement spirometer.
- **C.** A means of measuring gas concentrations—for example, oxygen and carbon dioxide analyzers or a mass spectrometer.
- **D.** A rebreathing source—for example, a 7-liter anesthesia bag.
- **E.** A carbon dioxide absorber contained within a plastic cylinder.
- **F.** A means of generating variable flow through the carbon dioxide absorber circuit—for example, a pump with a needle valve.
- **G.** A means of occluding the inspiratory side of the circuit rapidly without anticipation by the subject.
- **H.** A means of measuring effects of induced hypoxia on the actual saturation—for example, an ear oximeter.
- **I.** A recording device.
- **J.** If possible, a computer—calculator.
- **K.** Various valves, T-pieces, syringes, and tubing to complete the test circuit.

The greatest limitation to ventilatory response testing at present is the reliability of the generated data in reflecting output of various components quantitatively and reproducibly. Factors that affect the outcome may include the patient's effort and emotional state, various receptors in the lungs and chest wall, and changes in the hydrogen ion concentration, Pa_{O_2}, Pa_{CO_2}, and bicarbonate level as they affect peripheral receptors or the respiratory center and its output.

A test involving chemical stimulation is the hypercapneic response using the rebreathing method described by Read.[20] With this test, the subject rebreathes from a bag containing 5% to 7% carbon dioxide in oxygen, establishing equilibration between the bag, the alveoli, the arterial P_{CO_2}, and probably the cerebrospinal fluid P_{CO_2}.[14,23] The end point is the development of dyspnea, and end tidal carbon dioxide of 9%, or at the end of 4 minutes, maintaining hyperoxic conditions to eliminate any hypoxic contribution.

A modification of the rebreathing method is used to study the response to hypoxemia.[14,23] The subject rebreathes a mixture of 24% oxygen and 6% to 7% carbon dioxide in nitrogen. During this study one strives to maintain a normal P_{CO_2} level by regulating flow through the carbon dioxide absorber. One monitors the response in terms of change in oxygen saturation during this study. The end point involves an end tidal P_{O_2} of 40 mm Hg, a saturation of 60% to 70%, or distress by the subject.

The minute ventilation measured by these tests is limited by dependence on lung and chest wall mechanics. The presence of airway obstruction is a common example of this. One can analyze separately the tidal volume, respiratory frequency, and inspiratory and expiratory durations.

The inspiratory occlusion pressure at 100 msec (P_{100}) can be measured during room air, hypercapnic, or hypoxic conditions.[25] Without prior knowledge by the patient, the inspiratory line is occluded during the preceding expiration; thus a negative pressure is created during the subsequent inspiration relatively independent of compliance and resistance. This response is recorded on paper moving at a speed of 50 mm/sec.

One can also monitor neural activity from the respiratory muscle surface using, for example, an esophageal bipolar electrode to obtain the diaphragmatic electromyogram (EMG di). This can be analyzed as a moving average over a prescribed time interval by amplifying, filtering, and rectifying respiratory activity.[10,17]

- *Hypercapneic Response:* Minute ventilation expressed as liters/min BTPS is plotted on the Y axis versus mean PET_{CO_2} on the X axis. The slope ($\Delta\dot{V}E/\Delta PET_{CO_2}$) is determined by least squares regression analysis.[7] Normal values are found in the literature.[14,20]
- *Hypoxic Response:* Minute ventilation is plotted on the Y axis versus mean SaO_2% on the X axis. The slope is determined by least squares regression.[7] Normal values are published.[14,23]
- *Inspiratory Occlusion at 100 msec (P_{100}):* The negative inspiratory occlusion pressure at 100 msec is measured directly and plotted on the Y axis. The minute ventilation, PET_{CO_2} or saturation can be plotted on the X axis. Normal values are published.[25]

The mouth pressure transducer should respond linearly in a range of 0 to −30 cm H_2O by testing with a water manometer. Leaks can be checked by circulating air through the system with the valves in position for recirculation. When using high oxygen concentrations with the pneumotachograph, the conversion factor has to be reduced to 90% of the room air calibration value to correct for gas viscosity. The calibration of oxygen and carbon dioxide analyzers or a mass spectrometer is handled similarly to that described in the section on Exercise Testing and should include a range of 0 to 10% for carbon dioxide and 21% to 25% for oxygen. The ear oximeter can be tested against an arterial sample analyzed by a co-oximeter.

QUALITY CONTROL

Spirometry—Flow/Volume Measurements

The quality control of spirometry should include checks on volume, flow, and time measurement. Several devices are available for this purpose, including the volume syringe (Fig. A-9). These are built in the form of a cylinder with a hand-driven piston that pushes out a known volume of gas (usually around 3 liters). When using the volume syringe, one must be careful to bypass any BTPS conversion mechanism built into the spirometer being tested if the gas temperature within the syringe is identical to that within the spirometer. Otherwise an 8% or 10% error could result. Volume displacement types of spirometers should be checked with the syringe throughout the operating range, but this would not be necessary with pneumotach-based systems. However, both types of systems should be observed for zero drift.

Drift may be the result of several factors. In the case of a pneumotachometer-based system, it may be due to inadequate warmup time or misadjustment of the zero control. However, in a volume displacement

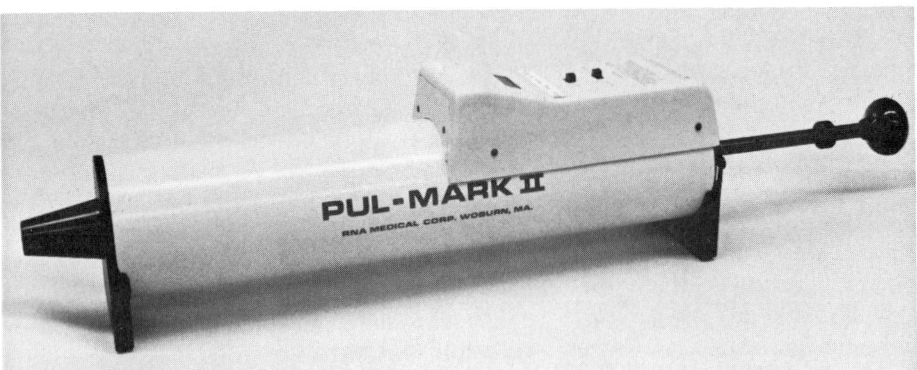

Fig. A-9. Example of a volume syringe for the quality control of spirometers adapted to measure the $FEF_{25-75\%}$.

device, it may be due to a mechanical problem or a leak in the circuit. In any case, drift problems should be corrected before other aspects of spirometer performance can be tested. The volume syringe should be used multiple times in order to check for reproducibility. Serial tests with the syringe should be performed at varying flow rates, especially with the pneumotachometer-based systems.

The average value of these determinations and the standard deviation should be computed and all data recorded in a permanent log. Some volume syringes have small electronic timers that can be used to compute the $FEF_{25\%-75\%}$ by measuring the elapsed time between 25% and 75% of the syringe volume. With this type of syringe, it is possible to check both volume and flow during a single maneuver. Some laboratories use precision flowmeters for quality control of flow measurement (Fig. A-10). These devices are usually driven by a 50 psi source of gas and can be ordered for a specific barometric pressure, room temperature, and gas viscosity and density. Some types can measure flows in excess of 10 liters/sec. These devices produce a constant flow that can be introduced into a system to check flow measurement over a variety of flowrates. These determinations should be made multiple times throughout the working range of the instrument, mean values and standard deviation computations performed, and all results permanently recorded in the laboratory log. Measuring a constant flow is generally easier than measuring a changing flow.

The most ideal way to check flow measurement would be to have a device that can generate a precise waveform similar to those generated by patients. The work by Gardner and Hankinson produced such a device with which they were able to evaluate commercially available equipment.[11] However, since this device is very expensive and not commercially available, it is impractical for use in the average laboratory. Perhaps the next best approach could be to use a series of standard curves that could be replayed into a system in the form of analogue signals as if they were actually being performed in the laboratory.[13] This procedure would bypass the basic sensor but would provide a check on computational methods. This could be useful to those with computer-automated systems.

Time measurement can be checked against a standard device such as a precision stopwatch. This check should also be conducted throughout the available range of the instrument and until a repeatable result is obtained.

Several other parameters should be considered when looking at spirometer performance characteristics, including the resistance to flow of the device and its frequency response. These factors are generally more difficult to quality control within the clinical environment than the characteristics already covered. Perhaps a reasonable approach to this would be to test a normal member of the laboratory staff regularly. Any sudden change in this person's results should indicate the need for more quality control tests.

Many systems use an X–Y or X–T recorder to provide a real time trace of the volume-time or flow-volume curve. In this case, the response characteristics of the recording device are just as important to accurate results as those of the spirometer or pneumotachometer and could be the source of any observed error.

Gas Analysis

One of the most important tests for gas analyzers is a linearity check. Many types of analyzers have built-in circuits to compensate for the inherently alinear response of the analyzer. There are two ways to check for this problem. The first is a serial dilution process in which the analyzer is first calibrated and checked for drift. Then a sample of the patient test gas is diluted by mixing nine parts of test gas with one part of air. Then a sample is prepared by mixing eight parts test gas and two parts of air, and so forth, until one has samples of gas that represent gas concentrations of 100%, 90%, . . . , 10%, and 0 of the testing gases used. This can be accomplished through the use of 50- or 100-cc glass syringes, stopcocks, tubing, and a test lung. All mixtures are then introduced, one at a time, into the analyzer and the resulting concentrations recorded. In this way, one can compare known to observed concentrations throughout the working range of the instrument.

The second way to perform this type of analysis is to purchase gas tanks with certified analysis for each of the test points. However, because of the ease with which gas samples can be prepared from a single tank, most laboratories generate their own samples. By using this technique, one can quality control two analyzers simultaneously if the tank used for sample preparation contains both gases. A common example of this application would be the single breath DL_{CO} measurement where both helium and carbon monoxide must be analyzed.

Probably the best way to represent the resulting data is in graph form where the x axis represents the observed values and the y axis the expected values. The ideal analyzer would show a straight line response where $Y = X$ for all values. If this is not the case, there will be a shifting away from the ideal response in the middle of the graph. In this event it might be advantageous to fit a quadratic, exponential, or other appropriate equation to the data in order to have a computational correction available. In addition, this type of quality control should be augmented through the testing of a normal subject at regular intervals.

Pressure Measurement

Pressure transducers can be checked for accuracy by comparison to several kinds of standards. These are frequently constructed out of tubing which, when filled with the appropriate liquid, will measure pressure by the change in the level of the liquid against a measuring scale. Examples of this kind of instrument are the common "U" tube or the mercury barometer used to measure barometric pressure. Pressure transducers may be either single-ended or differential in design. Single-ended transducers measure pressure with reference to some static pressure such as atmospheric pressure, whereas differential transducers measure the pressure difference between two sources of pressure.

Quality control of these transducers should include pressures throughout the entire working range of the instrument and should be performed multiple times as a check on reproducibility. "U" tube types of devices can be used to check the static measurement of pressure. Dynamic pressure measurement is a more difficult process but is important for the quality control of many types of tests. An oscillating pump that generates a constant pressure waveform with each stroke could be used to observe this type of re-

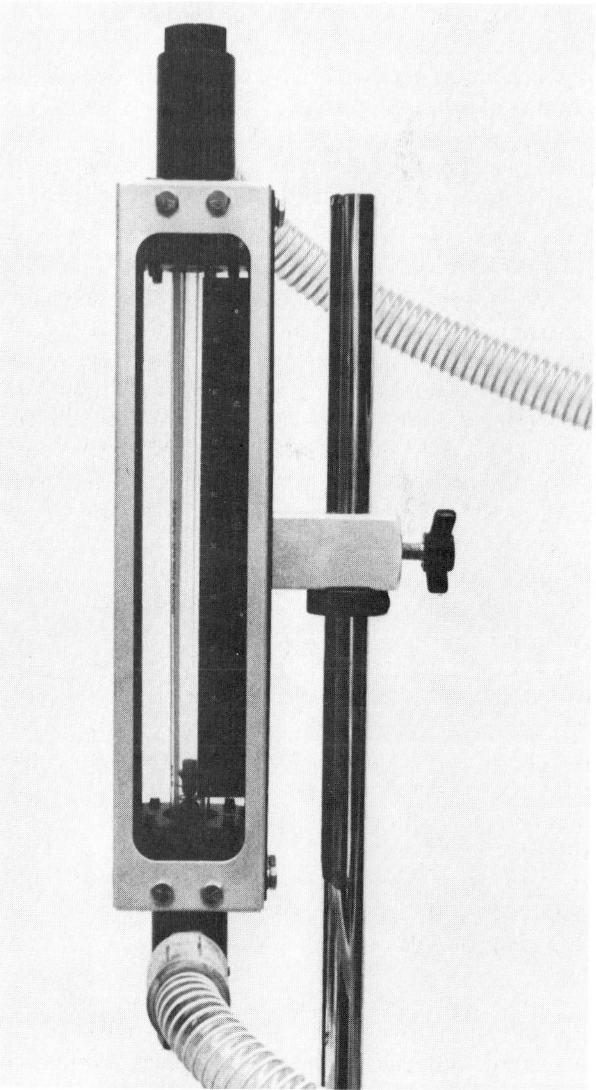

Fig. A-10. Example of a precision flowmeter for the quality control of flow measurements.

sponse. However, the observed output from most pressure transducers is not the direct transducer output but is instead a voltage coming from associated circuitry. Therefore, any observed problems may be the result of an error with calibration, transducers, electronic circuitry, or even the recording device used to capture the signal. Finally, quality control data, including raw waveforms, should be kept in a permanent log and reviewed at intervals for any unusual trends.

COMPUTERS

Most new laboratory equipment today uses computer technology. Generally, most of these systems are connected to spirometers, gas analyzers, and other devices that generate raw data or allow for automated control of equipment (Fig. A-11). The advantages to computerization are many and include increased laboratory efficiency, improved standardization or testing uniformity, and easier data base management.

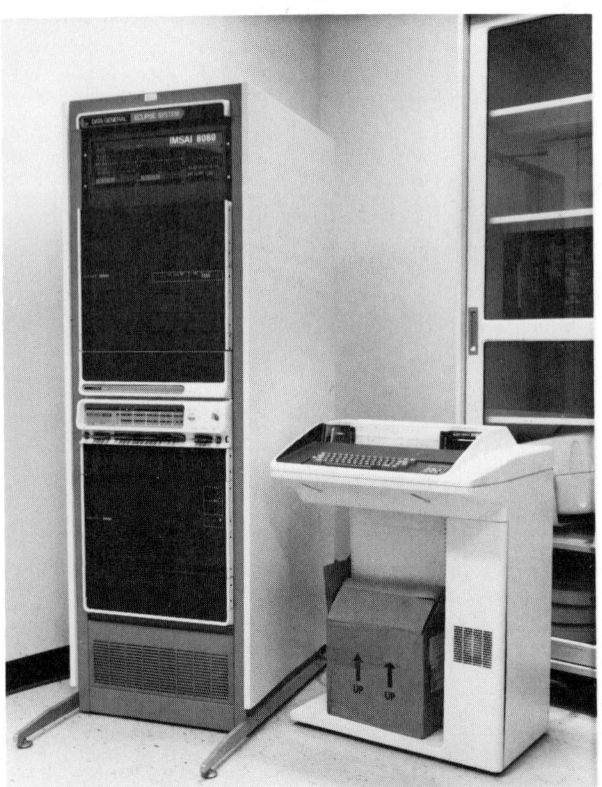

Fig. A-11. Example of a computer system and console printer used to perform real time pulmonary function testing and quality control procedures.

Most of the new computer systems have analogue to digital (A to D) conversion capability or automated waveform capture. This frees the operator from almost all manual entry and provides for almost instantaneous analysis of the data.

The resolution of the A to D conversion is determined by the number of parts into which a voltage change can be divided. This is usually specified by the number of bits (the smallest on/off unit in the digital computer) used during the conversion process. This means that an 8-bit converter will divide its maximum voltage change into 2 raised to the eighth power or 256 discrete numbers. Similarly, a 12-bit converter would break the same voltage change into 4096 parts. If the spirometer has a volume change of 10 liters and generates a voltage change equivalent to the maximum range of an 8-bit A to D converter, then the resolution of the system would be 10.0/256 or 0.039 liters. This means that the spirometer would move from empty to a volume of 39 ml without the A to D converter noticing any change in volume.

Another important factor of A to D boards is the sampling rate. During a slow vital capacity maneuver, a relatively slow sampling rate might be acceptable compared to the rate used during forced dynamic maneuvers. If the conversion time of the A to D board is changing, then a sample and hold option should be added to the converter. This will hold at a constant value the signal being sampled until conversion is complete. In addition, depending on how rapidly the sampled signal is changing and the resolution is desired in the captured waveform, the sample frequency will be determined. Most sources recommend a sampling rate of from 60 to 100 times a second for accurate analysis of forced exhalation. Each captured value must be evenly spaced in time with respect to other captured values.

Temperature drift and linearity are also concerns for the A to D board. The user's method of quality control for these devices will probably be a volume syringe, precision flowmeter, or both. Various waveforms should be used in the quality control procedure since the computer may analyze different waveforms in different ways.

NORMAL VALUES

For pulmonary function measurements to be useful clinically, they must be compared to a normal value for each test. Therefore each predicted value should be as accurate as possible to enhance the interpreter's ability to differentiate normal from abnormal. Normal pulmonary function values vary with each person studied and must therefore be indexed against the following factors to maximize accuracy: age, height, sex, race, lung volume, altitude, posture, and possibly other factors. In the past, the dividing line between normal and abnormal has often been to compare the patient's value to 80% of the predicted value for that patient. Today, however, many investigators are recommending the use of a 95% confidence interval. This approach assumes that there is normal variation within the population and that through the use of statistics a value can be computed that will represent more accurately the lowest limit of normal. A 95% confidence interval means that only 5% of all people studied in the normal population had values below this level, or alternately that 95% of all normal people have a value at or above this level. No similar claim can be made for the 80% of predicted method.

It has long been known that different types of testing equipment will produce significantly different results for a given patient. Therefore attention should be paid to the type of equipment used in a study of normal patients. These principles are best summarized in the article entitled "The ATS Snowbird Workshop Statement on the Standardization of Spirometry."[1] Testing procedure and computational methods may also significantly affect the resulting data and must be considered when deciding which normals to use. The methods of testing used and the derivation of equations for predicted normals may also affect the resulting data. For example, the vital capacity in normal persons increases for the first 23

Table A-1. Adult Normal Values

		LOWEST NORMAL VALUE*	REFERENCE
MALE			
FVC†	(0.06)(H) − (0.0214)(A) − 4.65	[1.115]	4
FEV_1†	(0.0414)(H) − (0.0244)(A) − 2.19	[0.842]	4
FEF 25%–75%	(0.0204)(H) − (0.038)(A) + 2.133	[1.666]	4
FEV_1/FVC	−(0.13)(H) − (0.152)(A) + 110.49	[8.28]	4
TLC†	(0.094)(H) − (0.015)(A) − 9.167	Not determined	12
RV†	(0.027)(H) + (0.017)(A) − 3.447	Not determined	12
FRC†	(0.081)(H) − (1.792)(S) − 7.11	Not determined	12
RV/TLC × 100	(0.343)(A) + 16.7	Not determined	12
$DL_{CO}SB$	(0.416)(H) − (0.219)(A) − 26.34	[8.2]	5
DL/VA	7.08 − (0.034)(A)	[1.4]	5
FEMALE			
FVC†	(0.0491)(H) − (0.0216)(A) − 3.59	[0.676]	4
FEV_1†	(0.0342)(H) − (0.0255)(A) − 1.578	[0.561]	4
FEF 25%–75%	(0.0154)(H) − (0.046)(A) + 2.683	[1.363]	4
FEV_1/FVC	−(0.202)(H) − (0.252)(A) + 126.58	[9.06]	4
TLC†	(0.079)(H) − (0.008)(A) − 7.49	Not determined	12
RV†	(0.032)(H) + (0.009)(A) − 3.9	Not determined	12
FRC†	(0.053)(H) − (0.017)(W) − 4.74	Not determined	12
RV/TLC	(0.265)(A) + 21.7	Not determined	12
$DL_{SB}CO$	(0.256)(H) − (0.144)(A) − 8.36	[6.0]	5
DL/VA	6.58 − (0.025)(A)	[1.31]	5

*The value which, when subtracted from the predicted value, yields the lower limit for the 95% confidence interval.

†Several studies have found these lung volume measurements in blacks to be 13% to 15% lower than those in whites matched for age, height, and sex.[3] H = height in cm; A = age in yr; W = weight in kg; S = body surface area in m^2.

to 27 years of life and then decreases with increasing age. Therefore a single straight line cannot possibly represent normal values accurately for this measurement. In order to do so, most studies have adopted the use of separate equations for adults and for pediatric populations.

Few studies have been performed that describe the normal rate of change of pulmonary function values; however, the use of exponential and other curvilinear methods has not generally worked significantly better than linear models, except in those equations that are used for all age groups. Probably the one single biggest factor is ensuring patient cooperation and repeatable values. In addition, the number of patients included in the study and their breakdown by sex and age categories should be observed for an even frequency distribution. In Tables A-1 and A-2, we present normal prediction equations for children and adults from those studies that we feel best adhere to the criteria outlined above.

Other commonly used normal prediction equations available may offer other advantages in certain situations.[2,16,18,22]

Table A-2. Pediatric Normal Values

		REFERENCE
BOYS		
FVC*	$(4.4 \times 10^{-3})(H)^{2.67}$	19
FEV_1*	$(2.1 \times 10^{-3})(H)^{2.8}$	19
FEF 25%–75%	$(2.621)(H) - 207.7$	19
TLC*	$(5.6 \times 10^{-3})(H)^{2.67}$	19
RV*	$(4.41 \times 10^{-3})(H)^{2.41}$	19
FRC*	$(0.75 \times 10^{-3})(H)^{2.92}$	19
GIRLS		
FVC*	$(3.3 \times 10^{-3})(H)^{2.72}$	19
FEV_1*	$(2.1 \times 10^{-3})(H)^{2.8}$	19
FEF 25%–75%	$(2.621)(H) - 207.7$	19
TLC*	$(4.0 \times 10^{-3})(H)^{2.73}$	19
RV*	$(4.41 \times 10^{-3})(H)^{2.41}$	19
FRC*	$(1.78 \times 10^{-3})(H)^{2.74}$	19

*Several studies have found these lung volume measurements in blacks to be 13% to 15% lower than those in whites matched for age, height, and sex.[3] H = height in cm.

REFERENCES

1. ATS Statement: Snowbird workshop on standardization of spirometry. Am Rev Respir Dis 119:831, 1979
2. Burrows B et al: Clinical usefulness of the single-breath pulmonary diffusing capacity test. Am Rev Respir Dis 84:789, 1961
3. Clausen JL: Pulmonary Function Testing: Guidelines and Controversies. New York, Academic Press, 1982
4. Crapo R, Morris A, Gardner R: Reference spirometric values using techniques and equipment that meet ATS recommendations. Am Rev Respir Dis 123:659, 1981
5. Crapo R, Morris A: Standardized single breath normal values for carbon monoxide diffusing capacity. Am Rev Respir Dis 123:185, 1981
6. Dinakara P et al: The effect of anemia on pulmonary diffusing capacity with derivation of a correction equation. Am Rev Respir Dis 102:965, 1970
7. Dorn WS, McCracken DD: Numerical Methods with Fortran IV Case Studies, pp 310–315. New York, John Wiley and Sons, 1972
8. DuBois A et al: A rapid plethysmographic method for measuring thoracic gas volume: A comparison with a nitrogen washout method for measuring functional residual capacity in normal subject. J Clin Invest 35:322, 1956
9. DuBois A, Botelho S, Comroe J: A new method for measuring airway resistance in man using a body plethysmograph: Values in normal subjects and in patients with respiratory disease. J Clin Invest 35:327, 1956
10. Evanich MJ, Lopata M, Lourenco RV: Analytic methods for the study of electrical activity in respiratory nerves and muscles. Chest 70:158, 1976
11. Gardner R, Hankinson J, West B: Evaluating commercially available spirometers. Am Rev Respir Dis 121:73, 1980
12. Goldman H, Becklake M: Respiratory function tests: Normal values at median altitudes and the prediction of normal results. Am Rev Tuberc 79:457, 1969
13. Hankinson J, Gardner R: Standard waveforms for spirometer testing. Am Rev Respir Dis 126:362, 1982
14. Hirshman CA, McCullough RE, Weil JV: Normal values for hypoxic and hypercapnic ventilatory drives in man. J Appl Physiol 38:1095, 1975
15. Jones NL, Campbell EJM: Clinical Exercise Testing, 2nd ed. Philadelphia, WB Saunders, 1982
16. Knudsen R et al: The maximal expiratory flow-volume curve: Normal standards, variability and effects of age. Am Rev Respir Dis 113:587, 1976
17. Lopata M, Evanich MJ, Lourenco RV: The electromyogram of the diaphragm in the investigation of human regulation of ventilation. Chest 70:162, 1976
18. Morris J, Koski A, Johnson L: Spirometric standard for healthy non-smoking adults. Am Rev Respir Dis 103:57, 1971
19. Polgar G, Promadhat V: Pulmonary Function Testing in Children: Techniques and Standards. Philadelphia, WB Saunders, 1971
20. Read DJC: A clinical method for assessing the ventilatory response to carbon dioxide. Australas Ann Med 16:20, 1967
21. Rebuck AS, Campbell EJM: A clinical method for assessing the ventilatory response to hypoxia. Am Rev Respir Dis 109:345, 1974

22. Schoenberg J, Beck G, Bouhuys A: Growth and decay of pulmonary function in healthy blacks and whites. Respir Physiol 33:367, 1978
23. Severinghaus JW: Proposed standard determination of ventilatory responses to hypoxia and hypercapnia in man. Chest (Suppl) 70:129, 1976
24. Wasserman K, Whipp BJ: Exercise physiology in health and disease. Am Rev Respir Dis 112:219, 1975
25. Whitelow WA, Derenne J, Milic–Emili J: Occlusion pressure as a measure of respiratory center output in conscious man. Respir Physiol 23:181, 1974

B

Methodology of Arterial Blood Gas Analysis

Linda Feenstra • James R. Dexter
John E. Hodgkin

The scope and the application of arterial blood gas analysis have taken giant steps forward during the last few years. With the advent of automated equipment, fast, accurate data analysis with a minimum of human interaction has become available. The complexity of the newer automated systems has not added to the accuracy of the sensors but has been applied to such things as autocalibration, membrane integrity checks, drift and stability checks, and calculation of secondary results. The P_{O_2}, pH, and P_{CO_2} electrodes remain relatively unchanged. Thus push-button simplicity in blood gas analysis does not yet exist, and the present level of sophistication in equipment should never be expected to compensate for unqualified or inexperienced personnel. The demands of the laboratory should determine whether a manual or automated system is most appropriate (Fig. B-1). In the following sections, we shall discuss the types of systems available and their respective applications.

Many factors affect the performance of the three electrodes involved in blood gas analysis. If calibration gases are introduced too rapidly or under too much pressure, the semipermeable membranes could be stretched, which would affect the electrodes' response time. After sampling, incomplete flushing of the cuvettes can cause contamination of the electrode membranes, which will also affect their response. Other factors, such as adjustment time, contamination of buffers, temperature, and electrode maintenance, will affect performance. These factors demonstrate the importance of consistency in calibration techniques and equipment maintenance. Automated equipment was developed to decrease the variability in calibration technique and equipment maintenance that occurs when humans perform these tasks.

OXYGEN ELECTRODE (CLARK ELECTRODE)

The first polarographic electrodes for the measurement of oxygen were developed in the late 1930s. However, the development in the 1950s of an electrode for measuring oxygen in blood and other solutions is attributed to Clark. Thus the P_{O_2} electrode is commonly referred to as a Clark electrode.

Both automated and manual systems use a Clark-type electrode for measuring P_{O_2} (Fig. B-2). The design is slightly different, but the principle for both systems is the same.

Measurements are made on whole blood that has been drawn or injected into a small chamber known as a cuvette. Blood is thus brought into contact with a thin plastic membrane (usually polypropylene), about 1 mm thick, which covers the tip of the electrode. This membrane has two functions: It serves as a barrier between the blood and the electrode, keeping the electrode and its electrolyte free of contamination; and it is a semipermeable barrier that allows for dif-

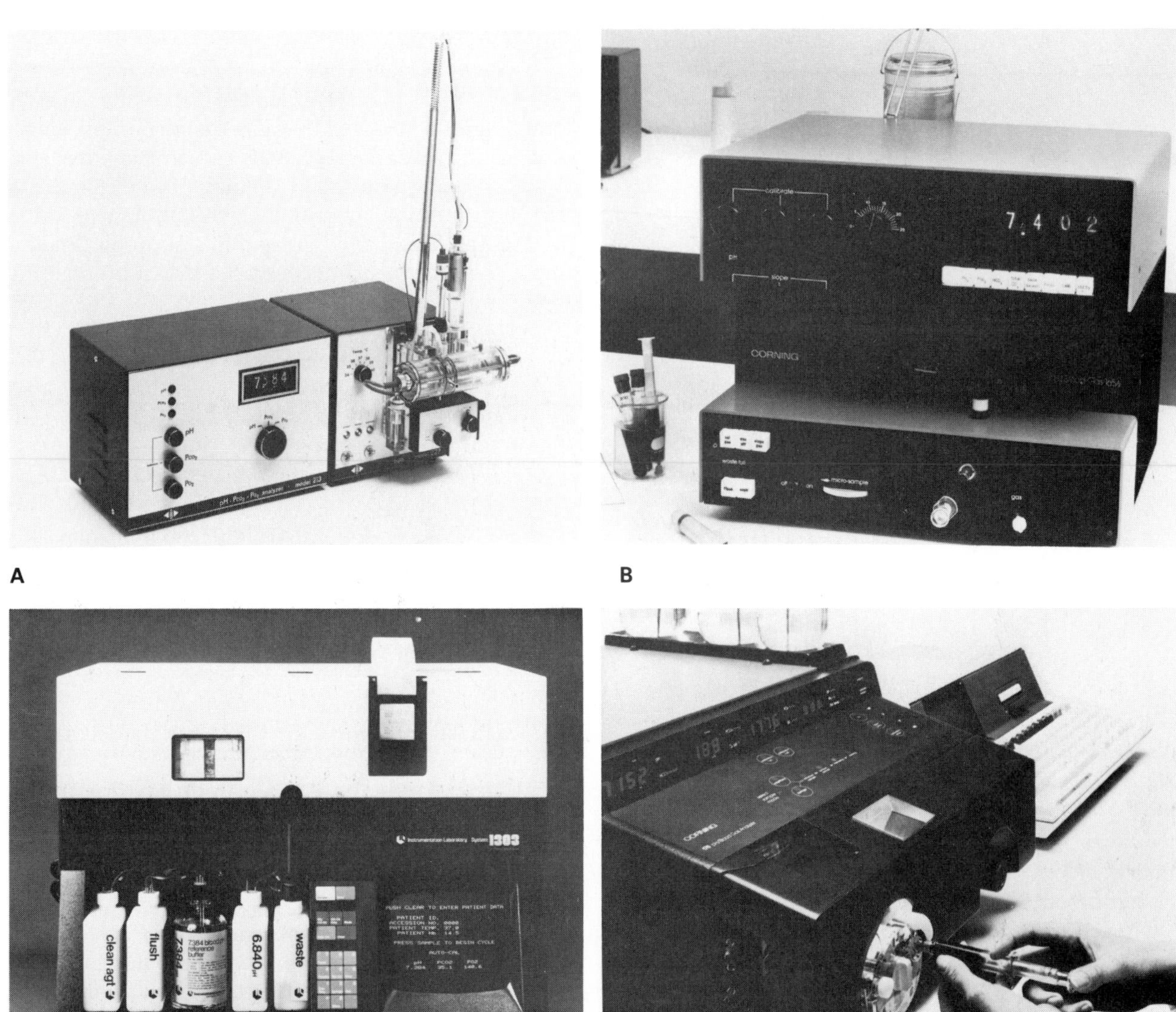

Fig. B-1. *(A, B)* Two examples of manual systems. Calibration and service procedures such as maintenance of liquid levels and flush procedures must be performed by the operator. *(C, D)*. Two examples of automated systems. Calibration and flush procedures are performed automatically at pre-set intervals. These procedures can be initiated by the operator but are still controlled by the instrument. Alarms warn the operator of service needs, electrode drift, and other mechanical or electronic malfunctions. (Corning and Instrumentation Laboratory, Inc.)

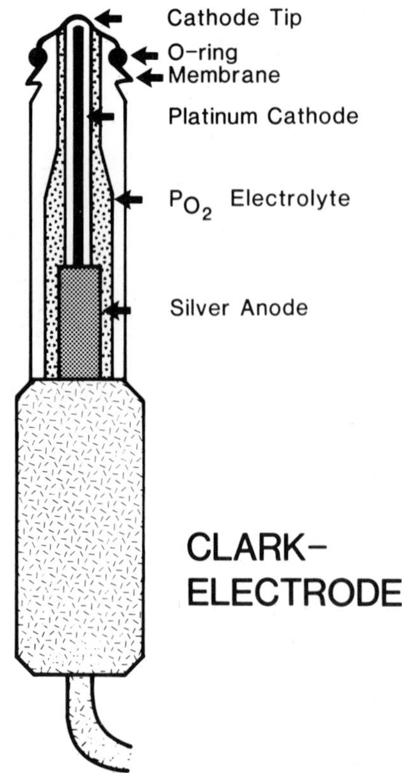

Fig. B-2. Schematic representation of the P_{O_2} (Clark) electrode.

fusion of oxygen molecules. Thus equilibration between blood and electrolyte occurs while variables such as temperature, contamination, and calibration can be closely controlled.

The cuvette is maintained at a thermostatically controlled temperature (usually 37°C), and the sample reaches this temperature within seconds of entry. Oxygen molecules present in the plasma diffuse through the semipermeable membrane until equilibrium between the plasma and the electrode solution occurs. A platinum cathode in contact with the electrolyte solution is supplied with a small voltage (about 700 mV), and oxygen molecules in contact with it undergo hydrolysis. The number of oxygen molecules present in the electrolyte determines the intensity of this reaction, which then determines the number of electrons (voltage) produced. Therefore, the reaction that takes place at the cathode produces a voltage proportional to the concentration of oxygen molecules present in the electrolyte solution (Fig. B-3). The more oxygen molecules present to take on electrons, the greater the electron flow or electrical current produced and the higher the P_{O_2} reading.

pH ELECTRODE

Most glass *p*H electrodes are of similar design. On one side of a *p*H-sensitive glass is a solution with a known *p*H (usually *p*H 6.840) and on the other side, a solution of unknown *p*H (blood). The difference in H^+ concentration between the two solutions produces a potential difference (voltage) that is proportional to the difference in *p*H between the two solutions (Fig. B-4).

The electrode is similar to two half cells with a liquid junction (saturated potassium chloride). One half cell is a silver/silver chloride measuring electrode in contact with a liquid of known *p*H (usually 6.840). Its function is to convey the potential difference across the *p*H-sensitive glass to the electronic circuitry. The other half cell is a mercury-mercurous chloride (calomel) reference electrode (anode) that supplies a constant reference voltage. The reference half cell is connected to the measuring half cell by the liquid junction or potassium chloride salt bridge that completes the circuit (Fig. B-5).

P_{CO_2} ELECTRODE (SEVERINGHAUS ELECTRODE)

The modern-type P_{CO_2} electrode was first developed by Stowe in the mid 1950s. It was further modified by Severinghaus in 1958. Therefore, the P_{CO_2} electrode is commonly referred to as the Severinghaus electrode.

Although physically resembling a P_{O_2} electrode, the P_{CO_2} electrode is, in principle, a *p*H electrode. The tip is covered by a membrane that acts as a diffusion barrier between the blood and the electrolyte. Blood is brought into contact with the membrane by means of a sampling cuvette similar to the P_{O_2} electrode. Carbon dioxide molecules diffuse across the membrane into the electrolyte solution and react with the buffer (Fig. B-6).

Diffusion proceeds until equilibrium has been reached. The resultant change in H^+ concentration in the buffer solution is measured by the *p*H-type electrode and is proportional to the amount of carbon dioxide that has diffused into the buffer (Fig. B-7).

ASTRUP EQUILIBRATION METHOD FOR DETERMINING P_{CO_2}

The Astrup method can be readily applied as a system of quality control on manual equipment. It in-

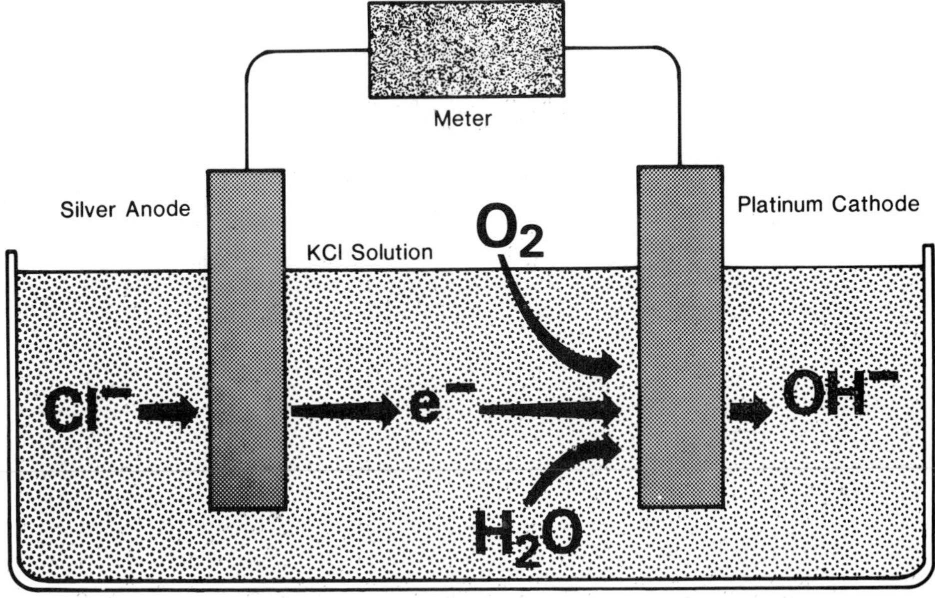

Fig. B-3. Chloride ion (Cl^-) reacts with silver anode to form silver chloride. This is an oxidation reaction that produces electrons (e^-). At the cathode, oxygen will react with platinum and water in a reduction reaction, thus using electrons generated at the anode. The resultant flow of electrons can be measured as a current. The more oxygen molecules present in the solution, the greater the flow of electrons (current).

corporates the relationship between *p*H and P_{CO_2} as depicted in the derivation of the Henderson–Hasselbalch equation and is expressed in the Astrup nomogram as a graphic demonstration of the linear relation between *p*H and log P_{CO_2} (Fig. B-8). The procedure consists of placing two small samples of well-mixed whole blood into two separate equilibration chambers known as tonometers. The tonometer is equipped with a motorized shaker so that the blood can be shaken and swirled completely. The blood in the tonometers is equilibrated with gases that contain two known concentrations of carbon dioxide (about 4% and 8%), with the balance being oxygen so that at the end of a 3-minute equilibration period, the blood in the tonometers will have taken on the partial pressure of the equilibrating gas. By measuring the resulting *p*H of each tonometered sample, one is essentially observing the buffering capacity of the blood. Since the P_{CO_2}s of the equilibrated samples are known and the *p*Hs measured, two x–y coordinates are available to be plotted on the nomogram. The two points plotted on the nomogram establish a buffer line that states the relationship for any P_{CO_2} and *p*H as determined by that particular blood sample. Thus the actual *p*H of the patient's whole blood, anaerobically maintained, can be located along this buffer line and the P_{CO_2} subsequently can be read off the vertical axis.

CALCULATION OF ADDITIONAL ACID–BASE PARAMETERS

Calculation of additional acid–base parameters based on *p*H and P_{CO_2} can be handled manually through the use of nomograms. These nomograms require simple plotting of data points, constructing a line between these points, and reading off the desired values at the appropriate intercepts, thus eliminating the need for mathematical computation.

The Siggaard–Anderson nomogram was originally devised empirically and graphically expresses relationships among *p*H, P_{CO_2}, buffer base, base excess, standard bicarbonate, and plasma bicarbonate. To use this nomogram, the Astrup equilibration technique is carried out, and the two sets of *p*H–P_{CO_2} coordinates are plotted on a graph (see Fig. B-8).

I

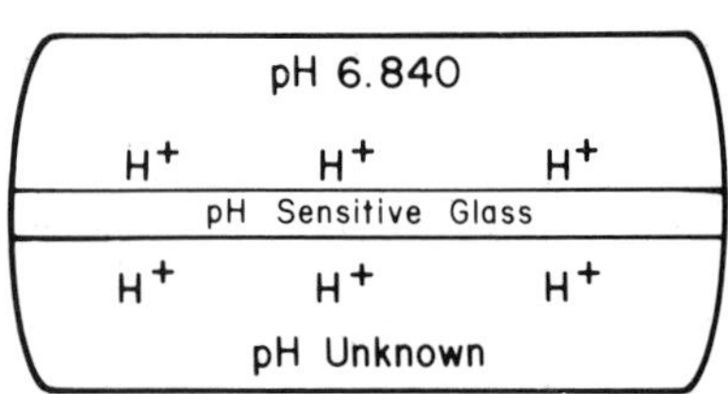

II

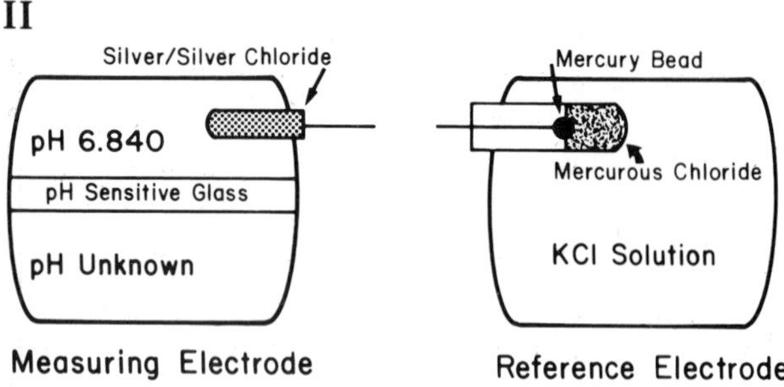

III

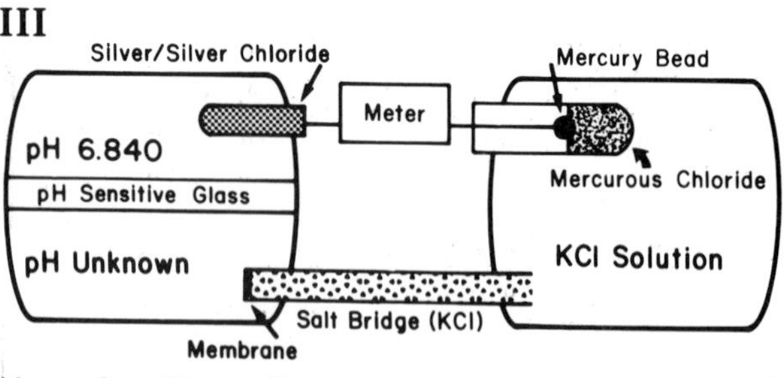

Fig. B-4. Principle of *p*H electrode. *I.* Voltage develops across *p*H sensitive glass when H^+ concentrations of the two solutions are unequal. *II.* Two half cells, a measuring electrode, and a reference electrode. *III.* Diagrammatic representation of a modern *p*H electrode.

Another Siggaard–Andersen nomogram, the alignment nomogram, requires only pH and P_{CO_2} measurements to determine base excess, total carbon dioxide, actual plasma bicarbonate, standard bicarbonate, base excess of the extracellular fluid (BE_{ECF}), and T_{40} bicarbonate (Fig. B-9). These and other similar nomograms have been adapted to slide-rule form, which provides quick and easy calculation of data. Use of a computer, of course, simplifies calculation of these additional values.

CO-OXIMETER FOR MEASURING OXYGEN SATURATION

Both Lavoisier and Priestly (in 1774) recognized that the color of blood and atmospheric oxygen were related. HoppeSeyler (in 1859) studied the spectra of blood and gave the colored pigment the name hemoglobin. Angström had described the absorbance spectrum of blood 2 years earlier. Vierodt (in 1873) was apparently the first to use the differences in the absorbance spectra of the species of hemoglobin to measure their concentration. Hufner (in 1900) extensively described a two wavelength photometric method to determine the percentages of oxyhemoglobin and carboxyhemoglobin.

Haldane (in 1900) developed the concept of oxygen saturation and oxygen capacity and devised a manometric instrument for their measurement. The standard gasometric method, still in use as a reference procedure, was described by Van Slyke and Neill in 1924.[4]

The normal oxyhemoglobin dissociation curve relating P_{O_2} and oxygen saturation is well documented for normal *p*H (7.4) and temperature (37°C). By use of proper correction factors, the oxygen saturation measurement can be corrected for curves shifted by varying *p*H or temperatures. Nomograms exist that allow these corrections to be determined quickly. However, these corrections do not allow for any change in the shape of the actual curve. Many factors can affect the relationship of hemoglobin to oxygen and alter the shape of the P_{O_2}–oxygen saturation curve. For example, a sample with an elevated carboxyhemoglobin level may have an actual oxygen saturation much lower than that predicted from the measured P_{O_2}. The curve may also be affected by factors such as 2,3 DPG, methemoglobin, and various congenital hemoglobins. Therefore, the ability to measure oxygen saturation accurately is preferable to reporting a calculated value.

Oxygen saturation measurements can be made by using a spectrophotometric device such as the IL 282 Co-Oximeter analyzer (Fig. B-10). With this instrument, whole blood is aspirated, mixed with diluent, and hemolyzed. It is then drawn into a cuvette where it is brought to a constant temperature. Monochromatic light at four specific wavelengths passes through the cuvette to a photodetector whose output is used to determine the absorbance pattern of the hemoglobin at these specific wavelengths (Fig. B-11). The instrument electronically computes total hemoglobin, percentage of oxyhemoglobin (O_2Hb), percent-

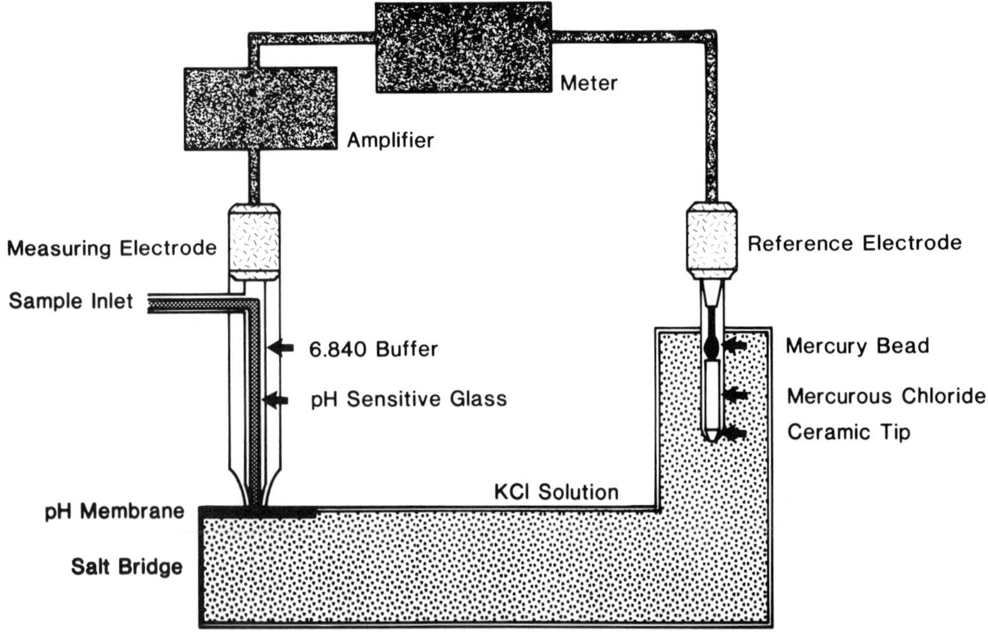

Fig. B-5. Schematic representation of a modern micro *p*H electrode.

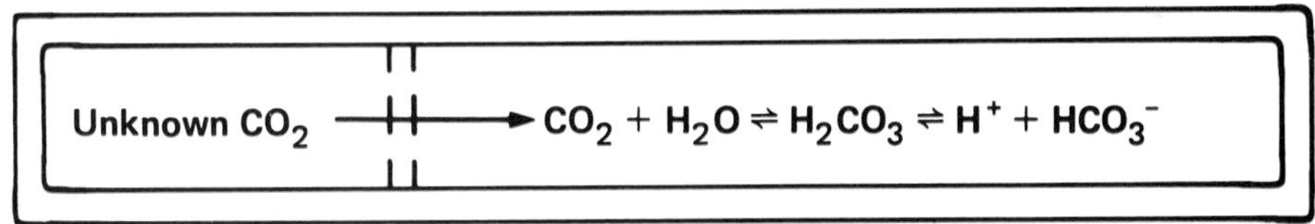

Fig. B-6. Diagrammatic representation of the reaction occurring within the P_{CO_2} electrode.

age of carboxyhemoglobin (COHb), percentage of methemoglobin (MetHb), oxygen content, and percentage of reduced hemoglobin (RHb). This assumes that RHb, O_2Hb, COHb, and MetHb are the only forms of hemoglobin present. Another form of hemoglobin that absorbs significantly at any of the specific wavelengths can introduce spectral interference—that is, sulfhemoglobin has an absorbance level similar to that of methemoglobin, and thus interference with absorbance at that specific wavelength would affect the measurement of methemoglobin. Other measurements might be affected, but the interference would probably be less because the absorption patterns are not as close as those for sulfhemoglobin and methemoglobin. Methemoglobin is the only measured form that exhibits significant pH sensitivity. For MetHb levels greater than 10%, this sensitivity can cause absorbance variations at the four wavelengths used, which can generate errors in all displayed values. For MetHb levels below 10%, a high degree of accuracy can be achieved for all parameters.

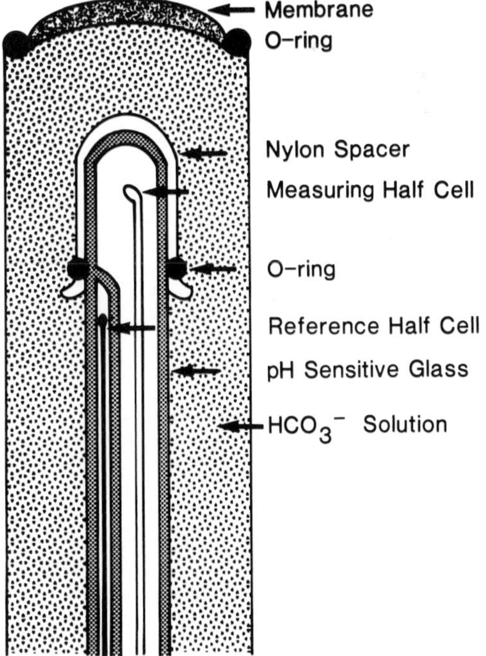

Fig. B-7. Schematic diagram of P_{CO_2} electrode.

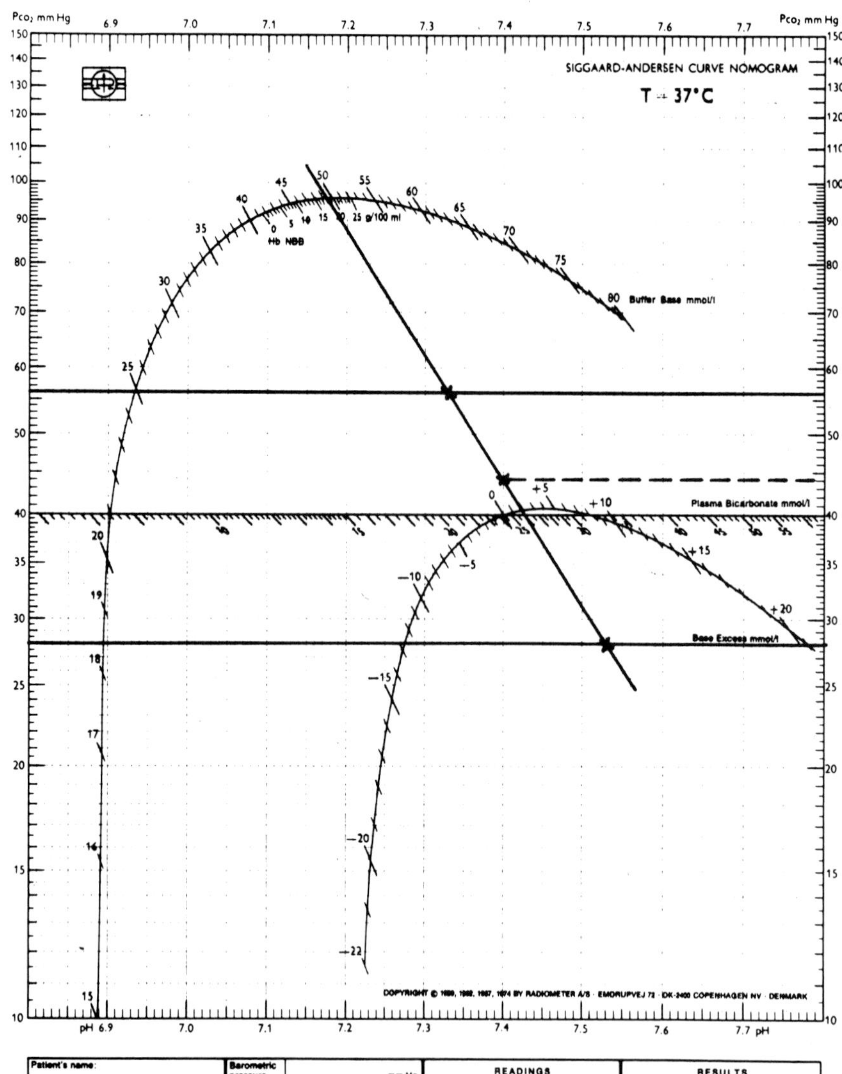

Patient's name:		Barometric pressure		mm Hg	READINGS			RESULTS	
		CO_2 percentage	Cylinder No 1:	%	Before equilibration	Actual pH:		Actual P_{CO_2}	mm Hg
Dept:	Sample No.:		Cylinder No 2:	%				Base Excess	mmol/l blood
Date:		CO_2 partial pressure	Cylinder No 1:	mm Hg	After equilibration	high P_{CO_2}	pH:	Buffer Base	mmol/l blood
Hour of Sampling:			Cylinder No 2:	mm Hg		low P_{CO_2}	pH:	Standard Bicarbonate	mmol/l plasma
Remarks:		Hemoglobin:		g/100 ml	Readings made by:			Actual Bicarb.	mmol/l plasma
		Oxygen Saturation:		percent	Signature:			Total CO_2	mmol/l plasma

CODE: 984-200

Fig. B-8. Siggaard–Andersen curve nomogram: [1] *p*H values are measured after equilibration, and the two points are plotted versus known P_{CO_2}; [2] a line is drawn between the two points and extended to intersect the buffer base and base excess curves (these values are read directly); [3] an approximate hemoglobin for purposes of quality control can be interpolated by subtracting the value of the BE curve from the BB curve reading directly below BB on the hemoglobin scale; [4] actual *p*H is plotted along this line, and the P_{CO_2} is read off the vertical axis; [5] the line itself intersects HCO_3^- at a P_{CO_2} of 40 mm Hg, thus indicating the standard HCO_3^-; [6] to determine actual plasma HCO_3^-, a 45° angle must be constructed through the actual *p*H until it intersects the HCO_3^- scale. Calculation of buffer base, base excess, and standard bicarbonate uses another modification of the Siggaard–Andersen nomogram. (Reproduced, with modifications, by permission of Siggaard–Andersen O and Radiometer A/S, Copenhagen, 1962)

SIGGAARD-ANDERSEN ALIGNMENT NOMOGRAM

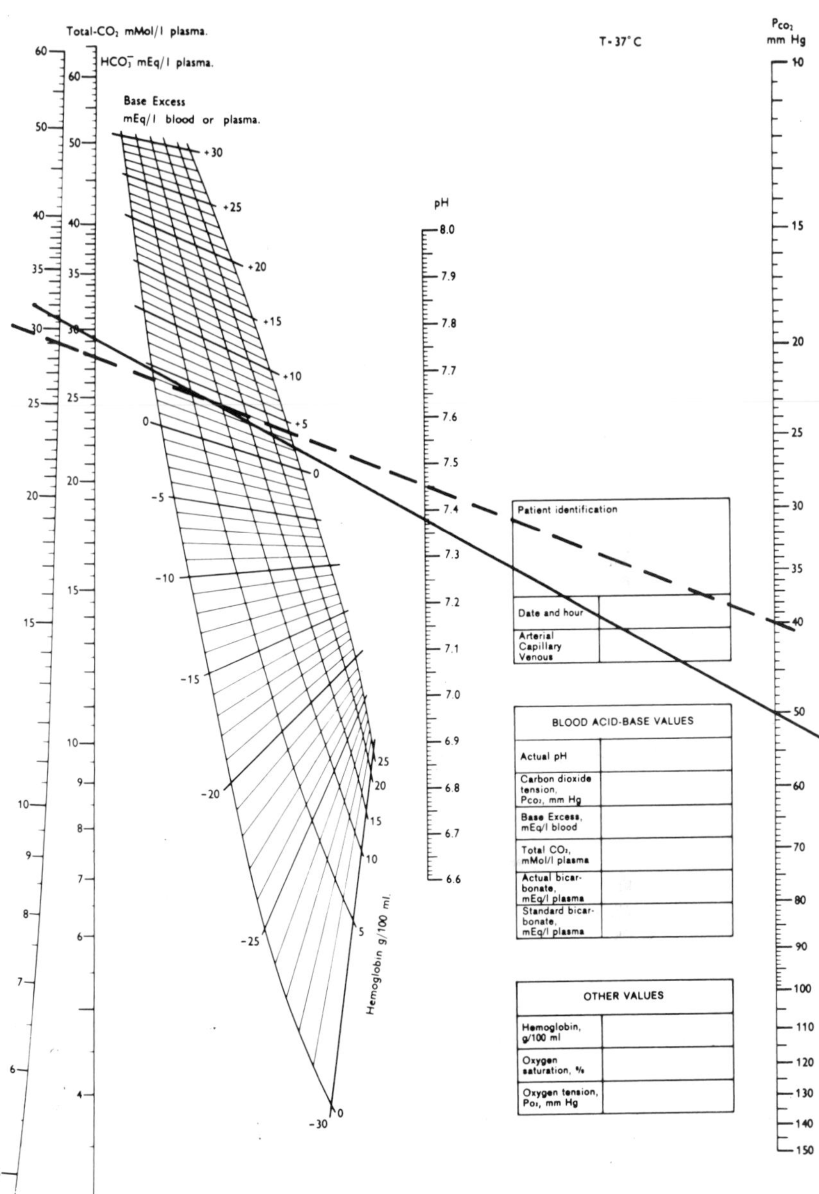

Fig. B-9. Siggaard–Andersen alignment nomogram: [1] a line is constructed between *p*H and P_{CO_2} [2] actual plasma HCO_3^- is read directly at the intersection of the line; [3] BE_b is hemoglobin-dependent and can be read at the intersection of the constructed line and the patient's Hb value; [4] standard HCO_3^- can be determined by constructing another line through the BE_b, Hb point, and a P_{CO_2} of 40 mm Hg, and by reading the HCO_3^- scale; [5] buffer base can be computed from the equation $BB = 41.7 + (0.42 \times Hb) + BE$; [6] BE_{ECF} is calculated similarly to the BE_b, but the BE_{ECF} is read off at the intersection of the constructed line and one third of the patient's Hb value; [7] T_{40} HCO_3^- can be determined by constructing another line through the BE_{ECF}, Hb/3 point, and a P_{CO_2} of 40 mm Hg, and by reading the HCO_3^- scale. (Reproduced, with modifications, by permission of Siggaard–Andersen O and Radiometer A/S, Copenhagen, 1963)

QUALITY CONTROL

As blood gas analysis continues to gain importance in the management of critically ill patients, the need for comprehensive quality control procedures becomes more crucial. Erroneous data are worse than no data. A quality control program encompasses [1] equipment maintenance, [2] calibration techniques, [3] standards and controls, and [4] sampling and analysis protocols. These procedures are all interdependent, and, if any are neglected, the accuracy of data analysis is affected.

EQUIPMENT MAINTENANCE

To help assure optimum performance, one should routinely maintain all instruments (manual or automated). This routine schedule should include all of the operator maintenance recommended for the specific instrument plus tubing change, membrane change, and electrode cleaning and rotating. The frequency with which the procedures should be performed is largely a function of the age of the instrument, its electrodes, and the work load of the laboratory. Poor electrode performance is often correctable by more frequent membrane changes or cleaning. Electrode banks are useful in extending the life of the electrodes and minimizing the "down time" of the instrument. The electrodes are stored "wet"—that is, with a membrane and electrolyte—and are rotated through the instrument routinely (monthly or biweekly). However, a new membrane and electrolyte should be applied when the electrode is put into service. This system keeps the operator aware of the condition of back-up as well as working electrodes. Log books are invaluable in evaluating instrument performance. For example, a sudden increase in membrane changes may indicate that an electrode needs cleaning or replacing, and this can be attended to before the situation becomes critical.

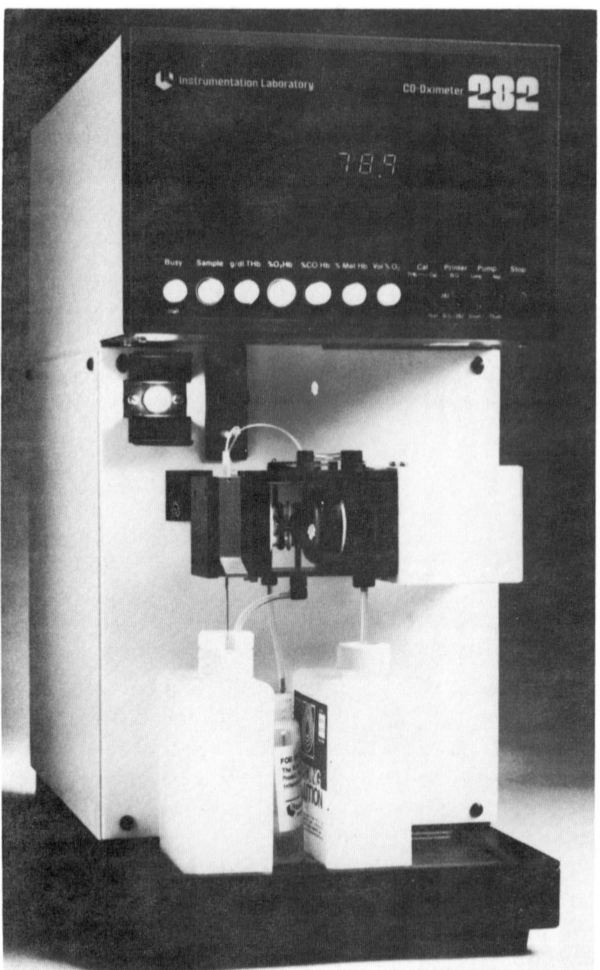

Fig. B-10. IL 282 CO-Oximeter Analyzer. (Instrumentation Laboratory, Inc.)

CALIBRATION TECHNIQUES FOR THE P_{O_2}, pH, AND P_{CO_2} ELECTRODES

An electrode's accuracy and performance are directly related to its calibration. Therefore, the accuracy of data analysis depends directly on exacting attention to detail in the calibration procedure. Each electrode should be calculated using two different known values: one above and one below the usual range of values measured. The selection of these points will determine the range and relative accuracy of the electrode. Traditionally, 4% to 5% carbon dioxide and 8% to 10% carbon dioxide are the gases used for calibrating the P_{CO_2} electrode. This provides a low calibration point of about 25 to 35 mm Hg and a high calibration point of about 55 to 69 mm Hg. These values are derived using the following formula and reflect the expected physiological ranges of carbon dioxide most frequently measured.

($P_B - 47$) × (% gas) = partial pressure in mm Hg (or torr)

P_B: barometric pressure in mm Hg

47: standard correction factor for water vapor pressure

% gas: The specific calibration gas used—that is, 4% CO_2 = 0.04

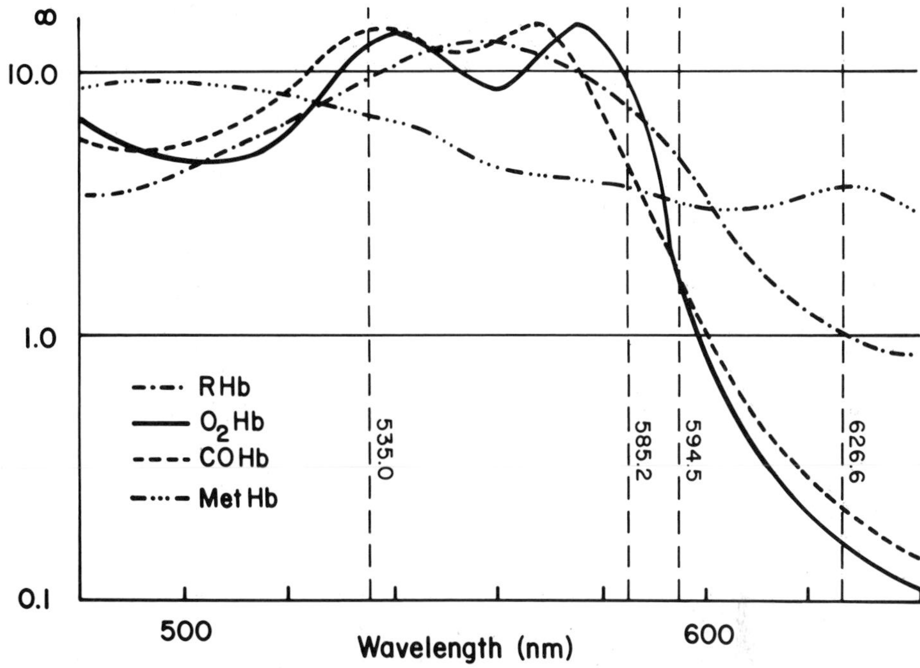

Fig. B-11. Many two-wavelength methods have been published for determining either carbon monoxide- or oxygen-bound hemoglobin. The wavelengths that are used vary. Typically, the wavelengths are either at an inflection or at an isosbestic point of two or more of the species. It is common to select one wavelength where the absorbance difference between species is at a maximum and the other where this difference approaches zero. Since the absorbance of these species generally changes differently and abruptly as a function of wavelength, the spectrophotometer must have the smallest possible bandwidth, and the center wavelength must be positioned accurately and reproducibly. This figure shows hemoglobin spectra for four species of hemoglobin. Further, in two wavelength methods, unmeasured species must be absent, or the wavelengths must be chosen to minimize spectral interference from unmeasured species. This has frequently been overlooked in determining oxyhemoglobin in the presence of small but varying levels of endogenous and environmentally generated carbon monoxide. (Instrumentation Laboratory, Inc. from the IL-282 Operators Manual)

Once the electrode has been calibrated using these two points, accuracy of measurement between those two points is assumed. Unfortunately, the linearity of the electrode will begin to decrease if measured values exceed the calibration points (Fig. B-12). The degree of nonlinearity depends on the age and maintenance history of the electrode. If blood samples that exceed the standard calibration points are to be analyzed, alternate gases should be used that allow recalibration above and below the expected unknowns. These same principles for calibration apply to the P_{O_2} electrode. These principles are diagrammatically represented in Figure B-12.

Calibration of the pH electrode involves the use of liquid buffers as opposed to the gases used for the P_{CO_2} and P_{O_2} electrodes. These must be certified buffers accurate to 0.005 pH units. Typically, the buffers used are 6.840 and 7.384. The pH electrode is stable enough and the physiological range small enough to guarantee linearity above and below these calibration points. However, if samples (*i.e.*, spinal fluid) with anticipated pHs of greater than 7.6 or less than 6.0 are to be measured, the pH electrode should be checked for its expected value. These instruments are designed to measure blood, and to attempt to use them for other purposes could adversely affect their performance by damaging pH-sensitive glass, dissolving membranes, and damaging hydrolics.

Automated machines calibrate themselves automatically at pre-set time intervals. In most machines, this function can be overridden, if desired. Consistency is maintained by introducing the gases and buffer solutions at controlled rates and pressures and by maintaining a constant equilibration time. If electrode response is not within acceptable limits, the performance is flagged as unacceptable and an alarm is activated on the instrument. The technician must then correct the situation before the machine will perform analysis with that electrode. Other functions, such as buffer levels, are also monitored and any service requirements indicated. Most automated instruments apply correction factors to the performance of their electrodes. These factors are derived statistically to compensate for the fact that the electrodes are calibrated with a gas but measure a liquid; however, the best indicator of precision and accuracy in any instrument is its performance on tonometry (to be discussed later).

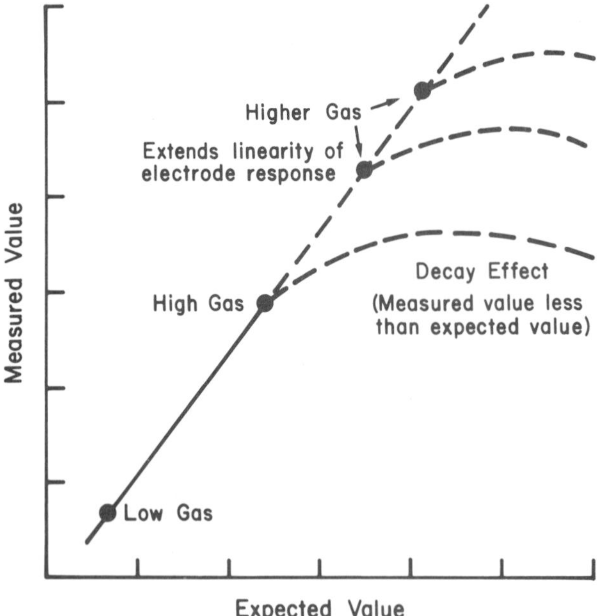

Fig. B-12. Diagrammatic representation of the nonlinearity of electrode behavior. If the value to be measured exceeds the high calibration point, the accuracy of that measurement cannot be guaranteed. Some electrodes will maintain their linearity past the high calibration point, whereas others will drop off dramatically. This is a function of the electrodes' age and maintenance and cannot be predicted. If the unknown to be measured is expected to exceed the high calibration point, the instrument should be recalibrated. This recalibration should be performed using a new slope gas that will provide a new high calibration point slightly exceeding the expected unknown. On some automated machines, resetting of the calibration points is not possible or the range is very limited. In these instances, accuracy past the high calibration point can be checked with tonometry. For example, if a shunt study is to be performed on a patient breathing 100% O_2 and the analyzer to be used cannot be recalibrated, blood tonometered with 100% O_2 can be used to check performance. The use of two samples, one at 50% O_2 and one at 100% O_2, would provide further assurance of analyzer performance. In instances such as shunt studies, where the unknowns to be analyzed could range from below 100 to above 500, a check of more than one point on the calibration curve is advisable to guarantee accuracy of results.

Calibration of manual equipment requires that the technician introduce the calibration gases into the P_{O_2} and P_{CO_2} cuvettes. Buffers must be introduced into the *p*H cuvette. To control drift of the electrodes, one should perform a complete two-point calibration every 8 hours and a single-point calibration before each sample is analyzed. If the single-point calibration indicates excessive drift between samples, complete recalibration or electrode maintenance is indicated. Strict attention to a standard calibration technique is critical for nonautomated equipment because it determines the accuracy and response time of the electrodes.

Typically, drift of all three electrodes is most marked just after the electrode membrane has been changed or a new electrode has been put into service. This problem lessens as the electrode is used. Maximum drift in a stabilized electrode should not exceed 1% to 2% of the reading in 5 minutes.

STANDARDS AND CONTROLS

The term "standards" refers to the gases or buffers with which the electronics of the instrument are set to read in a linear manner and over a reasonable physiological range. The gases that are used must be certified (guaranteed to be accurate), usually to within ± 0.5%. The buffers must be calibration buffers meeting the specifications of the specific instrument. Once the instrument has been properly calibrated using these standards, controls are used to verify the quality of performance. Many problems can go undetected unless the instrument's performance is verified with controls. For example, if the instrument or a portion of it were to become improperly thermostated and calibration were carried out, the electrodes would appear to calibrate properly but would be set inaccurately for the true concentration present in the standard. The *p*H buffers themselves are relatively insensitive to temperatures ranging from room temperature to body temperature, and in the event of heat loss from the analyzer the *p*H buffer may continue to produce the expected value. However, in an actual blood sample the *p*H is affected by the temperature of the analyzer; that is, if the analyzer is too cold or too hot, this will cause the carbon dioxide measurement to change, and the change in carbon dioxide will affect a change in *p*H. Thus, even though the buffer was measured correctly, the blood pH measurement could be incorrect if the temperature of the analyzer is incorrect. Similarly, faulty or contaminated standards or misuse of the standards (*i.e.*, poor technique in calibration) can lead to erroneous calibration of the electrodes, which will produce inaccurate blood gas values. Properly used, controls will detect such problems.

Commercially prepared controls are currently available. These controls provide a range of known values typical of those encountered in the clinical setting; pH values range from extreme acidosis to extreme alkalosis. The P_{O_2} and P_{CO_2} readings are represented in low, medium, and high ranges. Failure of the instrument to report the appropriate values will alert the user that a problem exists.

Tonometry is a method of equilibrating a gas of known concentration with a liquid. Tonometry for quality control can use either a buffer or whole blood. The choice of buffer or blood should be made after considering the advantages and disadvantages of each. Blood has the same viscosity and gas exchange properties as patient samples; however, because the buffering capacity (principally bicarbonate) of whole blood is unknown, it is impossible to predict how the change in P_{CO_2} and P_{O_2} will affect the pH of that same sample. Therefore, whole blood does not allow for control of pH. Buffers do provide a control for pH; because the bicarbonate is constant, the pH can be calculated. However, the viscosity and gas exchange properties of buffer solutions are different than those of whole blood. The gas used for tonometry must be checked for accuracy in the same manner as calibration gases. The chief disadvantage of tonometry is that it is technique-dependent and can vary from technician to technician. Small variations in such things as temperature, gas flow rate, sample size, and equilibration time will affect the results. Exacting attention to detail is needed to ensure that the procedure is done *exactly* the same way each time. To obtain reliable results with tonometry, the tonometer must be maintained at 37°C, the gas must be humidified, and the gas flow rate, the sample size, and equilibration time must be in accordance with the manufacturer's instructions. Before the sample is transferred from the tonometer to the blood gas analyzer, the sampling syringe must be purged with the tonometry gas to expel any room air from the syringe. Tonometry is performed at 37°C, which makes the tonometer and the solution in it an excellent culture medium. All equipment used for tonometry should be sterilized or disinfected to prevent bacterial growth. If previously analyzed patient samples are to be the source of blood for tonemetry, it may be advisable to add antibiotics to the tonometry system to prevent bacterial growth and its associated oxygen consumption before analysis. Some manufacturers use replacement cups to be disposed of with each sample to ensure cleanliness. Bacitracin and neomycin have been found effective in concentrations of 0.5 μg and 0.01 μg/ml blood, respectively. The expected tonometry value must be calculated daily using the daily barometer reading according to the following formula.

Sample value = (barometric pressure − 47) × % gas

47 = standard correction factor for water vapor

% gas = % CO_2 or % O_2 in the tonometry gas—that is, 8% CO_2 = 0.08

The results of all quality control analyses must be documented. This should include the values obtained, control limits, and any corrective action taken if the results were out of control limits. A specific log book should be used to record quality control records.

The control limits for a quality control sample are the range within which the control value is expected to fall. Typically, the accepted limit of tolerance is ± 2 standard deviations of an established mean, since, in a normal gaussian distribution, 95% of all observations will fall within this range. Each laboratory should establish its own statistics on its instrumentation for all levels of each new lot of material before it is put into routine use. This is necessary whether assayed commercial material, tonometry, or gas buffers are used. The mean and standard deviation should be established using a minimum of ten determinations.

A written protocol for the staff to follow should a quality control sample be out of range is invaluable. This helps to maintain consistency in equipment maintenance and troubleshooting.

Proficiency testing involves analyzing unknown samples provided by a vendor or professional organization. The analysis results are returned to the testing agency that provides statistical information on the laboratory's performance. The testing agency must provide the State Laboratory Licensing Board with the results in states where proficiency testing is required for laboratory licensure.

SAMPLING AND ANALYSIS PROTOCOLS

A standardized technique for obtaining and handling blood samples is essential for a good quality control program. Variables such as time between sampling and analysis, metabolism *in vitro*, air bubbles, and sample size can affect the sample before and during the analysis procedure. Any one or a combination of these factors can lead to results that do not reflect accurately the patient's true physiological state.

Samples should be analyzed as quickly as possible after sampling to expedite patient care and to reduce the risk of effects on the sample from air bubbles or metabolism. In blood samples iced immediately after sampling, there is no significant change in pH, P_{CO_2}, or P_{O_2} for up to 2 hours. The most dramatic change in noniced samples occurs during the first 15 minutes after the sample has been taken, and the value most dramatically affected is the P_{O_2}. The magnitude of change is impossible to predict because it depends on the initial level of P_{O_2} (values over 100 demonstrate the biggest change), white cell metabolism, and the diffusion properties of the sampling syringe.

An air bubble equivalent to 10% of the sample size has been demonstrated to induce a marked change in P_{O_2}.[3] Thus immediate removal of any air bubbles obtained during sample or analysis is important, that is, if verification of results were required owing to equipment failure and an air bubble had been left in the sample after the first analysis, the second analysis could be inaccurate.

Heparin dilution can affect all three measured blood gas values,[1,2] although its effect on P_{CO_2} is usually greater than on pH or P_{O_2}. Preventing adverse effects from heparin dilution is dealt with most effectively by controlling closely the amount of heparin used and the sample size. When using liquid heparin, one should evacuate the heparin from the sample syringe just before sample analysis. This will leave only the very tip of the syringe and the needle filled with heparin. The blood sample taken should fill at least one half of the volume of the sampling syringe—that is, 2.5- to 3-cc sample in a 5-cc syringe. The larger the sample, the less the dilutional affect of heparin. Very small samples are at higher risk for heparin dilution. In patient populations where small sample sizes are important (children and neonates), capillary tubes of 1-cc syringes that use crystalline heparin are advisable. This will keep the sample from clotting without the dilutional effects that could be expected with liquid heparin in such a small sampling device.

QUALITY CONTROL OF THE PATIENT SAMPLE

Even on a properly maintained, calibrated, and controlled blood gas analyzer, an incorrect measurement on any given sample is always possible. To eliminate any possibility of an erroneous reading owing to a temporary technical flaw (*i.e.*, an undetected air bubble in the cuvette), a further measure of quality control is needed to confirm blood gas accuracy. One approach is to analyze the sample simultaneously on two separate analyzers. The likelihood that the same error will occur on two instruments simultaneously is remote.

Another approach for pH and P_{CO_2} control is to compare the Astrup P_{CO_2} (*see* the section on the Astrup Equilibration Method) with the measured P_{CO_2}. Arrived at by two independent methods, this verifies the accuracy of both pH and P_{CO_2}. Another ingredient of quality control inherent in the Astrup method is verification of quality of slope of the buffer line on which all other calculations are based. Since hemoglobin is one of the principal blood buffers participating in establishing this buffer line, incorporated into the Siggaard–Anderson nomogram is a means of calculating the hemoglobin using the data obtained by the buffer line. This calculated hemoglobin can then be compared to the patient's observed hemoglobin, and the values should agree within 2 to 3 g/dl.

Another estimate of reliability can be obtained on routine P_{O_2} measurements when used in conjunction with an observed oxygen saturation value, such as that determined by the IL CO-Oximeter. The oxygen saturation, calculated from the patient's observed temperature, pH, and P_{O_2}, can be compared to the measured oxygen saturation. Appreciable discrepancy may suggest an error. If inspection and repetition verify the original measurement, this indicates that the patient either has a shifted oxyhemoglobin-disassociation curve or the presence of carboxyhemoglobin, methemoglobin, or sulfhemoglobin. In the hands of experienced technicians, using nomograms or blood gas slide rules, these comparisons can be made very quickly and, in terms of quality control, are well worth the time. For large numbers of procedures, even more desirable is the use of a computer program that can perform the calculations and corrections and present the data to the technician in seconds.

REFERENCES

1. Bageant RA: Variations in arterial blood gas measurements due to sampling techniques. Resp Care 20:565, 1974
2. Hansen JE, Simmons DH: Systematic error in the determination of blood P_{CO_2}. Am Rev Respir Dis 115:1061, 1977
3. Ishikawa S et al: The effects of air bubbles and time delay on blood gas analysis. Ann Allergy 33:72, 1974
4. Manual of Operations, IL 282, p 12. Instrumentation Laboratory, Lexington, Massachusetts, 1980

C

Sleep Apnea Syndromes

James R. Dexter • Gail A. Banasiak
Linda J. Corcoran • Linda Feenstra • Michael H. Bonnet

Improvements in polysomnographic technique during the last decade have produced a new appreciation for the relation between disorderd sleep and disease. This awareness has consequently formed the basis for a growing interest in the pulmonary sleep disorders and has been the impetus for development of clinical polysomnographic techniques in many medical centers. This section will deal specifically with the principles of sleep recording that have been responsible for the entry of polysomnography into clinical medicine, including an appreciation of the multifaceted nature of the sleep experience; an understanding of the immediate, if not the ultimate, causes of sleep apnea; and the development of technology for monitoring the sleeping subject in a relatively noninvasive manner.

SLEEP STAGES

Although the etiology of the human need to sleep is not understood, the mechanics of the sleep experience have been well defined. Clearly, sleep is a dynamic process during which the sleeper passes through an orderly, and rather stereotyped, sequence of transitions between the two major types of sleep: rapid eye movement (REM) and quiet, nonrapid eye movement (NREM) sleep. Figure C-1 demonstrates a typical sequence of sleep stages during a normal night's sleep.

Characteristic changes occur in the central nervous system (as evidenced in the EEG) and peripheral neuronal activity (as evidenced in the EMG), which distinguish active from quiet sleep and identify the stages of quiet sleep. Typical patterns for each stage are shown in Figure C-2.

These changes are the basis for sleep staging. Although the specific criteria for sleep staging are beyond the scope of this discussion, the major features of the sleep states are as follows.

1. Active sleep (REM) is associated with intense neuronal activity, dreaming, and bursts of rapid eye movement. In contrast with the intense CNS activity that is present, there is minimal ability to provide outgoing impulses to skeletal muscle, particularly in animals.[5,11] This allows a generalized muscular hypotonia that may result in uncoordinated or even paradoxical breathing.[8,12,16] The hypoxic drive to breathe remains intact, but the ventilatory response to hypercapnea is impaired.[13,14]
2. Quiet sleep (NREM) is not associated with rapid eye movement and is characterized by decreased neuronal activity despite a relatively intact ability to receive and transmit ner-

vous impulses. The stages of quiet sleep exhibit a progressive insensitivity to external stimuli and a decrease in the ability of the CNS to generate outgoing commands as sleep stages progress.[5,11]

SLEEP APNEA

The pulmonary sleep disorders are characterized by apneas and hypopneas. Apnea is defined as cessation of air flow for at least 10 seconds, whereas hypopnea is defined as a decrease in airflow to levels of less than one third of normal for at least 10 seconds. Three different types of apnea/hypopnea have been identified, although the ultimate etiology of each syndrome apparently resides in the central nervous system.[10,15]

1. *Obstructive apnea* is the most common apnea syndrome and is associated with a progressive loss of tone in the genioglossus muscle, allowing the posterior hypopharynx to collapse and occlude the airway at end expiration. Increasingly violent inspiratory efforts fail to provide airflow until the patient arouses and releases the obstruction with a resounding snort. Anatomical defects that increase resistance in the upper airway, such as tonsillar hypertrophy, micrognathia, acromegaly, and myxedema, predispose the patient to such episodes.[7]
2. *Central apnea* is caused by failure of the respiratory center to initiate an inspiratory effort. It is the least common apnea syndrome and is associated with abnormalities such as brain stem infarct, bulbar poliomyelitis, encephalitis, or cordotomy for intractable pain.[7]
3. *Mixed apnea* results from a combination of central and obstructive dysfunction and usually occurs when central apnea allows an obstruction to form, which then must be released by the same increasing respiratory effort seen in a simple obstructive apnea.

Figure C-3 portrays central, obstructive, and mixed apnea patterns.

Respiratory irregularity is common in normal persons, particularly in REM sleep. However, normal young adults average less than one period of apnea exceeding 10 seconds per hour of sleep. The pathologic condition sleep apnea syndrome requires an average of five apneic periods per hour of sleep during a night. Sleep apnea syndrome has been estimated to occur in 1% of the general population.[9] The syndrome increases with age and may be found in as many as 30% of people older than 65 years of age (although many of these people may be asymptomatic).*

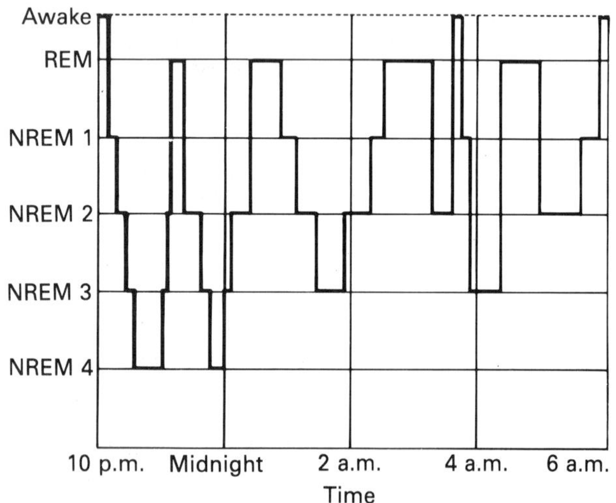

Fig. C-1. The typical sequence of transitions between active *(REM)* sleep and the stages of quiet *(NREM)* sleep experienced during a normal night's sleep. These transitions occur in a relatively stereotypic sequence throughout the night. (Kales A, Kales JD: Sleep disorders: Recent findings in the diagnosis and treatment of disturbed sleep. N Engl J Med 290:487, 1974.)

CLINICAL EVALUATION

Although Block[2] has demonstrated that some apparently healthy people exhibit sleep apnea, a number of specific clinical findings have been associated with sleep apnea and identify those patients who should be evaluated. These symptoms include excessive daytime sleepiness, morning headache and sore throat, frequent nighttime arousals, and complaints by the bed partner that the patient snores loudly or is unusually restless during sleep. Physical findings identifying the classic patient with obstructive apnea include the male sex (20:1 male:female ratio), an age range of 40 to 60 years with a "football player" body habitus (stocky frame and a short, thick neck), systemic hypertension, distended neck veins, edema, hyperactive gag reflex, and uvular petechiae.[4]

*Ancoli–Israel S, Kripke DF, Mason WJ, Kaplan OJ: A prevalence study of sleep disorders in seniors: 6-month results. Paper presented at the 22nd Annual Meeting of the Association for the Psychophysiological Study of Sleep, San Antonio, June 16–20, 1982.

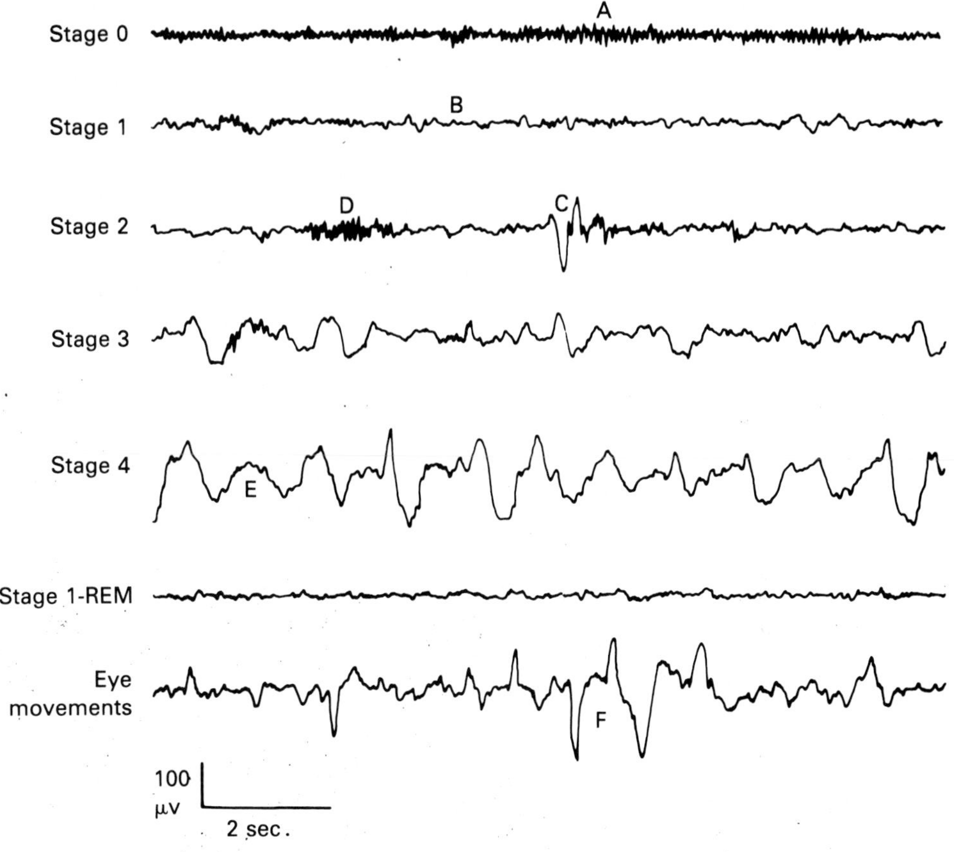

Fig. C-2. Characteristic EEG wave forms associated with the stages of quiet sleep (NREM) and active sleep *(REM),* and the rapid eye movemets as recorded by EOG (electrooculogram) wave forms associated with active sleep (REM). Stage identifiers include (A) alpha (awake); (B) low voltage fast activity (stage 1); (C) K complexes (stage 2); (D) sleep spindles (stage 2); (E) delta waves (stages 3 and 4); and (F) rapid eye movements (stage 1—REM sleep).

The consequences of the sleep apnea syndromes compose a spectrum ranging from minimal symptoms such as excessive snoring, morning headache, and mild daytime sleepiness to life-threatening cardiac arrhythmias and sudden death. Other consequences of the apnea syndromes include left and right ventricular failure, polycythemia, pulmonary hypertension, systemic hypertension, and mental ineptitude.[4] The severity of these complications correlates with the severity and duration of oxygen desaturation during sleep and is related to the total sleep time spent in apnea[4] (see Table C-1.)

TECHNICAL EVALUATION

Relatively specific protocols exist in Sleep Disorder Centers for evaluating respiratory disorders during sleep. However, most sleep centers may screen additionally for disease not related to respiration and may record functions differently. An excellent book on recording techniques has been published recently.[6]

A typical evaluation for suspected sleep apnea syndrome would include

1. an extensive sleep history to evaluate the length and severity of the problem; to determine the possibility of narcolepsy or seizure disorder; to determine the role of weight gain, drugs, or other events in the problem;
2. gathering sleep diary and sleepiness data over a 2-week period to determine baseline information;
3. administering psychological tests such as MMPI and Cornell Medical Index to ascertain the presence of psychopathology either as a causal agent or as a factor in later treatment choice;

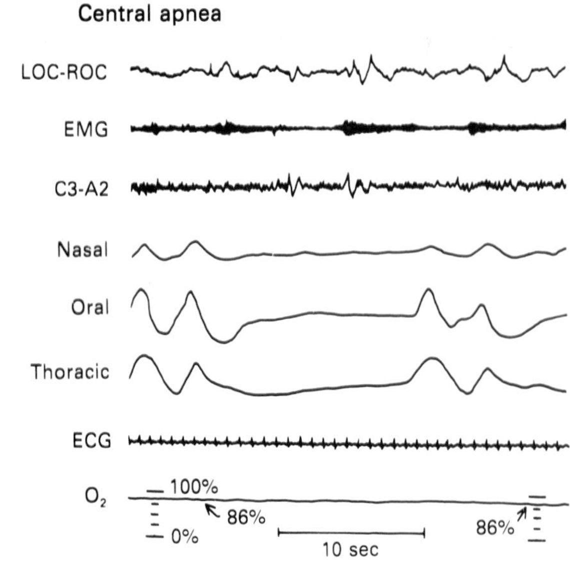

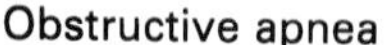

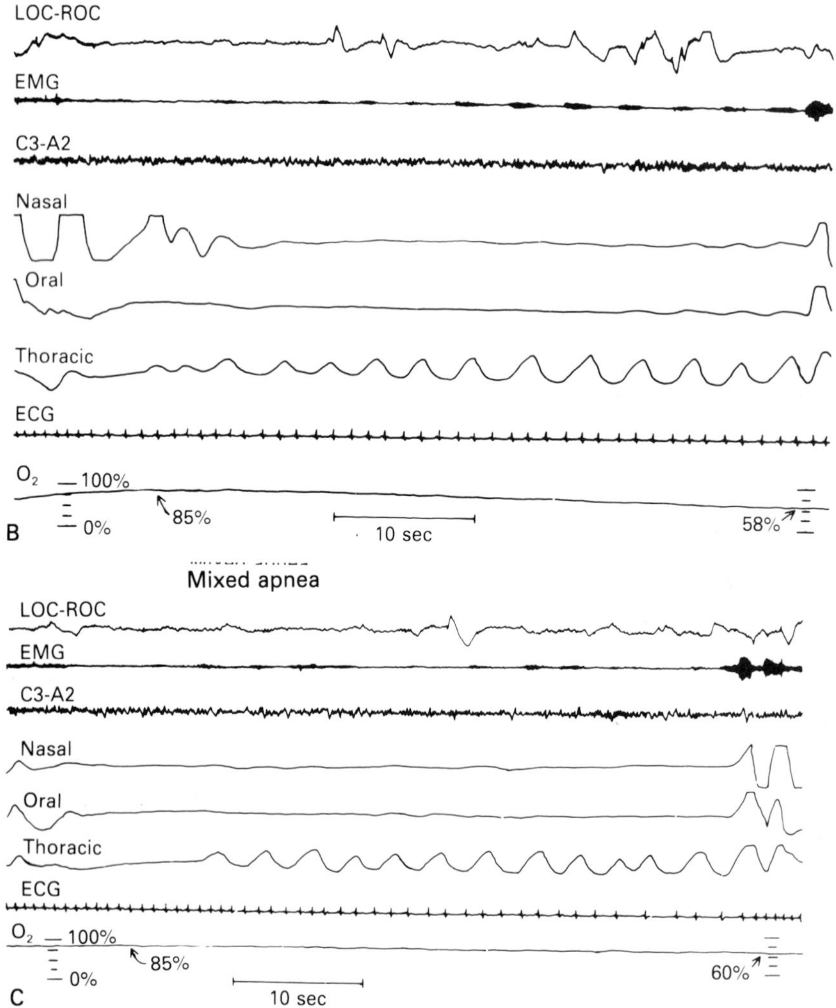

Fig. C-3. *(A)* Central apnea is caused by an absence of neurologic stimulation of the respiratory muscles; thus, chest movement ceases, air flow ceases, and oxygen saturation may fall. *(B)* Obstructive apnea is caused by a physical obstruction of the upper airway; thus, air flow is blocked, but chest wall movements increase in intensity as the patient attempts to breathe. Oxygen saturation falls coincidental with the cessation of air flow. *(C)* Mixed apneas usually begin with a central apnea and then develop into obstructive apneas before air flow is resumed. LOC-ROC = left eye channel-right eye EEG channel; EMG = chin EMG; C3-A2 = central EEG channel-central hemisphere to right ear; nasal and oral = airflow at the respective orifices; thoracic = thoracic chest movement; ECG = electrocardiogram; O_2 = blood oxygen saturation. (Remmers JE, Anch AM, de Groot WJ: Respiratory disturbances during sleep. Clin Chest Med 1:63, 1980)

Table C-1. Classification of the Severity of Sleep Apnea Syndrome by Frequency of Apneic Episodes and Corresponding Incidence of Cardiac Abnormalities

	CRITERIA		PERCENTAGE OF PATIENTS DEMONSTRATING	
CATEGORY	*Number of Episodes per Overnight Recording*	*Percentages of Total Sleep Time in Apnea*	*Left Ventricular Dysfunction**	*Right Ventricular Enlargement†*
Severe	300+	30	60	40
Moderate	60–299	7–29	50	10
Mild	30–59	6	7	7

(Modified from Clark RW: Sleep apnea. Primary Care 6:653, 1979)
*Abnormal pre-ejection period/left ventricular ejection time ratio on systolic time intervals.
†Determined by echocardiography or catheterization studies.

4. urine drug screens for barbiturates, benzodiazepines, amphetamines, and caffeine;
5. pulmonary function tests;
6. otolaryngologic consultation;
7. one full night polysomnographic recording (Fig. C-4), including
   - at least one channel for electroencephalographic (EEG) activity. The standard site is C_3/A_2 with C_4/A_1 attached as backup. If an additional channel is available, O_2/A_1 should be added;
   - at least one channel for electro-oculographic (EOG) activity. For one channel only, right eye/left eye is recommended; with two channels, right eye/A_2 and left eye/A_2 are recommended;
   - one channel for electromyographic (EMG) activity. Mental–submental EMG (above and below the chin) is standard. An additional backup electrode is sometimes added beneath the chin;
   - one channel for airflow from mouth and

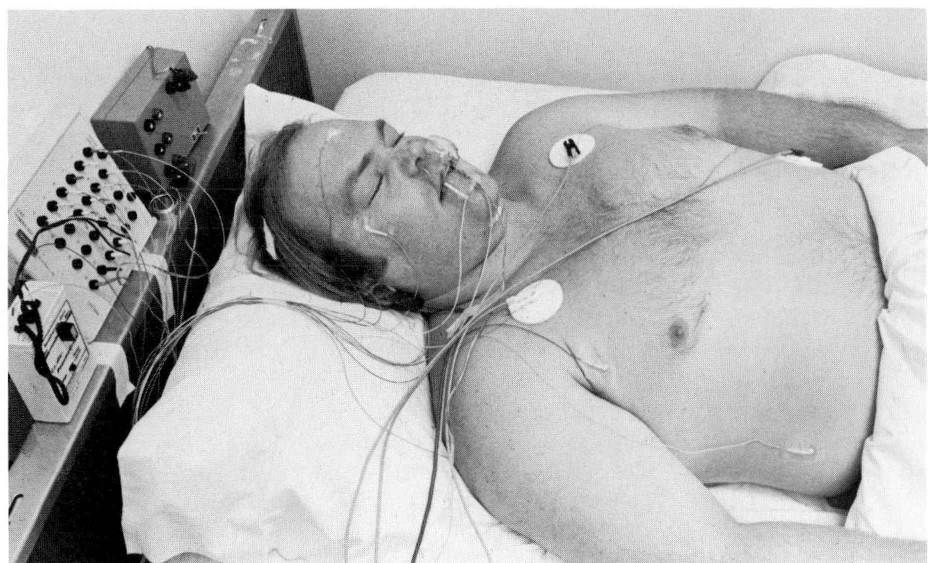

Fig. C-4. Patient being monitored with an ear oximeter for O_2 saturation; a chest impedance monitor for respiratory efforts; CO_2 sensor with mask for air flow; ECG for heart rate; EOG for rapid eye movement; EMG for relaxation of glossopharyngeal muscle; and EEG for sleep staging.

Table C-2. Essential Components of Polysomnography

Sleep staging	Electroencephalogram plus Electrooculogram plus Electromyogram
Detection of apnea	Thermistor at the nose and mouth or Measurement of oral and nasal CO_2 or Microphone over the larynx
Detection of respiratory effort	Chest and abdominal strain gauges or Inductance plethysmography or Chest magnetometer or Esophageal pressure
Detection of hypoxemia	Ear oximeter or Transcutaneous Po_2 monitor
Detection of arrhythmias	Electrocardiogram

nose. Air flow may be measured by linked thermisters taped in front of each nostril and the mouth. Alternatively, a mask and CO_2 analyzer can be used, whereas others have used a microphone over the larynx;

- two channels for chest movement. Current state-of-the-art measurement of respiration is best provided by a device called Respitrace (Respitrace Corporation, Ardsley, New York). The Respitrace has wide plethysmograph transducer coils placed around the rib cage and abdomen. When calibrated correctly, quantitative chest movement activity can be measured. In less demanding environments (where qualitative information is sufficient), respiratory movement may be measured by mercury strain gauges or pneumographs placed around the chest and abdomen, by devices sensitive to diaphragmatic EMG, or by devices that measure impedance (which changes with movement) across the chest and abdomen;
- one channel for an ECG lead;
- one channel for oxygen saturation. The Hewlett–Packard ear oximeter (HP 47201A) is currently the most widely used oximeter for adult patients. However, BTI has recently marketed an ear oximeter (BIOX IIA, BTI, Boulder, Colorado) that costs considerably less and features a significantly more comfortable earpiece. Transcutaneous oxygen monitors are typically used in small children; and

8. a series of five daytime naps (10 a.m., 12 noon, 2 p.m., 4 p.m., and 6 p.m.) following the nighttime recording to document the severity of daytime sleepiness (*see* Table C-2 for a list of essential components of polysomnography).

In an ideal setting, all parameters described for the polysomnographic recording are recorded simultaneously on a polygraph machine (e.g., Grass Model 7 or Beckman Model R612) at a paper speed of 10 mm/sec. Additional slow speed recordings of oxygen saturation or 25 mm/sec segments of ECG for clinical interpretation can be made on separate recorders as long as the technician carefully marks the position of each on the continuous recording.

It is important that patients be evaluated in surroundings that are as normal and as natural as possible. This consideration encompasses not only a dedicated bedroom in a quiet area of the hospital, but also the standard recording of nondrugged, nonsleep-deprived sleep during the normal nocturnal hours for an accurate picture of the many interacting functions. Sleep-inducing drugs, particularly barbiturates, and sleep deprivation increase the frequency of apnea and may lead to misdiagnosis. On the other hand, sleep during the day is fragmented and decreased in length. This, in addition to normal circadian changes that result in increased deactivation during the night, implies that daytime recordings generally underestimate the severity of respiratory disorders during sleep.

Individual cases warrant individual evaluation. Depending on patient history, other laboratory tests may be beneficial in delineating the source of excessive sleepiness. Some optional screening procedures include hemoglobin levels, Holter monitoring of cardiac rhythm, sleep cinefluoroscopy or bronchoscopy, hepatic profile, ECG, chest x-ray film, glucose tolerance test, and thyroid function tests. Optional measures that may be used during the polysomnogram itself in some patients include endoesophageal pressure, endoesophageal pH, and hemodynamic studies, including aortic and pulmonary arterial pressures, continuous measurement of arterial P_{O_2}, or intermittent blood gas samples.

DIAGNOSIS AND TREATMENT

The successful diagnosis and treatment of the disorders of sleep require a multidisciplinary approach in which many disparate sources of data must be collated and interpreted. Moderate amounts of apnea coupled with significant respiratory or cardiac disease may warrant vigorous treatment, whereas significant apnea in lieu of cardiac involvement or loss of daytime function may predispose the clinician to behavioral rather than surgical intervention. Generally, radical surgical procedures such as tracheostomy, for obstructive apnea, require 60 or more apneic periods per hour of sleep plus objective evidence of immediate cardiac risk or inability to function during the day—that is, inability to drive, loss of job, loss of spouse, and so forth. Pharyngoplasty may be beneficial if it can be documented that the tissue to be removed is indeed at the site of the obstruction. Pharyngoplasty, however, is useless if obstruction arises from an enlarged tongue or micrognathia, for example. In patients not at immediate risk, promising results have been reported for weight loss in obese patients, drug therapy, nocturnal oxygen therapy, and continuous positive airway pressure through the nose. Diaphragmatic pacing by means of phrenic nerve stimulation has been useful in cases of central apnea. One should avoid the temptation to perform expensive tests and to institute invasive therapy on asymptomatic patients.[4]

More detailed technical information on the evaluation and diagnosis of sleep disorders is available.[2,7] A recent federal educational program, Project Sleep,* has placed a slide–cassette program about sleep disorders and sleep-related breathing disorders in each medical school library in the United States.

*"Project Sleep" produced by Upjohn Company and University of Oklahoma Health Services.

REFERENCES

1. Association of Sleep Disorders Centers: Diagnostic classification of sleep and arousal disorders. Prepared by the Sleep Disorders Classification Committee (Roofwarg HP, chairman). Sleep 2:1, 1979
2. Block AJ et al: Sleep apnea, hypopnea and oxygen desaturation in normal subjects. N Engl J Med 300:513, 1979
3. Block AJ: Polysomnography: Some difficult questions. Ann Intern Med 95:644, 1981
4. Clark RW: Sleep apnea. Primary Care 6:653, 1979
5. Glenn LL, Routz AS, Dement WC: Membrane potential of spinal motoneurons during natural sleep in cats. Sleep 1:199, 1978
6. Guilleminault C (ed): Sleeping and waking disorders: Indications and techniques. Menlo Park, California, Addison–Wesley, 1982
7. Guilleminault C, Tilkian A, Dement WC: The sleep apnea syndromes. Annu Rev Med 27:465, 1976
8. Hairston LE, Sauerland EK: Electromyography of the human palate: Discharge patterns of the levator and tensor veli palatini. Electromyogr Clin Neurophysiol 21(2–3):287, 1981
9. Kripke D: Sleep apnea found more common than thought. Clin Psychiatry News 8:33, 1980
10. Martin RJ et al: Respiratory mechanics in timing during sleep and occlusive sleep apnea. J Appl Physiol 48:432, 1980
11. Nakamura Y et al: Intracellular analysis of trigeminal motoneuron activity during sleep in the cat. Science 19:204, 1978
12. Orem J, Netick A, Dement WC: Increased upper airway resistance to breathing during sleep in the cat. Electroenceph Clin Neurophysiol 43:14, 1977
13. Phillipson EA: Regulation of breathing during sleep. Am Rev Respir Dis 115(Suppl):217, 1977
14. Phillipson EA et al: Ventilatory and waking responses to hypoxia in sleeping dogs. J Appl Physiol 44:512, 1978
15. Remmers JE et al: Pathogenesis of upper airway occlusion during sleep. J Appl Physiol 44:931, 1978
16. Sauerland EK, Orr WC, Hairston LE: EMG patterns of oropharyngeal muscles during respiration in wakefulness and sleep. Electromyogr Clin Neurophysiol 21(2–3):307, 1981

D

Equations and "Rules of Thumb" for Management of Patients

John E. Hodgkin • Daniel B. Cress • Rodney A. Wertz

OXYGENATION

Calculation of Pa_{O_2} on Room Air Based on Age

- Predicted normal Pa_{O_2}, ages 14 to 84 years, supine[25]

$$Pa_{O_2} = 103.5 - (0.42 \times \text{age}) \pm 4$$

This was the formula from Sorbini's data, at 500-m elevation. When the data are corrected for a barometric pressure of 760 mm Hg, the formula for predicting the normal Pa_{O_2} at sea level becomes

$$Pa_{O_2} = 109 - (0.43 \times \text{age}) \pm 4.$$

- Predicted normal Pa_{O_2}, ages 15 to 75 years, seated[20]

$$Pa_{O_2} = 104.2 - (0.27 \times \text{age}) \pm 6$$

Calculation of PI_{O_2}

- PI_{O_2} (dry gas) = barometric pressure (PB) × FI_{O_2}
- PI_{O_2} (humidified gas)

1. PI_{O_2} = (barometric pressure − PH_2O) × FI_{O_2}

   PH_2O = 47 mm Hg (normal water vapor pressure for humidified gas)

2. A rough guide to calculating PI_{O_2} of humidified gas at or near sea level is as follows.

$$PI_{O_2} = (PB - PH_2O) \times FI_{O_2}$$

Since PB is 760 mm Hg at sea level and normal PH_2O is 47 mm Hg, then $PB - PH_2O$ = approximately 700. Thus,

$$PI_{O_2} = 700 \times FI_{O_2},$$

or $PI_{O_2} = 7 \times \%\ O_2$ in inspired gas.

Example: PI_{O_2} for an FI_{O_2} of 0.40 (40% O_2) is

$$PI_{O_2} = 7 \times 40 = 280$$

Calculation of PA_{O_2}

1. $PA_{O_2} = PI_{O_2} - (Pa_{CO_2} \times 1.25)$
   1.25 is a factor for respiratory quotient, assum-

ing a respiratory quotient of 0.8 where oxygen uptake equals 250 ml/min and CO_2 production equals 200 ml/min.

2. Simplified alveolar air equation at sea level, on room air

$$PA_{O_2} = 150 - Pa_{CO_2}$$

Calculation of Alveolar–Arterial Oxygen Tension Difference

1. $P(A\text{-}a)O_2 = PA_{O_2}$ (calculated) $- Pa_{O_2}$ (measured)
2. Calculation of approximate normal $P(A\text{-}a)O_2$, on room air, according to patient's age: The $P(A\text{-}a)O_2$ increases approximately 4 mm Hg for every increase of 10 years in age.
   Example: For an 80-year-old man, the $P(A\text{-}a)O_2$ should normally be ≤32 mm Hg.

Determination of the Cause of Hypoxemia

- If $P(A\text{-}a)O_2$ is normal, in the presence of hypoxemia, the cause is overall hypoventilation. A reduction in PI_{O_2} from high altitude will also, of course, reduce the Pa_{O_2}, with a normal $P(A\text{-}a)O_2$. The $P(A\text{-}a)O_2$ is increased when hypoxemia is due to $\dot{V}/\dot{Q}$ mismatch, diffusion defect, or shunt. The average $P(A\text{-}a)O_2$ in normal adults is 10 to 15 mm Hg; however, it widens normally with aging.
- The sum of the Pa_{O_2} and Pa_{CO_2} is between 110 and 130 mm Hg, on room air, when hypoxemia is due to overall hypoventilation. If the sum of the Pa_{O_2} and Pa_{CO_2} is <110, on room air *or* on supplemental O_2, the cause is $\dot{V}/\dot{Q}$ mismatch, diffusion defect, or shunt. The sum would also be <110 when a reduction in Pa_{O_2} occurs from the decreased PI_{O_2} of high altitude.

Determination If a Patient Is on Supplemental O_2

If the sum of the Pa_{O_2} and Pa_{CO_2} is >130 mm Hg, the patient is most likely on supplemental O_2. In young people, e.g., <16 years of age, the sum may approach 140 mm Hg, even though the subject is breathing only room air.

Determination of Predicted Normal Pa_{O_2} at Altitudes Above Sea Level[12,13,18]

$$a/A\ O_2 \text{ ratio} = \frac{\text{Predicted room air } Pa_{O_2} \text{ at sea level}}{PA_{O_2} \text{ at sea level}}$$

Example: If a patient had a predicted normal Pa_{O_2} of 87 mm Hg at sea level, with a PA_{O_2} of 100 mm Hg, the a/A O_2 ratio would be

$$\begin{aligned} a/A\ O_2 &= 87/100 \\ &= 0.87. \end{aligned}$$

At 5000 feet elevation, assuming a P_B of 632 mm Hg, the normal PA_{O_2} would be approximately 73 mm Hg. The predicted normal Pa_{O_2} for this patient, at 5000 feet elevation, would then be

$$\begin{aligned} Pa_{O_2} \text{ (normal at 5000 feet)} &= PA_{O_2} \text{ (at 5000 feet)} \\ &\quad \text{X a/A (at sea level)} \\ &= 73 \times 0.87 \\ &= 63.5 \text{ mm Hg.} \end{aligned}$$

Calculation of FI_{O_2} Needed to Achieve a Desired Pa_{O_2}, Having Determined an Initial Pa_{O_2}[12,13,18]

This assumes that such factors as cardiac output, $\dot{V}/\dot{Q}$ matchup, shunt, Pa_{CO_2}, and O_2 uptake remain constant.

Example: Knowing the patient's FI_{O_2}, Pa_{CO_2}, and Pa_{O_2}, one can calculate the PA_{O_2} and a/A O_2 ratio.

If a patient has a Pa_{O_2} of 50 mm Hg on an FI_{O_2} of 0.4, and a Pa_{CO_2} of 40 mm Hg at sea level, the PA_{O_2} = 235 mm Hg and the a/A O_2 ratio is 0.2127. If a Pa_{O_2} of 70 mm Hg is desired in this patient, the a/A O_2 ratio can be used to determine the PA_{O_2} and FI_{O_2} required to achieve this Pa_{O_2} for this patient.

$$\begin{aligned} PA_{O_2} \text{ (required)} &= \frac{Pa_{O_2} \text{ (desired)}}{a/A\ O_2 \text{ (calculated)}} \\ &= \frac{70}{0.2127} \\ &= 329 \text{ mm Hg} \end{aligned}$$

Assuming a respiratory quotient of 0.8, this can then be fitted into the alveolar air equation to solve for the FI_{O_2} needed to produce this PA_{O_2}.

$$\begin{aligned} PA_{O_2} &= PI_{O_2} - (Pa_{CO_2} \times 1.25) \\ PA_{O_2} &= (P_B - P_{H_2O})\, FI_{O_2} - (Pa_{CO_2} \times 1.25) \\ 329 &= (760 - 47)\, FI_{O_2} - (40 \times 1.25) \\ 329 &= (713)\, FI_{O_2} - 50 \\ FI_{O_2}\,(713) &= 379 \\ FI_{O_2} &= \frac{379}{713} \\ &= 0.53 \end{aligned}$$

If the FI_{O_2} is raised from 0.4 to 0.53, assuming things remain stable, the Pa_{O_2} should increase from 50 mm Hg to 70 mm Hg. Of course, the Pa_{O_2} must always be measured to determine the true Pa_{O_2} on the new FI_{O_2}.

Calculation of O_2 Uptake ($\dot{V}O_2$) or Cardiac Output ($\dot{Q}$) Using the Fick Equation

$$\dot{Q} = \frac{\dot{V}O_2}{(Ca_{O_2} - C\bar{v}_{O_2})\ 10}$$

$\dot{V}O_2$ is in ml/min, Ca_{O_2} and $C\bar{v}_{O_2}$ are in ml O_2/100 ml blood. The factor 10 is necessary to express $\dot{Q}$ in liters/min.

Calculation of Physiological Shunt

$$\frac{\dot{Q}s}{\dot{Q}T} = \frac{(Cc_{O_2} - Ca_{O_2})}{(Cc_{O_2} - C\bar{v}_{O_2})}$$

$\dot{Q}s/\dot{Q}T$ = ratio of shunt to cardiac output
Cc_{O_2} represents the end-pulmonary capillary O_2 content in ml O_2/100 ml blood

For calculation of O_2 content in arterial (Ca_{O_2}) and mixed venous ($C\bar{v}_{O_2}$) blood, use the following equations.[24]

$$\begin{aligned} O_2 \text{ content} &= \text{ml } O_2 \text{ bound to Hb/100 ml blood} \\ &\quad + \text{ml } O_2 \text{ dissolved/100 ml blood} \\ &= [\text{Hb (g/100 ml)} \times O_2 \text{ saturation} \times 1.39^*] + (Pa_{O_2} \times 0.003) \end{aligned}$$

For determination of Cc_{O_2}, it is best to take carboxyhemoglobin (HbCO) into account.[7] The PA_{O_2} should first be calculated. If the PA_{O_2} is greater than 150 mm Hg, the Pc_{O_2} is assumed to equal the PA_{O_2}, and the formula is

$$Cc_{O_2} = \text{Hb}\ [(1.0 - \text{HbCO})\ (1.39)] + (0.003 \times PA_{O_2}).$$

The following correction factors are recommended for a $PA_{O_2} \leq 150$ mm Hg.[7,24]

If $PA_{O_2} > 125$ and ≤ 150 mm Hg,
then $Cc_{O_2} = \text{Hb}\ [(1.0 - \text{HbCO}) - 0.01]\ (1.39) + (0.003 \times PA_{O_2})$

If $PA_{O_2} > 100$ and ≤ 125 mm Hg,
then $Cc_{O_2} = \text{Hb}\ [(1.0 - \text{HbCO}) - 0.02]\ (1.39) + (0.003 \times PA_{O_2})$

*Some use the factor 1.34 here; however, there is evidence that 1.39 is more accurate.

If HbCO (carboxyhemoglobin) is not measured directly, one could assume that the HbCO is approximately 1.5%.

Estimation of Shunt

If patient is on 100% O_2, there is a 5% shunt for every 100 mm Hg the Pa_{O_2} is below that expected.

> *Example:* For a patient at sea level, the Pa_{O_2} on 100% O_2 should be 550 mm Hg to 600 mm Hg normally. If the Pa_{O_2} is 300 mm Hg, one has a 15% shunt, *plus* the normal 3% to 4% shunt everyone has.

This rule of thumb works well down to a Pa_{O_2} of 100 mm Hg. Below this level, it is no longer accurate.

ACID–BASE

Calculation of Extracellular Fluid Base Excess (BE_{ECF})[9]

$$BE_{ECF} = \Delta HCO_3^- + 10\Delta pH$$

Where ΔHCO_3^- = actual HCO_3^- − 24 and ΔpH = actual pH − 7.4

Example: If the pH = 7.14 and plasma HCO_3^- = 28 mEq/liter, then

$$\begin{aligned} BE_{ECF} &= (28 - 24) + 10(7.14 - 7.40) \\ &= 4 + 10(-0.26) \\ &= 4 - 2.6 \\ &= 1.4 \text{ mEq/liter.} \end{aligned}$$

See Chapter 12, Blood Gas Analysis and Acid–Base Physiology, for a detailed explanation of extracellular fluid base excess.

In Acute Respiratory Acidosis

The plasma bicarbonate will increase, acutely, approximately 1 mEq/liter for every 15 mm Hg increase in the Pa_{CO_2} above 40 mm Hg as a result of the bicarbonate–carbonic acid buffer reaction.[2] This small increase in bicarbonate does not represent renal compensation for the CO_2 retention.

In Chronic Respiratory Acidosis

For each mm Hg ↑ in Pa_{CO_2}, the HCO_3^- ↑ 0.4 mEq/liter.[4,10,16,21]

In Acute Respiratory Alkalosis

The plasma bicarbonate will decrease, acutely, approximately 1 mEq/liter for every 5 mm Hg decrease in the Pa_{CO_2} below 40 mm Hg as a result of the bicarbonate–carbonic acid buffer reaction.[2] This decrease in plasma bicarbonate does not represent renal compensation for the acute hypocapnia.

In Chronic Respiratory Alkalosis

For each mm Hg ↓ in Pa_{CO_2}, the HCO_3^- ↓ 0.5 mEq/liter.[4,11,1]

In Maximally Compensated Metabolic Acidosis

The Pa_{CO_2} will decrease by about 1 mm Hg for every 1 mEq/liter decrease in plasma bicarbonate.[19]

The level of compensatory hypocapnia expected in metabolic acidosis can be calculated by the following formula.[1]

$$Pa_{CO_2} = 1.54 \times \text{plasma } HCO_3^- + 8.36 \pm 1.1$$

In Metabolic Alkalosis

For each mEq/liter ↑ in HCO_3^-, the Pa_{CO_2} ↑ 0.5 to 1.0 mm Hg.[5,8,21] The ventilatory response to metabolic alkalosis is less predictable than that seen with metabolic acidosis, and compensatory hypercapnia above 55 to 60 mm Hg is unusual.[5,14]

For Reasonably Accurate Conversion of *p*H to $[H^+]$[15]

pH	H^+ (nM/liter)
7.0	100
7.05	90
7.1	80
7.15	70
7.2	60
7.3	50
7.4	40
7.5	30
7.6	25
7.7	20
7.8	15
7.9	12.5
8.0	10

One might note that within the range of 7.2 to 7.5 there is a decrease of 0.01 in *p*H for every increase of 1 nM/liter in the H^+.

For Calculating H^+, P_{CO_2}, or Plasma Bicarbonate from the Other Two Values[17]

$$H^+ = 24 \times \frac{Pa_{CO_2}}{\text{Plasma } HCO_3^-}$$

To Determine Whether the Change in H^+ or *p*H Is Appropriate for Acute Respiratory Acidosis or Chronic Respiratory Acidosis

- In *acute* CO_2 retention

  One would expect an increase in H^+ of 0.8 nM/liter for every increase of 1 mm Hg in P_{CO_2}.

  The increase in $P_{CO_2} \times 0.008$ = the decrease in *p*H.[3]
- In *chronic* CO_2 retention

  One would expect an increase in H^+ of 0.3 nM/liter for every increase of 1 mm Hg in P_{CO_2}.

  The increase in $P_{CO_2} \times 0.003$ = the decrease in *p*H.[3]

Rough Guidelines for Pa_{CO_2} – *p*H Relationship in Acute Ventilatory Changes

For every 20 mm Hg ↑ in Pa_{CO_2} above 40 mm Hg, the *p*H ↓ approximately 0.10 unit.

For every 10 mm Hg ↓ in Pa_{CO_2} below 40 mm Hg, the *p*H ↑ appproximately 0.10 unit.

Pa_{CO_2}	pH
80	7.20
60	7.30
40	7.40
30	7.50
20	7.60

Determination of Plasma Bicarbonate from *p*H and Pa_{CO_2} (Assuming an Uncompensated Acid–Base Status)

$$\text{Plasma bicarbonate} = \frac{Pa_{CO_2} \times 24}{\text{difference of last two digits of pH and 80}}$$

Example

$pH = 7.30$

$Pa_{CO_2} = 50$

$$\text{Plasma bicarbonate} = \frac{40 \times 24}{80 - 30} = \frac{960}{50} = 19 \text{ mEq/liter}$$

Estimation of Base Excess from pH and Pa_{CO_2}[24]

1. Determine the difference between the measured Pa_{CO_2} and 40 mm Hg, then move the decimal point two places to the left.
2. If the Pa_{CO_2} is above 40 mm Hg, subtract one half of the number calculated in #1 above from 7.40. If the Pa_{CO_2} is below 40 mm Hg, add the difference to 7.40.
3. Determine the difference between the measured pH and the pH calculated in #2 above. Move the decimal point two places to the right and multiply by ⅔.

Example

Patient with Pa_{CO_2} of 75 mm Hg and pH of 7.30.

1. 75 − 40 = 35; moving the decimal two places to the left results in 0.35.
2. Since the Pa_{CO_2} is > 40 mm Hg, 7.40 − (½ of 0.35) = 7.22.
3. 7.30 − 7.22 = 0.08; moving the decimal point two places to the right and multiplying by ⅔, i.e., 8 × ⅔ = 5 mEq/liter base excess.

Determination of Bicarbonate Needed in Patients with Metabolic Acidosis

HCO_3^- needed* = Body wt (kg) × BE × 0.3. BE represents the deficit in buffer base. 0.3 is the factor that represents the extracellular space bicarbonate distribution.

MECHANICAL VENTILATION

Calculation of Respiratory System Compliance in Patients on a Ventilator

- Dynamic effective compliance

$$C_{RS}\,(dyn) = \frac{V_T}{\text{peak pressure}}$$

If on PEEP

$$C_{RS}\,(dyn) = \frac{V_T}{\text{peak pressure—PEEP}}$$

*Infuse one half of this amount i.v., recheck an ABG in 15 to 20 minutes, and repeat the calculation.

- Static effective compliance (eliminates airway resistance as a factor).

$$C_{RS}\,(st) = \frac{V_T}{\text{inflation hold pressure}}$$

If on PEEP

$$C_{RS}\,(st) = \frac{V_T}{\text{inflation hold pressure—PEEP}}$$

Determination of New Minute Ventilation ($\dot{V}_E$) Required to Achieve a Desired Pa_{CO_2}

- $$\text{New } \dot{V}_E = \frac{\text{present } \dot{V}_E \times \text{present } Pa_{CO_2}}{\text{desired } Pa_{CO_2}}$$

Example: Present $\dot{V}_E$ = 8 liters/min and Pa_{CO_2} = 50 mm Hg and a Pa_{CO_2} of 40 mm Hg is desired

$$\text{New } \dot{V}_E = \frac{8 \times 50}{40}$$

$$= 10 \text{ liters/min}$$

The new $\dot{V}_E$ can be achieved by either increasing the $\dot{V}_T$ or the respirator rate. Of course, the V_D/V_T ratio is a factor. If the V_T is kept constant and the ventilator rate is altered to achieve the new V_E, the above equation should be quite precise. If the V_T is increased, the V_D/V_T obviously changes, and the equation will not be quite as accurate (*see* III C below).

- Another method for estimating the change in ventilator rate needed to achieve a desired Pa_{CO_2} is as follows.[6]

$$\text{New ventilator rate} = \frac{\text{present ventilator rate} \times \text{present } Pa_{CO_2}}{\text{desired } Pa_{CO_2}}$$

Example

If the Pa_{CO_2} is 80 mm Hg on a ventilator rate of 12 breaths/min, and one desires a Pa_{CO_2} of 60 mm Hg, then the

$$\text{new ventilator rate} = \frac{12 \times 80}{60}$$

$$= 16 \text{ breaths/min.}$$

This method assumes, of course, that the tidal volume remains constant.

- Determination of new $\dot{V}_E$ required to achieve a desired Pa_{CO_2}, using alveolar ventilation ($\dot{V}_A$)[22]

$$\text{New } \dot{V}_A = \frac{\text{present } \dot{V}_A \times \text{present } Pa_{CO_2}}{\text{desired } Pa_{CO_2}}$$

Example: In a 200-pound (lean body weight) patient with a measured tidal volume of 600 cc and a ventilator rate of 10, the $\dot{V}_E$ is 600 cc. The anatomical deadspace in this patient would be assumed to be 200 cc (1 cc/lb lean body weight). 200 cc × 10 equals 2000 cc of anatomical deadspace ventilation per minute. 6000 cc—2000 cc represents 4000 cc alveolar ventilation per minute. If the measured Pa_{CO_2} in this patient is 60 mm Hg and a Pa_{CO_2} of 40 mm Hg is desired, then the

$$\text{new } \dot{V}_A = \frac{4000 \times 60}{40}$$

$$= 6000 \text{ ml.}$$

If the new $\dot{V}_A$ is to be achieved by increasing the V_T, the V_T would have to be increased from 600 cc to 800 cc, if the ventilator rate remains at 10/min, to achieve the new $\dot{V}_A$ required to alter the Pa_{CO_2} from 60 mm Hg to 40 mm Hg. An extra 200 cc of alveolar volume/breath × 10 = an ↑ in $\dot{V}_A$ of 2000 ml/min. In this example, the new $\dot{V}_E$ is 8000 ml.

If the new $\dot{V}_A$ is to be achieved by increasing the ventilator rate, the rate would have to be increased from 10/min to 15/min, if the V_T remains at 600 cc, to achieve the new $\dot{V}_A$ required to alter the Pa_{CO_2} from 60 mm Hg to 40 mm Hg. Since in this patient 400 cc of the 600-cc V_T is alveolar volume, then an extra 5 breaths/min will increase the $\dot{V}_A$ by 2000 ml/min. In this example, the new $\dot{V}_E$ is 9000 ml.

- Determination of new $\dot{V}_E$ required to achieve a desired Pa_{CO_2}, using the V_D/V_T[23]

The minute ventilation–Pa_{CO_2}–V_D/V_T graph depicted in Figure D-1 is used as follows.

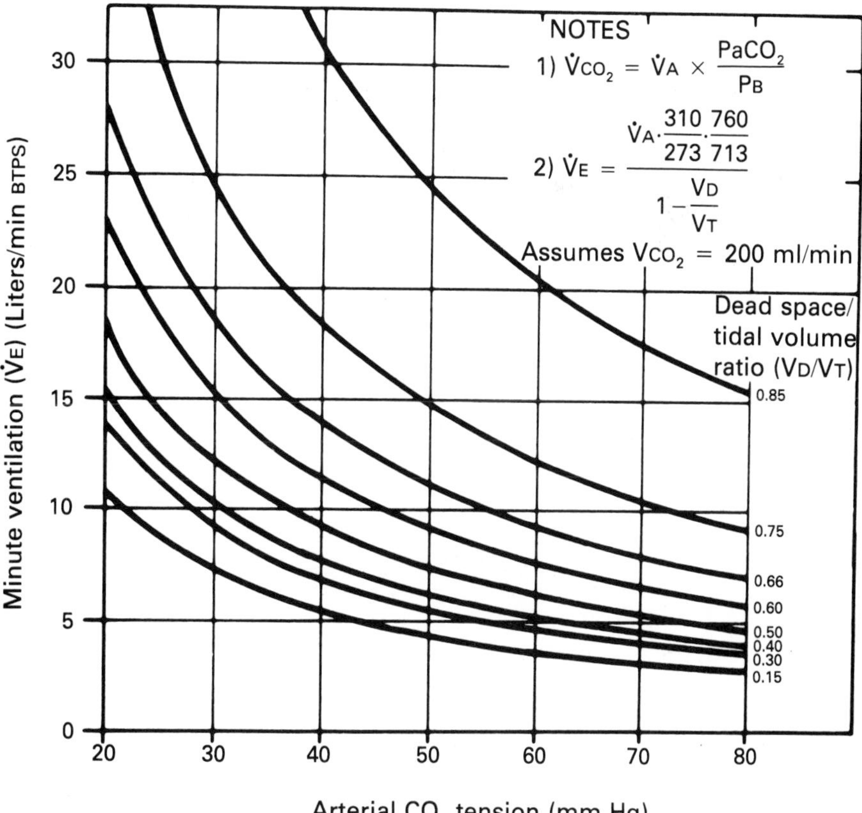

Fig. D-1. The relation between minute ventilation ($\dot{V}_E$) and arterial P_{CO_2} (Pa_{CO_2}) for various isopleths of the ratio of physiological dead space to tidal volume (V_D/V_T). The basic assumptions are noted in the upper right corner. $\dot{V}CO_2$ = CO_2 output; $\dot{V}_A$ = alveolar ventilation; P_B = atmospheric pressure. (Selecky PA et al: A graphic approach to assessing interrelationships among minute ventilation, arterial carbon dioxide tension, and ratio of physiologic dead space to tidal volume in patients on respirators. Am Rev Respir Dis 117:181, 1978)

1. Place patient on respirator at a minute ventilation ($\dot{V}E$) of 6 to 8 liters/min.
2. After 30 minutes of equilibration, measure the minute ventilation and obtain a simultaneous arterial CO_2 tension (Pa_{CO_2}).
3. The $\dot{V}E$ and corresponding Pa_{CO_2} are plotted on the graph. The deadspace-tidal volume ratio (VD/VT) is obtained by noting the isopleth that coincides with this point.
4. To obtain the $\dot{V}E$ required to achieve a desired Pa_{CO_2}, draw a vertical line from the desired Pa_{CO_2} on the abscissa to the VD/VT isopleth obtained in step 3. From this point, a horizontal line is drawn to the ordinate to obtain the required $\dot{V}E$.
5. The respirator is then adjusted by changing the tidal volume (VT) or frequency (f) to achieve the newly determined $\dot{V}E$ ($\dot{V}E = VT \times f$). (After 30 minutes at this new $\dot{V}E$ the Pa_{CO_2} should be remeasured).
6. As the patient's respiratory problem improves, the VD/VT will often decrease, indicating a need for a lower $\dot{V}E$. This new VD/VT can be calculated as in step 3 and an appropriate $\dot{V}E$ determined.

REFERENCES

1. Albert MD, Dell RB, Winters RW: Quantitative displacement of acid base equilibrium in metabolic acidosis. Ann Intern Med 66:312, 1964
2. Armstrong BW, Mohler JG, Jung RC, Remmers J: The in-vivo carbon dioxide titration curve. *Lancet* 1:759, 1966
3. Avery AG, Nicotra MB, Deaton WJ: Respiratory acid–base balance. Resp Therapy, p 59, May/June 1977
4. Bia M, Thier SO: Mixed acid base disturbances: A clinical approach. Med Clin North Am 65:347, 1981
5. Bone JM, Cowie J, Lambie A, Robson JS: The relationship between arterial PCO_2 and hydrogen ion concentration in chronic metabolic acidosis and alkalosis. Clin Sci Mol Med 46:113, 1974
6. Bone RC: Mechanical ventilation: Understanding the basics. J Respir Dis, p 57, January 1982
7. Cane RD et al: Minimizing errors in intrapulmonary shunt calculations. Crit Care Med 8:294, 1980
8. Cohen JJ, Kassirer JP: Acid base metabolism. In Maxwell MH, Kleeman CR (eds): Clinical Disorders of Fluid and Electrolyte Metabolism, pp 181–232. New York, McGraw–Hill, 1980
9. Collier CR, Hackney JD, Mohler JG: Use of extracellular base excess in diagnosis of acid–base disorders: A conceptual approach. Chest 61:6S, 1972
10. Engel K et al: Quantitative displacement of acid–base equilibrium in chronic respiratory acidosis. J Appl Physiol 24:288, 1968
11. Gennari FJ, Goldstein MB, Schwartz WB: The nature of the renal adaption to chronic hypocapnia. J Clin Invest 51:1722, 1972
12. Gilbert F, Keighley JF: The arterial/alveolar oxygen tension ratio: An index of gas exchange applicable to varying inspired oxygen concentrations. Am Rev Respir Dis 109:142, 1974
13. Gilbert R, Auchincloss J, Kuppinger M, Thomas MV: Stability of the arterial/alveolar oxygen partial pressure ratio. Crit Care Med 7:267, 1979
14. Goldring RM, Cannon PJ, Heinemann HO, Fishman AP: Respiratory adjustment to chronic metabolic alkalosis in man. J Clin Invest 47:188, 1968
15. Jones NL: Blood Gases and Acid–Base Physiology, p 87. New York, Brian C. Decker, 1980
16. Kaehny WD: Pathogenesis and management of respiratory and mixed acid–base disorders. In Schrier RW (ed): Renal and Electrolyte Disorders, pp 121–142. Boston, Little, Brown, 1976
17. Kassirer JP, Bleich HL: Rapid estimation of plasma carbon dioxide tension from pH and total carbon dioxide content. N Engl J Med 272:1067, 1965
18. Krider T: Clinical equations for oxygen therapy. In Eubanks DH (ed): AART 1981 Convention Lecture Series: Catch a Star. Dallas, American Association for Respiratory Therapy, 1982
19. Lennon EJ, Lemann J Jr: Defense of hydrogen ion concentration in chronic metabolis acidosis. Ann Intern Med 65:265, 1966
20. Mellemgaard K: The alveolar–arterial oxygen difference: Its size and components in normal man. Acta Physiol Scand 67:10, 1966
21. Narins RG, Emmett M: Simple and mixed acid–base disorders: A practical approach. Medicine 59:161, 1980
22. Rogers RM, Jeurs JA: Physiologic considerations in the treatment of acute respiratory failure. Basics of RD, Vol 3, (No 4). New York, American Thoracic Society, 1975
23. Selecky PA, Wasserman K, Klein M, Ziment I: A graphic approach to assessing interrelationships among minute ventilation, arterial carbon dioxide tension, and ratio of physiologic dead space to tidal volume in patients on respirators. Am Rev Respir Dis 117:185, 1978
24. Shapiro BA, Harrison RA, Walton JR: Clinical Application of Blood Gases, 3rd ed, pp 129, 222, 223. Chicago, Year Book Medical Publishers, 1982
25. Sorbini CA, Grassi V, Solinas E: Arterial oxygen tension in relation to age in healthy subjects. Respiration 25:3, 1968

E

Examples of Pulmonary Function and Arterial Blood Gas Data

John E. Hodgkin

EXAMPLES OF PULMONARY FUNCTION DATA

Patient 1. A 58-Year-Old White Woman with Dyspnea

		PREBRONCHODILATOR		POSTBRONCHODILATOR	
	PREDICTED	*Observed*	*% Predicted*	*Observed*	*% Predicted*
FVC, *liters*	2.63	1.81	69	1.57	60
2SVC, *liters*	2.63	1.74	66	1.66	63
ERV, *liters*	0.87	0.23	27	0.11	13
IC, *liters*	1.75	1.57	90	1.45	63
FEV_1, *liters*	1.95	1.46	75	1.50	77
FEV_3, *liters*	2.50	1.81	72	1.57	63
FEV_1/FVC, %	≥74	81		95	
FEV_3/FVC, %	≥95	100		100	
MVV, *liters/min*	79	34	43	34	43
$FEF_{25-75\%}$, *liters/sec*	2.4	1.5	62	2.0	66
FRC, *liters*	2.29	1.72	75		
RV, *liters*	1.42	1.06	75		
TLC, *liters*	4.05	3.04	75		
RV/TLC, %	35	35			
DL_{CO}, *ml/min/mm Hg CO*	18.4	9.3	51		

Interpretation and Discussion

The classic pattern for restrictive disease is present. The FVC and FEV_1 are reduced; however, the FEV_1/FVC% is normal. The reduction in $FEF_{25-75\%}$ is proportional to the reduction in VC. There is no improvement in spirometric data after inhalation of bronchodilator. All lung volumes are reduced; however, the RV/TLC is normal. The diffusing capacity (DL_{CO}) is reduced, in this case suggesting the presence of interstitial lung disease in light of the restrictive pattern. This group of findings is suggestive of many types of interstitial lung disease. The mediastinoscopy on this patient yielded lymph nodes that revealed noncaseating granulomas on the pathology sections, consistent with sarcoidosis.

Patient 2. A 73-Year-Old White Male Smoker with Shortness of Breath

		PREBRONCHODILATOR		POSTBRONCHODILATOR	
	PREDICTED	*Observed*	*% Predicted*	*Observed*	*% Predicted*
FVC, *liters*	2.95	2.08	70	2.02	68
2SVC, *liters*	2.95	2.07	70	2.04	69
ERV, *liters*	0.98	0.41	42	0.52	53
IC, *liters*	1.97	1.67	85	1.49	76
FEV_1, *liters*	2.01	0.70	35	0.64	32
FEV_3, *liters*	2.80	1.18	42	1.13	40
FEV_1/FVC, %	≥68	34		32	
FEV_3/FVC, %	≥95	57		56	
MVV, *liters/min*	76	29	38	31	42
$FEF_{25-75\%}$, *liters/sec*	2.3	0.2	9	0.2	9
FRC, *liters*	2.81	5.50	196		
RV, *liters*	1.83	5.09	278		
TLC, *liters*	4.78	7.17	150		
RV/TLC, %	38	71			
DL_{CO}, *ml/min/mm Hg CO*	23	8	35		

Interpretation and Discussion

This pattern demonstrates obstructive airway disease. The reduction in VC (FVC and 2SVC) suggests the possible presence of concomitant restrictive disease; however, the increased TLC indicates that the reduced VC is secondary to air-trapping and that there is no evidence for restrictive disease. No improvement occurs after bronchodilator inhalation. The marked reduction in diffusing capacity is compatible with loss of alveolar–capillary membrane owing to emphysema. The patient does have severe pulmonary emphysema.

Patient 3. A 37-Year-Old White Woman with a History of Rheumatic Heart Disease Who Now Complains of Dyspnea

		PREBRONCHODILATOR		POSTBRONCHODILATOR	
	PREDICTED	*Observed*	*% Predicted*	*Observed*	*% Predicted*
FVC, *liters*	3.10	1.45	47	1.54	50
2SVC, *liters*	3.10	1.67	54	2.02	65
ERV, *liters*	1.04	0.58	56	0.60	58
IC, *liters*	2.06	1.09	53	1.42	69
FEV_1, *liters*	2.42	1.30	54	1.37	57
FEV_3, *liters*	2.94	1.45	49	1.54	52
FEV_1/FVC, %	≥78	90		89	
FEV_3/FVC, %	≥95	100		100	
MVV, *liters/min*	84	59	70	63	75
$FEF_{25-75\%}$, *liters/sec*	2.7	2.0	75	2.1	79
FRC, *liters*	2.62	1.34	51		
RV, *liters*	1.58	0.76	48		
TLC, *liters*	4.68	2.43	52		
RV/TLC, %	34	31			
DL_{CO}, *ml/min/mm Hg CO*	20.6	14.4	70		

Interpretation and Discussion

These studies show a restrictive pattern. The FEV_1 and FVC are reduced; however, the FEV_1/FVC% is normal. The lung volumes are reduced, and the RV/TLC is normal. The diffusing capacity is slightly reduced. There is no significant improvement after inhalation of bronchodilator. This patient has mitral stenosis, resulting from rheumatic fever. Pulmonary interstitial edema is manifested by the reduction in TLC and diffusing capacity.

Patient 4. A 62-Year-Old White Woman with Cough and Shortness of Breath

		PREBRONCHODILATOR		POSTBRONCHODILATOR	
	PREDICTED	*Observed*	*% Predicted*	*Observed*	*% Predicted*
FVC, *liters*	2.35	2.05	87	2.24	95
2SVC, *liters*	2.35	2.11	90	2.22	94
ERV, *liters*	0.78	0.45	58	0.46	59
IC, *liters*	1.57	1.60	102	1.78	113
FEV_1, *liters*	1.74	0.73	42	0.84	48
FEV_3, *liters*	2.23	1.32	59	1.50	67
FEV_1/FVC, %	≥74	36		38	
FEV_3/FVC, %	≥95	64		67	
MVV, *liters/min*	58	28	48	32	55
$FEF_{25-75\%}$, *liters/sec*	2.2	0.3	15	0.3	18
FRC, *liters*	1.98	2.77	140		
RV, *liters*	1.20	1.72	143		
TLC, *liters*	3.55	4.22	119		
RV/TLC, %	34	48			
DL_{CO}, *ml/min/mm Hg CO*	17.8	16.0	90		

Interpretation and Discussion

This patient's spirogram shows marked obstruction to airflow. There is no improvement after inhalation of bronchodilator. Although the RV and FRC are increased, the TLC is only at the upper limits of normal. The diffusing capacity is normal, suggesting that the patient has predominantly chronic bronchitis, rather than anatomic emphysema. This patient does indeed have severe chronic obstructive lung disease, with chronic bronchitis as the predominant problem.

Patient 5. A 47-Year-Old White Woman Who Complained of Lethargy. She Was 63 Inches Tall and Weighed 247 Pounds.

		PREBRONCHODILATOR	
	PREDICTED	*Observed*	*% Predicted*
FVC, *liters*	2.77	3.15	114
2SVC, *liters*	2.77	3.28	118
ERV, *liters*	0.92	0.51	55
IC, *liters*	1.85	2.77	150
FEV_1, *liters*	2.11	2.67	127
FEV_3, *liters*	2.63	3.04	115
FEV_1/FVC, %	≥76	85	
FEV_3/FVC, %	≥95	96	
MVV, *liters/min*	101	68	67
$FEF_{25-75\%}$, *liters/sec*	2.8	3.1	111

Interpretation and Discussion

The spirographic data are normal, except for the reduction in ERV and MVV. This pattern is suggestive of centripetal obesity or variable effort. In this case the patient did indeed have prominent exogenous obesity.

Patient 6. A 52-Year-Old White Man with a 2-Month History of Chronic, Nonproductive Cough After a Severe Viral Pneumonia. His Cough Has Been Getting Progressively Better; He Is a Nonsmoker.

		PREBRONCHODILATOR		POSTBRONCHODILATOR	
	PREDICTED	*Observed*	*% Predicted*	*Observed*	*% Predicted*
FVC, *liters*	4.45	3.86	87	4.39	99
2SVC, *liters*	4.45	4.09	92	4.03	91
ERV, *liters*	1.48	1.40	94	0.49	33
IC, *liters*	2.97	2.69	91	3.54	119
FEV_1, *liters*	3.29	2.95	90	3.38	101
FEV_3, *liters*	4.23	3.38	80	4.14	98
FEV_1/FVC, %	≥74	77		77	
FEV_3/FVC, %	≥95	88		94	
MVV, *liters/min*	126	107	85	144	114
$FEF_{25-75\%}$, *liters/sec*	3.6	2.4	67	3.5	98

Interpretation and Discussion

The spirogram is normal, except for the reduced $FEF_{25-75\%}$ on the prebronchodilator study. The postbronchodilator spirometric data are normal. This patient had viral pneumonia and has a slowly resolving bronchiolitis secondary to that infection.

Patient 7. A 26-Year-Old White Man with Persistent "Wheezing" for 4 Months

		PREBRONCHODILATOR	
	PREDICTED	*Observed*	*% Predicted*
FVC, *liters*	4.89	5.33	109
2SVC, *liters*	4.89	5.28	108
ERV, *liters*	1.63	1.60	98
IC, *liters*	3.24	3.68	114
FEV_1, *liters*	4.01	1.54	38
FEV_3, *liters*	4.65	3.59	77
FEV_1/FVC, %	≥82	35	
FEV_3/FVC, %	≥95	67	
$FEF_{25-75\%}$, *liters/sec*	4.50	1.03	23

Interpretation and Discussion

The pattern suggests obstructive airway disease. Flow-volume curves demonstrated a plateau on both the forced inspiratory and expiratory loops, indicative of a fixed large airway obstruction. A bronchoscopy was performed that demonstrated a mass partially obstructing the trachea. Biopsy of the lesion showed a bronchial adenoma of the cylindroma type. Usual spirographic data do not differentiate between large airway and small airway obstruction. In this instance, the lesion was suggested by the characteristic shape of the flow-volume loop.

Patient 8. A 38-Year-Old White Man with a History of Intermittent Attacks of Shortness of Breath Associated with Wheezing

	PREDICTED	PREBRONCHODILATOR		POSTBRONCHODILATOR	
		Observed	*% Predicted*	*Observed*	*% Predicted*
FVC, *liters*	4.14	5.92	143	6.11	148
2SVC, *liters*	4.14	5.93	143	6.16	149
ERV, *liters*	1.38	1.66	120	1.84	133
IC, *liters*	2.76	4.41	160	4.55	165
FEV_1, *liters*	3.23	3.77	116	4.26	132
FEV_3, *liters*	3.93	5.42	138	5.71	145
FEV_1/FVC, %	≥78	64		70	
FEV_3/FVC, %	≥95	92		93	
MVV, *liters/min*	122	140	115	169	138
$FEF_{25-75\%}$, *liters/sec*	3.9	2.4	61	3.2	81

Interpretation and Discussion

The mechanics of ventilation are abnormal, demonstrating a reduction in the FEV_1/FVC% and in the $FEF_{25-75\%}$ in the prebronchodilator study. After inhalation of bronchodilator, the $FEF_{25-75\%}$ is normal. The finding of obstructive airway disease responsive to bronchodilator, in association with a history of intermittent attacks of wheezing along with symptom-free intervals, would be compatible with the diagnosis of bronchial asthma.

Patient 9. A 66-Year-Old White Man with a 15-Year History of Chronic Cough and Sputum Production. On Physical Examination He Had Severe Kyphoscoliosis.

	PREDICTED	PREBRONCHODILATOR		POSTBRONCHODILATOR	
		Observed	*% Predicted*	*Observed*	*% Predicted*
FVC, *liters*	3.69	2.11	57	2.12	57
2SVC, *liters*	3.69	2.22	60	2.05	56
ERV, *liters*	1.23	1.03	84	0.99	80
IC, *liters*	2.46	1.17	48	1.17	48
FEV_1, *liters*	2.62	1.05	40	1.09	42
FEV_3, *liters*	3.51	1.60	46	1.65	47
FEV_1/FVC, %	≥71	50		51	
FEV_3/FVC, %	≥95	76		78	
MVV, *liters/min*	87	31	36	40	46
$FEF_{25-75\%}$, *liters/sec*	2.9	0.5	17	0.5	17
FRC, *liters*	3.04	2.58	85		
RV, *liters*	1.81	1.56	86		
TLC, *liters*	5.02	3.56	71		
RV/TLC, %	36	44			

Interpretation and Discussion

The mechanics of ventilation are abnormal on the spirogram, suggesting possible combined obstructive and restrictive pulmonary disease. A TLC measurement is helpful to determine whether the reduction in vital capacity is due to air-trapping from severe obstructive airway disease or whether it does indeed represent the presence of concomitant restrictive disease. In this case the TLC is reduced, suggesting that the patient does indeed have restrictive pulmonary disease. The reduction in FEV_1/FVC%, along with the fact that the $FEF_{25-75\%}$ is reduced considerably more than the reduction in FVC, suggests that the patient definitely has obstructive airway disease. There is no significant improvement, after inhalation of bronchodilator, in the patient's expiratory flow rates. The patient's obstructive airway disease is due to combined chronic bronchitis and pulmonary emphysema. The restrictive pattern is secondary to the concomitant severe kyphoscoliosis.

EXAMPLES OF ARTERIAL BLOOD GAS DATA

Patient 10. A 56-Year-Old Woman Who, While on the Oncology Ward, Developed Shortness of Breath. She is Breathing Spontaneously on Room Air.

	ACTUAL VALUES	NORMAL VALUES
pH	7.48	7.35–7.45
P_{CO_2}, *mm Hg*	32	35–45
P_{O_2}, *mm Hg*	59	76–84
O_2 saturation, %	91.1	>93
O_2 content, *vol %*	13.4	16–20
$P(A-a)O_2$, *mm Hg*	49	<23
Plasma bicarbonate, *mEq/liter*	24	22–26
Standard bicarbonate, *mEq/liter*	25	22–26
Base excess (blood), *mEq/liter*	1	−2 to +2
Base excess (ECF), *mEq/liter*	1	−2 to +2

Interpretation and Discussion

The P_{O_2} is considerably lower than the predicted normal range for this patient's age, so that there is moderate hypoxemia on room air. The P_{O_2} would be even lower were it not for the patient's hyperventilation, as indicated by the reduced P_{CO_2}. The $P(A-a)O_2$ is increased, indicating the presence of ventilation/perfusion mismatch, diffusion defect, or shunt. The acid–base data are compatible with an uncompensated, mild respiratory alkalosis. A ventilation/perfusion lung scan was consistent with pulmonary embolism.

Patient 11. A 71-Year-Old Man Who Has Hypertension. He is Breathing Spontaneously on Room Air.

	ACTUAL VALUES	NORMAL VALUES
pH	7.5	7.35–7.45
P_{CO_2}, *mm Hg*	48	35–45
P_{O_2}, *mm Hg*	62	69–77
O_2 saturation, %	92.5	>93
O_2 content, *vol %*	16.7	16–20
$P(A-a)O_2$, *mm Hg*	29	<30
Plasma bicarbonate, *mEq/liter*	37	22–26
Standard bicarbonate, *mEq/liter*	35	22–26
Base excess (blood), *mEq/liter*	11	−2 to +2
Base excess (ECF), *mEq/liter*	14	−2 to +2

Interpretation and Discussion

Moderate hypoxemia is present on room air. The $P(A-a)O_2$ is normal for this patient's age, indicating that overall hypoventilation is the cause of the hypoxemia. The sum of the P_{O_2} and the P_{CO_2} on room air is 110 mm Hg, which would also suggest overall hypoventilation as the cause of the reduced P_{O_2}. The acid–base data are compatible with a partially compensated metabolic alkalosis. However, this is compatible with maximal compensation based on 95% confidence limit bands. The patient is being treated with diuretics for his hypertension, which has resulted in a metabolic alkalosis, and he now is hypoventilating in an attempt to compensate for the alkalosis.

Patient 12. An 80-Year-Old Woman with a History of Chronic Renal Disease. She Is Breathing Spontaneously on Room Air.

	ACTUAL VALUES	NORMAL VALUES
pH	7.36	7.35–7.45
P_{CO_2}, *mm Hg*	33	35–45
P_{O_2}, *mm Hg*	76	66–74
O_2 saturation, %	94.4	>93
O_2 content, *vol %*	7.3	16–20
$P(A-a)O_2$, *mm Hg*	31	<33
Plasma bicarbonate, *mEq/liter*	18	22–26
Standard bicarbonate, *mEq/liter*	19	22–26
Base excess (blood), *mEq/liter*	−6	−2 to +2
Base excess (ECF), *mEq/liter*	−6	−2 to +2

Interpretation and Discussion

The P_{O_2} is excellent on room air when compared to the predicted normal P_{O_2} for this patient's age. The P_{O_2} would be somewhat lower if the patient were not hyperventilating. The O_2 content, however, is markedly reduced, which is compatible with the patient's chronic anemia. The acid–base data are compatible with a compensated metabolic acidosis. The patient has chronic uremic acidosis. The severe anemia is due to the patient's chronic renal failure.

Patient 13. A 77-Year-Old Man Who Is Breathing Spontaneously on Room Air.

	ACTUAL VALUES	NORMAL VALUES
pH	7.36	7.35–7.45
P_{CO_2}, *mm Hg*	25	35–45
P_{O_2}, *mm Hg*	75	67–75
O_2 saturation, %	93.1	>93
O_2 content, *vol %*	12.7	16–20
$P(A-a)O_2$, *mm Hg*	43	<32
Plasma bicarbonate, *mEq/liter*	14	22–26
Standard bicarbonate, *mEq/liter*	17	22–26
Base excess (blood), *mEq/liter*	−10	−2 to +2
Base excess (ECF), *mEq/liter*	−10	−2 to +2

Interpretation and Discussion

The patient's P_{O_2} on room air is excellent; however, it would be lower were it not for the hyperventilation. The $P(A-a)O_2$ gradient is increased when compared to that predicted for this patient's age, which indicates the presence of ventilation/perfusion mismatch, diffusion defect, or shunt. Despite the excellent P_{O_2}, the O_2 content is reduced because of anemia. The acid–base data are compatible with a compensated metabolic acidosis. However, 95% confidence limit bands suggest the presence of metabolic acidosis with a superimposed respiratory alkalosis. In other words, for a base excess of −10 mEq/liter, one would not expect the patient to hyperventilate enough, in compensating for this acidemia, to return the pH to 7.36. This suggests that the patient has a reason for hyperventilation other than simply an attempt to compensate for the metabolic acidosis. The patient does have pneumonia in addition to diabetic ketoacidosis.

Patient 14. A 97-Year-Old Man Who Is Breathing Spontaneously on a 28% Ventimask Device.

	ACTUAL VALUES	NORMAL VALUES
pH	7.48	7.35–7.45
P_{CO_2}, *mm Hg*	22	35–45
P_{O_2}, *mm Hg*	51	59–67
O_2 saturation, %	88.8	>93
O_2 content, *vol* %	11.1	16–20
$P(A-a)O_2$, *mm Hg*	117	<47
Plasma bicarbonate, *mEq/liter*	16	22–26
Standard bicarbonate, *mEq/liter*	20	22–26
Base excess (blood), *mEq/liter*	−5	−2 to +2
Base excess (ECF), *mEq/liter*	−7	−2 to +2

Interpretation and Discussion

The P_{O_2} is barely adequate despite 28% O_2. The $P(A-a)O_2$ is significantly increased above that predicted for this patient's age and FI_{O_2}, indicating the presence of ventilation/perfusion mismatch, diffusion defect, or shunt. The O_2 content is markedly reduced, partly owing to the low P_{O_2}, but also to anemia. The acid–base data are compatible with a partially compensated respiratory alkalosis. This patient has severe pneumonia that has been present for several days.

Patient 15. A 25-Year-Old Man with a Complaint of Dyspnea. His Chest X-ray Shows Hilar Lymphadenopathy Bilaterally. He Is Breathing Spontaneously, with 3 liters/min Supplemental Oxygen via Nasal Cannula.

	ACTUAL VALUES	NORMAL VALUES
pH	7.51	7.35–7.45
P_{CO_2}, *mm Hg*	33	35–45
P_{O_2}, *mm Hg*	71	89–97
O_2 saturation, %	93.9	>93
O_2 content, *vol* %	21.3	16–20
$P(A-a)O_2$, *mm Hg*		
Plasma bicarbonate, *mEq/liter*	26	22–26
Standard bicarbonate, *mEq/liter*	28	22–26
Base excess (blood), *mEq/liter*	4	−2 to +2
Base excess (ECF), *mEq/liter*	3	−2 to +2

Interpretation and Discussion

Adequate oxygenation is present on 3 liters/min O_2 via nasal cannula. The $P(A-a)O_2$ cannot be calculated because the precise FI_{O_2} is unknown. However, the sum of the P_{O_2} and P_{CO_2} is less than 110 mm Hg, indicating the presence of ventilation/perfusion mismatch, diffusion defect, or shunt. The acid–base data are compatible with a combined respiratory and metabolic alkalosis. The plasma bicarbonate is normal because of the hypocapnia; however, the standard bicarbonate and base excess values are slightly increased. Mediastinoscopy provided biopsy evidence for a noncaseating granuloma compatible with sarcoidosis. Even though in this case the patient's chest x-ray film showed no evidence of lung parenchymal involvement, the diffusing capacity was 50% of predicted normal.

Patient 16. An 18-Year-Old Girl Who Presents to the Emergency Room in Coma. She Is Breathing Spontaneously on Room Air.

	ACTUAL VALUES	NORMAL VALUES
pH	7.21	7.35–7.45
P_{CO_2}, *mm Hg*	12	35–45
P_{O_2}, *mm Hg*	120	92–100
O_2 saturation, %	97.0	>93
$P(A-a)O_2$, *mm Hg*	16	<6
Plasma bicarbonate, *mEq/liter*	5	22–26
Base excess (blood), *mEq/liter*	−22	−2 to +2
Base excess (ECF), *mEq/liter*	−22	−2 to +2

Interpretation and Discussion

The P_{O_2} is supranormal for room air. A P_{O_2} this high is possible only if the patient has prominent hyperventilation. The P_{CO_2} is markedly decreased, so that indeed alveolar hyperventilation is present. A partially compensated metabolic acidosis is present; however, based on 95% confidence limit bands, this arterial blood gas would be compatible with a maximally compensated metabolic acidosis. The diagnosis is diabetic ketoacidosis.

Patient 17. A 28-Year-Old Male with a 3-Day History of Fever, Cough, and Shortness of Breath. He Is Breathing Room Air.

	ACTUAL VALUES	NORMAL VALUES
pH	7.56	7.35–7.45
P_{CO_2}, *mm Hg*	25	35–45
P_{O_2}, *mm Hg*	30	87–95
O_2 saturation, %	68	>93
$P(A-a)O_2$, *mm Hg*	90	<11
Plasma bicarbonate, *mEq/liter*	23	22–26
Base excess (blood), *mEq/liter*	+2	−2 to +2
Base excess (ECF), *mEq/liter*	0	−2 to +2

Interpretation and Discussion

The P_{O_2} is markedly decreased. The $P(A-a)O_2$ is increased, and the sum of the P_{O_2} and P_{CO_2} is less than 110 mm Hg indicating the presence of $\dot{V}/\dot{Q}$ disturbance, diffusion defect, or shunt as the cause of the hypoxemia. An uncompensated respiratory alkalosis is present. The diagnosis is influenzal pneumonia. Because of significant respiratory distress, the patient was intubated and placed on a volume ventilator with an FI_{O_2} of 1.0. Twenty minutes later, the following arterial blood gas data were obtained.

	ACTUAL VALUES	NORMAL VALUES
pH	7.46	7.35–7.45
P_{CO_2}, *mm Hg*	32	35–45
P_{O_2}, *mm Hg*	50	>580
O_2 saturation, %	85.7	100
$P(A-a)O_2$, *mm Hg*	631	<93
Plasma bicarbonate, *mEq/liter*	23	22–26
Base excess (blood), *mEq/liter*	0	−2 to +2
Base excess (ECF), *mEq/liter*	−1	−2 to +2

Interpretation and Discussion

Severe hypoxemia is still present. The $P(A-a)O_2$ is increased despite 100% oxygen, indicating that the cause of the hypoxemia is a right-to-left shunt. This is most likely a "physiologic shunt" rather than an anatomic shunt. A mild, uncompensated respiratory alkalosis is still present. In this patient with "adult respiratory distress syndrome," it would be appropriate to institute positive end-expiratory pressure (PEEP) in an attempt to reduce the FI_{O_2} and still maintain an adequate P_{O_2}.

Patient 18. A 16-Year-Old Girl Admitted to the Emergency Room in a Comatose State. She Is Breathing Spontaneously on Room Air.

	ACTUAL VALUES	NORMAL VALUES
pH	7.04	7.35–7.45
P_{CO_2}, *mm Hg*	85	35–45
P_{O_2}, *mm Hg*	45	93–101
O_2 saturation, %	60.1	>93
$P(A-a)O_2$, *mm Hg*	5	<6
Plasma bicarbonate, *mEq/liter*	22	22–26
Standard bicarbonate, *mEq/liter*	15	22–26
T_{40} bicarbonate, *mEq/liter*	19	22–26
Base excess (blood), *mEq/liter*	−12	−2 to +2
Base excess (ECF), *mEq/liter*	−7	−2 to +2

Interpretation and Discussion

Severe hypoxemia is present on room air. The $P(A-a)O_2$ is normal, and the sum of the P_{O_2} and P_{CO_2} is between 110 and 130 mm Hg on room air. Therefore, the cause of the hypoxemia is overall hypoventilation. The plasma bicarbonate is normal however, the T_{40} bicarbonate is reduced. The plasma bicarbonate is normal because the P_{CO_2} is markedly elevated. If the P_{CO_2} were normal (e.g., 40 mm Hg), the actual plasma bicarbonate would be 19 mEq/liter. Therefore, a combined respiratory and metabolic acidosis is present. The BE_{ECF} and T_{40} bicarbonate (based on *in vivo* data) more accurately portray the true level of metabolic acidosis in this case than do the BE (b) and standard bicarbonate (which are based on *in vitro* calculations). The diagnosis is drug overdose. The hypoventilation and severe respiratory acidosis are due to respiratory center depression. The metabolic acidosis is due to lactic acid accumulation secondary to inadequate tissue oxygenation resulting from the severe hypoxemia.

Patient 19. A 68-Year-Old Man with a Long History of Smoking, Cough, Sputum Production, and Shortness of Breath. Arterial Blood Gas Was Reportedly Drawn with the Patient on Room Air.

	ACTUAL VALUES	NORMAL VALUES
pH	7.30	7.35–7.45
P_{CO_2}, *mm Hg*	75	35–45
P_{O_2}, *mm Hg*	80	71–79
O_2 saturation, %	93.7	>93
Plasma bicarbonate, *mEq/liter*	38	22–26
T_{40} bicarbonate, *mEq/liter*	35.7	22–26
Base excess (blood), *mEq/liter*	+7	−2 to +2
Base excess (ECF), *mEq/liter*	+9	−2 to +2

Interpretation and Discussion

The P_{O_2} is excellent. There is a partially compensated respiratory acidosis. Plasma bicarbonate is increased slightly owing to the elevated P_{CO_2}. However, if the P_{CO_2} were 40 mm Hg the bicarbonate would still be elevated to 35.7 mEq/liters. The 95% confidence limit bands show that the data are compatible with a maximally compensated respiratory acidosis. The patient has chronic bronchitis with chronic respiratory failure. The sum of the P_{O_2} and P_{CO_2} is greater than 130 mm Hg. When this happens, one should suspect that the patient is not on room air, but rather on supplemental oxygen. The other possibility would be an error in either the P_{O_2} or P_{CO_2} measurements. Indeed, this patient was on 2 liters/min O_2 via nasal cannula (e.g., low-flow oxygen).

Patient 20. A 56-Year-Old Man Found to Be Somnolent and Cyanotic in the Postoperative Recovery Room While Breathing Room Air.

	ACTUAL VALUES	NORMAL VALUES
*p*H	7.14	7.35–7.45
P_{CO_2}, *mm Hg*	85	35–45
P_{O_2}, *mm Hg*	35	76–84
O_2 saturation, %	50	>93
O_2 content, *vol* %	10.5	16–20
$P(A-a)O_2$, *mm Hg*	8	<23
Plasma bicarbonate, *mEq/liter*	28	22–26
Standard bicarbonate, *mEq/liter*	21	22–26
T_{40} bicarbonate, *mEq/liter*	25	22–26
BB (blood), *mEq/liter*	44	46–50
BE (blood), *mEq/liter*	−4	−2 to +2
BE_{ECF}, *mEq/liter*	1.4	−2 to +2

Interpretation and Discussion

The severe hypoxemia is due to overall hypoventilation, as noted from the normal $P(A-a)O_2$ and the fact that the sum of the P_{O_2} and P_{CO_2} on room air is between 110 and 130 mm Hg. Respiratory acidosis is present. Plasma bicarbonate is slightly elevated; however, this is simply a result of the acute hypercapnia, as indicated by the normal T_{40} bicarbonate and normal BE_{ECF}. The standard bicarbonate, blood buffer base, and blood base excess values are low and thus misleading, since there is no metabolic acidosis present. This again points out the value of using calculations based on *in vivo* information (*i.e.*, T_{40} bicarbonate and BE_{ECF}) rather than on those based on *in vitro* measurements (*i.e.*, standard bicarbonate, BB_b, and BE_b). This patient's acute, uncompensated, respiratory acidosis and severe hypoxemia are a result of hypoventilation from respiratory center depression in a patient who has not yet recovered from the effects of his general anesthesia.

Patient 21. A 71-Year-Old Woman on the Surgery Unit. She Is Breathing 6 liters/min Oxygen Via Nasal Cannula.

	ACTUAL VALUES	NORMAL VALUES
*p*H	7.15	7.35–7.45
P_{CO_2}, *mm Hg*	35	35–45
P_{O_2}, *mm Hg*	95	69–77
O_2 saturation, %	94	>93
O_2 content, *vol* %	19.9	16–20
Plasma bicarbonate, *mEq/liter*	12	22–26
Base excess (ECF), *mEq/liter*	−15	−2 to +2

Interpretation and Discussion

Oxygenation is excellent on 6 liters/min O_2 by nasal cannula. The arterial blood analysis shows a prominent metabolic acidosis, with the P_{CO_2} at the lower limits of normal. This patient, 48 hours postlaparotomy, became cyanotic and unresponsive after an injection of morphine. The patient received i.v. levallorphan tartrate to reverse the respiratory center depression induced by the morphine. She now has excellent oxygenation on spontaneous breathing; however, she still has severe lactic acidosis resulting from tissue hypoxia during her period of acute hypoventilation.

F

Gas Laws and Certain Indispensable Conventions

George G. Burton • H. Frederic Helmholz, Jr.

Readers of this book will probably have learned, and then promptly forgotten, some of the basic physical laws and principles that undergird this profession unless they use them frequently in their day-to-day practice (e.g., in the pulmonary physiology laboratory). Accordingly, these laws and principles bear repeating, despite the caveat that their memorization (perish the thought!) can be relegated to an operative sequence of memory devices (mnemonics).[3] Detailed descriptions and discussions of this material have been published.[1,2,4–7]

FACTORS INFLUENCING THE BEHAVIOR OF GASES

Four basic variables affect gas volumetric relationships.

1. Temperature (T), when expressed as degrees Kelvin, indicates the level of energy of a gas sample and is referred to as absolute temperature, converted from temperature Centigrade or Celsius, or Fahrenheit.
2. Pressure (P), defined as absolute or total exerted pressure, is conventionally expressed in atmospheres, or as a given column of mercury or of water balancing the pressure (mm Hg, torr, or cm H_2O), or in pascals or kilopascals in the Systeme Internationale (SI) (*see* below under Standard Units.)
3. Volume (V) is expressed in cubic units, such as cubic meters or cubic centimeters, or in liters.
4. Relative mass of gas or number of molecules (n) is expressed in gram molecules (the molecular weight of the substance in grams).

For all physiological measurements the general (*"ideal") gas law* can be used without significant error (see a physical chemistry text for Van der Waal's equation, which includes the factor of space taken up by molecules and intermolecular forces.) The unit R is used to indicate the gas constant and perhaps should be designated R^g to differentiate it from R, which indicates exchange ratio of respired gases. The ideal gas law states that

$$PV = nR^gT$$

and is expressed in a conglomerate unit telling what units of pressure, volume, and temperature are used. The equation is better understood if one expresses it as follows.

$$\frac{PV}{nT} = \text{a constant,}$$

as long as energy equilibrium is obtained, when temperature is expressed on an absolute scale, pressure is absolute pressure, and uniform units are used for pressure, volume, and mass of material. Thus, as long as the amount of gas under consideration remains the same, the following powerful equation is available.

$$\frac{P_1V_1}{T_1} = \frac{P_2V_2}{T_2}.$$

This allows one to calculate the changes produced by changing conditions for any gas volume. The general gas law is actually composed of five separate but related laws.

1. *Boyle's law* states that volume varies inversely with absolute pressure (e.g., volume is reduced as pressure is increased), other factors remaining constant.

$$V_1P_1 = V_2P_2,$$

where T and n are constant.

2. *Charles' law* states that volume is directly proportional to temperature when it is expressed on an absolute scale, other factors remaining constant.

$$\frac{V_1}{T_1} = \frac{V_2}{T_2},$$

where P and n are constant.

3. *Gay–Lussac's law* expresses the same relationship but is stated as follows.

$$\frac{P_1}{T_1} = \frac{P_2}{T_2},$$

where V and n are constant. Thus the pressure of gases when volume is maintained constant is directly proportional to the absolute temperature for a constant amount of gas.

4. *Avogadro's law* states that equal volumes of gases under identical conditions contain equal numbers of molecules, or that the number of molecules is directly proportional to the volume, other factors remaining constant.

$$\frac{n_1}{V_1} = \frac{n_2}{V_2},$$

where P and T are constant.

5. *Dalton's law* states that gases in a mixture exert pressure equivalent to the pressure each would exert were it present alone in the volume of the total mixture, which means that each gas present in a mixture exerts a partial pressure equal to the fractional concentration (by volume) multiplied by the total pressure.

Taken together, Avogadro's law and Dalton's law indicate that in the gas phase, partial pressures will be proportional to molar concentrations, and volumetric expressions will indicate numbers of molecules if a standard is accepted.

By convention, numbers of molecules are indicated in physiology as follows: Whenever gas exchanges (uptake or utilization, or both, or elimination or production, or both) are being studied, volumes are corrected to agreed-on conditions that are standard conditions designated by the initials STPD (standard temperature is 0°C or 273°K; standard pressure is 1 atmosphere or 760 mm Hg or 14.69 psi; and D stands for a dry gas). One molecular weight of a true gas has a volume STPD (V^{stpd}) of 22.41 l.*

The number of molecules in 1 g molecular weight (mole) of a gas has been calculated at 6.06×10^{23}. This is fittingly called *Avogadro's number.*

Other conditions under which gases are often measured or in which volumes are expressed are indicated by the initials BTPS (body temperature and pressure saturated). Body temperature is 37°C or 310°K; body pressure is whatever pressure is ambient; and a gas saturated with water at body temperature contains 43.9 mg/liter and has a partial pressure of water vapor of 47 mm Hg. Volumes of gas (V^{btps}) at body temperature and pressure saturated are effective in washing carbon dioxide out of the pulmonary alveoli, and oxygen partial pressure under these same conditions is that which is effective at the alveolar level in causing diffusion into the blood.

ATPS refers to gas volumes at ambient temperature and pressure, saturated at ambient temperature. This would be the condition of gas in a measuring vessel in which expired air had been collected. ATP

*For CO_2, N_2O, and other gases, the critical temperatures of which are relatively high (near room temperature), this number is somewhat smaller but is not significantly different for purposes of respiratory therapy, and therefore the same "molecular volume" can be used for all gases. Thus one can calculate R^g using an expression such as

$$\frac{760 \times 22.41}{1 \times 273} = R,$$

with the notation that pressure is in mm Hg, volume in liters, temperature in degrees Kelvin, and n in moles.

alone is used to indicate the same as the above but without water vapor present. (ATPD is preferred for this condition.)

Since accurate tables of water vapor pressure at various temperatures are available, it is customary to use water vapor pressure in correcting volumes from wet to dry conditions. One may conclude from the above laws that the volume of a wet gas will bear the following relation to the volume of that gas where the water vapor has been removed (PB equals total or barometric pressure).

$$V_{dry} \times P_B = V_{wet} \times (P_B - P^T_{H_2O});$$

$$V_{dry} = V_{wet} \frac{P_B - P^T_{H_2O}}{P_B},$$

since the gas present exerts pressure in the wet gas equivalent to the total pressure minus the partial pressure of water vapor. Thus to correct a volume of gas BTPS to STPD, the following calculation can be given as an example.

$$V_{STPD} = V_{BTPS} \times \frac{P_B - 47}{760} \times \frac{273}{273 + 37}$$

$$= V_{BTPS} \times 0.8146$$

if PB = 760.

OTHER RELATIONS OF IMPORTANCE IN RESPIRATORY THERAPY

Flowing fluids (gases or liquids) obey certain important laws. Fluids flow only when acted on by a force, this force being proportional to a difference in pressure. Some of the laws are given below.

Poiseuille's law states that the flow of a fluid or gas that escapes through a tube (V) will be proportional to the pressure difference (ΔP) across the tube, to the fourth power of the radius (r) of the tube, and to time (t), and will be inversely proportional to the length of the tube (L) and the viscosity of the fluid (n).

$$\dot{V} = \frac{\Delta P \pi r^4 t}{8Ln}$$

The density of the fluid is not involved. This law holds only as long as the fluid flows in a laminar (orderly) fashion. Note that π and 8 are constants.

In the last century, Osborn Reynolds presented the concept that a nondimensional number could characterize a system in which there was fluid flow. This number is proportional to the density of the fluid, the velocity of the fluid flow, and the size of the system and is inversely proportional to the viscosity of the fluid. When this number exceeds a certain critical value (which depends on units used in expressing the determining variables), the fluid flow will become turbulent, and Poiseuille's law will no longer describe the situation. Under such circumstances, the flow will no longer increase directly as the differential in pressure increases but will increase only as the square root of the increase of pressure. In normal breathing there is little turbulence in the airway. The formula for the Reynolds' number is

$$N_R = \frac{\text{fluid density} \times \text{velocity} \times \text{size (of tube or particle)}}{\text{viscosity of fluid}}.$$

If the density of a fluid is reduced, and since viscosity is not affected by the density changes, the increase in velocity required to raise the *Reynolds' number* to a critical level is increased. Thus the less the density of the fluid, the greater the velocity it must obtain before the flow will become turbulent. The velocity at which any fluid will become turbulent will be characteristic of that fluid and is called the *critical velocity* of that fluid.

The relationships above have important implications for respiratory therapy.

1. In very small tubes of any length, the velocity of the gas cannot exceed the critical velocity at any pressure differential, and thus turbulent flow is impossible (e.g., in the small bronchi and bronchioles of the lung).
2. Since turbulent flow in the airways is essential for an effective cough, low-density gases (He-O_2) will make coughing ineffective. Moreover, the cough cannot effectively move secretions in peripheral airways.
3. Helium as a diluent for oxygen will effectively increase volume flows obtainable through short, narrowed segments of the major airways in which turbulence is present. This is particularly useful when there is turbulence during resting tidal flows.
4. Because aerosol particles are very small, their carriage and deposition are determined essentially by viscosity and kinetic factors alone.

Therefore, aerosols are delivered equally well by warm as by cold gases and by helium–oxygen mixtures as by oxygen or air.

5. During forced expiration, substitution of helium for nitrogen in the inhaled mixture will increase that part of the expiratory flow that was restricted by its turbulent character, which would be that in the larger airways—larynx, trachea, and the first few bronchial branchings.

Daniel Bernoulli noted that when the pressure drop across a tubing system was ignored, the total energy at points along the system remained constant. Thus the lateral pressure energy, the kinetic energy (energy of motion), and the potential energy (energy of position) added up to a constant, when one ignored the effect of friction.*

$$P + hdg + \frac{1}{2}dv^2 = \text{a constant},$$

where P = pressure; h = height above a reference plane; d = density; g = acceleration of gravity; and v = velocity. Thus decrease in pressure = $\frac{1}{2}dv^2$.

This theorem *(Bernoulli's principle)* explains the way jets of gas entrain materials brought to the side of a high-velocity stream, how the wings of an airplane work, and how water pumps on faucets work. When a fluid flows through a restricted portion of a tube, the velocity must increase; thus the energy of motion increases and the pressure energy (lateral wall pressure) *decreases*, so that at the edges of any high-velocity fluid stream pressures will be reduced. *(Note:* In a tube beyond the restriction, the lateral pressure again *rises.)* A high-velocity stream of gas escaping from a nozzle will be surrounded by an area of pressure below atmospheric, and any fluid in the area will be entrained. This explains the way a so-called Venturi-oxygen dilutor system works and how jet nebulizers and the Babbington nebulizer entrain fluids at the jets of gas.

Thomas Graham described *effusion*—the process by which a gas passes through an orifice. (An orifice is a hole with size, or area but no length.) The relative rates at which gases can be forced through an orifice are inversely proportional to the square root of the densities of the gases. Adolph Eugen Fick also showed that the rate of diffusion of a gas into another gas was inversely proportional to the square root of the molecular weight and thus the density. The above laws apply only to gas effusion and diffusion in gases. In the diffusion of a gas through other substances (in our frame of reference, aqueous media), the solubility of the gas in the medium directly influences the diffusion.

*Of course, to maintain flow, the total pressure at one end of any system in which a fluid is flowing must be greater than that at the other end.

Orders of magnitude should be considered. The diffusion of one gas into another is very rapid and is described by coefficients of "units" per second. When one considers diffusion in aqueous media, the coefficients are "units" of the same order of magnitude per 24 hours. The diffusion of gases in gas is at a rate at least 86,000 times that of gases in fluids. In the alveoli and alveolar ducts of the lung, diffusion maintains mixing without any need for gas movement. The process of diffusion is limiting only in the alveolar membrane and plasma, and primarily for oxygen because it is so much less soluble than carbon dioxide. In a gas, oxygen diffuses faster than carbon dioxide by a factor of 1.173, whereas in aqueous media carbon dioxide diffuses at least 20 times more rapidly than oxygen because it is more than 20 times more soluble.

STANDARD UNITS

For several years now there has been a movement to try to standardize units used in expressing laboratory data. The English, as they have converted to the metric system, have begun using the so-called International System of Units (Systeme Internationale d'Unites, or SI). This involves only a few changes from the metric-based system used in this country. The English recommend the substitution of joules for gram calories (c) and kilocalories (C) as units of energy; the substitution of the pascal and the kilopascal for centimeters of water or millimeters of mercury (torr) as units of pressure, and the substitution of the newton for the barye (1 dyne per square centimeter) as a unit of force (1 newton equals 100,000 baryes). They also advocate the use of the mole as the unit for amount of material instead of grams, milligrams, or other weights, and the substitution of moles per liter for grams percent, milligrams percent, and grams per liter. The use of concentrations as moles per liter is difficult in some situations (e.g., in regard to hemoglobin concentrations). Moreover, it is recommended that the very useful convention of expressing ionized materials in equivalents per liter, rather than moles per liter, be retained for physiological and biochemical expressions.

Table F-1. Method of Converting Between Usual Units and Metric or SI Units*

USUAL UNITS	CONVERSION FACTOR†	METRIC AND SI UNITS
inch (in)	2.54 →	centimeter (cm)
	← 0.3937	
foot (ft)	0.3048 →	meter (m)
	← 3.2808	
square inch (in^2 or si)	6.45 →	square centimeter (cm^2)
	← 0.155	
cubic foot (ft^3 or cu ft)	28.316 →	liters (l)
	← 0.0353	
cubic inch (in^3 or cu in)	16.39 →	cubic centimeters (cm^3 or cc)
	← 0.06102	milliliters (ml) essentially the same
pounds per square inch (psi)	51.7358 →	millimeters of mercury (mm Hg)
	← 0.01933	
pounds per square inch (psi)	70.0814 →	centimeters of water (cm H_2O)
(liquid)	← 0.01427	
inches of mercury (in Hg)	25.4 →	mm Hg
	← 0.0394	
millimeters of mercury (mm Hg)	0.13332 →	kilopascals (kPa)
	← 7.500	
centimeters of water (cm H_2O)	0.0984 →	kilopascals (kPa)
	← 10.160	
calories (gram calories) (c)	4.185 →	joule (J)
	← 0.2389	
calories (kilogram calories) (C)	4185.0 →	joule (J)
	← 0.0002389	kilojoule (kJ) preferable for metabolic data

*CF. Young DS: Standardized reporting of laboratory data: the desirability of using SI units. N Engl J Med 290:368, 1974; Study committee to evaluate changes in units of clinical chemistry tests. N Engl J Med 293:43, 1975.
†Example for using conversion factors: inches × 2.54 = centimeters; centimeters × 0.3937 = inches.

Some of the implications of the SI system are given in Table F-1, along with the conversion factors for units. All units, including the U.S. units, are based on the international prototype meter and the international prototype kilogram kept at the International Bureau of Weights and Measures in Sèvres, France.

In the metric system the dyne is the unit of force equal to the force required to give a free mass of 1 g an acceleration of 1 cm per second per second. In the SI system the newton is the unit of force equal to the force required to give a free mass of 1 kg an acceleration of 1 m per second per second. The pascal is suggested as the unit of pressure and is equal to a force of 1 newton acting over 1 m^2. This, however, is a very small unit, as is the barye of the usual metric system, and therefore it is suggested that the kilopascal be used as a unit of pressure for physiological data.

REFERENCES

1. Altman PL, Dittmer DS (eds): Respiration and Circulation. Bethesda, Maryland, Federation of American Societies for Experimental Biology, 1971
2. Bartels H et al: Methods in Pulmonary Physiology (Workman JM, trans) London, Hafna, 1963
3. Corrie D: Gas law mnemonics. Respir Care 20:1041, 1975
4. Egan DF: Fundamentals of Respiratory Therapy. St. Louis, CV Mosby, 1973
5. Handbook of Chemistry and Physics. Cleveland, Chemical Rubber Publishing Company, 1976
6. Standardization of definitions and symbols in respiratory physiology. Fed Proc 9:602, 1950
7. Young JA, Crocker D: Principles and Practice of Respiratory Therapy. Chicago, Year Book Medical Publishers, 1976

G

Terms and Symbols Used in Respiratory Physiology

John E. Hodgkin

The terms and symbols used in respiratory physiology, and their definitions, change from time to time. In an attempt to standardize these terms and symbols, the American Thoracic Society/American College of Chest Physicians Committee on Pulmonary Nomenclature published an initial report in 1975.[1] An American Thoracic Society Pulmonary Nomenclature Subcommittee on Respiratory Physiology subsequently revised the section dealing with terms and symbols used in respiratory physiology and published a portion of their report in Spring 1978.[2] This report is still undergoing revision and is reproduced as an interim document with permission from the American Thoracic Society. The editors and publishers have attempted to use this nomenclature through this edition of *Respiratory Care*.

GENERAL

P	Pressures in general
$\bar{X}$	Dash above any symbol indicates a mean value
$\dot{X}$	Dot above any symbol indicates a time derivative
$\ddot{X}$	Two dots above any symbol indicate the second time derivative
%X	Percent sign before a symbol indicates percentage of the predicted normal value
X/Y%	Percent sign after a symbol indicates a ratio function with the ratio expressed as a percentage. Both components of the ratio must be designated; e.g., $FEV_1/FEV\% = 100 \times FEV_1/FVC$
f	Frequency of any event in time; e.g., respiratory frequency: the number of breathing cycles per unit of time
t	Time
anat	Anatomical
max	Maximum

GAS PHASE SYMBOLS

Primary

V	Gas volume in general. Pressure, temperature, and percent saturation with water vapor must be stated
F	Fractional concentration in dry gas phase

Qualifying

I	Inspired
E	Expired
A	Alveolar
T	Tidal
D	Dead space
B	Barometric
STPD	Standard temperature and pressure, dry. These are the conditions of a volume of gas at 0° C, at 760 torr, without water vapor
BTPS	Body temperature (37° C), barometric pressure (at sea level = 760 torr), and saturated with water vapor
ATPD	Ambient temperature, pressure, dry
ATPS	Ambient temperature and pressure, saturated with water vapor
L	Lung

BLOOD PHASE SYMBOLS

Primary

$\dot{Q}$	Volume flow of blood
C	Concentration in blood phase
S	Saturation in blood phase

Qualifying

b	Blood in general
a	Arterial. Exact location to be specified in text when term is used
v	Venous. Exact location to be specified in text when term is used
$\bar{v}$	Mixed venous
c	Capillary. Exact location to be specified in text when term is used
c′	Pulmonary end-capillary

PULMONARY FUNCTION

Lung Volumes (Expressed as BTPS)

RV	Residual volume: volume of air remaining in the lungs after maximum exhalation
ERV	Expiratory reserve volume: maximum volume of air that can be exhaled from the end-tidal volume
V_T	Tidal volume: volume of gas inspired or expired during one ventilatory cycle
IRV	Inspiratory reserve volume: maximum volume that can be inspired from an end-tidal inspiratory level

V_L	Volume of the lung, including the conducting airways. Conditions of measurement must be stated
IC	Inspiratory capacity: volume that can be inspired from the end-tidal expiratory volume
IVC	Inspiratory vital capacity: maximum volume measured on inspiration after a full expiration
VC	Vital capacity: volume measured on complete expiration after the deepest inspiration but without respect to the effort involved
FRC	Functional residual capacity: volume of gas remaining in the lungs and airways at the end of a resting tidal expiration
TLC	Total lung capacity: volume of gas in the lung and airways after as much gas as possible has been inhaled
RV/TLC%	Residual volume to total lung capacity ratio, expressed as a percentage
V_D	Physiological dead space: calculated volume (BPTS), which accounts for the difference between the pressures of CO_2 in expired gas and arterial blood. Physiological dead space reflects the combination of anatomical dead space and alveolar dead space, the volume of the latter increasing with the importance of the nonuniformity of the ventilation/perfusion ratio in the lung
$V_{D_{anat}}$	Volume of the anatomical dead space (BTPS)
V_{D_A}	Alveolar dead-space volume (BTPS)

Forced Respiratory Maneuvers (Expressed as BTPS)

FVC	Forced vital capacity: the volume of gas expired after full inspiration, and with expiration performed as rapidly and completely as possible
FIVC	Forced inspiratory vital capacity: maximal volume of air inspired after a maximum expiration, and with inspiration performed as rapidly and completely as possible
FEV_1	Volume of gas exhaled in a given time interval during the execution of a forced vital capacity
FEV_1/FVC%	Ratio of timed forced expiratory volume to forced vital capacity, expressed as a percentage
PEF	Peak expiratory flow (liters/min or liters/sec)
$\dot{V}max_{XX\%}$	Maximum expiratory flow (instantaneous) qualified by the volume at which measured, expressed as percentage of the FVC that has been exhaled. (Example: $\dot{V}max_{75\%}$ is the maximum expiratory flow after 75% of the FVC has been exhaled and 25% remains to be exhaled)
$\dot{V}max_{XX\%TLC}$	Maximum expiratory flow (instantaneous) qualified by the volume at which measured, expressed as percentage of the TLC that remains in the lung. (Example: $\dot{V}max_{40\%TLC}$ is the maximum expiratory flow when 40% of the TLC remains in the lung)
FEF_{x-y}	Forced expiratory flow between two designated volume points in the FVC. These points may be designated as absolute volumes starting from the full inspiratory point or by designating the percentage of FVC exhaled
$FEF_{.1-1.2\,L}$	Forced expiratory flow between 200 ml and 1200 ml of the FVC; formerly called maximum expiratory flow
$FEF_{25\%-75\%}$	Forced expiratory flow during the middle half of the FVC; formerly called maximum mid-expiratory flow
MVV	Maximum voluntary ventilation: maximum volume of air that can be breathed per minute by a subject breathing quickly and as deeply as possible. The time of measurement of this tiring lung function test is usually between 12 and 30 sec, but the test result is given in liters (BTPS)/min
FET_x	Forced expiratory time required to exhale a specified FVC, e.g., $FET_{95\%}$ is the time required to deliver the first 95% of the FVC, $FET_{25\%-75\%}$ is the time required to deliver the middle half of the FVC
MIF_x	Maximum inspiratory flow (instantaneous). As in the case of the FET, appropriate modifiers designate the volume at which flow is being measured. Unless otherwise specified, the volume qualifiers indicate the volume inspired from RV at the point of measurement

Measurements of Ventilation

$\dot{V}\mathrm{E}$	Expired volume per minute (BTPS)
$\dot{V}\mathrm{I}$	Inspired volume per minute (BTPS)
$\dot{V}\mathrm{CO_2}$	Carbon dioxide production per minute (STPD)
$\dot{V}\mathrm{O_2}$	Oxygen consumption per minute (STPD)
R	Respiratory exchange ratio in general. Quotient of the volume of CO_2 produced divided by the volume of O_2 consumed
$\dot{V}\mathrm{A}$	Alveolar ventilation: physiological process by which alveolar gas is completely removed and replaced with fresh gas. The volume of alveolar gas actually expelled completely is equal to the tidal volume minus the volume of the dead space
$\dot{V}\mathrm{D}$	Ventilation per minute of the physiological dead space, BTPS
$\dot{V}\mathrm{D}_{anat}$	Ventilation per minute of the anatomical dead space, that portion of the conducting airway in which no significant gas exchange occurs (BTPS)
$\dot{V}\mathrm{D}_{A}$	Ventilation of the alveolar dead space (BTPS), defined by the equation $\dot{V}\mathrm{D}_A = \dot{V}\mathrm{D} - \dot{V}\mathrm{D}_{anat}$

Mechanics of Breathing (All Pressures Are Expressed Relative to Ambient Pressure Unless Otherwise Specified)

Pressure terms

Paw	Pressure at any point along the airways
Pao	Pressure at the airway opening, *i.e.*, mouth, nose, tracheal cannula
Ppl	Pleural pressure: the pressure between the visceral and parietal pleura relative to atmospheric pressure, in cm H_2O
Palv	Alveolar pressure
PL	Transpulmonary pressure: PL = Palv − Ppl, measurement conditions to be defined
PstL	Static recoil pressure of the lung; transpulmonary pressure measured under static conditions
Pbs	Pressure at the body surface
Pes	Esophageal pressure used to estimate Ppl
Pw	Transthoracic pressure: pressure difference between parietal pleural surface and body surface. Transthoracic in the sense used means "across the wall." Pw = Ppl − Pbs
Ptm	Transmural pressure pertaining to an airway or blood vessel
Prs	Transrespiratory pressure: pressure across the respiratory system. Prs = Palv − Pbs = PL + Pw

Flow-pressure relationships

R	Flow resistance: the ratio of the flow-resistive components of pressure to simultaneous flow in cm H_2O/liter/sec
Raw	Airway resistance calculated from pressure difference between airway opening (Pao) and alveoli (Palv) divided by the airflow, cm H_2O/liter/sec
RL	Total pulmonary resistance includes the frictional resistance of the lungs and air passages. It equals the sum of airway resistance and lung tissue resistance. It is measured by relating flow-dependent transpulmonary pressure to airflow at the mouth
Rrs	Total respiratory resistance includes the sum of airway resistance, lung tissue resistance, and chest wall resistance. It is measured by relating flow dependent transrespiratory pressure to airflow at the mouth
Rus	Resistance of the airways on the upstream (alveolar) side of the point in the airways where intraluminal pressure equals Ppl (equal pressure point), measured during maximum expiratory flow

Rds	Resistance of the airways on the downstream (mouth) side of the point in the airways where intraluminal pressure equals Ppl, measured during maximum expiratory flow
Gaw	Airway conductance, reciprocal of Raw
Gaw/VL	Specific conductance expressed per liter of lung volume at which Gaw is measured

Volume-pressure relationships

C	Compliance: the slope of a static volume-pressure curve at a point, or the linear approximation of a nearly straight portion of such a curve expressed in liter/cm H_2O or ml/cm H_2O
Cdyn	Dynamic compliance: the ratio of the tidal volume to the change in intrapleural pressure between the points of zero flow at the extremes of tidal volume in liter/cm H_2O or ml/cm H_2O
Cst	Static compliance, value for compliance based on measurements made during periods of cessation of airflow
C/VL	Specific compliance: compliance divided by the lung volume at which it is determined, usually FRC
E	Elastic: the reciprocal of compliance; expressed in cm H_2O/liter or cm H_2O/ml
Pst	Static components of pressure
W	Work of breathing: the energy required for breathing movements

Diffusing Capacity

DL	Diffusing capacity of the lung: amount of gas (O_2, CO, CO_2) commonly expressed as milliliters of gas (STPD) diffusing between alveolar gas and pulmonary capillary blood per torr mean gas pressure difference per minute Total resistance to diffusion for oxygen $\left(\frac{1}{DL_{O_2}}\right)$ and CO $\left(\frac{1}{DL_{CO}}\right)$ includes resistance to diffusion of the gas across the alveolar–capillary membrane, through plasma in the capillary, and across the red cell membrane (1/DM), and the resistance to diffusion within the red cell arising from the chemical reaction between the gas and hemoglobin, $(1/\theta V_c)$, according to the formulation $\frac{1}{DL} = \frac{1}{DM} + \frac{1}{\theta Vc}$
DM	The diffusing capacity of the pulmonary membrane
θ	The rate of gas uptake by 1 ml of normal whole blood per minute for a partial pressure of 1 torr
Vc	Average volume of blood in the capillary bed in milliliters
DL/VA	Diffusion per unit of alveolar volume. DL is expressed STPD, and VA is expressed in liters (BTPS)

Respiratory Gases

Pa_x	Arterial tension of gas x, torr (mm Hg)
PA_x	Alveolar tension of gas x, torr (mm Hg)
Sa_{O_2}	Arterial oxygen saturation (percent)
C	Concentration: e.g., Ca_{O_2} is the concentration of oxygen in a blood sample, including both oxygen combined with hemoglobin and physically dissolved oxygen, ordinarily expressed as ml O_2 (STPD)/100 ml blood, or mmol O_2/liter
PA-Pa	Alveolar–arterial gas pressure difference: the difference in partial pressure of a gas (e.g., O_2 or N_2) in the alveolar gas spaces and that in the systemic arterial blood, measured in torr. For oxygen, as an example, $PA_{O_2} - Pa_{O_2}$ Also symbolized AaD_{O2}
Ca-Cv	Arterial–venous concentration difference. For oxygen, as an example, $Ca_{O_2} - Cv_{O_2}$

Pulmonary shunts

$\dot{Q}s$	Shunt: vascular connection between circulatory pathways so that venous blood is diverted into vessels containing arterialized blood (right-to-left shunt, venous admixture) or *vice versa* (left-to-right shunt). Right-to-left shunt within the lung, heart, or large vessels due to malformations is more important in respiratory physiology. Flow from left to right through a shunt should be marked with a negative sign.

PULMONARY DYSFUNCTION

Altered breathing

Dyspnea	An unpleasant *subjective* feeling of difficult or labored breathing
Hyperventilation	An alveolar ventilation that is excessive relative to the simultaneous metabolic rate. As a result the alveolar P_{CO_2} is significantly reduced below normal for the altitude
Hypoventilation	An alveolar ventilation that is small relative to the simultaneous metabolic rate so that alveolar P_{CO_2} rises significantly above normal for the altitude

Altered blood gases

Hypoxia	Any state in which oxygen in the lung, blood, or tissues is abnormally low compared with that of a normal resting person breathing air at sea level
Hypoxemia	A state in which the oxygen pressure or concentration in arterial blood is lower than its normal value at sea level. Normal oxygen pressures at sea level are 85 to 100 torr in arterial blood. In adult humans the normal oxygen concentration is 17 to 23 ml O_2/100 ml arterial blood
Hypocapnia	Any state in which the systemic arterial carbon dioxide pressure is significantly below 40 torr, as in hyperventilation
Hypercapnia	Any state in which the systemic arterial carbon dioxide pressure is significantly above 40 torr. May occur when alveolar ventilation is inadequate for a given metabolic rate (hypoventilation) or during carbon dioxide inhalation

Altered acid–base balance

Acidemia	Any state of systemic arterial plasma in which the *p*H is significantly less than the normal value, 7.41 ± 0.02 in an adult man at rest
Alkalemia	Any state of systemic arterial plasma in which the *p*H is significantly greater than the normal value, 7.41 ± 0.02 in an adult man at rest
Base excess (BE)	Base excess: a measure of metabolic alkalosis or metabolic acidosis (negative values of base excess) expressed as the mEq of strong acid or strong alkali required to titrate a sample of 1 liter of blood to a *p*H of 7.40. The titration is made with the blood sample kept at 37° C, oxygenated, and equilibrated to P_{CO_2} of 40 torr
Acidosis	The result of any process that by itself adds excess CO_2 (respiratory acidosis) or nonvolatile acids (metabolic acidosis) to arterial blood. Acidemia does not necessarily result because compensating mechanisms (increase of HCO_3 in respiratory acidosis, increase of ventilation, and, consequently, decrease of arterial CO_2 in metabolic acidosis) may intervene to restore *p*H to normal
Alkalosis	The result of any process that, by itself, diminishes acids (respiratory alkalosis) or increases bases (metabolic alkalosis) in arterial blood. Alkalemia does not necessarily result because compensating mechanisms may intervene to restore plasma *p*H to normal

Other

Pulmonary insufficiency	Altered function of the lung that produces clinical symptoms usually including dyspnea
Acute respiratory failure	Rapidly occurring hypoxemia, hypercarbia, or both caused by a disorder of the respiratory system. The duration of the illness and the values of arterial oxygen tension and arterial carbon dioxide tension used as criteria for this term should be given. The term acute ventilatory failure should be used only when the arterial carbon dioxide tension is increased. The term pulmonary failure has been used to indicate respiratory failure specifically caused by disorders of the lung
Chronic respiratory failure	Chronic hypoxemia or hypercapnia caused by a disorder of the respiratory system. The duration of the condition and the values of arterial oxygen tension and arterial carbon dioxide tension used as criteria for this term should be given
Obstructive ventilatory defect	Slowing of air flow during forced ventilatory maneuvers
Restrictive ventilatory defect	Reduction of vital capacity *not* explainable by airflow obstruction
Impairment	A measurable degree of anatomical or functional abnormality that may or may not have clinical significance. Permanent impairment is that which persists for some period of time, e.g., 1 year after maximum medical rehabilitation has been achieved
Disability	A legally or administratively determined state in which a patient's ability to engage in a specific activity under certain circumstances is reduced or absent because of physical or mental impairment. Other factors, such as age, education, and customary way of making a livelihood, are considered in evaluating disability. Permanent disability exists when no substantial improvement of the patient's ability to engage in the specific activity can be expected

REFERENCES

1. Pulmonary terms and symbols. A report of the ACCP–ATS Joint Committee on Pulmonary Nomenclature. Chest 67:583, 1975
2. Updated nomenclature for membership reaction. Report from the ATS Pulmonary Nomenclature Subcommittee on Respiratory Physiology. ATS News 4:12, Spring 1978

H

Suctioning Protocol*

Sandra L. Caldwell • Kent N. Sullivan

The following steps are recommended for the effective implementation of suctioning.

1. Assemble equipment (*see* Chap. 21).
2. Prepare oxygenation apparatus (*e.g.*, non-self-inflating bag).
3. Wash hands with antimicrobial preparation except in emergencies (*see* Chap. 19).
4. Open catheter package; deposit catheter on sterile surface.
5. Hyperoxygenate patient with 6 to 7 breaths of 100% O_2.
6. Glove one hand with sterile glove.
7. Pick up tip of catheter with gloved hand; attach to vacuum connecting tubing.
8. Introduce the catheter into the tube orifice as far as it will go easily, with the suction *off*.
9. Apply suction as the catheter is removed. While removing the catheter, wrap the catheter around the first two fingers of the gloved hand and rotate the openings in the suction catheter, thus providing better suction of the trachea. *Suction should not be applied for more than 15 seconds.* Even though all secretions may not have been removed in that time, the patient should be hyperoxygenated again before any additional suctioning is performed. Wrapping the suction catheter around the fingers of the gloved hand as the catheter is removed also helps to prevent contamination of the catheter. As long as it has not been contaminated, it may be reinserted for additional suctioning. Turning the head from side to side may facilitate selective catheterization and suctioning, particularly of the left main bronchus.
10. *Note:* If the patient has tenacious secretions, 5 to 10 cc of sterile normal saline for injection should be instilled at the beginning of the suctioning procedure. This should be followed by bag breathing and sighing before suctioning is attempted. After the patient has been hyperoxygenated, another 15 seconds of suctioning may be accomplished. If, after suctioning this time, the patient seems to be clear of secretions, the non-self-inflating anesthesia bag should be used again to force the patient to sigh and to take several deep breaths held from 3 to 5 seconds and then released suddenly. Cough usually is induced, which may help to mobilize secretions that were not within reach on previous suctioning attempts.
11. Stop the suctioning at this point if no more

*For a more detailed discussion of suctioning, the reader is referred to Chapter 21.

secretions can be seen or heard, since the patient has been adequately suctioned. After the procedure has been completed, the catheter is wrapped around the fingers of the gloved hand. Taking the glove by the cuff and removing it inside out keeps the catheter inside the glove and will minimize contamination of the patient's surroundings. Once the catheter and glove have been disposed of, the vacuum connecting tube should be rinsed with sterile water and the cup discarded. Oxygen and the vacuum should be turned off and the bedside checked to be sure that all supplies are at hand for the next suctioning procedure.

Index

An f *following a page number represents a figure; a* t *indicates tabular material; page numbers in* **boldface** *represent glossary definitions.*